Cancer, Diet, and Nutrition
A Comprehensive Sourcebook

Reference Books Published by Marquis Professional Publications

Reference Books Published by
Marquis Professional Publications

Annual Register of Grant Support
Cancer, Diet, and Nutrition: A Comprehensive Sourcebook
Consumer Protection Directory
Directory of Medical Specialists
Directory of Publishing Opportunities
Directory of Registered Lobbyists and Lobbyist Legislation
Environmental Protection Directory
Family Factbook
Grantsmanship: Money and How to Get It
Marquis Who's Who Directory of Computer Graphics
Marquis Who's Who Directory of Online Professionals
Marquis Who's Who in Cancer: Professionals and Facilities
Marquis Who's Who in Rehabilitation: Professionals and Facilities
Music Industry Directory
NASA Factbook
NIH Factbook
NSF Factbook
Sourcebook of Equal Educational Opportunity
Sourcebook on Aging
Sourcebook on Death and Dying
Sourcebook on Food and Nutrition
Sourcebook on Mental Health
Standard Education Almanac
Standard Medical Almanac
Yearbook of Adult and Continuing Education
Yearbook of Higher Education
Yearbook of Special Education
Worldwide Directory of Computer Companies
Worldwide Directory of Federal Libraries

Forthcoming
Marquis Who's Who in Optical Science and Engineering

Cancer, Diet, and Nutrition
A Comprehensive Sourcebook

First Edition

Peter Greenwald, M.D., Dr.P.H.
Consulting Editor for Part 1

Abby G. Ershow, Sc.D.
Consulting Editor for Part 2

William D. Novelli
Consulting Editor for Part 3

Christine M. Benton
Research Editor

Marquis Who's Who, Inc.
Professional Publications Division
200 East Ohio Street
Chicago, Illinois 60611 U.S.A.

International Standard Book Number 0-8379-6801-1
Product Code Number 031140

Manufactured in the United States of America
1   2   3   4   5   6   7   8   9   10

Preface

Health professionals throughout the world are moving toward a major new strategy in the war against cancer. Within the next 15 years, their goal is to reduce the cancer mortality rate to half of what it is today, resulting in a saving of over 200,000 lives per year. This goal can be achieved by improvements in the development and dissemination of information on cancer treatment and by the application of new knowledge in cancer diagnosis and prevention. Their hope is that a larger number of people can be helped more quickly if medical, scientific, and media attention is focused on diet modification techniques and other preventive health measures.

The First Edition of *Cancer, Diet, and Nutrition: A Comprehensive Sourcebook* was compiled to present an overview of the research linking diet with the incidence of cancer. As a first edition, the *Sourcebook* addresses current research results and theories as well as studies undertaken in the past. A historical perspective is included to apprise readers of the progress of the research on cancer and diet/nutrition and to point to future directions in that research.

The identification of diet and nutrition as significant factors in cancer causation has given rise to a multidisciplinary approach to cancer prevention. Because dietary habits are inextricably tied to other sociological and cultural factors, it is no simple matter to elicit changes in those habits. However, any entity that influences food consumption patterns can effect dietary modification and thus play a role in the prevention of cancer. For this reason, we believe that individuals and institutions in all fields will find this *Sourcebook* both informative and thought provoking.

Cancer, Diet, and Nutrition: A Comprehensive Sourcebook has been compiled with attention to meeting the needs of physicians, cancer information specialists, medical librarians, cancer program and health care program directors, media health specialists, nutritionists, and others involved in a broad range of relevant medical disciplines. Medical and allied health professionals will find the *Sourcebook* to be a useful reference for up-to-date information on the state of cancer/diet research.

Since our goal was to review the progress of this research over the last 50 years, many of the articles included are review and overview papers, although some original research has been selected for illustrative purposes. Sources for selected articles are the most authoritative journals in the fields of cancer, nutrition, and epidemiology. These articles, written by highly respected investigators, include extensive reference sections. The increasingly rapid rate at which new cancer and diet/nutrition information becomes available makes it impractical for this or any work to be all-inclusive; rather, the *Sourcebook* identifies and explores major areas of current medical and scientific interest.

In reviewing the literature available on this broad subject, efforts generally focused on material published within the last five years. Some earlier articles are included in areas where research has not uncovered significant new information since their date of publication. We reviewed articles in over 200 journals, consulted several national databases, and conducted extensive interviews with authorities in the fields of cancer, epidemiology, and nutrition research to identify topics of major concern.

This project could not have been completed without the assistance of individuals at the National Cancer Institute, the American Cancer Society, the U.S. Department of Agriculture, and various branches of the National Institutes of Health. We sincerely appreciate their interest and cooperation.

Cancer, Diet, and Nutrition: A Comprehensive Sourcebook is divided into three sections. Part 1, "Scientific Evidence Linking Cancer to Diet and Nutrition," reviews research that demonstrates the roles diet and nutrition play in cancer etiology. This section begins with an overview of cancer as an avoidable risk, positions diet and nutrition as important factors in environmental causation, and summarizes current directions in the research. Articles in Part 1 review the dietary assessment and epidemiologic methods crucial to scientifically rigorous investigation; specific dietary and nutritional factors that have been linked to cancer causation and prevention; and the mechanisms of carcinogenesis and subsequent investigations into the role that dietary factors play in this process. Part 1 concludes with dietary guidelines recommended by the American Cancer Society and the National Cancer Institute.

Part 2, "Epidemiologic Support for the Link Between Cancer and Diet," presents epidemiologic data that, in conjunction with laboratory investigations, clarify the link between diet/nutrition and cancer. In this part we have included a selection of pertinent data obtained through studies of various geographic and demographic population groups. Part 2 also presents current information on dietary causation and prevention of cancer at specific sites where strong dietary links have been established.

Part 3, "Social Marketing and Dietary Cancer Prevention," reviews current social marketing techniques and theories as they apply to health promotion and disease prevention. This section defines social marketing and its role in health behavior modification and presents case studies of several dietary intervention programs that incorporate social marketing techniques.

Marquis Professional Publications, a division of Marquis Who's Who, Inc., continually strives to provide the professional community with comprehensive up-to-date information. Because much of the material included in the *Sourcebook* is of an interim nature, the editorial staff of Marquis Professional Publications encourages readers' comments and suggestions.

About the Consulting Editors

Peter Greenwald, M.D., Dr.P.H., is Director of the Division of Cancer Prevention and Control at the National Cancer Institute. After being certified in both Internal Medicine and Preventive Medicine, Dr. Greenwald earned his Dr.P.H. in Epidemiology at the Harvard School of Public Health. He currently serves on the National Research Council's Food and Nutrition Board and is Editor-in-Chief of the *Journal of the National Cancer Institute.* He has contributed extensively to the literature in cancer epidemiology.

Abby G. Ershow, Sc.D., is a staff fellow in the Epidemiology and Biostatistics Program, Division of Cancer Etiology, at the National Cancer Institute. Dr. Ershow earned her Sc.D. in Nutrition at the Harvard School of Public Health. A member of the American College of Epidemiology and a Registered Dietitian, she has written scientific papers and abstracts in the areas of clinical nutrition and cancer etiology.

William D. Novelli is President of Needham Porter Novelli, a marketing firm located in Washington, D.C. Mr. Novelli also serves as marketing consultant to the United Way of America and as a consultant for international marketing and preventive health care programs. He teaches graduate marketing management and health communication courses at the University of Maryland and is currently Vice Chairman of the Task Force on Professional Communications of the National Council on Patient Information and Education. Mr. Novelli has written and presented more than 30 papers on social marketing and health care promotion and serves on the Editorial Review Board of the *Journal of Health Care Marketing.*

Contents

Part 1: Scientific Evidence Linking Cancer to Diet and Nutrition

In 1982 the Committee on Diet, Nutrition, and Cancer, Assembly of Life Sciences, National Research Council released a comprehensive report entitled *Diet, Nutrition, and Cancer.* Included in the report were "Interim Dietary Guidelines," based on the research undertaken to date concerning a link between cancer and dietary and nutritional factors. Although the interim guidelines became an immediate subject of debate, with some disputing the validity of the recommendations, almost no one went so far as to argue against the necessity for examining a possible connection between cancer and diet. Indeed, the National Cancer Institute began a "Cancer Prevention Awareness Program" in 1984 and the American Cancer Society followed with a set of similar dietary recommendations aimed at cancer prevention. And today, both the NCI and the ACS, the two largest U.S. organizations dedicated to cancer research and information, are embarking on the most extensive prevention programs ever undertaken in this country to prevent this second leading cause of death.

The need for cancer prevention is considered self-evident by most authorities in the field. While it is not currently possible to pinpoint exactly what fraction of fatal cancers may truly be preventable, the fact remains that about one-fifth of all deaths in the U.S. are caused by cancer. No one can deny that cancer is the disease causing the greatest public concern in the U.S., and thus, a most appropriate subject of prevention research.

Research implicating environment as a causal factor in cancer etiology has been going on for more than 50 years, but it is only recently that such great emphasis has been placed on the role of lifestyle factors such as the food we eat. Many authorities now feel that nutrition and dietary habits play a far greater role in causation than the inadvertent environmental and occupational exposures to chemical carcinogens that have been the focus of past research. Recent studies have attributed as much as 90 percent of all human cancer to environmental factors, and many investigators have speculated that diet may be causative in as much as 30 to 40 percent. Because of such statistics, much current research focuses on the causal relationship between diet and cancer and, in turn, the possible chemopreventive role of various dietary components, both nutritive and nonnutritive. At this time, the precise nature of that relationship is not known, but investigators have made great inroads into increasing our knowledge of the mechanisms of carcinogenesis and the function of dietary factors in cancer causation and prevention.

It is important to understand the interim nature of our current knowledge on the link between diet and cancer and, thus, of any recommendations concerning changes in Western diets. Researchers stress that we are now at the point in our understanding of the cancer-diet link that we reached 20 years ago for the smoking-cancer link, at the time the first "Surgeon General's" report described a growing consensus on smoking and cancer. Therefore, while readers may rest assured that the papers in this section represent scientifically rigorous and up-to-date information, they should also be aware that the state of the field is changing constantly, and that new information is being uncovered rapidly.

The objective of the papers that follow is to provide an overview of the current information available on the link between cancer and diet. Since this is the first edition of *Cancer, Diet, and Nutrition: A Comprehensive Sourcebook,* the existing evidence presented includes both review articles and original research, current studies and examples of past studies that have laid the groundwork for present and future research.

The first section, "Overview," introduces the concept of cancer as an avoidable, and therefore potentially preventable, disease. Papers in this section also discuss the role of diet and nutrition in multifactorial cancer causation and raise some of the most pressing problems that investigators face in cancer-diet research, today and in the future.

In the second section, "Dietary Assessment and Epidemiologic Methods," readers will find a collection of articles assessing one of the most crucial issues of the research; namely, the strengths and limitations of methods used both to correlate rates of cancer incidence and mortality with causative factors and to measure and evaluate the diets of study subjects used in epidemiologic studies.

The following two sections, "Classic Experimental Studies" and "Dietary Factors Linked to Cause and Prevention of Cancer," present evidence collected over the course of the research that contributes to the theory of dietary chemoprevention and is the basis for prevention programs adopted by organizations such as the NCI and ACS. Emphasis in these sections is on topics of greatest interest to investigators today and on future areas of research, such as intervention programs now beginning to incorporate clinical trials. An attempt also has been made to stress research concerning cancers of certain sites, such as the colon, rectum, and breast, that are of particular interest to investigators because of their high incidence rates in the Western world. Readers should also refer to Part 2, "Epidemiologic Support for the Link Between Cancer and Diet," for further information on diet's role in these and other cancer sites.

Part 1 concludes with a review of "Recommendations for Dietary Change" that have been released by various organizations concerned with cancer and diet. Again, readers should keep in mind that these are generally intended to be interim guidelines and that they are likely to be updated in the future as new information on the cancer-diet link becomes available.

Peter Greenwald, M.D., Dr.P.H.
Director, Division of Cancer Prevention
    and Control
National Cancer Institute

Overview

The Causes of Cancer: Quantitative Estimates of Avoidable Risks of Cancer in the United States Today

by Richard Doll and Richard Peto

PREFACE

The percentage of today's fatal cancers that might, by suitable preventive measures, have been avoided is subject to some dispute. Indeed, the percentage avoidable by certain particular categories of preventive measure is subject to such vigorous dispute that the non-specialist (to whom the present review is addressed) may wonder whether research has yet discovered any solid facts at all about the avoidance of human cancer.

The truth seems to be that there is quite good evidence that cancer is largely an avoidable (although not necessarily a modern) disease, but, with some important exceptions, frustratingly poor evidence as to exactly what are the really important ways of avoiding a reasonable percentage of today's cancers. Perhaps because of this uncertainty, the number of different areas of current research into hypothetical ways of avoiding cancer is enormous. As a convenient framework in which to seek an overview of them all, we have divided the various hypothetical ways of increasing or decreasing cancer onset rates into a dozen groups, and for each such group we have attempted to review what is known about the percentage of current U.S. cancer deaths that might thereby be avoidable.

In some groups (e.g., smoking habits) the quantitative knowledge already available is quite reliable, whereas in others (e.g., dietary habits) it is not, and we have had to fall back on reviewing various current lines of research whose eventual outcome is still unknown. The "percentages" (of current cancer mortality thus avoidable) that we eventually cite for the separate groups are therefore not really comparable with each other. Some are fairly precisely known, whereas others are much less so. More importantly, some relate to quite specific preventive measures on which action would, at least in principle, be possible on present knowledge alone, whereas others relate to preventive measures (e.g., modification of dietary factors) where the changes that would be beneficial have not yet been reliably characterized. Moreover, even if two particular agents (e.g., asbestos and sunlight) happen to account for a similar percentage of all cancer deaths, that which is the more easily controlled is obviously of greater public health significance. Despite all these drawbacks, the "percentages" that we have attributed to each way or group of ways of avoiding cancer remain for us a useful summary of certain facts, and the estimation of those "percentages" remains a convenient way of structuring our review of the quantitative information that is already available or is emerging about the determinants of human cancer.

Our report consists of a review of the evidence that cancer is largely an avoidable disease, a review of recent upward or downward trends in the onset rates of various types of cancer, a review of our reasons for preferring an epidemiological rather than a laboratory-based approach to the quantitative attribution of human risk, and then a dozen separate sections, one on each of the possible ways or groups of ways of avoiding cancer. The final section then summarizes and brings together our principal conclusions. We have relegated most of our detailed discussions of trends and certain other matters to appendixes, for although these details might be of interest to the specialist our principal aim has been to explain matters to interested non-specialists. Of course some isolated pockets of detail remain in the text, but we have used paragraph subheadings fairly liberally throughout in the hope that wherever any reader feels the amount of detail excessive a few pages can be skipped without losing the general sense of our argument.

Richard Doll is Honorary Director, Imperial Cancer Research Fund, Cancer Epidemiology and Clinical Trials Unit, and Warden of Green College, Oxford, United Kingdom.

Richard Peto is Imperial Cancer Research Fund Reader in Cancer Studies, Nuffield Department of Clinical Medicine, University of Oxford, Radcliffe Infirmary, Oxford OX2 6HE, United Kingdom.

Finally, following Russell (1946), a few words of apology and explanation are called for, chiefly addressed to the specialists on the various subjects we touch on. Most of these subjects, with the possible exception of tobacco, are better known to some others than to us. If reports covering a wide field are to be written at all it is inevitable, since we are not immortal, that those who write them should spend less time on any one part than can be spent by someone who concentrates on a single subject. Some, whose scholarly austerity is unbending, will conclude that reports covering a wide field should not be written at all, or, if written, should consist of chapters by a multitude of authors. There is, however, something lost when many authors cooperate. If any balance is to be achieved between the findings in laboratory experiments and the distribution of disease that actually occurs in the population as a whole, and if the major and minor causes of death are to be seen in proper perspective, then the various aspects should be synthesized in a consistent way, which would have increased in difficulty exponentially with the number of authors.

ABSTRACT—Evidence that the various common types of cancer are largely avoidable diseases is reviewed. Life-style and other environmental factors are divided into a dozen categories, and for each category the evidence relating those particular factors to cancer onset rates is summarized. Where possible, an estimate is made of the percentage of current U.S. cancer mortality that might have been caused or avoided by that category of factors. These estimates are based chiefly on evidence from epidemiology, as the available evidence from animal and other laboratory studies cannot provide reliable human risk assessments. By far the largest reliably known percentage is the 30% of current U.S. cancer deaths that are due to tobacco, although it is possible that some nutritional factor(s) may eventually be found to be of comparable importance. The percentage of U.S. cancer deaths that are due to tobacco is still increasing, and must be expected to continue to increase for some years yet due to the delayed effects of the adoption of cigarettes in earlier decades.

Trends in mortality and in onset rates for many separate types of cancer are studied in detail in appendixes to this paper. Biases in the available data on registration of new cases produce apparent trends in cancer incidence which are spurious. Biases also produce spurious trends in cancer death certification rates, especially among old people. In (and before) middle age, where the biases are smaller, there appear to be a few real increases and a few real decreases in mortality from some particular types of cancer, but there is no evidence of any generalized increase other than that due to tobacco. Moderate increases or decreases due to some new agent(s) or habit(s) might of course be overlooked in such large-scale analyses. But, such analyses do suggest that, apart from cancer of the respiratory tract, the types of cancer that are currently common are not peculiarly modern diseases and are likely to depend chiefly on some long-established factor(s). (A prospective study utilizing both questionnaires and stored blood and other biological materials might help elucidate these factors.)

The proportion of current U.S. cancer deaths attributed to occupational factors is provisionally estimated as 4% (lung cancer being the major contributor to this). This is far smaller than has recently been suggested by various U.S. Government agencies. The matter could be resolved directly by a "case-control" study of lung cancer two or three times larger than the recently completed U.S. National Bladder Cancer Study but similar to it in methodology and unit costs; there are also other reasons for such a study.

A fuller summary of conclusions and recommendations comprises the final section of this report.—JNCI 1981; 66:1191–1308.

1. DEFINITION OF AVOIDABILITY OF CANCER

The various human cancers are diseases in which one of the many cells of which the human body is composed is altered in such a way that it inappropriately replicates itself again and again, producing millions of similarly affected self-replicating descendant cells, some of which may spread to other parts of the body and eventually overwhelm it.[1] Some cancers are easily curable; whereas others are almost always completely incurable by the time they are diagnosed, depending largely on the organ of the body (lung, larynx, large intestine, etc.) in which the first altered cell originated. The symptoms produced and the approach to treatment also vary with the site of origin, so that it has been customary for doctors to regard tumors originating from different organs as different diseases. Gradually, it has come to be realized that agents or habits which greatly increase or decrease the likelihood of one particular type of cancer arising (in humans or experimental animals) may have little effect on most other types of cancer, so that the prevention of each type also must be considered separately. This realization reinforces the need to consider cancers of different organs as largely independent diseases, just as we have to consider separately different infectious diseases such as syphilis, smallpox, and tuberculosis. When we consider them separately, we see at once that although there are several dozen different organs from which tumors may arise, cancers of three organs (lung, breast, and large intestine) are at present of outstanding importance as they currently account for half the U.S. cancer deaths (table 1). A substantial reduction in any of these three cancers, particularly lung cancer, would materially reduce total U.S. cancer death rates, whereas such reductions in any other type of cancer would have relatively little effect.

That the common fatal cancers occur in large part as a result of life-style and other environmental factors and are in principle preventable was recognized by an expert committee of the WHO in 1964. The committee, which had been appointed to consider how existing knowledge could be applied to prevent cancer, began its report (WHO, 1964) by stating that:

> The potential scope of cancer prevention is limited by the proportion of human cancers in which extrinsic factors are responsible. These [factors] include all environmental carcinogens (whether identified or not) as well as 'modifying factors' that favour neoplasia of apparently intrinsic origin (e.g., hormonal imbalances, dietary deficiencies and metabolic defects). The categories of cancer that are thus influenced, directly or indirectly, by extrinsic factors include many tumours of the skin and mouth, the respiratory, gastrointestinal and urinary tracts, hormone dependent organs (such as the breast, thyroid and uterus), haematopoietic and lymphopoietic systems, which, collectively, account for more than three-quarters of human cancers. It would seem, therefore, that the majority of human cancer is potentially preventible.

Many individuals had already expressed this belief previously, and the committee's report merely served to indicate that a consensus among most cancer research

TABLE 1.—*Numbers of deaths certified as being due to various types of tumor: United States, 1978*

Type of tumor	No. of deaths	Percent of all deaths from tumors
Cancer of the		
Lung[a]	95,086	24 ⎫
Large bowel (colon and rectum)	53,269	13 ⎬ 46
Breast	34,609	9 ⎭
Prostate	21,674	5
Pancreas	20,777	5 ⎫ 46
Stomach	14,452	4 ⎬
29 other types or categories,[b] each contributing less than 3% of deaths	128,705	32 ⎭
Other or unspecified tumors[c]	33,383	8
Total, all tumors	401,955	100

[a] The annual number of lung cancer deaths is changing rapidly and will probably be ≈105,000 by 1981. If it is, cancers of the lung, breast, and large intestine will account for just over half of all deaths from tumors where the site of origin of the tumor was specified on the death certificate (*see* footnote *c*).

[b] Including all leukemias as one category. (A detailed breakdown by sex and site is available in tables 17–19, pp. 1243–1244.)

[c] Comprising 4,963 deaths attributed to tumors of benign or unspecified histology, and 28,420 deaths attributed to cancer for which the site of origin was not specified; at least half of the latter probably originated from the six commonest sites.

workers had been achieved. In the years since that report was published, advances in knowledge have consolidated these opinions and few if any competent research workers now question its main conclusion. Individuals, indeed, have gone further and have substituted figures of 80 or even 90% as the proportion of potentially preventable cancers in place of the 1964 committee's cautious estimate of "the majority."

Unfortunately, the phrase "extrinsic factors" (or the phrase "environmental factors," which is often substituted for it) has been misinterpreted by many people to mean only "man-made chemicals," which was certainly not the intent of the WHO committee. The committee included, in addition to man-made or natural carcinogens, viral infections, nutritional deficiencies or excesses, reproductive activities, and a variety of other factors determined wholly or partly by personal behavior. To avoid similar misunderstandings, we shall refer throughout this report to the percentages of cancers that "might be avoidable" in various ways, rather than to the percentages that are due to various "extrinsic" or "environmental" factors, and have used the term "avoidable" in our title. We have had in mind throughout our report the avoidance of cancer only by means that might conceivably be socially acceptable, either now or in some plausible social atmosphere in the reasonably near future. (Potentially acceptable measures might, for example, include a continuation of the current decrease in cigarette smoking or tar yields, which would reduce the risk of lung cancer, but would not include a first pregnancy for most females by 15 years of age, though this would reduce the risk of breast cancer.) Even with this restriction, however, two ambiguities remain in what is meant by the "avoidability" of cancer.

First, by the year 2100 advances in basic research in biology may permit prevention of cancer by means now utterly unforeseen. No useful estimate of the likelihood of such progress can be made, and we have

---

[1] "Tumor" and "neoplasm" have similar meanings, but strictly the word "cancer" relates only to invasive solid tumors of certain tissues. However, most fatal tumors are "cancers" and we shall sometimes use this familiar term loosely to include both solid and diffuse malignant neoplasms plus sometimes even the fatal benign tumors as well.

therefore tried to restrict our attention chiefly to the avoidability of cancer by means whose effects on cancer risks are already reasonably certain or by means that might well be devised over the next decade or two rather than in the indefinite future. For this we have not assumed that the mechanisms underlying such means are known or will be known in the near future, but chiefly that it should be possible to identify those things which different groups of people already do, or have done to them, that account for the marked differences in cancer risk between or within communities and that this identification will in many instances lead to preventive strategies which are based either directly or indirectly on the ways in which some people already live and are therefore reasonably practical.

A second, more trivial, ambiguity in what we mean by the "avoidability" of cancer arises simply because everybody is bound to die sooner or later. (If there are about two million births per year in the United States, there are in the long run also bound to be about two million deaths per year.) If exactly half the cancer deaths that now occur were somehow magically prevented and nothing else changed, those people who would have died of cancer might live on for a further 5, 10, 20, or 30 more years (the average being 10 or 15 extra years), but they must eventually die of something and that something would for some of them be a second cancer. Even so, we would still describe such a change as a *halving* of the cancer rate. To take an opposite example, if every cause of death other than cancer were suddenly abolished then of course everyone would eventually die of cancer, although it might be misleading to describe such a change in terms of an increase in either the risk of cancer or the average age at death from cancer, especially if one were interested in the causes of cancer. The usual means of avoiding such absurdities is to avoid basing inferences on the percentage of people who "will eventually" die of cancer, on "crude" cancer rates, or on "the mean age at death from cancer." Instead, it is usual to restrict attention to "age-specific" or "age-standardized" cancer rates (*see* appendixes A and B). When we speak of the avoidance of a certain percentage of cancer, we therefore have in mind a reduction by that percentage in the age-standardized rates. (This may sound complicated, but it is merely the arithmetic equivalent of not advising people that the most reliable way of avoiding cancer is to commit suicide.)

In summary, the aim of our report is to review the established evidence and current research relating to each of several different possible ways or groups of ways of avoiding cancer and to estimate the percentage reduction in today's age-standardized U.S. cancer death rates that they might confer, now or in the medium-term future.

2. EVIDENCE FOR THE AVOIDABILITY OF CANCER

The evidence that much human cancer is avoidable can be summarized under four heads: differences in the incidence of cancer among different settled communities, differences between migrants from a community and those who remain behind, variations with time in the incidence of cancer within particular communities, and the actual identification of many specific causes or preventive factors. Genetic factors and age also affect cancer onset rates, of course, but this does not affect the conclusion that much human cancer is avoidable.

2.1 Differences in Incidence Between Communities

Evidence of differences in the incidence[2] of particular types of cancer between different parts of the world has accumulated slowly over the past 50 years. At first the only quantitative data available referred to mortality[2] rates in particular areas or, even more crudely, to the proportion of patients admitted to hospital suffering from different diseases. Such data were grossly affected by the age distribution of the population, the efficacy of treatment, and the frequency of other diseases. But even then data were sufficient to show that the incidence of some cancers among people of a given age in different parts of the world must vary by at least ten and possibly by a hundredfold. More recently, this evidence has been reinforced by the results of special surveys or by the establishment of registries in which records are consistently sought of all cases of cancer diagnosed in a defined population over a long period. Registry data also need care in interpretation owing to trends with time, or differences between different parts of the world, in the provision of medical services and in the extent to which they are used (especially by old people, among whom a large proportion of fatal cancers may never be diagnosed at all). Reasonably reliable comparisons between different areas are obtained only if comparisons are limited to men and women in middle life (or earlier, for some specific types of cancer), when a sufficient number of cases can be anticipated for onset rates to be reliably estimated and yet efforts at diagnosis are still likely to be thorough. The International Union Against Cancer (1970) and IARC (1976) have recommended that, for the cancers of adult life, attention be chiefly directed to the risks in the truncated age range of 35–64 years (and many artifacts of interpretation of trends in U.S. cancer data might be avoided if this simple precaution were generally adopted).

Table 2 shows for 19 common types of cancer their range of variation among those cancer registries that have produced data sufficiently reliable to be published for the purposes of international comparison by the IARC (1976) and the International Union Against Cancer (1966 and 1970). Types of cancer have been included if they are common enough somewhere to affect more than 1% of men (or women) by 75 years of age in the absence of other causes of death, and ranges of variation are shown for standardized incidence rates between 35 and 64 years of age.[3]

The range of variation (table 2) is never less than sixfold and is commonly much more. Some of this variation may be artifactual, due to different standards of medical service, case registration, and population enumeration, despite the care taken to exclude unreliable data; but in many cases the true ranges will be greater. First, large gaps remain in the cancer map of the world, and some extreme figures may have been

---

[2] Definition: The *incidence* (rate) depends on the total number of new cases of cancer (per year), while the *mortality* (rate), also called the death rate, ignores non-fatal cases.

[3] The incidence of most types of cancer increases with age so rapidly that it may be misleading to compare disease onset rates among people in one part of the world with those of people elsewhere if the proportions of people of different ages in the populations being compared are not the same. This particular difficulty may be circumvented by the use of age-standardized incidence rates (*see* appendix A), and the rates in table 2 are standardized as recommended by the IARC (1976).

TABLE 2.—*Range of incidence rates for common cancers among males (and for certain cancers among females)*

Site of origin of cancer	High incidence area	Sex	Cumulative incidence,[a] % in high incidence area	Ratio of highest rate to lowest rate[b]	Low incidence area
Skin (chiefly non-melanoma)	Australia, Queensland	♂	>20	>200	India, Bombay
Esophagus	Iran, northeast section	♂	20	300	Nigeria
Lung and bronchus	England	♂	11	35	Nigeria
Stomach	Japan	♂	11	25	Uganda
Cervix uteri	Colombia	♀	10	15	Israel: Jewish
Prostate	United States: blacks	♂	9	40	Japan
Liver	Mozambique	♂	8	100	England
Breast	Canada, British Columbia	♀	7	7	Israel: non-Jewish
Colon	United States, Connecticut	♂	3	10	Nigeria
Corpus uteri	United States, California	♀	3	30	Japan
Buccal cavity	India, Bombay	♂	2	25	Denmark
Rectum	Denmark	♂	2	20	Nigeria
Bladder	United States, Connecticut	♂	2	6	Japan
Ovary	Denmark	♀	2	6	Japan
Nasopharynx	Singapore: Chinese	♂	2	40	England
Pancreas	New Zealand: Maori	♂	2	8	India, Bombay
Larynx	Brazil, São Paulo	♂	2	10	Japan
Pharynx	India, Bombay	♂	2	20	Denmark
Penis	Parts of Uganda	♂	1	300	Israel: Jewish

[a] By age 75 yr, in the absence of other causes of death.
[b] At ages 35–64 yr, standardized for age as in IARC (1976). At these ages, even the data from cancer registries in poor countries are likely to be reasonably reliable (although at older ages serious underreporting may affect the data).

overlooked because no accurate surveys have been practicable in the least developed areas, these being just the areas that are likely to provide the biggest contrasts (both high and low) with Western society. Second, the rates cited in table 2 refer to cancers of whole organs, and in one particular organ such as the stomach, liver, or skin there may be many different types of cells that are affected differently by different carcinogens or protective factors; for example, in the skin the few cancers arising from the cells that are responsible for the manufacture of the dark pigment melanin in blacks or in suntanned whites are called "melanomas," and differ greatly in etiology and prognosis from the many "non-melanoma skin cancers." Third, various anatomic parts of one single organ such as the colon or skin may be affected differently by different factors; for example, cancers of the skin have different principal causes in the populations where they are common depending on whether they chiefly appear on the face, abdomen, forearm, or legs. Finally, although cancers of the skin are so common in certain parts of the world that they outnumber all other cancers, most are so easily cured that they engender little medical interest and are commonly not reported to, or in some cases sought by, even some of the best cancer registries. For these reasons and because the extremes of variation in skin cancer incidence between different communities are affected by skin color as well as by the means of avoidance which chiefly interest us, skin cancers (other than melanomas) are perhaps of less interest than any other type of cancer in table 2.

Variation in incidence is not, of course, limited to the types of cancer that are common enough somewhere in the world to have been included in table 2. For example, Burkitt's lymphoma has nowhere been found in over 0.1% of the population, but even so is 100 times less common in North America than in the West Nile district of Uganda. Also, Kaposi's sarcoma, which is extremely rare in most of the world, is so common in parts of Central Africa that it accounted for more than 10% of all tumors seen in the (mostly young) males in one hospital (Cook and Burkitt, 1971).

Some few rather rare types of cancer, such as the nephroblastoma of childhood, may perhaps eventually be shown to occur with approximately the same frequency in all communities; but no common types of cancer will be found to do so. In the absence of other causes of death, cancer of the breast would affect about 6% of U.S. women before the age of 75 years as against only 1% of non-Jewish Israeli women, and it is possible that an even lower percentage would be affected in certain other populations where reliable cancer registries do not yet exist. With breast cancer as the only possible exception, for each type of cancer a population exists where the cumulative incidence by the age of 75 years is well under 1%. In other words, every type of cancer that is common in one district is rare somewhere else.

Most of the figures in table 2 refer to the incidence of cancer in different communities defined by the area in which they live. Communities can, however, be defined in other ways and no matter how they are defined (whether by ethnic origin, religion, or economic status) similar or sometimes even greater differences will be found. Of particular interest are some of the differences that have been observed in the United States between members of different religious groups.[4] For example, in comparison with members of other religious groups living in the same States, the Mormons of Utah and the Seventh-day Adventists and Mormons of California experience low incidence rates for cancers of the respiratory, gastrointestinal, and genital systems.

Of course, it is unlikely that any one single community will by chance have the highest rates in the world for every single type of cancer, just as it is unlikely that any one single community will by chance have the lowest rates in the world for every single type of cancer. Consequently, when we consider total cancer

---

[4] See, for example, the papers from the recent workshop on "Cancer and Mortality in Religious Groups": Lyon et al., 1980a; Lyon et al., 1980b; Enstrom, 1980; West et al., 1980; Phillips et al., 1980; Martin et al., 1980; King and Locke, 1980a.

rates, which are obtained by adding the rates for each separate type of cancer, in various communities we find less extreme variation (only threefold) between communities around the world than was found for many separate single types of cancer. However, there is if anything still *more* variation in these total cancer incidence rates than would have been expected if for each community the rates for the separate single types of cancer had been picked at random from the corresponding rates around the world for single types of cancer (Peto J: Unpublished calculations based on IARC, 1976). Consequently, the relative constancy of total cancer incidence rates around the world does not suggest that if one cancer is prevented another will tend to replace it;[5] it merely shows that if many things are added up, irregularities will tend to be averaged out.

Apart from cancer of the skin, the risk of which is much greater for whites than for blacks (and possibly also apart from the consistent lack among people of Chinese or Japanese descent of certain lymphoproliferative conditions) it does not seem likely that most of the large differences in cancer onset rates between communities could be chiefly due to genetic factors (*see* section 2.5), and such factors certainly cannot explain the differences observed on migration or with the passage of time that are described in the following sections.

2.2 Changes in Incidence on Migration

Evidence of a change in the incidence of cancer in a migrant group (from that in the homeland they have left toward that of their new country of residence) provides good evidence of the importance of life-style or other environmental factors in the production of the disease. That such changes have occurred and are occurring is beyond reasonable doubt, but strictly controlled quantitative evidence comparing incidence rates in the three populations (original country, migrant group, and new country) is hard to come by. Black Americans, for example, experience cancer incidence rates that are generally much more like those of white Americans than like those of the black population in West Africa from which they were originally drawn, as is indicated for selected sites[6] in table 3. From the strict scientific point of view, this comparison is unsatisfactory because the ancestors of black Americans would have come from many different parts of (chiefly West) Africa, some of which are likely to have cancer rates somewhat different from those observed in Nigeria. Nevertheless, the contrast is so great that there can be little doubt that new factors were introduced with migration. These, it would appear, are not chiefly the result of genetic dilution by interbreeding, for at most major sites the differences between

black and white Americans in defined areas seem largely independent of the degree of admixture of white-derived genes among the blacks in those areas (Petrakis, 1971).

A similar comparison can be made between the Japanese and Caucasian residents in Hawaii and the Japanese in two particular prefectures of Japan (table 4). The close approximation of the rates in the two prefectures gives some justification for believing that they may be typical of the areas from which the Japanese migrants to Hawaii (or their ancestors) originated, although the migrants will have come from other parts of Japan as well. For every type of cancer except cancer of the lung, the rates for the migrants are more like those for the Caucasian residents than for those in Japan.

Other groups for which data are available include Indians who went to Fiji and South Africa (and lost their high risk of developing oral cancer), Britons who went to Fiji (and acquired a high risk of skin cancer), and Central Europeans who went to North America and Australia. Data for some of these groups were reviewed in 1969, under the auspices of the International Agency for Research on Cancer (Haenszel, 1970; Kmet, 1970), and recent data on cancer patterns in different ethnic groups within the United States were reviewed in 1980 under the auspices of the National Cancer Institute (Kolonel, 1980; King and Locke, 1980b; Locke and King, 1980; Lanier et al., 1980).

2.3 Changes in Incidence Over Time

Changes in the incidence of particular types of cancer with the passage of time provide conclusive evidence that extrinsic factors affect those types of cancer. Such changes are, however, notoriously difficult to estimate reliably, chiefly because it is difficult to compare the efficiency of case finding at different periods and partly because few incidence data have been collected for a sufficiently long time, so that we have to compare mortality rates, which record only fatal cases and thus may be influenced by changes in treatment. There are no uniform rules for deciding which of the many apparent changes in cancer incidence are real. Each set of incidence data and each type of cancer must be assessed individually. It is relatively easy to be sure about changes in the incidence of cancer of the esophagus, because the disease can be diagnosed without complex investigations and its occurrence is nearly always recorded, at least in middle age, for it is nearly always fatal. It is much more difficult to be sure about changes in the incidence of many other types of cancer. The common basal cell carcinomas of the skin, for example, are also easy to diagnose but are often not registered at all, as they seldom cause death and may be treated effectively outside the hospital. What appears to be a change in incidence may, therefore, be a change only in the completeness of registration. Cancer of the pancreas, by contrast, is almost always fatal but is easily misdiagnosed, perhaps as cancer of some other organ, unless it is specially looked for. What appears to be an increased incidence may, therefore, be wholly or partly due to improvements in diagnosis, in the availability of medical services, or (as for all other types of cancer) in the readiness of physicians to inform cancer registries of any cancers they find. Such changes are particularly likely to affect the cancer incidence rates recorded for people over 65 years of age, as many terminally ill old people used not to be intensively investigated (some-

---

[5] The suggestion that environmental and life-style factors do not usually have much effect on whether or when an individual gets cancer, but merely affect the site at which a (hypothetically) predestined cancer will appear, has recurred from time to time for half a century ever since Cramer (1934) overlooked the fact that the coefficient of variation of total cancer rates must of necessity be less than that of individual cancer rates. It is easily disproved by noting that people exposed to hazards (e.g., carcinogens in industry or cigarette smoke: Doll, 1978) which affect specific types of cancer do not have reduced risks of cancer of any other type. The same is, of course, true among experimental animals.

[6] We omitted data for cancer sites for which the Ibadan rates resemble the U.S. white rates (e.g., esophagus and stomach).

TABLE 3.—*Comparison of cancer incidence rates*[a] *for Ibadan, Nigeria, and for two populations of blacks and whites in the United States*

Primary site of cancer	Patients' sex[c]	Annual incidence/million people[b]		
		Ibadan, Nigeria, 1960–69	United States[d]	
			Blacks	Whites
Colon	♂	34	349	294
			353	335
Rectum	♂	34	159	217
			248	232
Liver	♂	272	67	39
			86	32
Pancreas	♂	55	200	126
			250	122
Larynx	♂	37	236	141
			149	141
Lung	♂	27	1,546	983
			1,517	979
Prostate	♂	134	724	318
			577	232
Breast	♀	337	1,268	1,828
			1,105	1,472
Cervix uteri	♀	559	507	249
			631	302
Corpus uteri	♀	42	235	695
			208	441
Lymphosarcoma[e] at ages <15 yr	♂	133	10	4
			5	3

[a] From IARC (1976).
[b] Ages 35–64 yr, standardized for age as in IARC (1976).
[c] For brevity, wherever possible only the male rates have been presented, and sites for which the rates among U.S. whites resemble those in the country of origin of the non-white migrants have been omitted.
[d] For each type of cancer, upper entry shows incidence in San Francisco Bay area, 1969–73; lower entry shows incidence in Detroit, 1969–71.
[e] Including Burkitt's lymphoma. The cited rates are the average of the age-specific rates at ages 0–4, 5–9 and 10–14 yr.

TABLE 4.—*Comparison of cancer incidence rates*[a] *in Japan and for Japanese and Caucasians in Hawaii*

Primary site of cancer	Patients' sex[c]	Annual incidence/million people[b]		
		Japan[d]	Hawaii, 1968–72	
			Japanese	Caucasians
Esophagus	♂	150	46	75
		112		
Stomach	♂	1,331	397	217
		1,291		
Colon	♂	78	371	368
		87		
Rectum	♂	95	297	204
		90		
Lung	♂	237	379	962
		299		
Prostate	♂	14	154	343
		13		
Breast	♀	335	1,221	1,869
		295		
Cervix uteri	♀	329	149	243
		398		
Corpus uteri	♀	32	407	714
		20		
Ovary	♀	51	160	274
		55		

[a] From IARC (1976).
[b] Ages 35–64 yr, standardized for age as in IARC (1976).
[c] Male only, wherever possible; sites selected as in table 3.
[d] For each type of cancer, upper entry shows incidence in Miyagi prefecture, 1968–71; lower entry shows incidence in Osaka prefecture, 1970–71.

times, it must be admitted, to their advantage).

As most cancers are commoner among the old than among the young, these spurious changes in old age are liable to distort overall rates quite considerably and (if attention is not restricted to people under 65 years of age) may conceal a stable or even a decreasing incidence at younger ages at which cancer has been reasonably well diagnosed for several decades. Despite these difficulties, some changes during periods when no large improvements in relevant diagnostic technology were introduced have been so gross that there can be no doubt about their reality. These changes include the increase in esophageal cancer in the black population of South Africa, the continued increase in lung cancer throughout most of the world, the increase in mesothelioma of the pleura in males in industrialized countries, and the decrease in cancer of the tongue in Britain and in cancers of the cervix uteri and stomach throughout Western Europe and North America. Worldwide changes in the mortality attributed to cancers of the lung and stomach in the last 25 years are given in table 5. Detailed U.S. data for these and many other types of cancer are discussed in section 4.1 and in appendixes C, D, and E.

2.4 Identification of Causes

The simplest evidence of the preventability of cancer would be the demonstration by scientific experiment that a particular action actually leads to a reduction in the incidence of the disease. Even where such evidence could in principle have been sought by means of randomized trials, this has not in general been done, and so we often have to be content with the type of strong circumstantial evidence that would be sufficient to obtain a conviction in a court of law. Action, based on such evidence, has in practice often been followed by the desired result—for example, a reduction in the incidence of bladder cancer in the chemical industry has been seen since stopping the manufacture and use of 2-naphthylamine, while the progressive increase in lung cancer risk that regular cigarette smokers suffer is avoided by people who give up the habit of smoking. Cancer research workers throughout the world have therefore accepted that the type of human evidence that has been obtained, sometimes but by no means invariably (*see* section 4.2) combined with laboratory evidence that some suspect agent is carcinogenic in animals, is strong enough to justify the conclusion that a means of avoiding some cases of human cancer has been identified. There are, of course, many borderline instances where reasonable differences of opinion exist, while even for the well-established causes a few critics can always be found who will argue that causality is not established. A majority of students of the subject agreed that a few dozen agents or circumstances have already been shown to cause or prevent cancer in humans and that, in a number of other instances, the conditions that give rise to an increased incidence of cancer have been closely defined without a specific agent having yet been identified (IARC Working Group, 1980). These agents and conditions are listed in table 6. Exposure to some agents, it will be noted, has been on only a small scale, as in the case of a drug introduced briefly for the treatment of a rare disease, whereas exposure to others has been intensive and widespread, and hundreds of thousands of cancers have been caused each year. The extent to which these listed agents and conditions are now affecting the incidence of cancer in the United States is discussed in Section 5.

TABLE 5.—*International changes since 1950 in death certification rates for cancers of stomach and lung*

Country	Period	Percent change in mortality[a] from cancer of:	
		Stomach	Lung
Australia	1950–51 to 1975	−53	+146
Austria	1952–53 to 1976	−53	−8
Chile	1950–51 to 1975	−56	+38
Denmark	1952–53 to 1976	−62	+87
England and Wales	1950–51 to 1975	−49	+33
West Germany	1952–53 to 1975	−50	+36
Ireland	1950–51 to 1975	−54	+177
Israel	1950–51 to 1975	−49	+58
Japan	1950–51 to 1976	−37	+408
The Netherlands	1950–51 to 1976	−60	+89
New Zealand	1950–51 to 1975	−54	+137
Norway	1952–53 to 1975	−59	+118
Scotland	1950–51 to 1975	−46	+44
Switzerland	1952–53 to 1976	−64	+72
United States	1950–51 to 1975	−61	+148

[a] Average of ♂ and ♀ rates at ages 35–64 yr, standardized for age as in IARC (1976).

2.5 Role of Genetic Factors, Luck, and Age

Some people of a given age will develop cancer in the near future, and some will not. The determinants of who will and who will not develop cancer are best divided into three categories, not only the usual "nature" and "nurture" but also "luck," or the play of chance. "Nature" relates to a person's genetic makeup at conception, and this certainly affects the risk of some types of cancer. For example, other things being equal, a white-skinned person is more likely to develop skin cancer in response to sunlight than is a black-skinned person, while people who have inherited xeroderma pigmentosum, a very rare genetically determined inability to repair the normal effects of sunlight on the skin (Robbins et al., 1974), are likely to develop several skin cancers per person. "Nurture," which is the subject of this whole report, relates to what people do or have done to them (in the womb, in childhood, or in adult life) and is of public interest as a determinant of cancer risk because it is the only thing that can be influenced by personal or political choice.[7]

Finally, "luck" takes care of the remaining differences in outcome that both observation and theory lead us to expect (Peto, 1977b), perhaps by determining the concatenation of events that brings about specific changes in particular molecules in individual cells at particular times. Somewhat similarly, luck involves some of us but not others in traffic accidents. Even among genetically identical laboratory animals kept under conditions that are as closely uniform as possible, some will die of cancer in middle age, while others will live on into old age with no cancer. (Analogously, the fact that some

people die of lung cancer at 40 years of age while other people live on in apparently similar circumstances to 80 does not *of itself* provide any suggestion at all as to whether or not there are any genetic factors which affect lung cancer risks, for variation in age at onset of disease would be expected in either case.)

Nature and nurture affect the probability that each individual will develop cancer, and luck then determines exactly which individuals will actually do so. However, although for each single individual the role of luck is enormous, in a population of a hundred thousand or more (e.g., the population covered by one particular cancer registry) the role of luck is smaller, and in determining the annual number of cancers in the whole United States luck has a completely negligible effect, for the larger the population the more the good and bad luck will tend to average out. Consequently, in the comparison of national cancer rates only nature and nurture are important. Much of the evidence outlined above (changes of cancer incidence with migration, changes over the decades within one country, and the identification of particular causes of cancer) points to an important role for "nurture." However, this does not deny an equally important role for "nature." For example, the stomach cancer risks in certain countries differ markedly from each other, and most are decreasing rapidly (table 5), both of which observations point to the relevance of nurture. However, in both high-risk and low-risk countries people whose "ABO" blood group (a factor that is determined purely genetically) is of type "A" have a stomach cancer risk some 20% greater than that of their compatriots of type "O." In this instance, as for skin cancer, nature and nurture seem to multiply each other's effects. If many other genetic factors are relevant to stomach cancer, then maybe two compatriots chosen at random would be likely to differ quite widely in their genetic susceptibility to the external causes of stomach cancer, although it is still possible that there is much less individual genetic variation than many people suppose.[8] Whether most Americans are of similar susceptibility or whether there is typically wide variation in susceptibility makes little difference to the net effects of changes in nurture on the total number of cases in the nation as a whole and is therefore of little immediate public health relevance. (In either case, if the causes of stomach cancer are halved, then the stomach cancer rates will be roughly halved, as has been happening every 20 years.) Moreover, even if individuals do vary widely in their genetic susceptibility to stomach cancer, this does not suggest that different countries will vary widely in the averages of the genetic susceptibilities of their citizens, for in each

---

[7] One difficulty of terminology with the distinction between nature and nurture is where to classify a genetically inherited tendency to behave in certain ways (e.g., to overeat or undereat). From a public health point of view it is probably most appropriate to attribute the net results of tendency-plus-behavior to "nurture," since few such compulsions can be so rigid that social factors will not also affect the behavior pattern. Another difficulty in identifying "nurture" as "that which might be avoidable" is that some day selective abortion (or, more speculatively, selective conception) may be possible to avoid the birth of a few babies with a near certainty of death from cancer.

---

[8] It is sometimes suggested that because a percentage of smokers do not get lung cancer, there must be other causes, or genetic variability. The conclusion may or may not be correct, but the argument for it is bogus. Conversely, it is often argued that because the relatives of patients with a particular type of cancer have only moderate rather than marked excess risks of that type of cancer (although no excess of cancer in general), the amount of simply inherited genetic susceptibility must also be moderate rather than marked. This argument sounds reasonable, but in fact quite marked genetic variation usually leads to surprisingly moderate excess risks in relatives (Peto J, 1980), so this argument too is bogus unless the analysis is of people with two or more relatives affected by one particular type of cancer (and makes due allowance for familial similarities in life-style and environment). At present, the relevance of genetic susceptibility to the common types of cancer remains obscure.

TABLE 6.—*Established human carcinogenic agents and circumstances*[a,b]

Agent or circumstance	Exposure[c]			Site of cancer
	Occupational	Medical	Social	
Aflatoxin			+	Liver
Alcoholic drinks			+	Mouth, pharynx, larynx, eosphagus, liver
Alkylating agents:				
Cyclophosphamide		+		Bladder
Melphalan		+		Marrow
Aromatic amines:				
4-Aminodiphenyl	+			Bladder
Benzidine	+			"
2-Naphthylamine	+			"
Arsenic[d]	+	+		Skin, lung
Asbestos	+			Lung, pleura, peritoneum
Benzene	+			Marrow
Bis(chloromethyl) ether	+			Lung
Busulphan		+		Marrow
Cadmium[d]	+			Prostate
Chewing (betel, tobacco, lime)			+	Mouth
Chromium[d]	+			Lung
Chlornaphazine		+		Bladder
Furniture manufacture (hardwood)	+			Nasal sinuses
Immunosuppressive drugs		+		Reticuloendothelial system
Ionizing radiations[e]	+	+		Marrow and probably all other sites
Isopropyl alcohol manufacture	+			Nasal sinuses
Leather goods manufacture	+			Nasal sinuses
Mustard gas	+			Larynx, lung
Nickel[d]	+			Nasal sinuses, lung
Estrogens:				
Unopposed		+		Endometrium
Transplacental (DES)		+		Vagina
Overnutrition (causing obesity)			+	Endometrium, gallbladder
Phenacetin		+		Kidney (pelvis)
Polycyclic hydrocarbons	+	+		Skin, scrotum, lung
Reproductive history:				
Late age at 1st pregnancy			+	Breast
Zero or low parity			+	Ovary
Parasites:				
Schistosoma haematobium			+	Bladder
Chlonorchis sinensis			+	Liver (cholangioma)
Sexual promiscuity			+	Cervix uteri
Steroids:				
Anabolic (oxymetholone)		+		Liver
Contraceptives		+		Liver (hamartoma)
Tobacco smoking			+	Mouth, pharynx, larynx, lung, esophagus, bladder
UV light	+		+	Skin, lip
Vinyl chloride	+			Liver (angiosarcoma)
Virus (hepatitis B)			+	Liver (hepatoma)

[a] Expanded from IARC working group, 1980.
[b] By restricting this table to firmly established causes, we undoubtedly have omitted some of the more important determinants of human cancer. (A few borderline cases might not command uniform agreement; e.g., we have on balance just included cadmium and just excluded beryllium.)
[c] A plus sign indicates that evidence of carcinogenicity was obtained.
[d] Certain compounds or oxidation states only.
[e] For example, from X-rays, thorium, thorotrast, some underground mining, and other occupations.
Note: Occupational exposure to phenoxyacid/chlorophenal herbicides (or their impurities) is a reasonably well established cause of soft tissue sarcomas or perhaps lymphomas.

such average all the large variations between compatriots will be ironed out. For a few types of internal cancer the differences between countries may be chiefly due to large differences in genetic susceptibility (e.g., the shortfall of chronic lymphocytic leukemia among the Chinese and Japanese or the excess of cancer of the nasopharynx among the southern Chinese), but this seems likely to be the exception rather than the rule. For example, taking the three types of cancer which are currently commonest in the United States (lung, colorectal, and breast cancers), lung cancer was less than half as common a quarter of a century ago, which shows that most cases are avoidable, while for both breast and colorectal cancers there are striking correlations between the rates in particular countries and

various aspects of those countries' life-style (e.g., fat consumption; text-fig. 1). It is most implausible that international variations in daily fat consumption are chiefly determined genetically, and if it is accepted that they are not, then the striking correlations between dietary factors and the onset rates of certain types of cancer show that the large international differences in onset rates are not chiefly genetic in origin. [Note that these correlations merely suggest that these cancers are largely avoidable (except perhaps among those few people with the extremely rare genetic conditions of a strong predisposition to colon cancer or to breast cancer at an early age) but do not mean that avoidance of dietary fat would achieve this.]

Turning finally to the role of age itself, it is

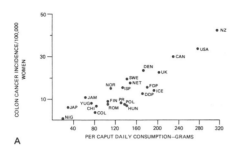

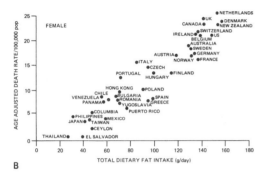

TEXT-FIGURE 1.—A) Correlation between colon cancer incidence in various countries and meat consumption (Armstrong and Doll, 1975a; reprinted with permission of *British Journal of Preventive and Social Medicine* and R. Doll). B) Correlation between breast cancer mortality in various countries and fat consumption (Carroll, 1975; reprinted with permission of *Cancer Research* and K. K. Carroll).

These striking age-standardized correlations do not necessarily suggest that either meat or some type of fat are major determinants of either colon or breast cancer, but they do suggest that manipulable determinants of these cancers do exist.

sometimes suggested that because cancer is ten or a hundred times more likely to arise in the coming year in old people than in young people, aging per se should be thought of as an important determinant of cancer. We rather doubt whether this viewpoint is a scientifically fruitful one (Doll, 1971; Peto et al., 1975), and in any case we are concerned in this report with avoidable causes of cancer, among which we can hardly count old age.

3. PROPORTION OF U.S. CANCERS THAT ARE KNOWN TO BE AVOIDABLE

If the foregoing is accepted as justifying the belief that much human cancer is avoidable, then a crude estimate of the proportion of cases that might be avoided in any one community can be obtained by comparing for each separate type of cancer the incidence in that community with the lowest reliable incidence that is recorded elsewhere. For this purpose, the calculation is best confined to figures for men and women under 65 years of age, because the data on older people are unreliable (*see also* Appendix C). The proportion of avoidable cancers in older people is best estimated indirectly (*see below*). For certain types of tumor we have also thought it wise to omit rates for those communities that are believed to have low rates largely because of genetic insusceptibility. Finally, we have omitted the common non-melanoma skin cancers entirely as, although they vary in incidence even more widely than most other types of cancer, reliable figures for their incidence are not generally available and they

are, in any case, easily treated and seldom fatal.

Before incidence rates in different communities can be compared meaningfully, however, they must first be corrected for the fact that some communities have a higher proportion than others of young people (among whom cancer is everywhere extremely rare). This is allowed for by "age standardization," which we have done by calculating what the incidence in each community would have been expected to be if the proportions of young people in each had been the same as in the respondents to the 1970 U.S. census. Details are given in appendix A, and age-standardized rates for different communities can differ only if the incidence rates observed among people *of a given age* really differ between the different communities.

To estimate the proportion of all cancers that might have been avoided, we have taken, as an example, the population under 65 years of age in Connecticut during 1968–72 and have compared the incidence of each type of cancer (other than non-melanoma skin cancer) in that population with the incidence rates recorded in the populations listed in table 7. For example, the age-standardized rate for cancer of the esophagus among men under 65 years of age in Connecticut was 34.6 per million, while that in rural Norway was only 6.5 per million. Similar calculations were made for 37 other types (or groups of types) of cancer in men and for 40 types (or groups of types) in women. In selecting low rates, we confined ourselves to data from about 1968 to 1972 from registries selected by the IARC (1976) as being reasonably reliable.

The results are shown in table 7, and the total of these low incidence rates is contrasted with the corresponding totals for all types of cancer (except non-melanoma skin cancer) in Connecticut and in many other parts of the United States in table 8. The comparisons in table 8 suggest that in most parts of the United States in 1970 about 75 or 80% of the cases of cancer in both sexes might have been avoidable. The proportion could be more, as the lowest rates that have been used almost certainly include some avoidable cancers, especially since some of the countries that differ most markedly in various ways from the United States do not have a good cancer registry and so have not been used in table 7. (Moreover, the proportion in 1980 will probably be about one percentage point larger than that in 1970 due to the steady increase in tobacco-induced lung cancer in the United States.) However, the proportion that might by practicable means be avoidable may well be somewhat less than is suggested by tables 7 and 8, partly because in a developed area such as the United States some lumps may have been counted that, although histologically "cancer," were biologically benign (appendix C), but, more importantly, because even if means of modification of cancer risks can be identified, these may not be socially acceptable. This might obviously be a serious limitation if preventive measures had perforce to be limited to ways whereby different countries already differ, for affluent people will not be persuaded to adopt certain aspects of the life-style of the impoverished. But there may be many different simple or highly technical ways of preventing the same cancer (*see* subsequent sections), some of which have not been inadvertently adopted by any country with a good cancer registry, at least one of which ways may be both practicable and acceptable.

About half of the cancers diagnosed in the United States are found among people 65 or more years old, and we have made no explicit estimate in table 7 of

TABLE 7.—*Cancer rates[a] in selected low-incidence areas among people under 65 years of age[b,c]*

Type of cancer	Male rates in: Connecticut registry	Male rates in: Low-incidence registry	Registry with lowest reliable incidence for: Males	Registry with lowest reliable incidence for: Females	Female rates in: Connecticut registry	Female rates in: Low-incidence registry
Lip	11.8	4.1	United Kingdom, southern metropolitan region	United Kingdom, Birmingham	0.8	0.4
Tongue	19.8	4.1	New Mexico: Spanish	Israel: ♀ Jews	6.7	2.7
Salivary gland	7.3	2.3	Japan, Miyagi	Japan, Miyagi	6.7	1.2
Mouth	31.3	0.8	" "	" "	11.8	2.4
Oropharynx	13.9	1.1	" "	" "	6.0	0.8
Nasopharynx	5.6	2.4	East Germany	East Germany	1.1	1.1
Hypopharynx	10.7	1.4	" "	" "	2.9	0.2
Esophagus	34.6	6.5	Norway, rural	Norway, rural	8.3	1.8
Stomach	66.2	28.0	New Mexico: whites	United States, Iowa	26.7	16.6
Small intestine	6.4	3.0	Israel: Jews	Israel: ♀ Jews	5.0	2.5
Colon	137.2	13.7	Nigeria, Ibadan	Nigeria, Ibadan	140.7	11.6
Rectum	98.6	14.1	" "	" "	66.1	17.2
Liver	11.8	6.0	United Kingdom, southern metropolitan region	United Kingdom, Oxford	5.3	1.0
Gallbladder, plus ducts	9.0	3.3	Norway, rural	Norway, rural	11.2	6.7
Pancreas	45.1	21.0	Nigeria, Ibadan	Nigeria, Ibadan	30.9	14.9
Nose	3.2	2.2	United States, Iowa	United States, Iowa	2.4	1.5
Larynx	54.7	11.5	Japan, Miyagi	Japan, Miyagi	8.2	0.4
Bronchus	325.8	9.0	Nigeria, Ibadan	Nigeria, Ibadan	96.9	8.7
Bone	9.3	7.3	Puerto Rico	United States, Iowa	7.5	5.2
Connective tissue	20.0	12.5	United Kingdom, Birmingham	United Kingdom, southern metropolitan region	14.6	6.4
Melanoma	40.8	8.0	United Kingdom, Liverpool	United Kingdom, Liverpool	38.6	18.4
Breast	3.5	1.7	Finland	Israel: ♀ non-Jews	593.7	100.9
Cervix	—	—	—	Israel: ♀ Jews	90.4	42.5
Choriocarcinoma	—	—	—	United Kingdom, Oxford	1.2	0.2
Other uterine cancers	—	—	—	Japan, Miyagi	150.6	11.1
Ovary	—	—	—	" "	104.8	25.9
Other female genital organs	—	—	—	" "	16.0	2.3
Prostate	92.3	5.3	Japan, Miyagi	—	—	—
Testis	26.6	7.1	" "	—	—	—
Penis	2.0	0.2	Israel: Jews	—	—	—
Bladder	113.1	17.8	Japan, Miyagi	Japan, Miyagi	32.8	7.3
Kidney	59.6	9.0	Nigeria, Ibadan	Nigeria, Ibadan	23.2	2.5
Eye	4.3	2.0	Japan, Miyagi	Japan, Miyagi	4.3	0.5
Brain and CNS	54.9	12.2	" "	" "	35.2	8.9
Thyroid	12.4	3.6	United Kingdom, southern metropolitan region	United Kingdom, Oxford	34.0	8.8
Other endocrine cancers	2.5	1.4	Puerto Rico	Puerto Rico	2.2	0.6
Lymphosarcoma	39.8	13.1	" "	" "	25.5	6.4
Hodgkin's disease	37.4	6.2	Japan, Miyagi	Japan, Miyagi	28.1	3.5
Other reticuloses	11.3	1.8	Israel: Jews	Israel: ♀ Jews	7.6	1.9
Myeloma	15.1	1.8	Japan, Miyagi	Japan, Miyagi	9.6	3.3
Leukemia	57.9	40.8	New Mexico: Spanish	" "	41.1	36.3
Polycythemia	4.8	0.6	Japan, Miyagi	" "	1.6	0.3
All other cancers	89.9	33.7	New Zealand: whites	New Zealand: whites	74.6	23.5
Total, all cancers	1,590	321			1,775	408

[a] For all tumors except those of benign or unspecified malignancy and non-melanoma skin cancers (which, collectively, accounted for <2% of all cancer deaths in the United States in 1978).
[b] From IARC (1976).
[c] Annual rates/million people <65 yr old, standardized for age as described in appendix A.

what proportion of these might be avoidable. This is because data from cancer registries become very unreliable in old age, not so much in the United States nowadays as in those countries where the contrasts with the U.S. life-style and environment may be greatest. Consequently, any similar analysis of rates among older people might be severely biased. There is, however, little reason to suppose that the proportion of U.S. cancers that would be preventable differs greatly above and below the age of 65 years as long as lung cancer (which is relatively slightly more common among the old) and other cancers are considered separately (*see* section 5.1 and appendix E). Paradoxically, therefore, the most reliable available estimate of the proportion of cancer among older people that is avoidable may simply be the proportion that is avoidable among middle-aged people.

The foregoing estimates refer to all malignant tumors, both fatal and non-fatal (excluding only non-melanoma skin cancer). Direct estimation by similar methods (but on the basis of national death certification rates instead of, as in tables 7 and 8, registered incidence rates) of the proportion of fatal cancers that are avoidable might be misleading. This is because many

TABLE 8.—*Comparison of total tumor incidence rates*[a,b] *observed in various American cancer registries, circa 1970*

Area in United States covered by tumor registry[d]	Male tumor incidence		Female tumor incidence	
	Observed	Minimal,[c] as % of observed	Observed	Minimal,[c] as % of observed
Alameda, Calif. (W)	1,589	20	2,103	19
San Francisco, Calif. (W)	1,668	19	2,137	19
Connecticut	1,590	20	1,775	23
Iowa	1,422	23	1,594	26
Detroit, Mich. (W)	1,498	21	1,737	23
New Mexico (W)	1,469	22	1,784	23
New York, upstate	1,372	23	1,481	28
El Paso, Tex. (W)	1,245	26	1,682	24
Utah	1,215	26	1,464	28
"Ten areas" from TNCS (a study covering a moderately representative tenth of the whole United States)				
TNCS White	1,519	21	1,702	24
TNCS Non-white	1,906	17	1,721	24
TNCS White and non-white	**1,557**	**21**	**1,705**	**24**

[a] Annual rates/million people <65 yr old, standardized for age as described in appendix A.
[b] *See* table 7, footnote *a*, for excluded tumors.
[c] The total of the lowest reliable rates for each type of cancer listed in table 7 was 321 (♂) and 408 (♀), which is a crude indication of the minimal incidence that might be achieved.
[d] W = whites only.

underdeveloped countries enumerate causes of death so inaccurately that comparison of their certified death rates from particular types of cancer with the corresponding rates in the United States might overestimate the proportion of U.S. cancer deaths that is avoidable. However, the two types of cancer (lung and large intestine) that currently kill the largest numbers of Americans have incidence rates that vary particularly widely between the United States and certain other countries and the U.S. deaths from these two types are therefore largely avoidable. The same is true of many other types of cancer that currently kill large numbers of Americans, and it is reasonable to suppose that the proportion of fatal cancers whose onset could have been avoided will be approximately the same as the avoidable proportion of all cancers discussed above, i.e., more than 75 or 80% in principle but perhaps less in practice for many years to come.

4. ATTRIBUTION OF RISK

4.1 Increases and Decreases in U.S. Cancer Rates

If there were currently an "epidemic" of cancer in the United States (by which we mean rapid increases in the probability of people *of a given age* developing most particular types of cancer), this might suggest that the search for avoidable causes for the cancers that we observe today should be directed chiefly toward various aspects of the modern environment that were much less widespread half a century or more ago. If, conversely, most of the cancers that are now common have been common for many decades, then, although this would not be evidence as to whether our new habits will eventually increase or decrease future cancer risks, it might suggest that the cancers that are currently common, and that will continue to be common unless we do something about them, have been largely determined by long-established aspects of the American life-style or environment.

Practical Difficulties in Gauging Cancer Trends

Cancer is certainly much more noticeable nowadays than it was a decade or two ago, but this is not in itself evidence that cancer rates are increasing as there are several factors that influence public awareness about cancer. First, especially when active treatment is being undertaken, the friends and relatives of cancer patients (or the general public, if the patient is a public figure) may discuss the disease openly, whereas previously such matters often used to be hushed up and the diagnosis perhaps withheld even from the victim. Second, some cancers are now diagnosed that might previously have gone unnoticed in the medical treatment (and subsequent death certification) of dying people, especially of the elderly. Third, cancer has become *relatively* more common as a cause of death chiefly because of the prevention or cure of so many other diseases. This is nicely illustrated by the data for females in 1935 and 1975 (table 9). The non-respiratory cancer death rates decreased substantially, but the death rates from all other causes decreased even more substantially. Therefore, the *percentage* of female deaths attributable to non-respiratory cancer is actually greater now than it was 40 years ago, even though among women of a given age the *absolute* cancer risks are lower nowadays. If attention had been restricted to people under the age of 65 years (text-fig. 2), then the contrast between declining absolute rates and increasing percentages would have been even more marked. Fourth, there is a larger proportion of old people nowadays, and cancer risks are ten or a hundred times greater among old people than among young people. Finally, cancer has become a highly political issue, and consequently discoveries (perhaps using modern ultrasensitive analytical methods) of even quite small amounts of carcinogens in various everyday contexts attract vigorous media coverage, as do various other aspects of cancer research.

We shall therefore review in this section, and in our appendixes C, D and E, some of the objective evidence concerning the upward and downward trends in the U.S. death rates from, and incidence rates of, various cancers. Epidemic increases in lung cancer are clearly taking place, as would be expected as a result of

TABLE 9.—*Death certification rates/1,000 Americans,*[a] *1935 and 1975*

Sex	Years	All causes except neoplasms		All neoplasms[b] except respiratory cancers		Respiratory tract cancers		All causes	
		Rate	%[c]	Rate	%[c]	Rate	%[c]	Rate	%[c]
Male	1933–37	15.12	91.0	1.42	8.5	0.09	0.5	16.63	100
	1973–77	8.91	81.0	1.41	12.8	0.69	6.2	11.01	100
Female	1933–37	11.92	87.6	1.65	12.1	0.03	0.2	13.60	100
	1973–77	4.96	78.8	1.17	18.6	0.16	2.5	6.29	100

[a] All ages, standardized for age to U.S. 1970 census (*see* appendix A). For most scientific purposes, separate examination of the trends above and below the age of 65 is preferable (*see* appendixes C and D), since many deaths from cancer half a century ago may have been miscertified as due to other causes, particularly among older people.
[b] Benign and malignant tumors are included in this table, as elsewhere throughout this text.
[c] Rate as percent of corresponding all-causes rate in last column.

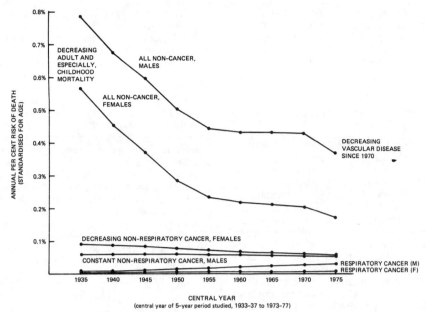

TEXT-FIGURE 2.—Annual age-standardized death rates, 1933–77, among Americans under 65 years of age.

the widespread adoption of cigarette smoking earlier this century, but apart from this we can see no good evidence of a cancer "epidemic" in the above sense.

Unfortunately, both cancer *registration* rates (a "cancer registry" tries to count all the new cancer onsets in a particular area, such as the State of Connecticut) and cancer *death certification* rates are subject to large errors; more unfortunately, these errors are not constant with time so that artifactual trends in the registered incidence or certified mortality rates for particular cancers may be superimposed on the true trends. The problem with any comparisons of cancer rates in different decades is that these artifactual trends may be of the same order of magnitude as the trends in real cancer onset rates that one wishes to study. The chief sources and likely magnitudes of such biases are discussed in appendix C.

Reduction of Bias: Trends in Mortality in Middle Age

The data suggesting moderate improvements in relative 5-year survival rates (e.g., from 60 to 68% for breast cancer) are also discussed in appendix C (*see* table C2 on page 1278), where it is suggested that part at least of these moderate apparent improvements is artifactual, due to progressively more complete enumeration of the non-fatal cases. Changes in treatment for many types of cancer have chiefly improved palliation rather than cure of the disease, and the true cure rates for many of the common types of cancer have probably changed very little since 1950. For these types of cancer the trends in death certification rates among people under 65 years of age, at which ages treatment of the curable and medical investigation of the causes of death of the incurable have for decades been reasonably careful, may paradoxically yield a much more reliable (and representative) indication of the real trends in cancer onset rates than can the superficially more attractive study of any of the currently available data on registered incidence rates. The need to restrict attention to death certification rates for people *under* the age of 65 years

arises because many people who died of cancer in past years never had their disease diagnosed and might have been certified as dying of pneumonia, senility, or the wrong type of cancer. Progressive correction of such errors over the past several decades has resulted in large artifactual trends (some upward, some downward) in the death certification rates for certain types of cancer, especially during the first half of this century or, since 1950, especially among old people. (These and various additional biases also affect the trends in disease registration rates, where a registry tries to count both all fatal and non-fatal cases of cancer: *see* appendix C.) However, for most types of cancer the trends since the **1950's** among **middle**-aged American death certification rates seem likely to yield a reasonable indication of the true underlying trends in the corresponding real disease onset rates.

Increase in Middle-Aged Mortality From Respiratory Cancer

Either by examining the lower lines in text-figure 2 with a magnifying glass, or by referring to appendix tables D1 and D2 (pp. 1282–1283) from which text-figure 2 was derived, it can be seen that male respiratory cancer death rates appear to have been rising steadily for at least half a century and that female respiratory cancer death rates started to rise a quarter of a century ago and are now increasing alarmingly rapidly. The trends in respiratory cancer are discussed in more detail in appendix E, where we conclude that before 1950 almost the whole of the apparent increase in female lung cancer and some of the apparent increase in male lung cancer were artifactual, due to more accurate detection of lung cancer, but that some of the pre-1950 male increase and virtually all of the more recent increases in both sexes are real and are largely or wholly caused by the delayed effects of the adoption, decades ago, of the use of cigarettes (*see also* section 5.1). (The long delay between cause and full effect arises because even among people who have smoked regularly throughout most of their adult lives the degree of exposure of the lungs to cigarette smoke during their late teens or early twenties remains a surprisingly important determinant of lung cancer risks in middle or old age. *See* text-fig. E1 on page 1292.)

Lack of Generalized Increase in Middle-Aged Mortality From Non-respiratory Cancer

Text-figure 2 and tables D1 and D2 (pp. 1282-1283) also indicate that the aggregate of all non-respiratory cancers has taken a fairly constant toll among males for half a century (with about a 10% decrease among younger men in the past decade), but that the total non-respiratory cancer death rate among females has been decreasing rapidly for half a century, due not chiefly to improved treatment but rather to decreased onset rates among women of a given age. For age-specific details, *see* text-figs. C1 and C2 on page 1272. (All the overall comparisons we make are based on "age-standardized" rates, which can change only because of changes in the risk of cancer among people of a given age; increases or decreases in the proportions of old people will not affect them. This is not true of "crude" cancer rates nor of "percentages of all deaths attributable to cancer," and these should never be used to characterize trends: *see* appendix A.) However, non-respiratory cancer is an aggregate of many completely different types of cancer, some of which are increasing and some of which are decreasing.

Text-figures 3 and 4 describe, for males and for females, respectively, changes in mortality (or, more strictly, death certification rates) during the past quarter century for various types of cancer. More detailed data are presented in table D3 on page 1284, together with a separate discussion of the apparent changes in mortality from various particular types of cancer among people under 65 years of age. Corresponding details for people aged 65 years and over appear in table D4 on page 1285. All the changes are small in comparison

with the large increases in the smoking-related cancers of the respiratory and upper digestive tracts, although the decreases in mortality from cancers of the stomach and uterus are also important.

In appendix D we also present the recent (1968-78) trends in death certification rates among Americans in *early* middle life (35-44 years of age), as it is here that the first effects of any changes for better or worse in the causes of cancer might first be clearly evident. Reassuringly, no unexpected upward trends emerge (*see* table D6 on page 1287), while significant downward trends are seen in mortality from many types of cancer. For males, the sites where there are now significant decreases in mortality at ages 35-44 years include the pancreas, lungs (presumably chiefly due to decreasing tar yields per cigarette: *See* appendix E), and genitalia. For females, they include the intestines, genitalia, reproductive system, and breast (the latter decrease due perhaps to a protective effect of early childbirth on the mothers of the 1950's glut of babies). Overall, cancer mortality among young adults in the United States is decreasing quite rapidly, and much of the decrease cannot plausibly be attributed to improved therapy.

Trends in Incidence, as Assessed by Cancer Registry Data

Turning (with some trepidation, because of the greater likelihood of bias) from trends in certified mortality to trends in registered incidence, we are immediately confronted with the problem of exactly which incidence data to study—those from particular cancer "registries" that have operated for decades, trying to list all the cases, fatal or otherwise, of cancer in New York or Connecticut, those from comparison

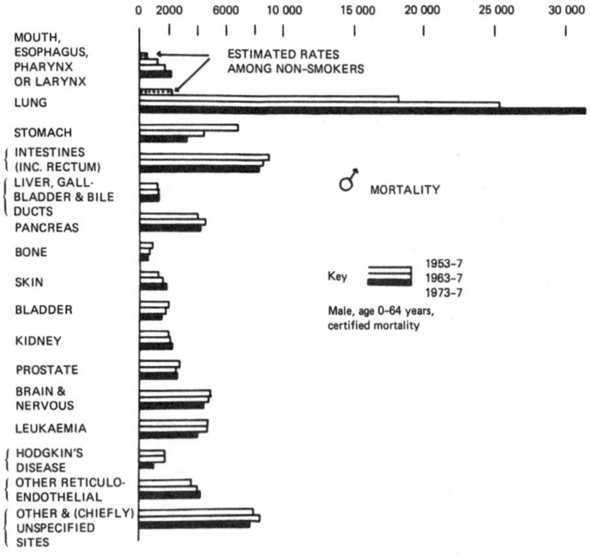

TEXT-FIGURE 3.—Certified mortality per 100 million males, ages 0–64 years (standardized for age to U.S. 1970 population as described in appendix A).

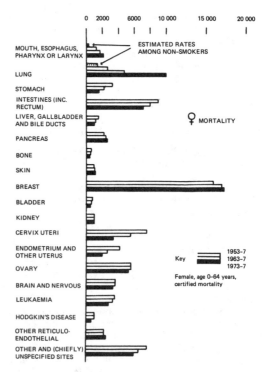

TEXT-FIGURE 4.—Certified mortality per 100 million females, ages 0–64 years (standardized for age to U.S. 1970 population as described in appendix A).

of the Second National Cancer Survey (SNCS) in 1947 or 1948 with the Third National Cancer Survey (TNCS) in 1969–71, or those from comparison of the TNCS with the Surveillance, Epidemiology, and End Results (SEER) program of the mid-1970's? (SNCS, TNCS, and SEER all tried to monitor cancer incidence in about one-tenth of the entire U.S. population.) Unfortunately, many of the above comparisons suffer from such large artifactual irregularities and biases (*see* discussion in appendix C and text-figs. C3 to C5, pp. 1274–1276) that for most types of cancer they yield much less reliable information about long-term trends in real disease onset rates than the mortality data do.

The only one of these comparisons of cancer incidence rates that is at all compatible with the mortality data is that of the SNCS (in 1947 or 1948) with the TNCS (in 1969–71). This comparison has been described by Devesa and Silverman (1978, 1980). From their 1978 paper we have abstracted text-figures 5 and 6, describing the changes in registered incidence rates for each of the major types of cancer. The overall pattern of change indicated by these text-figures is, of course, roughly similar to that indicated by the mortality data, for this was why we selected this particular comparison of incidence rates for study. Consequently, we would not strongly disagree with anyone who argued that even the comparison of incidence rates in text-figures 5 and 6 is so uninformative that it would be preferable to rely chiefly on mortality data (although some of the striking differences between certain of the trends in incidence may be informative as, for example, the apparent decrease in cancer of the cervix but not of the endometrium).

However, even if the detail of the incidence trends is uncertain, the general picture is clear: *a*) the most important absolute increases have been in cancer of the lung, *b*) the most important absolute decreases have been in cancers of the stomach and uterine cervix, and *c*) less reliably, there seem to be no large changes in the aggregate of the incidence of all nonrespiratory cancer[9] (for which the age-standardized incidence registration rates decreased between 1947–48 and 1969–71 by 3% for males and by 19% for females.)

Comparison With Interpretations by Others

In summary, the trends since 1950 in mortality in middle age, somewhat reinforced by the trends in incidence between the Second and Third National Cancer Surveys, suggest that, apart from the effects of smoking (and perhaps asbestos: *See* section 5.6), there are no major epidemic increases in cancer. Unfortunately, our conclusion is not shared by all commentators. Epstein (1981b), whose book, *The Politics of Cancer*[10] (Epstein, 1978, 1979), was based on the assumption that Americans live in an era of genuinely and rapidly increasing cancer rates over and above the

---

[9] We have excluded, since the surveys did not attempt to register it, non-melanoma skin cancer. Non-melanoma skin cancer is diagnosed more commonly than any other type of cancer, but it is nearly always so easily cured that it is one of the least common fatal cancers.

[10] For a wide-ranging comment on Epstein's (1978, 1979, 1981a, 1981b) perspective on the causes of cancer, which will make clear our reasons for not drawing on it in our present report, *see* Peto, 1980. The particular question of the role of occupational factors will be dealt with in section 5.6 and appendix F, where strong reasons for distrusting Epstein's (1981a,b) sources are given.

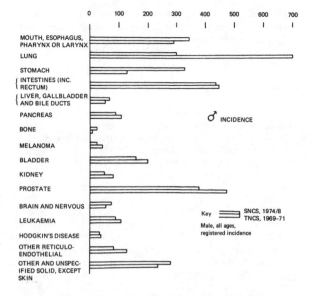

TEXT-FIGURE 5.—Registered incidence rates per million males, all ages (standardized for age to U.S. 1950 population and for race to 90% white).

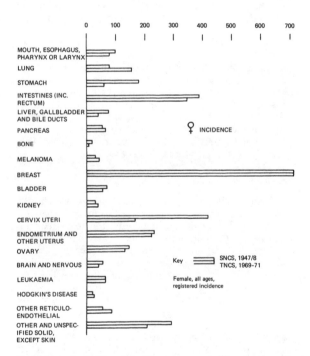

TEXT-FIGURE 6.—Registered incidence rates per million females, all ages (standardized for age to U.S. 1950 population and for race to 90% white).

increase due to tobacco, rejects it out of hand without acknowledging or explaining why the trend in U.S. mortality from non-respiratory cancer in middle age is actually downward, and without serious discussion of the potential biases in trends in death certification rates among older people (or, still more so, in trends in the registered incidence rates of tumors) that we have emphasized in appendixes C, D, and E. The Toxic Substances Strategy Committee (TSSC) in their 1980 report to the U.S. President also came to a conclusion directly opposite to ours, namely, that "even after adjustments for age . . . recent figures show that both incidence (new cases) and mortality (deaths) rates are increasing," and later that "when the effects of cigarette smoking are corrected for, the recent trends in incidence show an increase." Their conclusions about rising incidence rates were based on the data of Pollack and Horm (1980) and on the interpretation of these data by Schneiderman (1979) and rested heavily on a comparison of the incidence rates recorded in the TNCS during 1969–71 with those recorded in the ongoing SEER program that began in 1973. In appendix C we show that this particular comparison yields estimates of trends in real disease onset rates that are grossly discrepant with more reliable data.

An even more serious error in the TSSC (1980) report is the committee's peculiar method of "allowing" for the effects of cigarette smoking on the recent trends in lung cancer (and in certain other types of cancer) when it tries to estimate the residual effects of toxic substances other than cigarette smoke. The committee completely overlooked the fact that even if national exposure to cigarette smoke had remained constant throughout the 1960's and 1970's and all other relevant exposures had been constant throughout this century, large increases in lung cancer during this period would still have occurred due to the delayed effects of the large increases in cigarette consumption some decades before (*see* appendix E).

From this review of trends and from our more detailed review of trends in appendixes C, D, and E, we conclude that although a small part of the current morbidity from cancer may be due to new processes and products, it appears that changes in the American life-style, diet, or environment have also helped to reduce some old hazards, and (apart from lung cancer) most of the types of cancer that are common today in the United States must be due mainly to factors that have been present for a long time.

Implications

When seeking means to prevent cancer, we should certainly pay special attention to those types that are increasing in incidence, not only for fear that the increase may herald the onset of a new epidemic but also because the fact of the increase indicates that the cause (or causes) must have been introduced during this century and can presumably be eliminated. However, our review of trends obviously offers no guarantee that future risks may not be importantly affected by current exposure to some new factor(s) whose effects have yet to appear. To concentrate on a search for new agents to the exclusion of other causes is, however, to ignore the possibility of preventing that mass of present-day cancers which are due to avoidable factors that must have been prevalent in the Western world at least throughout this century or before.

4.2 Prediction From Laboratory Experiments

Over the past quarter of a century, various laboratory methods have been developed for predicting which particular chemicals would be likely to cause cancer if humans were acutely exposed to high doses or were chronically or intermittently exposed to low or moderate doses. An excellent review of the main methods and their relative merits has recently been compiled by the International Agency for Research on Cancer (IARC,

1980; *see also* Hollstein et al., 1979). The most favored methods now include not only "long-term" tests (in which the test chemical is usually fed at very high doses for a substantial part of the life-span of a few dozen rats or mice or some other small, short-lived animal to see if there is any marked excess of tumors of some particular type) but also various "short-term" tests, which are intended to be much quicker and cheaper than the long-term tests.

Different Types of Short-Term Test

The most attractive (IARC, 1980) short-term tests currently available fall into the following three main classes.

Effects on the genetic material (DNA) of cultured cells.—The test chemical may be applied, perhaps together with certain of the enzymes, etc., to which it would presumably be exposed in the human body (in case it is thereby "metabolically activated," i.e., converted from an inactive to an active form[11]), to suitably modified bacteria or mammalian cells growing freely in culture. The aim is to see whether the action of the test chemical or its metabolite(s), perhaps followed quickly by a round or two of cell replication, can cause the cellular DNA to suffer either a permanent change (i.e., one that is likely to be inherited by both daughters when changed cells divide and that can be detected by allowing selective proliferation of changed cells) or damage of a type which, although perhaps not directly detectable, causes particular cellular side effects[12] that can be detected. If bacteria are used (as in the "Ames test") then the whole test takes only a few days, but some important effects detectable only in mammalian cells may be missed, and vice versa. Even at the cost of somewhat increasing the number of "false-positive" findings, the use of both mammalian and bacterial short-term tests seems prudent for the more important chemicals.

Effects on DNA in the cells of living animals.—The test chemical may be administered in one very large dose to a few animals that are killed a few hours later, ground up exceedingly finely, and then examined (by alkaline elution) to see if the DNA extracted from any particular organ(s) shows breaks due to recent chemical attack. (Search in the urine of animals treated briefly with the test agent for excreted by-products of DNA repair has been proposed by various people but is not yet validated.) Alternatively, in the "mouse spot test," pregnant mice of appropriate genotype are treated with the test agent to see whether, 5 weeks later, their offspring will have a few spots on their fur due to chemical alteration in the fetal mice of the genetic information in a few single coat color cells (which proliferated during the intervening 5 weeks into a clone of descendants large enough to be seen as a spot of altered color). Finally, alterations in the sperm or other cells from animals may be sought. This latter technique, which is developing rapidly, may apply directly to putatively exposed human populations.

Compared with tests on the DNA of cultured cells,

---

[11] No "metabolic activation" system seems perfect for use in short-term tests, but the most widely used system consists of microsomes extracted from fragmented cells from either rat or, preferably, human liver (IARC, 1980).

[12] Definitions of the side effects that may be sought, such as prophage induction, chromosomal "breakage," sister chromatid exchange, or "unscheduled" DNA synthesis, may be found in IARC (1980), but are not necessary for our present discussion.

tests on the DNA of cells in intact animals usually suffer from less uncertainty as to what form of metabolic activation is appropriate but more uncertainty as to the concentration of the test agent that reaches the target cells.

Effects on the behavior of cultured cells.—The test chemical may be applied (perhaps with some metabolic activation) to semi-normal cultured mammalian cells to see if it alters a few of them into cancerous-looking cells with a selective advantage, after a few weeks of growth in culture, over their unaltered neighbors.

Advantages of Short-Term Tests

The enormous advantage of the use of short-term tests is that they take only a few days or weeks and cost only a few hundred or a few thousand dollars (even if enough duplicate assays are done to achieve statistically reliable estimates of potency), whereas long-term tests take a few years and cost a few hundred thousand dollars (and the data may even then be subject to appreciable random or even systematic[13] statistical uncertainty unless a very striking carcinogenic effect occurs). Moreover, clear positive results in several short-term tests may yield the intangible but important benefit of conceptual clarification; for example, although we still do not know the cellular mechanism(s) whereby damage to DNA increases the likelihood of cancer, progress in understanding the mode of action of a carcinogen such as dimethylnitrosamine that damages DNA in many short-term tests is likely to be much more rapid than for carcinogens such as the halogenated hydrocarbons that are inactive in many short-term tests. Indeed, short-term tests have now developed to such a point that any serious scientific investigators who are responsible for initiating a careful long-term animal test on a particular chemical should themselves also routinely assume responsibility for ensuring that the results from the careful and competent execution of several short-term tests will be available to them before the final animal study report is prepared, for this increase of a few percent in the total amount spent will in most cases yield a very substantial increase in the scientific understanding of the biological effects of the test agent. No single short-term test can be relied on to pick up all effects of potential interest, which is why a combination of several such tests is advisable. (IARC, 1980, provides an excellent introduction to the selection of suitable short-term tests.)

Laboratory tests can be used either "exogenously" or "endogenously" to try to identify preventable causes of human cancer. First and most obvious, "exogenously," the additives, main components and contaminants of our drugs, drinks, diet, etc., may be separately screened in short- or long-term tests. Second, "endogenously," crude fractions of the feces (Bruce et al., 1979), blood, urine (Yamasaki and Ames, 1977), breast secretions, pancreatic juices, bile, etc. from several different individuals may be analyzed for moderate activity using

some short-term method such as the Ames test which may be sensitive to very small amounts of active chemicals. If detectable activity is found in any sample, then that sample may be further fractionated in various ways, repeatedly using the short-term test activity as an assay to decide which fractions to throw away and which to subfractionate, until the active chemical(s) are located and characterized. Either before or after this, one may be able to experiment for a few days at a time with the few people whose fluids show the most pronounced activity, to find which aspects of their normal work, diet, drinks, drugs, diseases, medicaments, etc. chiefly determine the variation in total short-term test activity within individuals. Such findings may direct attention toward fruitfully testable specific epidemiological hypotheses which would not otherwise have occurred to the investigators.

Limitations of Short-Term Tests: Factors Affecting "Later Stages" of Carcinogenesis

From the above brief account of the nature and possible uses of laboratory cancer tests, it will be apparent that most of today's short-term tests rely heavily on the hypothesis that chemical agents which damage cellular DNA can cause cancer if they can gain access to the DNA in the "stem" cells of our bodies.[14] Most scientists find this claim plausible, but there is much less evidence for the converse claim that all of the really important determinants of human cancer are such agents. Quite apart from any possible inhibitors of carcinogenesis, there may be whole classes of chemicals that are human carcinogens but which are not likely to be detected by any of today's short-term tests.

One fundamental reason for this is that alteration of a completely normal cell into the seed of a growing cancer may usually require at least two qualitatively different types of change, and the chief causes of one type may not be important causes of the other type, and vice versa (Peto, 1977, 1979). A cell that has undergone the "early" change(s) and is therefore now at risk of the "late" change(s) is, if it divides, likely to produce two daughter cells which are *both* at risk of the "late" change(s). So agents may in principle increase the likelihood of cancer in various completely different ways, perhaps by facilitating the early change(s), by conferring a selective advantage on partially altered cells relative to their normal unaltered neighbors, by facilitating the later change(s) (among partially altered cells descended from a stem cell that has undergone the early change(s)), or by interfering with any hypothetical host defense factors that may exist to restrain fully cancerous cells from proliferating.

Different cancer research workers tend to emphasize the relevance of different links in this chain, but none of the groups of processes are well understood. One class of chemicals called "initiators," which seem

---

[13] If, as is often the case, the test agent materially reduces the life expectancy of the heavily dosed group(s) of animals, then exact statistical correction for the effects of this on the yields of hepatomas or of any other moderately lethal type of tumor is impossible unless the cost-free precautions against bias recommended in the statistical annex to IARC (1980) are built into the conduct of the experiment. Omission of this may occasionally lead to unnecessary errors of interpretation of results which are of marginal statistical significance.

[14] The human body is composed of many cells that are incapable of any further division (e.g., many of the cells in our muscles, brains, and blood) plus many cells that appear capable only of a strictly limited number of further divisions, all the descendants of which will be inert or gone within the next few days or months, plus, most importantly of all, a few "stem" cells whose descendants will still be dividing a year or more hence and which are presumably the cells most at risk of cancerous alteration. Cairns (1975) has discussed the possible cellular basis of the differences between stem and other cells and has speculated that interference with the mechanisms which maintain these differences may be of critical importance in human carcinogenesis.

chiefly to affect the early stages, is reasonably well characterized, although the extent to which the "early" processes of the currently common human cancers are caused by such initiators is still unknown. Another class of chemicals called "promoters," which seem chiefly to affect either the selective proliferation of partially altered cells or the "late" processes (or, perhaps by separate mechanisms, both), is becoming reasonably well characterized, but again although promoters will undoubtedly be important tools for studying some particular mechanism(s) whereby cells *can* become cancerous, the common human cancer may not usually arise by such mechanisms (or, if they do, those mechanisms may have been triggered by accidents or agents unrelated to "promoters").

Perhaps the currently emerging understanding of "initiators" will turn out to be substantially correct, with the current short-term tests picking out all the important exogenous chemicals which currently cause human cells to undergo the "early" stages of carcinogenesis (and being useful tools in the search for the preventable determinants of the endogenous synthesis of such chemicals). However, "promotion" is still very poorly understood, as are almost all the other intracellular processes involved in transforming a partially altered cell into a fully cancerous cell. [One molecular biologist whose recent discoveries chiefly relate to "early," DNA-damaging carcinogens commented, "The key to carcinogenesis lies in understanding the later stages of the process; the early stages are just trivial molecular biology" (Cairns J: Personal communication). For review articles on the later stages of carcinogenesis, *see* Slaga et al., 1980.] Moreover, such "late" processes may turn out to be of much greater relevance to carcinogenesis in large-bodied animals like man that have to avoid cancer for 75 years than in the small, short-lived animals that laboratory workers must necessarily study (Peto, 1979). If cells must independently undergo first "early" and then "late" processes before cancer can develop, then a 50% reduction in *either* class of processes would halve the eventual risk of cancer (Peto, 1977), and the only determinant of which class is more "important" is which is more easily halved.

Implications of, and Interrelationships Between, Results From Different Types of Tests

Some evidence bearing indirectly on the reliability of long-term tests comes from the correlation between the findings in mice and rats. Purchase (1980) found 248 compounds that had been tested in both species, and in each species about half these compounds were significantly carcinogenic and half were not. If the results in each species were of no predictive value whatever, one might expect 50% agreement and 50% disagreement by chance alone, whereas in fact Purchase found 85% agreement and only 15% qualitative disagreement.[15]

However, the similarities between rats and mice are obviously greater than the similarities between rats and humans, so the percentage of correct answers if rat carcinogenicity were used to predict human carcinogenicity in a similar range of chemicals would presumably be less than 85%. (For comparison, remember that, given the real data on carcinogenicity among mice for each compound, deciding whether to call that compound "a rat carcinogen" merely on the flip of a coin should yield 50% "concordance" between the two species!) Considerably more direct evidence that both short-term and long-term tests are moderately reliable is provided by the observation that most chemicals that have been found to be carcinogenic in *both* rats *and* mice also exhibit marked DNA-damaging activity in one or more of the short-term bacterial mutagenicity tests, whereas most chemicals that have been tested and found not to cause any significant excess of cancers in *either* rats *or* mice are inactive in all such tests.[16]

Turning to more directly relevant correlations, of the 39 established human carcinogenic agents or circumstances which were listed in table 6 on page 1203 a mere *one third* are well-characterized individual chemicals which might have been picked up as clearly carcinogenic in *routine* feeding experiments in mice and rats, while the remaining two-thirds are not. Of those which are not, some are chemicals which although able to cause cancer in humans have not been found to be carcinogenic in any animal experiment thus far devised or have been found to be carcinogenic in animals only if given intrapleurally or subcutaneously, but not if given in their diet.[17] However, some of the factors listed in table 6 as affecting human cancer are not chemicals at all (e.g., various forms of radiation or immunosuppression, certain infective agents, and various physiological changes caused by pregnancy or hormonal alteration), although of course it is just as important to recognize these as to recognize carcinogenic chemicals. In others of the listed carcinogenic circumstances the responsible chemicals have not been identified with certainty (e.g., certain manufacturing processes and also two extremely important causes of human cancer, betel chewing and tobacco smoking). The study of cigarette smoke exemplifies the practical difficulties in using laboratory tests to predict human cancer risks. In developed countries tobacco may be the most important single cause of cancer, currently accounting for about one-third of all U.S. cancer deaths

---

[15] Some of these apparent discrepancies may have been due merely to chance fluctuations in the outcomes of certain particular experiments causing false-positive or false-negative results that would have been avoided had larger groups of animals been studied. Ideally, a mere tenfold discrepancy between the carcinogenic potency of a chemical in two different species should not be considered a qualitative discrepancy, although it might appear to be so if there were no statistically significant effect in the hardier species. Practically, however, the false-positives and false-negatives that inevitably arise by chance in realistic animal tests are an important inherent limitation of the method.

---

[16] The quantitative details of the correlations of results between short-term and long-term tests are subject to vigorous dispute (e.g., Ames and McCann, 1980; for a review and extensive bibliography, *see* IARC, 1980), which is why no percentages are cited. When there is eventual agreement as to how accurately short-term tests do predict which among a thousand particular chemicals are carcinogenic for rodents, it would be reasonable to hope for a similar degree of accuracy in predicting which of these thousand will be carcinogenic to man, for the differences between bacteria and humans are not obviously greater than the differences between bacteria and small, short-lived laboratory animals (unless, to keep our large human bodies free of cancer for our long human life-span, we rely much more heavily than do rodents on some cellular mechanisms which have no analog in bacteria).

[17] Most insoluble dust particles that people inhale are ultimately transferred, via the respiratory tract mucus, down the digestive tract, so even for asbestos dust feeding studies might have been thought relevant but would probably have failed to detect the hazard. Studies of chronic inhalation of the various physical forms of dust to which humans are exposed would have discovered rat lung tumors in response to asbestos dust (Wagner et al., 1974).

(section 5.1), but for many years cigarette smoke failed to produce malignant tumors in routine animal inhalation tests (a fact used in those years to deny the relevance of the human lung cancer data!). By persistent modification of the experimental circumstances malignant tumors were eventually produced by animal inhalation of cigarette smoke, and repeated application of certain components of cigarette smoke to the skins of laboratory mice can easily be shown to cause cancers. However, despite a quarter of a century of intensive study in a variety of animal and other laboratory systems, it remains unclear which of the many components of cigarette smoke "tar" are the most important causes of human cancer, and so the relative carcinogenicity for humans of tobacco "tars" of various different compositions cannot be predicted with confidence, nor can it be stated with confidence that everything other than the "tar" is innocuous. (Likewise, cigarette smoke is an important cause of both vascular and respiratory disease, but for both the causative components of the smoke remain uncertain.)

On this evidence, animal feeding studies have great value in certain circumstances but may not offer an uncomplicated and straightforward means of discovering preventable causes for the majority of human cancers, and at the very least it certainly does not seem likely that they can offer a reliable means of estimating quantitative human hazards.

There is, however, an important sense in which examination of table 6 is not a fair way to assess the extent to which human carcinogens can be detected by routine rodent feeding tests on particular chemicals, for by definition table 6 excludes the greatest successes of animal feeding tests, i.e., the instances where these detect human carcinogens that epidemiology has not detected. (Nitrosamines exemplify this possibility.) But this may be counterbalanced by the fact that table 6 also excludes by definition any "false positives," i.e., agents which confer no material risk in the circumstances in which humans are exposed to them but which are significantly carcinogenic in laboratory animals, either due to random fluctuations[18] or due to important differences between mice and men. (Phenobarbital may be an example of such an agent: *See* Clemmesen and Hjalgrim-Jensen, 1977.)

Overlooking Important Determinants of Human Cancer

The trouble with all the foregoing attempted correlations, however, is that they depend rather critically on the range of chemicals that one chooses to study. Part of this trouble can be circumvented arithmetically [by expressing the results in terms of an "odds ratio" $(x/1-x)/(y/1-y)$, where x and y are the respective probabilities that agents active and agents inactive in a short-term test will be carcinogenic in a long-term test], but the more important troubles still remain. A nearly perfect screening system that picked up all currently known occupational carcinogens other than asbestos might be of less public health value than a lousy system that picked up asbestos but missed nearly everything else, simply because asbestos causes such a

large percentage of occupational cancers. Likewise, a lousy research system that nevertheless identified one important preventable cause of breast cancer but which missed nearly everything else might be of more public health value for women than an ideal battery of long- and short-term tests for exogenous DNA-binding carcinogens. In other words, what we really need as the most relevant measure of the value of a laboratory test is a *weighted* correlation, in which the ability to predict the major ways whereby human cancer can be prevented counts for much more than the ability to predict minor causes and in which the identification of carcinogens to which humans are not and will not be seriously exposed is irrelevant.

Because this ideal measure of quality is unknowable, it is necessary to fall back on studying the correlations between the results of different tests, even though this may lead to a self-reinforcing over-valuation of the merits of the currently available test procedures. It is too soon to known which, if either, of the "exogenous" and the "endogenous" uses of today's testing technology will prove really fruitful in searching out previously unrecognized preventable causes of human cancer. Tobacco smoke is certainly active in many test systems, which is encouraging. But apart from tobacco, the avoidance of all human exposure to all the other exogenous and endogenous chemicals that are active in long-term animal studies or in today's short-term tests might have prevented surprisingly few of the cancers of today whose causes still elude us,[19] or perhaps avoidance of such exposure would have prevented most of them. Possibly, misleading conclusions are being drawn from over-emphasis on the spectrum of chemicals found active in mutagenicity tests and in chronic carcinogenicity studies in rodents. For example, the authors of official guidelines on how to do long-term tests usually emphasize the importance of concurrent controls and the need for strictly identical diet, handling, heat, light, stress, and infection in the treated and control animals. Why? Can minor details of the lifestyle of the animals really be important determinants of the animals' "spontaneous" tumor yields? And, if so, might not the same also be true for humans? In experimental animals, quite minor details of the total quantity of food and of the vitamins, fats, and carbohydrates (Jose, 1979; Roe and Tucker, 1974; Tucker, 1979; Conybeare, 1980; Roe, 1981) in the food can certainly be enormously important determinants of spontaneous tumor yields. But, because the mecha-

---

[18] If statistical significance is assessed incautiously, the number of such "false positives" may be large, for in separate analysis of tumor rates in many organs in two sexes of two species many possibilities of a false-positive result will arise. For discussion of how moderate degrees of statistical significance in animal feeding tests should be interpreted, *see* the statistical annex to IARC (1980).

---

[19] Cairns (personal communication) has noted that exposure of the whole body of a smoker to a marked excess of Ames-test-positive mutagens (Yamasaki and Ames, 1977) results in only a moderate excess of urinary and pancreatic cancers and in no large excess of leukemias, lymphomas, or solid cancers at other sites distant from the respiratory tract. Cairns (1981) and German (1979) have also noted that although xeroderma pigmentosum patients are grossly defective in their ability to repair DNA damage due to almost all of the currently recognized Ames-positive mutagens, the very limited data available do not demonstrate an excess risk of cancer at any internal site. Finally, although the contents of the colon may be strikingly mutagenic in the Ames test (Bruce et al., 1979), this activity has not yet been evaluated as an important determinant of colon cancer, and since there can be similar mutagenic activity both in the human small intestine (where cancer is rare) and in the colons of many different species of animal, its significance remains open. It may turn out to be one of the most important observations yet made by any such methods, or alternatively if mutagenic feces have been common for millions of years then perhaps mammalian intestines have evolved effective defenses against them.

nisms are not understood, short-term tests for the possible relevance to humans of these processes do not exist, and these phenomena are typically viewed as a potential nuisance to serious investigators who want to study the carcinogenicity of some trace environmental contaminant rather than as being themselves a potentially fruitful area of inquiry.

Difficulties in Quantitating Human Risks From Laboratory Data

Many promising lines of laboratory research into the development and use of various tests for carcinogenicity exist, but although there is every hope that current lines of laboratory research will draw attention to at least some of the preventable causes of human cancer, there is little reason to expect from them, at least in the near future, any *quantitative* predictions of human risk which are reliable to within a factor of ten or even, perhaps, a hundred. Quantitative extrapolations (e.g., of the dose in mg/kg/day which halves the lifelong probability of remaining tumorless) from animals to humans *may* already be giving us approximately correct assessments of human risk. Conversely, however, they may suggest risks that are wildly misleading in one or another direction. At present (*pace* Meselson and Russell, 1977) there seems to be quantitative human data on the risks from too few chemicals to know. The IARC (1980) review concluded that we are not even at the point yet where useful quantitative estimates of animal risk in long-term feeding studies can be derived from the findings in the various short-term tests, and, whether or not this is true, quantitation of human risk must therefore be a still more remote goal. Even if the potencies of different members of one particular family of chemicals are assessed for their activity in one short-term test and in one particular strain of animals, the correlation may be poor (Bartsch et al., 1980), so estimation of even the animal potency of a member of a previously untested class of chemicals may be still less reliable. Despite this unfortunate uncertainty, the quantitative data from laboratory tests (especially short-term tests) are, for many occupational, environmental, and dietary contaminants, the only information likely to be available in the next few years, and even tenfold or hundredfold uncertainties may be dwarfed by the millionfold variations between chemicals in their apparent potency and in the degree of human exposure to them.

Use of Laboratory Data for "Priority Setting" But Not for "Risk Assessment"

If our perspective on both short-term and animal tests is accepted, then quantitative human "risk assessment," as currently practiced, is so unreliable, suffering not only from random but also probably from large systematic errors of unknown direction and magnitude, that it should definitely be given another name: "Priority setting" might perhaps be a more honest, although less saleable, name. So many thousands of chemicals are active to some extent or other in one laboratory test or another that it is difficult to know what, if any, practicable regulations to enact on the basis of laboratory tests. For some tests it has been recommended that the regulations which are promulgated should be based only on whether or not the chemical being tested is active, irrespective of the quantitative degree of activity of that chemical. But, if no explicit use is to be made of the degree of activity of each chemical, then instead

of effective reduction of the total of all human cancer the chief result may be complete paralysis (either of the regulators or of the "regulatees").

A more proper use of each particular laboratory test might be to multiply the potency of each chemical studied in that test by whatever crude estimate is available of the degree of human exposure to that chemical, to yield some sort of index of human hazard according to that one laboratory test. When this has been done, it is likely that, for long-term tests and for each separate short-term test, one or a few chemicals will stand out head and shoulders above the rest with respect to these indices of human hazard. The best use of the various laboratory tests might be to identify, study, and if possible reduce these few apparently most extreme human hazards with respect to each particular test (together with any more moderate exposures that can be cheaply controlled) without necessarily requiring direct human evidence of harm. Although in many cases the benefits might be illusory, a few prudent restrictions against the apparent extremes with respect to each type of test might be nearly as effective as a broad action against all apparently active chemicals. This is true, however, only if before priorities are established a serious effort has been made to seek out as many sources of exposures as possible to agents active in that test (including endogenous formation of mutagens and other active agents in the gastrointestinal tract and exogenous absorption of such agents from involuntary or deliberate inhalation of smoke).[20] In the absence of direct evidence of the exact quantitative relevance to humans of the findings in long-term animal tests or in any of the short-term tests, blanket restrictions on very large numbers of minor chemical pollutants may be unacceptably expensive, and the approach we have suggested might turn out to be a socially acceptable alternative way of setting a few priorities.

The conclusion that laboratory studies can be useful for priority setting but not for risk assessment is also prominently featured as one of the few major recommendations for change made by the National Academy of Science's recent committee of enquiry into the methods currently used by the Environmental Protection Agency to regulate pesticides (Committee on Prototype Explicit Analyses for Pesticides, 1980). Their thorough and thoughtful report addresses very nicely both the theoretical and the practical difficulties in regulating pesticides.

Returning to our present limited purpose of estimating the percentages of today's cancers that could be prevented by various particular means, we conclude that the great uncertainty inherent in quantitative estimation of human risks from currently available

---

[20] For example, in deciding how rigorously to regulate one particular source of environmental contamination by dioxins, it may be helpful to bear in mind the "background" extent to which such agents may be formed anyway wherever organic matter is burned (Bumb et al., 1980); in deciding how rigorously to regulate one particular source of dietary nitrosamines, it may be helpful to bear in mind the "background" extent to which nitrosamines are formed anyway in the human digestive tract (section 5.3); and in deciding how rigorously to regulate some other source of inhaled or ingested mutagens, it may be helpful to bear in mind the "background" extent to which the blood and urine of cigarette smokers are contaminated by such agents anyway (Yamasaki and Ames, 1977), for massive regulatory efforts against quantitatively unimportant targets may in their total effects be diversionary.

laboratory test results means that in what follows we must of necessity rely chiefly on quantitative epidemiological findings, merely reinforced in some of our final judgments about what is, and what is not, a real cause-and-effect relationship by laboratory findings.

4.3 Use of Epidemiological Observations

We concluded from previous sections that to estimate the percentages of current U.S. cancer deaths that might be avoidable in various ways, we must of necessity base our estimates chiefly on observations of the patterns of disease that are actually found in humans rather than on laboratory studies of particular chemicals, thus avoiding the many pitfalls, reviewed in section 4.2, inherent in extrapolation from laboratory studies to human experience. In this section we shall discuss some further advantages, disadvantages, and pitfalls of epidemiology. First, observations of the vagaries of human behavior may suggest ideas that might never occur to a laboratory investigator. Historically, they provided the starting point for a large part of all cancer research by pinpointing the risks associated with exposure to the combustion products of coal, sunlight, X-rays, asbestos, and many chemical agents. They drew attention to the hazards associated with chewing various mixtures of betel, tobacco, and lime and with smoking tobacco, and they suggested lines of research based on a hitherto unsuspected role for some type(s) of dietary fiber and on the relevance to breast cancer of the hormonal factors associated with pregnancy. Second, study of national trends in age-specific mortality from particular diseases may direct attention fruitfully toward diseases that are deserving of special further study (as happened in the 1940's with cancer of the lung), while study of the evolution of cancer rates among occupational or other groups in which an excess of cancer was present for reasons that were incompletely understood provides a monitoring system to check whether any hygienic measures that have been instituted have effectively reduced exposure to the actual causes of disease. Third, positive epidemiological observations (e.g., on radiation carcinogenesis) provide quantitative data relating directly to some of the doses to which humans are actually exposed. By so doing, they avoid or reduce the pitfalls in the extrapolation not only from one species to another but also from one dose level to another extremely different level and so provide estimates of the human risks associated with low exposure levels that are reliable enough for rational comparison of risks and benefits. Fourth, epidemiologists can sometimes study such large numbers of people that direct evidence of very small effects can be obtained. Humans feed themselves, house themselves, and arrange their own medical care at no cost to the epidemiologist. Observations can, therefore, be made on hundreds of thousands of individuals, whereas studies of comparable numbers of laboratory animals would be prohibitively expensive. No practicable experiment, for example, could have shown that doses of X-rays of the order of 1 rad to a fetus in its mother's abdomen could result in 1 cancer in every 2,000 individuals during childhood, as was shown in Great Britain by Stewart et al. (1958) and in the United States by MacMahon (1962).

Epidemiological observations, however, also have serious disadvantages that limit their value. First, they can seldom be made according to the strict requirements of experimental science, and consequently the available observations may be open to a variety of interpretations. A particular factor may be associated with some disease merely because of its association with some other factor that causes that disease, or the association may be an artifact due to some systematic bias in the information collection. Second, the observations that can be made on humans are limited to the conditions that have actually occurred. Except perhaps for the study of some putatively protective factor(s), the observations cannot be repeated at the command of the investigator with people exposed, for example, to another dose. Moreover, although large numbers of people may have been exposed to a moderate dose of some agent (e.g., an air or water pollutant), no comparable study groups may be available that have been consistently exposed to doses different enough for a measurably large difference in risk to arise (*see* below). Third, it may not be possible to detect the effects of a carcinogen on people until it has been in use for many years. Long induction periods are common for cancer, and hazards that are undetectably small after 10 years' exposure may be major after 30 years. By the time effects are clearly evident to the epidemiologist irreversible damage may have been done to large numbers of people, so that even after exposure is recognized and stopped cancers may continue to occur for many years.

These disadvantages limit the value of observations on humans, but they do not outweigh the major advantages that have been described. No one would choose to obtain evidence of the existence of a hazard by observing the appearance of a disease in humans if other practicable means were available, but until we know exactly how cancer is caused and how some factors are able to modify the effects of others, the need to observe imaginatively what actually happens to various different categories of people will remain.

Interpreting Epidemiology: Need for Comparison of Individuals, and Not Only of Large Groups

Trustworthy epidemiological evidence, it should be noted, always requires the demonstration that a relationship holds for individuals (or perhaps small groups) within a large population as well as between large population groups. Correlation between the incidence of cancer in whole towns or whole countries and, for example, the consumption of particular items of food can, at the most, provide hypotheses for investigation by other means. Attempts to separate the role of causative and confounding factors by the statistical techniques of multiple regression analysis have been made often, but evidence obtained in this way is, at best, of only marginal value.[21]

---

[21] It is commonly, but mistakenly, supposed that multiple regression, logistic regression, or various forms of standardization can routinely be used to answer the question: "Is the correlation of exposure (*E*) with disease (*D*) due merely to a common correlation of both with some confounding factor (or factors) (*C*)?" The trouble is that unless the confounding factor is something (such as age or sex) that can be estimated with negligible measurement error, adjustment by any standard statistical techniques of the correlation of *E* with *D* for the *measured* values of *C* will reduce *but will not extinguish* the correlation between *E* and *D* even if, given the error-free (but unknown) values of *C*, no correlation between *E* and *D* would remain. (*See* appendix B14: Two properties of multiple regression analysis *in* Fletcher et al., 1976.) Moreover, it is obvious that multiple regression cannot correct for important variables that have not been recorded at all.

In practice, the danger of reaching a wrong conclusion from epidemiology is slight when observations are made on individuals rather than on whole populations and when the risk of disease is increased many times by exposure to the agent under suspicion. In these circumstances, risks have been detected that are quite small in absolute terms (affecting perhaps only one exposed person in 1,000) and some have been detected after only a handful of cases of a rare type of cancer have occurred in all.

Limitations of Epidemiology

The situation is, however, very different when the induced disease is as common as cancer of the lung or cancer of the breast is now. In these circumstances, human studies will be able to detect a specific risk only if the absolute risk of death is quite large. Even risks that will ultimately kill, for instance, 1% or more of the exposed population may be overlooked or attributed to chance unless a very large-scale investigation is undertaken. In these circumstances, too, when the cancer rates among exposed people are only a moderate multiple of those among the unexposed (e.g., when the relative risk lies between 1 and 2, as for kidney cancer among smokers or breast cancer among women who have been treated with reserpine; for an excellent discussion of the latter example, *see* Labarthe, 1979), problems of interpretation may become acute, and it may be extremely difficult to disentangle the various contributions of biased information, confounding of two or more factors, and cause and effect.

In short, unless epidemiologists have studied reasonably large, well-defined groups of people who have been heavily exposed to a particular substance for two or three decades without apparent effect, they can offer no guarantee that continued exposure to moderate levels will, in the long run, be without material risk. For this reason, prudent restrictions on occupational or public exposure to various substances often have to be based on indirect inference from laboratory studies of the agent being examined, without any direct evidence concerning its actual effect on humans. That is not to say that human evidence can ever be dispensed with. It is always relevant, but the weight that can be given to it varies greatly with the duration and intensity of the exposure experienced by individuals. Positive evidence (unless due to confounding) is always important. Negative human evidence may mean very little, unless it relates to prolonged and heavy exposure. If, however, it does, and is consistent in a variety of studies (correlation studies over time, cohort studies of exposed individuals, and case-control studies of affected patients), whereas the laboratory evidence is limited in its scope to, for instance, a particular type of tumor in a few species, negative human evidence may justify the conclusion that for practical purposes the agent need not be treated as a human carcinogen. In practice it is, of course, not usual for such perfect negative human evidence to be available, but even less conclusive negative human evidence may help determine priorities between different courses of action.

Advantages of Epidemiology

Our present purpose, however, is not to predict the future effect of new agents, but to make estimates of the proportions of today's cancers that are attributable to various avoidable causes, and for this purpose epidemiology, influenced by laboratory investigation, is far superior to the latter alone. Epidemiology has at present an undeservedly low reputation among people who have first artificially limited themselves to wondering which environmental pollutants to restrict and who then find that almost none of the few thousand chemicals they are worried about have been adequately studied by epidemiologists. This is, however, to condemn epidemiology for failing to achieve ends that it does not have. Epidemiology starts not with the 10,000 chemicals polluting a particular city but with the 10,000 annual cancer deaths in that city, and it tries to determine the major causes of these actual deaths. Epidemiology is, admittedly, more likely to overlook many undetectably small effects of various chemicals than laboratory studies might do, but it is much less likely to overlook the large determinants of contemporary cancer rates and trends, especially if these are not simple environmental pollutants or dietary contaminants.

Environmental Carcinogenesis: Misconceptions and Limitations to Cancer Control

by John Higginson, M.D., and Calum S. Muir, M.B.

Most cancers are associated to some degree with environmental factors. Unfortunately, people often assume that a similar proportion of cancers are preventable now through simple regulatory control directed predominantly at industrial pollution and man-made chemicals (*1, 2*). Consequently, scientists and public health authorities are criticized both for failure to develop effective prevention measures and for inadequate and misdirected research on environmental carcinogenesis, because the scientific and nonscientific limitations to effective control of many human cancers are not always recognized (*3, 4*). Thus we have thought it worthwhile to summarize our views on the current state of environmental carcinogenesis and the possibilities of primary cancer prevention.

The objectives of this paper are: 1) to stress that extensive information is already available on cancer causation in man and to summarize additional inferences concerning possible carcinogenic mechanisms and etiology that may be drawn from epidemiologic data; 2) to emphasize the complexities inherent in the concept of "environment," particularly, "carcinogenic risk factors" and "life-style," and their significance for cancer prevention; and 3) to propose that more research is needed in human cancer on the role of cocarcinogenesis, including promotion.

DEVELOPMENT OF ENVIRONMENTAL CARCINOGENESIS

The concept of chemical carcinogenesis arose from the demonstration of occupational hazards followed by the isolation of pure chemical carcinogens. These

John Higginson, M.D., and Calum S. Muir, M.D., are with the International Agency for Research on Cancer, 150, Cours Albert-Thomas, 69372 Lyon, Cedex 2, France.

historic developments and the growth of the petrochemical industry have focused attention on synthetic chemicals as the major potential carcinogenic stimuli in the human environment. However, as early as 1950, leading workers in epidemiology and experimental carcinogenesis concluded that although geographic variations in cancer incidence in man were largely related to the environment, the environment included not only discrete chemical carcinogens but also ill-defined life-style factors such as dietary, social, and cultural habits (*5*). By the mid-1970's, such diverse environmental factors as cigarette smoking and alcoholic beverages as well as occupational and iatrogenic hazards had been identified and evaluated. In addition, most of the hypotheses on the basic mechanisms of chemical carcinogenesis had been promulgated (*6*). The statement that environmental, chemical carcinogenesis, and life-style factors have been ignored is not true.

Nature of Cancer-Causing Factors in Man

Clinical cancer is the end result of numerous influences at the cellular level, many of which cannot be investigated easily in epidemiologic studies, even though such studies may provide clues as to the mechanisms involved. The concept of a defined carcinogenic stimulus (chemical or physical) is widely understood irrespective of the mode of action (*7*). Initiators are regarded as mutagenic and irreversible in action in contrast to promoters that may also operate at an epigenetic level (*8–10*) and may be reversible. The distinction in practice, however, is not easy as illustrated by cigarette smoke, a human carcinogen, but one in which the relative importance of initiation and promotion is still unclear. Moreover, not all carcinogens may be mutagens nor is initiation always extrinsic or "complete."

Reprinted with permission from *Journal of the National Cancer Institute*, Vol. 63, No. 6, December 1979, pp. 1291-1298.

Several factors, however, are associated with an increased cancer risk. These include absence of fiber, excess of dietary fat, obesity, and such behavior patterns as age at first marriage or age at first pregnancy, which cannot be defined at present as carcinogens in the sense described above. Carcinogenic risk factor is a convenient label for such factors, without implication of an understanding of the biologic mechanisms involved. Evidence shows, however, that many factors may be describable eventually in terms of cocarcinogenic theory, with use of the concept in a wide sense, because not only is there increasing evidence for cocarcinogenesis in man but also many promoting, enhancing, and inhibiting factors have been identified in the human environment (11, 12). However, appropriate technology for field studies will be essential for such investigations.

Multifactorial Causation and Predominant Factors

A carcinogenic factor may be so predominant that a particular cancer would not manifest in its absence without necessarily precluding a contributory role for other factors. The multifactorial etiology of cancer must be considered not only in terms of initiators but also in terms of cocarcinogenesis (10). This premise is illustrated by the enhancing effect of asbestos on cigarette-induced lung cancer (13) or possibly maternal hepatitis B infection in aflatoxin-induced liver cancer (14, 15). In such situations, determination of which factors should be considered predominant becomes a matter of judgment. In practice, this risk would probably be that in the absence of which the greater number of cancers would not occur, e.g., cigarette smoking in lung cancer in asbestos workers or asbestos in mesothelioma. For carcinogenic risk factors the question is often more difficult; thus age at first pregnancy, family history, and diet may all contribute to breast and endometrial cancer, but none seems predominant (16). In contrast, estrogen therapy is clearly a predominant factor for endometrial cancer in some women over 50 years of age (17).

EVIDENCE FOR ENVIRONMENTAL ETIOLOGY OF HUMAN CANCER

The evidence for attribution of a high proportion of human cancers to environmental factors has been reviewed elsewhere (18, 19) and relates to the following two categories.

Cancers Caused by Well-Defined Exogenous Factors

These tumors generally occur in adults and are epithelial, involving the skin, respiratory organs, and upper digestive tract. Most of the tumors are asso-

ciated with such personal habits as smoking, sunbathing, betel quid chewing, and excess alcohol consumption. A small proportion of the tumors is related to specific occupation or iatrogenic exposures. In general, a sufficient amount is known about etiology of these tumors to permit proposals for effective control and they will not be discussed further. The monographs of the International Agency for Research on Cancer (20) evaluate the literature on over 400 chemicals and related industrial processes suspected to be human hazards.

Cancers of Suspected but Unproved Environmental Etiology

This group comprises cancers, notably of the gastro-intestinal and endocrine-dependent systems, for which the *most rational interpretation of the epidemiologic data* indicates an association with environmental factors (18). However, controversy surrounds the nature of the factors and mechanisms involved that have implications for the selection of approaches to cancer research and control. Some authors (2, 21) emphasize low-dose exposures to numerous chemical carcinogens, mostly industrial, in the general environment, whereas others (5, 8, 10, 12, 19) believe that cocarcinogenic mechanisms (including promotion) associated with life-style-related risk factors are of greater significance. For the reasons discussed next, practical suggestions for the effective control of these tumors are not yet possible.

Cancer in Industrialized Societies

The effects of high-level or point-source occupational exposures are usually relatively easy to investigate, but evaluation of low-dose exposures, single or multiple, to man is more difficult, as illustrated by the polycyclic aromatic hydrocarbons (22) and the nitrosamines (23), which are diffusely and widely distributed in the environment. Often people assume that industrial and urban environments are more heavily contaminated by such agents as chemical carcinogens, mutagens, and promoters and that comparison with nonindustrial areas should provide a measure of their effect. However, these comparisons are complicated by widespread pollution by such chemicals as pesticides and herbicides occurring in modern agricultural societies as well as by behavioral and dietary variables.

Time trends.—Environmental contamination by such carcinogens as polycyclic aromatic hydrocarbons is long-standing, and industrialization, which began in many countries over 100 years ago, has not been homogeneous, with resultant geographic variations in pollution and life-styles.

Since 1950 morbidity statistics in the United States

have become reasonably reliable and show that despite long-standing industrialization, a rapidly expanding petrochemical industry, and increasing awareness of occupational hazards, the overall cancer rates are decreasing in black and white females and in white males if tumors related to alcohol and tobacco are excluded. The remaining increase observed in black males is largely attributable to cancer of the prostate gland and esophagus (24). Trends in Western Europe are similar. Although fairly rapid increases in cancer of the colon and slower increases in cancer of the breast and prostate gland have been observed in Japanese migrants to the United States, no changes of comparable degree have been reported in industrialized Japan (25–28).

Residence.—Attempts have been made to correlate cancer patterns with place of residence, industrialization, and population density, especially in the United States (29, 30). Although urban–rural differences have been reported in several countries, they are not consistent. When population groups with a homogeneous life-style are examined (e.g., Mormons), urban–rural differences largely disappear (31). Few cancers can be attributed to air pollution per se, though air pollution may potentiate the cancer effects of cigarette smoke (32). However, the possibility that some delayed effect, perhaps environmental pollution, which requires elucidation, can be important is suggested by the fact that migrants from the United Kingdom to New Zealand and South Africa show that, despite comparable smoking habits, lung cancer patterns between country of origin and those of the new country are intermediate.

Inconsistencies are also observed in the incidence of individual cancers in different countries (19). Thus whereas bladder cancer has been associated with the presence of chemical and allied industries in the United States (33), no industrial association has been found in Japan (34). Prostate cancer is twice as frequent in blacks in the United States as in whites residing in the same counties, and in both groups the frequency is much higher than in the industrialized United Kingdom and many times more frequent than in Japan. Even if lung cancer is excluded, cancer patterns within Europe show no correlation with industrialization. Thus the incidence in nonindustrialized Geneva, Switzerland, is as high as that in urbanized England (35). Although many experimental carcinogens cause liver cell cancer, such tumors in man appear related either to alcoholic beverage ingestion or mycotoxins, and possibly to hepatitis B (14, 15), rather than to general or limited industrial exposures. Associations of cancer with general water pollution (36) or fluoridization have not withstood statistical scrutiny.

Although teratogens have been regarded as crude indices for environmental carcinogens, congenital malformations show very slight variations in time and place and cannot be correlated with adult cancer patterns, though these malformations are reported to be increased in the offspring of smoking mothers. Childhood cancers, which globally tend to be similar in incidence, do not correlate with industrialization.

Occupation.—Studies from England and Wales (37) have shown that, whereas certain occupations are associated with a greater or less cancer risk than the population average, nearly 90% of such variation can be eliminated if comparison is made between individuals of similar habits and social class (38). Although the cause of the residual risk may be studied in such high-risk groups, detection and analysis of the same cause at much lower levels in the general population would clearly be difficult because of greater confounding by life-style and other factors.

Thus the general pattern of cancer observed in North America and Europe with a high frequency of cancer of the lung, large intestine, breast, and uterus suggests some common factors in the environment as compared to the very different patterns seen in Africa and Asia. However, it is unjustified to link simply the modest geographic and secular changes observed at several sites (e.g., breast, colon, uterus, ovary, pancreas, and prostate gland) in Europe and North America to recent food additives or pollutants or to changes in ambient environmental pollution and industrialization; other explanations appear more plausible. Thus variations in cancer of the breast, ovary, and uterus can be related at least partly to changes in reproductive patterns. These data are inconsistent with the view that present cancer patterns only present a demonstrable accumulation of multiple chemicals, mutagens or carcinogens, in the ambient environment.

Life-Style and Cocarcinogenesis in Human Cancer

In addition to smoking, alcohol, and occupational exposures, other aspects of life-style may have significant influence on tumors of the gastrointestinal and endocrine-dependent systems. Of these aspects, diet and behavior seem to be the most significant.

Diet.—Diet should not be considered only in terms of food additives or ingested carcinogens. In 1950, Kennaway wrote: "Response of any tissue to a carcinogen depends on both the more recent and less recent quantitative and qualitative characteristics of the diet. This subject requires both experimental work on animals and observations on human populations living under a great variety of conditons" (39). Dietary variables include a) preformed potential carcinogens, e.g., aflatoxin and pyrolysates (40, 41); b) carcinogen precursors, e.g., secondary amines and nitrates (41); c) type and relative proportion of nutrients, e.g, ratio of saturated to nonsaturated fats, and trace elements; d) nonnutrients, not carcinogens per se, whether relatively inert, e.g., fiber, or biologically active, e.g., goitrogens, steroids, enzyme inducers, promoters, inhibitors, and antibiotics (11, 42, 43); and e) nonspecific effects, e.g., calorie intake (8).

Whereas the association is defined between specific

dietary items and cancer, e.g., aflatoxin and liver cancer (*15*) and alcoholic beverages and esophageal cancer, for other cancers and items of diet results have been inconsistent and difficult to interpret. Thus studies relating cancers of the breast and colon to meat, fat, and calorie intake have not been supported by other studies of Mormons and nuns (*31, 44-47*). Studies on the roles of fecal flora and steroid content and transit time in cancer of the large bowel conflict. The correlation between dietary fiber and colon cancer has only been adequately demonstrated in a few studies (*48*).

Behavior.—Investigations of migrants, religious groups, and geographic variations (*25-28*) have confirmed that tumors of the endocrine-dependent system are dependent on environmental factors, the effects of which, though considerable, may only become apparent over several generations. These environmental factors include such carcinogenic risk factors as age at first intercourse or marriage, number of children, celibacy, and other behavioral patterns that reflect the cultural setting. Although one is tempted to explain part of the action of such culturally determined factors on the basis of subtle changes in hormone status, other factors, such as dietary fat, have been correlated with cancer of the breast. Diet is also a significant factor in the determination of height, weight, and age at menarche, all of which have been described as risk factors for cancer of the breast and endometrium. Thus before rational control measures can be suggested, a better understanding of the complex interplay of diet and cultural factors will be necessary. In this context, Miller (*16*) emphasized the value of the use of risk factors, such as age at first pregnancy, as a source for developing and testing hypotheses on the relative role of hormones and other factors. The correlation between obesity as a risk index for certain endocrine-dependent tumors may possibly be explained by its association with increased formation of extraglandular estrogen.

Cocarcinogenesis, including promotion, may be especially relevant to endocrine-dependent tumors (*12*). Therefore, the observation that the frequency of "small" latent prostate cancers is much the same in populations with contrasting incidence of clinical cancer, even though "large" latent tumors are common in countries having a high incidence (*49*), strongly suggests promotion and progression. Similarly, the relatively rapid change in endometrial cancers observed in residents of San Francisco (*17*) and related to steroid therapy for the menopause again suggests promotion rather than initiation. Accordingly, high priority must be given to developing research to measure and express life-style or carcinogenic risk factors in biochemical and physiological terms. This task will not be easy because migrant studies indicate that such factors may have greatest impact early in life and require more than 1 generation to affect cancer patterns [e.g., cancer of the breast and prostate gland (*25-28*)].

PROPORTION OF CANCERS RELATED TO VARIOUS ASPECTS OF THE ENVIRONMENT

In the selection of control and research priorities, evaluation of the relative importance of known or suspected etiologic factors is desirable, covering a spectrum of environments.

It is not possible to give, with any precision, an upper limit to the sum of all attributable risks, which may be well above 100%, for the total cancer burden in a community. However, the degree to which a predominant factor may contribute to the total cancer incidence may be estimated in the sense that in the absence of the factor, that proportion of all related cancers would not occur. Thus tobacco smoking is responsible for about 85% of lung cancer whether in the general population or in asbestos-exposed workers in the United Kingdom.

In the establishment of the proportion of cancers related to environmental factors, two approaches are possible: One method would be to estimate the number of persons exposed in the entire population and calculate the number of resulting cancers to be expected from knowledge of the effect of various dose levels and durations of exposure. Such calculations are not currently possible for any population, even for such a common risk factor as smoking for which large populations have been studied. Even if a profile of all exposures were available for each individual, allowance for every synergistic or antagonistic effect would be impossible.

The second and currently most fruitful approach is to examine cancer risk site by site for a given population and assess the proportion of cancers due to known or suspected predominant causes and cancers considered due to life-style. The residue may be assumed to be due to factors as yet unidentified. For some of these cancers, there may be sound epidemiologic evidence that certain stimuli are unlikely to be involved, e.g., occupation in breast cancer.

In the United Kingdom, 80-85% of lung cancer is due to the predominant risk—tobacco, and no more than 15-20% could be caused by other factors. For cancer of the male bladder in the United States, estimates for occupation range from 15 to 30%, cigarettes probably account for 50%, and coffee has been suggested to be related to a further 20%. The remaining causes may be due to unidentified risks (*50*). Miller (*16*) ascribes 25% of breast cancer to age at first pregnancy, 20% to family history, and 17% to dietary fat intake.

This second approach is exemplified by analysis, which takes local conditions into account, of an English population (Birmingham and West Midlands) and an Indian (Bombay) population (text-figs. 1-4). In the former population, a long-established industrial community, less than 2% are employed in agriculture and over 60% are employed in industry; in the latter

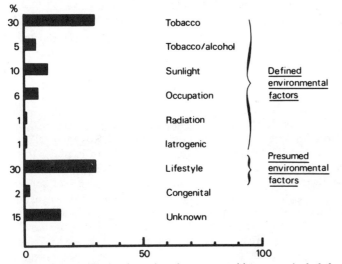

TEXT-FIGURE 1.—Proportion of male cancers, skin cancer included (*35*), in the Birmingham and West Midland region of England in 1968–72, attributed to causes listed. (For method of computation and discussion on various categories, *see* text.)

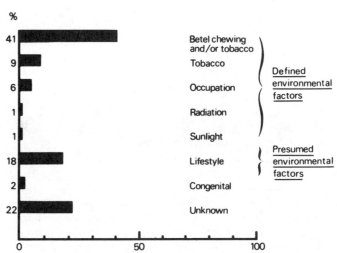

TEXT-FIGURE 3.—Proportion of male cancers, skin cancer included (*35*), in Greater Bombay, India, in 1968–72, attributed to the causes listed.

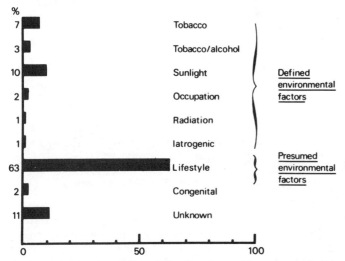

TEXT-FIGURE 2.—Proportion of female cancers, skin cancer included (*35*), in the Birmingham and West Midland region of England in 1968–72, attributed to causes listed.

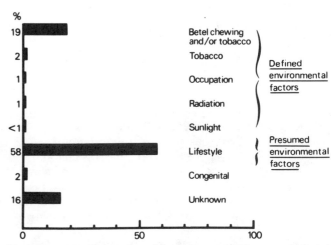

TEXT-FIGURE 4.—Proportion of female cancers, skin cancer included (*35*), in Greater Bombay, India, in 1968–72, attributed to the causes listed.

population, over 50% are industrial workers, many of whom are migrants from elsewhere in India (*35*).

Data from many sources, summarized in (*51*), were used in the preparation of these estimates; they included analytical and correlation studies, sex ratios, changes in population migration, and geographic risk differences. For example, for each site cancer incidence in females provides a reference point for the evaluation of the impact of these environmental exposures mainly affecting males, e.g., heavy industry. In contrast, the identical incidence of colon cancer in both sexes in Birmingham suggests common exposures. A similar approach can be used to evaluate geographic differences. Assignment to a given cause does not mean that other factors are not concerned; the assignment only means that the factor listed is probably the predominant cause.

The histograms are clearly approximations, and the proportions ascribed to different causes selected may vary according to the population studied; thus in some parts of Africa over 40% of cancers (liver) might be attributed to mycotoxins, with hepatitis virus being considered as a promoting, but not a predominant, factor.

Personal Habits

Tobacco.—In the United Kingdom, 80–85% of lung cancers are thought to be caused by cigarette smoking. Smoking is also implicated in cancer of the mouth, larynx, pharynx, esophagus, cardiac end of the stomach, the bladder, and probably the pancreas. The proportion of cancers due to cigarette smoking is somewhat lower in Bombay, where tobacco use appears to have its impact through the betel quid on the oral cavity, pharynx, and upper esophagus.

Tobacco-alcohol.—In the United Kingdom, excessive alcohol consumption causes cancer of the mouth, pharynx, esophagus, and liver. Inasmuch as most persons with cancers of the mouth and esophagus both smoke and drink heavily, they have been assigned to the tobacco-alcohol category. Findings in nonsmoking, "teetotal" Mormons and Seventh-Day Adventists in the United States support these estimates. Alcohol consumption is relatively rare in Bombay.

Sunlight.—Although sunlight is regarded as the major cause of skin cancer, changing social conditions make it difficult to distinguish between occupational and leisure exposures. Skin cancer is rare in India due to protective skin pigment.

Occupation.—Computation of the amount of occupational cancer relating to point-source exposures in a population is dependent on assessment of the *excess* risk for a given site for exposed individuals. Case-control studies show that the lung and the bladder are the sites most often involved in occupational cancer. National figures on occupational mortality are essentially confined to those from England and Wales (*37*). The analysis is complex, inasmuch as it requires evaluation of both on-the-job exposures and life-style factors (*37, 38*) and takes tobacco and alcohol habits into consideration. Cultural habits and life-style were not taken into account in the recent estimates by the National Cancer Institute and the National Institute of Environmental Health Sciences (*52*).

To avoid underestimating the potential importance of occupational exposures, we have considered that for both sexes the low risk of lung cancer in nonsmoking women and physicians (*53*) represents a background level unassociated with either smoking or occupation. Accordingly, after allowing for smoking and background, we have attributed the remainder (10%) of all lung cancers to occupation. All mesotheliomas (0.1% of all male cancers) in Birmingham were attributed to occupation, as was 30% of male bladder cancer and, under the assumption that all of the male-female difference is due to occupation, 30% of leukemia. Other investigators might wish to attribute more of these cancers to smoking or other factors. The proportion of occupational cancer in Bombay is more difficult to estimate because much industry is artisanal, but a 6% estimate is probably too high.

Job-associated cancers are attributed to their suspected etiology; for example, esophageal cancer in bartenders is assigned to alcohol consumption.

Iatrogenic causes and radiation.—There is no evidence that more than 1% of cancers are due to radiation, including diagnostic exposures. In the United States, where estrogen therapy has been widespread, the proportion of iatrogenic cancers in women could be higher (*17*).

Life-style.—For the aforementioned reasons, we have attributed most tumors of the gastrointestinal tract and endocrine-dependent organs to life-style. Although some carcinogenic risk factors have been identified, these are ill defined and are insufficient to explain the large geographic and temporal differences in incidence of cancer between Birmingham and Bombay and some other parts of the world (e.g., prostate cancer and breast cancer in Japan). That these estimates are reasonable is suggested by studies on Mormons and Seventh-Day Adventists, in whom lower rates are observed for cancers of the breast and gastrointestinal tract as well as for the tobacco- and alcohol-related tumors (*31, 54*). As yet, to attribute precise proportions of cancer incidence to diet and to cultural and behavioral patterns is not possible.

Congenital, Hereditary, and Unknown Factors

A role for individual general susceptibility to cancer is not excluded. We agree with Knudson (*55*) that no more than 2% of cancers can be related to hereditary or congenital causes alone. Unknown cancers are cancers for which at present we have no reasonable hypothesis as to the etiology.

We stress that these estimates are population averages, and the pattern for small groups within these large areas may be quite different.

POSSIBLE FUTURE TRENDS IN CANCER PATTERNS

The aforementioned estimates relate only to past and present patterns. However, the forecast of future patterns is of considerable health importance to both the scientific community and to the public. Such estimates are by necessity based on the extrapolation of present trends. However, we do not know that the incidence of stomach cancer will continue to decrease or that breast cancer will continue to increase in many countries, because future exposures and changes in behavioral patterns cannot be readily predicted.

Interpretation of time trends in terms of ambient general pollution, workplace exposures, or smoking is difficult, as illustrated by the incidence of bladder cancer which is slowly rising in males living in the United States but is falling in females dwelling there. Whether the decline in rectal cancer and the comparable increase in colon cancer in whites of both sexes living in the United States are due to changes in assignment of the rectosigmoid neoplasms, life-style changes, or other factors (*24*) is unknown.

The need for prudent interpretation of even short-term changes is demonstrated by the experience in the United States in 1975, during which a rapid increase in cancer mortality was widely interpreted as heralding an epidemic due to environmental chemical pollution. Upon closer examination, the increase proved largely artifactual (*21*).

For future trends, the greatest controversy surrounds asbestos (*52, 56*), to which many workers have been exposed. Because the fiber remains in the tissues, fear exists that an ever-increasing number of cancers will appear even in nonsmokers. In the United Kingdom, a decrease in lung cancer incidence has been demonstrated in an asbestos factory (*57*) after control measures were instituted, but future trends are difficult to forecast due to the long latency period involved. Recent reports (*58*) indicate that general ambient asbestos exposures have not caused a public health problem so far for the general population in Europe.

Almost certainly new industrial and iatrogenic hazards will be discovered after they enter the environment; hence appropriate surveillance systems must be created for their identification.

CONCLUSIONS

The role of the environment in human cancer has been recognized for many years, and the criticism that the scientific community has failed to study these problems has little justification. However, part of that community, as well as the public, has refused to accept the fact that the major causal factors so far identified in human cancer relate to personal habits and lifestyle. Although some consensus exists as to control of some of these factors, many tumors of undoubted environmental origin, but for which no definite cause has been identified, exist in people living in all countries, especially in females.

The preceding discussion suggests that most cancers of presumed environmental etiology cannot readily be ascribed to industrial exposures, either point-source or general, or to identified cultural habits such as smoking or drinking.

Experimental work is consistent with the view that the life-style associations described in man, such as lack of dietary fiber, excess fat and caloric intake, and possibly hormone carcinogenesis, imply multifactorial origin. This view agrees with Berenblum's hypothesis (*8*) that initiation, extrinsic or intrinsic, is often incomplete and that cocarcinogenic mechanisms, including promotion, are involved.

If correct, this theory has important implications for the selection of research approaches and priorities. Acceptance of the role of cocarcinogenesis and other factors as of considerable significance suggests that the impact on the total cancer burden of systematic testing programs, directed only to the identification of initiators, either in animals or in vitro mutagenic systems, might be less than anticipated. Such testing programs are essential for the identification of existing initiators and for the control of new hazards. However, as Berenblum pointed out (*8*), the practical difficulties of

identifying, evaluating, and controlling the vast number of all potential carcinogens in the environment are immense. Furthermore, the data suggest that apart from high-risk situations, the effect of such control on present life-style-associated cancer patterns will be difficult to detect.

In the interim, until the etiology of such cancers is better understood, prudence is advisable in the advocacy of marked changes in dietary customs apart from the avoidance of obviously unhealthy habits such as overeating. Thus the Finnish diet, which is associated with a low risk of large-bowel cancer (*48*), is apparently associated with high risks of cardiovascular disease (*59*). No evidence indicates that low risks of cancers in Norway are due to a "better" or "wiser" nutrition than in Geneva, Switzerland, where cancer occurs more frequently. Even where carcinogenic risk factors have been described, their control does not necessarily lead to prevention. Thus early sexual intercourse increases the risk of cancer of the cervix uteri, whereas early pregnancy protects against breast cancer.

Although the difficulties involved in the investigation of multifactorial mechanisms in man should not be underrated (*60-62*), it is undesirable that we are unable to explain adequately the cause of approximately 40% of cancers in males and 60% of cancers in females in nearly all countries, industrialized or not. Obviously, human carcinogenesis implies a wider approach than the study only of initiation at the target cell level. Thus events before or after initiation may be fundamental to neoplastic development, especially when the initiating factor is very weak. This view has significant implications whether they relate to legislative controls or to extrapolating to man from simpler systems. However, as indicated by Berenblum (*8*), the multistage hypothesis offers an intellectual base for future research.

These conclusions and comments are not original and have been previously discussed by us (*62*) and by others (*5-12*). Nevertheless, in view of the recent concentration by toxicologists on environmental chemicals and carcinogens, largely of industrial origin, we believe that the neglect of a balanced program of basic and epidemiologic research on other carcinogenic mechanisms, including cocarcinogenesis and promotion, may be dangerous, especially for life-style-related cancers in females.

REFERENCES

(*1*) WHELAN E: Cancer: The enemy is us. Int Herald Tribune, 2 September 1978, p 6
(*2*) EPSTEIN SS: The Politics of Cancer. San Francisco: Sierra Club Books, 1978, 583 pp
(*3*) ASHBY LORD: Protection of the environment: The human dimension (Jephcott lecture). Proc R Soc Lond [Biol] 69:721-730, 1976
(*4*) BATES R: Regulation of carcinogenic food additives and drugs in the U.S. In Proceedings of IARC/INSERM Symposium on Carcinogenic Risks-Strategies for Intervention (Davis W, Rosenfeld C, eds). IARC Sci Publ No. 25 and INSERM Sym-

posia Series, vol 74. Lyon: IARC, 1979, pp 93-100

(5) CLEMMESEN J, ed: Symposium on Geographical Pathology and Demography of Cancer, Oxford, England, 1950. Paris: Council Int Org Med Sci, 1950, 150 pp

(6) MILLER E: Some current perspectives on chemical carcinogenesis in humans and experimental animals: Presidential address. Cancer Res 38:1479-1496, 1978

(7) IARC Working Group: Polychlorinated Biphenyls and Polybrominated Biphenyls. IARC Monogr Eval Carcinog Risk Chem Man 18:1-140, 1978

(8) BERENBLUM I: Theoretical and practical aspects of the two-stage mechanism of carcinogenesis. *In* Carcinogens: Identification and Mechanisms of Action (Griffin AC, Shaw CR, eds). New York: Raven Press, 1979, pp 25-36

(9) WEINSTEIN B, YAMASAKI H, WIGLER M, et al: Molecular and cellular events associated with the action of initiating carcinogens and tumor promoters. *In* Carcinogens: Identification and Mechanisms of Action (Griffin AC, Shaw CR, eds). New York: Raven Press, 1979, pp 399-418

(10) SIVAK A: Mechanisms of tumor promotion and cocarcinogenesis. *In* Carcinogenesis—A Comprehensive Survey (Slaga TJ, Sivak A, Boutwell RK, eds), vol 2. New York: Raven Press, 1978, pp 553-564

(11) WATTENBERG LW: Inhibition of chemical carcinogenesis. J Natl Cancer Inst 60:11-18, 1978

(12) WYNDER EL, HOFFMANN D, MCCOY D, et al: Tumor promotion and co-carcinogenesis as related to man and his environment. *In* Carcinogenesis: A Comprehensive Survey (Slaga TJ, Sivak A, Boutwell RK, eds), vol 2. New York: Raven Press, 1978, pp 59-77

(13) SELIKOFF IJ, HAMMOND EC, CHURG J: Asbestos exposure, smoking and neoplasia. JAMA 204:106-112, 1968

(14) LAROUZÉ B, BLUMBERG BS, LONDON WT, et al: Forecasting the development of primary hepatocellular carcinoma by the use of risk factors: Studies in West Africa. J Natl Cancer Inst 58:1557-1561, 1977

(15) LINSELL CA, PEERS FG: Aflatoxin and liver cell cancer. Trans R Soc Trop Med Hyg 71:471-473, 1977

(16) MILLER AB: An overview of hormone-associated cancers. Cancer Res 38:3985-3990, 1978

(17) AUSTIN DF, ROE KM: Increase in cancer of the corpus uteri in the San Francisco–Oakland standard metropolitan statistical area, 1960-75. JNCI 62:13-16, 1979

(18) HIGGINSON J, MUIR CS: Détermination de l'importance des facteurs environnementaux dans le cancer humain: Rôle de l'épidémiologie. Bull Cancer (Paris) 64:365-384, 1977

(19) HIGGINSON J: Perspectives and future developments in research on environmental carcinogenesis. *In* Carcinogens: Identification and Mechanisms of Action (Griffin AC, Shaw CR, eds). New York: Raven Press, 1979, pp 187-208

(20) TOMATIS L, AGTHE C, BARTSCH H, et al: Evaluation of the carcinogenicity of chemicals: A review of the monograph program of the International Agency for Research on Cancer (1971 to 1977). Cancer Res 38:877-885, 1978

(21) CHIAZZE L, SILVERMAN DT, LEVIN DL: The cancer mortality scare. JAMA 236:2310-2312, 1976

(22) IARC Working Group: Some Polycyclic Aromatic Hydrocarbons and Heterocyclic Compounds. IARC Monogr Eval Carcinog Risk Chem Man 3:1-271, 1973

(23) WALKER EA, CASTEGNARO M, GRICIUTE L, et al, eds: Environmental aspects of N-nitroso compounds. IARC Sci Publ 19:1-566, 1978

(24) DEVESA SS, SILVERMAN DT: Cancer incidence and mortality trends in the United States: 1935-74. J Natl Cancer Inst 60:545-571, 1978

(25) HAENSZEL W: Cancer mortality among the foreign-born in the United States. J Natl Cancer Inst 26:37-132, 1961

(26) HAENSZEL W, KURIHARA M: Studies of Japanese migrants. I. Mortality from cancer and other diseases among Japanese in the United States. J Natl Cancer Inst 40:43-68, 1968

(27) BUELL P, DUNN JE: Cancer mortality among Japanese Issei and Nisei of California. Cancer 18:656-664, 1965

(28) BUELL P: Changing incidence of breast cancer in Japanese-American women. J Natl Cancer Inst 51:1479-1483, 1973

(29) HAENSZEL W, LOVELAND DB, SIRKEN MG: Lung-cancer mortality as related to residence and smoking histories. I. White males. J Natl Cancer Inst 28:947-1001, 1962

(30) HAENSZEL W, TAEUBER KE: Lung-cancer mortality as related to residence and smoking histories. II. White females. J Natl Cancer Inst 32:803-838, 1964

(31) LYON JL, KLAUBER MR, GARDNER JW, et al: Cancer incidence in Mormons and non-Mormons in Utah, 1966-1970. N Engl J Med 294:129-133, 1976

(32) CEDERLOF R, DOLL R, FOWLER B, et al, eds: Air pollution and cancer: Risk assessment of methodology and epidemiological evidence (report of a task group). Environ Health Perspect 22:1-12, 1978

(33) MASON TJ, MCKAY FW, HOOVER R, et al: Atlas of Cancer Mortality for U.S. Counties: 1950-1969. Washington, D.C.: U.S. Govt Print Off, 1975, pp 1-103

(34) OHNO Y, AOKI K: Epidemiology of bladder cancer deaths in Japan. Gan 68:715-729, 1977

(35) WATERHOUSE J, MUIR CS, CORREA P, et al, eds: Cancer Incidence in Five Continents. IARC Sci Publ 15:1-584, 1976

(36) DEROUEN TA, DIEM JE: The New Orleans drinking water controversy: A statistical approach. Am J Public Health 65:1060-1062, 1975

(37) Office of Population Censuses and Surveys: Occupational Mortality. The Registrar General's Decennial Supplement for England and Wales, 1970-1972, series DS No. 1. London: HM Stat Off, 1978, pp 1-224

(38) FOX AJ, ADELSTEIN AM: Occupational mortality: Work or way of life? J Epidemiol Community Health 32:73-78, 1978

(39) KENNAWAY EL: Forms of cancer in man suitable for investigation. *In* Symposium on Geographical Pathology and Demography of Cancer, Oxford, England, 1950 (Clemmesen J, ed). Paris: Council Int Org Med Sci, 1950, pp 122-124

(40) SUGIMURA T, NAGAO M, KAWACHI T, et al: Mutagen-carcinogens in food, with special reference to highly mutagenic pyrolytic products in broiled foods. *In* Cold Spring Harbor Conferences on Origins of Human Cancer (Hiatt HH, Watson JD, Winsten JA, eds), vol 4. Cold Spring Harbor, N.Y.: Cold Spring Harbor Lab, 1977, pp 1561-1577

(41) WEISBURGER JH, COHEN LA, WYNDER EL: On the etiology and metabolic epidemiology of the main human cancers. *In* Cold Spring Harbor Conferences on Origins of Human Cancer (Hiatt HH, Watson JD, Winsten JA, eds), vol 4. Cold Spring Harbor, N.Y.: Cold Spring Harbor Lab, 1977, pp 567-602

(42) CONNEY AH, PANTUCK EJ, HSIAO KC, et al: Regulation of drug metabolism in man by environmental chemicals and diet. Fed Proc 36:1647-1652, 1977

(43) BORGSTROM A, GENELL S, OHLSSON K: Elevated fecal levels of endogenous pancreatic endopeptidases after antibiotic treatment. Scand J Gastroenterol 12:525-529, 1977

(44) GRAY GE, PIKE MC, HENDERSON BE: Breast cancer incidence and mortality rates in different countries in relation to known risk factors and dietary practices. Br J Cancer 39:1-7, 1979

(45) ENSTROM JE: Cancer and total mortality among active Mormons. Cancer 42:1943-1951, 1978

(46) KINLEN LJ: Cancer mortality in certain meat-abstaining groups. Presented at Symposium No. 14, 12th Int Cancer Congress, Buenos Aires, Argentina, Oct 5-11, 1978. In press

(47) GRAHAM S, METTLIN C: Diet and colon cancer. Am J Epidemiol 109:1-20, 1979

(48) IARC Microecology Group: Dietary fiber, transit-time, fecal bacteria, steroids and colon cancer in two Scandinavian populations. Lancet 2:207-211, 1977

(49) BRESLOW N, CHAN CW, DHOM G, et al: Latent carcinoma of prostate at autopsy in seven areas. Int J Cancer 20:680-688, 1977

(50) COLE P: A population-based study of bladder cancer. *In* Host Environment Interactions in the Etiology of Cancer in Man (Doll R, Vodopija I, eds). Lyon: IARC, 1973, pp 83-87

(51) HIGGINSON J, MUIR CS: Epidemiology. *In* Cancer Medicine

(Holland JF, Frei E, eds). Philadelphia: Lea & Febiger, 1973, pp 241-306

(52) BRIDBORD K, DECOUFLE P, FRAUMENI JF, et al: Estimates of the Fraction of Cancer in the United States Related to Occupational Factors. National Cancer Institute-National Institute of Environmental Health Sciences-National Institute of Occupational Safety and Health: Bethesda, Md.: 1978, pp 1-50

(53) DOLL R, PETO R: Mortality in relation to smoking: 20 years' observations on male British doctors. Br Med J 2:1525-1536, 1976

(54) PHILLIPS RL: Role of lifestyle and dietary habits in risk of cancer among Seventh-Day Adventists. Cancer Res 35:3513-3522, 1975

(55) KNUDSON AG: Genetic predisposition to cancer. *In* Cold Spring Harbor Conferences on Origins of Human Cancer (Hiatt HH, Watson JD, Winsten JA, eds), vol 4. Cold Spring Harbor, N.Y.: Cold Spring Harbor Lab, 1977, pp 45-52

(56) IARC Working Group: Asbestos. IARC Monogr Eval Carcinog Risk Chem Man 14:1-106, 1977

(57) PETO J, DOLL R, HOWARD SV, et al: A mortality study among workers in an English asbestos factory. Br J Ind Med 34:169-173, 1977

(58) Anon: Asbestos. Lancet 2:1211-1212, 1977

(59) FURBERG C, ROMO M, LINKO E, et al: Sudden coronary death in Scandinavia. A report from Scandinavian coronary heart disease registers. Acta Med Scand 201:553-557, 1977

(60) MARX JL: Tumor promoters: Carcinogenesis gets more complicated. Science 201:515-518, 1978

(61) HIGGINSON J, OETTLÉ AG: Cancer incidence in the Bantu and "Cape Colored" races of South Africa: Report of a cancer survey in the Transvaal (1953-55). J Natl Cancer Inst 24:589-671, 1960

(62) HIGGINSON J: Present trends in cancer epidemiology. *In* Proceedings of the Eighth Canadian Cancer Conference, Honey Harbour, Ontario, Canada, 1968 (Morgan JF, ed). Toronto: Pergamon Press, 1969, pp 40-75

Executive Summary from *Diet, Nutrition, and Cancer*

*by the Committee on Diet, Nutrition, and Cancer of the
National Academy of Sciences.*

Scientific pronouncements are usually viewed by the public as carrying a rather high level of certainty. Therefore, scientists must be especially careful in their choice of words whenever they are not totally confident about their conclusions. For example, it has become absolutely clear that cigarettes are the cause of approximately one-quarter of all the fatal cancers in the United States. If the population had been persuaded to stop smoking when the association with lung cancer was first reported, these cancer deaths would now not be occurring. Twenty years ago the "stop-smoking" message required some rather cautious wording. Today, the facts are clear, and the choice of words is not so important.

The public often demands certain kinds of information before such information can be provided with complete certainty. For example, weather forecasting is often not exact; nevertheless, the public asks that the effort be made, but has learned to accept the fact that the results are not always reliable.

The public is now asking about the causes of cancers that are not associated with smoking. What are these causes, and how can these cancers be avoided? Unfortunately, it is not yet possible to make firm scientific pronouncements about the association between diet and cancer. We are in an interim stage of knowledge similar to that for cigarettes 20 years ago. Therefore, in the judgment of the committee, it is now the time to offer some interim guidelines on diet and cancer.

Approximately 20% of all deaths in the United States are caused by cancer. Although the number of cancer cases is steadily increasing as the population grows, the age-adjusted total cancer incidence and mortality rates for sites other than the respiratory tract (cancers of which are primarily due to cigarette smoking) have as a whole remained stable during the last 30 to 40 years.

The search for the causes of cancer has been an important branch of cancer research. Considerable effort has been devoted to

---

This material is excerpted from *Diet, Nutrition, and Cancer*. As such, it contains references to portions of *Diet, Nutrition, and Cancer* not present here.

---

studying the influence of both environmental and genetic factors on the incidence of cancer. In the course of this research, it has become clear that most cancers have external causes and, in principle, should therefore be preventable. For example, blacks and Japanese residing in the United States develop the spectrum of cancers that is typical for the United States but different from that in Africa and Japan.

But what might these external causes be? Many factors in our environment are potential causes of cancer. They include substances in the air we breathe, the water we drink, the regions in which we work and live, and the foods we eat. Our exposure to some of these factors varies in ways that can be precisely measured. For most factors, however, the measurement of the exposures and the assessment of their effects are neither precise nor straightforward. Among the factors whose precise effects are difficult to assess are the diets consumed by different groups of people. The measurements are difficult not only because it is hard to learn what people eat but also because the foods comprising their diets are so complex.

Studies of the association between diet and cancer have focused on cancers of the gastrointestinal tract, the breast and other tissues susceptible to hormonal influence, and, to a lesser extent, the respiratory tract and the urinary bladder. After assessing the resultant literature, the committee concluded that the differences in the rates at which various cancers occur in different human populations are often correlated with differences in diet. The likelihood that some of these correlations reflect causality is strengthened by laboratory evidence that similar dietary patterns and components of food also affect the incidence of certain cancers in animals.

Chapters 16 and 17 provide information about the trends in cancer incidence and the relationship between diet and the incidence of cancer at specific sites.

Epidemiologists have found it rela-

tively easy to demonstrate a correlation between diets consumed in modern affluent societies and the incidence of cancers in such organs as the breast, colon, and uterus. But it has proved to be much more difficult to establish causal relationships and to determine which, if any, of the dietary components is responsible.

Similarly, difficulties are encountered in laboratory experiments. Like humans, most animals have a significant incidence of cancer in old age, and the rates of these cancers often tend to be affected by changes in diet. However, the influence of diet on spontaneous and experimentally induced cancers is not easily investigated because the underlying mechanisms and molecular biology of the cancers are still not fully understood. Indeed, the effects of diet were often regarded as a nuisance--i.e., yet another variable standing between the investigators and their measurement of carcinogenicity. As a consequence, researchers have only recently returned to the study of diet as a factor in carcinogenesis.

It is possible that research in progress will generate more definitive information that will be useful in formulating dietary recommendations to minimize the risk of cancer. In the meantime, the committee believes that the evidence at hand justifies certain interim guidelines. These guidelines appear at the end of this chapter following a summary of the committee's findings and the conclusions it believes can be drawn from the scientific evidence.

SUMMARY AND CONCLUSIONS

Dietary Patterns and Components of Food

Since the turn of the century, new methods of processing and storage have resulted in a proliferation of the kinds and numbers of food items available to the U.S. population. Unfortunately, little is known about the ways in which such innovations have altered the specific composition of the diet. The only components of food that have been monitored regularly are the nutrients. The dietary levels of most nutrients have changed relatively little over the past 80 years.

Attempting to determine which constituents of food might be associated with cancer, epidemiologists have studied population subgroups, including migrants to the United States, to examine the relationship between specific dietary patterns or the consumption of certain foods and the risk of developing particular cancers. In general, the evidence suggests that some types of diets and some dietary components (e.g., high fat diets or the frequent consumption of salt-cured, salt-pickled, and smoked foods) tend to increase the risk of cancer, whereas others (e.g., low fat diets or the frequent consumption of certain fruits and vegetables) tend to decrease it. The mechanisms responsible for these effects are not fully understood, partly because nutritive and nonnutritive components of foods may interact to exert effects on cancer incidence.

In the laboratory, investigators have attempted to shed light on the mechanisms by which diet may influence carcinogenesis. They have examined the ability of individual nutrients, food extracts, or nonnutritive components of food to enhance or inhibit carcinogenesis and mutagenesis, thereby providing epidemiologists with testable hypotheses regarding specific components of the diet. Because the data from both types of studies are generally grouped according to dietary constituents, the committee found it advantageous to organize its report in a similar fashion.

Total Caloric Intake

The committee reviewed many studies in which the variable examined was the total amount of food consumed by humans or animals, rather than the precise composition of the diet. This review is contained in Chapter 4, which is entitled "Total Caloric Intake," even thought the studies did not indicate

whether the observed effects resulted from the changes in the proportion of specific nutrients in the diet or from the modification of total caloric intake.

Since very few epidemiologists have been able to examine the effect of caloric intake per se on the risk of cancer, their reports have provided largely indirect evidence for such a relationship, and much of it is based on associations between body weight or obesity and cancer.

In laboratory experiments, the incidence of tumors is lower and the lifespan much longer for animals on restricted food intake than for animals fed ad libitum. However, because the intake of all nutrients was simultaneously depressed in these studies, the observed reduction in tumor incidence might have been due to the reduction of some specific nutrient, such as fat. It is also difficult to interpret experiments in which caloric intake has been modified by varying dietary fat or fiber, both of which may by themselves exert effects on tumorigenesis.

Thus, the committee concluded that neither the epidemiological studies nor the experiments in animals permit a clear interpretation of the specific effect of total caloric intake on the risk of cancer. Nonetheless, the studies conducted in animals show that a reduction in total food intake decreases the age-specific incidence of cancer. The evidence is less clear for human beings.

Lipids (Fats and Cholesterol)

Many epidemiological and laboratory studies have been conducted to examine the association between cancer and intake of lipids, i.e., total dietary fat, saturated fat, polyunsaturated fat, and cholesterol.

Fats. Epidemiological studies have repeatedly shown an association between dietary fat and the occurrence of cancer at several sites, especially the breast, prostate, and large bowel. In various populations, both the high incidence of and mortality from breast cancer have been shown to correlate strongly with higher per capita fat consumption; the few case-control studies conducted have also shown this association with dietary fat. Like breast cancer, increased risk of large bowel cancer has been associated with higher fat intake in both correlation and case-control studies. The data on prostate cancer are more limited, but they too suggest that an increased risk is related to high levels of dietary fat. In general, it is not possible to identify specific components of fat as being clearly responsible for the observed effects, although total fat and saturated fat have been associated most frequently.

The epidemiological data are not entirely consistent. For example, the magnitude of the association of fat with breast cancer appears greater in the correlation data than in the case-control data, and several reports on large bowel cancer fail to show an association with fat. Possible reasons for these discrepancies are apparent. These are discussed in Chapter 5 (see pages 5-5 and 5-18).

Like epidemiological studies, numerous experiments in animals have shown that dietary lipids influence tumorigenesis, especially in the breast and the colon. An increase in fat intake from 5% to 20% of the weight of the diet (i.e., approximately 10% to 40% of total calories) increases tumor incidence in various tissues; conversely, animals consuming low fat diets have a lower tumor incidence. When the intake of total fat is low, polyunsaturated fats appear to be more effective than saturated fats in enhancing tumorigenesis. However, this distinction becomes less prominent as total fat intake is increased.

Dietary fat appears to have a promoting effect on tumorigenesis. For example, some studies suggest that the development of colon cancer is enhanced by the increased secretion of certain bile steroids and bile acids that accompanies high levels of fat intake. Nonetheless, there is little or no knowledge concerning the specific mechanisms involved in tumor promotion. This lack of understanding contributes to our overall uncertainty about the mechanisms that underlie the effect of diet on carcinogenesis. Although most of the data suggest that dietary fat has promoting activity, there is not enough evidence to warrant the complete exclusion of an effect on initiation.

The committee concluded that of all the dietary components it studied, the combined epidemiological and experimental evidence is most suggestive for a causal relationship between fat intake and the occurrence of cancer. Both epidemiological studies and experiments in animals provide convincing evidence that increasing the intake of total fat increases the incidence of cancer at certain sites, particularly the breast and colon, and, conversely, that the risk is lower with lower intakes of fat. Data from studies in animals suggest that when fat intake is low, polyunsaturated fats are more effective than saturated fats in enhancing tumorigenesis, whereas the data on humans do not permit a clear distinction to be made between the effects of different components of fat. In general, however, the evidence from epidemiological and laboratory studies is consistent.

Cholesterol. The relationship between dietary cholesterol and cancer is not clear. Many studies of serum cholesterol levels and cancer mortality in human populations have demonstrated an inverse correlation with colon cancer among men, but the evidence is not conclusive. Data on cholesterol and cancer risk from studies in animals are too limited to permit any inferences to be drawn.

Chapter 5 contains a more detailed discussion of these studies.

Protein

The relationship between protein intake and carcinogenesis has been studied in human populations as well as in the laboratory. These studies are discussed in Chapter 6.

Results of epidemiological studies have suggested possible associations between high intake of dietary protein and increased risk for cancers at a number of different sites, although the literature on protein is much more limited than the literature concerning fats and cancer. In addition, because of the very high correlation between fat and protein in the diets of most Western countries, and the more consistent and often stronger association of these cancers with fat intake, it seems likely that dietary fat is the more active component. Nevertheless, the evidence does not completely preclude the existence of an independent effect of protein.

In most laboratory experiments, carcinogenesis is suppressed by diets containing levels of protein at or below the minimum required for optimal growth. Chemically induced carcinogenesis appears to be enhanced as protein intake is increased up to 2 or 3 times the normal requirement; however, higher levels of protein begin to inhibit carcinogenesis. There is some evidence to suggest that protein may affect the initiation phase of carcinogenesis and the subsequent growth and development of the tumor.

Thus, in the judgment of the committee, evidence from both epidemiological and laboratory studies suggests that high protein intake may be associated with an increased risk of cancers at certain sites. Because of the relative paucity of data on protein compared to fat, and the strong correlation between the intakes of fat and protein in the U.S. diet, the committee is unable to arrive at a firm conclusion about an independent effect of protein.

Carbohydrates

As discussed in Chapter 7, information concerning the role of carbohydrates in the development of cancer in humans is extremely limited. Although some studies suggest that a high intake of refined sugar or starch increases the risk of cancer at certain sites, the results are insufficient to permit any firm conclusions to be drawn.

The data obtained from studies in animals are equally limited, providing too little evidence to suggest that carbohydrates (possibly excluding fiber) play a direct role in experimentally induced carcinogenesis. However, excessive carbohydrate consumption contributes to caloric excess, and this in turn has been implicated as a modifier of carcinogenesis.

Dietary Fiber

Considerable effort has been devoted to studying the effects of dietary fiber and fiber-containing foods (such as certain vegetables, fruits, and whole grain cereals) on the occurrence of cancer (see Chapter 8).

Most epidemiological studies on fiber have examined the hypothesis that high fiber diets protect against colorectal cancer. Results of correlation and case-control studies of dietary fiber have sometimes supported and sometimes contradicted this hypothesis. In both types of studies, correlations have been based primarily on estimates of fiber intake obtained by grouping foods according to their fiber content. In the only case-control study and the only correlation study in which total fiber consumption was quantified rather than estimated from the consumption of high fiber foods, no association was found between high fiber intake and a lower risk of colon cancer. However, the correlation study indicated that the incidence of colon cancer was inversely related to the intake of one fiber component--the pentosan fraction, which is found in whole wheat products and other food items.

Laboratory experiments also have indicated that the consumption of some high fiber ingredients (e.g., cellulose and bran) inhibits the induction of colon cancer by certain chemical carcinogens. However, the results are inconsistent. Moreover, they are difficult to equate with the results of epidemiological studies because most laboratory investigations have focused on specific fibers or their individual components, whereas most epidemiological studies have been concerned with fiber-containing foods whose exact composition has not been determined.

Thus, the committee found no conclusive evidence to indicate that dietary fiber (such as that present in certain fruits, vegetables, grains, and cereals) exerts a protective effect against colorectal cancer in humans. Both epidemiological and laboratory reports suggest that if there is such an effect, specific components of fiber, rather than total fiber, are more likely to be responsible.

Vitamins

In recent years, there has been considerable interest in the role of vitamins A, C, and E in the genesis and prevention of cancer. In contrast, less attention has been paid to the B vitamins and others such as vitamin K. Chapter 9 contains more detailed information on the evidence summarized below.

Vitamin A. A growing accumulation of epidemiological evidence indicates that there is an inverse relationship between the risk of cancer and the consumption of foods that contain vitamin A (e.g., liver) or its precursors (e.g., the carotenoids in green and yellow vegetables). Most of the data do not show whether the effects are due to carotenoids, to vitamin A itself, or to some other constituent of these foods. In these studies, investigators found an inverse association between estimates of "vitamin A" intake and carcinoma at several sites, e.g., the lung, the urinary bladder, and the larynx.

Studies in laboratory animals indicate that vitamin A deficiency generally increases susceptibility to chemically induced neoplasia and that an increased intake of the vitamin appears to protect against carcinogenesis in most, but not all cases. Because high doses of vitamin A are toxic, many of these studies have been conducted with its synthetic analogues (retinoids), which lack some of the toxic effects of the vitamin.

Retinoids have been shown to inhibit chemically induced neoplasia of the breast, urinary bladder, skin, and lung in animals.

The committee concluded that the laboratory evidence shows that vitamin A itself and many of the retinoids are able to suppress chemically induced tumors. The epidemiological evidence is sufficient to suggest that foods rich in carotenes or vitamin A are associated with a reduced risk of cancer. The toxicity of vitamin A in doses exceeding those required for optimum nutrition, and the difficulty of epidemiological studies to distinguish the effects of carotenes from those of vitamin A, argue against increasing vitamin A intake by the use of supplements.

Vitamin C (Ascorbic Acid). The epidemiological data pertaining to the effect of vitamin C on the occurrence of cancer are not extensive. Furthermore, they provide mostly indirect evidence since they are based on the consumption of foods, especially fresh fruits and vegetables, known to contain high concentrations of the vitamin, rather than on actual measurements of vitamin C intake. The results of several case-control studies and a few correlation studies suggest that the consumption of vitamin-C-containing foods is associated with a lower risk of certain cancers, particularly gastric and esophageal cancer.

In the laboratory, ascorbic acid can inhibit the formation of carcinogenic N-nitroso compounds, both in vitro and in vivo. On the other hand, studies of its inhibitory effect on preformed carcinogens have not provided conclusive results. In recent studies, the addition of ascorbic acid to cells grown in culture prevented the chemically induced transformation of these cells and, in some cases, caused reversion of transformed cells.

Thus, the limited evidence suggests that vitamin C can inhibit the formation of some carcinogens and that the consumption of vitamin-C-containing foods is associated with a lower risk of cancers of the stomach and esophagus.

Vitamin E (α-Tocopherol). Because vitamin E is present in a variety of commonly consumed foods (particularly vegetable oils, whole grain cereal products, and eggs), it is difficult to identify population groups with substantially different levels of intake. Consequently, it is not surprising that there are no epidemiological reports concerning vitamin E intake and the risk of cancer.

Vitamin E, like ascorbic acid, inhibits the formation of nitrosamines in vivo and in vitro. However, there are no reports about the effect of this vitamin on nitrosamine-induced neoplasia. Limited evidence from studies in animals suggests that vitamin E may also inhibit the induction of tumorigenesis by other chemicals.

The data are not sufficient to permit any firm conclusion to be drawn about the effect of vitamin E on cancer in humans.

The B Vitamins. No specific information has been produced by epidemiological studies, and there have been only a few inadequate laboratory investigations to determine whether there is a relationship between various B vitamins and the occurrence of cancer. Therefore, no conclusion can be drawn.

Minerals

Of the many minerals present in the diet of humans, the committee reviewed the evidence for nine that have been suspected of playing a role in carcinogenesis. The assessment was severely limited by a paucity of relevant studies on all but two minerals--selenium and iron. Where data on dietary exposure and carcinogenesis were insufficient, the committee used information from studies of occupational exposure or laboratory experiments in which the animals were exposed through routes other than diet. Chapter 10 contains more detailed information on the evidence summarized below.

Selenium. Selenium has been studied to determine its role in both the causation and the prevention of cancer. The epidemiological evidence is derived from a few geographical correlation studies, which have shown that the risk of cancer is inversely related to estimates of per capita selenium intake, selenium levels in blood specimens, or selenium concentrations in water supplies. It is not clear whether this relationship applies to all types of cancer or only to cancer at specific sites such as the gastrointestinal tract. There have been no case-control or cohort studies.

Experiments in animals have also demonstrated an antitumorigenic effect of selenium. But the relevance of these results to cancer in humans is not apparent since the selenium levels used in most of the studies far exceeded dietary requirements and often bordered on levels that are toxic. Earlier reports suggesting that selenium was carcinogenic in laboratory animals have not been confirmed.

Therefore, both the epidemiological and laboratory studies suggest that selenium may offer some protection against the risk of cancer. However, firm conclusions cannot be drawn from the limited evidence. Increasing the selenium intake to more than 200 μg/day[1] by the use of supplements has not been shown to confer health benefits exceeding those derived from the consumption of a balanced diet. Such supplementation should be considered an experimental procedure requiring strict medical supervision and is not recommended for use by the public.

Iron. Iron deficiency has been related to an increase in the risk of Plummer-Vinson syndrome, which is associated with cancer of the upper alimentary tract. Some evidence suggests that iron deficiency may be related to gastric cancer, also through an indirect mechanism. Although epidemiological reports have suggested that inhalation exposures to high concentrations of iron

---

[1]The upper limit of the Range of Safe and Adequate Daily Dietary Intakes published in the Recommended Dietary Allowances (see Chapter 10).

increase the risk of cancer, there is no evidence pertaining to the effect of high levels of dietary iron on the risk of cancer in humans. The limited evidence from animal experiments suggests that a deficiency of dietary iron may increase susceptibility to some chemically induced tumors.

The data are not sufficient for a firm conclusion to be drawn about the role of iron in carcinogenesis.

Copper, Zinc, Molybdenum, and Iodine. Some epidemiological studies suggest that dietary zinc is associated with an increase in the incidence of cancer at certain sites; others suggest that blood and tissue levels of zinc in cancer patients are lower, and those of copper are higher, than in the controls. Results of experiments in animals are also inconclusive. Different levels of dietary zinc either enhance or retard tumor growth, depending on the specific test design. High levels of copper have been observed to protect against chemical induction of tumors.

There is some epidemiological evidence that a deficiency of molybdenum and other trace elements is associated with an increased risk of esophageal cancer. Limited experiments in animals suggest that dietary molybdenum supplementation may reduce the incidence of nitrosamine-induced tumors of the esophagus and forestomach.

Studies conducted in Colombia, Iceland, and Scotland indicated that iodine deficiency, and also excessive iodine intake, may increase the risk of thyroid carcinoma. These observations have not been confirmed in other countries or in other studies. In general, the results of studies in animals support the association between iodine deficiency and thyroid cancer.

The committee concluded that the data concerning dietary exposure to zinc, copper, molybdenum, and iodine are insufficient and provide no basis for conclusions about the association of these elements with cancer risk.

Arsenic, Cadmium, and Lead. Occupational exposure to these elements is associated with an increased risk of cancer at several sites. Exposure to high concentrations of arsenic in drinking water has been linked with skin cancer. However, the evidence for cancer risk resulting from exposure to the normally low levels of these elements in the diet is not conclusive. No carcinogenic effects of dietary cadmium and arsenic have been observed in laboratory experiments, whereas high intakes of certain lead compounds appear to increase the incidence of cancer in mice and rats.

On this basis, the committee believes that no firm conclusions can be drawn about the risk of cancer due to normal dietary exposure to arsenic, cadmium, and lead.

Inhibitors of Carcinogenesis

Foods and numerous nutritive and nonnutritive components of the diet have been examined for their potential to protect against carcinogenesis. In epidemiological studies, investigators have attempted to correlate the intake of specific foods (and by inference, certain vitamins and trace elements) and the incidence of cancer. In laboratory experiments, vitamins, trace elements, nonnutritive food additives, and other organic constituents of foods (e.g., indoles, phenols, flavones, and isothiocyanates) have been tested for their ability to inhibit neoplasia (see Chapter 15).

The committee believes that there is sufficient epidemiological evidence to suggest that consumption of certain vegetables, especially carotene-rich (i.e., dark green and deep yellow) vegetables and cruciferous vegetables (e.g., cabbage, broccoli, cauliflower, and brussels sprouts), is associated with a reduction in the incidence of cancer at several sites in humans. A number of nonnutritive and nutritive compounds that are present in these vegetables also inhibit carcinogenesis in laboratory animals. Investigators have not yet established which, if any, of these compounds may be responsible for the protective effect observed in epidemiological studies.

Alcohol

The effects of alcohol consumption on cancer incidence have been studied in human populations. In some countries, including the United States, excessive beer drinking has been associated with an increased risk of colorectal cancer, especially rectal cancer. This observation has not been confirmed in other studies. There is limited evidence that excessive alcohol consumption causes hepatic injury and cirrhosis, which in turn may lead to the formation of hepatomas (liver cancer). When consumed in large quantities, alcoholic beverages appear to act synergistically with inhaled cigarette smoke to increase the risk for cancers of the mouth, larynx, esophagus, and the respiratory tract. The studies of alcohol consumption and cancer are discussed in Chapter 11.

Naturally Occurring Carcinogens

In addition to nutrients, a variety of nonnutritive substances (e.g., hydrazines) are natural constituents of foods. Furthermore, metabolites of molds (e.g., mycotoxins such as the potent carcinogen aflatoxin) and of bacteria (e.g., carcinogenic nitrosamines) may contaminate foods. Many of these are occasional contaminants, whereas others are normal components of relatively common foods. In Chapter 12, the committee examines evidence linking consumption of some of these substances to carcinogenesis.

The committee concluded that certain naturally occurring contaminants in food are carcinogenic in animals and pose a potential risk of cancer to humans. Noteworthy among these are mycotoxins (especially aflatoxin) and N-nitroso compounds, for which there is some epidemiological evidence. Studies in animals indicate that a few nonnutritive constituents of some foods, such as hydrazines in mushrooms, are also carcinogenic.

The compounds thus far shown to be carcinogenic in animals have been reported to occur in the average U.S. diet

in small amounts; however, there is no evidence that any of these substances individually makes a major contribution to the total risk of cancer in the United States. This lack of sufficient data should not be interpreted as an indication that these or other compounds subsequently found to be carcinogenic do not present a hazard.

Mutagens in Foods

Mutagens are substances that cause heritable changes in the genetic material of cells. If a chemical is mutagenic to bacteria or other organisms, it is generally regarded as a suspect carcinogen, although carcinogenicity must be confirmed in long-term tests in whole animals.

As is evident from the discussion in Chapter 13, considerable attention has recently been directed toward mutagenic activity in foods. Many vegetables contain mutagenic flavonoids such as quercetin, kaempferol, and their glycosides. Furthermore, some substances found in foods can enhance or inhibit the mutagenic activity of other compounds. Mutagens in charred meat and fish are produced during the pyrolysis of proteins that occurs when foods are cooked at very high temperatures. Mutagens can also be produced during normal cooking of meat at lower temperatures. Smoking of foods as well as charcoal broiling results in the deposition of mutagenic and carcinogenic polynuclear organic compounds such as benzo[a]pyrene on the surface of the food.

Most mutagens detected in foods have not been adequately tested for their carcinogenic activity. Thus, the committee believes that it is not yet possible to assess whether such mutagens are likely to contribute significantly to the incidence of cancer in the United States.

Food Additives

In the United States, nearly 3,000 substances are intentionally added to foods during processing. Another estimated 12,000 chemicals (e.g., vinyl chloride and acrylonitrile, which are used in food-packaging materials) are classified as indirect (or unintentional) additives, and are occasionally detected in some foods. Large amounts of some additives, such as sugar, are consumed by the general population, but the annual per capita exposure to most indirect additives represents only a minute portion of the diet. Although the Food Safety Provisions and, in many cases, the "Delaney Clause" of the Federal Food, Drug, and Cosmetic Act[2] prohibit the addition of known carcinogens to foods, only a small proportion of the substances added to foods have been tested for carcinogenicity according to protocols that are considered acceptable by current standards. Moreover, except for the studies on nonnutritive sweeteners, only a few epidemiological studies have been conducted to assess the effect of food additives on cancer incidence.

Chapter 14 contains detailed information on certain additives, i.e., selected nonnutritive sweeteners, antioxidants, and additives used in packaging or for promoting the growth of animals used for food. Particular attention is given to substances to which humans are widely exposed.

Of the few direct food additives that have been tested and found to be carcinogenic in animals, all except saccharin have been banned from use in the food supply. Only minute residues of a few indirect additives that are known either to produce cancer in animals (e.g., acrylonitrile) or to be carcinogenic in humans (e.g., vinyl chloride and diethylstilbestrol) are occasionally detected in foods.

The evidence reviewed by the committee does not suggest that the increasing use of food additives has contributed significantly to the overall risk of cancer due to their lack of carcinogenicity, to the relatively recent use of many of these substances, or to the inability of epidemiological techniques to detect the effects of additives against the background of common cancers from other causes.

Environmental Contaminants

Very low levels of a large and chemically diverse group of environmental contaminants may be present in a variety of foods. The dietary levels of some of these substances are monitored by the Market Basket Surveys conducted by the Food and Drug Administration. Many of them have been extensively tested for carcinogenicity.

In Chapter 14, the committee has summarized the evidence concerning exposure of humans to, and the carcinogenicity of, selected pesticides, some industrial chemicals, and other environmental contaminants. As with food additives, consideration was given primarily to compounds to which humans are widely exposed.

The results of standard chronic toxicity tests indicate that a number of environmental contaminants (e.g., some organochlorine pesticides, polychlorinated biphenyls, and polycyclic aromatic hydrocarbons) cause cancer in laboratory animals. The committee found no epidemiological evidence to suggest that these compounds individually make a major contribution to the risk of cancer in humans. However, the possibility that they may act synergistically and may thereby create a greater carcinogenic risk cannot be excluded.

Contribution of Diet to Overall Risk of Cancer

By some estimates, as much as 90% of all cancer in humans has been attributed to various environmental factors, including diet (see Chapter 18). Other investigators have estimated that diet is responsible for 30% to 40% of cancers in men and 60% of cancers in women.

---

[2]Sec. 402(a)(2)(C) and Sec. 409(c)(1)(A), respectively.

Recently, two epidemiologists suggested that a significant proportion of the deaths from cancer could be prevented by dietary means and that dietary modifications would have the greatest effect on the incidence of cancers of the stomach and large bowel and, to a lesser extent, on cancers of the breast, the endometrium, and the lung.

The evidence reviewed by the committee suggests that cancers of most major sites are influenced by dietary patterns. However, the committee concluded that the data are not sufficient to quantitate the contribution of diet to the overall cancer risk or to determine the percent reduction in risk that might be achieved by dietary modifications.

INTERIM DIETARY GUIDELINES

It is not now possible, and may never be possible, to specify a diet that would protect everyone against all forms of cancer. Nevertheless, the committee believes that it is possible on the basis of current evidence to formulate interim dietary guidelines that are both consistent with good nutritional practices and likely to reduce the risk of cancer. These guidelines are meant to be applied in their entirety to obtain maximal benefit.

1. There is sufficient evidence that high fat consumption is linked to increased incidence of certain common cancers (notably breast and colon cancer) and that low fat intake is associated with a lower incidence of these cancers. The committee recommends that the consumption of both saturated and unsaturated fats be reduced in the average U.S. diet. An appropriate and practical target is to reduce the intake of fat from its present level (approximately 40%) to 30% of total calories in the diet. The scientific data do not provide a strong basis for establishing fat intake at precisely 30% of total calories. Indeed, the data could be used to justify an even greater reduction. However, in the judgment of the committee, the suggested reduction (i.e., one-quarter of the fat intake) is a moderate and practical target, and is likely to be beneficial.

2. The committee emphasizes the importance of including fruits, vegetables, and whole grain cereal products in the daily diet. In epidemiological studies, frequent consumption of these foods has been inversely correlated with the incidence of various cancers. Results of laboratory experiments have supported these findings in tests of individual nutritive and nonnutritive constituents of fruits (especially citrus fruits) and vegetables (especially carotene-rich and cruciferous vegetables).

These recommendations apply only to foods as sources of nutrients--not to dietary supplements of individual nutrients. The vast literature examined in this report focuses on the relationship between the consumption of foods and the incidence of cancer in human populations. In contrast, there is very little information on the effects of various levels of individual nutrients on the risk of cancer in humans. Therefore, the committee is unable to predict the health effects of high and potentially toxic doses of isolated nutrients consumed in the form of supplements.

3. In some parts of the world, especially China, Japan, and Iceland, populations that frequently consume salt-cured (including salt-pickled) or smoked foods have a greater incidence of cancers at some sites, especially the esophagus and the stomach. In addition, some methods of smoking and pickling foods seem to produce higher levels of polycyclic aromatic hydrocarbons and N-nitroso compounds. These compounds cause mutations in bacteria and cancer in animals, and are suspected of being carcinogenic in humans. Therefore, the committee recommends that the consumption of food preserved by salt-curing (including salt-pickling) or smoking be minimized.

4. Certain nonnutritive constituents of foods, whether naturally occurring or introduced inadvertently (as contaminants) during production, processing, and storage, pose a potential

risk of cancer to humans. The committee recommends that efforts continue to be made to minimize contamination of foods with carcinogens from any source. Where such contaminants are unavoidable, permissible levels should continue to be established and the food supply monitored to assure that such levels are not exceeded. Furthermore, intentional additives (direct and indirect) should continue to be evaluated for carcinogenic activity before they are approved for use in the food supply.

5. The committee suggests that further efforts be made to identify mutagens in food and to expedite testing for their carcinogenicity. Where feasible and prudent, mutagens should be removed or their concentration minimized when this can be accomplished without jeopardizing the nutritive value of foods or introducing other potentially hazardous substances into the diet.

6. Excessive consumption of alcoholic beverages, particularly combined with cigarette smoking, has been associated with an increased risk of cancer of the upper gastrointestinal and respiratory tracts. Consumption of alcohol is also associated with other adverse health effects. Thus, the committee recommends that if alcoholic beverages are consumed, it be done in moderation.

* * *

The committee suggests that agencies involved in education and public information should be encouraged to disseminate information on the relationship between dietary and nutritional factors and the incidence of cancer, and to publicize the conclusions and interim dietary guidelines in this report. It should be made clear that the weight of evidence suggests that what we eat during our lifetime strongly influences the probability of developing certain kinds of cancer but that it is not now possible, and may never be possible, to specify a diet that protects all people against all forms of cancer. The cooperation of the food industry should be sought to help implement the dietary guidelines described above.

Since the current data base is incomplete, future epidemiological and experimental research is likely to provide new insights into the relationship between diet and cancer. Therefore, the committee suggests that the National Cancer Institute establish mechanisms to review these dietary guidelines at least every 5 years.

A Comparison of Dietary Methods in Epidemiologic Studies[1]

by R. W. Morgan,[2] M. Jain,[3] A. B. Miller,[3] N. W. Choi,[4]
V. Matthews,[5] L. Munan,[6] J. D. Burch,[3] J. Feather,[5] G. R. Howe[3]
and A. Kelly[6]

Morgan, R. W. (Dept. of Preventive Medicine, U. of Toronto, Ontario M5S
1A8, Canada), M. Jain, A. B. Miller, N. W. Choi, V. Matthews, L. Munan, J. D.
Burch, J. Feather, G. R. Howe and A. Kelly. **A comparison of dietary methods
in epidemiologic studies.** *Am J Epidemiol* 107:488–498, 1978.

Three methods of estimating group and individual dietary consumption
have been developed and assessed in a case-control study of diet and breast
cancer. The methods comprised a 24-hour recall, a detailed quantitative diet
history directed to the most recent two-month period and the two-month
period six months before, and a four-day diet diary. There is a high degree of
correlation between the estimates of food consumption for the controls using
each of the methods. The highest estimate was obtained from the diet
history, with a slightly higher estimate in the period six months before than
the current period, while the lowest is found in the 24-hour recall. The latter
corresponds with the same method in a Nutrition Canada Survey. It is
concluded that all methods are applicable to case-control studies, but the
diet history is preferred when current food intake may be influenced by a
disease.

Geographic differences corresponding to
regional variations in calorie and fat intake (1–3), animal experiments (4), and a
need to explain racial or geographic differ-

ences in urinary estrogens (5), have raised
the possibility that breast cancer may be
caused by nutritional factors (6). This paper describes the rationale and techniques
for collection and use of dietary data in a
case-control study of breast cancer.

Many methods of dietary assessment
traditionally are applied to current, rather
than past intake but little is known concerning the relationship of present food
intake to the diet of previous decades (7).
This is an important deficiency because of
the demonstrated relationship of early reproductive events to later development of
breast cancer (8).

The effect of diet on breast cancer risk
might be measured most accurately in a

Received for publication May 2, 1977, and in final
form January 3, 1978.

[1] This study was supported by the National Cancer Institute of Canada and in part under National
Health Research and Development Project No. 613-
1047-30 of Health and Welfare Canada.

[2] University of Toronto.

[3] Epidemiology Unit, National Cancer Institute
of Canada.

[4] University of Manitoba.

[5] University of Saskatchewan.

[6] University of Sherbrooke.

Reprint requests to Dr. Morgan, Departments of
Preventive Medicine and Biostatistics, U. of Toronto, McMurrich Building, Toronto, Ontario M5S
1A8, Canada.

cohort study but such an approach would be difficult, expensive and require prolonged follow-up. Out of these considerations, we elected to use a case-control approach, with the assumption (neither questioned nor supported by data) that individual dietary patterns have sufficient constancy to allow recent intake to serve as an indicator of prior practices. We considered it important to validate the methods of dietary data collection to ensure, as far as possible, that the data collected were as representative as possible of true intake. For this reason, we developed and used three different instruments. We have also developed food composition tables and computer programs to convert dietary data to nutritional components suitable for testing our major hypotheses.

The present paper describes these methods and presents results for four samples of 100 healthy subjects without breast cancer from the provinces of Manitoba, Saskatchewan, Quebec and Ontario.

Previous work in nutritional methods as applied to epidemiology

Collection of nutrient data by methods requiring weighing and laboratory analysis is impractical for survey research. Dietary history, observation, and recording of food intake have, therefore, been used most frequently. This section will be concerned with methods useful for field investigations to study dietary characteristics of large groups.

Food Frequency Interview. The Food Frequency Interview inquires about usual intake, in terms of the frequency of consumption of various food items. The respondent may be asked the frequency of consumption of an item in terms of relative or actual frequency per day, week or month. Abramson et al. (9) concluded that this method should be considered where evidence is sought of an association with diet in general, rather than with specific nutrients. It may, therefore, be of use in the "clue seeking" stage of a study. Frequency data have been used in several studies investigating possible associations between diet and health (10–17) and in nutritional programs to search for individuals likely to require more detailed dietary investigation (18). Graham et al. (19) in a

study of diet and gastric cancer considered the frequency interview approach most feasible in the early stages of dietary research; reliability checks on their frequency data gave a mean agreement of 81 per cent. In another study (11) an average reproducibility of 90 per cent was found depending on the frequency of consumption and the type of food.

Quantitative Research Dietary History. The Quantitative Research Dietary History developed by Burke (20) is directed towards a subject's usual pattern of eating, with food consumed recorded in common household measures. For example, the subject is asked, "What do you usually eat for breakfast?" Frequency and usual size of portions, as well as the kinds of food are recorded. An important step in this kind of history is known as the "cross check." The cross check form lists all the food groups. The frequency and amount of consumption of these food groups is assessed against the information given for the usual intake.

Few epidemiologic studies have used this type of dietary history as a research tool. Most studies have used a modified version (21–28). In the Framingham study (26), the interview was not structured; that is, the questions were not written or asked by rote. The subjects gave their usual daily frequency of food intake. An absence of a definitive pattern of questions may have failed to elicit all the required information and also might have introduced interviewer bias as regards the persistency and depth of probing used. In the Israel Ischemic Heart Disease study (9) only a moderate correlation was found between the data from a Burke type history and the short questionnaire developed in the study.

The Burke type dietary history has also been used in nutritional studies to characterize nutrient intakes of individuals over long periods of time. Beal (29) used it to assess the nutrient intake of normal children from infancy through adolescence. In addition, a dietary history can be used to quantify specific items in a diet Thus, Nutrition Canada (30) has used a dietary history in its National Nutrition Survey to assess the non-nutritive additives to food. Attempts have been made to assess the reliability of the method and it has been found that an error of 12–35 per cent in calorie assessment may be introduced depending on the type of respondent (31). Reed and Burke (32) tested reliability by correlating protein intake with the rate of growth of muscle in the lower leg of children and concluded that the dietary history is not in error more than 10 gm protein per day. Tests for reliability showed no significant differences in the values obtained within two years for a dietary history and seven-day food records (33, 34). It appears that a dietary history properly taken for research purposes serves a very useful purpose and is of greater value than is generally appreciated.

Diet Record. The Diet Record is usually used for collection of individual dietary data (35–37). This written record of all foods and beverages consumed by the respondent is directed to current intake. Since the actual recording is performed by the respondent, the method can only be used for literate persons. Also, the method is inappropriate when symptoms or treatment of a condition affect the diet. A dietary record covering seven consecutive days or 20 consecutive meals has been considered to be the shortest period of time feasible for validity (38–41). However, Tinsley (42) recommended that if a week of record keeping is not practical, three days represent the minimum time to give a fair picture of food intake. Darby (43) reached similar conclusions.

Diet-Recall Interview. In this method food consumption for a specified period of time is recalled in as much detail as possible. The recall period may vary from one day to weeks, though long periods are presumably subject to substantial defects of memory. The 24-hour period is most commonly used (6, 30). Although it may not give correct data on the usual food consumption of an individual since the menu on the day recalled may be atypical, the method is believed to give fairly reliable data on the current food consumption of the group. Frequently a combination of 24-hour recall and a history of frequency of consumption of various foods has been used to obtain a more accurate estimate of a respondent's usual diet (44, 45).

Comparison of different methods. Young et al. (46–49) found that the diet history estimated a higher mean intake than a seven-day diet record and 24-hour recall. They also found that it was not possible to predict the intake of an individual from a seven-day record or from the dietary history. They concluded that the three methods could not be used interchangeably in describing the intake of an individual. Similar conclusions have been reported by others (50–52). Trulson (53) concluded that of the three main methods, no one method is more reliable, but she preferred the dietary history interview since it might reveal long-range dietary practices. Agreement in the results of a 24-hour recall and dietary history improves with increasing level of subject education (54).

Ohlson et al. (55) studied the dietary intake of 18 women, 48–77 years of age, by means of three 24-hour recall interviews and 10 days of unrestricted weighed dietary intake. The apparent mean intake of all nutrients was greater when measured by the recall method. Similar results were reported by Pekkarinen et al. (50) though contrary findings have been reported by others (53, 56–58). Hankin et al. (59) found that a seven-day quantitative recall of particular food items has considerable validity when compared with a seven-day diary and is a reasonable choice of method for studies of large groups concerning the role of particular food items in the etiology of cancer. The estimated quantitative intakes tended to be higher for the diary than the recall method due to the higher values of recorded frequencies than those recalled.

METHODS

In designing the study, we attempted to select methods that would quantify the "characteristic diet" of an individual in the hope that this would reflect life-long dietary intake. Thus, an important objective of the study was to develop and standardize dietary methods for use in future epidemiologic studies of cancer.

It is evident from the cited review that our requirements could be met by the use of a Burke type dietary history and a four-day diet record. We also added the 24-hour recall to help train respondents to complete the four-day diet record. To standardize interviewing procedures, interviewers from all study areas were trained simultaneously at Saskatoon. A detailed interviewer's manual was prepared and used in all centers throughout the study. Quality control was also achieved by visits to study areas to assess fieldwork procedures. The interview included a questionnaire on personal and medical history, with questions to elicit information about changes in past diet over any appreciable time. This was administered immediately prior to the dietary history and 24-hour recall. All interviews were administered in the respondent's home.

Dietary History Questionnaire

The purpose of this questionnaire was to describe, quantitatively, the respondent's usual or average diet. It does not record precisely what she has eaten in a given day or week, but should show her usual pattern of food intake. The respondent describes kinds of foods eaten, frequency of consumption in a day, week or month, their preparation and amount.

As it is difficult for people to recall details about what they ate or drank all their life, we limited recall to two periods stretching over approximately eight months. First, the respondent was asked to report frequency and amount of foods usually eaten in the last two months. Then, for the same item, the respondent was asked to think back six months and report on the two preceding months before that date. For example, for an interview conducted on December 1, 1974 with a patient diagnosed as having breast cancer on August 12, 1974, Time I would comprise October and November 1974 while Time II would be April and May 1974, thus avoiding the period immediately before or after the diagnosis of cancer.

A series of items covering the entire range of consumable foods and drinks are listed on the questionnaire. Interviewers were trained not to suggest answers, but to ask the questions in the manner specified in the Interviewer's Manual. A structured interview of this nature reduces the bias which might occur as a consequence of differences in the depth and persistence of interviewer probing. Instructions for probing appeared in parentheses on the questionnaire, for example, "type," "variety," "brand." Specific reminder words such as "broiled," "fried," "poached" were also used to signify the need to describe the method of preparation of the particular food item. Similar food items were grouped together to reduce interview time; for example, corn, peas and beans formed one group. Some listed items were followed by "add" which required recording anything that a respondent adds to the item, e.g., butter on vegetables. The use of such specified instructions ensured uniformity of administration of the instrument.

The respondent was asked the amount of food consumed at each sitting. Interviewers concentrated on the respondent's personal intake to avoid confusion with the family's consumption. The respondent's estimate of portion size was assisted by a set of simulated food models representing a range of alternative portion sizes. The respondent's estimates of food portions in common household terms or measures were not accepted. The food models used in this study were a refinement of those developed and modified in studies elsewhere (30). Actual weights or measurements were not recorded on the models to avoid respondent bias. Other units were used for foods like eggs, apples, oranges, etc., or foods in standard packaging, e.g., a pat of butter, pack of jam or marmalade, or a cube of sugar.

After recording the information on frequency and amounts of food eaten, the respondent was asked about the method of preparation and any unusual recipes were recorded. Since fats and oils are normally not served or taken as food items by themselves and these were important nutrients to test the study hypotheses, the questionnaire was designed so that the interviewer asked about them in conjunction with all other food items.

24-Hour Recall Questionnaire

The 24-hour recall questionnaire was administered to the respondent after the dietary history. A description of everything consumed in the 24-hour period from midnight to midnight of the day before the interview was requested. Food models were used sparingly; the main emphasis being on measuring with standard measuring cups and spoons the household utensils from which foods and beverages were taken the day before. Foods and beverages were described in the same detail as in the diet history and space was provided for recording the recipes of all mixed dishes, unusual desserts, etc.

Four-Day Diet Record

The interview was concluded by leaving the respondent with a Four-Day Diet Record. The respondent was asked to complete the record over the next four days, including a Sunday. The respondent was directed not to change what she normally consumed while keeping the record and to record all meals and snacks eaten at home or elsewhere. The amount of detail required for any food item was the same as for the diet history and 24-hour recall. Use of weighing scales might have increased accuracy, but could also influence eating patterns. Therefore, the respondent was encouraged to report the quantities in terms of household measures, cups, spoons and dimensions. Some of these were measured by the interviewer and a sheet indicating their equivalence in standard measures was left with the respondent. Distinction was made between fluid ounces and weight ounces. Unless the respondent bought the food in weight ounces, she was encouraged to report all the food items in fluid ounces or dimensions. On its completion the Four-Day Diet Record was retrieved by the interviewer who then checked with the respondent the description, amount and preparation of all foods recorded before leaving. In some instances, due to either extreme weather conditions, or distance, the respondent mailed the completed diary to the local Study Center.

Food composition tables

Food composition tables from the US Department of Agriculture (60) were modified and considerably extended by us to include items characteristically Canadian or specific to the individual study areas. Sources for these additions included food composition tables (30, 61–63), commercial firms, cook books and recipes obtained directly from study participants. Values

on a number of items were obtained from food composition tables prepared by Home Economists at the Exercise Laboratory, Department of Medicine, University of Saskatchewan.

Cooking fat is estimated to form approximately 22 per cent of total daily fat intake per person in a North American diet (64). We used the respondent's data, cookbooks and research papers in addition to certain food tables available (65–69) to calculate the amount of fat/oil used for cooking. The basic food composition tables containing 2929 food items were thus expanded to include 319 of the original foods in each of the 22 fat and oil combinations, to yield a total of 9947 separate items.

In order to convert amounts reported in terms of the volume of the food models, density measurements were also included for most items.

Coding

Coding was done for all areas by a coder trained and supervised by one of the authors (M.J.). An extensive and detailed manual for coding dietary and non-dietary information was prepared. The dietary history and the 24-hour recall were designed for coding directly on the questionnaire. Some food items on the dietary history were also pre-coded. A separate code sheet was designed to transfer information from the four-day diet record.

Many food items are not commonly marketed and differ from the homemade recipes reported in the US Department of Agriculture Handbook No. 8 (60). In such instances, rules of procedure for uniform handling were applied. When the actual recipes could be obtained from the respondent, the ingredients were separately assigned codes from the food composition tables.

RESULTS

Response. In each area 100 neighborhood controls were admitted to the study (for details of their selection in each area see reference 70). Each person completed a 24-hour recall questionnaire and diet history questionnaire. However, only 87 per cent of respondents completed the four-day diet record. Reasons for non-completion of records were various. Some respondents left soon after the interview for vacation, some blamed ill-health, some did not feel committed to complete the diet record.

Comparison of methods by group mean values. The mean values and standard errors for the daily intake of the control respondents, as obtained for each nutrient are presented in table 1, for the separate areas and all areas combined. There was very close concordance between the different segments of the diet history, although for each area and for each nutrient, diet history II, comprising the two months period six months before the interview, gave slightly higher values. In addition, the diet history produced a higher estimate of average daily intake than either the 24-

hour recall or the four-day record. Again this was consistent for each area, and for each nutrient.

For the other two methods, with only three exceptions, the four-day record gave higher average daily intake than the 24-hour recall. The exceptions were calories and saturated fat in area 4 and linoleic acid in area 1.

With the exception of the histories at times I and II, these differences were significant at the 5 per cent level. The consistency of these differences is emphasized in table 2 for all areas combined, the average daily intakes for each of the methods being recorded as a percentage of the history at time II. It will be noted that

TABLE 1

Average daily intake of control subjects* in the diet and breast cancer study

Dietary method used	Area I†		Area II		Area III		Area IV		All areas	
	Mean	SE‡	Mean	SE	Mean	SE	Mean	SE	Mean	SE
Calories										
24-hour recall	1646	66	1449	56	1621	67	1743	140	1615	44
Diet history I§	2019	64	1967	74	2391	114	2302	75	2170	43
Diet history II¶	2208	109	2020	82	2430	113	2478	92	2284	50
4-day record	1792	55	1680	57	1909	60	1739	60	1780	29
Total fat (gm)										
24-hour recall	78.8	4.9	67.0	3.7	63.6	3.6	74.9	5.2	71.2	2.2
Diet history I	90.7	3.7	85.1	4.0	95.0	4.9	103.2	4.5	93.5	2.2
Diet history II	96.5	4.6	88.4	4.5	96.9	5.0	111.0	5.1	98.2	2.4
4-day record	82.5	3.7	76.6	3.6	81.2	3.0	77.5	3.2	79.6	1.7
Saturated fat (gm)										
24-hour recall	30.0	1.9	24.9	1.6	23.8	1.6	30.3	2.3	27.3	0.9
Diet history I	35.8	1.7	31.7	1.6	34.8	2.0	40.0	1.8	35.6	0.9
Diet history II	37.9	2.0	32.8	1.8	35.6	2.1	43.4	2.0	37.4	1.0
4-day record	32.1	1.6	29.6	1.5	30.8	1.3	30.3	1.4	30.7	0.7
Oleic (gm)										
24-hour recall	32.5	2.2	27.5	1.5	25.2	1.6	29.2	2.3	28.6	0.9
Diet history I	35.2	1.6	34.6	1.7	37.2	1.9	39.1	1.8	36.6	0.9
Diet history II	37.3	1.8	35.7	1.8	37.8	1.9	41.6	2.0	38.1	0.9
4-day record	33.2	1.5	31.4	1.5	33.1	1.3	31.3	1.3	32.3	0.7
Linoleic (gm)										
24-hour recall	9.0	0.8	7.1	0.6	6.8	0.5	7.3	0.7	7.6	0.3
Diet history I	11.0	0.6	10.0	0.6	11.7	0.7	13.2	0.9	11.5	3.7
Diet history II	11.7	0.7	10.6	0.7	11.9	0.7	14.7	1.0	12.2	0.4
4-day record	8.7	0.5	7.6	0.5	7.8	0.4	8.2	0.5	8.1	0.2
Cholesterol (mg)										
24-hour recall	336.6	21.4	277.4	20.9	276.3	27.9	327.0	25.2	304.3	12.0
Diet history I	470.4	27.5	386.7	19.2	408.6	22.7	450.4	21.2	429.0	11.8
Diet history II	488.1	29.0	393.1	19.4	417.0	23.1	470.3	26.5	442.2	12.5
4-day record	387.1	17.9	343.8	15.6	374.2	17.5	362.4	18.7	367.2	8.7

* Number of subjects: (a) For 24-hour recall and diet history: 100 per area. (b) For four-day record: Area I – 95; Area II – 90; Area III – 85; Area IV – 77.

† Area I – Winnipeg; Area II – Saskatoon; Area III – Sherbrooke; Area IV – Toronto.

‡ Standard error.

§ Current two months.

¶ Two-month period six months before the interview.

when expressed in this way the discrepancy between methods is greatest for linoleic acid but least for oleic acid.

Comparison with Nutrition Canada Survey. In table 3 caloric intake measured by 24-hour recall in the present study and as reported for the corresponding province by Nutrition Canada, using a 24-hour recall method, is given. There is good agreement between the Nutrition Canada results and those in the present study. The 24-hour recall in the present study estimated a higher mean intake than the Nutrition Canada study in area 1 and area 4, but a lower mean intake in area 2 and area 3. The difference was greatest in area 1, the most predominantly rural area.

Comparison of nutrients – individual data. Simple correlation coefficients between the various nutrients for all areas combined were calculated for each of the methods. The correlation coefficients were very similar for each method, all nutrients being highly correlated (the data are not tabulated here). The greatest discrepancies between the different nutrients were for the comparisons involving linoleic acid and cholesterol. These nutrients also gave the greatest discrepancy between methods. The closest individual correlations were between calories and total fat, saturated fat and oleic acid.

Comparison of methods – individual data. Table 4 shows simple correlation coefficients for the data from all areas combined for each nutrient between the various methods. All values are positive, the highest correlation for each nutrient being between the two components of diet history.

DISCUSSION

An important aspect of the present study was the development of methods to quantify individual consumption of dietary items. It is of course not possible to be certain that the estimates of consumption derived from any of the methods used correctly reflect the actual food intake of the respondents. Such confirmation is almost impossible to obtain as the actions necessary to validate food consumption, for example, weighing or direct observation, will have an indirect or subconscious effect on the diet consumed for the period of the study. Such an influence may not be entirely absent from diet diaries and this together with the difficulty in obtaining 100 per cent cooperation make this particular method less satisfactory for epidemiologic studies.

TABLE 2

Comparison of dietary methods

Average daily intake expressed as % of history at time II				
Nutrient	24-hour recall	4-day record	History I	History II
Calories	70.7	77.9	95.0	100
Total fat	72.5	81.1	95.2	100
Saturated fat	73.0	82.1	95.2	100
Oleic	75.1	84.8	96.1	100
Linoleic	62.3	66.4	94.3	100
Cholesterol	68.8	83.1	97.1	100

TABLE 3

Comparison of areas: caloric intake as estimated in present study and Nutrition Canada Survey by 24-hour recall method

	Area 1	Area 2	Area 3	Area 4
Present study	1646	1449	1621	1743
Nutrition Canada Survey	1557	1473	1681	1695

TABLE 4

Simple correlation coefficients between the various dietary methods used for all areas combined

Dietary method used	Diet history I	Diet history II	4-day record
Calories			
24-hour recall	0.287	0.219	0.322
History I		0.871	0.339
History II			0.267
Total fat			
24-hour recall	0.287	0.238	0.249
History I		0.917	0.361
History II			0.307
Saturated fat			
24-hour recall	0.322	0.263	0.244
History I		0.923	0.402
History II			0.337
Oleic			
24-hour recall	0.271	0.241	0.222
History I		0.923	0.386
History II			0.339
Linoleic			
24-hour recall	0.331	0.314	0.345
History I		0.891	0.380
History II			0.318
Cholesterol			
24-hour recall	0.265	0.231	0.324
History I		0.874	0.421
History II			0.340

The respondents were instructed to report their usual dietary pattern in the diet histories. Although there is a high correlation between the current history intake and that measured by the history directed to the period six months before, the current history estimates a lower intake than the past history. This may reflect the fact that less is eaten now than previously because of increasing concern with the hazards associated with overweight and obesity. The fact that current history is better correlated than past history with both 24-hour recall and four-day record suggests that all three methods when directed to the same period measure the same thing although the estimates vary in quantity. It also suggests that a reduced intake actually exists in the current period.

Nevertheless, the relatively low individual correlation between the three basic methods suggests that the 24-hour recall does not adequately predict the diet as recorded by the four-day record, and that these do not predict the diet as estimated by the diet histories. The implication is that although each may be satisfactory for comparing group values, the decision as to which, if any, is satisfactory for individual values has to be made on other grounds. We believe that both the 24-hour recall and the four-day diary are inherently less reliable for individual estimates of usual intake, and that when such estimates are required, the diet history should be used. Further, as in this study there is reason for concern that current history is influenced by the diagnosis or treatment of breast cancer, the past history is to be preferred, and is therefore reported (71).

The observation that current history produces higher mean intakes than 24-hour recall methods has been made before (53, 56–58). Ohlson et al. (55) also reported higher mean intakes when measured by three 24-hour recalls as compared to 10 days of unrestricted weighed food records. This reflects the fact that weighing and recording imposes a reduced dietary intake to avoid such time consuming procedures. By not asking respondents to weigh, we overcame this difficulty and that may explain why our four-day estimates are higher than the 24-hour recall.

The only external assessment of the accuracy of any of the methods used in the present study is the comparison of the results of the 24-hour recall in the present study with the 24-hour recall as administered in the same province at about the same time period in the Nutrition Canada study. Although the population studied was somewhat different, the correspondence in the results tends to confirm the validity of our group estimates.

It should be noted that the 24-hour recall and four-day record methods are disadvantageous if, in a case control situation, the disease affecting the cases may be expected to have an effect on current diet. In the present study, care was taken when arranging interviews with cases that these were administered when all treatments that might have interfered with current diet were at an end. However, such adjustments may be impossible, for example, in case-control studies of gastrointestinal cancer when recent dietary changes may have occurred both as a result of the presence of the disease and of surgery given as treatment. Thus, diet history methods are more applicable in this situation and also give a more representative measure of normal diet than intake determined for a brief specific period.

Although results are given only for calorie intake and various aspects of fat consumption, our methods permit quantification of other nutrients. Aspects which may be particularly relevant in studies of some cancers include intake of protein, fiber, vitamins and minerals. The close correlation between the various nutrients as measured in the present study was not unexpected as a similar high correlation has been noted for animal protein consumption and fat intake (4). The implication of this high degree of correlation, however, is that when looking for dietary differences between cases and controls, it may be difficult to separate the effects of various nutrients with precision.

REFERENCES

1. Lea AJ: Dietary factors associated with death rates from certain neoplasma in man. Lancet 2:332–333, 1966
2. Carroll KK, Gammal EB, Plunkett ER: Dietary fat and mammary cancer. Can Med Assoc J 98:590–594, 1968

3. Hill MJ, Goddard P, Williams REO: Gut bacteria and the etiology of cancer of the breast. Lancet 2:472–473, 1971
4. Carroll KK, Khor HT: Dietary fat in relation to tumorigenesis. Prog Biochem Pharmacol 10:308–353, 1975
5. MacMahon B, Cole P, Brown JB, et al: Urine estrogen profiles of Asian and North American women. Int J Cancer 14:161–167, 1974
6. Miller AB: Role of nutrition in the etiology of breast cancer. Cancer 37:2704–2708, 1977
7. Ohlson MA, Harper LJ: Longitudinal studies of food intake and weight of women from ages 18 to 56 years. J Am Diet Assoc 69:626–631, 1976
8. MacMahon B, Cole P, Brown J: Etiology of human breast cancer, a review. J Natl Cancer Inst 50:21–42, 1973
9. Abramson JH, Some C, Kosovsky C: Food frequency interview as an epidemiological tool. Am J Public Health 53:1093–1101, 1963
10. Weiss RL, Trithart AH: Between-meal eating habits and dental caries experience in preschool children. Am J Public Health 53:1097–1104, 1960
11. Acheson ED, Doll R: Dietary factors in carcinoma of the stomach. A study of 100 cases and 200 controls. Gut 5:126–131, 1964
12. Higginson J: Etiological factors in gastrointestinal cancer in man. J Natl Cancer Inst 37:527–545, 1966
13. Hirayama T: The epidemiology of cancer of the stomach in Japan with special reference to the role of diet. *In*: Proceedings of the 9th International Cancer Congress, Tokyo, October 1966; Panel Discussion. UICC Monograph Series—Vol 10. Edited by RJC Harris. Berlin, Germany, Springer-Verlag, pp 37–48, 1967
14. Choi NW, Entwistle DW, Michaluk W, et al: Gastric cancer in Icelanders in Manitoba. Israel J Med Sci 7:1500–1508, 1971
15. Graham S, Schotz W, Martino P: Alimentary factors in the epidemiology of gastric cancer. Cancer 30:927–938, 1972
16. Bjelke E: Epidemiologic studies of cancer of the stomach, colon and rectum with special emphasis on the role of the diet. Scand J Gastroenterol 9:Suppl 31, 1974
17. Haenszel W, Correa P, Cuello C, et al: Gastric cancer in Colombia. II. Case control epidemiologic study of precursor lesions. J Natl Cancer Inst 57:1021–1026, 1976
18. Babcock MJ, Gates LO: Rapid survey of eating habits—a stimulus to nutrition education. School Science and Mathematics 54:601–611, 1954
19. Graham S, Lilienfeld AM, Tidings JE: Dietary and purgation factors in the epidemiology of gastric cancer. Cancer 20:2224–2234, 1967
20. Burke BS: The dietary history as a tool in research. J Am Diet Assoc 23:1041–1046, 1947
21. Wynder EL, Kmet J, Dungal N, et al: An epidemiological investigation of gastric cancer. Cancer 16:1461–1496, 1963
22. Wynder EL, Kajitani T, Ishikawa S, et al: Environmental factors of cancer of the colon and rectum. II. Japanese epidemiological data. Cancer 23:1210–1220, 1969
23. Haenszel W, Kurihara M, Segi M, et al: Stomach cancer among Japanese in Hawaii. J Natl Cancer Inst 49:969–988, 1972
24. Haenszel W, Kurihara M, Locke FB, et al: Stomach cancer in Japan. J Natl Cancer Inst 56:265–274, 1976
25. Segi M, Fukushima I, Fujisaku S, et al: An Epidemiological Study on Cancer in Japan. The Report of the Committee for Epidemiological Study on Cancer, sponsored by the Ministry of Welfare and Public Health. Gann 48 (Suppl):1–63, 1957
26. Mann GV, Pearson G, Gordon T, et al: Diet and cardiovascular disease in the Framingham Study. I. Measurement of dietary intake. Am J Clin Nutr 11:200–225, 1962
27. Hankin JH, Stallones RA, Messinger HB: A short dietary method for epidemiological studies. III. Development of questionnaire. Am J Epidemiol 87:285–298, 1967
28. Browe JH, Gofstein MR, Morlley DM, et al: Diet and heart disease study in the Cardiovascular Health Centre. I. A questionnaire and its application in assessing dietary intake. J Am Diet Assoc 48:95–100, 1966
29. Beal VA: Nutritional intake of children: Calories, carbohydrates, fat and protein. J Nutr 50:223–234, 1953
30. Nutrition Canada National Survey: A Report by Nutrition Canada to the Department of National Health and Welfare. Information Canada, Ottawa, 1973
31. Campbell VA: Review of dietary methodology and evaluation. (unpublished data)
32. Reed RB, Burke BS: Collection and analysis of dietary intake data. Am J Public Health 44:1015–1026, 1954
33. Trulson MF, McCann MB: Comparison of dietary survey methods. J Am Diet Assoc 35:672–676, 1959
34. Dawber TR, Pearson G, Anderson P, et al: Dietary assessment in the epidemiologic study of coronary heart disease: The Framingham Study. II. Reliability of measurement. Am J Clin Nutr 11:226–234, 1962
35. Hankin JH, Huenemann R: A short dietary method for epidemiologic studies. I. Developing standard methods for interpreting seven-day measured food records. J Am Diet Assoc 50:487–492, 1967
36. Moore LB, Gremillion L, Lopez's A: Serum lipids, dietary intakes and physical exercise in medical students. J Am Dietet Assoc 64:43–46, 1974
37. Peckos PS, Ross ML: Longitudinal study of the calorie and nutrient intake of individual twins. I. Calorie, protein, fat and carbohydrate intakes. J Am Dietet Assoc 62:399–403, 1973
38. Wait B, Roberts LJ: Studies in food requirements of adolescent girls. II. Daily variations in the energy intake of the individual. J Am Diet Assoc 8:323–331, 1932
39. Anderson RK, Sandstead HR: Nutritional appraisal and demonstration program of the U.S. Public Health Service. J Am Diet Assoc 23:101–107, 1947
40. Leverton RM, Marsh AG: Comparison of food intakes for weekdays and for Saturday and Sunday. J Home Econ 31:111–114, 1939
41. Gray CE, Blackman NR: More high school student diets evaluated. J Home Econ 39:505–506, 1947
42. Tinsley WV: Development of instruments for evaluating food practices, nutrition information and school lunch programs and their use in nutrition education at the elementary level. Doctor's Thesis. St Paul, MN, University of Minnesota, 1947

43. Darby WJ: The influence of some recent studies on the interpretation of the findings of nutrition surveys. J Am Diet Assoc 28:43–48, 1952

44. Larsen LB, Dodds JM, Massoth DM, et al: Nutritional status of children of Mexican American migrant families. J Am Diet Assoc 64:29–35, 1974

45. Gaines EG, Daniel WA: Dietary iron intakes of adolescents, relation of sex, race and sex maturity ratings. J Am Diet Assoc 65:275–280, 1974

46. Young CM, Chalmers FW, Church HN, et al: A comparison of dietary study methods. I. Dietary history vs. seven-day record. J Am Diet Assoc 28:124–128, 1952

47. Young CM, Trulson MF: Methodology for dietary studies in epidemiological surveys. II. Strengths and weaknesses of existing methods. Am J Public Health 50:803–814, 1960

48. Young CM: The interview itself. J Am Diet Assoc 35:677–681, 1959

49. Young CM, Hogan GC, Tucker RE, et al: A comparison of dietary study methods. II. Dietary history vs. seven-day record vs. 24-hour recall. J Am Diet Assoc 28:218–221, 1952

50. Pekkarinen M, Kivioja S, Jortikka L: A comparison of the food intake of rural families estimated by one-day recall and precise weighing methods. Voeding 28:470–476, 1967

51. Hartog CD, Schaik TFSM, Dalderup LM, et al: The diet of volunteers participating in a long-term epidemiological food survey on coronary heart disease at Zutphen, the Netherlands. Voeding 26:184–208, 1965

52. Huenemann R, Turner D: Methods of dietary investigation. J Am Diet Assoc 18:562–568, 1942

53. Trulson MF: Assessment of dietary study methods. I. Comparison of methods for obtaining data for clinical work. J Am Diet Assoc 30:991–995, 1954

54. Stevens HA, Bleiler RE, Ohlson MA: Dietary intake of five groups of subjects. 24-hour recall diets vs. dietary patterns. J Am Diet Assoc 42:387–393, 1963

55. Ohlson MA, Jackson L, Boek J, et al: Nutrition and dietary habits of aging women. Am J Public Health 40:1101–1108, 1963

56. Bransby RE, Daubney CG, King J: Comparison of results obtained by different methods of individual dietary surveys. Br J Nutr 2:89–110, 1948

57. Morrison SD, Russell FC, Stevenson J: Estimating food intake by questioning and weighing: A one-day survey of eight subjects. Br J Nutr (Abs) 3:V, 1949

58. Combe GF, Wolfe AC: Methods used in dietary survey of civilians in Ecuador. Public Health Rep 75:707–716, 1960

59. Hankin JH, Rhoads GG, Glober GG: A dietary method for an epidemiological study of gastrointestinal cancer. Am J Clin Nutr 28:1055–1060, 1975

60. US Department of Agriculture, Agriculture Research Service, Composition of Foods: Raw, Processed, Prepared. Agriculture Handbook No 8, 1968, Expansion (March 1972)

61. US Department of Agriculture: Nutritive Values of Foods. Home and Garden Bulletin No 72, 1971

62. Bowes A de P: Food Values of Portions Commonly Used. 11th edition. Revised by CF Church, HN Church. JB Lippincott Co, 1970

63. Health and Welfare Department: Nutrient Value of Some Common Foods. Canada, 1971

64. US Department of Agriculture: Report No 6, 1966

65. US Department of Agriculture, Agriculture Research Service: Proximate Composition of Beef from Carcass to Cooked Meat; Method of Derivation and Tables of Values. Home Economics Res Rep No 31, 1965

66. US Department of Agricultrue, Agriculture Research Service: Food Yields: Summarized by different stages of preparation. Agriculture Handbook No 102, 1956

67. US Department of Agriculture: Procedures for calculating nutritive values of home prepared foods, as used in A H-8. ARS 62–13, March 1966

68. Leverton RM, Odell GV: The nutritive value of cooked meat. MP-49, Oklahoma State University, 1959

69. US Department of Agriculture: Fatty Acids in Food Fats. Home Economics Res Rep No 7

70. Choi NW, Howe GR, Miller AB, et al: An epidemiological study of breast cancer. Am J Epidemiol 107:510–521, 1978

71. Miller AB, Kelly A, Choi NW, et al: A study of diet and breast cancer. Am J Epidemiol 107:499–509, 1978

Nutrition and Cancer[1]

by A. B. Miller, with Gio B. Gori, Ph.D., Saxon Graham, Ph.D.,
Takeshi Hirayama, M.D., Michael Kunze, M.D., Bandaru S.
Reddy, Ph.D., John H. Weisburger, Ph.D.

The evidence from high and low incidence populations worldwide, the corresponding correlations with fat and caloric intake, the picture that has emerged from migrant studies and studies of singular populations—such as the Seventh Day Adventists, the analyses of trends in incidence and dietary changes in certain well-characterized populations, and emerging evidence from case-control and other studies on specific dietary factors, all provide defensible arguments for dietary implications in the causation of certain major human cancers, stomach, breast, and colon specifically, and for dietary recommendations toward prevention. The evidence is reinforced by experimental animal studies that have shown data supportive of the epidemiologic studies, and provided clues to the possible mechanisms of action. Thus, there would seem to be sufficient evidence to propose modifying the diet of Western countries to reduce total fat and increase dietary fiber on the lines of the prudent diet, and to introduce certain protective factors, such as an increase in green vegetables and Vitamin C.

INTRODUCTION

The current scientific evidence indicates that nutrition is associated with certain cancers, but the mechanisms by which diet affects the development of cancer are as yet not fully understood. Diet could exert an effect in a number of different

A. B. Miller is with the National Cancer Institute of Canada, Epidemiology Unit, University of Toronto, Toronto, Ontario M5S 1AB, Canada.

Gio B. Gori, Ph.D., is with the Division of Cancer Cause and Prevention National Cancer Institute.

Saxon Graham, Ph.D., is with the Department of Social and Preventive Medicine, State University of New York at Buffalo.

Takeshi Hirayama, M.D., is with the Epidemiological Section, Japanese National Cancer Center, Research Institute.

Michael Kunze, M.D., is with the Hygiene-Institute der Universitat Wien, Vienna, Austria.

Bandaru S. Reddy, Ph.D., is with the Naylor Dana Institute, American Health Foundation.

John H. Weisburger, Ph.D., is with the Naylor Dana Institute, American Health Foundation.

[1] Presented at the American Health Foundation/Deutsche Krebshilfe Conference on the Primary Prevention of Cancer: Assessment of Risk Factors and Future Directions, N.Y., N.Y., June 7–8, 1979.

ways: (a) carcinogens as components of food, either naturally or as additives, (b) carcinogens as contaminants of food, (c) carcinogens produced in food through processing or cooking, (d) carcinogens produced in the body (for example in the stomach or intestine) from food constituents, (e) the indirect effects of undernutrition or malnutrition, (f) the indirect effects of overnutrition, and (g) the protective effect of certain dietary factors.

This paper summarizes the accumulating evidence from a number of different types of studies showing that nutrition is related to cancer in several sites, and attempts an estimation of the contribution of nutrition to cancer etiology.

In general, the evidence suggests that nutritional factors include promotional and initiating agents. This is advantageous, as preventive approaches based on nutritional factors might have more immediate effects if they were based on prevention of exposure to promoters rather than to initiating agents. However, in prevention, it makes little difference by what mechanism an agent operates, providing that its elimination or reduction can be shown to lead to a decline in cancer incidence.

STUDIES CORRELATING INCIDENCE OR MORTALITY OF CANCER WITH NUTRITIONAL FACTORS

In several studies dietary variables were found to be strongly correlated geographically with several types of cancer (1, 6, 24). Cancer of the breast, corpus uteri, and colon have now been found to be strongly associated with total protein and total fat, particularly meat and animal fat. Positive correlations with dietary variables were also found for cancer of the small intestine, pancreas, ovary, and bladder and negative associations with gastric cancer and cancer of the cervix uteri (1). Causal relationships were suggested between alcohol intake and cancer of the mouth and larynx, total fat intake and cancer of the large intestine and breast, and beer intake and cancer of the rectum (24). An association has been found in Japan between fat intake and consumption of pork and breast cancer mortality in different prefectures (21).

A disadvantage of this type of study is that current dietary factors are correlated with current information on incidence and mortality whereas a more appropriate time relationship might be to take dietary information some 20 or 30 years ago and correlate this with current incidence or mortality rates. Further, the relationship between dietary fat and cancer occurrence has recently been challenged with significant positive correlations reported for the United States for total fat and vegetable fat with breast and colon mortality and negative or no correlation for animal fat (14). However, the authors of this report seem likely to have ignored the fact that in all human studies the strongest correlation is with total fat, while in experimental studies this is true for breast cancer, providing there is a small amount of unsaturated fat present (7).

Reductions in incidence and mortality from stomach cancer have been occurring in most countries for several decades. These changes have been correlated with changing dietary practices in Japan (21), and similar factors are believed responsible in technically advanced countries. The relevant factors probably include reduction in use of salt pickling, lower consumption of smoked foods, increased use of refrigeration, increased consumption of milk, green vegetables, and fruit. The relevant mechanism may be a greatly reduced opportunity for the production of nitrosamines in the gastric contents (37), and possibly reduced exposure to other carcinogens in food. Pickled fish has been shown to contain mutagens which cause cancer of the glandular stomach, like that seen in man, in a rat model (38). Formation of the mutagen can be completely blocked by Vitamin C, mimicking the human situation and emphasizing the protective action of fresh fruits, salads, and vegetables. Nevertheless, gastric cancer still remains an important cause of death from cancer and further evaluation of dietary factors is required.

STUDIES IN WHICH INDIRECT INDICATORS OF NUTRITIONAL STATUS ARE FOUND TO BE ASSOCIATED WITH VARIOUS CANCERS

Indirect indicators of nutritional status include height and weight. Both have been reported to be associated with breast cancer (12) with a recent concentration on body mass as the relevant variable (11). An association with height would be important as it would indicate the relevance of nutritional factors early in life. Improvements in nutrition resulting in earlier age at menarche could be one indirect mechanism whereby breast cancer rates might increase through hormonal factors (9, 15). An association with weight could indicate the relevance of dietary factors at any time in life. These associations have not invariably been confirmed in other studies and require further evaluation (8, 27, 40). Nevertheless, in one study, breast cancer incidence and mortality rates were found to be correlated with height, weight, and age at menarche (17). There were, however, correlations with total fat and animal protein consumption even after controlling for the three anthropometric variables. This suggests that, while some of the effects of diet on breast cancer rates may be mediated through effects on these known risk factors, there may be more direct effects as well.

Obesity has been found to be associated with endometrial cancer in many investigations (27). However, it is unlikely that obesity per se is the risk factor, rather, specific nutritional factors such as high fat diet which directly increase both cancer risk and result in obesity.

Other indirect indicators of the importance of nutrition come from changing incidence and mortality rates in populations that could be related to acculturation and, particularly, changes in dietary factors. Such factors may explain the increasing mortality from breast cancer in Iceland which appears to be directly related to environmental changes in successive cohorts and not to reproductive factors such as age at first pregnancy (2). The nature of changes in breast cancer mortality rates appear to reflect acculturation of migrants in the western United States and Canada, in Hawaii, as well as in Japan (5). Changes in migration suggest that if dietary factors are important they may operate early in life for breast cancer but at more recent time periods for colon cancer. Other changes in the migrant and native Japanese include decreasing rates of stomach cancer, and increasing rates for prostate cancer. Other migrant groups showing changes in cancer incidence consistent with dietary changes are Polish migrants to the U.S., migrants to Israel and Hong Kong, and migrants from rural to urban areas in Colombia. Studies of migrants support the importance of environmental variables (such as nutritional factors) rather than genetic factors as the main explanation of international differences.

Further indirect evidence in man derives from comparison of cancer incidence patterns in the United States between Seventh Day Adventists and non-Adventists in California (31), and Mormons and non-Mormons in Utah (25). The most distinct feature in the Seventh Day Adventists lifestyle is their unique vegetarian diet, substantially lower in protein and higher in fiber and unrefined carbohydrates than that of the U.S. population.

DIRECT STUDIES OF DIETARY FACTORS IN ASSOCIATION WITH CANCER EITHER THROUGH THE CASE CONTROL OR COHORT MECHANISM

Direct studies of the effect of dietary factors are acknowledged to be difficult. However, problems such as errors in recall and bias may be minimized by careful research design. Although it is almost impossible to ascertain dietary information directly over long time periods, current diet may be a sufficient reflection of past diet to determine relevant dietary factors for cancer causation (30). Use of a quantitative dietary questionnaire in a case control study of breast cancer has indicated a weak association for total fat intake in both pre- and post-menopausal women (28), and an unpublished study of colon cancer showed a stronger association for total fat, fat of animal origin, and animal protein. An association has also been identified by a study using a diet frequency questionnaire between lack of use of vegetables of the brassica variety and colon and rectal cancer (16). An association in a case–control study with lack of use of foods containing dietary fiber with colon but not with rectal cancer has also been noted (29), as has an association between colon cancer and the intake of beef and other dietary items in Hawaiian-Japanese (18). A case–control study of diet in American Blacks showed a high colon cancer risk associated with a high intake of saturated fats and low intake of fiber-containing foods (10). A number of case control studies of gastric cancer have been largely unrewarding though some have suggested a protective effect of green vegetables and specifically lettuce, in Buffalo, Hawaii, Japan, Norway, and Columbia (4).

Some cohort studies have also evaluated the effect of dietary factors. Thus, an association between low vitamin C intake and lung cancer has been noted (3), an association between lung cancer and lack of consumption of green and yellow vegetables (22), and an apparent protective effect of milk consumption on gastric cancer in Japan (21). Animal experiments and *in vitro* studies show a protective effect of retinoids in epithelial tumors (35). There is also experimental evidence that antioxidants and constituents of green vegetables such as brussels sprouts, cabbage, and cauliflower affect the metabolism of chemical carcinogens in a way which would support a protective effect in the diet (36). Further, a case–control study of lung cancer has shown a protective effect of Vitamin A among smokers and nonsmokers (26).

Coffee drinking may play a minor role in the etiology of bladder cancer. Although a low risk has been demonstrated in a number of studies, no dose–response relationship has been seen.

LABORATORY EVIDENCE ALLIED TO EPIDEMIOLOGIC STUDIES OF DIFFERENT POPULATIONS

Laboratory evidence in association with epidemiologic studies has been sought for a number of associations between nutrition and cancer. This approach has been named "metabolic epidemiology." Such studies have shown the importance of the interaction of high fat diet and the production of bile acids and biliary steroids in the etiology of colon cancer (19, 33, 34). High fat diet has been shown to be associated with secretion of prolactin and thus indirectly to breast cancer (20). Other studies have also indicated differences in fiber consumption in the diet in Scandinavian populations that appear to correlate well with incidence and mortality for colon cancer (23). In Finland the low incidence of colon cancer in spite of a high dietary fat intake can probably be attributed to a high intake of dietary fiber (32). These studies thus suggest that both a high intake of fat and a low intake of fiber may be necessary for the full expression of risk to colon cancer and possibly also to breast cancer.

AMOUNT OF CANCER ATTRIBUTABLE TO NUTRITION

Calculations of the extent to which cancer in a number of sites may be attributed to nutritional factors have been made imprecise by imprecision in estimation of dietary differences. Thus, an attributable risk for breast cancer for total fat intake in Canada of 27% is almost certainly an underestimate due to a combination of difficulties with the dietary methodology and possibly to overmatching with the control series (27). It has, however, been estimated that about one-half of the differences in the incidence of breast cancer between Holland and Japan can be attributed to differences in body mass in postmenopausal women (13). Other specific estimates have not yet been attempted although it has been estimated, on the basis of a number of considerations, that possibly as much as 50% of common cancers may be attributable to dietary factors (39).

Table 1 shows the result of an exercise in which the range of mortality for a number of cancers in which there is evidence for dietary associations is used to derive an estimate for the extent of the differences that can be attributed to environmental factors including, and for many sites almost exclusively due to, dietary factors. However, such estimates have to be regarded with caution, particularly for the sites where the evidence for dietary associations is only suggestive. Only a determined effort to change dietary factors will eventually provide firm data on which such estimates can be based with precision.

In conclusion, there would seem to be sufficient evidence to propose modifying the diet of Western countries to reduce total fat and increase dietary fiber on the lines of the prudent diet, and to introduce certain protective factors, such as an increase in green vegetables and Vitamin C. Although further research is required, such measures are unlikely to be hazardous and can be advocated with a strong hope for benefits in the population.

TABLE 1
AGE-ADJUSTED MORTALITY RATES FOR POTENTIAL NUTRITIONALLY RELATED CANCERS[a]

	Lowest rate		Highest rate		U.S. (white)	
	Male	Female	Male	Female	Male	Female
Breast	—	4.0 Japan	—	26.5 Netherlands	—	22.0
Prostate	1.8 Japan	—	22.7 U.S.[d]	—	12.6	—
Colon	3.5 Japan	3.4 Japan	15.4 Scotland	15.0 Scotland	13.7	12.8
Stomach	8.5 U.S.	4.4 U.S.	66.8 Japan	34.6 Japan	8.5	4.4
Endometrium[c]	—					
Ovary (fallopian tube, broad ligament)	—	1.9	—	11.1	—	7.4
Pancreas	4.2 Italy	2.5 Italy	9.9 U.S.[d]	6.1	8.4	4.9
Thyroid	0.2 New Zealand	0.4 Australia	1.6 Switzerland	1.5 Austria	0.3	0.5
Liver (and biliary passages)	2.8 Norway	2.5 New Zealand	14.7 Japan	20.2 Germany (FR)	4.5	4.0
Bladder (and other urinary)	2.4 Japan	1.0 Japan	7.9 S. Africa	2.7 U.S.[d]	5.1	1.7

[a] From Segi, M., and Kurihara, M. Cancer mortality, 24 countries. Nagoya, Japan Cancer Society No. 6, 1972.
[b] 3, Excellent; 2, good; 1, suggested.
[c] National mortality rates not available.
[d] U.S. nonwhite.

REFERENCES

1. Armstrong, B., and Doll, R. Environmental factors and cancer incidence and mortality in different countries, with special reference to dietary practices. *Int. J. Cancer* 15, 617–631 (1975).
2. Bjarnason, O., Day, N., Snaedal, G., and Tulinuis, H. The effect of year of birth on the breast cancer age incidence curve in Iceland. *Int. J. Cancer* 13, 689–696 (1974).
3. Bjelke, E. Dietary vitamin A and human lung cancer. *Int. J. Cancer* 15, 561–565 (1975).
4. Bjelke, E. Dietary factors and the epidemiology of cancer of the stomach and large bowel, *in* ''Aktuell Probleme der Klinischen Diatetik'' (H. Kaspar, Ed.), p. 10. Thieme, Stuttgart, 1978.
5. Buell, P. Changing incidence of breast cancer in Japanese-American women. *J. Nat. Cancer Inst.* 51, 1479–1483 (1974).
6. Carroll, K. K. Experimental evidence of dietary factors and hormone-dependent cancers. *Cancer Res.* 35, 3374–3383 (1975).
7. Carroll, K. K., and Hopkins, G. J. Dietary polyunsaturated fat versus saturated fat in relation to mammary carcinogenesis. *Lipids* 14, 155–158 (1979).
8. Choi, N. W., Howe, G. R., Miller, A. B., Matthews, V., Morgan, R. W., Munan, L., Burch, J. D., Feather, J., Jain, M., and Kelly, A. An epidemiologic study of breast cancer. *Amer. J. Epidemiol.* 107, 510–521 (1978).
9. Cole, P., and Cramer, D. Diet and cancer of endocrine target organs. *Cancer* 40, 434–437 (1977).
10. Dales, L. G., Friedman, G. D., Ury, H. K., Grossman, S., and Williams, S. R. A case–control study of relationships of diet and other traits to colorectal cancer in American Blacks. *Amer. J. Epidemiol.* 109, 132–144 (1979).
11. de Waard, F. Breast cancer incidence and nutritional status with particular reference to body weight and height. *Cancer Res.* 35, 3351–3356 (1975).

| Germany (Federal Republic) | | Percentage difference | | | | Dietary etiological factors and strength of evidence[b] |
| | | Maximum | | U.S. high | | |
Male	Female	Male	Female	Male	Female	
—	18.0	—	84.9	—	81.8	High total fat (2); fried foods (1)
13.3	—	92.1	—	85.7	—	High total fat (1); fried foods (1)
10.6	9.4	77.3	77.3	74.5	73.4	High total fat, low fiber (2); fried foods (1)
34.8	19.3	87.3	87.3	0	0	High carbohydrate, low fresh fruit and veg. (2); high nitrate (1) Excessive calories (2); high total fat (1)
—	—	—	82.9	—	74.4	High total fat (1)
6.0	3.9	57.6	59.0	50.0	49.0	High total fat (1)
0.5	0.8	87.5	73.3	33.0	20.0	Iodine deficiency (2)
8.8	10.2	80.9	75.7	38.8	37.5	Nutritional deficiency (B Vitamins) (1); mycotoxins (aflatoxin) (3)
—	—	69.6	63.0	52.9	41.1	High protein, high fat, tryptophan metabolites, coffee (1)

12. de Waard, F., and Baanders-van Halewjyn, E. A. A prospective study in general practice on breast cancer risk in postmenopausal women. *Int. J. Cancer* 14, 153–160 (1974).

13. de Waard, F., Cornelis, J. P., Aoki, K., and Yoshida, M. Breast cancer incidence according to weight and height in two cities of the Netherlands and Aichi prefecture, Japan. *Cancer* 40, 1269–1275 (1977).

14. Enig, M. G., Munn, R. J., and Keeney, M. Dietary fat and cancer trends—a critique. *Fed. Proc.* 37, 2215–2220 (1978).

15. Frisch, R. E., Hegsted, D. M., and Yoshinaga, K. Body weight and food intake at early estrus of rats on a high-fat diet. *Proc. Nat. Acad. Sci. USA* 72, 4172–4176 (1975).

16. Graham, S., Dayal, H., Swanson, M., Mittleman, A., and Wilkinson, G. Diet in the epidemiology of cancer of the colon and rectum. *J. Nat. Cancer Inst.* 61, 709–714 (1978).

17. Gray, G. E., Pike, M. C., and Henderson, B. E. Breast cancer incidence and mortality rates in different countries in relation to known risk factors and dietary practices. *Brit. J. Cancer* 39, 1–7 (1979).

18. Haenszel, W., Berg, J. W., Segi, M., Kurihara, M., and Locke, F. B. Large-bowel cancer in Hawaiian Japanese. *J. Nat. Cancer Inst.* 51, 1765–1779 (1973).

19. Hill, M. J. Metabolic epidemiology of dietary factors in large bowel cancer. *Cancer Res.* 35, 3398–3402 (1975).

20. Hill, P., and Wynder, E. L. Diet and prolactin release. *Lancet* 2, 806 (1976).

21. Hirayama, T. Changing patterns of cancer in Japan with special reference to the decrease of stomach cancer mortality, *in* "Origins of Human Cancer," pp. 55–75. Cold Spring Harbor Laboratory, Cold Spring Harbor, N.Y., 1977.

22. Hirayama, T. Presentation at the 12th International Cancer Congress, Buenos Aires, October, 1978.

23. IARC Microecology group. Dietary fibre, transit-time, faecal bacteria, steroids and colon cancer in two Scandinavian populations. *Lancet* 2, 207–211 (1977).

24. Knox, E. G. Foods and diseases. *Brit. J. Soc. Prev. Med.* 31, 71–80 (1977).

25. Lyon, L. J., Klauber, R. M., Gardner, J. W., and Smart, C. R. Cancer incidence in Mormons and non-Mormons in Utah, 1966–1970. *New Engl. J. Med.* 294, 129–133 (1976).

26. Mettlin, C., Graham, S., and Swanson, M. Vitamin A and lung cancer. *J. Nat. Cancer Inst.* 62, 1435–1438 (1979).

27. Miller, A. B. An overview of hormone-associated cancers. *Cancer Res.* 38, 3985–3990 (1978).

28. Miller, A. B., Kelly, A., Choi, N. W., Matthews, V., Morgan, R. W., Munan, L., Burch, J. D., Feather, J., Howe, G. R., and Jain, M. A study of diet and breast cancer. *Amer. J. Epidemiol.* 107, 499–509 (1978).

29. Modan, B., Barell, V., Lubin, F., Modan, M., Greenberg, R. A., and Graham, S. Low-fiber intake as an etiologic factor in cancer of the colon. *J. Nat. Cancer Inst.* 55, 15–18 (1975).

30. Morgan, R. W., Jain, M., Miller, A. B., Choi, N. W., Matthews, V., Munan, L., Burch, J. D., Feather, J., Howe, G. R., and Kelly, A. A comparison of dietary methods in epidemiologic studies. *Amer. J. Epidemiol.* 107, 488–498 (1978).

31. Phillips, R. L. Role of life-style and dietary habits in risk of cancer among Seventh Day Adventists. *Cancer Res.* 35, 3513–3522 (1975).

32. Reddy, B. S., Hedges, A., Laakso, K., and Wynder, E. L. Metabolic epidemiology of large bowel cancer, fecal bulk and constituents of high-risk North American and low-risk Finnish population. *Cancer* 42, 2832–2838 (1978).

33. Reddy, B. S., Mastromarino, A., and Wynder, E. L. Further leads on metabolic epidemiology of large bowel cancer. *Cancer Res.* 35, 3403–3406 (1975).

34. Reddy, B. S., Weisburger, J. H., and Wynder, E. L. Colon cancer. Bile salts as tumor promotors, *in* "Carcinogenesis" (T. J. Tsaga, A. Swak, and R. K. Boutwell, Eds.), Vol. 2, p. 453. Raven Press, New York, 1978.

35. Sporn, M. B. Vitamin A and its analogs (retinoids) in cancer prevention. *Curr. Concepts Nutr.* 6, 119–30 (1977).

36. Wattenberg, L. W. Effect of dietary constituents on the metabolism of chemical carcinogens. *Cancer Res.* 35, 3326–3331 (1975).

37. Weisburger, J. H., and Raineri, R. Dietary factors and the etiology of gastric cancer. *Cancer Res.* 35, 3469–3474 (1975).

38. Weisburger, J. H., Marquardt, H., Hirota, N., Mori, H., and Williams, G. M. Induction of glandular stomach cancer in rats with an extract of nitrite treated fish. *J. Nat. Cancer Inst.*, in press.

39. Wynder, E. L., and Gori, G. B. Contribution of the environment to cancer incidence: An epidemiologic exercise. *J. Nat. Cancer Inst.* 58, 825–833 (1977).

40. Wynder, E. L., MacCornack, F. A., and Stellman, S. D. The epidemiology of breast cancer in 875 United States caucasian women. *Cancer* 41, 2341–2354 (1978).

Assessing the Risks of Cancer

by Peter N. Lee

ABSTRACT Recent claims that there is a growing epidemic of cancer caused by chemical and physical agents in the environment are shown to be weakly based. After smoking and diagnostic changes have been taken into account, trends in cancer mortality rates are not suggestive of any marked increases due to occupational factors. Estimates indicating that past occupational exposure to asbestos will cause large increases in cancer rates are shown to be markedly in error. Evidence that nutritional factors are likely to be much more important than occupational factors is summarized.

INTRODUCTION

In recent years it has increasingly been suggested that we are having an "epidemic" of deaths from cancer. This "epidemic," it is suggested, is overwhelmingly caused by chemical and physical agents in the environment, some of which are self-inflicted, as in smoking, but the majority of which are external and beyond the control of the individual. This suggestion has been given particular publicity in the United States by Epstein [1] and more recently in the United Kingdom by the ASTMS union [2].

Is this claim scientifically justified? The objective of this paper is to examine the truth of it by a) quantifying the loss of life due to cancer; b) assessing whether or not cancer rates are increasing; and c) looking at the relative importance of the different causes of cancer.

MAGNITUDE OF THE PROBLEM

In England and Wales, about 20% of male and 20% of female deaths are due to cancer (Table I). Though the percentage of deaths due to cancer is higher in those dying before age 65 than in those dying after age 65, especially in women, the majority, almost two-thirds, of cancer deaths still occur in the over 65 group (Table II).

It might be thought by the statistically uninitiated that because life expectation is around 70 years and because 20% of all deaths are caused by cancer, removal of cancer as a cause of death would add about 14 years (= 20% of 70) to our life expectation. In fact this is not so at all. Because most of cancer deaths occur in the old, and because death rates from other causes are also high then, life expectation for the population at large would only go up by slightly less than 3 years if the whole of cancer deaths were suddenly to disappear overnight. This compares with an increase

Address reprint requests to Peter N. Lee, 25 Cedar Road, Sutton, Surrey, SM2 5DG, England

TABLE I. Percentage of Deaths Due to Cancer by Age (England and Wales, 1974)

	Age group							
	0–14	15–34	35–64	0–64	65–74	75 +	65 +	All ages
Male	4	19	28	25	26	16	21	22.3% = 66,000 deaths
Female	5	23	41	36	25	11	15	19.3% = 56,000 deaths

TABLE II. Percentage of All Cancer Deaths Occurring at Different Ages (England and Wales, 1974)

	Age group							
	0–14	15–34	35–64	0–64	65–74	75 +	65 +	All ages
Male	0.6	1.4	34	36	39	25	64	100% = 66,000 deaths
Female	0.5	1.3	35	37	30	34	63	100% = 56,000 deaths

of almost 30 years in life expectation since the beginning of this century due predominantly to the conquering of infectious diseases.

This does not, of course, mean that great efforts should not be made to prevent or to cure cancer. After all, the person who actually dies of cancer has on average quite a substantial life expectation at the time he dies, almost 15 years. Rather, the figure of less than 3 years illustrates that we should not overestimate the loss of life due to cancer in the population as a whole, nor become overly hopeful of the magnitude of the benefits to be gained from preventing it.

IS THIS PROBLEM INCREASING?

It is certainly easy to produce figures that suggest cancer incidence and mortality have been rising sharply—for instance, cancers were responsible for only 7% of male deaths and 9% of female deaths at the time of World War I, whereas they are responsible for 20% now. However, such comparisons are misleading for two major reasons. First, the age structure of the population at risk has changed dramatically over this century, such that far more people nowadays survive to ages at which cancer is common. Secondly, diagnosis of cancer for some sites has improved considerably since the beginning of the century. This is particularly clear for lung cancer where, at the turn of the century, it has been estimated [3] that the percentage of correct diagnosis was only 5%. Recently, the Royal College of Physicians [4] presented in graphical form estimates that suggested that though *recorded* male lung cancer death rates rose by a factor of 40 between 1916 and 1951, *actual* death rates probably only rose by a factor of 3 or 4. In other words improvements in diagnostic standards have resulted in a detection rate 10 or more times better.

Of course, even an increase in the true lung cancer rate by a factor of three or four is a large one. However, there are clear indications that this increase, which has been attributed to the mass adoption of the cigarette smoking habit around the time of World War I by men and some 30 years later by women, is now coming to an end. Indeed, as Table III shows, lung cancer rates are now falling in men at all ages under 70 and in women at ages under 45, probably due in part to the prevailing switch to filter cigarettes with reduced tar deliveries [5]. The fact that rates are still rising in the oldest age groups probably reflects a duration-of-smoking effect, the 80-year-old group now containing a larger proportion who have smoked for a relatively long time than the 80-year-old group of five years ago, say. This is illustrated more clearly by considering a hypothetical population, all of whom took up smoking in 1915 or at age 15 if they were born after 1900 (Table IV). It can be seen that the rises are likely to die out soon for men. Indeed during very recent years overall male lung cancer rates in England and Wales appear to have been static and should fall soon. It has been estimated that female rates will flatten out eventually at about a third of those for males [6].

What are the recent trends in age-specific cancer rates generally? Table V (men) and Table VI (women) list percentage changes in overall cancer rates between 1966–1970 and 1971–1975 by site, presenting the data in terms of the relative frequency of the different types of cancer. Longer-term trends, over the period 1951–1955 to 1971–1975, are summarized in Table VII.

TABLE III. Recent Changes in Lung Cancer Death Rates in England and Wales

Age group	Percentage change in rate 1966–1970 to 1971–1975	
	Men	Women
35–39	− 22	− 16
40–44	− 17	− 17
45–49	− 4	+ 16
50–54	− 7	+ 17
55–59	− 6	+ 24
60–64	− 5	+ 30
65–69	− 2	+ 23
70–74	+ 9	+ 23
75–79	+ 21	+ 24
80–84	+ 26	+ 31
85 +	+ 26	+ 26
All ages	+ 7	+ 27

TABLE IV. Trends in Lung Cancer Risk for a Hypothetical Population All of Whom Took up Smoking in 1915, or at Age 15 for Those Born After 1900

Age at year stated	Duration of smoking at year:						Risk increases up to year
	1930	1940	1950	1960	1970	1980	
40	15	25	25	25	25	25	1940
50	15	25	35	35	35	35	1950
60	15	25	35	45	45	45	1960
70	15	25	35	45	55	55	1970
80	15	25	35	45	55	65	1980
90	15	25	35	45	55	65	1990

Assumptions: 1) Risk increases with increased duration of smoking; 2) no change in cigarettes; 3) non-smoking-related factors ignored.

TABLE V. Recent Trends in Age-Specific Cancer Death Rates in Men (England and Wales)

ICD (8th rev)	Site	% of all neoplasms rate, 1966–1970	Age-standardized death rates per million		
			1966–1970	1971–1974	% Change
162,163	Bronchus	38.8	953	983	+ 3%
151	Stomach	11.9	293	270	− 8%
153	Large intestine	6.5	159	163	+ 3%
185	Prostate	6.4	156	156	Nil
154	Rectum	5.0	122	119	− 2%
188	Bladder	4.2	103	105	+ 2%
157	Pancreas	4.2	103	106	+ 3%
204–207	Leukemia	2.7	66	65	− 2%
150	Esophagus	2.6	63	68	+ 8%
	All others	17.8	436	444	+ 2%
140–239	Total	100.0	2454	2479	+ 1.0%
	Total (excluding bronchus)	61.2	1501	1496	− 0.3%

TABLE VI. Recent Trends in Age-Specific Cancer Death Rates in Women (England and Wales)

ICD (8th rev)	Site	% of all neoplasms rate, 1966–1970	Age-standardized death rates per million		
			1966–1970	1971–1974	% Change
174	Breast	20.5	385	409	+ 6
153	Large intestine	10.5	197	196	− 1
151	Stomach	10.0	187	163	− 13
162,163	Bronchus	9.7	182	217	+ 19
180–182	Uterus	7.8	147	137	− 7
183	Ovary	5.3	131	132	+ 1
154	Rectum	4.9	92	88	− 4
157	Pancreas	4.2	79	83	+ 5
204–207	Leukemia	2.7	50	49	− 2
150	Esophagus	2.3	43	45	+ 5
188	Bladder	1.9	36	37	+ 3
	All others	18.6	349	362	+ 4
140–239	Total	100.0	1878	1918	+ 2.1
	Total (excluding bronchus)	90.3	1696	1701	+ 0.3

TABLE VII. Percentage Changes in Age-Standardized Death Rates 1951–1955 to 1971–1974 (England and Wales)

Site	Males	Females
Bronchus, etc	+ 49	+ 115
Stomach	− 29	− 41
Large intestine	− 16	− 19
Rectum	− 25	− 17
Bladder	+ 19	+ 6
Pancreas	+ 29	+ 26
Leukemia	+ 23	+ 14
Oesophagus	+ 3	+ 15
Prostate	+ 4	—
Breast	—	+ 13
Uterus	—	− 20
Ovary	—	+ 16
All others	+ 2	+ 8
Total	+ 12	+ 2
Total (excluding bronchus)	− 7	− 5

The tables illustrate that when all sites except the bronchus are considered together the short-term picture is of no overall change in the age-standardized death rate, whereas looking at longer-term rates there is a small decrease. Some sites show a clear decrease (stomach, large intestine, rectum, and uterus) and some show a clear increase (bladder, pancreas, leukemia, esophagus, breast, and ovary). When one considers that there have been marked increases in the ability to diagnose pancreatic cancer and leukemia accurately and when one also notes that bladder and esophageal cancer have been linked to smoking [7], and that the rise in breast cancer is consistent with the hypothesis that it is related to low fertility, it is clear that the grounds for believing there to be an explosion of occupationally linked cancers from this evidence is weak. Of course the fact that some cancers may be related to smoking does not exclude them being also related to occupational factors. Therefore, we will next go on to look at recent scientific estimates of the role of different factors in cancer etiology.

Before doing so, however, we will note parenthetically that improvements in cancer cure rates have only been marked for some rarer forms of cancer (such as Hodgkin disease, choriocarcinoma, or Wilms tumour). Those arguing in favor of a growing cancer epidemic cannot therefore argue that we have a situation where improving cancer cure is being counterbalanced by increasing cancer incidence.

ROLE PLAYED BY DIFFERENT FACTORS IN CANCER

Last year the American Health Foundation organized a conference on the primary prevention of cancer, a specific aim of which was to assess the role played by different risk factors in cancer. Their conclusions, which accord quite well with earlier estimates given by Higginson [8], are summarized in Table VIII.

In looking at this table one should bear in mind that it is unrealistic to assume that cancer is always caused by a single agent. Not only is there evidence that smoking and alcohol have a synergistic effect in relation to cancer of the upper aerodigestive tract [9] and that smoking similarly reacts synergistically with asbestos and other occupational hazards to cause lung cancer [8] but also it is clear that in a number of cases, genetic, endocrine, nutritional, and immunologic factors substantially modify the response to chemical or physical carcinogens. For this reason, and also because the smoking estimate by Hammond and Seidman [10] on which the figures in Table VIII are based ignores recent changes in the type of cigarette smoked, the percentages attributed to smoking in the table are likely to be on the high side, a view that is reinforced by the observation by other workers in the UK [11,12] that general air pollution may play a rather larger role in lung cancer etiology than indicated by the Hammond and Garfinkel [13] estimates used in Table VIII.

The most striking differences between the conclusions of the AHF conference and those of Epstein [1] lie in their estimates of the relative contribution of occupationally related factors and of nutritional factors to the total.

The major contribution to Epstein's estimate of occupationally related cancer came from a document by Bridbord et al that was widely circulated in the United States but was never published [14]. This document estimated that between 8 million and 11 million US workers had been employed since World War II in environments with significant asbestos exposure and that as a result 2.15 million of these workers would ultimately get cancer. This encouraged Califano, the former Health, Education and Welfare Secretary in Washington, to make the assertion that as many as half of these 8–11 million workers would develop serious diseases related to their exposures. As has been noted previously [15,16], the method of calculation was subject to two major flaws, both of which had the effect of greatly increasing the estimates of the numbers of cancers attributable to occupational factors. The first was that estimates of risk for exposed workers were taken from studies of workers exposed in the 1920s to the 1950s, ignoring the fact that workplace conditions for known carcinogens and for many other chemicals also, have improved considerably since then. The second is that the document used exposed population figures based on the National Occupational Hazard Survey, a survey that did not measure levels of exposure and in fact included actual, potential, or inferred exposures as well as part-time exposures.

The gross weakness of their estimation procedure is highlighted by the fact that detailed studies of deaths related to asbestos exposure at work [17] show that about 1 in 8 of all excess deaths and about 1 in 5 of all excess cancer deaths are due to mesothelioma. The Bridbord estimate thus implies something over 400,000 mesothelioma deaths are likely to occur in these workers, or, since most of these cancers should be seen in the next 30–35 years, over 10,000 mesotheliomas per year. When one considers that total annual deaths from mesothelioma are currently less than

TABLE VIII. Assessment of Risk Factors for Cancer (conclusions from AHF conference, 1979)

Major factors	Risk attributable
Nutrition	Up to 50% of common cancer
Smoking	25–35% of male cancers in USA, 5–10% of females
Minor factors	
Alcohol	3% of all US cancers
Occupation	6% of male and 2% of female cancers in UK
Ionizing radiation	Less than 3% of cancers in USA (half background radiation) and 40% or more diagnostic X-rays
Ultraviolet radiation	Less than 2% of cancer deaths in USA
Factors contributing little to overall risk	Other factors
Food additives and contaminants	Genetic factors—may affect susceptibility in
Drugs	10–25% of cases
General air pollution	
Water pollution	Viruses—no common cancer shown to be virus-
Immunological factors	associated

1,000 in the United States (and less than 300 in the UK) it is clear that the estimates used by Califano and Epstein are at least an order of magnitude too high.

Nutritional factors are scarcely considered at all by Epstein but are well documented as having a major association with cancer incidence [18]. Two of these associations are particularly worthy of mention. The first is the striking correlation between fat consumption in different countries and their breast and colon cancer rates (Fig. 1). This is not explicable in terms of dietary fat being a vehicle for fat-soluble pesticides and industrial chemicals, as Epstein [1] suggests, because it ignores the fact that countries with high chemical use do not stand out from the general cancer-fat relationship [16].

The other nutrition-cancer relationship demanding particular attention is the dramatic relationship seen in animal experiments between total calorie intake and tumor rates. One example of this can be seen in the experiment of Conybeare [19], where a 25% reduction in total dietary intake caused a dramatic reduction in incidence of a whole range of tumors in untreated control mice (Table IX). This, and similar findings by Tucker [20], have been reviewed by Roe [21], who notes that it is certain that this effect could not be due to a 25% lower intake in one or more toxicants or carcinogens in the diet, for this would assume an incredibly steep dose-response curve. Roe suggests that a possible explanation is that rats or mice who see an empty food hopper suffer stress because of the absence of food, this stress resulting in a consequent rise in plasma corticosteroid levels. He postulates that a daily rise in plasma corticosteroid levels may be protective against the development of many kinds of tumors.

Although much of the data implicating nutrition as a major factor in carcinogenesis are relatively "soft," reflecting in part the difficulties of studying dietary factors accurately in human populations, and the estimates of percentage of cancers attributable to nutrition are subject to considerable uncertainty, the importance and the great need for further study are obvious.

CONCLUSIONS

Our look at the evidence does not all suggest the existence of any raging epidemic of cancer related to exposure to physical and chemical agents in the environment. In fact, though one cannot

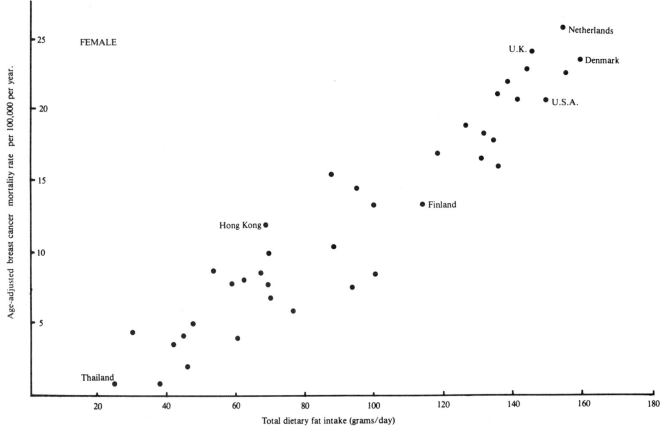

Fig. 1.   Breast cancer mortality and dietary fat consumption in 39 countries.

TABLE IX. Effect of Simple Dietary Restriction on Tumor Incidence in Mice

Sex	Type of tumor	Ad lib	Restricted to 75% of ad lib	% Reduction in incidence
			% incidence	
Male	Lung	30	19	−37
	Liver	47	12	−74
	Lymphoma	4	1	−75
	Other	8	4	−50
	Any tumor	71	36	−49
	Any malignant tumor	17	7	−59
Female	Lung	24	8	−67
	Liver	7	1	−86
	Lymphoma	11	4	−64
	Other	12	4	−67
	Any tumor	50	17	−66
	Any malignant tumor	23	7	−70

be encouraged at the slow progress made in conquering cancer, there is no evidence of any overall rise in non-smoking-related cancer at all in recent years. The look at causes of cancer suggests that relatively too much attention is being given to occupational carcinogens and not enough to cancers associated with nutrition.

REFERENCES

1. Epstein SS. The Politics of Cancer. Sierra Club Books, 1978.
2. ASTMS. The Prevention of Occupational Cancer. London: Association of Scientific, Technical and Managerial Staffs, 1980.
3. Rigdon RH, Kirchoff H. Cancer of the lung from 1900 to 1930. Surg, Gynecol Obstet 1958; 107:105–118.
4. Royal College of Physicians. Smoking or health. The third report from the Royal College of Physicians of London. London: Pitman Medical, 1977.
5. Lee PN, Garfinkel L. Mortality and type of cigarette smoked. J Epidemiol Community Health. 1981;35:16–22.
6. Office of Population Censuses and Surveys. Trends in mortality 1951–1975, London. Series DHI No. 3 London: Her Majesty's Stationery Office, 1978.
7. Doll R, Peto R. Mortality in relation to smoking; 20 years observation on male British doctors. Br Med J 1976;2:1525–1536.
8. Higginson J. Cancer and environment. Higginson speaks out. Science 1979;205:1363–1366.
9. Rothman KJ. The proportion of cancer attributable to alcohol consumption. Prev Med 1980;9:174–179.
10. Hammond EC, Seidman H. Smoking and cancer in the United States. Prev Med 1980;9:169–173.
11. Adelstein AM. Trends with particular reference to lung cancer and smoking. National Cancer Records. Paper read to the Marie Curie Foundation Symposium on Cancer, Royal College of Surgeons, London, 1976.
12. Dean G, Lee PN, Todd GF, Wicken AJ. Report on a second retrospective mortality study in North-East England, Part II: Changes in lung cancer and bronchitis mortality and in other relevant factors occurring in areas of North-East England, 1963–1972. London: Tobacco Research Council, 1978.
13. Hammond EC, Garfinkel L. General air pollution and cancer in the United States. Prev Med 1980;9:206–211.
14. Bridbord K et al. Estimates of the fraction of cancer in the United States related to occupational factors. Prepared by the National Cancer Institute, National Institute of Environmental Health Sciences and the National Institute for Occupational Safety and Health, September 18th, 1978.
15. American Industrial Health Council. A reply to "Estimates of the fraction of cancer in the United States attributable to occupational factors," October 23rd, New York, 1978.
16. Peto R. Distorting the epidemiology of cancer: The need for a more balanced overview. Nature 1980;284:297–299.
17. Advisory Committee on Asbestos. Final report of the Advisory Committee Health and Safety Commission. London: Her Majesty's Stationery Office, 1979.
18. Miller AB. Nutrition and cancer. Prev Med 1980;9:189–196.
19. Conybeare G. Effect of quality and quantity of diet on survival and tumour incidence in outbred Swiss mice. Food Cosmet Toxicol 1980;18:65–75.
20. Tucker MJ. The effect of long-term food restriction on tumours in rodents. Int J Cancer 1979;23:803–807.
21. Roe FJC. Food and cancer. J Hum Nutr 1979;33:405–415.

A Review of Validations of Dietary Assessment Methods

by Gladys Block

In recent years epidemiologists and other medical researchers have become increasingly interested in the effects that diet may have on health and disease. The chief impediment to research on nutritional causes of disease has been uncertainty about the validity of existing dietary assessment methods and the consequent uncertainty about the results obtained with them. Numerous studies over the past 30 years have tried to establish the reliability or validity of various methods, but the methods themselves have been variable, and the criteria against which they were judged were also variable, with the result that until recently one would have been hard pressed to make a statement with any confidence about any of them.

However, recent work has led to some clarification. This review will describe the dietary intake assessment methods in use, discuss the meaning of validation in this context, and review the studies which have addressed reliability or validity of the methods.

In evaluating the methods and valida-

Gladys Block, Ph.D., is a Staff Fellow, Operations Research Branch, Division of Cancer Prevention and Control, National Cancer Institute, Blair Building, 9000 Rockville Pike, Bethesda, MD 20205.

tions described below, it is useful to bear in mind two important dimensions which affect both dietary research and investigations of its methodology. The first is the dichotomy of group vs. individual. Nutritionists and clinicians would like, of course, a method which could give accurate results for each individual; that is, Patient A's dietary assessment accurately reflects Patient A's intake. Assessment methods have sometimes been faulted for failing to achieve this goal. Yet such accuracy at an individual level is not essential in order to produce valid and useful research on diet and disease. Indeed, similar situations are fairly common in medical research. Single random blood pressure measurements have questionable validity on an individual level, yet their usefulness at the group level has contributed greatly to our understanding of the relationship of blood pressure and disease.

The second important distinction in dietary research is that of quantitative precision vs. classification or ranking of individuals. Most research to date on dietary methodologies has been performed by nutritionists whose goal has been to assess intake in precise quantities—in milligrams of vitamin C, or international units of vitamin A. Yet once again, such precision is not essential for useful epidemiologic research. Less precise methods which locate individuals on the distribution in broad categories of low, medium and high intake would still permit the examination of nutritional hypotheses and the assessment of dose-response relationships.

With respect to assessment methods, four general approaches have been used in dietary studies. Each has its strengths and weaknesses. One widely accepted technique is the *dietary history* approach developed by Burke and Stuart (1), who in the 1940s proposed the principle that what is important in nutrition research is the long-term history or pattern of usual intake. Their method, subsequently modified and used in many studies, is an attempt to elicit such a usual intake pattern. It requires an extensive interview by a trained nutritionist.

The *24-hour recall* method may be administered by persons with less training, in a shorter time. The subject is asked to recall his exact intake in the last 24 hours. In its favor, memory of recent intake may be more precise and quantities may be estimated with greater accuracy. On the other hand, individual diets vary greatly from day to day (25–29), so that a single day's intake may not be representative.

The *seven-day recall* method is an attempt to achieve greater representativeness. However, memories of intake may fade rather quickly beyond the most recent day or two, so that loss in accuracy may exceed gain in representativeness.

A more common approach, and one that appears to rest on firmer ground, is the *seven-day record* of actual intake, with either weighing, measuring or estimation of portion sizes. Such a method should give a reasonably accurate measurement of actual intake, and an average of seven days is more representative of usual intake than a single day. The chief objection is that it is impractical for clinical or epidemiologic studies since it demands a high degree of cooperation on the part of subjects, and the number who could be induced to participate may be a small and unrepresentative sample.

Since the 1960s there have been a number of efforts to develop a method which would be easier and quicker to administer than the seven-day record or history methods, but which would achieve a more representative result than the 24-hour recall method. These have involved a number of different approaches, which are here considered together as *short-cut methods*.

VALIDATION

Validation, the demonstration that a method measures what it is intended to measure, requires that the truth be known, and for dietary intake that is the difficulty. For any method which purports to measure usual intake over a prolonged period of time, knowing the true intake either presents overwhelming practical difficulties (direct observation of many individuals over a long time) or is actually impossible (if the meaning of "usual" is not limited in time).

Twenty-four hour recall methods can be validated on one level if the actual intake is observed, and preferably measured, surreptitiously during the 24-hour period. Similarly, observations over periods of seven days are theoretically possible, although the practical problems may be severe. However, a demonstration of validity at this level is necessary but not sufficient. The ability to gather valid information about the past 24 hours must be coupled with a demonstration that the 24-hour recall method accurately reflects the usual diet of an individual or group over an extended time. And at this level of validation, the 24-hour recall and record methods join the history method in being theoretically difficult or impossible to validate.

This dilemma has been faced by all investigators of dietary assessment methods. There appears to be no wholly satisfactory solution. Since "the truth" is not available to them, investigators have therefore had to use other criteria. Some of the investigators to be discussed below have "validated" their method against some other method which has greater acceptance but which nevertheless has not been validated against the truth. Others have attempted to demonstrate that a method elicits a usual intake by showing that it can produce similar results on two different occasions. "Reliability" studies of this sort are clearly fraught with conceptual difficulties, making results difficult to interpret. Since we do not know whether what is being measured remains unchanged, we do not know whether dissimilar results on two occasions reflect an unreliable measure or reflect a reliable measure which is measuring a changed condition.

Again, there is no perfect way around this. At the least, investigators performing such methodologic studies should make every attempt to determine whether or not the diet has in fact changed from one occasion to the next. Objective indicators would include weight changes and intentional behavior changes such as cutting down on animal fats. This information would permit the separate analysis of diets with and without such objective evidence of diet change. Lacking some such objective indications, the meaning of correlations between two administrations of the same dietary assessment will remain unclear.

To return to the question of validity, how then are we to assess the validity of a measure for which it is difficult or impossible to know the truth? First, we may have to accept the approach of relative validation, which uses as the reference criterion a method which has greater face validity or physical and other evidence of validity.

Second, a more tolerant attitude toward this situation might be appropriate. Epidemiologists have tended to demand clear evidence of validity in dietary studies, whereas absence of absolute validation is not an uncommon situation in other areas of medical research. There are a number of conditions for which self-reports are the only reasonable sources of information. In other situations, the existence of a condition is ultimately a matter of judgment, usually a physician's or a pathologist's. And in still other instances, the existence of a condition is unknowable without heroic efforts such as autopsying every death, or is unknowable by present methods of detection. Yet, for research purposes, we sometimes must accept mortality statistics based on death certificates when no autopsy data or hospital data are available, knowing that they are compiled by fallible human beings on the basis of imperfect knowledge.

Finally, it should be pointed out that validation must be viewed in the context of what inferences are to be drawn from any research done with these methodologies. For example, if inferences are to be made about the mean intake of a group or several groups, then validation can be directed toward whether a mean value arrived at by a new method accurately reflects the "true" group mean, by whatever definition. However, if inferences are to be made about individuals, then validation must be directed toward whether any individual's value by the new method accurately reflects his "true" intake as indicated by a reference method. Many of these methods meet the first test but fail the second. At still another level, a method may be used to place individuals in the upper or lower ends of distribution, and validation would be directed toward the extent to which a method can do this accurately. Few of the validation studies address this point at all, and few present the data which would make it possible for a reviewer to address it. From the point of view of epidemiologic studies, however, it is clearly of great importance.

In their attempts to assess the worth of the various dietary assessment methods, researchers have used various reference methods to represent the truth. In addition, they have variously used group means, individual values or classifications within a distribution as the outcome of interest. The discussion below considers each dietary method separately and groups together those studies which used similar reference methods.

HISTORY METHOD

The method originally developed by Burke and Stuart (1) has been modified by many investigators and often includes the presentation of food models to facilitate quantitation. For purposes of this review, the history method includes any method which consists of an extensive interview designed to elicit the usual or customary diet.

The papers by Burke and associates (1–3) do not describe an attempt to validate the method. However, Burke (3, p. 1044) says the method produces "a surprisingly representative picture of the individual's average intake." As discussed above, probably no true validation is possible. Burke and associates and other investigators have attempted relative validations in several ways.

Agreement between history method and seven-day or longer record of intake

A number of investigators have compared the results obtained using the history method and those obtained from a seven-day diary or record of intake, and many have found that the history method yields higher values than the seven-day record. Young et al. (4) compared these two methods in six types of subjects, including children and pregnant women and with numbers ranging from 49 to 164 per group. They concluded that the mean values given by diet history and subsequent seven-day unweighed record were different, with history giving higher values. Paul et al. (5) also found that the history gave higher values than the record, as did Hartog et al. (6) and Jain et al. (7). Jain et al. used the approach of having a wife or other household member record the diet of her husband for 30 days. For all nutrients the history method gave a higher value, with mean values being significantly higher for some nutrients.

It seems clear that the two methods do not reliably yield the same values for nutrient intakes. This fact is of great importance to nutritionists seeking precise intake data. However, it may not be nearly so serious for epidemiologic research, since while precise agreement has not been found, several different approaches have demonstrated a relationship.

In 1942 Huenemann and Turner (8) compared the group means resulting from diet history and 10–14-day weighed records for 25 children. They found that the means given by the two methods were within ±20 per cent of each other for most nutrients. Using regression techniques, a number of more recent investigators have found a significant association between the two methods. (Association is often reported as the correlation coefficient between the test and the criterion measure or between the first and second test. Rarely is the statistical significance of the coefficient reported, but is often high enough to yield significance based on the number of subjects. The operationally useful level of correlation is, of course, another question.) Hart and Cox (9), examining individual nutrient values given by the two methods, found an $r = 0.46$ for calories, and $r = 0.61$ for calcium. Lubbe (10) found that for calories, protein and carbohydrate $r = 0.6$ to 0.8, while for fat and various vitamins $r = 0.3$ to 0.85. Jain et al. (7) found significant regression and correlation coefficients for most nutrients. They concluded that although the diet history method gave higher values than did the 30-day record, there was sufficient association between the two that "the diet history is a reasonable measure for at least seven of the 13 nutrients," and several of the other nutrients aproached significance.

A third approach has been to ask whether the history method could place individuals into the same part of the distribution of intake values as could the record method. Huenemann and Turner (8) found that 56 per cent of the children were placed in the same extreme thirds of the calorie intake distribution by the two methods, and 18 per cent were placed into the opposite third, hereafter referred to as "grossly misclassified." For vitamin C, 70 per cent were in the same extreme thirds by the two methods, and none were grossly misclassified. Hart and Cox (9) and Lubbe (10) found a similar ability to classify calorie intakes using the two methods, and Jain et al. (7) found similar results for calories, protein and total fat.

Agreement between results of repeated histories

This approach may be viewed as a test of reliability, although with the conceptual difficulties alluded to in the introduction. If two histories disagree, is the method unreliable or has the intake changed? Lacking an absolute truth, conclusions drawn from such comparisons must be based on the consistency of the results after taking into consideration the evidence bearing on whether the individuals' diets had indeed changed.

In the Framingham study, Dawber et al. (11) reported high correlation coefficients for individuals and no significant differences between mean nutrient values when interviews were two years apart. However, after a four-year interval the means were significantly different for calories, fat and plant protein, although not for animal protein. Similarly, after two years no one who had been in the lower third of the distribution was placed in the upper third by the second interview, but after four years 10 per cent were in the opposite extreme third of the distribution for fat intake. These variations may indicate unreliability in the method; however, there were concurrent changes in weight in the group, presumably the result of changes in calorie and fat intake. Thus, these results may indicate a reliable method reflecting actual changes in the diet over time, although this cannot be determined definitely without more objective information. Trulson and Mc-Cann (12), McCann et al. (13) and Reshef and Epstein (14) conducted repeat interviews over intervals ranging from six months to two years, and found no significant differences in the means of major nutrients. Reed and Burke (15) studied 103 children in several repeated interviews and found "a reliability approaching anthropometric observations."

Jain et al. (7) interviewed 26 pairs of bowel cancer patients and neighborhood controls, obtaining a diet history for the time period immediately preceding the interview and for the time period six months earlier. After six months all subjects were reinterviewed and similar diet histories obtained. For controls, correlation coefficients between the two administrations were statistically significant for all 13 nutrients ($r = 0.45$ to 0.81) when the histories referred to intake during the same period of calendar time. When the histories referred to time periods six months apart, the correlation coefficients were statistically significant for all nutrients except vitamin C, which has been shown to vary by season.

Results for the bowel cancer patients were also instructive. When the two diet histories referred to periods six months apart, for cases the correlation coefficients were significant for only four of the nutrients. The investigators interpret this to be an indication that the actual dietary intake of these patients changed between the time of diagnosis of their bowel cancer and the period six months later. Again, differences in reported dietary history may reflect not an unreliable measure, but one which is accurately reporting changes in actual intake.

Agreement between history method and clinical criteria

Though not strictly validation, this approach could be viewed as corroborative. Burke and associates (1, 2) classified diets into categories ranging from very poor through excellent, on the basis of their diet history method. They found that no pregnant women with a diet classified as good or excellent by that method had pre-eclampsia, while almost 50 per cent of those with poor or very poor diets had pre-eclampsia. There were similarly good associations with the health of the resulting baby and with actual biochemical analyses such as plasma vitamin C. Reed and Burke (15) examined relationships between protein intake classification as indicated by diet history and growth of muscle in 103 young children. They found a correlation coefficient of 0.46 for girls, 0.68 for boys, a highly statistically significant result.

Conclusions regarding the history method

It might be well to point out, first, that all evaluations of the history method, except for the clinical associations examined by Burke et al. (1−3), were based on numeric values, whereas Burke herself (3, p. 1045) indicated that exact figures "give an unjustified impression of accuracy of the data," and recommended the use of the method only to derive a scale for rating nutrients from excellent to very poor with regard to some criterion like the Recommended Dietary Allowances (16). The concordance of the method used in this way, either with repeated measurements or with other criteria, has rarely been examined. More recent investigators (e.g., 14, 24), however, have used food models and other methods to create a firmer basis for quantitation.

Because of the difficulty of establishing the truth in the assessment of usual diet, investigators attempting validation have rather addressed themselves to reliability on repeated interviews and to agreement with the diet record method. Most investigators have found that while diet history and diet record do not yield identical mean nutrient intake values, and while some individuals may be classified quite differently on the distribution of values, by and large the two methods do yield a similar relationship between individuals with regard to nutrient intake. That is, significant positive correlations between results given by the two methods have been found, ranging from 0.4 to 0.9, and individuals who are low on the distribution by one method tend to be low by the other method.

The reliability of the method based on repeated administrations has been found by most investigators to be very good. When one considers weight changes and other objective indications about diet stability, there appears to be some justification for concluding that the method is reflecting the usual diet and changes in it.

We cannot know, based on the approaches reported above, whether the diet history method is valid in the sense of accurately and precisely reflecting the truth. It does seem justifiable to conclude, however, that it is reflecting some reasonably stable marker which is similarly revealed by different methods and on different occasions, and which bears some relationship to clinical criteria.

24-HOUR RECALL METHOD

Unlike the other methods, the 24-hour recall method is more easily susceptible of direct validation. That is, the truth is knowable. Since the time covered is limited and short, direct observation and measurement of intake is possible and even practical.

Agreement with known or recorded intake

Madden et al. (17) compared 24-hour recall with observed and weighed duplicate meals for 76 elderly persons who consumed an institutional lunch. The group mean values by the two methods were found to be similar for all nutrients except calories. Furthermore, while Madden et al. and other investigators have found significant underreporting of intake by the recall method (18–20), analysis of variance revealed a highly significant relationship between actual and recalled values for all nutrients. Gersovitz et al. (21) also compared recall with actual weighed amounts for 31 elderly persons at congregate meal sites, and again found that mean reported intake values were not significantly different from weighed values for nine of 10 nutrients.

Young et al. (22) compared a 24-hour recall with the average value from a seven-day diary of intake recorded by the subjects. They found that the group means given by the two methods were "interchangeable" if the number was greater than 50. Both this result and that of Thomsom (20) may be somewhat weakened, however, by the possibility that self-recording may influence recall.

Agreement of 24-hour recall with diet history

As with the comparison between diet history and diet record, this involves the use of one unvalidated method as the reference method for another. Nevertheless, the data on the history method suggest that it may have validity, and proponents of this approach argue that it is an appropriate way to assess the representativeness of the 24-hour recall.

Young et al. (22) and Stevens et al. (23) studied several disparate groups, including children, pregnant women, and older persons. Stevens et al. found the mean values given by history and recall to be similar for most nutrients. Young et al., on the other hand, found that the means given by the history method were higher for two groups, lower for the third, and concluded that the two methods gave inconsistent results. Morgan et al. (24) obtained a dietary history and 24-hour recall at the same sitting for 400 persons. They found the mean values for calories and fat to be significantly different and correlations, though significant, were low.

Balogh et al. (25) used the approach of averaging the results of several 24-hour recalls obtained over a 12-month period, and comparing that average with a shortened version of the dietary history. They found that group means given by these two approaches were very similar, and correlations for calories, fat, protein and carbohydrate ranged from 0.6 to 0.8. These results suggest that it is possible to obtain similar results by the two methods, and that perhaps both are reflecting a reasonably stable marker. However, it should be noted that the 24-hour recall figure used by Balogh et al. actually refers to the average of eight monthly recalls so that the method, even if valid, may be of practical use only in some situations.

Variations in intake from day to day

The recall of one day's intake is of interest only because of the implicit assumption that a single day is somewhat representative of a usual pattern of intake. Thus, the extent to which this is true must be one aspect of any validation of the method.

Heady (26) had 116 English male bank employees record their intake for seven days. He found that the mean intake of the group was not significantly different from day to day, with the exception of certain culturally determined dietary patterns, such as intake of eggs and cake. For individuals, however, he found large variations from day to day for any one man. Hankin et al. (27) found similar results for 93 men.

Balogh et al. (25) studied day-to-day variations within individuals by repeated 24-hour recalls over a 12-month period. They found that day-to-day variation within individuals is very high. In order to have 95 per cent probability of being within ± 20 per cent of a person's true year-long mean for calories, it would be necessary to obtain four 24-hour recalls for the least variable half of the population, and nine 24-hour recalls for 90 per cent of the population. Similar results were reported by White et al. (28) and Liu et al. (29).

Conclusions regarding the 24-hour recall method

Further validation, perhaps in the form of biochemical studies which analyzed the degree to which reported intake is reflected in serum or urine values (1, 30), would contribute to our confidence that the measure accurately reflects intake in the past 24 hours. Such studies would not, however, resolve the question of whether intake in the past 24 hours adequately represents the usual intake over an extended period of time. Indeed, Balogh et al. (25) and a number of other studies have shown that it does not, and that in fact a very large number of 24-hour recalls over an extended period of time would be necessary to represent adequately the average or usual value for an individual. Thus, it seems clear that a single 24-hour recall is not an appropriate tool for assessing the usual diet of an individual.

Its value in assessing the average intake of a group has considerable support, however. Madden et al. (17), Gersovitz et al. (21) and others showed clear relationships between reported and weighed group mean values, and Heady (26) and Hankin et al. (27) found that group mean values do not vary significantly from day to day. Thus, although some attention should be given to the question of the misclassifications which are inevitable, the value of this method in establishing the average intake levels of groups seems reasonably well established.

SEVEN-DAY RECALL

In the hope of achieving less variation in individual records, some investigators have asked subjects to recall their intake for the past seven days. Adelson (31) obtained seven-day recalls from 59 professional men. They compared the results with values obtained from a seven-day weighed record obtained during the following week. This study is noteworthy in that the wives of the men participated in the recall. They found that group mean values of nutrient intakes were within ±5 per cent of each other by the two methods, with no significant differences. For individuals, agreement of the two methods within ±20 per cent of each other varied; 90 per cent of the men's values agreed this closely for calories, while only 40 per cent had this much agreement for riboflavin.

Flores et al. (32) weighed the food consumed by 16 rural Guatemalan women, and compared the results with a seven-day recall. Between 60 and 70 per cent could be classified into the same extreme thirds of the distribution by the two methods. It should be noted that the diets of these women were very monotonous, and recall would presumably present more of a problem in a society with a more varied diet.

Conclusions regarding the seven-day recall method

It would seem that here again the method may be adequate for characterizing the means of groups, but its accuracy in characterizing an individual's value, i.e., his position in the distribution, is less certain, and varies depending on the nutrient in question.

SEVEN-DAY RECORD

A seven-day record should replace errors of memory with errors of recording, and subdue somewhat the fluctuations of a single day's intake by substituting the average of seven days. An ideal validation would be one which compared the intake indicated by the record with the actual weighing and analysis of food eaten by a free-living population. However, such a procedure would necessarily involve such intrusion into people's lives that the results might nonetheless be suspect because of the observer effect. Another attractive validation might be the comparison of recorded intake with biochemical analysis of output. This analysis, however, is itself plagued with problems of validity, and does not in any case address doubts about the representativeness of a seven-day record. Consequently, we must again rely on analyses of different elements of the question.

Agreement with known values

Gersovitz et al. (21) attempted to validate the seven-day record against actual known intake. Forty-four elderly persons kept a seven-day intake diary, and during that week the investigators surreptitiously weighed the amount of food consumed during a lunch at a congregate meal site. Group means once again agreed well with known values. For eight of 10 nutrients, mean values reported for a meal were not significantly different from amounts actually consumed. For individual data, regression analysis revealed a significant association of actual and recorded values in the first two days, but suggested that accuracy of recording deteriorates in the last three days. Numbers were small (11 cases for the first two days) and the subjects were elderly (mean age 71.7).

Agreement of the results of two different seven-day records

Chappell (33) recorded her diet for 70 weeks and found that a standard error of 20–25 per cent of the average value can be expected with samples of only one week. A standard error of only 5 per cent can be obtained by three one-week records throughout the year, for most nutrients. Of course, these estimates must be conservative since they are based on data from one person. Individuals may vary in their variability, as shown by Yudkin (34), who had six dietetics students record their diets for four weeks. One student had a high-calorie day only 2 per cent higher than her low-calorie day, while another's was 68 per cent higher. Other nutrients were even more variable.

Adelson (31) studied the agreement of two consecutive weeks' records of 39 professional men. They found that mean values were not significantly different, and paired difference tests revealed no significant differences for individuals, except for vitamin C. Heady (26) and Morris et al.

(35) compared the records of bank employees repeated after an interval of one to nine months. They found that for most nutrients the records agreed quite well, with $r = 0.70$ to 0.85. They concluded that the correlations are high enough to make it probable that if a person had a high value one week, he will probably have a high value in a later week. They also point out that the correlation coefficient underestimates the stability of intake, since "the odd individual has a disproportionate effect on the correlation coefficient." Thomson (20), Huenemann and Turner (8) and Hankin et al. (36) compared two seven-day records obtained after intervals of six weeks to two years. They all found correlation coefficients in the range of 0.7 to 0.9 for most nutrients.

Trulson and McCann (12) also compared records two years apart, for 11 professors. The correlation coefficients for calories, protein and carbohydrates were 0.4 to 0.5, and for fat, only 0.33. However, these men were participants in a cholesterol-modifying experiment, so it would be expected that those values would be poorly correlated. Keys et al. (37) provide another example of poor correlations after a long interval. Among 42 rural Greek men, with records three years apart, they found $r = 0.3$ for calories. Marr (38) points out that their work was seasonal and varied, and that their diets may have varied as a result.

Conclusions regarding the seven-day record method

The results of Gersovitz et al. (21) suggest good agreement with actual known intake for mean values, and even good agreement for individual values during the first few days of the recorded week.

It is difficult to attempt to draw inferences about the validity of the method from those studies which compared two different seven-day records. Agreement may reflect a consistent diet and an accurate method, or may reflect the tendency of people to give the same responses at different times; disagreement may reflect a changing diet and an accurate method, or may reflect a consistent diet and an unreliable method. Nevertheless, the extent and precision of the required record argue in favor of accepting apparent reliability as a proxy measure for validity. The seven-day record method involves a detailed record of all food consumed and measurements of portion size, and consistency unrelated to intake would require that the respondent invent a detailed diet and measurements consistent over two 21-meal records. A suggestion that this is not what is occurring may be derived from the fact that certain nutrients are reported to be consumed in different amounts at different seasons (26, 35), and the fact that agreement is often found to be poorer among respondents whose weight has changed and whose diets one would expect therefore to have been different (11, 12).

These arguments, though not conclusive, lend credence to a belief that agreement between records indicates an accurate reflection of a consistent diet, in the absence of objective evidence of dietary change. Most of the studies reported in this section have found good agreement between mean values obtained on two different occasions (8, 20, 26, 31, 35, 36). Investigators who have found poor agreement have been those working with individuals on special diets or other special circumstances (12, 37). Thus, it may be reasonable to conclude that there is an underlying truth which these repeated measures are consistently recording.

This conclusion is supported by the results of Gersovitz et al. (21), described earlier, who found good agreement between the mean values obtained by seven-day record and by actual weighing of intake. However, as with the 24-hour recall method, the validity of this method may be limited to group mean values, since individuals' records may become unreliable after the first few days.

SHORT-CUT METHODS

Drawbacks of the other methods have been mentioned. Histories and seven-day records may be valid, but are time-consuming and require much training on the part of the interviewer or cooperation on the part of the subject. Twenty-four hour recalls are valid for group values but are not valid enough for individuals. As a result, a number of investigators have attempted to develop methods which would be cheaper and easier to administer, but which would nevertheless have validity. One approach attempts to produce exact quantitation of nutrient intake, as the longer methods do. This is described below as the prediction equation approach. Other approaches have tended to emphasize more qualitative measures such as frequency of consumption, and these are grouped together and described as frequency questionnaires below.

Methods involving frequency and other brief questionnaires

Questionnaires which ask only the frequency with which specified foods were eaten in a given interval are capable of being administered quickly in person or by mail to large numbers of people, and so lend themselves to large-scale epidemiologic research. Consequently, Graham, Hankin, and a number of other investigators have attempted to develop such methods (24, 39–43, 46, 49). Abramson et al. (40) compared the results from a 30-minute segment of an interview on frequency and usual intake with those from the longer interview. Correlation coefficients between estimated quantity and number of times per week an item was consumed were between 0.50 and 0.96 for various foods. Morgan et al. (24) also found a food frequency interview to provide reliable results. However, in both cases the short-cut method and the criterion against which it was judged both came from the same interview, which could have contributed to the correlations. Similarly, Balogh et al. (41) compared a 15-minute frequency interview with values obtained by a Burke history, and obtained correlation coefficients of 0.80 to 0.95. However, less than 24 hours had elapsed between the long and short interview, so similar values are less surprising, though reassuring.

The same authors also compared the 15-minute frequency interview with values obtained on a seven-day weighed record performed months later. Although in this part of their study there were only 14 subjects, the correlation coefficients are impressive, between 0.70 and 0.95. Browe et al. (42) compared values obtained by a self-administered questionnaire with those obtained by a Burke history, on 29 men involved in a cardiovascular study. Correlations ranged from 0.66 to 0.81. As before, one cannot be sure which if either of these methods reflects the true value. Nevertheless, this degree of agreement with a widely accepted research method is impressive.

In an attempt to determine whether a frequency questionnaire could accurately detect foods previously eaten and recorded, Hankin et al. (43) had 50 subjects record the relative amounts and frequencies of their consumption of 33 specific foods for seven consecutive days. On the eighth day they were asked to recall whether they had eaten those specific foods in the past 24 hours and in the past seven days. Agreement between record and recall ranged from 78 to 100 per cent, although it should be remembered that this type of agreement statistic is influenced by prevalence and a high level of agreement would be expected for foods eaten either commonly or rarely in this population (44, 45). In a similar study of a food checklist, Nomura et al. (46) found good agreement between recalling having eaten a food recently on two widely separated occasions.

Investigations of proxy respondents also shed some light on the question of the validity of the method. Making the assumption that subjects' responses to a food frequency questionnaire could be used as the criterion for the truth for spouses' responses, both Marshall et al. (47) and Kolonel et al. (48) investigated the accuracy of spouse responses. Both investigators found good agreement between spouses, at a level similar to that found on repeat administrations to the same respondent.

Methods involving prediction equations

Heady (26) in England, Hankin (36, 39) and Phillips (50) in the United States, and associates, have devoted great effort to the development of a short quantitative method for dietary research. Their methods began with a preliminary study to develop scores which could then be used as coefficients in an equation. Once such an equation was developed, it was hoped that the results of a simple frequency-of-consumption questionnaire could be plugged in as factors, and that these coefficents and factors could be used to calculate precise levels of nutrients in the diet.

Heady (26) used seven-day records to derive coefficients by regression. He then developed a mailable seven-day menu record which he administered to 41 bank employees. Using the previously derived coefficients and the menu record, he calculated a score for each nutrient and then compared it with a subsequent seven-day weighed record. However, only two nutrients appeared to give promising results using this method.

Hankin et al. (36) used a similar technique, deriving a prediction equation and then applying it to frequencies obtained from a mailable seven-day recall. They termed the results "disappointing." Correlations between predicted and measured values ranged from 0.4 to 0.6, and only 20–40 per cent of the values were within ±10 per cent of each other. Later Hankin et al. (39) attempted to perfect this approach. One hundred five women kept a diary for four days. The amounts and frequencies recorded by 53 of these women were used to derive prediction equations for calories and five nutrients. These equations were then tested by applying them to the frequencies on the food records of the other 52 women. Predicted mean values based on frequency of consumption were significantly different from recorded amounts for two of six nutrients. Correlations between predicted and recorded amounts were approximately 0.5, except for protein for which $r = 0.26$. The authors conclude that there is a "substantial lack of agreement between individual observed and predicted intakes" (39, p. 358).

Considerable work is still being conducted on this approach. However, its usefulness would appear to be limited to the population for which it was developed, since one would not expect detailed prediction equations based on the diets of British bankmen or Hawaiian Japanese-Americans to be readily generalizable.

Conclusions regarding short-cut methods

Methods involving frequencies or other types of short questionnaires offer the possibility of great usefulness in epidemiologic studies. However, most studies which utilized prediction equations to permit quantitation on the basis of short questionnaires have involved considerable effort, questionable generalizability and a disappointing level of predictive ability. On the other hand, studies using brief frequency interviews or questionnaires have found good correlations with more extensive diet histories. Some of these methods do not yield precise milligrams of nutrients; nevertheless, for epidemiologic purposes the ability to classify individuals into categories of intake would be of great value.

CONCLUSIONS

Most of the methods described above appear to have some degree of validity when measured against one another. Some epidemiologists may be reluctant to term this validity, yet the situation is common in medical science. Frequently we accord to one such measurement the aura of truth, and use it as a standard against which to judge other instruments of measurement. But ultimately, in most cases, all such validations are simply comparisons of one method with another. In the final analysis, the judgment must be made on the basis of the consistency of the evidence from various lines of investigation—the agreement among different methods, the repeatability of methods in many populations, the lack of repeatability in groups for which there is evidence of change in diet, the agreement with available clinical and biochemical evidence and, as Graham (49) has pointed out, the ability to show dose-response relationships. While any single approach may be inconclusive, the entire pattern suggests that several of these methods are valuable.

Nevertheless, further attempts to perfect and validate the methods are desirable, particularly with regard to short-cut approaches suitable for large-scale studies. In doing so, it is important to gather as much information as possible on weight change and changes in eating behavior, so as to evaluate agreement or lack of it. Furthermore, the analyses should permit the examination of validity at both group and individual levels and at varying levels of precision.

Finally, it would be appropriate to take a close look at the precision of information which is necessary to conduct valuable research on nutrition and disease. Rather than focussing on a method's ability to yield precise and accurate numbers of milligrams of a nutrient, it may be more important to produce and evaluate a method which can simply place individuals into broad categories along the distribution of intake, from very little to very much. This is an approach which has not been emphasized in most of the work described above. Epidemiologists have been captured by the nutritionists' dream of developing a method which will yield precise and accurate quantitative amounts of nutrients. This may be an appropriate goal for nutritionists who would like, for example, to be able to set quantitative standards for nutrient intake. And it may ultimately be a reasonable goal for epidemiologists. But at the present level of knowledge about the relationship between nutrition and disease, such precision may be unnecessary. Many questions are answerable with crude instruments. John Snow did not need to know the exact dose of the organism necessary to cause cholera. In fact, he did not even need to know about the organism at all in order to produce a tremendous. advance in public health. If nutritional assessment methodology is at a similar stage—and it may in fact be more advanced—it is still possible to ask and answer some important questions.

REFERENCES

1. Burke BS, Stuart HC. A method of diet analysis. J Pediatr 1938; 12:493-503.
2. Burke BS, Beal MA, Kirkwood SB, et al. Nutrition studies during pregnancy. Am J Obstet Gynecol 1943;46:38-52.
3. Burke BS. The dietary history as a tool in research. J Am Diet Assoc 1947;23:1041-6.
4. Young CM, Chalmers FW, Church HN, et al. A comparison of dietary study methods. I. J Am Diet Assoc 1953;28:124-8.
5. Paul O, Lepper MH, Phelan WH, et al. A longitudinal study of coronary heart disease. Circulation 1963;28:20-3.
6. den Hartog C, van Schaik TFSM, Dalderup LM, et al. The diet of volunteers participating in a long term epidemiological field study on coronary heart disease at Zutphen, The Netherlands. Voeding 1965;26:184-208.
7. Jain M, Howe GR, Johnson KG, et al. Evaluation of a diet history questionnaire for epidemiologic studies. Am J Epidemiol 1980;111:212-9.
8. Huenemann RL, Turner D. Methods of dietary investigation. J Am Diet Assoc 1942;18:562-8.
9. Hart ML, Cox AG. A comparison of dietary analysis methods using a computer. Nutrition 1967;21:146-50.
10. Lubbe AM. A survey of the nutritional status of white school children in Pretoria: description and comparative study of two dietary survey techniques. S Afr Med J 1968;42:616-22.
11. Dawber TR, Pearson G, Anderson P, et al. Dietary assessment in the epidemiologic study of coronary heart disease: The Framingham study. II. Reliability of measurement. Am J Clin Nutr 1962;11:226-34.
12. Trulson MF, McCann MB. Comparison of dietary survey methods. J Am Diet Assoc 1959;35:672-6.
13. McCann MB, Trulson MF, Stare FJ. Follow-up of serum cholesterol, diet and physical findings of Italian American factory workers. Am J Clin Nutr 1961;9:351-5.
14. Reshef A, Epstein LM. Reliability of a dietary questionnaire. Am J Clin Nutr 1972;25:91-5.
15. Reed RB, Burke BS, Collection and analysis of dietary intake data. Am J Public Health 1954;44:1015-26.
16. National Research Council Food and Nutrition Board, Committee on Dietary Allowances. Recommended Dietary Allowances. 9th revised ed, 1980. Washington, DC: National Academy of Sciences, 1980.
17. Madden JP, Goodman SJ, Guthrie HA. Validity of the 24-hour recall. Analysis of data obtained from elderly subjects. J Am Diet Assoc 1976; 68:143-7.
18. Emmons W, Hayes M. Accuracy of 24-hour recalls of young children. J Am Diet Assoc 1973;62:409-15.
19. Campbell VA, Dodds ML. Collecting dietary information from groups of older people. J Am Diet Assoc 1967;51:29-33.
20. Thomson AM. Diet in pregnancy. I. Dietary survey technique and the nutritive value of diets taken by primigravidae. Br J Nutr 1958;12: 446-61.
21. Gersovitz M, Madden JP, Smiciklas-Wright H. Validity of the 24-hour dietary recall and seven-day record for group comparisons. J Am Diet Assoc 1978;73:48-55.
22. Young CM, Hagan GC, Tucker RE, et al. A comparison of dietary study methods. II. Dietary history vs. seven-day record vs. 24-hour recall. J Am Diet Assoc 1952;28:218-21.
23. Stevens HA, Bleiler RE, Olhson MA. Dietary intake of five groups of subjects. J Am Diet Assoc 1963;42:387-92.
24. Morgan RW, Jain M, Miller AB, et al. A comparison of dietary methods in epidemiologic studies. Am J Epidemiol 1978;107:488-98.

25. Balogh M, Kahn H, Medalie JH. Random repeat 24-hour dietary recalls. Am J Clin Nutr 1971;24:304-10.
26. Heady JA. Diets of bank clerks. Development of a method of classifying the diets of individuals for use in epidemiologic studies. J Roy Stat Soc Series A 1961;124:336-61.
27. Hankin JH, Reynolds WE, Margen S. A short dietary method for epidemiologic studies. II. Variability of measured nutrient intakes. Am J Clin Nutr 1967;20:935-45.
28. White EC, McNamara DJ, Ahrens EH Jr. Validation of a dietary record system for the estimation of daily cholesterol intake in individual outpatients. Am J Clin Nutr 1981;34:199-203.
29. Liu K, Stamler J, Doyer A, et al. Statistical methods to assess and minimize the role of intra-individual variability in obscuring the relationship between dietary lipids and serum cholesterol. J Chronic Dis 1978;31:399-418.
30. Horwitt MK, Harvey CC, Hills OW, et al. Correlation of urinary excretion of riboflavin with dietary intake and symptoms of ariboflavinosis. J Nutr 1950;41:247-64.
31. Adelson S. Some problems in collecting dietary data from individuals. J Am Diet Assoc 1960;36:453-61.
32. Flores M, Flores Z, Lara MY. Estimation of family and mothers' dietary intake comparing two methods. Trop Geogr Med 1965;17:135-45.
33. Chappell G. Long-term individual dietary surveys. Br J Nutr 1955;9:323-39.
34. Yudkin J. Dietary surveys: variation in weekly intake of nutrients. Br J Nutr 1951;5:177-94.
35. Morris JN, Marr JW, Heady JA, et al. Diet and plasma cholesterol in 99 bankmen. Br Med J 1963;1:571-6.
36. Hankin JH, Messinger HB, Stallones RA. A short dietary method for epidemiologic studies. IV. Evaluation of questionnaire. Am J Epidemiol 1970;91:562-7.
37. Keys A, Aravanis D, Sdrin H. The diets of middle-aged men in two rural areas of Greece. Voeding 1966;27:575-84.
38. Marr JW. Individual dietary surveys: purposes and methods. World Rev Nutr Diet 1971;13:105-64.
39. Hankin JH, Rawlings V, Nomura A. Assessment of a short dietary method for a prospective study on cancer. Am J Clin Nutr 1978;31:355-9.
40. Abramson JH, Slome C, Kosovsky C. Food frequency interviews as an epidemiologic tool. Am J Public Health 1963;53:1093-101.
41. Balogh M, Medalie JH, Smith H, et al. The development of a dietary questionnaire for an ischaemic heart disease survey. Israel J Med Sci 1968;4:195-203.
42. Browe JH, Gofstein RM, Morlley DM, et al. Diet and heart disease study in the cardiovascular health center. J Am Diet Assoc 1966;48:95-108.
43. Hankin JH, Rhoads GG, Glober GA. A dietary method for an epidemiological study of gastrointestinal cancer. Am J Clin Nutr 1975;28:1055-60.
44. Fleiss JL. Statistical methods for rates and proportions. New York: John Wiley & Sons, 1973.
45. Lee J. Alternate approaches for quantifying aggregate and individual agreements between two methods for assessing dietary intakes. Am J Clin Nutr 1980;33:956-64.
46. Nomura A, Hankin JH. The reproducibility of dietary intake data in a prospective study of gastrointestinal cancer. Am J Clin Nutr 1976;29:1432-6.
47. Marshall J, Priore R, Haughey B, et al. Spouse-subject interviews and the reliability of diet studies. Am J Epidemiol 1980;112:675-83.
48. Kolonel LN, Hirohata T, Nomura AMY. Adequacy of survey data collected from substitute respondents. Am J Epidemiol 1977;106:476-84.
49. Graham S. Diet and cancer. Am J Epidemiol 1980;112:247-52.
50. Phillips RL, Kuzma JW. Estimating major nutrient intake from self-administered food frequency questionnaires. Am J Epidemiol 1976;104:354-5 (abstract).

Assessing Human Epidemiologic Data on Diet as an Etiologic Factor in Cancer Development*

by James E. Enstrom, Ph.D.

T he epidemiology of cancer among human populations is an observational, not an experimental science. The closest that an epidemiologist comes to experimental data is a randomized controlled trial, very difficult to conduct because of practical and ethical considerations. Consequently, epidemiologists are limited primarily to interpreting naturally occurring phenomena. Before specifically examining the relationship between diet and cancer, it is useful to recall the five criteria used in 1964 by the Surgeon General's Advisory Committee on Smoking and Health in establishing a "causal" association between cigarette smoking and lung cancer.[1] The first is consistency, which implies that diverse methods of approach, such as retrospective and prospective studies, lead to the same conclusion. The second is strength, which measures the relative risk and can yield a judgment on the size of the effect of an etiologic factor and whether this factor is important in producing the disease. Third is specificity, which implies the precision with which a factor predicts the occurrence of a disease in a given individual. Fourth is temporal relationship, which means that exposure to a causal agent must precede in time the onset of the disease it produces. Fifth is coherence, which means that all major data are compatible with a genuine association. It is possible to

* Presented as part of a *Symposium on Assessing Therapeutic Dietary Claims* held by the Section on Clinical Nutrition of the New York Academy of Medicine at the Academy February 28, 1981.

This research has been supported by American Cancer Society Grants No. PDT-51A and PDT-51B and by National Cancer Institute Grant No. IR26 CA25157.

James E. Enstrom, Ph.D., is with the School of Public Health, University of California at Los Angeles.

conclude that cigarette smoking "causes" lung cancer because these five criteria are supported by such a vast amount of data, especially the fact that the lung cancer rate is so much higher in cigarette smokers than in nonsmokers.

However, this conclusion is not yet possible with the existing data relating diet and cancer in spite of the fact that some investigators believe as much as 40% of male cancer and 60% of female cancer is related to diet.[2,3] Any given dietary theory is advocated by citing evidence that supports the theory and ignoring contradictory evidence.

I would like to begin my assessment by examining what I think are the two most obvious facts about cancer that one must face. First is the strong exponential relationship between the cancer death rate and aging.[4,5] During a one-year period, about 0.2% of all people will die of cancer, but this varies from 0.01% for people under age 25 to about 2% for people above age 85—a 200-fold difference. So, in practical terms, cancer is primarily a disease associated with aging. Second is the relative constancy of the age-adjusted cancer death rate since the beginning of the century.[4,5] Although the age-adjusted total death rate has continuously declined throughout this century, from about 17.8 deaths/1,000 in 1900 to about 5.9 per 1,000 in 1980, including declines in essentially all the major diseases, the overall cancer rate has remained almost constant at around 1 death/1,000,[4,5] as seen in Figure 1. However, the nature of the cancer problem has changed in the sense that stomach cancer has declined from about 40% to about 3% of all cancer deaths and lung cancer has risen from essentially 0% to 25% of cancer deaths. Excluding lung cancer, the remaining cancer rate has moderately declined during recent decades. Further, the cancer rate has been declining gradually in people under age 45 and only three out of eight cancer deaths now occur in people under age 65.

Probably the best established relationship involving diet and cancer is between alcohol consumption and upper alimentary tract cancer in most

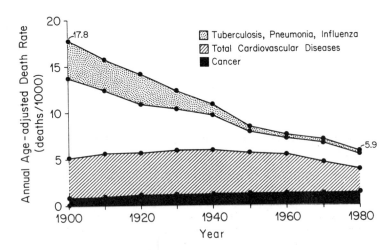

Fig. 1. Annual age-adjusted death rate for U.S. population by major cause every 10 years, 1900-1980, standardized to the 1940 U.S. population.

Western countries.[6] However, the primary dietary factors of current interest are fat, fiber, vegetables, and vitamins. The primary "diet-related" cancers are generally considered to be stomach, colorectal, and breast cancer.[2,3]

Retrospective case-control studies date back to those of Percy Stocks[7] and Frederick Hoffman[8] during the 1930s. Since then there have been at least 20 major case-control studies and three prospective cohort studies, primarily focused on diet and cancer.[6,9] These studies have taken place in England, Finland, Israel, Norway, Canada, Japan, Hawaii, and several areas within the continental United States. Several individual dietary items have been implicated with a risk factor of the order of 2 to 3. For instance, high consumption of meat, beef, fat, and beer, low consumption of fiber, various groups of vegetables, and dietary vitamins A and C, and low serum levels of vitamin A and cholesterol have all been associated with increased cancer risk in one or another of these studies. But, integrating the studies yields substantial conflicting findings: beef consumption was associated with colon cancer in Hawaiian Japanese,[10] but not in three groups of native Japanese.[11,12] Probably the most consistent finding is the association observed for the past several years between low levels of vitamin A (generally below the recommended dietary allowance) and increased risk of cancer, particularly lung cancer.[13] This relationship is somewhat unexpected because lung cancer is already so strongly linked with cigarette smoking. In any case, no dietary factor yet satisfies the five criteria for causality.

Because the retrospective and prospective studies have been inconsistent and inconclusive, the "strongest" available epidemiologic data relating diet to cancer are international geographical correlations between, for instance, per capita fat consumption and age-adjusted colon and breast cancer rates.[14,15] But there are many weaknesses in these correlations. For example, fat consumption for each country is usually estimated from the national sales and disappearance of food stuffs but often does not agree with fat consumption obtained from direct dietary surveys such as the 1971-1974 U.S. Health and Nutrition Examination Survey conducted by the National Center for Health Statistics.[16] Note that the data in often cited Figures 2 and 3 are not consistent in fat-consumption levels. Figure 2 shows that American men consume 55 grams per day,[14] whereas the Survey indicates 100 grams per day.[16] Figure 3 shows that American women consume 150 grams per day,[15] whereas the survey indicates 67 grams per day.[16] Further, correlations between cancer rates and fat intake in 64 areas within the United States, based on survey data, are essentially zero[17] as shown in Figure 4; this is far different from the strong international correlations. In other words, there is a large variation in colon cancer rates with essentially constant fat intake throughout the United States.

Another form of epidemiologic evidence involves migrant studies. Japanese who migrate from Japan to the United States have increased rates for colon and breast cancer relative to rates in Japan.[18,19] These increased rates are frequently attributed to the substantially increased fat intake of

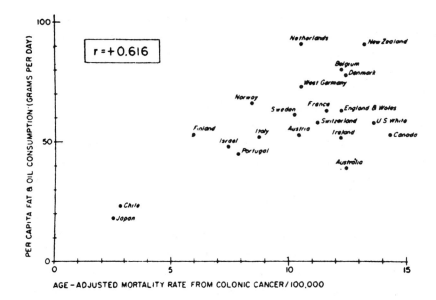

Fig. 2. Large-bowel cancer mortality (1966 to 1967) and dietary fat and oil consumption (1964 to 1966) in males. Reproduced by permission from Wynder, E. L.: The epidemiology of large bowel cancer. *Cancer Res. 35:*3389, 1975.

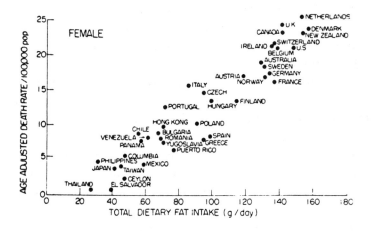

Fig. 3. Correlation between per capita consumption of dietary fat and age-adjusted mortality from breast cancer in different countries. The values for dietary fat are averages for 1964 to 1966 and those for cancer mortality are for 1964 to 1965, except in a few cases where data were available only for 1960 to 1961 or 1962 to 1963. Reproduced by permission from Carroll, K. K.: Experimental evidence of dietary factors and hormone-dependent cancers. *Cancer Res. 35:*3379, 1975.

Japanese migrants relative to native Japanese.[2,3] However, this is selective use of data. In spite of increases in colon and breast cancer, the total cancer rate among Japanese-Americans remains essentially unchanged and their total death rate decreases and remains lower than that of native Japanese.[18,20] American-born Japanese are especially healthy. Based on survey data, American Japanese appear to have almost the same dietary fat intake as American whites, about 80 grams per day—comprising about 40% of total caloric intake[16]—and yet their overall death rates remain relatively low. In summary, the 1970 standardized mortality ratio

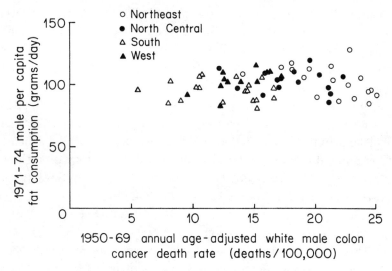

Fig. 4. Mortality and fat consumption in males in 64 areas within the U.S.

for Japanese-Americans compared with American whites is about 50% for all causes, 80% for total cancer, 75% for colon cancer, and 30% for breast cancer (see table).[19,20] These and other data indicate that Japanese are the healthiest race in America in spite of an "Americanized" diet.[20]

In addition to Japanese-Americans, at least two American white sub-populations have relatively low "diet-related" cancer rates without any obvious relationship to diet. Mormons, for instance, advocate abstention from tobacco, alcohol, and caffeine-containing beverages, as well as dietary moderation. The average standardized mortality ratio for active Mormons in California and Utah is about 60% for total cancer, 65% for colon cancer, and 80% for breast cancer.[21] Mexican-Americans, defined as American whites born in Mexico, have a standardized mortality ratio of about 95% for total cancer, only 45% for colon cancer, and 60% for

1968-72 STANDARDIZED MORTALITY RATIOS RELATIVE TO 1970 U.S. WHITES[19,20]

Cause of death	Japanese Males	Japanese Females	Total Males	Total Females	Issei (Japanese born) Males	Issei (Japanese born) Females	Nisei (American born) Males	Nisei (American born) Females	U.S. Whites Males	U.S. Whites Females
Breast cancer	—	20	—	31	—	15	—	40	100	100
Colon cancer	31	32	75	79	67	84	84	72	100	100
Rectum cancer	115	136	113	87	120	86	105	89	100	100
Colorectal cancer	53	51	85	80	80	84	90	75	100	100
Stomach cancer	846	882	351	408	409	410	287	404	100	100
Total cancer	93	87	84	73	105	87	66	61	100	100
All causes	~90	~100	~50	~50					100	100

breast cancer.[22] The diets of Mormons and Mexican-Americans need to be studied in much greater detail, but, based on the data now available, including the Health and Nutrition Examination Survey and the U.S. Department of Agriculture Nationwide Food Consumption Survey, they do not appear to differ noticeably from other white Americans with respect to fat consumption or other major dietary variables including intake of total calories, protein, carbohydrates, calcium, iron, magnesium, and vitamin intake from foods.[21,23] Other dietary variables such as intake of total fiber and vitamin and mineral supplements are not yet quantified.

Another way of looking at this is to compare Mormons to Seventh-Day Adventists, who abstain from tobacco, alcohol, and caffeine, and, in addition, eat very little meat. Mormons and Adventists have essentially identical cancer rates, which are both about 60% of the American white rate.[21,23] These rates are also similar to those of specially selected cohorts of health conscious nonsmokers such as those in the American Cancer Society Cancer Prevention Study.[24] From this comparison, the Adventist diet per se appears to confer no lower risk of cancer among already low risk cohorts. However, this may not be as good a test as one thinks because, in spite of the low meat intake of Adventists, their total fat intake is not much lower than 40% of total calories.[23]

The rigorous way to assess the effect of a so-called "prudent" diet on subsequent cancer occurrence is to conduct randomized controlled trials on human subjects. Such trials have already been conducted for cholesterol-lowering diets and show no significant change in either cancer or total mortality rates.[25,26] Trials involving fat-lowering diets remain to be done in order properly to evaluate the low fat hypothesis.

In lieu of these dietary trials, probably the best epidemiologic evidence that can be hoped for is that an unusually low rate of cancer can be demonstrated in a group which adopts and maintains a diet different from the typical American diet. In an effort to find an optimum diet, as many variations as possible should be explored. For instance, it would be very valuable to locate people on long-term, low fat, high fiber, high vegetable, and/or high vitamin diets and examine their cancer rates. It may be difficult to locate many genuine vegetarians because the Health and Nutrition Examination Survey showed that only 0.1% of Americans never use meat, poultry, or fish.[16] But people with unusual diets can be found. In this spirit, I am currently examining a group of very health-conscious persons who use supplements of vitamins and minerals far in excess of the recommended dietary allowance. So far, I do not yet have enough data to show any specific relationship between their diet and cancer rate, but the group is worth further study.

In summary, epidemiologic studies as a whole have not yet uncovered any "causal" relationship between diet and cancer and have not yet demonstrated any specific diet which in and of itself leads to a greatly reduced cancer death rate. Further, it appears there are substantially lower than average cancer rates among several groups of nonsmokers with a fairly average American diet. However, a number of interesting leads should be vigorously pursued with the goal of precisely determining an optimum diet.

Properly understanding the dramatic decline in stomach cancer deaths would be a great accomplishment for cancer prevention. Before people get their hopes up that a new diet will prevent cancer, it should first be demonstrated that lung cancer can be prevented by smoking cessation. In the meantime, Americans can take some comfort in the fact that, even though their diet may not be optimal, they are currently experiencing the lowest total death rate and highest life expectancy in American history.[5]

Questions and Answers

QUESTION: Please explain Figures 2 and 3. The data seem misleading.

DR. ENSTROM: I presented Figures 2 and 3 as examples. These two published figures demonstrate the difficulties in using gross food-consumption data from various countries rather indiscriminantly. For example, such data indicate that the cancer rates in countries such as Thailand and El Salvador are almost zero, but I don't believe that the true cancer death rates in those countries are that low. What generally happens in such countries is that the disease is not reported on death certificates.

QUESTION: What is the source of your data on comparative death rates?

DR. ENSTROM: The comparison of death rates from 1900 to 1980 is based on available data published by the National Center for Health Statistics. In 1900 only 40% of the country's population was in the death-registration area, which included mainly such eastern states as Massachusetts and New York. Cancer was probably underreported in those early days. Some of the increase during the early decades of the century was probably due to increased reporting of cancer deaths and this would make the total cancer death rate curve even flatter.

Since 1940 the diagnostic methods and the coverage over the entire United States have been consistent and there has only been about a 10% increase in the entire cancer death rate. This indicates that, relatively speaking, there have been vast changes in mortality from certain other diseases but not from cancer.

REFERENCES

1. U.S. Public Health Service: *Smoking and Health—Report of the Advisory Committee to the Surgeon General of the Public Health Service.* Public Health Service Publication No. 1103. Washington, D.C., Govt. Print. Off., 1964.
2. Wynder, E. L. and Gori, G. B.: Contribution of the environment to cancer incidence: an epidemiological exercise. *J. Nat. Cancer Inst. 58:* 825-32, 1977.
3. Weisburger, J. H., Reddy, B. S., Hill, P., et al.: Nutrition and cancer—On the mechanisms bearing on causes of cancer of the colon, breast, prostate, and stomach. *Bull. N.Y. Acad. Med. 56:* 673-96, 1980.
4. Linder, F. E. and Grove, R. D.: *Vital Statistics Rates in the United States, 1900-1940.* Bureau of the Census. Washington, D.C., Govt. Print. Off., 1943.
5. U.S. Department of Health and

Human Services: *Health—United States. 1980.* DHHS Publication No. (PHS) 81-1232. Washington, D.C., Govt. Print. Off., 1980.

6. Doll, R.: Nutrition and cancer: A review. *Nutr. Cancer 1*(3): 35-45, 1979.

7. Stocks, P. and Karn, M. N.: A co-operative study of the habits, home life, dietary and family histories of 450 cancer patients and of an equal number of control patients. *Ann. Eug. 5:* 237-80, 1933.

8. Hoffman, F. L.: *Cancer and Diet.* Baltimore, Williams and Wilkins, 1937.

9. Bjelke, E.: Epidemiological Studies of Cancer of the Stomach, Colon, and Rectum, with Special Emphasis on the Role of Diet. Unpublished Ph.D. thesis, University of Minnesota, 1973.

10. Haenszel, W., Berg, J. W., Segi, M., et al.: Large-bowel cancer in Hawaiian Japanese. *J. Nat. Cancer Inst. 51:* 1765-79, 1973.

11. Haenszel, W., Locke, F. B., and Segi, M.: A case-control study of large-bowel cancer in Japan. *J. Nat. Cancer Inst. 64:* 17-22, 1980.

12. Hirayama, T.: Diet and cancer. *Nutr. Cancer 1*(3): 67-81, 1979.

13. Peto, R., Doll, R., Buckley, J. D., and Sporn, M. B.: Can dietary beta-carotene materially reduce human cancer rates? *Nature 290:* 201-08, 1981.

14. Wynder, E. L.: The epidemiology of large bowel cancer. *Cancer Res. 35:* 3388-94, 1975.

15. Carroll, K. K.: Experimental evidence of dietary factors and hormone-dependent cancers. *Cancer Res. 35:* 3374-83, 1975.

16. National Center for Health Statistics: *Health and Nutrition Examination Survey (HANES I) 1971-1974. Dietary Frequency and Adequacy.* Advance data No. 54 and Catalog Number 4701. Hyattsville, Md., National Center for Health Statistics, 1979.

17. Enstrom, J. E. Colorectal cancer and beer drinking. *Br. J. Cancer 35:* 674-83, 1977 and to be published.

18. Haenszel, W. and Kurihara, M.: Studies of Japanese migrants. I. Mortality from cancer and other diseases among Japanese in the United States. *J. Nat. Cancer Inst. 40:* 43-68, 1968.

19. Locke, F. B. and King, H.: Cancer mortality risk among Japanese in the United States, *J. Nat. Cancer Inst. 65:* 1149-56, 1980.

20. U.S. Department of Health, Education and Welfare: *Health—United States. 1979.* DHEW Publication No. (PHS) 80-1232. Washington, D.C., Govt. Print. Off., 1980.

21. Enstrom, J. E.: Health and Dietary Practices and Cancer Mortality Among California Mormons. In: *Banbury Report 4: Cancer Incidence in Defined Populations.* Cairns, J., Lyon, J. L., and Skolnick, M., editors. Cold Spring Harbor, Cold Spring Harbor Laboratory, 1980, pp. 3-67, 69-92 (related articles by other authors on pp. 3-67).

22. Lilienfeld, A. M., Levin, M. L., and Kessler, I. I.: *Cancer in the United States.* Cambridge, Mass., Harvard University Press, 1972.

23. Enstrom, J. E. and Phillips, R. L.: In preparation.

24. Garfinkel, L.: Cancer mortality in nonsmokers: Prospective study by the American Cancer Society. *J. Nat. Cancer Inst. 65:* 1169-73, 1980.

25. Ederer, F., Leren, P., Turpeinen, O., and Frantz, I. D., Jr.: Cancer among men on cholesterol-lowering diets. Experience from five clinical trials. *Lancet 2:* 203-06, 1971.

26. Turpeinen, O.: Effect of cholesterol-lowering diet on mortality from coronary heart disease and other causes. *Circulation 59:* 1-7, 1979.

Understanding the Results of Epidemiologic Studies

by Gladys Block and Anne M. Hartman

"EPIDEMIOLOGY can be regarded as a sequence of reasoning concerned with biological inferences derived from observations of disease occurrence and related phenomena in human population groups."[1] While laboratory experiments can elucidate mechanisms and animal studies can demonstrate effects in animals, only studies in human populations address the health questions of interest: Does it work that way in humans? Is the relationship found in the laboratory both real and strong enough to be observable in a human population?[2] In order to answer these questions, epidemiologists have developed methods designed to permit valid inferences in the face of the complexity of interactions among physiologic factors, environmental insult, biologic response, psychosocial modulators, and chance.

Epidemiologic research progresses, in theory if not always in practice, from observations in large populations, through studies in carefully characterized groups of individuals, to experimental trials with deliberate manipulation of the study conditions. Each of these types of investigation has different implications for the type of inference that can be drawn and the degree of certainty that should be attached to it.

OBSERVATION AND CORRELATION

The first stage in this progression consists of observational and correlational studies in large

populations. Vital statistics data revealing a high incidence of a given cancer in some counties in the United States and a low incidence in other counties,[3] for example, arouse our curiosity and lead to the development of hypotheses. Statistical tests may then help us to distinguish between observations that are likely to be the result of random fluctuations and those for which some etiologic hypothesis other than chance warrants investigation. It may then be possible to refine the hypothesis by using other published population data (the distribution of industries in US counties,[4] for example) to produce leads and etiologic hypotheses that can then be investigated in more definitive studies. The chief drawback here is that much of the data of interest, such as exposure data on potential etiologic agents and confounding factors like smoking or diet, are not routinely collected or published.

Some population data on food consumption and mortality are available and have had a considerable impact on the development of the diet-cancer hypothesis. For example, the analysis in Fig. 1[5] is often presented as supporting evidence of a relationship between breast cancer and dietary intake of fat. Such international correlations may be supportive of a hypothesis, but they should be interpreted cautiously for several reasons.

First, the dietary data are based not on actual individual intake information but on food disappearance data. Such aggregate data are computed by calculating the total food production in a country (number of acres in corn, for example) plus total food imports, subtracting total food exported, and dividing by the population.[6,7] This

Gladys Block and Anne M. Hartman are with the Operations Research Branch, Division of Cancer Prevention and Control, National Cancer Institute, Blair Building, 9000 Rockville Pike, Bethesda, MD 20205.

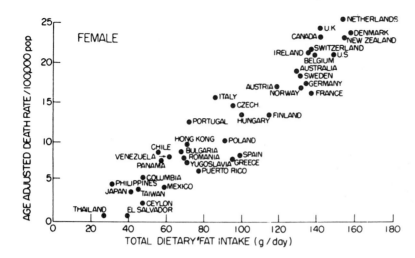

Fig. 1. Correlation between per capita consumption of dietary fat and age-adjusted mortality from breast cancer in different countries. The values for dietary fat are averages for 1964 to 1966 and those for cancer mortality are for 1964 to 1965, except in a few cases where data were available only for 1960 to 1961 or 1962 to 1963. Reprinted with permission.[5]

is the quantity that presumably "disappeared" into consumption. In addition to the relative crudity of such a measure, there may be differences from country to country in the accuracy with which all of the parameters are known, or in the criteria by which they are calculated.

Second and more serious from a methodologic point of view, correlation studies fail to take into account the numerous other factors that might influence or even cause the observed effect. In so doing, they encourage an etiologic inference without actually providing strong support. The countries mentioned in Fig. 1, for example, may also differ in their level of economic development, in genetic factors and associated cultural patterns, or in general nutritional status. The latter influences age at menarche, which may affect cancer incidence, while differences in economic development and socioeconomic status are associated with a vast array of differences in exposures and behavior that may be related to breast cancer risk. Lacking the ability to examine or control for these factors, it is important to be cautious about inferences based on any observed relationship.

A third limitation on the certainty of our inference from correlational studies is the fact that they are based on data from populations rather than individuals. The relationship between fat consumption figures and breast cancer incidence in populations is only of interest because of the implicit assumption that the relationship is true for individuals; that is, that the women who develop cancer are indeed the same women who tend to have a high fat intake. This always remains an assumption in international correlation studies. Thus, epidemiology turns to case-control and prospective studies, in which exposure and outcome are measured in the same individuals, to obtain a better test of the hypothesis.

PROSPECTIVE AND CASE-CONTROL STUDIES

Yerushalmy and Palmer[8] (based on the work of Henle and Koch) proposed the following principles for evaluating causality: (1) individuals with a given characteristic or exposure should develop the disease more frequently than those without the chracteristics; (2) individuals with the disease should have the characteristic or exposure more frequently than those without the disease; and (3) an inference of a causal relationship is stronger if a given characteristic is specific for a given disease. The first criterion underlies the prospective study, while the second forms the logical basis for the case-control approach. The third criterion, whose roots lie in the investigations of infectious disease, proffers to chronic disease epidemiology the requirement that hypotheses make biologic sense and be specific enough to be disprovable.

Other criteria commonly used to evaluate whether or not an association is a causal one include the following:[9–11] strength of the association; existence of a dose-response relationship; an appropriate temporal relationship; consistency of the observation across different studies and approaches; coherence of the observation with known biologic facts and mechanisms; and finally, reduction of a harmful factor, or introduction of a protective one, should be observed to reduce the incidence of the disease. Just as Yerushalmy and Palmer's first two criteria underlie the prospective and case-control approaches, the last criterion mentioned above underlies the clinical trial.

The prospective study examines the hypothesis that individuals with a putatively harmful exposure or characteristic will have a higher incidence of a disease than those without that exposure (or in the case of a supposed protective factor, that they will have a lower incidence). In this approach, individuals with and without the characteristic are identified and their subsequent disease outcome tracked. Such tracking may involve frequent monitoring and examination of health status, as in the Framingham study, or may involve an initial measurement followed by later ascertainment of their vital status and cause of death. Nonconcurrent designs are also possible, if the exposure was measured and recorded in the past.

The measure of association for prospective studies is the relative risk (RR), usually defined as the ratio of the incidence in the exposed group to the incidence in the unexposed group. The farther from 1.00 this ratio is (in either direction), the stronger the association. For some types of prospective studies, the risk ratio is calculated as the ratio of the observed incidence in the exposed group to that which would have been expected on the basis of the experience of the unexposed group, adjusted for the differences in other risk factors between the exposed and unexposed groups.

An example of a prospective study involving dietary factors and cancer may be seen in the investigation, in Norway, of the relationship between reported dietary intake of vitamin A and subsequent lung cancer.[12] In 1967, 16,713 people responded to a mailed survey on dietary habits, and from their responses an index of vitamin A intake was calculated for most individuals. In addition, information regarding demographic characteristics, occupation, and smoking history had previously been obtained for these individuals. Subsequently, outcome information regarding all cases through 1978 and the specific site and histologic type of tumor for most cases was obtained.

Some of the results are shown in Table 1. Over the 11½-year followup period, the risk of lung cancer was lower for individuals with the highest vitamin A index at baseline than for those with the lowest vitamin A index; the estimated ratio of these risks was 0.62, statistically significant at $P < 0.04$.

Furthermore, there is an indication that Yerushalmy and Palmer's third criterion, specificity, is at work here. Among histologically confirmed squamous-cell carcinomas, the apparently protective effect of a high vitamin A index is even stronger than in the total series, with a risk ratio of 0.28. On the other hand, there is no indication of a protective effect against adenocarcinomas, where the ratio is actually in the other direction, 1.21, with a probability of 0.80 that this result could have occurred by chance alone. The authors' comment on the biologic plausibility of this result, "Our finding of a particularly strong negative association between our index of vitamin A intake and the subset of squamous-cell carcinomas is thus in accord with animal data on the effect of vitamin A on epithelial cell differentiation."[12]

An important problem in prospective as well as retrospective studies of diet is the adequacy of the dietary assessment instrument. Some types of

Table 1. Lung Cancer by Vitamin A Index—Observed and Expected Distribution (O/E) and Trend Statistics† for Histologic Subtypes*

Vitamin A Index Scores		<5 (0)	5–6 (1)	7–9 (2)	≥10 (3)	Total	b† ± SE (b)	R^3‡	P
Total series	O/E	65/54.6	43/44.1	33/36.2	12/18.1	153	−0.16 ± 0.08	0.62	0.04
Cases with histological verification of primary tumour, total	O/E	45/36.4	31/30.1	21/25.1	7/12.4	104	−0.22 ± 0.10	0.52	0.02
Squamous and small-cell carcinomas	O/E	32/22.4	19/18.7	11/15.7	3/8.1	65	−0.38 ± 0.14	0.32	0.003
Squamous-cell carcinomas	O/E	23/15.5	13/12.9	7/10.9	2/5.8	45	−0.43 ± 0.17	0.28	0.006
Small-cell carcinomas	O/E	9/7.0	6/5.8	4/4.8	1/2.4	20	−0.27 ± 0.24	0.44	0.22
Adenocarcinomas	O/E	4/6.1	7/4.6	4/3.6	1/1.7	16	0.06 ± 0.25	1.21	0.80
Other and unspec. carcinomas	O/E	9/7.9	5/6.7	6/5.7	3/2.6	23	0.00 ± 0.21	1.00	0.99

*Adjusted for sex, age, region, and urban/rural place of residence.
†b = logistic slope.
‡R^3 = relative odds estimate, index ≥ 10 v < 5. Two-tailed P values.
Reprinted with permission.[12]

assessment are inappropriate for classifying individuals with respect to their usual intake.[13] For example, the variability (particularly for micronutrient intake) of an individual's diet from day to day makes the use of a single 24-hour recall questionable for prospective or retrospective studies in which individuals will be classified with respect to dietary exposures. Thus, for this purpose investigators either use multiple 24-hour recalls,[14] extensive dietary interview,[15] or, more commonly in these studies, shorter food frequency questionnaires.[16] The study described above used such a questionnaire.

Whatever method is used, inaccuracies in the assessment and dietary changes over time will doubtless result in misclassification; such misclassification, if random, weakens the ability to detect a real effect. Failure to find an association may be due to the inadequacy of the dietary instrument, and, therefore, confidence in such a negative result should await confirmation with more precise techniques.

Prospective studies permit the actual assessment of risk in each of the exposure categories, as well as an assessment of exposure unbiased by an individual's memory and knowledge of his disease outcome. However, because incidence of any given disease is usually low, prospective studies also require long periods of time and large numbers. Case-control studies minimize both of these requirements by approaching the question from the perspective of Yerushalmy and Palmer's second principle: if there is a causal relationship between an exposure and a disease, then patients with the disease should be found to have the factor more often than those without the disease. In addition to this theoretical basis, it can be shown statistically that if a disease is rare, the results of this approach closely approximate what would be found if the prospective approach were used.

This case-control method is a common epidemiologic approach to investigations of the role of diet and cancer. Individuals with and without a given disease are selected and their exposure to various dietary factors is assessed. A study of vitamin A and lung cancer by Mettlin, Graham, and Swanson[16] is an example of this approach. These investigators compared 292 patients with histologically confirmed lung cancer with 801 control patients with neither cancer nor respiratory disease. The vitamin A index was based on the results of questionnaires completed by the patients prior to diagnosis and referred to the period 1 year prior to the onset of symptoms. The results are shown in Table 2, by age and smoking status. This table indicates, for example, that among men 60 years or older who smoked more than one pack of cigarettes a day, patients with lung cancer were much more likely to report a low vitamin A intake than were controls. This information, allows us to estimate an RR of 4.0.

Estimated RRs in studies such as this are typically reported with respect to a low-risk reference category. That is, in this example the risk for individuals in the ≥125 vitamin A category is arbitrarily set at 1.0, and the risks in the other categories are compared to that. Thus, one may infer a relationship between the level of vitamin A intake and the occurrence of lung cancer, and a high-risk ratio implies a strong relationship. It should be noted, however, that the risk attributable to a factor, and the benefit to be obtained from eliminating it from the population, is a function not only of the strength of the association but also the proportion of the population that has the risk factor, the incidence of the disease, and of course, whether or not the observed relationship is a causal one.

In case-control studies of cancer, one might question the accuracy of the retrospective assessment of diet. This subject is being investigated

Table 2. Lung Cancer RR Associated With Vitamin A Index by Smoking Status and Age*

| | One Pack of Cigarettes or Less | | | | | | | More Than One Pack of Cigarettes | | | | | | | |
| | <60 | | | ≥60 | | | | <60 | | | ≥60 | | | | Age- and Smoking-Adjusted RR |
Vitamin Level†	Lung Cancer Patients	Controls	RR	Lung Cancer Patients	Controls	RR	Age-Adjusted RR‡	Lung Cancer Patients	Controls	RR	Lung Cancer Patients	Controls	RR	Age-Adjusted RR‡	
≤74	38	122	1.5	59	204	1.4	1.4	28	38	1.8	32	17	4.0§	2.4§	1.7§
75–124	19	81	1.1	35	95	1.8	1.4	17	31	1.3	11	9	2.6	1.6	1.5
≥125	16	77	1.0	17	81	1.0	1.0	13	31	1.0	7	15	1.0	1.0	1.0
Total	73	280		111	380			58	100		50	41			

*RR = relative risk. Food items included in the index and their vitamin A content (in IU/100 g edible portion) are cabbage (130), sauerkraut (50), coleslaw (130), brussels sprouts (520), kale (8,000), cauliflower (60), broccoli (2,500), red cabbage (40), kohlrabi (20), parsnips (30), carrots (11,000), rutabaga (550), cucumber (100), pickles (100), beets (20), tomatoes (900), lettuce (330), beef (50), chicken (200), fruit (517), and milk (340 IU/cup).

†Estimate of monthly intake in thousands of IU.

‡Mantel-Haenszel pooled RR.

§Differs from RR of 1.0 ($P \leq 0.05$); χ^2 test.

Reprinted with permission.[16]

under the auspices of the National Cancer Institute; pending a final answer, some reassurance may be found in evidence of consistency in an individual's diet over time[17,18] and in the consistency of results from many different investigations. Further, one may ask whether the long latency period for cancer does not require that we assess the diets of individuals 20, 30, or 40 years ago. This might well be the case if dietary factors affected only the initiation step. However, if they interrupt later-stage events, it is not the diet at the time of initiation but diet at the time of promotion or progression that is relevant. Indeed, substantial laboratory evidence exists that some inhibitory agents, notably the retinoids, do act to interrupt the late-stage promotion event.[19–21]

Because of the complexity of behavior, exposure, disease, and causation in human populations, inferences from both observational and intervention studies are strong only to the degree that the studies are as free as possible of bias and spurious associations due to confounding. Confounding is "the effect of an extraneous prognostic factor or variable that wholly or partially accounts for the apparent effect of the study exposure, or that masks an underlying true association."[22] In addition to confounding, problems in interpretation may arise when the risk depends on the level of a second factor. For example, the relationship between a dietary factor and cancer may be different for smokers and nonsmokers. This is called interaction or effect modification. Potential confounders or effect modifiers such as cigarette smoking, sex, age, place of residence, and socioeconomic level were considered in the studies previously discussed.[12,16]

In the design phase, confounding may also be controlled by randomization or by matching cases and controls (or exposure groups in a prospective study) on important factors. Matching may be done on an individual basis (ie, for each case, match a control on the relevant factors) or by category (ie, select controls from the corresponding subgroups of the relevant factors in proportion to the number of cases in these subgroups).[22,23]

Confounding and interaction may be considered in the analysis phase. There is a large body of literature that deals with these phenomena.[22,24,25] Stratified analysis is one technique that aids in the examination of interaction and the control of confounding. In stratified analysis, subjects are classified by levels of potentially important factors (such as smoking status), and the estimated RR for each of the strata is calculated. Examination of the resulting risks for each stratum helps to reveal the presence or absence of interaction, and holds confounding factors constant. If the risks are consistent over the strata, a summary risk estimate adjusting for the confounding factors may be calculated by using appropriate statistical methods. The previously cited study by Mettlin et al[16] uses these techniques.

Other techniques can be used when the number of factors makes impractical a simple stratified analysis for control of confounding and examination of interaction. One such technique, logistic modeling, involves the development of a mathematical model that gives a simplified description of the relationship between several risk factors and the probability of disease. Kvale et al[12] used a form of this approach to derive the estimates of relative risk reported in Table 1.

The measures described above for the control of confounding permit a clearer evaluation of the existence and strength of a relationship between a factor and an outcome. In order to evaluate whether or not that relationship is a causal one, the examination of the dose-response relationship is of central importance. The data in Table 2 present "a pattern suggestive of a dose-response relationship,"[16] since the RRs for lung cancer tend to increase with decreasing vitamin A level. In the study by Kvale et al,[12] such a dose response was found to be statistically significant.

It is important to bear in mind, for all of the types of studies discussed above, that although a relationship may have been shown, causality has not. It is possible, for instance, that another factor associated with vitamin A intake is in fact the cause of the observed association with lung cancer. Careful analysis of as many other factors as possible may minimize, but does not eliminate, this possibility. Thus, the final step in evaluation of a hypothesis is often the controlled clinical trial.

EXPERIMENTAL STUDIES

Since this area of epidemiology is most familiar to the clinician, only a few points relevant to diet trials of prevention will be highlighted here. The reader is referred to several general reviews on clinical trials for more specific details.[26–32]

Several factors are essential in order to ensure a high probability of identifying the better procedure, if one is actually better, and to convince others of the validity of the conclusions. (This latter motive is crucial if interventions such as major dietary changes may be introduced on a large scale. Trials of such agents must pass the test of public and professional scrutiny.) Randomization is of central importance since it eliminates bias from the assignment of intervention groups, tends to balance treatment groups as to important prognostic factors, and is necessary for the validity of the statistical tests used in the comparison of groups. It does not guarantee comparability on all factors, however, and therefore consideration should be given to randomizing within strata defined by important prognostic factors, as well as to techniques of adjustment in the analysis.[29,30,32,33] In diet trials, individuals may resist randomization because they have an opinion about the efficacy of the diet regimen. This may introduce accrual problems, while on the other hand, failure to randomize may result in bias with regard to the type of individual in the two groups.

In addition, cancer prevention trials related to diet and nutrition must give special attention to issues such as the compliance of the intervention group, the adoption by the control group of similar protective behaviors, and lag time to maximum effectiveness. Eating behavior is difficult to change, and noncompliance may be high over the course of a long trial. Conversely, population trends toward more "healthful" diets and lifestyles may cause the control group to converge on the treatment group in both diet and outcome. All of these factors, in addition to the low incidence of cancer, can have a serious impact on the projected sample size and, subsequently, on the actual outcome of a trial.

It is not possible, even in an experimental design, to have complete control over the study conditions when human populations are involved. At all levels of epidemiologic research, inference ultimately rests on the coherence of the evidence from many disciplines, the strength of the evidence each supplies, and the consistency of results across many investigations.

REFERENCES

1. Lilienfeld AM, Lilienfeld DE: Foundations of Epidemiology (ed 2). Oxford, Oxford University Press, 1980.

2. Hegsted DM: The relevance of animal studies to human disease. Cancer Res 35:3537–3539, 1975

3. Mason TJ, McKay FW, Hoover R, et al: Atlas of Cancer Mortality for U.S. Counties: 1950–1969. U.S. Department of Health, Education & Welfare, DHEW publication no. 75–780, 1975

4. US Bureau of the Census: Census of Manufacturers, 1963, vol I and II. Washington, DC, US Government Printing Office, 1966

5. Carroll KK: Experimental evidence of dietary factors and hormone-dependent cancer. Cancer Res 35:3374–3383, 1975

6. Economic Research Service: Major statistical series of the U.S. Department of Agriculture: How they are constructed and used, no. 5, Consumption and utilization of agricultural products: Agriculture Handbook 365

7. Welsh SL, Marston RM: Review of trends in food use in the United States, 1909–1980. JADA 81:120–125, 1982

8. Yerushalmy J, Palmer CE: On the methodology of investigations of etiologic factors in chronic diseases. J Chronic Dis 10:27–40, 1959

9. Lilienfeld AM: On the methodology of investigations of etiologic factors in chronic disease—some comments. J Chronic Dis 10:41–46, 1959

10. Surgeon General, Advisory Committee of the USPHS: Smoking and Health. PHS publication no. 1103. Washington, DC US GPO, 1964

11. Evans AS: Causation and disease: A chronological journey. Am J Epidemiol 108:249–258, 1978

12. Kvale G, Bjelke E, Gart JJ: Dietary habits and lung cancer risk. Int J Cancer 31:397–405, 1983

13. Block G: A review of validations of dietary assessment methods. Am J Epidemiol 115:492–505, 1982

14. Beaton GH, Milner J, McGuire V, et al: Source of variance in 24-hour dietary recall data: Implications for nutrition study design and interpretation. Carbohydrate sources, vitamins, and minerals. Am J Clin Nutr 37:986–995, 1983

15. Mann GV, Pearson G, Gordon T, et al: Diet and cardiovascular disease in the Framingham Study. I. Measurement of dietary intake. Am J Clin Nutr 11:200, 1962

16. Mettlin C, Graham S, Swanson M: Vitamin A and lung cancer. JNCI 63:1435–1438, 1979

17. Dawber TR, Pearson G, Anderson P, et al: Dietary assessment in the epidemiologic study of coronary heart disease: The Framingham Study. II. Reliability of measurement. Am J Clin Nutr 11:226–234, 1962

18. Hankin JH, Messinger HB, Stallones RA: A short dietary method for epidemiologic studies. IV. Evaluation of questionnaire. Am J Epidemiol 91:562–567, 1970

19. Sporn MB, Dunlop NM, Newton DL, et al: Prevention of chemical carcinogenesis by vitamin A and its synthetic analogs (retinoids). Fed Proc 35:1332–1338, 1976

20. DiPalma JR, McMichael R: The interaction of vitamins with cancer chemotherapy. CA 29:280–286, 1979

21. Sporn MB, Newton DL: Chemoprevention of cancer with retinoids. Fed Proc 38:2528–2534, 1979

22. Schlesselman JJ: Case-Control Studies: Design, Conduct, Analysis. New York, Oxford University Press, 1982

23. Karon JM, Kupper LL: In defense of matching. Am J Epidemiol 116:852–866, 1982

24. Breslow NE, Day NE: The analysis of case-control studies: Statistical Methods in Cancer Research, vol 1. IARC scientific publication no. 32. Lyon, International Agency for Research on Cancer, 1980

25. Kleinbaum DG, Kupper LL, Morgenstern H: Epidemiologic Research: Principles and Quantitative Methods. Belmont, California, Lifetime Learning Publications, Wadsworth, Inc, 1982

26. Byar DP, Simon RM, Friedewald WT, et al: Random-

ized clinical trials—perspectives on some recent ideas. N Engl J Med 295:74–80, 1976

27. Friedman LM, Furberg CD, DeMets DL: Fundamentals of Clinical Trials. Boston, John Wright, PSG Inc, 1981

28. Green SB: Randomized clinical trials: Design and analysis. Semin Oncol 8:417–423, 1981

29. Peto R, Pike MC, Armitage P, et al: Design and analysis of randomized clinical trials requiring prolonged observation of each patient. I. Introduction and design. Br J Cancer 34:585–612, 1976

30. Peto R, Pike MC, Armitage P, et al: Design and analysis of randomized clinical trials requiring prolonged observation of each patient. II. Analysis and examples. Br J Cancer 35:1–39, 1977

31. Shapiro SH, Louis TA (eds): Clinical Trials. Issues and Approaches. Statistics: Textbooks and Monographs, vol 46. New York, Marcel Dekker, Inc, 1983

32. Simon R: Restricted randomization designs in clinical trials. Biometrics 35:503–512, 1979

33. Armitage P: Importance of prognostic factors in the analysis of data from clinical trials. Controlled Clin Trials 1:347–353, 1981

Classic Experimental Studies

The Genesis and Growth of Tumors: III. Effects of a High-Fat Diet

by Albert Tannenbaum, M.D.

Watson and Mellanby (10) have found that feeding mice a diet containing 12.5 to 25 per cent butter fat causes a definite increase in the incidence of skin tumors produced by tarring. The results of Baumann and his associates (1, 2, 5, 6) are in the same direction. In numerous experiments they have shown that skin tumors of the mouse, induced either by ultraviolet light or carcinogenic hydrocarbons, are formed in greater numbers and at an earlier time in mice receiving a high-fat diet than in control mice consuming the basal rations. In contrast to these results, the same investigators have found that the production of sarcomas by carcinogenic hydrocarbons is not significantly altered by a high-fat diet.

This communication is a report of the effects of dietary fat on both the genesis and growth of tumors. The tumors utilized were the spontaneous breast tumor, induced skin tumor, induced sarcoma, and primary lung tumor of the mouse. The investigations demonstrate that increasing the fat content of a basic ration exerts diverse effects on the formation of different types of tumors; these effects range from a striking augmentation of the formation of spontaneous breast tumors to a possible inhibition of the formation of sarcomas induced by a carcinogenic hydrocarbon. An attempt has also been made to clarify the mechanism by which fat affects the genesis of tumors.

This investigation was aided by a grant from the National Cancer Institute.

The late Dr. Albert Tannenbaum was with the Department of Cancer Research, Michael Reese Hospital, Chicago, Illinois, at the time this article was written.

METHODS

In all experiments pure strain mice were used, obtained from the Roscoe B. Jackson Memorial Laboratory or derived from their stock. They were divided into groups equivalent as to age, weight, and sex, usually 50 for the experimental group and 50 for the control group. Each animal was numbered and a separate record of its progress was kept. The animals were inspected for tumors biweekly, at which time they were weighed unless they bore skin carcinomas or subcutaneous tumors. Postmortem examination was performed when the tumors became large, at the death of the animal, or at the termination of the experiment. The lesions were recognized as tumors by their appearance and progressive growth; the type of tumor was established by gross examination and sectioning. Histological examinations were made of many tumors, selected at random, and of all those lesions about which doubt existed; the results of the histological studies indicated that the gross examinations were reliable. Percentages of tumor formation were computed on the basis of the number of animals alive at the time the first tumor appeared in either group of the experiment (effective total). The "tumor count" refers to the number of animals which developed tumors.

All animals were fed ad libitum and had free access to water. In each experiment the control group was fed a basic ration relatively low in fat, but adequate for growth, while the second group was fed the same basic ration modified by the substitution of fat.[1] Two basic rations were employed, modified

[1] Hydrogenated cottonseed oil (kremit), generously furnished by Armour and Company.

in such a way that 3 experimental high-fat diets resulted. The diets were prepared by mixing the dry components with sufficient water to form an easily molded mash, which was cut into equal blocks, each containing a definite amount of the dry mixture. The actual average food consumption per animal was obtained each week by weighing back the food left in the cages. These values were not obtained in our earlier experiments.

Diet 1.—The control diet (1c) was a basic ration consisting of cracked spring wheat, 145; Purina dog chow meal, 40; skimmed milk powder, 15; and white milled flour, 25. The high-fat diet (1f) was prepared from the basic ration by substituting 25 parts of fat for 25 of wheat, and 5 parts of vitamin-free casein for 5 of flour. On Sunday an equivalent amount of Purina dog chow checkers was fed to both the control and high-fat groups. The approximate compositions of the diets were as follows:

	Control (1c), per cent	High-fat (1f), per cent
Protein	17	17
Fat	3	12
Carbohydrate	64	58
Ash	3	3

Diet 2.—The control basic ration (2c) was the same as in diet 1. The high fat diet (2f) was made by substitution, in a manner similar to that used in preparing high-fat diet 1f, but differing in that 75 parts of fat replaced 50 of wheat. Otherwise, the method of preparation of the diets, daily feeding, and Sunday feeding were the same as with diet 1. The approximate compositions of the diets were as follows:

	Control (2c), per cent	High-fat (2f), per cent
Protein	17	15
Fat	3	28
Carbohydrate	64	46
Ash	3	3

Diet 3.—Experience and refinement of technic resulted in diet 3. The control diet (3c) consisted of 1.4 gm. Purina dog chow meal, 0.9 gm. skimmed milk powder, and 1.9 gm. cornstarch. This amount was fed daily to each animal. The high-fat diet (3f) was prepared by substituting an isocaloric amount (0.9 gm.) of hydrogenated cottonseed oil for the 1.9 gm. of starch. Thus equicaloric amounts of the 2 diets contained equal quantities of protein, vitamins, and minerals, and differed only in the fat and carbohydrate content. The approximate compositions of the diets in grams per mouse per day were as follows:

	Control (3c), gm.	High-fat (3f), gm.
Protein	0.62(15%)	0.62(19%)
Fat	0.08(2%)	0.98(31%)
Carbohydrate	2.92(70%)	1.22(38%)
Ash	0.16(4%)	0.16(5%)

It is to be noted that the fat content of the 3 high-fat diets was 12 to 31 per cent in comparison with a fat content of 2 to 3 per cent for the 2 control rations.

RESULTS

Effects of a High-Fat Diet on the Formation of Spontaneous Breast Tumors

Experiment 1.—The control and experimental groups were each composed of 44 female dba mice, matched as to their birth dates, number of litters, and litter dates (12 in each group were virgin). At an average age of 38 weeks (range, 32 to 48 weeks) they were placed on their respective diets: diet 1c, control, and the corresponding high-fat diet (1f) described under "Methods." The experiment was continued until all the animals had died. There was no observable difference in the general health and appearance of the mice in the 2 groups, and the rate of nontumor deaths was approximately the same in both groups.

The results as shown in Table I and Fig. I A reveal that more tumors were formed in the high-fat group. Twenty-four tumors (55 per cent) arose in the F11 group receiving the high-fat diet in contrast to 14 tumors (32 per cent) in the F12 group fed the basic diet. The tumors in the high-fat group arose at a mean age of 70 ± 3.1 weeks in comparison with 72 ± 5.7 weeks for those of the control group.

Experiment 2.—Experiment 1 was repeated on 2 groups of 50 virgin dba mice. At an average age of 24 weeks (range, 18 to 32), they were placed on the control (1c) and high-fat (1f) diets. The experiment was terminated when the mice had attained an average age of 2 years, at which time only 3 of the control group (F22) and 2 of the high-fat group (F21) were alive and without tumors.

The results are shown in Table II, and the cumulative tumor counts are graphically represented in Fig. 1 B. Thirty-two spontaneous breast tumors (64 per cent) arose in the high-fat group in comparison with 16 tumors (32 per cent) in the control group. The tumors in the high-fat group appeared at a mean age of 62 ± 1.8 weeks, compared with 74 ± 3.1 for those of the control group. Thus, the high-fat diet caused the formation of twice as many tumors and a significant shortening of the mean age of appearance. As in experiment 1, there was no observable difference in the general health and appearance of the 2 groups, and the rates of nontumor deaths were approximately the same.

The definite increase in the incidence of spontaneous breast tumors brought about by a fat-enriched diet is significant, and this effect is the most striking result obtained in our studies with various types of tumors. Also, the tumors appeared at an earlier time. There are certain quantitative differences in the results of the 2 experiments. The control groups of both experiments had 32 per cent tumors while

TABLE I: THE EFFECTS OF A HIGH-FAT DIET ON THE FORMATION OF SPONTANEOUS BREAST TUMORS IN DBA MICE

Average age, weeks	F12: control, diet 1c			F11: high-fat, diet 1f		
	Mean weight, gm.	Animals alive and tumor-free	Cumulative tumor count	Mean weight, gm.	Animals alive and tumor-free	Cumulative tumor count
38	29	44	0	28	44	0
46	30	43	1	31	39	3
54	31	40	3	33	36	5
62	31	34	6	34	32	7
70	31	28	8	34	26	9
78	28	24	10	33	19	14
86	28	13	11	32	5	22
94	28	9	11	..	0	24
102	—	2	13	..	..	..
110	..	0	14	..	..	..

* Average age of mice at beginning of experiment (May 17, 1938): 38 weeks.

TABLE II: THE EFFECTS OF A HIGH-FAT DIET ON THE FORMATION OF SPONTANEOUS BREAST TUMORS IN DBA VIRGIN MICE

Average age, weeks	F22: control, diet 1c			F21: high-fat, diet 1f		
	Mean weight, gm.	Animals alive and tumor-free	Cumulative tumor count	Mean weight, gm.	Animals alive and tumor-free	Cumulative tumor count
24	27	50	0	26	50	0
32	30	50	0	31	50	0
40	31	50	0	34	49	1
48	33	50	0	36	44	5
56	34	47	2	38	36	13
64	33	38	5	37	25	20
72	32	26	7	33	15	28
80	31	14	14	34	8	30
88	28	8	15	—	4	32
96	—	5	15	—	3	32
102	—	3	16	—	2	32

* Average age of mice at beginning of experiment (June 30, 1938): 24 weeks.

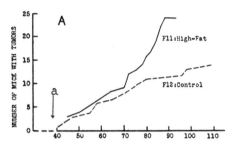

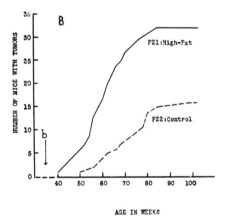

AGE IN WEEKS

Fig. 1.—Effects of a high-fat diet on the formation of spontaneous breast tumors in dba female mice. Curve of cumulative number of tumors. (a) Diets instituted at 38 weeks. (b) Diets instituted at 24 weeks.

the high-fat groups of experiments 1 and 2 had 55 per cent and 64 per cent respectively. Furthermore, in experiment 1, the high-fat diet did not significantly decrease the mean age at which the tumors appeared, while in experiment 2 the mean age of appearance of the tumors was shortened by about 3 months. The mice of experiment 2 were approximately 14 weeks younger than those of experiment 1 at the beginning of these experiments and were, there-fore, subjected to the dietary differences for a longer period. It is suggested that if mice be fed a high-fat diet throughout their early adult life a more decided augmentation and acceleration of tumor formation occurs. When the animals of experiments 1 and 2 were classified into smaller subgroups, according to the age at which the diets were instituted, it appeared that the augmentation of tumor formation through the high-fat diet was less pronounced in the older subgroups.

EFFECTS OF A HIGH-FAT DIET ON THE FORMATION OF INDUCED EPITHELIAL TUMORS

These experiments were performed with 3 different strains of mice. The skin tumors were induced by a 0.3 per cent benzene solution of 3,4-benzpyrene. Twice weekly, in general, one drop of the solution, containing about 0.05 mgm. of the carcinogen, was applied to the interscapular region by means of a dropping pipette. Tumors were recorded as papillomas or carcinomas, but since most of the papillomas eventually became carcinomas, and the exact time of conversion was not always recognizable, the tumor counts include both types.

Experiment 3.—Two groups, each containing 45 JAX Swiss females, were placed on their respective control and high-fat diet 2 when they were about 10 weeks of age. They received 32 applications of the benzpyrene solution during the following 20 weeks. The average daily food consumption for the high-fat group (K1) was 3.0 gm. per mouse compared with 3.3 gm. for the control animals (K2). The experiment was continued for 42 weeks following the initial application of the carcinogen.

The results are shown in Table III. Twenty-eight skin tumors (67 per cent) were formed in the high-fat group and 22 tumors (51 per cent) in the control

TABLE III: THE EFFECTS OF A HIGH-FAT DIET ON THE FORMATION OF INDUCED SKIN TUMORS IN MALE SWISS MICE

Weeks after first application *	K2: control, diet 2c			K1: high-fat, diet 2f		
	Mean weight, gm.	Animals alive and tumor-free	Cumulative tumor count	Mean weight, gm.	Animals alive and tumor-free	Cumulative tumor count
1	21	45	0	20	45	0
11	25	43	0	26	40	2
15	27	37	3	28	36	6
19	29	32	7	30	34	7
23	31	30	8	32	25	15
27	33	21	17	35	16	23
31	33	19	19	35	14	25
35	32	19	19	38	11	27
39	34	16	21	38	10	28
42	35	15	22	39	9	28

* Thirty-two applications of benzpyrene solution beginning March 10, 1939.

TABLE IV: THE EFFECTS OF A HIGH-FAT DIET ON THE FORMATION OF INDUCED SKIN TUMORS IN MALE C57 BLACK MICE

Weeks after first application *	So: control, diet 3c			S1: high-fat, diet 3f		
	Mean weight, gm.	Animals alive and tumor-free	Cumulative tumor count	Mean weight, gm.	Animals alive and tumor-free	Cumulative tumor count
†	24	49	0	24	50	0
0	28	49	0	28	50	0
13	34	49	0	36	50	0
17	35	47	2	38	45	4
21	38	46	2	40	43	5
25	39	43	4	41	40	6
29	38	42	4	42	38	7
33	40	39	6	44	36	9
37	40	35	6	44	31	11
41	39	26	10	42	24	14
45	38	21	11	40	21	15
49	—	19	13	—	15	17

* Twenty-six semiweekly applications of benzpyrene solution beginning Aug. 2, 1940.

† Diets started on June 24, 1940, 6 weeks before first application of carcinogen.

group. The mean time of appearance of the tumors in the high-fat group was 23 ± 1.3 weeks, compared with 24 ± 1.7 for those of the control group.

Experiment 4.—Two groups of 50 C57 black male mice, all born within a span of 3 weeks, were transferred to their respective control and high-fat diet 3 when they were 10 weeks of age. At 16 weeks of age they received the first of 26 semiweekly applications of the benzpyrene solution. The animals of the control group (So) consumed an average of 3.5 gm. per day in comparison with 3.0 gm. per day for the high-fat group (S1). It is to be noted that these amounts of food contained approximately the same quantities of essential dietary components (protein, vitamins, and minerals) and were approximately isocaloric.

The results are given in Table IV and the tumor counts are graphically presented in Fig. 2 A. In the high-fat group (S1), 17 mice (35 per cent) developed tumors compared with 13 (27 per cent) in the corresponding control group (So). The mean time of appearance of the tumors in the high-fat group was 31 ± 2.8 weeks, compared with 34 ± 3.0 in the control group. Toward the end of the experiment skin ulcerations occurred in approximately equal numbers in both groups.

Experiment 5.—Two groups of 50 mice each were made up of dba male mice born within a span of 6 weeks. At 10 weeks of age the groups were placed on their respective control and high-fat diet 3. Four weeks later the first of 19 semiweekly applications of the benzpyrene solution was begun. The average daily food intake per mouse was 4.0 gm. for the control group and 3.1 for the high-fat group. Again, as in the previous experiment, the animals were fed ad libitum; yet the 2 groups consumed isocaloric amounts of food containing approximately equal quantities of essential dietary components.

The results are shown in Table V and Fig. 2 B.

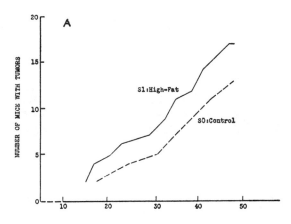

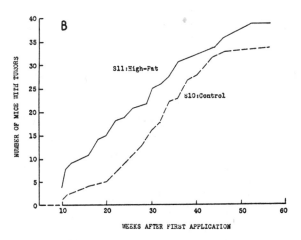

FIG. 2.—Effects of a high-fat diet on the formation of induced epithelial tumors. Curve of cumulative number of tumors.

Thirty-nine skin tumors (78 per cent) were formed in the high-fat group, in comparison with 34 tumors (68 per cent) in the control group. The mean time of appearance of these tumors was 27 ± 2.2 and 31 ± 1.8 weeks respectively.

It should be noted from the tables and figures that in the stage of each experiment when only a few tumors had formed (21 to 24 weeks) the percentage difference in the incidence of tumors in the 2 groups was relatively large. However, by the time the experiments were terminated (42 to 56 weeks) larger numbers of tumors had formed in both groups, resulting in smaller relative differences in the incidence of tumors. These facts in no way alter the interpretation of the results, but do indicate that the magnitude of the effect appears to be greater in the early stages of the experiments.

In 2 experiments on JAX ABC mice comparable results were obtained when the fat content of the basic ration was increased by the addition of 10 per cent wheat germ oil, instead of hydrogenated cottonseed oil.

Thus, all 5 experiments with induced skin tumors show the same results: A high-fat diet produced a definite increase in the incidence of skin tumors and shortened the mean time of appearance of these tumors. Although the differences in any one experiment are

TABLE V: THE EFFECTS OF A HIGH-FAT DIET ON THE FORMATION OF INDUCED SKIN TUMORS IN MALE DBA MICE

Weeks after first application *	S10: control, diet 3c			S11: high-fat, diet 3f		
	Mean weight, gm.	Animals alive and tumor-free	Cumulative tumor count	Mean weight, gm.	Animals alive and tumor-free	Cumulative tumor count
†	23	50	0	23	50	0
0	26	50	0	25	50	0
8	29	50	0	29	50	0
16	32	46	4	31	38	11
24	30	40	9	31	30	19
32	32	31	18	34	23	26
40	31	20	28	32	18	31
48	—	8	33	33	11	36
56	—	3	34	—	7	39

* Nineteen semiweekly applications of benzpyrene solution beginning Sept. 7, 1940.

† Diets started Aug. 10, 1940, 4 weeks before first application of carcinogen.

not of significant magnitude statistically, the results are remarkably consistent and are in qualitative agreement with those obtained by other workers (2, 5, 6, 10).

EFFECTS OF A HIGH-FAT DIET ON THE FORMATION AND GROWTH OF INDUCED SARCOMAS

Experiment 6.—Two groups, each of 40 JAX Swiss female mice 10 weeks of age, were given a single subcutaneous injection of 0.15 mgm. of 3,4-benzpyrene in 0.2 cc. of lard in the interscapular area. At that

time they were placed on their respective control and high-fat diet 2. The control group (L30) consumed a daily average of 3.0 gm. per mouse compared with 3.4 gm. for the high-fat group (L1).

Fewer tumors were formed in the high-fat group. The results are given in Table VI and Fig. 3 B. Twelve sarcomas (30 per cent) arose in the high-fat group in comparison with 19 sarcomas (49 per cent) in the control group. The mean time of appearance of the tumors was 25 ± 2.7 and 25 ± 1.4 weeks respectively.

The rate of growth of the tumors in the 2 groups

TABLE VI: THE EFFECTS OF A HIGH-FAT DIET ON THE FORMATION OF INDUCED SARCOMAS IN FEMALE SWISS MICE

Weeks after injection *	L30: control, diet 2c			L1: high-fat, diet 2f		
	Mean weight, gm.	Animals alive and tumor-free	Cumulative tumor count	Mean weight, gm.	Animals alive and tumor-free	Cumulative tumor count
0	19	40	0	19	40	0
8	24	40	0	26	40	0
16	28	37	1	32	38	2
24	30	27	1	36	32	7
32	31	18	18	40	27	9
40	31	17	19	42	21	12
48	34	15	19	43	18	12
52	34	15	19	42	16	12

* Single injection of 3,4-benzpyrene on May 22, 1939.

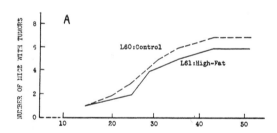

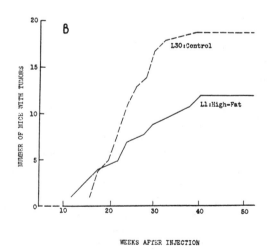

FIG. 3.—Effects of a high-fat diet on the formation of induced sarcomas. Curve of cumulative number of tumors.

did not differ. The 13 tumors measured in the normal group (L30) had a mean growth index [2] of 13 ± 1.1 compared with 13 ± 2.3 for the 9 tumors measured in the high-fat group (L1).

Experiment 7.—At 9 weeks of age 40 JAX ABC mice were placed in the control group (L60) and 37 mice in the high-fat group (L61). A single subcutaneous injection of 0.1 mgm. of 3,4-benzpyrene in 0.2 cc. of lard was given in the interscapular region. Diets 2c and 2f were again utilized. The daily average food consumption per mouse was 3.6 and 3.3 gm. for the control and high-fat groups respectively.

In Table VII and Fig. 3 A the results of this experiment are given. Six sarcomas (16 per cent) were formed in the high-fat group, 7 (18 per cent) in the control group. The mean time of appearance of these tumors was 29 ± 3.9 and 28 ± 3.5 weeks respectively.

TABLE VII: THE EFFECTS OF A HIGH-FAT DIET ON THE FORMATION OF INDUCED SARCOMAS IN FEMALE ABC MICE

Weeks after injection *	L60: control, diet 2c			L61: high-fat, diet 2f		
	Mean weight, gm.	Animals alive and tumor-free	Cumulative tumor count	Mean weight, gm.	Animals alive and tumor-free	Cumulative tumor count
0	18	40	0	18	37	0
7	25	40	0	27	37	0
15	32	39	1	34	36	1
23	35	38	2	41	35	1
31	38	33	5	44	31	4
39	39	31	6	45	30	5
47	40	30	7	44	29	6
51	40	29	7	42	25	6

* Single injection of 3,4-benzpyrene on May 27, 1939.

As in the previous experiment, growth rates of tumors were studied. No appreciable difference was found between the mean growth indices of the tumors in the control and high-fat groups: 14 ± 1.3 (6 tumors) and 13 ± 2.7 (4 tumors) respectively.

Thus, a high-fat diet definitely does not increase the formation of induced sarcomas; under selected conditions of carcinogenesis it may even inhibit their formation. The results of these 2 experiments with induced sarcomas are in decided contrast to those obtained with spontaneous breast tumors (considerable increase) and induced epithelial tumors (moderate increase).

EFFECTS OF A HIGH-FAT DIET ON THE FORMATION OF PRIMARY LUNG TUMORS

Three of the experiments reported (experiments 3, 6, and 7) were performed on strains of mice that

[2] Growth index $= \dfrac{\text{Change in size of tumor}}{\text{Interval in days}} \times 10$

Size of tumor = Length plus breadth in millimeters as measured by calipers; estimated error less than 10 per cent.

normally develop primary lung tumors. At the termination of these investigations it seemed expedient to utilize the postmortem examination records to study the effects of the high-fat diet on the formation of primary lung tumors. Primary epithelial lung tumors were found in relatively equal numbers in the control and high-fat groups. However, one must consider that these results were observed in animals which were not much over one year of age, well before the maximum number of lung tumors is expected. The tumors in both groups were, on the average, from 1 to 3 mm. in diameter. Table VIII shows the results of this study. It is evident that a high-fat diet has no significant effect upon the genesis of primary lung tumors. Watson and Mellanby (10) reported that there was a slight increase in the number of lung tumors in their high-fat groups. However, it is difficult to compare our finding with theirs since they considered only lung tumors in animals with tumors of the skin while we considered only those of animals free from other tumors. They stated that the lung tumors in their animals were both metastatic tumors and primary lung tumors, and it is probable that the metastatic tumors were more numerous in the high-fat animals since their skin tumors were formed earlier.

TABLE VIII: THE DIVERSE EFFECTS OF A HIGH-FAT DIET ON THE FORMATION OF DIFFERENT TYPES OF TUMORS

Type of tumor	Group experiment number	Number of mice (effective total)	Tumors, per cent	Mean time of appearance, weeks
Spontaneous breast carcinoma	F12: control	44	32	72 ± 5.7 *
	F11: high-fat	44	55	70 ± 3.1
	F22: control	50	32	74 ± 3.1
	F21: high-fat	50	64	62 ± 1.8
Induced skin tumors	K2: control	43	51	24 ± 1.7 †
	K1: high-fat	42	67	23 ± 1.3
	S0: control	49	27	34 ± 3.0
	S1: high-fat	50	35	31 ± 2.8
	S10: control	50	68	31 ± 1.8
	S11: high-fat	50	78	27 ± 2.2
Induced sarcomas	L30: control	39	49	25 ± 1.4 †
	L1: high-fat	40	30	25 ± 2.7
	L60: control	40	18	28 ± 3.5
	L61: high-fat	37	16	29 ± 3.9
Primary lung tumors	K2: control	15	52	52 ‡
	K1: high-fat	9	44	
	L30: control	15	27	62
	L1: high-fat	16	25	
	L60: control	29	34	60
	L61: high-fat	25	36	

* Mean age of mice.
† Mean time after first application of carcinogen.
‡ Mean age of mice at time of examination.

DISCUSSION

The most striking result of these investigations is the diversity of effects produced by a high-fat diet: The incidence of spontaneous breast carcinoma in the mouse was significantly increased; the formation of induced skin tumors was also increased, but probably to a lesser extent; the primary lung tumor incidence was unaffected; and the formation of induced sarcomas was unaffected or actually inhibited. Furthermore, whenever an increase in the incidence of tumors occurred, there was also a shortening of the mean time of appearance. The results, summarized in Table VIII, are the outcome of investigations in which: (a) at least 2 experiments were performed with each type of tumor; (b) various strains of mice were used; (c) adequate numbers of animals were employed; (d) the experiments were continued for a sufficiently long period; (e) the general health of both the control and experimental groups was good; and (f) the number of nontumor deaths was not unusual and was of the same order in both groups.

Some investigators have reported that fat-enriched diets produced a decided greasiness of the skin in their animals. We have noted only the slightest oiliness of the skin in animals on the diets containing 31 per cent fat, and none in the animals on the diet containing 12 per cent fat. The animals on the high-fat diets were heavier, in general, and had a greater proportion of fat, as well as more, in the fat depots (subcutaneous, genital, perirenal, mesenteric, etc.).

The assumption is made that in a qualitative sense the diverse effects of a fat-enriched diet observed in these experiments are essentially real, and dependent on the type of tumor. There is no reason to believe that fat must act in only one way. It seems to us that the effects reported in this communication may be the resultant of two properties of fat: (a) "solvent action" on the carcinogen; and (b) "cocarcinogenic action" on the developing tumor cell. Under certain conditions solvent action may concentrate the carcinogen in a particular area, while under other conditions it may remove the carcinogen, as from a site of injection. Cocarcinogenic action may be considered to be a metabolic stimulation of carcinogenesis. In the light of this hypothesis the effect of a high-fat diet on the genesis of the tumors studied will be discussed.

Spontaneous breast tumors.—It is possible that a high-fat diet increases the formation of spontaneous breast tumors principally through the action of larger quantities of estrogenic hormone held in solution in the larger amounts of adipose tissue surrounding the breasts of mice on a fat-enriched diet. For this type of tumor the solvent action and cocarcinogentic action may act together to produce the augmentation observed.

Induced skin tumors.—According to Beck and Peacock (3) chemical carcinogens disappear from the surface of mouse skin within a few days. Using simi-lar methods we have found that the carcinogen tends to disappear somewhat more rapidly from the surface of the skin of mice that are on a high-fat diet. This suggests that the carcinogen may be carried into the skin more rapidly in such mice. There is at least one fact, however, that argues against solvent action as the cause of the observed augmentation of tumor formation: Experiments in which fat-enriched diets were fed during various phases of the tumor process (6, 8) suggest that fat feeding in the period *following* the application of the carcinogen is more effective in increasing the formation of tumors. This fact, however, is compatible with the view that the increased tumor incidence is due to cocarcinogenic action.

Induced sarcomas.—Baumann, Jacobi, and Rusch (2) carried out experiments with large dosages of carcinogen (0.5 to 1.25 mgm.), obtaining high percentages of tumors in both the control and high-fat groups. There was no significant difference in tumor formation. On the other hand, our experiments were carried out with 0.1 and 0.15 mgm. of 3,4-benzpyrene and resulted in what may be an inhibition of tumor formation. It is possible that this lack of agreement may be due to different dosages [3] of carcinogen.

It is generally believed that the injected carcinogen gradually disappears from the animal's body. It is probably removed from the injected solvent by a partition between the solvent and the subcutaneous tissue (fat) of the animal. Through increased solvent action a given amount of carcinogen, dissolved in a medium such as lard, would probably be removed at a faster rate if injected into subcutaneous tissue containing large amounts of fat (high-fat group) than if injected into subcutaneous tissue of normal animals (control group). Under these conditions a comparatively smaller "effective dose" (in contrast to the amount injected) would remain at the injection site in the high-fat animals, resulting in fewer tumors. This view is given credence since: (a) in our high-fat animals the lard cysts disappeared more rapidly, suggesting that there may also be a more rapid removal of the carcinogen from the injection site; and (b) Peacock and Beck (7) have shown that groups of mice in which the carcinogen was retained at the site of injection for a shorter time developed fewer tumors.

The difference between the removal rates of carcinogen in the control and the high-fat group may result, depending on the original dose of carcinogen, in diverse effects. It is probable that the rate of

---

[3] It is now generally believed that a dose of carcinogen large enough to produce tumors in practically 100 per cent of the animals employed may mask or override the effect of an experimental procedure. A smaller dose might permit the effect to be disclosed. The effectiveness of a given quantity of carcinogen is dependent on many factors. In referring to a dose as "high" we imply that in a particular experimental procedure this dose produced tumors in practically all the animals; a "low" dose, on the other hand, is one that produces only a small percentage of tumors even when the experiment is permitted to continue throughout the life span of the animals.

removal of carcinogen from an injection site is proportional to the original dose of carcinogen. Bryan and Shimkin (4) have shown that if the percentage of tumors induced by a given dose of carcinogen is plotted against the logarithm of the dose, an ʃ-shaped curve is obtained. Consequently, it may be expected that proportionate decreases (due to a high-fat diet) in the effective dosage of carcinogen would result in a lesser effect on tumor incidence when the injected dose is either high or low (at the extremities of the ʃ-curve) than when the carcinogen is injected in intermediate amounts (middle of the ʃ-curve). This hypothesis would explain the negative results of Baumann, Jacobi, and Rusch (2), in which high dosages were used, the negative results of our own experiment 7, in which a low dosage was used, and the decrease in tumor incidence observed in our experiment 6, in which an intermediate dosage was employed.

Primary lung tumors.—The incidence of this type of tumor is unaffected by a high-fat diet. This may be due to the fact that fat is not deposited in the lung; thus, neither the solvent action nor the cocarcinogenic action of fat would be expected to exert any effect on the formation of primary lung tumors.

Growth of tumors formed in animals on a high-fat diet.—Baumann, Jacobi, and Rusch (2) found that the growth rate of tumors of the ear in mice, induced by ultraviolet light, appears to be unaffected by a high-fat diet. In our experiments with induced sarcomas there was no significant difference in the mean growth rate of tumors developing in animals of the control and fat-enriched groups. These results are not unexpected since it is probable that only dietary changes which drastically affect the health and weight of a tumor-bearing animal will significantly alter the growth rate of its tumor.

Significance.—The same factors which lead to an increased incidence of cancer in mice on a high-fat diet may be responsible for the increased incidence of cancer observed in overweight human subjects (9). It should also be pointed out that these investigations indicate the danger of generalizing from the results of an experimental procedure on only one type of tumor.

SUMMARY

1. By utilizing the spontaneous breast carcinoma, induced skin tumor, induced sarcoma, and primary lung tumor of the mouse, the effects of a high-fat diet on the genesis of tumors were studied.

2. The most striking result of these investigations is the diversity of effects produced by a high-fat diet: (a) The incidence of the spontaneous breast carcinoma was significantly increased. (b) The incidence of the induced skin tumor was increased. (c) The incidence of the primary lung tumor was unaffected. (d) The incidence of the induced sarcoma was unaffected or actually inhibited.

3. A high-fat diet not only produced a definite increase in the incidence of spontaneous breast and induced skin tumors, but also shortened the mean time of appearance of these tumors.

4. The mean growth rate of sarcomas arising in the high-fat group was not significantly different from that of sarcomas arising in the control group.

5. A twofold action of a high-fat diet (solvent action and cocarcinogenic action) is postulated to explain the diverse effects on tumor formation.

REFERENCES

1. BAUMANN, C. A., and RUSCH, H. P. Effect of Diet on Tumors Induced by Ultraviolet Light. Am. J. Cancer, 35:213-221. 1939.
2. BAUMANN, C. A., JACOBI, H. P., and RUSCH, H. P. The Effect of Diet on Experimental Tumor Production. Am. J. Hyg., Sect. A, 30:1-6. 1939.
3. BECK, S., and PEACOCK, P. R. The Latent Carcinogenic Action of 3:4 Benzpyrene; Results of Intermittent Applications to the Skin of Mice. Brit. J. Exper. Path., 21:227-230. 1940.
4. BRYAN, W. R., and SHIMKIN, M. B. Quantitative Analysis of Dose-Response Data Obtained with Carcinogenic Hydrocarbons. J. Nat. Cancer Inst., 1:807-833. 1941.
5. JACOBI, H. P., and BAUMANN, C. A. The Effect of Fat on Tumor Formation. Am. J. Cancer, 39:338-342. 1940.
6. LAVIK, P. S., and BAUMANN, C. A. Dietary Fat and Tumor Formation. Cancer Research, 1:181-187. 1941.
7. PEACOCK, P. R., and BECK, S. Rate of Absorption of Carcinogens and Local Tissue Reaction as Factors Influencing Carcinogenesis. Brit. J. Exper. Path., 19:315-319. 1938.
8. TANNENBAUM, A. Unpublished data.
9. TANNENBAUM, A. Relationship of Body Weight to Cancer Incidence. Arch. Path., 30:509-517. 1940.
10. WATSON, A. F., and MELLANBY, E. Tar Cancer in Mice. II: The Condition of the Skin When Modified by External Treatment or Diet, as a Factor in Influencing the Cancerous Reaction. Brit. J. Exper. Path., 11:311-322. 1930.

The Influence of a Hypervitaminosis on the Effect of 20-Methylcholanthrene on Mouse Prostate Glands Grown *in Vitro*

*by Ilse Lasnitzki**

From the Strangeways Research Laboratory, Cambridge.

EXPERIMENTS suggest that vitamin A influences the direction and type of differentiation in the epidermis and mucous epithelium. Thus lack of the vitamin was found to produce squamous keratinising epithelium in organs which normally are lined by mucous producing ciliating cells, as in the respiratory tract of rats and guinea-pigs (Wolbach and Howe, 1925, 1928) while in vitamin A deficient rats the prostate glands showed squamous metaplasia of the alveolar epithelium (Bern, 1952).

On the other hand, high doses of the vitamin given either systemically (Studer and Frey, 1949) or locally (Sabella, Bern and Kahn, 1951) caused a thickening of the epidermis in rats, particularly of the stratum granulosum. Recently, Fell and Mellanby (1953) grew embryonic chick ectoderm in the presence of excess vitamin A *in vitro* and found that keratinisation was suppressed and mucous-producing ciliating epithelium, histologically similar to that of the nasal mucosa, differentiated instead.

It has been shown in previous work (Lasnitzki, 1951) that 20-methylcholanthrene added to the medium of mouse prostate glands *in vitro* induces hyperplasia and squamous metaplasia of the alveolar epithelium, changes which become more pronounced after withdrawal of the carcinogen. It seemed possible that high doses of vitamin A might alter the response of the tissue to 20-methylcholanthrene and in the present investigation the influence of excess vitamin A on the carcinogenic effect was studied.

Three groups of experiments were made. In the first, vitamin A alone was added to the medium, in the second excess vitamin was given simultaneously with 20-methylcholanthrene, and in the third it was administered to cultures previously treated with the carcinogen. Two concentrations of vitamin and of 20-methylcholanthrene were used.

---

* Sir Halley Stewart Fellow.

MATERIAL AND TECHNIQUE.

The explants consisted of the ventral prostate glands of C3H mice of 3 months of age. They were grown by the watchglass technique (Lasnitzki, 1951, 1954) on clots consisting of a mixture of fowl plasma, rat plasma, chick embryo extract and human serum containing the carcinogen. The total amount of medium per watchglass was 0·5 ml.

One half of the paired gland was grown with excess vitamin A, alone or with the carcinogen added either simultaneously or subsequently, while the other half was kept as a control in normal medium or with 20-methylcholanthrene alone (Me control). The period of cultivation was either 10 or 20 days, and the explants were transferred to a fresh medium every 3–4 days. In all, 102 explants, corresponding to 51 whole ventral prostate glands, were grown.

The fowl plasma used for the experimental cultures contained either 2000 or 3000 i.u. per 100 ml. of added vitamin A in alcoholic solution. Its strength was such that the final plasma contained 0·2 per cent or less ethanol. In each experiment the same quantity of ethanol was added to the control plasma. Most of the vitamin in the artificially reinforced plasma was in a fat soluble form in contrast to the natural vitamin which is water soluble (Fell and Mellanby, 1952). Since the fowl plasma constituted one half of the total medium the final concentrations amounted to 1000 or 1500 i.u. per 100 ml. The vitamin A content of normal fowl plasma is 200–300 i.u./100 ml. while that of normal mouse plasma is 20–60 i.u./100 ml. The concentration in the normal control medium was therefore slightly hypervitaminotic for the mouse prostate gland.

The carcinogen was suspended in human serum ; 0·06 ml. or 0·15 ml. of a 0·3 per cent solution of 20-methylcholanthrene in acetone was shaken into 4 ml. of serum. 0·025 ml. or one drop of this suspension containing 1 μg. or 2·5 μg. were added to the culture medium bringing the final concentrations to 2μg. or 5 μg./ml.

The experiments were arranged as follows :

I. *Vitamin A alone.*

Experimental cultures were grown with (1) 1000 i.u. and (2) 1500 i.u. of vitamin A for 11 days ; the two sets of controls were kept in normal medium for the same period.

II. *20-methylcholanthrene combined with vitamin A.*

(*a*) Control cultures were kept in medium containing 2 μg. of 20-methylcholanthrene alone for 10 days and then fixed (Me controls).

(*b*) Experimental cultures were treated with 2 μg. of 20-methylcholanthrene and 1000 i.u. of vitamin A for the same period and then fixed.

(*c*) Control cultures (Me controls) were kept in medium containing (1) 2 μg. and (2) 5 μg. of 20-methylcholanthrene per ml. for 11 days followed by cultivation in normal medium for 9 days.

(*d*) Experimental cultures were kept in medium containing (1) 2 μg of 20-methylcholanthrene and 1000 i.u. of vitamin A and (2) 5 μg of 20-methylcholanthrene and 1500 i.u. of vitamin A for 11 days followed by cultivation in normal medium for 9 days.

III. *20-methylcholanthrene followed by vitamin A.*

(*a*) Control cultures (Me controls) received (1) 2 μg. and (2) 5 μg. of 20-methylcholanthrene for 11 days followed by cultivation in normal medium for 9 days.

(*b*) Experimental cultures were grown for 11 days with (1) 2 μg. and (2) 5 μg. of 20-methylcholanthrene followed by cultivation in media containing (1) 1000 i.u., and (2) 1500 i.u. of vitamin A for 9 days.

At the end of the experimental period the explants were fixed in 2 per cent acetic Zenker's fluid for 30 minutes, washed in distilled water, dehydrated, embedded in paraffin and serial sections of 6 μ thickness were cut. The sections were stained with haematoxylin-eosin, or by the periodic-acid Schiff method with diastase digestion.

The symbols $+$ and $++$ are used in Tables I, II and III to give a measure of the incidence and extent of hyperplasia and metaplasia in treated cultures. Hyperplasia $+$ signifies that up to half the total number of alveoli in the explant show epithelial proliferation to form 3–6 layers of cells ; hyperplasia $++$ signifies that half or more of the total number of alveoli are hyperplastic with partial or complete occlusion of the lumen in half the hyperplastic alveoli. Metaplasia $+$ means squamous changes in up to half the number of hyperplastic alveoli, $++$ in half to all hyperplastic alveoli.

RESULTS.

The ventral prostate gland of a 3-month-old mouse consists of alveoli lined with one row of cuboidal or cylindrical epithelium (Fig. 1) which is rarely folded, in contrast to that from younger animals. The lumina are fairly wide and the secretory epithelium often shows pycnosis and is shed into the lumen.

Control cultures.—Two types of growth can be distinguished *in vitro.* The proliferation of unorganised fibroblasts which surround the explant and are removed at every transfer and the development of differentiated alveoli which are carried over at subcultivation (Fig. 2). The newly formed alveoli resemble those *in vivo,* are lined with one layer of cuboidal or cylindrical secretory epithelium the free surface of which is usually covered by a thin homogeneous layer of PAS positive material. Occasionally reserve cells are seen between the lining epithelium and the basement membrane. The epithelium *in vitro* is more folded and the lumen is narrower than *in vivo* and degeneration is absent in the layer bordering the lumen. The connective tissue is slightly increased as compared with the gland *in vivo* and alveoli are surrounded by concentric strands of collagenous fibres, while fibroblasts and thinner fibres diffusely fill the interalveolar spaces.

I. *Vitamin A alone.*

Explants grown for 10 days with 1000 i.u. of vitamin A alone show no changes as compared with their untreated controls. The folding and height of the alveolar epithelium and the amount of connective tissue are similar in both sets of cultures. In explants treated with the higher dose (1500 i.u.), however, more PAS positive material can be distinguished, which is deposited in coarse granules between and in front of the secretory cells.

II. *20-methylcholanthrene combined with Vitamin A.*

The effect on prostatic epithelium of 20-methylcholanthrene alone has been described in detail elsewhere (Lasnitzki, 1951), so need be only briefly recapitulated here and those points emphasized which are of importance in connection with the action of vitamin A.

Since 1951 many prostate cultures from mice of different ages have been treated with the carcinogen and the results obtained confirmed those of the earlier experiments. Application of the carcinogen is followed by increased proliferation of the reserve cells resulting in many layers of densely crowded cells, which partially or completely occlude the alveolar lumen. At the beginning of treatment these cells are round or columnar with distinct spherical or oval basophilic nuclei. Between the 10th and 20th day of growth, i.e. after withdrawal of the carcinogen which is discontinued after the 10th or 11th day, hyperplasia becomes more extensive and stratification and squame formation of the hyperplastic epithelium begins (Fig. 3). In hyperplastic alveoli the periphery is occupied by actively dividing cells corresponding to the basal cells in stratified epithelium, and an inner layer of prickle cells. There is a gradual increase in cell size towards the centre due to enlargement of the cytoplasm which stains pink with eosin. In such cells the nuclei are usually shrunk and stain very faintly with haemotoxylin-eosin. The original secretory epithelium degenerates, is shed and replaced by flat cells orientated with their long axis parallel to the lumen. In some cultures keratin is formed from such cells, in others they degerate without cornifying and are sloughed (Fig. 4). The onset of squamous metaplasia and the proportion of basal to prickle and cornifying cells is related to the concentration of the carcinogen : after a lower dose there are usually more basal cells and squamous changes occur later, whereas after the higher dose more squamous cells are formed and the onset of metaplasia is accelerated.

Of six explants treated for 10 days with 20-methylcholanthrene three show slight and one more extensive hyperplasia, while squamous changes have not yet begun (Table I, Column 1).

Addition of 1000 i.u. per 100 ml. of vitamin A to the medium does not modify these effects of the carcinogen. Thus, in 4 out of 7 treated explants there is mild hyperplasia but no squamous metaplasia (Table I, Column 2).

Explants grown with 2 μg. of 20-methylcholanthrene for 11 days and maintained in normal medium for a further 9 days, show hyperplasia which is extensive in 3 and less so in 4 cultures, while marked metaplasia appears in 4 explants. After 5 μg., both hyperplasia and squamous metaplasia are more pronounced than after the lower concentration (Table II, Column 1).

Application of 1000 and 1500 i.u. of the vitamin simultaneously with 20-methylcholanthrene for 11 days followed by cultivation in normal medium for 9 days does not alter the incidence or extent of epithelial hyperplasia (Table II, Column 2), but the hyperplastic epithelium presents significantly different features from those of the (Me) controls (Fig. 5). At both concentrations only 2 out of 6 glands show mild squame formation which, moreover, is confined to a very small number of alveoli. In other hyperplastic alveoli the epithelium consists either of heaped up small round or oval cells, which towards the centre sometimes, but not always, assume columnar shape (Fig. 6), or stratification takes place in such a

TABLE I.—*Comparison of the Effect of 20-methylcholanthrene Alone and of 20-methylcholanthrene and Excess Vitamin A combined for 10 days.*

Treatment.	2 μg. Me + 1000 i.u. A	
	Hyperplasia.	Squamous metaplasia.
Me 10 days {	1 + + (6)* 3 + .. 2 − ..	.. 6 − ..
Me + A 10 days {	4 + (7) 3 − ..	7 − ..

* Figure in brackets gives number of treated explants.

TABLE II.—*Comparison of the Effect of (1) 20-methylcholanthrene Alone and of 20-methylcholanthrene Combined with Excess Vitamin A for 11 days, followed by Cultivation in (2) Normal Medium and (3) maintained with Excess Vitamin A followed by Normal Medium.*

Treatment.	2 μg. Me.		5 μg. Me.	
	Hyperplasia.	Squamous metaplasia.	Hyperplasia.	Squamous metaplasia.
(1) Me 11 days normal medium 9 days {	3 + + (7) 4 + ..	4 + + 2 + 1 −	5 + + (6) 1 + ..	5 + + 1 + ..
	2 μg. Me + 1000 i.u. A		5 μg. Me + 1500 i.u. A.	
(2) Me + A 11 days normal medium 9 days {	2 + + (6) 4 +	2 + 4 −	4 + + (6) 2 +	2 + 4 −
(3) Me + A 11 days, A 3 days, normal medium 6 days {	4 + (6) 2 − ..	6 −	1 + + (6) 4 + 1 −	6 − .. ..

way that the small peripheral cells are associated with layers first of columnar and then hexagonal cells ; both types show intercellular cytoplasmic bridges (Fig. 7). In contrast to the prickle cells in carcinogen-treated cultures, the cytoplasm and nuclei of these hexagonal cells are basophilic. At the lumen they are joined by cytoplasmic bridges with the innermost layer of cylindrical secretory epithelium. In Me controls the secretory epithelium usually degenerates, is sloughed and replaced by a layer of flat cells. After 2 μg. of 20-methylcholanthrene keratin is formed at the lumen ; after 5 μg., no keratin appears and instead the innermost layer of flat cells degenerates (Fig. 4). Addition of the vitamin completely suppresses the keratin formation or degeneration of the innermost layer, while the secretory epithelium is preserved in most of them. Cell divisions can be observed in all cell layers including the secretory epithelium in contrast to Me controls in which mitosis is confined to the basal cells (Fig. 8 and 9).

In glands treated with the vitamin for 3 days after withdrawal of the carcinogen followed by 6 days' cultivation in normal medium the differentiation of the hyperplastic epithelium is similarly altered. In addition, squame formation is entirely absent and the incidence of hyperplasia reduced (Table II, Column 3). Slides stained with PAS show increased mucin production in unchanged alveoli and in those with early hyperplasia, but in alveoli showing marked hyperplasia only faint traces of mucin can be distinguished in the secretory lining.

III. 20-methylcholanthrene followed by vitamin A.

Application of the vitamin for a further 9 days to explants treated for 11 days with the carcinogen inhibits or suppresses squamous changes and significantly decreases the incidence of hyperplasia (Table III, Column 2). Thus, metaplasia is missing in all, and hyperplasia found in only 2 of 6 cultures treated with 2 μg. of 20-methylcholanthrene followed by 1000 i.u. of vitamin A ; after the higher concentration 2 out of 7 cultures show slight squamous changes and 6 mild hyperplasia (Fig. 10). Stratification with squamous changes is confined to very few alveoli ; elsewhere it is absent and the hyperplastic epithelium consists of a few rows of small round or columnar cells (Fig. 11).

TABLE III.—*The Effect of Excess Vitamin A on Explants Treated Previously with 20-methylcholanthrene.*

Treatment.	2 μg. Me.		5 μg. Me.	
	Hyperplasia.	Squamous metaplasia.	Hyperplasia.	Squamous metaplasia.
(1) Me 11 days normal medium 9 days	2++ (6)	4+	9++ (10)	9++
	2+	2—	1+	1—
	2—	..	..	..
	2 μg. Me + 1000 i.u. A.		5 μg. Me + 1500 i.u. A.	
(2) Me 11 days A 9 days	2+ (6)	6—	6+ (7)	2+
	4—	..	1—	5—

DISCUSSION.

Excess vitamin A added alone to the medium of mouse prostate glands does not influence the normal development of the epithelial structures although the higher concentration causes a slight increase in the production of mucin. Simultaneous addition of the vitamin with the carcinogen, however, reduces squamous changes, suppresses keratin formation and prevents the degeneration of the secretory lining epithelium.

This result again indicates that the vitamin is an important factor in the control of both keratin- and mucin-formation. In recent experiments on spayed rats Kahn (1954) showed that vitamin A applied locally prevented cornification of the vagina after oestrogen treatment and produced stratified cuboidal epithelium instead. Dziewiatowsky (1954) provided direct experimental proof that the vitamin promotes mucin production ; thus the incorporation of S^{35} as sulphate sulphur into mucopolisaccharides was increased in A deficient rats treated with vitamin A. Similarly, Fell, Mellanby and Pelc (1954) found that the mucous metaplasia of embryonic chick ectoderm grown *in vitro* with excess vitamin A was associated with a marked uptake of S^{35} sulphate.

It is probable that the action of the vitamin is exerted primarily on the reserve or basal cells which at this stage may be capable of both types of differentiation : squamous or columnar. An interesting feature is the appearance in stratified alveoli of cytoplasmic bridges between columnar and hexagonal cells, but particularly those joining the luminal epithelium with the cell layer underneath. Cell bridges do not normally occur in columnar epithelium. The hexagonal cells resemble the prickle cells of the epidermis save for their basophily, and may be considered either not fully differentiated precursors of the eosinophilic prickle cells or a variation of the columnar cell type.

The presence of cytoplasmic bridges between the luminal epithelium and the layer of hexagonal cells suggests that the secretory elements are derived by differentiation from the former. On the other hand, since cell divisions are observed among the luminal cells it is possible that they grow independently and in spite of the stratification going on beneath them.

Administration of the vitamin to explants treated previously with 20-methylcholanthrene not only suppresses squamous changes but reduces the increased cell multiplication due to the carcinogen. The greater effectiveness of the vitamin in this group of experiments may be due to its increased uptake in the absence of competition from the carcinogen.

The reduction in hyperplasia is difficult to interpret since the mechanism by which it is brought about is, as yet, unknown. Two facts are clear however. It is unlikely to be due to a direct inhibition of mitosis since the author has shown (Lasnitzki, 1955) that excess vitamin A added to the medium of chick fibroblasts *in vitro* increases the mitotic rate as well as cell migration. Further, it is not affected by destruction of the hyperplastic epithelium like that which follows oestrone treatment of mouse prostate glands *in vitro* pretreated with 20-methylcholanthrene (Lasnitzki, 1954). It seems probable that the effect is an indirect one and that the vitamin affects the mechanism controlling the ratio of cell multiplication and differentiation. It may thus restore the normal balance of the two processes by reversing the disturbance due to the carcinogen. How this is brought about is not known.

The results suggest that the vitamin A level may have some influence on the rate of development of epithelial tumours. A slight increase above the normal may accelerate tumour growth by suppressing squamous changes, while higher concentrations, by antagonising the action of the carcinogen, may retard it.

SUMMARY.

Ventral prostate glands from 3-month-old C3H mice were grown *in vitro* by the watchglass technique with (1) excess vitamin A alone and (2) with a combination of 20-methylcholanthrene and excess vitamin applied simultaneously and successively. Two concentrations of carcinogen and vitamin were studied.

The addition of the vitamin alone does not influence growth and development of the prostatic epithelium, but the higher concentration slightly increases mucin production.

Addition of 20-methylcholanthrene alone induces hyperplasia and squamous metaplasia of the alveolar epithelium.

Simultaneous addition of vitamin A and 20-methylcholanthrene followed by cultivation in normal medium does not alter the incidence and extent of epithelial hyperplasia but suppresses keratin formation and prevents degeneration of the secretory lining epithelium. The hyperplastic epithelium consists of small basal cells, columnar elements and hexagonal basophilic cells with intercellular bridges. The latter are considered either not fully differentiated precursors of eosinophilic prickle cells or atypical columnar epithelium.

Addition of excess vitamin A to glands previously treated with 20-methylcholanthrene likewise prevents keratinisation, but it also decreases significantly the incidence and degree of hyperplasia.

I am greatly indebted to the late Sir E. Mellanby, F.R.S. for the provision of the plasma used in these experiments. I should also like to thank Dr. Honor B. Fell, F.R.S. for constructive criticism in the preparation of the manuscript, Mr. R. J. C. Stewart, chief technician at the Nutrition Building, National Institute for Medical Research, for preparing the blood plasma, and Mr. G. C. Lenney, Strangeways Research Laboratory, for the microphotographs.[1]

REFERENCES.

BERN, H. A.—(1952) *Cancer Res.*, **12**, 85.

DZIEWIATKOWSKI, D. D.—(1954) *J. exp. Med.*, **100**, 11.

FELL, H. B. AND MELLANBY, E.—(1952) *J. Physiol*, **116**, 320.—(1953) *Ibid.*, **119**, 470.

Iidem AND PELC, S. R.—(1954) *Brit. med. J.*, ii, 611.

KAHN, R. H.—(1954) *Amer. J. Anat.*, **95**, 309.

LASNITZKI, I.—(1951) *Brit. J. Cancer*, **5**, 345.—(1954) *Cancer Res.*, **14**, 632,—(1955) *Exp. Cell Res.*, **8**, 121.

SABELLA, J. D., BERN, H. A. AND KAHN, R. H.—(1951) *Proc. Soc. exp. Biol., N.Y.*, **76**, 499.

STUDER, A. AND FREY, J. R.—(1949) *Schweiz. med. Wschr.*, **79**, 382.

WOLBACH, S. B. AND HOWE, P. R.—(1925) *J. exp. Med.*, **42**, 753.—(1928) *Arch. Path.*, **5**, 239.

---

[1]Microphotographs were not included in this reprinting.

Dietary Factors Linked to Cause
and Prevention of Cancer

Mechanisms of Chemical Carcinogenesis

by Elizabeth C. Miller, Ph.D., and James A. Miller, Ph.D.

Of the known carcinogenic agents (viruses, ultraviolet and ionizing radiations, and chemicals), chemicals appear to be of major importance in the induction of human cancers. The known chemical carcinogens include a wide range of structures. Their common feature is that their ultimate forms are electrophilic reactants; in most cases, these reactants arise through metabolism *in vivo*. Carcinogenesis by chemicals is a multistage process. The first stage, initiation, occurs rapidly and appears to be irreversible. The available data indicate that initiation generally results from one or more mutations of cellular DNA. Covalent reactions of electrophilic derivatives of carcinogens with DNA are the major cause of these mutations. The second stage, promotion, occurs over a longer period of time. Promotion is a complex process, for which the early stages are largely reversible. The critical events appear to be epigenetic. Complete carcinogens have both initiating and promoting activities, but the ratios of these two activities for various chemicals may differ greatly. This knowledge of the mechanisms of carcinogens by chemicals provides a useful basis for approaches to the prevention of human cancer.
Cancer **47: 1055–1064, 1981.**

OUR KNOWLEDGE OF THE FACTORS involved in the development of human cancers, although incomplete, has increased greatly over the past few decades and, especially, in the past two decades.[16,19,25] In view of these advances and the increased concern about approaches to the prevention of human cancer, this conference on prevention and early detection is most timely. Detailed knowledge on the causes of human cancers and on the mechanisms involved in their development provides the strongest baseline from which the prevention of human cancers can be approached.

Presented at the American Cancer Society National Conference on Cancer Prevention and Detection, Chicago, Illinois, April 17–19, 1980.

From the McArdle Laboratory for Cancer Research, University of Wisconsin Medical School, Madison, Wisconsin.

Supported by Grant No. CA-07175 and CA-22484 of the National Cancer Institute, USPHS.

Address for reprints: McArdle Laboratory for Cancer Research, University of Wisconsin Medical School, 450 N. Randall Ave., Madison WI 53706.

Etiologic Agents for Cancer

Studies in experimental animals and observations on the human have demonstrated three classes of agents with the property of being carcinogenic, *i.e.*, able to induce tumors. The abilities of certain chemicals, of ultraviolet light with a wave-length of about 3000 Å, and of ionizing radiations to cause cancers in both experimental animals and humans have been documented for many years.[19,25] Exposure to ultraviolet light of the sun filtered through the stratosphere appears to be responsible for most cancers of the skin and melanomas of the skin among light-skinned individuals.[79] Although exceptional exposures to ionizing radiations have been correlated with increased incidences of certain cancers, background ionizing radiations do not appear to be a major factor in the overall incidences of human cancers.[78]

The horizontal transmission of some cancers by infectious viruses is possible in experimental animals under the special conditions available in the laboratory, but these cancers are usually not infectious under ordinary circumstances. However, horizontal transmission of leukemia occurs readily among household cats,[20] and Marek's disease, a viral leukemia, is infectious in chickens.[47] Similarly, infectious papillomas and fibromas occur in several species.[18] The possible roles of viruses as etiologic agents for human cancers are not clear. There are virally transmissible human warts,[18] and correlations have been reported between the occurrence of antibodies to hepatitis B antigens and the development of hepatocellular carcinoma in some parts of Africa and the Far East.[6] Likewise, correlations have been observed between the development of antibodies to Epstein-Barr virus antigens in certain populations and the likelihood of development of Burkitt's lymphoma or nasopharyngeal carcinoma.[87] However, in other parts of the world, infection with hepatitis B or Epstein-Barr virus is not correlated with the development of cancers, and infectious viruses are not known to play major roles as carcinogenic agents for the human.

The importance of an understanding of chemical carcinogenesis is emphasized by the known associations between human exposures to certain chemicals and the likelihood for the development of certain cancers[28] (Table 1). Thus, in specific cases, exposures in the work place have been correlated with increased cancer risks. The increased incidences of cancer of the urinary bladder in workers heavily exposed to certain aromatic amines have been recognized since the early part of this century; strong epidemiologic data clearly implicate benzidine, 2-naphthylamine, and 4-aminobiphenyl as causative factors.[28] Industrial exposures to the alkylating agents bis(chloromethyl)ether and bis(2-chloroethyl)sulfide and to certain inorganic substances (chromium and nickel compounds and asbestos) have been associated with increased risks of development of respiratory cancers.[28]

Increased cancer incidences have also resulted from the use of certain medicinal products (Table 1). These include *in utero* exposures to massive doses of diethylstilbestrol, which gave rise to increased incidences of vaginal carcinomas,[29] and to the apparent increase in the number of second primary cancers (primarily of lymphoid origin) among patients treated with large doses of some alkylating agents.[29] However, the most important of the known causes of cancer in the number of potential cancer patients and the possibility of avoidance appear to be the carcinogens to which persons are exposed as a consequence of societal habits. In this part of the world, the epidemic of lung cancer that has followed the increase in cigarette smoking in both sexes is a particularly serious problem.[22]

Evidence is accumulating that other chemicals in some human environments may also contribute to increased cancer incidences. One example is aflatoxin B_1, a product of some strains of *Aspergillus flavus* that can contaminate foods stored under warm, moist conditions. Strong correlations have been reported between the intake of this hepatotoxin and the incidence of hepatocellular carcinoma in some areas of Africa and the Far East.[50,81] Exposures to aflatoxin B_1 or related mold toxins and hepatitis B virus may interact in the causation of these cancers.[6] Evidence also points to N-nitroso derivatives formed in the gastrointestinal tract as possible etiologic agents for some human cancers.[11,76] The

TABLE 1. Chemicals Generally Recognized as Carcinogenic in Humans*

	Sites of tumor formation	Reference
Industrial exposures		
2-Naphthylamine	Urinary bladder	28, vol. 4
Benzidine	Urinary bladder	28, vol. 1
4-Aminobiphenyl	Urinary bladder	28, vol. 1 and 4
Bis(chloromethyl)ether	Lungs	28, vol. 4
Bis(2-chloroethyl)sulfide (mustard gas)	Respiratory tract	28, vol. 9
Vinyl chloride	Liver mesenchyme	28, vol. 7
Certain tars, soots, and oils	Skin, lungs	28, vol. 3
Chromium compounds	Lungs	28, vol. 2
Nickel compounds	Lungs, nasal sinuses	28, vol. 2 and 11
Asbestos	Pleura, peritoneum (lungs when combined with cigarette smoking)	28, vol. 2 and 14
Benzene	Lymphoid tissue	29, p. 24
Medical exposures		
N,N-bis(2-Chloroethyl)-2-naphthylamine (chlornaphazin)	Urinary bladder	28, vol. 4
Diethylstilbestrol	Vagina	29, p. 32
Inorganic arsenic compounds	Skin	28, vol. 2
Melphalan	Lymphoid tissue	29, p. 44
Societal exposures		
Cigarette smoke	Lungs, urinary tract, other	22
Betal nut and tobacco quid	Buccal mucosa	46

* This is a conservative list of human carcinogens for which relatively extensive data are available. Some other chemicals are also suspected of having induced cancer in humans, but the data are more limited.

etiologic agents implicated in human cancers are discussed in more detail in other papers from this symposium.

Multistage Nature of Carcinogenesis

Carcinogenesis is now generally recognized as a multistage process (Fig. 1).[71] The first stage is termed *initiation*, and the product is termed an "initiated cell." These initiated cells appear not to be tumor cells, and they cannot be recognized directly. They are known to exist in that a subsequent stage, known as *promotion*, causes them to develop into tumor cells that replicate to yield gross tumors. Although promotion is often considered to be a single stage, it requires a prolonged period and probably comprises more than one process.

The classic system for the demonstration of initiation and promotion is the induction of skin tumors in the mouse[8,9,80] (Fig. 2). Thus, as first observed in the 1940's by Rous and Kidd,[62] Mottram,[45] and Berenblum and Shubik,[4] the administration of an appropriate low dose of an initiating agent (which can be a chemical, ultraviolet light, or ionizing radiation) to mouse skin results in few or no tumors during the life span of the animal. Histologically, the treated skin appears essentially normal. However, the subsequent administration of repetitive doses over several months of a promoting agent causes the appearance of large numbers of papillomas per mouse. Continuation of the promoting treatment results at about one year in the development of carcinomas of the skin. 12-O-Tetradecanoylphorbol-13-acetate from the oil of croton seeds is an especially potent promoting agent for epidermal tumors of the mouse.[23,80] Tumors do not develop when only the initiating or only the promoting agent is administered in appropriate doses. Furthermore, tumors do not result if the promoting agent is applied before, rather than after, the initiating agent. The essentially irreversible nature of initiation is indicated by the finding that a high yield of tumors is obtained even if application of the promoting agent is delayed for many months after the administration of the initiator.[9,80] The promotion step appears to be at least partially reversible. Thus, doses of a promoter that are too low or too widely spaced render the promoter less effective, even though the total dose would be adequate for strong promotion with other dosage schedules.[8]

A two-stage system of hepatic tumor induction in rats was introduced by Peraino *et al.*[51] in 1971. They showed that the limited administration of the carcinogen 2-acetylaminofluorene and subsequent long-term administration of phenobarbital resulted in a high incidence of relatively highly differentiated hepatic carcinomas. By analogy to the skin tumor system, this limited dose of

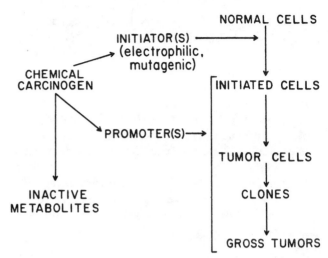

FIG. 1. A simplified scheme for the steps in the induction of cancer by a chemical.

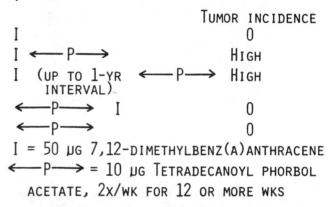

FIG. 2. Diagrammatic representation of the two-stage induction of tumors in the skin of the mouse. Typical initiators are the polycyclic aromatic hydrocarbons, ethyl carbamate, and certain alkylating agents. The most potent promoting agent known is 12-O-tetradecanoylphorbol-13-acetate. Papillomas develop in about 12–20 weeks, and carcinomas develop within one year.

2-acetylaminofluorene induced few tumors, and phenobarbital by itself was ineffective. Pitot[55] has since shown that a single dose of diethylnitrosamine or 7,12-dimethylbenz(a)anthracene administered to rats during the period of DNA synthesis after a partial hepatectomy initiates hepatic cells that give rise to gross tumors on subsequent treatment with phenobarbital. These livers, as well as livers treated by other regimens that include a dose of an initiating agent and some system for promotion,[17,44,55,63] contain large numbers of foci of hepatic cells that can be recognized by certain histochemical stains before they are readily demonstrable by staining with hematoxylin and eosin. The evidence suggests that these foci of hepatic cells are precursors of hepatic tumors, but whether or not some of the cells in these foci are neoplastic has not been determined.

Two-stage models of carcinogenesis of the urinary bladder have been devised by Hicks *et al.*[26] and by

Cohen *et al.*[13] The former group used a single small dose of N-methyl-N-nitrosourea as the initiating agent and long-term administration of high levels of sodium cyclamate or saccharin as the promoter. Cohen *et al.* showed that prolonged treatment with saccharin or tryptophan in rats previously given a marginally carcinogenic dose of N-[4-(5-nitro-2-furyl)-1-thiazolyl]formamide greatly increased the incidence of bladder carcinomas. Multiple stages in experimental carcinogenesis of the mammary gland,[1,60] thyroid,[21] and colon[60] have also been demonstrated. Similarly, separable initiation and promotion steps have been demonstrated for the malignant transformation of fibroblasts in culture by chemicals or ultraviolet light.[33,42,43]

Structural Features of Chemical Carcinogens

The known carcinogens include several groups of chemicals. There are strong structural similarities within groups but little or none between groups. Thus, there is a relatively large group of direct alkylating agents, as well as a much smaller group of direct acylating agents, that can induce tumors at sites of application (Fig. 3). There is also a large group of carcinogenic polycyclic aromatic hydrocarbons, which can be formed as products of incomplete combustions, and which can induce tumors in a wide variety of tissues (Fig. 4). The aromatic amide and amine carcinogens can produce tumors in a variety of tissues, but they are frequently most active in the induction of hepatic, urinary bladder, and mammary tumors. The N-nitrosamines and N-nitrosamides comprise a large group of versatile and potent carcinogens, many of which are active in a wide variety of species and tissues. Unlike the other examples shown in Figure 4, ethyl carbamate and ethionine appear to be structurally unique carcinogens.

The approximately 30 known chemical carcinogens that are products of plants and microorganisms are illustrated by the varied structures shown in Figure 5.[39,64] These include the potent hepatic carcinogen aflatoxin B_1, which was noted above as a possible factor in the high levels of hepatocellular carcinoma in some areas of the world. There is no evidence for a role in human cancer of any of the other known naturally occurring carcinogens, although cyasin and the pyrrolizidine alkaloids with an α,β-unsaturated ester are potent experimental hepatocarcinogens. By contrast, safrole is a relatively weak hepatocarcinogen.

Electrophilic Reactivity as a Requirement for Initiating Activity

It was early recognized that chemical carcinogens are metabolized to a variety of products that lack the ability

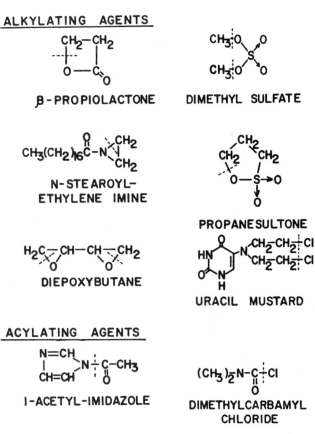

FIG. 3. Examples of direct-acting chemical carcinogens.

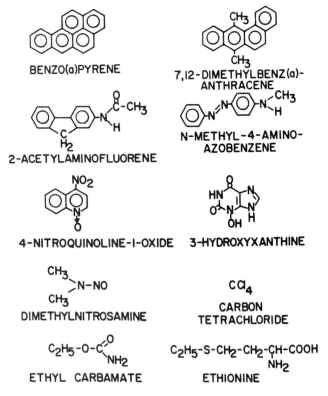

FIG. 4. Examples of the variety of synthetic chemical carcinogens that require metabolic activation.

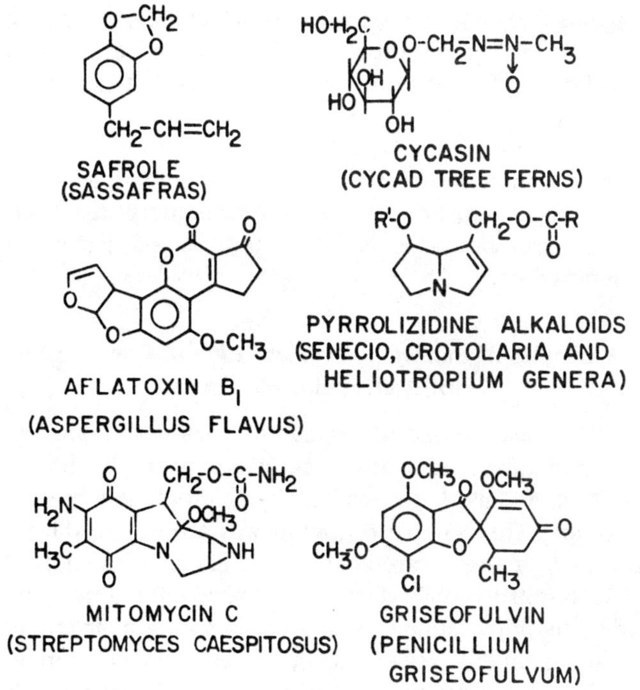

FIG. 5. The structures of some chemical carcinogens that are products of plants and microorganisms.

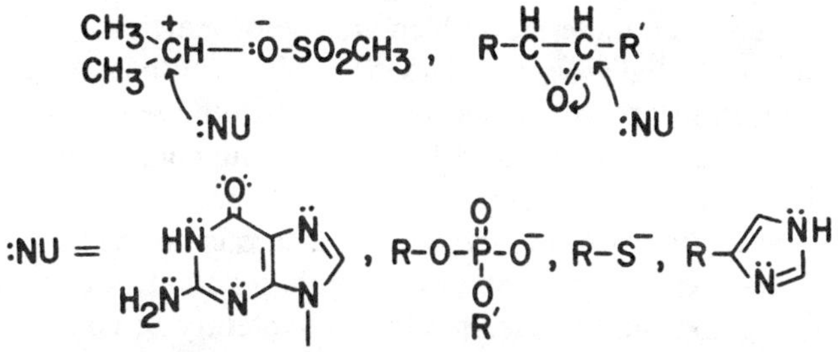

FIG. 6. Examples of strong electrophilic reactants and their reactions with nucleophiles (:NU) through sharing of electron pairs of electron-rich atoms.

to induce tumors (Fig. 1). In the past 20 years, it has also become evident that most chemical carcinogens, other than the direct alkylating and direct acylating carcinogens, must be metabolically activated *in vivo* to derivatives that we have termed "ultimate carcinogens", *i.e.*, the derivatives that are actually involved in the induction of tumors.[36,40] The balance between metabolism to active and inactive metabolites is one of the critical factors in the carcinogenic potencies of chemicals. Further, unless the test system provides initiating or promoting activity from some other source, chemicals that will be recognized as carcinogenic must have both initiating and promoting activity either directly or through one or more metabolites.

An initiating chemical has the special property of being a strong electrophilic reactant and thus of being able to combine chemically with nucleophilic sites in the target cells, including the informational macromolecules DNAs, RNAs, and proteins (Fig. 6).[36,40] The electrophilic reactivity depends on the presence of uncharged or positively charged electron-deficient atoms. Electrophiles react nonenzymatically to form covalent bonds through the sharing of electron pairs from nucleophilic atoms. Because of the metabolism of some precarcinogens to more than one ultimate electrophilic form and because of the multiple nucleophilic sites in the macromolecules, multiple DNA-, RNA-, and protein-bound derivatives of many carcinogens have been observed when the studies have been sufficiently detailed.

Although epigenetic processes are not excluded, initiation apparently occurs primarily through genetic events.[36,84] The genetic basis of initiation is suggested by the rapid, irreversible nature of the event and by the reaction of electrophilic carcinogens with DNA to yield carcinogen-DNA adducts. In some cases, the formation of certain adducts has been correlated with the occurrence of mutations in appropriate systems.[49,86] The persistence of the altered bases in DNA and the fixation of errors by erroneous base-pairing during replication of the DNA (*i.e.*, the development of mutations) appear to be critical factors in the process of initiation.[49] Further support for the genetic basis of carcinogenesis by chemicals has come from the development of stable, revertible temperature-sensitive malignant transformants of BHK cells on treatment with certain chemical carcinogens.[7] The development of malignant cells by transfection with DNA from cells malignantly transformed by chemicals[67] appears to be an important approach to the demonstration of the mutagenic basis of initiation. However, the recent report of the malignant transformation of cells by transfection with small pieces of DNA from normal cells[15] indicates that the interpretation of the experiments with DNA from chemically transformed cells may be complicated.

Overall, the data are quite compelling in suggesting that most tumors are probably initiated through one or more changes in the informational content of the DNA. However, other data suggest that some cancer cells may arise by epigenetic mechanisms.[35,41,54] The most convincing of these is the experimental observations of Mintz and her colleagues[41] and others on the ability of individual mouse teratocarcinoma cells implanted in mouse blastoceles to differentiate and to give rise to a variety of apparently normal somatic cells. These experiments indicate that the teratocarcinoma cells have genetic information that is consistent with normal controlled growth, at least under some circumstances.

Properties Associated with Promotion

The essential natures of tumor promoters and the basic interactions essential to the promotion of tumors are less well understood than are the properties of initiators and the process of initiation.[14,80] As noted earlier, promotion appears to occur over a prolonged period and to be at least partially reversible. The potent tumor promoter 12-O-tetradecanoylphorbol-13-acetate appears to be active without metabolism. There is no evidence for its conversion to an electrophilic reactant, it is not mutagenic, and it does not bind covalently to cellular macromolecules.[5,23,73] 12-O-Tetradecanoylphorbol-13-acetate causes a wide variety of pleiotropic responses both in cultured cells and in epidermal cells of the whole animal. In mouse epidermis, these effects include rapid increases in phospholipid synthesis, RNA synthesis, and induction of ornithine decarboxylase activity; enhancement of DNA synthesis and the mitotic rate follow within 24 hours.[9,14,80] In addition to the above responses, the phorbol esters and several related macrocyclic plant diterpenes cause increases in specific proteases, alterations in the degree of terminal differentiation, alterations in growth properties, and modifications of the membranes of cells grown in culture.[14,77,80,83] None of the individual responses has been unequivocally identified as critical to the tumor-promoting activity. However, the ability to induce these responses has generally correlated well with tumor-promoting activity within this class of promoting agents, and it seems likely that the primary target may be the cell membrane.[83] Where tested, other chemically unrelated compounds (e.g., anthralin, Tween 80, and acetic acid) that show weaker promoting activity for mouse skin cause qualitatively similar, but smaller, changes as compared with those observed after application of the phorbol esters to the skin.[48]

Chemicals, such as phenobarbital and certain chlorinated lipophilic hydrocarbons,[51,56] that are promoters for hepatic carcinogenesis similarly do not appear to require conversion to electrophilic or mutagenic intermediates for activity.[57,65] To the extent that they have been studied, these hepatic tumor promoters do not cause effects on the differentiation of cells similar to those characteristic of the phorbol esters.[32] However, unlike the phorbol esters, they cause the induction of increased levels of some species of cytochrome P-450 and their associated oxygenase activities both in the liver and other tissues.[58,65,72] They also cause increased synthesis of certain other enzymes.[58,65,72]

Both the promoters for skin tumor formation and those for hepatic tumor formation cause hyperplasia of the target tissues.[9,65] It is possible that hyperplasia is critical to the promoting activity, but not all hyperplastic agents have shown tumor-promoting activity.

For carcinogenesis by a chemical that has both initiating and promoting activities (*i.e.*, a complete carcinogen), the ultimate initiating and ultimate promoting agents from a given precarcinogen can theoretically be the same or different metabolites of the carcinogen. Although the known promoting agents that lack initiating activity are not electrophilic reactants, it is possible, and even likely, that in some situations electrophilic metabolites may be involved in promotion as well as in initiation. For their promoting activity, reactions with proteins and RNA's may be of particular importance.

Examples of the Metabolic Activation of Carcinogens to Electrophilic Reactants

The best studied of the carcinogens with regard to their metabolic activation and reactivity are the donors of simple alkyl groups, such as ethyl and methyl groups. The N-nitroso compounds are important examples of these carcinogens. Metabolic activation of the N-nitroso-dialkylamines, typified in Figure 7 by dimethylnitrosamine, is catalyzed by a cytochrome P-450-dependent oxygenase in the endoplasmic reticulum.[34] Oxidative removal of one N-alkyl group yields the corresponding monoalkylnitrosamine. These derivatives are unstable and rearrange spontaneously to electrophilic alkyldiazonium ions. The N-nitrosamides, on the other hand, do not require enzymatic activation, since their nonenzymatic reaction with water or other cellular nucleophiles under physiologic conditions results in the formation of the same alkyldiazonium ion.[34] This ion apparently initiates carcinogenesis by alkylation of some critical nucleophilic sites on the DNA.

For these simple alkylating agents, correlative data on the levels of alkylation of the oxygen at carbon-6 of guanine in DNA, on the persistence of this alkylated base in the DNA, and on the induction of tumors suggest that alkylation of the O^6 atoms of guanine residues in DNA may be one of the critical reactions involved in

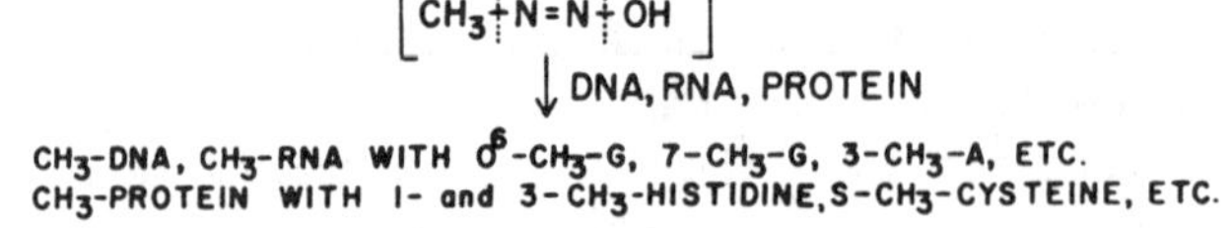

CH$_3$-DNA, CH$_3$-RNA WITH O^6-CH$_3$-G, 7-CH$_3$-G, 3-CH$_3$-A, ETC.
CH$_3$-PROTEIN WITH I- and 3-CH$_3$-HISTIDINE, S-CH$_3$-CYSTEINE, ETC.

FIG. 7. The *in vivo* conversion of dimethylnitrosamine and of N-methyl-N-nitrosourea to a reactive electrophile and its reaction with cellular macromolecules.

tumor initiation by these compounds.[49] Some exceptions to these correlations have been reported. Whether these exceptions provide evidence that the O^6-alkylation may not be a key factor or whether lower tumor induction than expected for the levels of O^6-alkylguanines in DNA was due to other causes, such as the lack of an adequate promotion system, is not clear. Information on the levels and persistence of O-alkyl derivatives of cytosine and thymine in DNA is also essential, since the formation of these derivatives appears to parallel the alkylation of O^6 of guanine residues in DNA.[70] Like O^6-alkylguanines, O^4-alkylthymines are proven promutagenic lesions,[49] and recent evidence has been presented for persistence of O^2-ethylthymidine in DNA.[74]

2-Acetylaminofluorene: 2-Acetylaminofluorene is one of the more complex carcinogens for which the metabolic activation has been worked out for one tissue in some detail. The first step in its activation in the rat liver is N-hydroxylation by the cytochrome P-450 system in the endoplasmic reticulum with the formation of N-hydroxy-2-acetylaminofluorene[40] (Fig. 8). This proximate carcinogen is further metabolized by a soluble liver sulfotransferase activity to form the ester 2-acetylaminofluorene-N-sulfate, which appears to be a major ultimate carcinogenic metabolite in rat liver. Thus, the sulfuric acid ester is a very strong electrophile with the ability to modify the informational content of DNA, as evidenced by its high mutagenic activity in a bacterial transforming DNA system.[40] Further, the level of hepatic sulfotransferase activity has been correlated with susceptibility to hepatic tumor formation,[40] and the hepatotoxicity and hepatocarcinogenicity of N-hydroxy-2-acetylaminofluorene for the rat were decreased when the diet was manipulated to reduce the amount of available sulfate *in vivo*.[85]

The multiplicity of electrophilic metabolites of potential importance in carcinogenesis that can be generated from a given precarcinogen has been exemplified by the studies on 2-acetylaminofluorene. In addition to the N-sulfate, three other pathways catalyzed by mammalian enzymes are known for the generation of electrophilic metabolites[38] (Fig. 9). N-Acetoxy-2-acetylaminofluorene, another reactive ester, and 2-nitrosofluorene arise through a dismutation of a nitroxide free radical, which is a product of a peroxidative attack on N-hydroxy-2-acetylaminofluorene.[3] The strong electrophilic ester N-acetoxy-2-aminofluorene is a product of a reaction catalyzed by an acetyl transferase found in many tissue.[2,31] Some studies have implicated this electrophile or N-hydroxy-2-aminofluorene as an important intermediate in the mutagenicity of N-hydroxy-2-acetylaminofluorene for *Salmonella typhimurium* strains.[66,82] The O-glucuronide, a major metabolite of N-hydroxy-2-acetylaminofluorene, is also electrophilic,

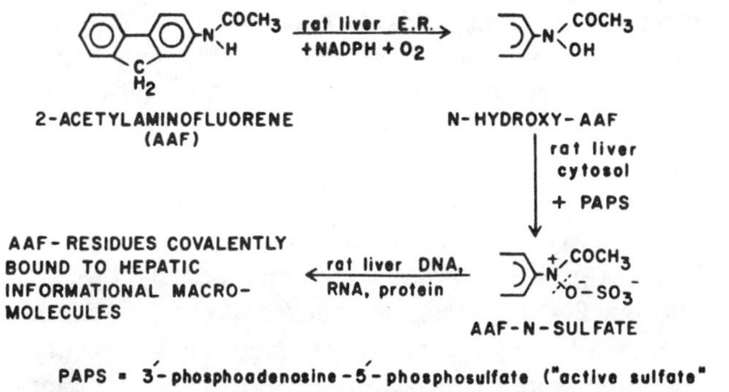

FIG. 8. The major pathway for the metabolic activation of 2-acetylaminofluorene for carcinogenesis in the rat liver. E.R.: endoplasmic reticulum.

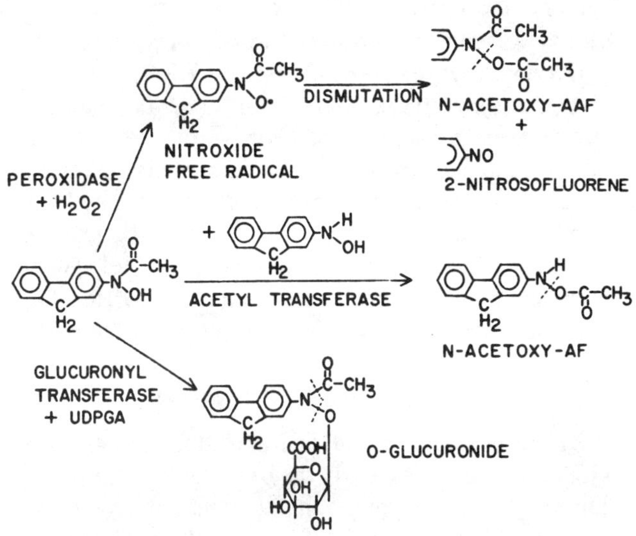

FIG. 9. Pathways, in addition to the formation of the sulfuric acid ester, for the metabolism of N-hydroxy-2-acetylaminofluorene to electrophilic reactants in rat liver. N-ACETOXY-AAF: N-acetoxy-2-acetylaminofluorene; N-ACETOXY-AF: N-acetoxy-2-amino fluorene; UDPGA: uridine diphosphoglucuronic acid.

although much weaker than the other metabolites just mentioned.[37]

Polycyclic aromatic hydrocarbons: The metabolism of the polycyclic aromatic hydrocarbons has been a subject of detailed study in many laboratories. As early as 1950, Boyland[10] suggested that the metabolically formed phenols and dihydrodiols then known might be secondary products and that the primary oxidation products might be epoxides. Derivatives in which the epoxides were in the K-region were the first to be synthesized and studied. These K-region epoxides are electrophilic, mutagenic, and able to cause malignant transformation of cells in culture.[24,68] However, based on differences between the properties of the DNA-adducts formed from nonenzymatic reaction of these K-region epoxides *in vitro* and those found in cells treated with the parent hydrocarbons,[24] seminal studies by Sims, Grover, and their colleagues[69,75] with benz(a)anthracene and benzo(a)pyrene first focused attention on the formation *in vivo* of dihydrodiol epoxides of the hydrocarbons.[52]

The dihydrodiol epoxides are formed in a three-step reaction, as shown for benzo(a)pyrene (Fig. 10). With benzo(a)pyrene, epoxidation catalyzed by the cytochrome P-450 system first occurs at the 7,8-position. The resulting epoxide is very susceptible to hydrolysis by an epoxide hydrase in the endoplasmic reticulum, and the resulting 7,8-dihydrodiol is a substrate for further epoxidation at the 9,10-position in a stereoselective manner. The very high electrophilic reactivity of this dihydrodiol epoxide, its very high mutagenic activity, and its strong activity for the initiation of lung adenomas when administered to newborn mice makes (+)7β,8α-dihydroxy-9α,10α-epoxy-7,8,9,10-tetrahydrobenzo(a)pyrene the major candidate as an ultimate carcinogenic metabolite of benzo(a)pyrene.[12] Studies with a number of other polycyclic aromatic hydrocarbons indicate that the formation of similar dihydrodiol epoxides, in which the epoxide is in the "bay region" formed by the angular rings, may be a relatively general mechanism for the enzymatic activation of the polycyclic aromatic hydrocarbons for carcinogenesis.[30]

Perspectives for Prevention

Where possible, avoidance or reduction of contact with carcinogens is clearly the best strategy for prevention of cancer. The generalization that strong electrophilic reactivity is a basic requirement for the initiation of carcinogenesis and detailed knowledge of the enzyme systems involved in the metabolic activation and deactivation of many chemicals are providing important tools for recognition of potential carcinogens. Such

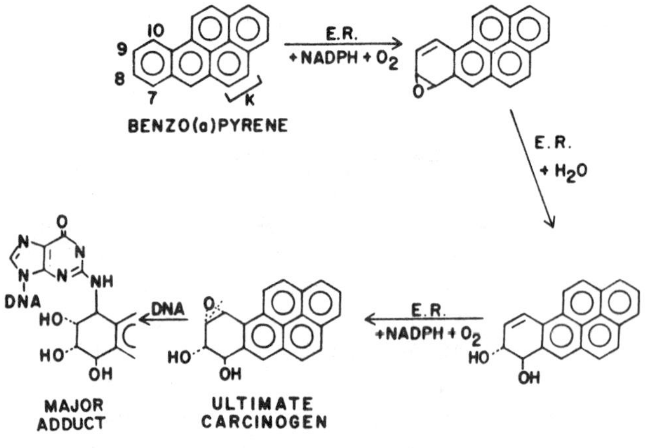

FIG. 10. The major route for the metabolic activation of benzo(a)pyrene and the major adduct formed on reaction of the ultimate carcinogen with DNA. E.R.: endoplasmic reticulum.

recognition can be followed by development of procedures for reduction of exposure. However, at present only limited predictions can be made of the potential electrophilic reactivity of a chemical or its metabolites, and therefore of its possible initiating or carcinogenic activities, from structural and metabolic analyses and analogies to known carcinogens. The best current rapid test systems are various assays for mutagenic activity; these must frequently be fortified with tissue preparations for metabolic activation. These assays are being used widely to screen chemicals for potential electrophilic activity.[27,59,61]

Malignant transformation of mammalian cells in culture, sometimes supplemented with tissue preparations for the metabolic activation of test chemicals, also provides useful assay systems.[53,59] These systems are more rapid than conventional whole animal bioassays for carcinogenic activity and have an advantage over mutagenicity assays since formation of cancer cells is the endpoint of the assay. Furthermore, the use of human tissues for conventional metabolism studies, for activation of chemicals for mutagenicity or transformation assays, and for other assays that provide indications of DNA damage (e.g., DNA repair assays, sister chromatid exchange) is beginning to provide information on the metabolic similarities and differences of human and animal cells and tissues.

In spite of the great advances that have occurred through the use of mutagenicity, malignant transformation, and other short-term assays for indicating chemicals of special interest, the abilities of high doses of chemicals to induce cancers in the whole animal are the closest approach currently available for the evaluation of the potentials of chemicals for causing human cancer. However, dependence on the administration of high levels of a single chemical for long periods in the conventional life-time assays must be reconsidered in view of the need to recognize agents that have strong initiating or strong promoting activity, even though they may have little complete carcinogenic activity. Furthermore, we are faced with the difficult problems of extrapolation of carcinogenicity data from species to species, especially from high doses in relatively small experimental populations to much lower doses in very large human populations.

The possible, and probable, exposures of humans for their lifetimes to a wide variety of chemicals including complete carcinogens, initiating agents, promoters, and some chemicals that modify the metabolism of other chemicals provide additional difficulties. To all of these complexities are added those that may result from various hormonal environments, immunologic factors, possible interactions with oncogenic viruses, and other biologic responses. Thus, the quantitative assessments of both experimental and epidemiologic data with regard to the risks of development of human cancers will be a difficult problem for some time. Resolution of this problem will require much further research, especially with the ethical use of human cells, tissues, organs, and body fluids and excreta. It also seems likely that new concepts with heuristic value will be necessary for further far-reaching progress.

REFERENCES

1. Armuth V, Bereblum I. Promotion of mammary carcinogenesis and leukemogenic action by phorbol in virgin female Wistar rats. *Cancer Res* 1974; 34:2704–2707.

2. Bartsch H, Dworkin M, Miller JA, Miller EC. Electrophilic N-acetoxyaminoarenes derived from carcinogenic N-hydroxy-N-acetylaminoarenes by enzymatic deacetylation and transacetylation in liver. *Biochim Biophys Acta* 1972; 286:272–298.

3. Bartsch H, Hecker E. On the metabolic activation of the carcinogen N-hydroxy-N-2-acetylaminofluorene. III. Oxidation with horseradish peroxidase to yield 2-nitrosofluorene and N-acetoxy-N-2-acetylaminofluorene. *Biochim Biophys Acta* 1971; 237:567–578.

4. Berenblum I, Shubik P. A new quantitative approach to the study of the stages of chemical carcinogenesis in the mouse's skin. *Br J Cancer* 1947; 1:383–391.

5. Berry DL, Bracken WM, Fisher SM, Viage A, Slaga TJ. Metabolic conversion of 12-O-tetradecanoylphorbol-13-acetate in adult and newborn mouse skin and mouse liver microsomes. *Cancer Res* 1978; 38:2301–2306.

6. Blumberg BS. Australian antigen and the biology of hepatitis B. *Science* 1977; 197:17–25.

7. Bouck N, diMayorca G. Somatic mutation as the basis for malignant transformation of BHK cells by chemical carcinogens. *Nature* 1976; 264:722–727.

8. Boutwell RK. Some biological aspects of skin carcinogenesis. *Progr Exp Tumor Res* 1964; 4:207–250.

9. Boutwell RK. The function and mechanism of promoters of carcinogenesis. *CRC Crit Rev Toxicol* 1974; 2:419–443.

10. Boyland E. The biological significance of metabolism of polycyclic compounds. *Biochem Soc Sympos* 1950; 5:40–54.

11. Bruce WR, Varghese AJ, Wang S, Dion P. The endogenous production of nitroso compounds in the colon and cancer at that site. In: Miller EC, Miller JA, Takayama S, Sugimura T, Hirono I, eds. Naturally Occurring Carcinogens-Mutagens and Modulators of Carcinogenesis, Tokyo: Japan Scientific Society Press and Baltimore: University Park Press, 1979:221–228.

12. Buening MK, Wislocki PG, Levin W, *et al*. Tumorigenicity of the optical enantiomers of the disastereomeric benzo[a]pyrene 7,8-diol-9,10-epoxides in newborn mice: exceptional activity of (+)-7β,8α-dihydroxy-9α,10α-epoxy-7,8,9,10-tetrahydrobenzo[a]pyrene. *Proc Natl Acad Sci USA* 1978; 75:5358–5361.

13. Cohen SM, Arai M, Jacobs JB, Friedell GH. Promoting effect of saccharin and DL-tryptophan in urinary bladder carcinogenesis. *Cancer Res* 1979; 39:1207–1217.

14. Colburn NH. Tumor promotion and preneoplastic progression. In: Slaga TJ, ed. Carcinogenesis, vol. 5, Modifiers of Chemical Carcinogenesis. New York: Raven Press, 1980:33–56.

15. Cooper GM, Okenquist S, Silverman L. Transforming activity of DNA of chemically transformed and normal cells. *Nature* 1980; 284:418–421.

16. Emmelot P, Kriek E, eds. Environmental Carcinogenesis: Occurrence, Risk Evaluation, and Mechanisms. Amsterdam: Elsevier/North Holland, 1979.

17. Farber E, Cameron R. The sequential analysis of cancer development. *Adv Cancer Res* 1980; 31:125–226.

18. Fenner F, McAuslan BR, Mims CA, Sambrook J, White DO. The Biology of Animal Viruses, 2nd ed. New York: Academic Press, 1974:480–481, 486–487.

19. Fraumeni JF Jr, ed. Persons at High Risk of Cancer. An Approach to Cancer Etiology and Control. New York: Academic Press, 1975.

20. Grant CK, Essex M, Gardner MB, Hardy WD Jr. Natural feline leukemia virus infection and the immune response of cats of different ages. *Cancer Res* 1980; 40:832–839.

21. Hall WH, Bielschowsky F. The development of malignancy in experimentally induced adenomata of the thyroid. *Br J Cancer* 1949; 3:534–541.

22. Hammond EC. Tobacco. In: Fraumeni JF, ed. Persons at High Risk of Cancer. An Approach to Cancer Etiology and Control. New York: Academic Press, 1975:131–137.

23. Hecker E. Structure-activity relationships in diterpene esters irritant and cocarcinogenic to mouse skin. In: Slaga TJ, Sivak A, Boutwell RK, eds. Carcinogenesis, vol. 2, Mechanisms of Tumor Promotion and Cocarcinogenesis, New York: Raven Press, 1977: 11–48.

24. Heidelberger C. Chemical carcinogenesis. *Ann Rev Biochem* 1975; 44:79–121.

25. Hiatt HH, Watson JD, Winsten JA, eds. Origins of Human Cancer. Cold Spring Harbor, NY: Cold Spring Harbor Laboratory, 1977.

26. Hicks RM, Wakefield J St J, Chowaniec J. Evaluation of a new model to detect bladder carcinogens or co-carcinogens; results obtained with saccharin, cyclamate, and cyclophosphamide. *Chem-Biol Interact* 1975; 11:225–233.

27. Hollstein M, McCann J, Angelosanto FA, Nichols WW. Short-term tests for carcinogens and mutagens. *Mutat Res* 1979; 65: 133–226.

28. IARC. Monographs on the evaluation of carcinogenic risk of chemicals to man, vols. 1–21. Lyon: International Agency for Research on Cancer, 1972–1979.

29. IARC. Monographs on the evaluation of carcinogenic risk of chemicals to man, supplement 1. Lyon: International Agency for Research on Cancer, 1979:32, 37, 44.

30. Jerina DM, Lehr R, Schaefer-Ridder M, et al. Bay-region epoxides of dihydrodiols: a concept explaining the mutagenic and carcinogenic activity of benzo(a)pyrene and benzo(a)anthracene. In: Hiatt HH, Watson JD, Winsten JA, eds. Origins of Human Cancer, Cold Spring Harbor Laboratory, 1977:639–658.

31. King CM. Mechanism of reaction, tissue distribution, and inhibition of arylhydroxamic acid acyltransferase. *Cancer Res* 1974; 34:1503–1515.

32. Knutson JC, Poland A. 2,3,7,8-Tetrachlorodibenzo-p-dioxin: failure to demonstrate toxicity in twenty-three cultured cell types. *Toxicol Appl Pharmacol* 1980; 54:377–383.

33. Lasne C, Gentil A, Chouroulinkov I. Two-stage malignant transformation of rat fibroblasts in tissue culture. *Nature* 1974; 247: 490–491.

34. Magee PN, Montesano R, Preussmann R. N-Nitro compounds and related carcinogens. In: Searle CE, ed. Chemical Carcinogens. ACS Monograph 173. Washington: American Chemical Society, 1976:491–625.

35. Markert CL. Cancer: the survival of the fittest. In: Saunders GF, ed. Cell Differentiation and Neoplasia, New York: Raven Press, 1978:9–26.

36. Miller EC. Some current perspectives on chemical carcinogenesis in humans and experimental animals: presidential address. *Cancer Res* 1978; 38:1479–1496.

37. Miller EC, Lotlikar PD, Miller JA, Butler BW, Irving CC, Hill JT. Reactions *in vitro* of some tissue nucleophiles with the glucuronide of the carcinogen N-hydroxy-2-acetylaminofluorene. *Mol Pharmacol* 1968; 4:147–154.

38. Miller EC, Miller JA. The metabolism of chemical carcinogens to reactive electrophiles and their possible mechanisms of action in carcinogenesis. In: Searle CE, ed. Chemical Carcinogens. American Chemical Society Monograph No. 173. Washington: American Chemical Society, 1976:737–762.

39. Miller EC, Miller JA. Naturally occurring chemical carcinogens that may be present in food. In: Neuberger A, Jukes TH, eds. International Review of Biochemistry, Biochemistry of Nutrition 1A, vol. 27. Baltimore: University Park Press, 1979:123–165.

40. Miller JA. Carcinogenesis by chemicals. An overview. G.H.A. Clowes Memorial Lecture. *Cancer Res* 1970; 30:559–576.

41. Mintz B. Genetic mosaicism and in vivo analysis of neoplasia and differentiation. In: Saunders GF, ed. Cell Differentiation and Neoplasia, New York: Raven Press, 1978:27–53.

42. Mondal S, Brankow DW, Heidelberger C. Two-stage chemical oncogenesis in cultures of C3H/10T1/2 cells. *Cancer Res* 1976; 36:2254–2260.

43. Mondal S, Heidelberger C. Ultraviolet light in the oncogenic transformation of cultured C3H/10T1/2 mouse embryo cells. *Natl Cancer Inst Monogr* 1978; 50:71–74.

44. Moore MM, Drinkwater NR, Miller EC, Miller JA, Pitot HC. Quantitative analysis of the time-dependent development of glucose-6-phosphatase-deficient foci in the livers of mice treated neonatally with diethylnitrosamine. *Cancer Res* (submitted).

45. Mottram JC. A developing factor in experimental blastogenesis. *J Pathol Bacteriol* 1944; 56:181–187.

46. Muir CS, Kirk R. Betel, tobacco, and cancer of the mouth. *Br J Cancer* 1960; 14:597–608.

47. Nazerian K. Marek's disease: a neoplastic disease of chickens caused by a herpesvirus. *Adv Cancer Res* 1973; 17:279–315.

48. O'Brien TG. The induction of ornithine decarboxylase as an early, possibly obligatory, event in mouse skin carcinogenesis. *Cancer Res* 1976; 36:2644–2653.

49. O'Connor PJ, Saffhill R, Margison GP. N-Nitroso compounds: biochemical mechanisms of action. In: Emmelot P, Kriek E, eds. Environmental Carcinogenesis: Occurrence, Risk Evaluation, and Mechanisms. Amsterdam: Elsevier/North Holland, 1979:73–96.

50. Peers FG, Gilman GA, Linsell CA. Dietary aflatoxins and human liver cancer. A study in Swaziland. *Int J Cancer* 1976; 17:167–176.

51. Peraino C, Fry RJM, Staffeldt E. Reduction and enhancement by phenobarbital of hepatocarcinogenesis induced in the rat by 2-acetylaminofluorene. *Cancer Res* 1971; 31:1506–1512.

52. Phillips DH, Sims P. Polycyclic aromatic hydrocarbon metabolites: their reactions with nucleic acids. In: Grover PL, ed. Chemical Carcinogens and DNA, vol. 2 Boca Raton, Florida: CRC Press, 1979:29–57.

53. Pienta RJ, Poiley JA, Lebherz WB III. Morphological transformation of early passage golden Syrian hamster embryo cells derived from cryopreserved primary cultures as a reliable *in vitro* bioassay for identifying diverse carcinogens. *Int J Cancer* 1977; 19:642–655.

54. Pierce GB. Differentiation of normal and malignant cells. *Fed Proc* 1970; 29:1248–1254.

55. Pitot HC. Drugs as promoters of carcinogenesis. In: Estabrook RW, Lindenlaub E, eds. The Induction of Drug Metabolism. Stuttgart/New York: F.K. Schattauer Verlag, 1979:471–483.

56. Pitot HC, Goldsworthy T, Campbell HA, Poland A. Quantitative analysis of the promotion by 2,3,7,8-tetrachlorodibenzo-p-dioxin of hepatocarcinogenesis from diethylnitrosamine. *Cancer Res* 1980; 40:3616–3620.

57. Poland A, Glover E. An estimate of the maximum *in vivo* covalent binding of 2,3,7,8-tetrachlorodibenzo-p-dioxin to rat liver protein, ribosomal RNA, and DNA. *Cancer Res* 1979; 39:3341–3344.

58. Poland A, Kende A. The genetic expression of aryl hydrocarbon hydroxylase activity: evidence for a receptor mutation in nonresponsive mice. In: Hiatt HH, Watson JD, Winsten JA, eds. Origins of Human Cancer. Cold Spring Harbor, NY: Cold Spring Harbor Laboratory, 1977:847–867.

59. Purchase IFH, Longstaff E, Ashby J, et al. An evaluation of 6 short-term tests for detecting organic chemical carcinogens. *Br J Cancer* 1978; 37:873–959.

60. Reddy BS, Cohen LA, McCoy GD, Hill P, Weisburger JH, Wynder EL. Nutrition and its relation to cancer. *Adv Cancer Res* 1980; 32:237–345.

61. Rinkus SJ, Legator MS. Chemical characterization of 465 known or suspected carcinogens and their correlation with mutagenic activity in the *Salmonella typhimurium* system. *Cancer Res* 1979; 39:3289–3318.

62. Rous P, Kidd JG. Conditional neoplasms and subthreshold neoplastic states: a study of the tar tumors of rabbits. *J Exp Med* 1941; 73:365–390.

63. Scherer E, Emmelot P. Foci of altered liver cells induced by a single dose of diethylnitrosamine and partial hepatectomy: their contribution to hepatocarcinogenesis in the rat. *Eur J Cancer* 1975; 11:145–154.

64. Schoental R. Carcinogens in plants and microorganisms. In: Searle CE, ed. Monography No. 173. Chemical Carcinogens. Washington: American Chemical Society, 1976:626–689.

65. Schulte-Hermann R. Induction of liver growth by xenobiotic compounds and other stimuli. *CRC Rev Toxicol* 1974; 2:97–158.

66. Schut HAJ, Wirth PJ, Thorgeirsson SS. Mutagenic activation of N-hydroxy-2-acetylaminofluorene in the *Salmonella* test system: the role of deacetylation by liver and kidney fractions from mouse and rat. *Mol Pharmacol* 1978; 14:682–692.

67. Shih C, Shilo B-Z, Goldfarb MP, Dannenberg A, Weinberg RA. Passage of phenotypes of chemically transformed cells via transfection of DNA and chromatin. *Proc Natl Acad Sci USA* 1979; 76: 5714–5718.

68. Sims P, Grover PL. Epoxides in polycyclic aromatic hydrocarbon metabolism and carcinogenesis. *Adv Cancer Res* 1974; 20: 166–274.

69. Sims P, Grover PL, Swaisland A, Pal K, Hewer A. Metabolic activation of benzo(a)pyrene proceeds by a diol-epoxide. *Nature* 1974; 252:326–328.

70. Singer B. All oxygens in nucleic acids react with carcinogenic ethylating agents. *Nature* 1976; 264:333–339.

71. Slaga TJ, Sivak A, Boutwell RK, eds. Mechanisms of Tumor Promotion and Cocarcinogenesis. New York: Raven Press, 1978.

72. Smith SJ, Liu DK, Leonard TB, Duceman BW, Vesell ES. Molecular biology of phenobarbital actions and interactions. *Ann NY Acad Sci* 1976; 281:372–383.

73. Soper CJ, Evans FJ. Investigations into the mode of action of the cocarcinogen 12-O-tetradecanoylphorbol-13-acetate using auxotrophic bacteria. *Cancer Res* 1977; 37:2487–2491.

74. Steward AP, Scherer E, Emmelot P. Formation of relatively persistent O²-ethylthymidine by diethylnitrosamine in rat liver DNA. *FEBS Letters* 1979; 100:191–194.

75. Swaisland AJ, Hewer A, Pal K, et al. Polycyclic hydrocarbon epoxides: The involvement of 8,9-dihydro-8,9-dihydroxybenz(a)-anthracene 10,11-oxide in reactions with the DNA of benz(a)anthracene-treated hamster embryo cells. *FEBS Letters* 1974; 47:34–39.

76. Tannenbaum SR. Endogenous formation of nitrite and N-nitroso compounds. In: Miller EC, Miller JA, Sugimura T, Takayama S, Hirono I, eds. Naturally occurring carcinogens—mutagens and modulators of carcinogenesis, Tokyo: Japan Scientific Society Press and Baltimore: University Park Press, 1979:211–220.

77. Troll W. Blocking tumor promotion by protease inhibitors. In: Magee PN, Takayama S, Sugimura T, Matsushima T, eds. Fundamentals in cancer prevention. Baltimore: University Park Press, 1976:41–55.

78. Upton AC. Radiation effects. In: Hiatt HH, Watson JD, Winsten JA, eds. Origins of Human Cancer, Cold Spring Harbor, NY: Cold Spring Harbor Laboratory, 1977:477–500.

79. Urbach F, Rose DB, Bonnem M. Genetic and environmental interactions in skin carcinogenesis. In: M.D. Anderson Hospital and Tumor Institute, ed. Environment and Cancer, Baltimore: Williams and Wilkins, 1972:354–371.

80. Van Duuren BL. Tumor-promoting and co-carcinogenic agents in chemical carcinogenesis. In: Searle CE, ed. Chemical Carcinogens. ACS Monograph 173. Washington: American Chemical Society, 1976:24–51.

81. Van Rensburg SJ, Van der Watt JJ, Purchase IFH, Pereira Coutinho L, Markham R. Primary liver cancer rate and aflatoxin intake in a high cancer area. *S Afr Med J* 1974; 48:2508a–2508d.

82. Weeks CE, Allaben WT, Louie SC, Lazea EJ, King CM. Role of arylhydroxamic acid acyltransferase in the mutagenicity of N-hydroxy-N-2-fluorenylacetamide in *Salmonella typhimurium*. *Cancer Res* 1978; 38:613–618.

83. Weinstein IB, Lee LS, Fisher PB, Mufson A, Yamasaki H. Cellular and biochemical events associated with the action of tumor promoters. In: Miller EC, Miller JA, Hirono I, Sugimura T, Takayama S, eds. Naturally Occurring Carcinogens-Mutagens and Modulators of Carcinogenesis. Tokyo: Japan Scientific Societies

Press and Baltimore: University Park Press, 1979:301–314.

84. Weinstein IB, Yamasaki H, Wigler M, *et al*. Molecular and cellular events associated with the action of initiating carcinogens and tumor promoters. In: Griffin AC, Shaw CR, eds. Carcinogens: Identification and mechanisms, New York: Raven Press, 1979:399–418.

85. Weisburger JH, Yamamoto RS, Williams GM, Grantham PH, Matsushima T, Weisburger EK. On the sulfate ester of N-hydroxy-N-2-fluorenylacetamide as a key ultimate hepatocarcinogen in the rat. *Cancer Res* 1972; 32:491–500.

86. Yang LL, Maher VM, McCormick J. Error-free excision of the cytotoxic and mutagenic N^2-deoxyguanosine DNA adduct formed in human fibroblasts by ($\pm$)-7β,8α-dihydroxy-9α,10α-epoxy-7,8,9,10-tetrahydrobenzo(a)pyrene. *Proc Natl Acad Sci USA*, 1980; 77: 5933–5937.

87. zur Hausen H. Oncogenic Herpes viruses. *Biochim Biophys Acta* 1975; 417:25–53.

Nutrition and Cancer: Mechanisms of Genotoxic and Epigenetic Carcinogens in Nutritional Carcinogenesis*

by John H. Weisburger, Ph.D., M.D., and Clara Horn, B.A., M.T.

ENVIRONMENT AND CANCER

THE majority, or as much as 70–90%, of human cancers, have been associated with environmental causes.[1-4] Our complex environment is often misunderstood as consisting primarily of ubiquitous chemicals, and, more specifically, those due to modern technology and industrial development. It is true that a number of food additives, pesticides, insecticides, and industrial chemicals introduced commercially during the last 40 years have exhibited carcinogenic properties in animal models.[2,5] Historically, chemical exposure due to occupation or to drugs has led to human cancers.[2,6] However, most of the chief human cancers in the Western world do not stem from intentional or even inadvertent chemical contaminants in the environment. Thus, it is important to identify the real, actual causes of cancer, as a rational, effective basis for prevention.

Cancer represents many different diseases, and insight into the complex causes of cancer requires detailed analysis of factors inherent in the occurrence of each specific type of cancer. From worldwide statistics on the incidence of diverse cancers as well as the altered risk for migrants from areas of high to low incidence over several generations and the corresponding analysis of data obtained under controlled conditions in animal models, a picture emerges that permits delineation of the multiple etiologic factors involved in each of the main human cancers.[2,7]

*Presented as part of a *Symposium on Assessing Therapeutic Dietary Claims* held by the Section on Clinical Nutrition of the New York Academy of Medicine at the Academy February 28, 1981.

This research was supported in part by USPHS Grants CA-12376 and CA-29602 from the National Cancer Institute, and CA-15400, CA-16382, and CA-24217 through the National Large Bowel Cancer Project; and Grant OH-0611 from the National Institute of Occupational Health.

This essay is dedicated to the founder of the American Health Foundation, Dr. Ernst L. Wynder, on the occasion of the 10th Anniversary of the Naylor Dana Institute for Disease Prevention.

Address for reprint requests: Dr. John Weisburger, American Health Foundation, Valhalla, New York 10595

John H. Weisburger and Clara Horn are with the American Health Foundation, Naylor Dana Institute for Disease Prevention, Valhalla, New York, 10595.

MECHANISMS OF CARCINOGENESIS

New knowledge of the mechanisms of carcinogenesis has been developed in recent decades. Thus, neoplasia may stem from a somatic mutation involving a change in normal cells at the level of the genetic material.[8-12] This has been quite a controversial area for more than 100 years, but multidisciplinary approaches and various lines of evidence provide an adequate scientific basis for this concept.

Genotoxic phenomena. A change in genetic material can be visualized as arising through several mechanisms. In one, genetic material can be changed through direct attack by radiation, chemicals, or viruses. Radiation or chemicals can damage genetic material at a number of loci along the DNA chain that are converted to permanent alterations by mispairing of bases during replication of damaged regions. With viruses, a more specific insertion of DNA segments or, through reverse transcriptase of RNA sequences, takes place through the operation of specific polymerases and hence yields an abnormal DNA containing new information.[13]

Other mechanisms, such as faulty operation of DNA polymerase during DNA synthesis resulting in inaccurate transcription of the parent DNA segment, can produce abnormal DNA. Certain carcinogenic metal ions may have this effect.[14] Abnormal DNA can also ensue, especially during postreplicative DNA synthesis, through errors introduced by specific DNA polymerases concerned with DNA repair.[15-17]

The infidelity of DNA polymerases may lead to further abnormalities in DNA produced during replication of early tumor cells, and thus may represent a means whereby tumor cells progress to less differentiated, more malignant cancer types during their growth and development.

Epigenetic phenomena. Production of abnormal DNA by any of the above mechanisms is only the first step in a long sequence of events terminating in a malignant invasive neoplasm. An important element is the ability of an abnormal cell population to achieve a selective growth advantage in the presence of surrounding normal cells. The cell-duplication process depends on a number of endogenous and exogenous controlling elements. Two key controlling elements are promoters or inhibitors of growth which either enhance or retard the process.

As numerous experiments documenting this phenomenon indicate, promoters do not lead to the production of an invasive cancer in the absence of antecedent cell change.[11,18-20] Thus, in exploring the causes of any specific human cancer, consideration must be given both to agents leading to an abnormal genome and to any other agents possibly involved in the growth and development of the resulting abnormal neoplastic cells, and their further progression to clinical malignancy.

Chemical carcinogens, accounting for the majority of human cancers, have been classified by Weisburger and Williams[11,21] into eight classes that, in turn, belong to two main groups: genotoxic carcinogens and agents, including promoters, operating by epigenetic pathways (Table I). This classification, in relation to an understanding of the relevant mechanisms, is important in dissecting the complex causes of diverse kinds of

TABLE I. CLASSIFICATION OF CARCINOGENIC CHEMICALS

Type	Mode of action	Example
Genotoxic		
Direct-acting	Electrophile, organic compound genotoxic, interacts with DNA	Ethylene imine, bis (chloromethyl) ether
Procarcinogen	Requires conversion through metabolic activation by host or in vitro to type 1	Vinyl chloride, benzo-(a)pyrene, 2-naphthyl-amine, dimethylnitro-samine
Inorganic carcinogen	Not directly genotoxic, leads to changes in DNA by selective alteration in fidelity of DNA replication	Nickel, chromium
Epigenetic		
Solid-state carcinogen	Exact mechanism unknown; usually affects only mesenchy-mal cells and tissues; physical form vital	Polymer or metal foils, asbestos
Hormone	Usually not genotoxic; mainly alters endocrine system balance and differentiation; often acts as promoter	Estradiol, diethyl-stilbestrol
Immuno-suppressor	Usually not genotoxic; mainly stimulates "virally induced," transplanted, or metastatic neoplasms	Azathioprine, antilym-phocytic serum
Cocarcinogen	Not genotoxic or carcinogenic, but enhances effect of type 1 or type 2 agent when given at the same time. May modify conversion of type 2 to type 1	Phorbol esters, pyrene catechol, ethanol, n-dodecane, SO_2
Promoter	Not genotoxic or carcinogenic, but enhances effect of type 1 or type 2 agent when given subsequently	Phorbol esters, phenol anthralin, bile acids, tryptophan metabolites, saccharin

Reproduced by permission from Weisburger, J.H. and Williams, G.M.: Chemical Carcinogenesis. In: *Toxicology: The Basic Science of Poisons*, 2nd ed., Doull, J., Klaassen, C., and Amdur, M., editors. New York, Macmillan, 1980, p. 84.

cancer and arriving at a specification of the role of each agent—genotoxic carcinogen, cocarcinogen, or promoter—in the overall carcinogenic process for each kind of cancer.

NUTRITION LINKED CANCERS

Pickled (nitrate-nitrite treated) fish or beans—origin of genotoxic carcinogens for stomach cancer? Alkylnitrosoureido compounds such as N-methyl-N'-nitro-N-nitrosoguanidine (MNNG) have been specific tools to induce glandular stomach cancer in animal models.[22] Kinetics of the reaction of the nitrosation of such alkylamides as methylurea has been studied by Mirvish,[23] who also made the important discovery that ascorbic acid inhibits the nitrosation of methylurea and alkylamines.

We have found that treating Sanma mackerel, a fish commonly eaten in Japan, or the type of beans eaten in Latin America with nitrite at pH 3, mimicking gastric conditions, yields high levels of mutagenic activity for Salmonella typhimurium TA1535.[25] Yano[24] recently found alkylating activity in fish treated likewise with nitrite. Formation of the mutagen was inhibited by the simultaneous presence of vitamin C. When this mutagenic activity from the reaction of nitrite and Sanma was given to Wistar rats by gavage, it induced adenocarcinomas of the glandular stomach.[25] The nature of the mutagen(s) obtained from the reaction is as yet unknown, but the mode of formation and inhibition, along with mutagenicity/carcinogenicity, suggest a possible alkylnitrosoureido compound.[26,27]

Nitrite is essential for the formation of such gastric carcinogens. Nitrate in foods is converted to nitrite during storage at room temperature for 24 hours, a reaction inhibited by cold storage or refrigeration, and nitrate can be reduced efficiently to nitrite by the oral bacterial flora.[28]

Thus, various lines of evidence[25] suggest that genotoxic carcinogens for human gastric cancer may arise from consumption of salted, pickled foods, that the active agent or agents has the properties of alkynitrosoureido compounds formed from nitrite and undefined substrates, and, importantly, that the formation of the carcinogen may be blocked by vitamin C or by vitamin E (Table II).

Cancer of the glandular stomach is an important neoplasm in Japan, Iceland, mountainous interior regions of Central and Western Latin America, and some Eastern European countries. In contrast, Western Europe, many Anglo-Saxon countries (except Wales), and the United States have a low incidence. In fact, during the last 50 years the gastric cancer rate in the United States has declined appreciably from 30 to 3.7/100,000 for men and 22 to 7.5/100,000 for women.[29]

Dietary risk factors with positive correlations among high risk populations include high consumption of dried salted fish, pickled vegetables, smoked fish, and fewer vegetables and a lowered vitamin C intake particularly on a seasonal basis.[30-32] Another correlation has been reported between elevated levels of nitrate in foods and drinking water due to high levels in the soil and water supply.[33] This correlation that holds only in the periodic absence of fresh vegetables as sources of the vitamin C, an antagonist of nitrite.[25] Now that better transport makes such foods more

TABLE II. NUTRITIONAL FACTORS INVOLVED IN CERTAIN HUMAN CANCERS

Source of genotoxic carcinogen	Epigenetic enhancing factors*	Inhibiting factors	Organs affected
Nitrite + specific foods (fish, beans, *not* meats)	Salt	Vitamin C, vitamin E, pyrogallol.	Stomach
Fried foods	Fat	Fiber, vitamins vitamins (?), minerals (Se salts, Zn ion, others?), microwave cooking, antioxidants or soy protein in cooking	Colon, breast, prostate, pancreas.

*Mechanisms discussed in text

widely available, measurement of urine nitrate alone fails to correlate with risk.[34] Crude salt or saltpeter used to preserve certain foods such as fish may also contain nitrate. On the other hand, Japanese migrants in Hawaii with a higher intake of such uncooked vegetables as celery, lettuce, tomatoes, and fresh fruit juices had a low gastric cancer risk as compared to indigenous Japanese and to first generation Japanese migrants to Hawaii.[30,32]

Thus, intake of foods containing vitamin C with each meal all year long from childhood onward may inhibit the formation of gastric carcinogens, and may account for the sharp decline in the incidence of gastric cancer in the United States, a decline also beginning to be apparent in other areas of the world where gastric cancer is still high.

Lower salt use would have similar benefits, and, further, reduce the risk of hypertension. In the MNNG-induced gastric cancer model, Tatematsu et al.[35] found that salt (sodium chloride) had a promoting effect. This observation may also mimic the human environment, for Joossens et al.[36] document a parallelism in international trends between gastric cancer and hypertension.

Mutagens and mode of cooking—origins of genotoxic carcinogens for cancer in colon, pancreas, breast, or prostate? Until recently there were no data nor even ideas as to the genotoxic carcinogens responsible for nonoccupational human cancer in the general public in western countries, except for those found in tobacco smoke.[2,37,38] This is especially so for such nutritionally-linked cancers as colon, pancreas, breast, or prostate.

An important clue to the nature of such carcinogens came from demonstration that charcoal broiling of meat or fish yielded mutagenic activity for *Salmonella typhimurium* TA-98.[7,39,40] Since mutagenic activity often indicates carcinogenic activity, the development of mutagenic activity as a function of mode and temperature of cooking was studied under typical realistic cooking conditions.[7] Frying meat mixed with soy protein flour or a small amount of the antioxidant BHA yielded less mutagenic activity.[41]

The principal mutagenic compounds from fried beef were resolved into two major fractions (those from fried fish could be separated into more fractions), and included small amounts of compounds such as the amino acid pyrolysates TRP-1 and TRP-2.[7,39] One of the main components in fried sardines is identical to one of the mutagens in beef. Its structure, 2-amino-3-methylimidazo-[4,5-d]quinoline, is similar sterically and structurally to known homocyclic carcinogenic arylamines, such as 3,2'-dimethyl-4-aminobiphenyl, which are colon, mammary gland, and prostate carcinogens in rodents.[7] The main mutagens in fried meat or fish most likely do not derive only from pyrolysis of amino acids or peptides but from formation of heterocyclic compounds from carbohydrate components and amino acids under similar conditions. This concept was tested in a model system for browning reactions. Thus, the reaction of sugars with ammonium ions yielded compounds with strong mutagenic activity with mobilities in high pressure chromatography systems similar to those in fried meat.[7] These reactions, which produce pyrazine derivatives, are base-catalyzed and can be inhibited by the antioxidant propyl gallate.[42] Thus, the reactions leading to mutagens during frying may be akin to those that take place during the browning reactions.[42,43]

Whether this mutagenic activity is relevant to human disease is the subject of current research. That such antioxidants as propyl gallate or BHA are effective inhibitors of mutagen formation, as was soy protein during the frying of meat, may provide practical ways to reduce mutagen formation which may be associated with disease risk (Table II).

EPIGENETIC AGENTS IN NUTRITIONALLY LINKED CANCERS

We have discussed the question of genotoxic carcinogens for cancers in the gastrointestinal tract and endocrine-sensitive organs. Of great potential importance is delineation of epigenetic promoting effects relevant for these cancers. It would appear that for cancer of the stomach salt exerts definite, but minor, promoting effects, and that the major element in gastric carcinogenesis is the long-lasting direct action of genotoxic carcinogens, as witnessed by the fact that migrants from such high risk areas as Japan or Poland, for example, to a lower risk area such as the United States or Australia maintain the risk of gastric cancer.[2,4,31,32,44-46] In respect to the other nutritionally linked cancers, especially in the colon, breast, and prostate, however, promoting effects appear to be more important. Whether or not overt invasive disease develops depends a great deal on epigenetic promoting factors. In the case of prostrate cancer, *in situ* lesions have been found in diverse populations but clinically invasive disease is observed only in populations consuming higher levels of dietary fat. Thus, the conclusion that promoting stimuli are important for the occurrence of invasive disease is strong.

The following discussion will emphasize the rationale for epigenetic actions for cancers of the colon, breast, and prostate.

Colon cancer. Large bowel or colon cancer needs to be considered as distinct from rectal cancer on the basis of several lines of evidence, including international and intranational incidence patterns, sex ratio, and age distribution. Not much is known about risk factors for rectal cancer; ale or stout is one element incriminated.[47] For colon cancer, diet appears to be a major etiologic factor[48] judging by variations in incidence for different regions of the world and the altered risk of migrant populations (Table III).

Specific dietary elements documented as relevant through studies in man and in animal models are the amount of dietary fat and fiber (Table IV). In fact, one of the best arguments for these concepts is the changing incidence of colon cancer in Japan during recent years as the Japanese nutritional intake progressively became westernized.[30] In addition, in many areas of the world, an association exists between colon cancer and coronary heart disease, where the amount of dietary fat and cholesterol have been shown to relate to risk for heart disease. A key exception to this rule is Finland, where the risk for heart disease is high and that of colon cancer is low, and we[48] as well as the International Agency for Research on Cancer[49,50] have obtained some evidence that the lower risk of Finnish people for colon cancer despite a high fat

TABLE III. CURRENT CONCEPTS ON COLON CANCER CAUSATION AND DEVELOPMENT

Risk factors: Diets high in fat, cholesterol, fried foods, and low in fiber

Established mechanisms

High fat ──────────► High cholesterol biosynthesis ──┐
                                      High dietary cholesterol ──┘ ──► High gut bile acid levels

Low fiber ──────────► High concentration of gut bile acids (low dilution through lack of bulk)

High bile acid concentration ──────────► Promoting effect in colon carcinogenesis

Mechanisms under study

Fried food ──────────► Mutagens ──────────► Colon carcinogens?

Role of micronutrients (vitamins and minerals) and different types of fiber in production and metabolism of carcinogens, bile acids, promoters?

Mechanisms of promotion?

Reproduced by permission from Winawer, S.J., Schottenfeld, D., and Sherlock, P., editors: *Colorectal Cancer: Prevention, Epidemiology, and Screening.* New York, Raven, 1980.

intake is related to their consumption of foods high in fiber, especially cereal bran fiber.

Laboratory research by a number of groups, particularly by Reddy et al.[48] and Nigro,[51] has provided an explanation for the effect of fat in promoting colon cancer risk and of fiber in inhibiting colon carcinogenesis. The main effect of dietary fat appears to reside in a direct association between endogenous cholesterol biosynthesis, in turn leading to increased bile acid biosynthesis. Bile acids have been shown to be effective promoters for colon cancer. Thus, they act as epigenetic agents in the overall carcinogenic process. The effect of dietary fiber is to increase intestinal and stool bulk, thereby reducing the *concentration* of promoters, and hence effectively

TABLE IV. COMPARISON OF HIGH AND LOW RISK DIETARY FACTORS FOR CANCER IN SPECIFIC ORGANS.

Organ	Population Lower risk	Dietary factors Lower risk	Population High risk	Dietary factors High risk
Stomach	USA	Fresh fruit, salad, vitamins C and E	Japan, Chile, Colombia	Salted, pickled food, nitrate
Colon	Japan	Low fat	USA, Western Europe, New Zealand, Australia, Scandinavia	High fat, low fiber, fried food.
Colon	Mormons	Higher fiber	USA in general	Idem.
Colon	Seventh Day Adventists	Low or no fried food, higher fiber	USA in general	Idem.
Colon	Finland	Higher fiber, lower fried food	USA in general Denmark	Idem.
Breast	Japan	Low fat	USA, Western Europe, New Zealand, Australia	High fat
Prostate	Japan	Low fat	USA, Scandinavia, Western Europe	High fat

lowering the risk for development of colon cancer. This concept may account for the lower colon cancer risk of such populations as the Mormons and the Finns who consume fried meat and other sources of genotoxic carcinogens and promoters but who also eat sizable amounts of cereal grains, which consequently lowers the risk (Table IV).

Breast cancer. Epidemiologic studies show that premenopausal American and Japanese women have comparable rates of breast cancer as a function of age, although Japanese women have a somewhat lower incidence compared to American women. The incidence among Japanese woman reaches a plateau at menopause and then decreases. In contrast, the incidence in Americans increases sharply during and following menopause, the curve showing a characteristic "hook". This biphasic incidence of breast cancer in pre- and postmenopausal women possibly reflects two independent disease factors.[52,53] An important distinction between environmental factors in Japan and the United States is dietary, and the main variable is the quantity of dietary fat. High-risk populations consume a higher proportion of dietary fat, the percentage of which has been increasing over the past 50 years.[54] This change may be related to the slight but definitely increased incidence of breast cancer among Western women during the same time span. De Waard[55] reported that obesity was a promotional factor in Dutch women, but this does not appear to play a role in North American Caucasian women.[56,57] First-generation Japanese migrants to a high-incidence area such as the United States have only a slight increase in breast cancer, and not until the second generation is a risk similar to that of the long-term residents in the high-incidence region attained. This is in contrast to the colon cancer risk incurred by migrants to high-risk areas where first-generation migrants from low-risk regions have an appreciable increase in risk of colon cancer. This aspect deserves further documentation because it suggests that, for breast cancer, residence in a high-risk area at the time of puberty and breast development is critical.[58] Female Sprague-Dawley rats are more sensitive to a single dose of hydrocarbon carcinogen at or around puberty than are older or younger animals, a susceptibility that seems to be correlated with the rate of cell division and serum prolactin levels.[59]

Useful animal models have been those based on the induction of breast cancer in rats by specific chemicals — dimethylbenz(a)-anthracene (DMBA) and N-nitrosomethylurea (NMU). Using the DMBA model, Carroll et al.[60] demonstrated that diets with a fat content between 10% to 20% (by weight) significantly increased the frequency of breast cancer, as compared to diets containing 0.5% to 5% fat. The effect was found to be exerted primarily on the promotional phase of breast cancer development, and diets rich in polyunsaturated fats were more effective tumor promoters than were diets rich in saturated fats. Cohen et al.[61] extended Carroll's finding in an N-nitrosomethylurea model and showed that fat can increase carcinogenesis in ovariectomized rats, a model for postmenopausal human breast cancer (Figure 1).

Evidence from experimental and epidemiologic investigations in breast cancer has reached sufficient proportions to warrant more systematic explora-

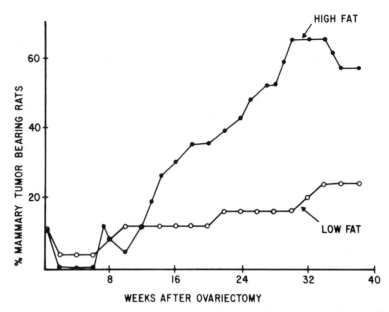

Cumulative tumor incidence curves for animals fed high- and low-fat diets. Female Charles River rats were given a single dose of 10 mg. 7,12-dimethylbenz(a)anthracene at age 50 days. Eighty days later a bilateral ovariectomy was performed on all rats, when 6/50 had palpable mammary tumors. After seven days, 25 rats were placed on a low fat (0.5%) or a high fat (20% lard) diet. Forty weeks after ovariectomy, all rats were killed, autopsied, and tumors examined histologically. Tumor incidence was significantly different ($P<0.05$) by X^2 test, at all time points from 18 weeks to 40 weeks post-Ovx. Reproduced by permission from Cohen, L.A., Chan, P.C., and Wynder, E.L.: A high fat diet enhances the development of mammary tumors in ovariectomized rats. *Cancer 47*:66-71, 1981.

tions into mechanisms. Postulated mechanisms by which dietary fat may influence breast cancer fall into two basic categories: those involving direct effects on host metabolism, especially the endocrine balances, and those related to effects on membrane components.

We have focused on the possibility that dietary fat elicits its tumor-enhancing effects by altering host endocrine metabolism—in particular, that component of the endocrine system that regulates prolactin secretion. Our interest in a fat-prolactin-breast cancer relationship was prompted by two facts: prolactin is a known classic promoter in a number of murine breast tumor systems, and prolactin is a liporegulatory hormone in birds and lower mammals, rodents, and possibly man. In addition, there is no question but that other hormones are involved in control of growth of the mammary gland through general action and specific receptor systems. Thus, the problem is to define the nutritionally-linked hormonal balances characteristic of high or low risk situations. In any case, it is clear that the dietary effect involves epigenetic promoting mechanisms which remain to be explored.

Prostate cancer. Epidemiology has provided data on the incidence of prostate cancer as a function of a number of factors such as race, age, area of residence, and diet. [62-64] Thus, Caucasians in the Western world have a higher incidence of prostatic cancer than Japanese. First-generation Japanese migrants to the United States retain their low risk, but later generations exhibit a higher risk.[65] However, native Japanese have *in situ* lesions, and it has been suggested that the difference in proliferative types of prostatic carcinoma seen in Western men is due to promotion by environmental factors, among which diet deserves primary consideration (Tables II, III).

For unknown reasons, the risk for prostate cancer is higher among American blacks than American whites. Nonetheless, it is clear that, as a rule, population groups with a high risk of breast, colon, and endometrial cancer also have a high risk of prostate cancer.[46] Since, for the former types, an association with diet has been documented not only in epidemiologic studies, but in metabolic and physiologic approaches, it is probable that dietary fat plays a role in the etiology of prostate cancer.[66] For breast and colon cancer, dietary fat hypothesis is further supported by such detailed studies in animal models as those described above. At present, there has not been available a reliable and realistic animal model involving specific chemical carcinogens for prostate cancer amenable to mechanistic studies. However, we have developed one such model involving a systemically acting chemical carcinogen, 3,2′-dimethyl-4-aminobiphenyl,[67] and at this time are exploring the effect of such dietary modulators as the level of fat, zinc, cadmium, and the like.

Concluding Remarks

The concepts outlined in this paper, based on various lines of evidence and multidisciplinary approaches, suggest that nutrition and specific nutritional components, as well as dietary habits, in various parts of the world may play an important role in the causation and development of a number of important cancer types. Nutrition may relate directly to the occurrence of 30-40% of cancers in men and 50-60% of cancers in women in the United States and other Western countries.[7] Because of the rapid Westernization of nutritional customs in Japan, parallel alterations have occurred in the incidence of specific cancers due to this change.[30] We have dissected the overall carcinogenic process into a number of sequential steps, all of which are needed for the development of clinically invasive cancer. This sequence has been demonstrated in numerous studies in animal models and there is no reason to assume that this sequence would not also hold for the initiation, development, and progression of human cancers.

We have presented the concept that the early lesions are the result of neoplastic change caused by genotoxic carcinogens for cancer of the colon, breast, prostate, and perhaps even pancreas. (The pancreas may be subject also to carcinogens from tobacco smoke[68] and possibly from coffee.[69,70]) We have noted that mutagens which may be such carcinogens are seen at the surface of fried or broiled foods such as meat or fish. It is clear that this concept needs further validation through research being performed in a number of laboratories in Japan and in the United States. Gastric cancer, on the other hand, appears to have a totally distinct element, namely, pickled and salted fish or beans and residence in areas with geochemical or agricultural sources of nitrate intake, not balanced by the presence of vitamin C, vitamin E, or certain phenolic antioxidants and nitrite traps such as pyrogallol or tannins. The possible genotoxic carcinogen is postulated as an alkylnitrosamide type. The formation of such compounds is inhibited by vitamin C, vitamin E, and certain antioxidants. This fact can be used deliberately to decrease the risk for gastric cancer, as has been discussed.

Epigenetic agents play a major role in the development of cancer of the colon, breast, and prostate. These stem from the intake of appreciable amounts of dietary fat that are responsible for the endogenous production of specific epigenetic agents associated with increased risk. Modulators, such as stool bulk due to adequate fiber intake, reduce the risk of colon cancer. More research is also needed on modulators and inhibitors such as micronutrients, vitamins, and minerals that would eventually find application in lowering human disease risk.

These facts are excellent evidence for the thesis presented in this paper, namely, that the mode of cooking and the level of dietary fat and fiber are associated with the occurrence of cancer of the colon, breast, and perhaps of the prostate and pancreas. It is hoped that, as further evidence accumulates from human studies through metabolic epidemiology and from experimental systems, a convincing case can be made for relatively minor alterations in dietary habits, involving mainly a somewhat lower fat intake and a higher fiber consumption.

Because these elements operate through epigenetic mechanisms, their action is by definition dose and time dependent. Thus, a reduction in effective dose, by whatever means, would be expected to lead to rather rapid lowering of risk, and hence of incidence. This applies even to patients with such diseases, where dietary intervention promises to be an effective adjuvant therapy. When the postmenopausal use of estrogen drugs such as premarin was discontinued, endometrial cancer rapidly declined, witness that epigenetic phenomena are reversible.

If current research does further document that the mode of cooking, especially frying and broiling, does yield carcinogens for these kinds of cancers, means to prevent formation of such carcinogens may be found, and would eventually yield a lower risk. Along these lines, research on optimal levels of vitamins, minerals, antioxidants, and other micronutrients in the current diet would provide a broad basis for chemoprevention. Over the last several years, research has provided new perspectives on the causes and modifiers of the main premature killing diseases. Data in this paper specifically record experimentation designed to yield understanding of underlying mechanisms as a sound reliable basis to prevent many important kinds of human cancer and for the long-term goals of disease prevention generally.

REFERENCES

1. Wynder, E. L. and Gori, G. B.: Contribution of the environment to cancer incidence: An epidemiologic exercise, *J. Nat. Cancer Inst. 58:*825, 1977.
2. Hiatt H. H., Watson J. D., and Winsten J. A., editors: *Origins of Human Cancer.* Cold Spring Harbor, New York, Cold Spring Harbor Lab., 1977.
3. Higginson, J.: Environmental Carcinogenesis: A Global Perspective. In: *Environmental Carcinogenesis: Occurrence, Risk Evaluation and Mechanisms,* Emelot, P. and Kriek, E., editors. Amsterdam, Elsevier/No. Holland Biomedical Press, 1979, p. 9.
4. Doll, R., Peto, R., The causes of can-

cer: Quantitative estimates of avoidable risks of cancer in the United States today, *J. Nat. Cancer Inst.* 66:1191, 1981.

5. IARC Monographs. On the evaluation of the carcinogenic risk of chemicals to humans. Lyon, France, International Agency for Research on Cancer, 1971-1980, vol. 1-25.

6. Nelson, N.: A personal view of occupational cancer and its prevention. *J. Nat. Cancer Inst.* 67:227-31, 1981.

7. Weisburger, J. H., Reddy, B. S., Hill, P., et al.: Nutrition and cancer—On the mechanisms bearing on causes of cancer of the colon, breast, prostate, and stomach. *Bull. N.Y. Acad. Med.* 56:673, 1980.

8. Griffin, A. C. and Shaw, C. R., editors: *Carcinogens: Identification and Mechanisms of Action.* New York, Raven, 1979.

9. Emmelot P. and Kriek E., editors: *Environmental Carcinogenesis: Occurrence, Risk Evaluation and Mechanisms.* Amsterdam, Elsevier/No. Holland, 1979.

10. Grover, P. L., editor: *Chemical Carcinogens and DNA.* Boca Raton, Fla., CRC Press, 1979, vols. 1, 2.

11. Weisburger, J. H. and Williams, G. M.: Chemical Carcinogenesis. In: *Toxicology: The Basic Science of Poisons,* 2nd ed., Doull, J., Klaassen, C., and Amdur, M., editors. New York, Macmillan, 1980, p. 84.

12. Straus, D. S.: Somatic mutation, cellular differentiation, and cancer causation. *J. Nat. Cancer Inst.* 67:233-41, 1981.

13. Berg, P.: Dissection and reconstruction of genes and chromosomes. *Science* 209:296-303, 1981.

14. Tkeshelashvii, L. K., Shearman, C. W., Zakour, R. A., et al.: Effects of arsenic, selenium, and chromium on the fidelity of DNA synthesis. *Cancer Res.* 40:2455, 1980.

15. Roberts, J. J.: Carcinogen-induced DNA damage and its repair, *Br. Med. Bull.* 36:25, 1980.

16. Setlow, R. B.: Different basic mechanisms in DNA repair, *Arch. Toxicol.* (Suppl.)3:217, 1980.

17. Cleaver, J. E.: DNA damage, repair systems and human hypersensitive diseases. *J. Environ. Pathol. Toxicol.* 3:53, 1980.

18. Slaga, T. J., Sivak, A., and Boutwell, R. K., editors: *Mechanisms of Tumor Promotion and Cocarcinogens.* New York, Raven, 1978.

19. Weinstein, I. B., Lee, L. S., Fisher, P. B., et al.: The Mechanisms of Action of Tumor Promoters and a Molecular Model of Two Stage Carcinogenesis. In: *Environmental Carcinogenesis: Occur-*

rence, Risk Evaluation and Mechanisms, Emmelot, P. and Kriek, E., editors. Amsterdam, Elsevier/No. Holland, 1979, p. 265.

20. Pitot, H. and Sirica, A.: The stages of initiation and promotion in hepatocarcinogenesis. *Biochem. Biophys. Acta* 605:191, 1980.

21. Williams, G. M. and Weisburger, J. H.: Systematic carcinogen testing through the decision point approach, *Ann. Rev. Pharmacol. Toxicol.* 21:393, 1981.

22. Sugimura, T. and Kawachi, T.: Experimental Stomach Carcinogenesis. In: *Gastro-intestinal Tract Cancer,* Lipkin, M. and Good, R., editors. New York, Plenum, 1978, p. 327.

23. Mirvish, S., Karlowski, K., Birt, D., and Sams, J. P.: Dietary and other factors affecting nitorsomethylurea (NMU) formation in the rat stomach. *IARC Sci. Pub.* 31:271, 1980.

24. Yano, K.: Alkylating activity of processed fish products treated with sodium nitrite in simulated gastric juice. *GANN* 72:451-54, 1981.

25. Weisburger, J. H., Marquardt, H., Mower, H. F., et al.: Inhibition of carcinogenesis: Vitamin C and the prevention of gastric cancer. *Prev. Med.* 9:352, 1980.

26. Mirvish, S. S.: Inhibition of the Formation of Carcinogenic N-nitroso Compounds by Ascorbic Acid and Other Compounds. In: *Cancer: Achievements, Challenges and Prospects for the 1980s,* vol. 1, Burchenal, J. H. and Oettgen, H. F., editors. New York, Grune & Stratton, 1981, pp. 557-87.

27. Weisburger, J. H.: N-Nitroso compounds: Diet and Cancer Trends. An Approach to the Prevention of Gastric Cancer. In: *N-Nitroso Compounds.* Washington, D.C., American Chemical Society Symposium Series, 1981.

28. Tannenbaum, S. R., Weisman, N., and Fett, D.: The effect of nitrate intake on nitrite formation in human saliva. *Food Cosmet. Toxicol.* 14:459, 1976.

29. Silverberg, E.: Cancer statistics, 1981. *Ca-A Cancer J. Clin.* 31:20, 1981.

30. Hirayama, T.: Diet and cancer. *Nutr. Cancer* 1:67, 1979.

31. Bjelke, E.: Epidemiologic studies of cancer of the stomach, colon and rectum with special emphasis on the role of diet. *Scand. J. Gastroenterol.* (Suppl. 32)9:1-235, 1974.

32. Stemmerman, G. N.: Gastric cancer in the Hawaiian Japanese. *GANN* 68:525, 1977.

33. Zaldivar, R. and Wetterstrand, W. H.: Nitrate nitrogen levels in drinking water of urban areas with high and low risk populations from stomach cancer: An

environmental epidemiology study. *Z. Krebsforsch.* 92:227, 1978.

34. Armijo, R., Gonzalez, A., Orellana, M., et al.: Epidemiology of gastric cancer in Chile: II—Nitrate exposures and stomach cancer frequency. *Int. J. Epidemiol. 10:*57-62, 1981.

35. Tatematsu, M., Takashashi, M., Fukishima, S., et al., Effects in rats of sodium chloride on experimental gastric cancers induced by N-methyl-N'-nitrosoguanidine or 4-nitro-quinoline-1-oxide, *J. Nat. Cancer Inst. 55:*101, 1975.

36. Joossens, J. V., Kesteloot, H., and Amery, A.: Salt intake and mortality from stroke, *N. Engl. J. Med. 300:*1396, 1979.

37. Wynder, E. L. and Hoffman, D.: Tobacco and health. A societal challenge. *N. Engl. J. Med. 300:*894, 1979.

38. Shigeaki, S., Seino, Y., Ohka, T., et al.: Mutagenicity of smoke condensates from cigarettes, cigars, and pipe tobacco. *Cancer Lett. 3:*1-8, 1977.

39. Sugimura, T., Kawachi, T., Nagav, M. and Yahagi, T.: Mutagens in Food as Causes of Cancer. In: *Nutrition and Cancer: Etiology and Treatment,* Newell, G. R. and Ellison, N. M., editors. New York, Raven, 1981, p. 59.

40. Shelby, M. D. and Matsushima, T.: Mutagens and carcinogens in the diet and digestive tract. *Mutation Res.* 85:177, 1981.

41. Wang, Y. Y., Spingarn, N. E., Vuolo, L. L., et al.: Effects of fat and soy protein on mutagen production during frying of beef. *Proc. Ann. Meeting Amer. Assoc. Cancer Res. 22:*115, 1981.

42. Spingarn, N. E. and Garvie, C. T.: Formation of mutagens in sugar-ammonia model systems. *J. Agric. Food Chem.* 27:1319, 1979.

43. Shibamoto, T., Nishimura, O., and Mihara, S.: Mutagenicity of products obtained from a maltol-ammonia browning model system. *J. Agric. Food Chem.* 29:641-46, 1981.

44. Fraumeni, J. F., Jr., editor: *Persons at High Risk of Cancer.* New York, Academic, 1975.

45. McMichael, A. J., McCall, M. G., Hartsthorne, J. M., et al.: Patterns of gastro-intestinal cancer in European migrants to Australia: The role of dietary change. *Int. J. Cancer 25:*431-37, 1980.

46. Armstrong, B. and Doll, R.: Environmental factors and cancer incidence and mortality in different countries, with special reference to dietary factors. *Int. J. Cancer 15:*617, 1975.

47. Editorial: Beer and bowel cancer. *Lancet 1:*1396-97, 1981.

48. Reddy, B. S., Cohen, L. A., McCoy, G. D., et al.: Nutrition and its relationship to cancer, *Adv. Cancer Res. 32,* 237, 1980.

49. Jensen, O. M. and McLennan, R.: Dietary factors and colorectal cancer in Scandinavia. *Isr. J. Med. Sci. 15:*329, 1979.

50. I.A.R.C. Intestinal Microecology Group: Dietary fiber, transit time, fecal bacteria, and steroids in two Scandinavian populations. *Lancet 2:*207, 1977.

51. Nigro, N. D.: Animal studies implicating fat and fecal steroids in intestinal cancer, *Cancer Res. 41:*3769-70, 1981.

52. DeWaard, F.: Premenopausal and postmenopausal breast cancer: One disease or two? *J. Nat. Cancer Inst. 63:*549, 1979.

53. Vorherr, H.: *Breast Cancer.* Baltimore-Munich, Urban & Schwarzenberg, 1980, pp. 1-487.

54. Gortner, W. A.: Nutrition in the United States. *Cancer Res. 35:*1900, 1975.

55. DeWaard, F.: Breast cancer incidence and nutritional status with particular reference to body weight and height. *Cancer Res. 35:*3351, 1975.

56. Wynder, E. L., McCoy, G. D., Reddy, B. S., et al.: Nutrition and Metabolic Epidemiology of Cancers of the Oral Cavity, Esophagus, Colon, Breast, Prostate, and Stomach. In: *Nutrition and Cancer,* Newell, G. R. and Ellison, N. M., editors. New York, Raven, 1981.

57. Armstrong, B. K.: Diet and hormones in the epidemiology of breast and endometrial cancers. *Nutr. Cancer 1:*90-95, 1979.

58. Weisburger, J. H.: Mechanism of action of diet as a carcinogen. *Cancer 43:*1987, 1979.

59. Yanai, R. and Nagasawa, H.: Effects of pituitary graft and 2-bromo-α-ergocryptine on mammary DNA synthesis in mice in relation to mammary tumorigenesis. *J. Nat. Cancer Inst. 56:*1055, 1976.

60. Carroll, K. K.: Experimental evidence of dietary factors and hormone-dependent cancers. *Cancer Res. 35:*3374, 1975.

61. Cohen, L. A., Chan, P. C., and Wynder, E. L.: A high fat diet enhances the development of mammary tumors in ovariectomized rats. *Cancer 47:*66-71, 1981.

62. Wynder, E. L., Mabuchi, K., and Whitmore, W. F.: Epidemiology of cancer of the prostate. *Cancer 28:*344, 1971.

63. Guileyardo, J. M., Johnson, W. D., Welsh, R. A., et al.: Prevalence of latent prostate carcinoma in two U.S. popula-

tions. *J. Nat. Cancer Inst. 65:*311, 1980.

64. Hirayama, T.: Epidemiology of prostate cancer with special reference to the role of diet. *Nat. Cancer Inst. Monogr. 53:*149, 1979.

65. Akazaki, K. and Stemmermann, G. N.: Comparative study of latent carcinoma of the prostate among Japanese in Japan and Hawaii. *J. Nat. Cancer Inst. 50:*1137, 1973.

66. Hill, P., Wynder, E. L., Garnes, H., and Walker, A. R. P.: Environmental factors, hormone status, and prostatic cancer. *Prev. Med. 9:*657, 1980.

67. Fiala, E. S., Weisburger, J. H., Katayama, S., et al.: The effect of disulfiram on the carcinogenicity of dimethyl-4-aminobiphenyl in Syrian Golden hamsters and rats. *Carcinogenesis.* In press.

68. Wynder, E. L.: An epidemiological evaluation of the causes of cancer of the pancreas. *Cancer Res. 35:*2228, 1975.

69. MacMahon, B., Yen, S., Trichopoulos, D., et al.: Coffee and cancer of pancreas. *N. Engl. J. Med. 304:*630, 1981.

70. Nagao, M., Takahashi, U., Yamanaka, H., et al.: Mutagens in coffee and tea. *Mutation Res. 68:*101-06, 1979.

71. Winawer, S. J., Schottenfeld, D., and Sherlock, P., editors: *Colorectal Cancer: Prevention, Epidemiology, and Screening.* New York, Raven, 1980.

Diet and Cancer—An Overview (First of Two Parts)

by Walter C. Willett, M.D., and Brian Macmahon, M.D.

ALTHOUGH laboratory workers have known for decades that tumor incidence in animals can be affected by nutritional manipulation,[1] the possibility that diet may be important in the cause and prevention of cancer in human beings has received major attention only recently. Since knowledge in this area is developing rapidly, we will outline processes by which hypotheses relating dietary factors to cancer are formulated and tested. In addition, we will discuss the limited available data that are relevant to some hypotheses that have attracted particular interest. An exhaustive review of the literature is contained in *Diet, Nutrition, and Cancer*, published by the National Research Council, which has served as the basis for a series of preliminary dietary recommendations[2] as well as indicating directions for future research.[3]

Interest in the relation between diet and cancer in human beings has been stimulated by international studies in which large differences in cancer incidence rates have been found between countries.[4,5] For example, age-adjusted rates of breast and colon cancer in many areas of the world are less than one fifth those in the United States. Moreover, very strong nutritional correlates exist for many specific cancers. Two correlations that are often cited are those between the total fat intake per capita and the national rate of breast-cancer mortality among women

From the Department of Epidemiology, Harvard School of Public Health; the Channing Laboratory, Department of Medicine, Harvard Medical School; and Brigham and Women's Hospital.

Supported by a Career Development Award (HL-01018) from the National Heart, Lung and Blood Institute and a program project grant (CA-06373) from the National Cancer Institute.

(r = 0.89) and between per capita fat intake and mortality from colon cancer (r = 0.85 for men and 0.81 for women).[4,6]

The central problem in interpreting these correlational studies is that many factors other than dietary differences distinguish countries with a high incidence of cancer from those with a low incidence. For example, with a few notable exceptions such as Japan, countries with a low incidence of breast and colon cancer tend to be relatively undeveloped economically. Therefore, any variable related to economic development will be similarly correlated with incidence of breast cancer. Indeed, the correlation between gross national product and breast-cancer mortality rate[4] is 0.72.

Genetic predisposition cannot account for the major international variations in cancer incidence rates. This is demonstrated by studies of migrant populations and of secular trends within countries. In general, populations migrating from an area with its own pattern of cancer incidence rates acquire rates characteristic of their new location[7,8] although, for a few tumor sites, this change occurs only in later generations.[9,10] Furthermore, there have been large changes in incidence rates for many types of cancer within genetically stable populations. Examples include the dramatic decrease in gastric cancer within the United States[11] and a substantial increase in the incidence of breast cancer in Iceland.[12]

The differences between the highest and lowest national cancer incidence rates for specific cancer sites have been used to arrive at an estimate that approximately 90 per cent of cancers in the United States are environmentally determined[13] and thus potentially avoidable. Doll and Peto have recently conducted an extensive review to estimate quantitatively the specific environmental determinants of cancer.[14] Stressing the limitations of current knowledge, they estimated that 35 per cent of cancers in the United States (with a possible range of 10 to 70 per cent) may be caused by components of the diet. If correct, this estimate would make diet second only to cigarette smoking as a determinant of cancer in this country. The challenge for researchers addressing the relation between diet and cancer is to identify the specific dietary determinants of cancer and to quantify their effects. Several approaches are being used.

RANDOMIZED TRIALS

The most scientifically rigorous approach is the randomized trial, optimally conducted as a double-blind experiment. However, experiments among human beings are justifiable only after considerable nonexperimental data have been collected, to ensure both that benefit is reasonably probable and that an adverse outcome is unlikely. Experimental studies can be practical for evaluating hypotheses that minor components of the diet, such as trace elements or vitamins, can prevent cancer.

Even if feasible, randomized trials of dietary factors and cancer are likely to encounter several problems. The time between change in exposure to a dietary factor and any expected change in cancer incidence is uncertain. Therefore, trials must be of long duration, and it is difficult in practice to eliminate the possibility that a lack of observed difference between treatment groups may merely mean that the trial has not run long enough. Compliance with the treatment diet is likely to decrease during an extended trial, particularly if treatment involves a real change in food intake, and the control group may well adopt the dietary behavior of the treatment group if the treatment diet is thought to be beneficial. Such trends, which were found in the Multiple Risk Factor Intervention Trial (MRFIT) of prevention of coronary heart disease,[15] may obscure a real benefit of the treatment. Several trials addressing hypotheses that relate diet and cancer are being conducted, but none has been completed. Because of their importance, randomized trials should be employed whenever feasible, despite their expense and difficulty.

LABORATORY EXPERIMENTS

Many substances that cause mutations among microorganisms also cause cancer in animals and human beings.[16] This observation underlies the usefulness of microbial mutagenicity tests (such as the Ames test), which have been widely used to study components of human diets. They are attractive because results are available in only days and at a relatively low cost. Although these tests are unquestionably helpful in di-

recting human research and elucidating mechanisms of action, they cannot by themselves provide information that is directly relevant to human beings. For example, there are many substances, such as asbestos, that influence the risk of cancer but are not mutagenic. They may act, for example, by affecting the permeability of host tissues to carcinogens, by altering hormonal balances that inhibit or promote tumor growth, or by changing the immune response of the host. Since these higher-level functions are not replicated in bacterial testing systems, false-negative and false-positive results will appear.

Experimental exposure of laboratory animals to substances that may influence cancer incidence is more likely to simulate the effect of a chemical or food on the incidence of cancer in human beings. However, high doses of potential carcinogens that do not reflect human experience are generally used, and species often differ in the way their enzymatic systems activate or deactivate potentially carcinogenic substances. Such factors preclude direct extrapolation of findings from animal experiments to human beings.

METABOLIC AND BIOCHEMICAL STUDIES

Another approach involves metabolic or biochemical studies in human beings. For example, Goldin and co-workers have studied the effect of diet on estrogen profiles,[17] which in turn are thought to be related to the risk of breast cancer. These studies do not address the relations between dietary intake and the occurrence of cancer directly.

EPIDEMIOLOGIC STUDIES

Epidemiologic studies of diet and cancer constitute a relatively new area of research. Until recently, many nutritionists and epidemiologists have thought that the difficulties of assessing the diets of free-living human beings over extended periods of time made large-scale studies impossible. However, a number of useful methods for assessing dietary intake have been developed.[18] These include the use of food diaries in which subjects record all the foods they eat on a meal-by-meal basis,[19] interviews about previous dietary intake,[20] short-term recall,[21] and questionnaires relating to the usual frequency of consumption of a selected list of foods.[22]

Although each method has advantages in particular applications, the food-frequency approach is most practical for large studies. This method has typically been used to categorize subjects in one of several levels of relative intake, such as quintiles, rather than to obtain an absolute quantification of intake. Questions usually relate to customary intake over an extended period of time, such as a year. Such a time interval is more likely to be relevant to cancer causation than are periods of a few days or weeks, which are the periods assessed with traditional dietary methods. Results obtained with food-frequency questionnaires are reproducible[23] and correlate with intakes determined by more detailed dietary methods,[19,22,24] with independent assessments of intake obtained from spouses,[25] and with biochemical indexes of nutrient intake.[26] However, differences in the methods and thoroughness of collecting dietary data may explain some of the apparent discrepancies in studies of diet and cancer.

The precision of dietary questionnaires or interviews varies considerably among nutrients, and for some nutrients such methods may be useless. Cholesterol intake, for example, can be reasonably assessed by a simple frequency questionnaire, since it is largely derived from a fairly small number of foods with a reasonably constant cholesterol composition. By contrast, the concentration of selenium in foods depends largely on the soils in which they are produced. Since people are generally unaware of the source of their food, intakes of selenium and of some other trace elements may not be meaningfully measured by questionnaires or interviews.

The refining and testing of methods for measuring dietary intakes in epidemiologic studies are currently in progress; the precision and limitations of these methods should be better defined during the next several years. Although most epidemiologic research has thus far related change in risk of cancer to relative scales of nutrient intake, future work should attempt to quantify these relations further. For example, one would really like to know the change in age-specific incidence of colon cancer, given a specified change in daily cholesterol intake — say from 400 to 200 mg. In addition, it would be highly desirable to be able to specify at which points in a person's lifetime each dietary factor exerts its effect on the occurrence of cancer. This will generally be difficult to determine except when a change in diet is associated with a major event, such as religious conversion, or in the case of vitamin or mineral supplements, since the dates when subjects start and stop taking them can be determined with some precision.

In some instances analyses of biologic specimens may substitute for information on dietary intake. Unfortunately, only a few nutrients have corresponding biochemical indexes that have been documented to reflect dietary intake. For example, levels of serum cholesterol, glucose, and sodium reflect dietary intakes of these substances poorly or not at all. Therefore, dietary cholesterol may be better assessed by questionnaires than by serum levels. On the other hand, serum levels of carotene and vitamin E are sensitive to dietary intake[26] and can therefore be used to study the relation of intakes of these nutrients with cancer. Serum samples that were collected over the past 20 years as part of prospective cardiovascular studies are now proving useful for biochemical measurements of nutritional indexes that can be related to cancer rates among cohort members.[27] The utility of such specimen collections could be enhanced by further work

defining the relations of nutrient intakes to their corresponding blood levels.

Although epidemiologic studies can address the relations of diet to cancer in human beings directly, the interpretation of these studies is often difficult. Investigators often collect information on a large number of foods or nutrients, and several "statistically significant" relations may emerge on the basis of chance alone. Furthermore, in studies in which the previous diets of patients with cancer are compared with the diets of persons who do not have cancer, the patient's recall may be biased by knowledge of his illness or loss of appetite secondary to the cancer or its treatment. Interviewers who are aware of a hypothesis may also interpret responses in cases and controls differently.

In addition, dietary factors are likely to be associated with other possible determinants of cancer, including other dietary variables. This problem (confounding) can be handled in the data analysis if information on the potentially confounding variables is available. However, confounding by an unmeasured variable is impossible to deal with.

Nutrient interactions may introduce further complexity. For example, an effect of low intake of vitamin E may be observed only when the intakes of other antioxidants are also low. Finally, studies that fail to show a relation between cancer and a specific nutrient may do so only because of the imprecision of the nutritional measurement or because there is insufficient variability of exposure in the population that was studied.

For the many diet–cancer associations that cannot be addressed with randomized trials, no single study or methodologic approach will definitively establish a cause–effect relation. Ultimately, dietary recommendations should be based on a synthesis of consistent observational investigations that are supported by laboratory experiments and metabolic studies. The observational studies should include investigations that examine all major health outcomes simultaneously, since it is possible that a dietary factor that reduces the incidence of cancer could increase the risk for other diseases.

SPECIFIC EXAMPLES OF POSSIBLE DIET AND CANCER RELATIONS

The possible combinations of dietary factors and cancer sites for which there are hypothetical relations are too extensive to discuss in a single review. We have therefore chosen to discuss possible relations, both causal and protective, that relate to common cancers and for which there is relevant information. We have chosen to avoid discussion of the effects of alcohol,[28] coffee,[29] microbial contamination of food,[30] food additives,[31] environmental contamination,[2] and the effects of food processing and cooking.[32] For the associations described we will discuss, whenever possible, studies comparing disease rates among populations, epidemiologic studies in individual subjects, experiments in vitro and in animals, and investigations of possible mechanisms.

Preformed Vitamin A and Carotene

A major physiologic role of vitamin A is to control cell differentiation. Since loss of cell differentiation is a basic feature of cancer, there is ample reason to suspect that intake of vitamin A may be related to cancer incidence. In the first major epidemiologic study relating vitamin A intake to cancer, Norwegian men whose vitamin A consumption was above average had less than half the rate of lung cancer of men whose consumption was below average.[33] Similar findings for vitamin A and lung cancer have been reported from Japan,[34] Singapore,[35] and the United States,[36] and in an update of the Norwegian study.[37] An inverse relation has also been found between vitamin A intake and cancers of the bladder,[38] upper gastrointestinal tract,[39] and breast.[40]

The interpretation of these studies of vitamin A and cancer is complicated by the diversity of vitamin A sources. Natural preformed vitamin A is found only in foods from animal sources. Plants, principally green and yellow vegetables, contain not preformed vitamin A but a series of carotenoid compounds, some of which can be metabolized to form retinol, the physiologically active form of vitamin A. Beta carotene, the most plentiful carotenoid with potential vitamin A activity, is a dimer that is partially cleaved after absorption to form two molecules of retinol. Since the questionnaires employed in most studies of vitamin A and cancer have inquired primarily about plant rather than animal sources of vitamin A, these investigations provide stronger support for a protective effect of beta carotene than for one of preformed vitamin A itself.[41] In a prospective study that attempted to differentiate intake of beta carotene from that of preformed vitamin A, a protective effect was found for the former but not the latter.[42] Unfortunately, the primary dietary data for this study were lost, which necessitated making a rather crude distinction between carotene and preformed vitamin A. This and previous studies could thus be interpreted as providing support for the hypothesis that carotene protects against cancer but not as furnishing evidence against an association between preformed vitamin A intake and cancer. To add to the confusion, in a recent British study an inverse relation between intake of preformed vitamin A and risk of lung cancer was found among men but not women.[43]

Although the majority of the studies that have examined the relation between carotene intake and cancer have found a protective effect of carotene, this observation has not been entirely consistent. A recent reanalysis of an Israeli study of gastrointestinal cancer found no effect of beta carotene.[44] Some of the apparently discrepant findings among studies could be explained if beta carotene were not equally protective for all cancer sites. A protective effect against lung cancer is currently the most strongly supported relation.[33-35,37,42,43]

In studies employing a different epidemiologic approach, retinol levels of subjects in whom cancer subsequently developed were measured in serum samples that had been collected and frozen before diagnosis, and were compared with retinol levels of subjects without subsequent cancer.[27,45] In the two initial studies, overall cancer rates were highest among persons with the lowest levels of serum retinol, even though those levels were within what is generally considered the normal range for serum retinol. Although the size of these studies did not allow stable estimates to be made of the association between retinol levels and site-specific cancer rates, the largest differences between cases and controls were for lung cancer. In contrast to the apparently protective effect of serum retinol in these two studies, no relation with cancer incidence was observed according to a preliminary report from a study in Germany[46] or in a recent multicentered study in the United States.[47] Because of their potential importance, these studies need to be replicated. However, it will be essential to ensure that specimens from cancer patients and controls are handled identically, since it is conceivable that the thawing and refreezing of specimens from patients but not of those from controls may have affected the findings in one of the original reports.[45]

Although it appears that higher levels of serum retinol may be advantageous, little is known about factors that influence these levels within well-fed populations. Evidence suggests that even massive vitamin A or beta carotene supplements will not materially increase serum retinol levels[48] except in cases of frank vitamin A deficiency. Thus, the issue of whether low serum retinol levels increase the risk of cancer is not directly related to observations that a reduced intake of foods containing vitamin A is associated with lower cancer rates. Additional data that address the independent relations of intakes of preformed vitamin A and carotene with cancer incidence are clearly needed.

Concurrently with the epidemiologic studies of vitamin A, carotene, and cancer, a large number of related experiments have been conducted in animals.[49] These studies have generally found that retinol and some retinoids (synthetic analogues of retinol) decrease the incidence of cancers that are induced by a variety of agents and that occur at many sites. This inhibitory effect is present even when retinol is administered after the cancer has been induced[50] — a feature of major potential epidemiologic and public-health importance. The effect of beta carotene on animal tumor models has not been intensively studied. However, it has been suggested that beta carotene protects mice against skin tumors induced by ultraviolet light and chemical carcinogens,[51] and against chemically induced gastrointestinal tumors.[52]

Another line of laboratory investigation has been to pursue mechanisms whereby vitamin A or carotene may exert an anticancer effect. As already noted, vitamin A regulates cell differentiation, but it may also favorably influence host immunologic defenses.[53] However, carotene itself may protect against oxidative reactions by quenching singlet oxygen and trapping free radicals,[54,55] thus limiting damage to DNA.

Although the epidemiologic evidence relating dietary carotene intake to cancer incidence appears promising and is supported by some laboratory evidence, it is possible that constituents of green and yellow vegetables other than carotene actually reduce cancer incidence. Fortunately, it is possible in this instance to employ the optimal investigative approach, a randomized trial, because beta carotene is without known serious side effects, even in doses so high as to cause an obvious orange skin coloration. The National Institutes of Health has thus funded a placebo-controlled trial of beta carotene in which all male American physicians 40 to 85 years of age have been invited to participate as subjects.[56]

Vitamin C

Considerable public attention has been drawn to the possibility that vitamin C (ascorbic acid) reduces the risk of cancer.[57] It has been pointed out that regions of Great Britain in which there is low vitamin C intake have high overall cancer rates.[58] Low vitamin C consumption has been associated with an elevated incidence of gastric cancer in Iceland[59] and high rates of esophageal cancer in Iran.[60] However, the meaning of these anecdotal observations is questionable.

Studies in individual subjects relating vitamin C intake to cancer have likewise been inconclusive. A case–control investigation of laryngeal cancer found protective associations for both vitamin A and vitamin C intake.[61] However, since the vitamin A effect was stronger, and since many foods contain both vitamin A and vitamin C, the apparent beneficial effect of vitamin C could have been due to the former. The same authors found no relation between vitamin C intake and oral cancer.[62] Among a group of black American men, those with the lowest intake of vitamin C had twice the risk of esophageal cancer of men with the highest intake, but again it was not clear that this effect was independent of other dietary variables.[63]

In a U.S. study, some vegetables were found to be associated with a decreased risk of gastric cancer, although citrus fruits, which are a major source of vitamin C, showed no such relation.[64] Similarly, in a case–control study of gastric cancer among Japanese Americans, highly salted foods were positively associated with gastric cancer, but important sources of vitamin C had little relation to cancer.[9] Among Norwegians, the risk of gastric cancer increased in a dose–response manner with decreasing levels of vitamin C intake, most strongly among persons under 60 years of age.[65] This protective effect of vitamin C could not be accounted for on the basis of confounding by other dietary factors. The same author found a similar relation between vitamin C intake and gastric cancer among Scandinavians living in the United States, although he observed only a suggestive association between vitamin C intake and colonic cancer.[65] No relations were seen between vitamin C intake and incidence of colon cancer in a case–control study among Canadians.[66] Recently, women with cervical dysplasia were found to consume less vitamin C than control women.[67]

Overall, there is minimal epidemiologic evidence supporting an important role for vitamin C in the prevention of cancer. On the other hand, because of the limitations of available data, there is no strong evidence against such an association. Most studies of cancer were not designed to examine the role of vitamin C specifically, and such studies have therefore not generally determined the intake of major sources of this vitamin, such as multiple vitamins, vitamin C pills, and citrus fruit. In addition, most studies have not measured vitamin C intake from multiple foods and have not controlled for the possible confounding effects of beta carotene and other nutrients.

Studies of vitamin C and cancer incidence in animals have also been equivocal. Early work suggested that vitamin C may actually stimulate the growth of sarcoma in rodents.[68] More recent experiments using guinea pigs with established tumors have shown a similar effect: animals given 1 g of ascorbic acid per kilogram of body weight daily had more rapid tumor growth than those receiving 10 mg per kilogram daily.[69] Although some data suggest that induced tumors in guinea pigs appear earlier if the animals are deficient in vitamin C,[70] other experiments have shown that large supplements have little if any effect on carcinogenesis.[71,72] In tissue culture, vitamin C increases the survival of ovarian tumor cells that are exposed to radiation[73] and reverses malignant changes in hamster lung cells that are induced by tobacco or marijuana smoke.[74]

Despite the paucity of empirical data demonstrating an anticancer effect of vitamin C in either human beings or animals, many possible mechanisms for such an effect have been proposed.[57] These include an influence on maintenance of the integrity of the intercellular matrix, enhancement of immune mechanisms, promotion of tumor encapsulation, and an antioxidative effect. Vitamin C blocks the conversion of nitrates and nitrogen-containing compounds to carcinogens under conditions found in the stomach[75] and in food stored under normal conditions.[76] This inhibition of carcinogen formation may be especially important with respect to gastric cancer.[77]

In summary, there is little empirical evidence that vitamin C provides protection against cancer in human beings. However, there are ample theoretical reasons to explore such relations further. In this process it will be important to determine whether it is only persons with very low intakes (say, below 60 mg per day) who are at an increased risk of cancer, or whether large supplements greatly exceeding the usual dietary intake from natural sources (from 60 to 200 mg per day) provide additional benefit.

Vitamin E

Like vitamin C, vitamin E has received popular attention as a possible inhibitor of cancer. However, relevant epidemiologic data are limited; in one preliminary report no relation was observed between vitamin E levels in prospectively collected serum samples and risk of cancer at all sites combined.[47] Although an inhibitory effect has been seen in a small number of experiments in animals,[78-80] such an effect has not been observed consistently.[81,82] Since vitamin E is an important intracellular antioxidant[83] that reduces mutations in some bacterial testing systems,[84] it deserves further study as a potential inhibitor of carcinogenesis.

REFERENCES

1. Tannenbaum A. The genesis and growth of tumors. III. Effects of a high-fat diet. Cancer Res 1942; 2:468-75.
2. Committee on Diet, Nutrition and Cancer; National Research Council. Diet, nutrition, and cancer. Washington, D.C.: National Academy Press, 1982.
3. Committee on Diet, Nutrition and Cancer; National Research Council. Diet, nutrition, and cancer: directions for future research. Washington, D.C.: National Academy Press, 1983.
4. Armstrong B, Doll R. Environmental factors and cancer incidence and mortality in different countries with special reference to dietary practices. Int J Cancer 1975; 15:617-31.
5. Schrauzer GN, White DA, Schneider CJ. Cancer mortality correlation studies. III. Statistical associations with dietary selenium intakes. Bioinorgan Chem 1977; 7:23-31.
6. Carroll KK. Experimental evidence of dietary factors and hormone-dependent cancers. Cancer Res 1975; 35:3374-83.
7. Staszewski J, Haenszel W. Cancer mortality among the Polish-born in the United States. JNCI 1965; 35:291-7.
8. Adelstein AM, Staszewski J, Muir CS. Cancer mortality in 1970-1972 among Polish-born migrants to England and Wales. Br J Cancer 1979; 40:464-75.
9. Haenszel W, Kurihara M, Segi M, Lee RKC. Stomach cancer among Japanese in Hawaii. JNCI 1972; 49:969-88.
10. Buell P. Changing incidence of breast cancer in Japanese-American women. JNCI 1973; 51:1479-83.
11. Haenszel W. Variation in incidence of and mortality from stomach cancer, with particular reference to the United States. JNCI 1958; 21:213-62.
12. Bjarnason O, Day N, Snaedal G, Tulinius H. The effect of year of birth on the breast cancer age-incidence curve in Iceland. Int J Cancer 1974; 13:689-96.
13. MacMahon B. International studies in the epidemiology of cancer. Jpn J Public Health 1964; 11:193-209.
14. Doll R, Peto R. The causes of cancer: quantitative estimates of avoidable risks of cancer in the United States today. JNCI 1981; 66:1191-308.
15. Multiple Risk Factor Intervention Trial Research Group. Multiple Risk Factor Intervention Trial: risk factor changes and mortality results. JAMA 1982; 248:1465-77.
16. Ames BN, Lee FD, Durston WE. An improved bacterial test system for the detection and classification of mutagens and carcinogens. Proc Natl Acad Sci USA 1973; 70:782-6.
17. Goldin BR, Adlercreutz H, Gorbach SL, et al. Estrogen excretion patterns and plasma levels in vegetarian and omnivorous women. N Engl J Med 1982; 307:1542-7.
18. Block G. A review of validations of dietary assessment methods. Am J Epidemiol 1982; 115:492-505.
19. Heady JA. Diets of bank clerks: development of a method of classifying the diets of individuals for use in epidemiologic studies. J R Stat Soc (A) 1961; 124:336-61.
20. Burke BS. The dietary history as a tool in research. J Am Diet Assoc 1947; 23:1041-6.
21. Beaton GH, Milner J, Corey P, et al. Sources of variance in 24-hour dietary recall data: implications for nutrition study design and interpretation. Am J Clin Nutr 1979; 32:2546-59.
22. Stefanik PA, Trulson MC. Determining the frequency intakes of foods in large group studies. Am J Clin Nutr 1962; 11:335-43.
23. Acheson ED, Doll R. Dietary factors in carcinoma of the stomach. Gut 1964; 5:126-31.
24. Balogh M, Medalie JH, Smith H, Groen JJ. The development of a dietary questionnaire for an ischemic heart disease survey. Isr J Med Sci 1968; 4:195-203.
25. Marshall J, Priore R, Haughey B, Rzepka T, Graham S. Subject-spouse interviews and the reliability of diet studies. Am J Epidemiol 1980; 112:675-83.
26. Willett WC, Stampfer MJ, Underwood BA, Speizer FE, Rosner B, Hennekens CH. Validation of a dietary questionnaire with plasma carotenoid and α-tocopherol levels. Am J Clin Nutr 1983; 38:631-9.
27. Wald N, Idle M, Boreham J, Bailey A. Low serum-vitamin-A and subsequent risk of cancer: preliminary results of a prospective study. Lancet 1980; 2:813-5.
28. Tuyns AJ. Epidemiology of alcohol and cancer. Cancer Res 1979; 39:2840-3.
29. MacMahon B, Yen S, Trichopoulos D, Warren K, Nardi G. Coffee and cancer of the pancreas. N Engl J Med 1981; 304:630-3.
30. Miller EC, Miller JA. Naturally occurring carcinogens that may be present in foods. In: Neuberger A, Jukes TH, eds. Biochemistry of nutrition I. Baltimore: University Park Press, 1979:135-45.
31. Fairweather FA, Swann CA. Food additives and cancer. Proc Nutr Soc 1981; 40:21-30.
32. Sugimura T, Nagao M, Kawachi T, et al. Mutagen-carcinogens in food, with special reference to highly mutagenic pyrolytic products in broiled foods. In: Hiatt HH, Watson JD, Winsten JA, eds. Origins of human cancer. Cold Spring Harbor, N.Y.: Cold Spring Harbor Laboratory, 1977:1561-77.
33. Bjelke EA. Dietary vitamin A and human lung cancer. Int J Cancer 1975; 15:561-5.
34. Hirayama T. Diet and cancer. Nutr Cancer 1979; 1(3):67-81.
35. MacLennan R, Da Costa J, Day NE, Law CH, Ng YK, Shanmugaratnam K. Risk factors for lung cancer in Singapore Chinese, a population with high female incidence rates. Int J Cancer 1977; 20:854-60.
36. Mettlin C, Graham S, Swanson M. Vitamin A and lung cancer. JNCI 1979; 62:1435-8.
37. Kvåle G, Bjelke E, Gart JJ. Dietary habits and lung cancer risk. Int J Cancer 1983; 31:397-405.
38. Mettlin C, Graham S. Dietary risk factors in human bladder cancer. Am J Epidemiol 1979; 110:255-63.
39. Mettlin C, Graham S, Priore R, Marshall J, Swanson M. Diet and cancer of the esophagus. Nutr Cancer 1980; 2:143-7.
40. Graham S, Marshall J, Mettlin C, Rzepka T, Nemoto T, Byers T. Diet in the epidemiology of breast cancer. Am J Epidemiol 1982; 116:68-75.
41. Peto R, Doll R, Buckley JD, Sporn MD. Can dietary beta-carotene materially reduce human cancer rates? Nature 1981; 290:201-8.
42. Shekelle RB, Lepper M, Liu S, et al. Dietary vitamin A and risk of cancer in the Western Electric Study. Lancet 1981; 2:1185-90.
43. Gregor A, Lee PN, Roe FJC, Wilson MJ, Melton A. Comparison of dietary histories in lung cancer cases and controls with special reference to vitamin A. Nutr Cancer 1980; 2:93-7.
44. Modan B, Cuckle H, Lubin F. A note on the role of dietary retinol and carotene in human gastro-intestinal cancer. Int J Cancer 1981; 28:241-4.
45. Kark JD, Smith AH, Switzer BR, Hames CG. Serum vitamin A (retinol) and cancer incidence in Evans County, Georgia. JNCI 1981; 66:7-16.
46. Stähelin HB, Buess E, Rösel F, Widmer LK, Brubacher G. Vitamin A, cardiovascular risk factors, and mortality. Lancet 1982; 1:394-5.
47. Willett WC, Polk BF, Underwood BA, et al. Relation of serum vitamins A and E and carotenoids to the risk of cancer. N Engl J Med 1984; 310:430-4.
48. Willett WC, Stampfer MJ, Underwood BA, Taylor JO, Hennekens CH. Vitamins A, E, and carotene: effects of supplementation in their plasma levels. Am J Clin Nutr 1983; 38:559-66.
49. Sporn MB, Dunlop NM, Newton DL, Smith JM. Prevention of chemical carcinogenesis by vitamin A and its synthetic analogs (retinoids). Fed Proc 1976; 35:1332-8.
50. McCormick DL, Burns FJ, Albert RE. Inhibition of Benzo[a]pyrene-induced mammary carcinogenesis by retinyl acetate. JNCI 1981; 66:559-64.
51. Mathews-Roth MM. Antitumor activity of β-carotene, canthaxanthin and phytoene. Oncology 1982; 39:33-7.
52. Seifter E, Wong F, Stratford F, Levenson SM, Rettura G. Vitamin A and β-carotene: actions in 7,12-dimethylbenz(a)anthracene (DMBA) tumor prevention. Presented at the 183rd National Meeting of the American Chemical Society Divison of Medical Chemistry, Las Vegas, March 28-April 2, 1982.
53. Jurin M, Tannock IF. Influence of vitamin A on immunological response.

Immunology 1972; 23:283-7.

54. Krinsky NI. Carotenoid protection against oxidation. Pure Appl Chem 1979; 51:649-60.

55. Krinsky NI, Deneke SM. The interaction of oxygen and oxy-radicals with carotenoids. JNCI 1982; 69:205-10.

56. Hennekens CH, Physicians Health Study Research Group. Strategies for a primary prevention trial of cancer and cardiovascular disease among U.S. physicians. Am J Epidemiol 1983; 118:453-4. abstract.

57. Cameron E, Pauling L, Leibovitz B. Ascorbic acid and cancer: a review. Cancer Res 1979; 39:663-81.

58. Knox EG. Ischaemic-heart-disease mortality and dietary intake of calcium. Lancet 1973; 1:1465-7.

59. Dungal N, Sigurjonsson J. Gastric cancer and diet: a pilot study on dietary habits in two districts differing markedly in respect of mortality from gastric cancer. Br J Cancer 1967; 21:270-6.

60. Hormozdiari H, Day NE, Aramesh B, Mahboubi E. Dietary factors and esophageal cancer in the Caspian Littoral of Iran. Cancer Res 1975; 35:3493-8.

61. Graham S, Mettlin C, Marshall J, Priore R, Rzepka T, Shedd D. Dietary factors in the epidemiology of cancer of the larynx. Am J Epidemiol 1981; 113:675-80.

62. Graham S, Dayal H, Rohrer T, et al. Dentition, diet, tobacco, and alcohol in the epidemiology of oral cancer. JNCI 1977; 59:1611-8.

63. Pottern LM, Morris LE, Blot WJ, Ziegler RG, Fraumeni JF Jr. Esophageal cancer among black men in Washington, D.C. I. Alcohol, tobacco, and other risk factors. JNCI 1981; 67:777-83.

64. Graham S, Schotz W, Martino P. Alimentary factors in the epidemiology of gastric cancer. Cancer 1972; 30:927-38.

65. Bjelke E. Epidemiologic studies of cancer of the stomach, colon, and rectum; with special emphasis on the role of diet. Scand J Gastroenterol [Suppl] 1974; 31:1-235.

66. Jain M, Cook GM, Davis FG, Grace MG, Howe GR, Miller AB. A case-control study of diet and colo-rectal cancer. Int J Cancer 1980; 26:757-68.

67. Wassertheil-Smoller S, Romney SL, Wylie-Rosett J, et al. Dietary vitamin C and uterine cervical dysplasia. Am J Epidemiol 1981; 114:714-24.

68. Brunschwig A. Vitamin C and tumor growth. Cancer Res 1943; 3:550-3.

69. Migliozzi JA. Effect of ascorbic acid on tumour growth. Br J Cancer 1977; 35:448-53.

70. Russell WO, Ortega LR, Wynne ES. Studies on methylcholanthrene induction of tumors in scorbutic guinea pigs. Cancer Res 1952; 12:216-8.

71. Abul-Hajj YJ, Kelliher M. Failure of ascorbic acid to inhibit growth of transplantable and dimethylbenzanthracene induced rat mammary tumors. Cancer Lett 1982; 17:67-73.

72. Reddy BS, Hirota N, Katayama S. Effect of dietary sodium ascorbate on 1, 2-dimethylhydrazine- or methylnitrosourea-induced colon carcinogenesis in rats. Carcinogenesis 1982; 3:1097-9.

73. O'Connor MK, Malone JF, Moriarty M, Mulgrew S. A radioprotective effect of vitamin C observed in Chinese hamster ovary cells. Br J Radiol 1977; 50:587-91.

74. Leuchtenberger C, Leuchtenberger R. Protection of hamster lung cultures by L-cysteine or vitamin C against carcinogenic effects of fresh smoke from tobacco or marihuana cigarettes. Br J Exp Pathol 1977; 58:625-34.

75. Mirvish SS, Wallcave L, Eagen M, Shubik P. Ascorbate-nitrite reaction: possible means of blocking the formation of carcinogenic N-nitroso compounds. Science 1972; 177:65-8.

76. Raineri R, Weisburger JH. Reduction of gastric carcinogens with ascorbic acid. Ann NY Acad Sci 1975; 258:181-9.

77. Correa P, Haenszel W, Cuello C, Tannenbaum S, Archer M. A model for gastric cancer epidemiology. Lancet 1975; 2:58-60.

78. Jaffe WG. The influence of wheat germ oil on the production of tumors in rats by methylcholanthrene. Exp Med Surg 1946; 4:278-82.

79. Haber SL, Wissler RW. Effect of vitamin E on the carcinogenicity of methylcholanthrene. Proc Soc Exp Biol Med 1962; 111:774-5.

80. Cook MG, McNamara P. Effect of dietary vitamin E on dimethylhydrazine-induced colonic tumors in mice. Cancer Res 1980; 40:1329-31.

81. Epstein SS, Joshi JS, Andrea J, Forsyth J, Mantel N. The null effect of antioxidants on the carcinogenicity of 3, 4, 9, 10-dibenzpyrene to mice. Life Sci 1967; 6:225-33.

82. Wattenberg LW. Inhibition of carcinogenic and toxic effects of polycyclic hydrocarbons by phenolic antioxidants and ethoxyquin. JNCI 1972; 48:1425-30.

83. Bieri JG, Corash L, Hubbard VS. Medical uses of vitamin E. N Engl J Med 1983; 308:1063-71.

84. Shamberger RJ, Corbett CL, Bearman KD, Kasten BL. Antioxidants reduce the mutagenic effect of malonaldehyde and β-propiolactone. IX. Antioxidants and cancer. Mutat Res 1979; 66:349-55.

Diet and Cancer—An Overview (Second of Two Parts)

by Walter C. Willett, M.D., and Brian Macmahon, M.D.

Selenium

Selenium is an essential trace element that has a key role in the activity of glutathione peroxidase, an enzyme that protects against oxidative tissue damage on a cellular level.[85] Both internationally[5] and within the United States[86] geographic areas with low selenium levels in the soil or in pooled blood-bank serum samples generally have higher cancer rates than areas with higher selenium levels. In a study that examined selenium intake in relation to site-specific cancer rates, the strongest inverse correlations were with breast cancer (r = 0.8) and colon cancer (r = 0.7).[5] Although these correlational studies are useful for stimulating further research, they are far from conclusive because of their inability to control for potentially confounding variables. For example, the high-selenium areas in the United States are primarily the sparsely populated western plains regions and are different in many respects from the low-selenium areas, which include the major population centers of the United States.

Blood selenium levels are usually depressed in patients with cancer,[87-89] and one small case–control study found serum selenium levels among women with breast cancer that were significantly lower than levels among a series of controls.[90] Although these observations are consistent with the hypothesis that lower selenium levels are causally related to the occurrence of cancer, it is also possible that attendant wasting and depressed food intake caused the lower selenium levels.[91] These methodologic problems were largely circumvented in a recent analysis that used serum samples that were collected and stored up to five years before the diagnosis of cancer to compare selenium levels of cancer cases with those of matched controls.[92] Although the number of cases did not allow detailed analyses by site, the overall risk of cancer for those in the lowest quintile for serum selenium level was twice that of those in the highest quintile. This apparent protective effect of selenium was especially pronounced among subjects with low serum levels of retinol.

Further studies of selenium and cancer in human beings will need to employ the measurement of levels in biologic specimens as indicators of intake; dietary questionnaires are not likely to be useful for this purpose (see Part I). Blood levels reflect intake over an extended period, since they are sensitive to dietary intake and also have a relatively long half-life.[93,94] Similarly, since keratin structures, such as hair[95,96] or nails,[97] concentrate selenium and reflect its dietary intake, such specimens could be useful to evaluate further the relation between selenium intake and cancer incidence.

A large number of in vitro studies and studies in animals support the hypothesis that increased intake of selenium reduces the risk of cancer in human beings. Selenium decreases the mutagenic activity of a variety of known carcinogens in the Ames test.[98,99] In tissue culture, selenium reduces the metabolic activation of certain carcinogens, altering the patterns of degradation to favor less toxic metabolites.[100] Selenium has a protective effect in a large number of animal tumor models employing a variety of inducing agents.[101-106] In addition, adding 2 parts per million of selenite to the drinking water of C3H mice (a strain with a very high rate of "spontaneous" mammary cancer) reduced the incidence from 82 to 10 per cent.[107]

From the Department of Epidemiology, Harvard School of Public Health; the Channing Laboratory, Department of Medicine, Harvard Medical School; and Brigham and Women's Hospital.

Supported by a Career Development Award (HL-01018) from the National Heart, Lung, and Blood Institute and a program project grant (CA-06373) from the National Cancer Institute.

Like retinol, selenium has been protective even when it has been administered well after the carcinogen,[108] suggesting that it has an inhibitory effect on the later stages of carcinogenesis.

Possible mechanisms of selenium's action may relate to its antioxidant activity, which is mediated through the activity of glutathione peroxidase[85] and probably other pathways.[109] As is consistent with an antioxidant function, the inhibition of mammary cancer by selenium was greatest in rats fed a diet high in polyunsaturated fat,[110] which normally increases intracellular peroxidation.[111] In addition, selenium may have a favorable effect on carcinogen metabolism[112] and enhance immune defenses.[113]

In summary, selenium reduces the occurrence of some cancers in animals, and descriptive statistics suggest a possible benefit in human beings. If this or some other trace element in food is ultimately found to reduce the incidence of cancer in human beings, it would have major potential public-health implications. As compared with efforts that require major changes in people's personal habits, supplementation would be a relatively simple maneuver. However, at very high intakes not presently defined, selenium is toxic, producing apparently reversible changes in hair, skin, and mood.[114] We need not only a simple positive or negative answer regarding the effect of selenium on the occurrence of cancer in human beings, but a quantification of the dose–response relationship.

Fiber and Colon Cancer

Interest in the relation between fiber intake and colon cancer is largely the result of Dr. Denis Burkitt's observation of low rates of colon cancer in areas of Africa where fiber consumption and stool bulk were high.[115] Although fiber was originally seen simply as providing bulk to dilute potential carcinogens and speed their transit through the colon, current data suggest that the relation between fiber intake and colon cancer, if any, may be more complex than that.

Western countries have rates of colon cancer that are up to eight times those of many developing countries,[4] and migrants from areas of high incidence to those of low incidence generally attain rates of colon cancer similar to those of their new environment.[116] Although fiber intake is generally higher in low-incidence countries, the differences between developing and industrialized countries are myriad and include other important dietary variables, such as meat and fat consumption. Liu et al.[117] have suggested that the inverse relation between fiber intake and incidence of colon cancer is secondary to higher cholesterol consumption in high-incidence nations. Rates of colon cancer according to region within the United Kingdom are inversely associated with intake of pentose polymer, a fiber constituent of grains, but not with overall intake of dietary fiber.[118]

In Norway,[119] New York,[120] and Greece,[121] higher ingestion of fruits and vegetables (which are major sources of fiber as well as of several vitamins) was associated with a lower risk of colon cancer. Case–control studies in Israel[122] and among American blacks[123] have shown a protective effect of fiber. However, in a case–control study among Canadians[66] there was no such association, and Puerto Ricans with colon cancer actually reported greater fiber intake than did controls.[124]

Some of the inconsistency in findings about fiber may relate to the extremely heterogeneous nature of "crude fiber," which is the term traditionally used by nutritionists. Crude fiber is empirically defined as the residue of a chemical digestion process. A definition of dietary fiber has been espoused by Southgate[125] that attempts to characterize more completely the carbohydrates that are not digested in the human gastrointestinal tract. However, even this definition of dietary fiber encompasses a diverse collection of carbohydrates that are unlikely to have identical physiologic effects. The fiber hypothesis has been further complicated by the finding that transit time is apparently not consistently increased by the addition of fiber to the diet,[126] although some forms of fiber do increase the quantity of stool.[127] Fiber may have effects that are mediated by the binding of carcinogenic substances, rendering them less active,[128] or by the altering of intraluminal colonic flora, which may be involved in transforming substances that are less carcinogenic to those that are more so[129] (see below).

Although studies in animals of the effects of fiber have been somewhat inconsistent,[130-132] Reddy et al.[133] recently reported that both wheat bran and fiber from citrus fruits protect rats against chemically induced colon cancer. In their review of previous experiments on the effects of fiber in laboratory animals, the authors suggest that prior studies that failed to show a protective effect of fiber may have used doses of chemical carcinogens that were too powerful to be inhibited by dietary factors. It is of interest that the addition of dioctyl sodium sulfosuccinate, a commonly used nonfibrous enhancer of stool bulk, also decreased the number of induced colon tumors in rats.[134]

Although the available epidemiologic data are not entirely consistent, the weight of evidence generally supports the hypothesis that fiber protects against colon cancer. Some difficulty in interpreting simple relations between fiber intake and cancer occurs because foods that are high in fiber may contain other substances that are related to cancer. For example, it has been suggested that the apparent protective effect of certain vegetables may relate to their content of indoles, a series of compounds that reduce the incidence of cancer in animals.[120,135]

Dietary Fat, Cholesterol, and Colon Cancer

There is some evidence that diets high in fat increase the risk of large-bowel cancer, and it is possible that high fat and low fiber intakes act synergistically.[136] The associations between per capita consumptions of total fat, saturated fat, and cholesterol and national incidence rates of colon cancer are remarkably strong,[4] with correlation coefficients as high as 0.85. In Japan recent increases in fat consumption[137] have been associated with a striking increase in rates of colon cancer.[138]

However, epidemiologic studies of fat intake and colon cancer in individual subjects have been quite inconsistent. Case–control studies of colon cancer in Israel[122] and the United States[120] failed to find any material association. In a recent Canadian study,[66] patients with colon cancer reported higher intake of total fat, saturated fat, and cholesterol than controls, with the strongest association being with saturated fat. However, findings in this study are difficult to interpret because patients consumed more total calories, even though they were not more obese than controls; this suggests that they were more physically active, that they were less metabolically efficient, or that there was bias in the ascertainment of food intake. Similarly, in a Puerto Rican case–control study, patients with colon cancer reported not only higher intakes of fat than controls but also higher consumption of fiber and all other food groups examined.[124]

Consumption of meat, an important source of fat, was associated with large-bowel cancer among Japanese Hawaiians in a study by Haenszel et al.,[139] but the same authors could not confirm this relation in a study conducted in Japan.[140] Meat intake was strongly related to risk of colorectal cancer in a recent Greek study; subjects with high consumption of meat and low intake of vegetables had an eightfold increase in risk as compared with those who had a low meat and high vegetable intake.[121] The exceptionally strong associations with both vegetable and meat intake seen in this study may relate to the wide diversity of diets within Greece.

Subjects in clinical trials who were treated with drugs to promote cholesterol excretion have had higher rates of large-bowel cancer,[141] suggesting that increased excretion of cholesterol metabolites through the colon may increase the risk of colon cancer. The reasonably consistent finding in prospective studies that persons with lower levels of serum cholesterol have elevated rates of colon cancer[142-144] is not necessarily in conflict with the hypothesis that increased dietary cholesterol and saturated fatty acids cause colon cancer. It is possible that, at a given level of dietary intake of cholesterol and saturated fatty acids, persons with low levels of blood cholesterol may have more efficient excretion of cholesterol metabolites into the biliary system and, thus, higher rates of colon cancer. Observations that cholecystectomy, which increases the colonic concentration of secondary bile acids, is associated with higher rates of right-sided colon cancer[145,146] are consistent with the hypothesis that bile acids and dietary fat are related to this disease.

Among animals, increased intake of saturated fat,[147,148] unsaturated fat,[148] and cholesterol[149,150] increase the incidence of chemically induced colon cancer, although there is some suggestion that unsaturated fats may have a stronger effect.[149] The effect of dietary fat is present even when it is given weeks after tumor induction,[151] suggesting that the mechanism may be one of tumor promotion. In human beings[152-154] as well as in animals,[154,155] diets that are high in fat cause an increase in the excretion of bile acids. Higher levels of dietary cholesterol increase the concentration of fecal neutral sterols,[152,156] which are metabolites of cholesterol, and probably cause a modest increment in the excretion of bile acids.[157] Increased fecal concentrations of bile acids and neutral steroids have been found in populations with higher rates of colon cancer,[154,158] in individual patients with colon cancer,[159,160] and in patients with colonic polyps.[161] However, such findings are not entirely consistent,[162,163] and it is not yet proved that increased levels of bile acids or neutral sterols or both precede the occurrence of cancer. In animal models bile acids act as tumor promoters.[164,165] Evidence suggests that their tumor-enhancing effect, which may be mediated by increasing the turnover of intestinal mucosal cells,[166] is increased after they are enzymatically modified by intestinal bacteria to form secondary bile acids.[167] Colonic flora with an increased enzymatic capacity for transforming bile acids to potential carcinogens have been found in populations with high rates of colon cancer and in omnivores as compared with vegetarians.[154,168]

Epidemiologic studies of dietary intakes among individual subjects currently provide inconsistent support for the hypothesis that fat intake is related to colon cancer. However, the negative findings may be due to difficulty in categorizing subjects according to fat intake (see below). In spite of these methodologic difficulties, epidemiologic studies of dietary fat and colon cancer should be pursued because experiments in animals and data relating to the effects of bile acids suggest that such a relation may exist. Since meat is the most important source of dietary fat in the United States, it will be important to determine whether it has any relation with colon cancer that is independent of its fat content; at present there is little such evidence.

Dietary Fat and Breast Cancer

Japan, other far eastern countries, and most undeveloped nations have rates of breast cancer that are as low as one-fifth those of the United States and northern Europe.[169] The offspring of immigrants from Japan to the United States, but not the immigrants themselves, have breast-cancer rates that are similar to those of the general American population.[10] However, Polish women who migrate to the United Kingdom or the United States themselves attain rates of breast cancer that are similar to the higher rates among women born in these countries,[7,8] suggesting that the delayed effect among Japanese-Americans may be due to a slower acculturation process. Interest . in dietary fat as a possible explanation of these differences in rates has been stimulated by the very strong correlation between national per capita consumption of fat and age-adjusted rates of breast cancer.[4]

Other studies of breast-cancer rates in population groups provide an inconsistent picture. A positive correlation between per capita consumption of dairy fat and breast-cancer rates has been noted for geographic areas within England, but fat intake from other sources was inversely related to breast-cancer rates.[170] Although rates of breast cancer were initially reported to be lower than average among Seventh-Day Adventists, who consume relatively small amounts of fat,[171] a more recent study by the same group found that this difference was largely explainable by differences in socioeconomic status.[172] Likewise, rates of breast cancer among orders of nuns who consume little or no meat were similar to those among the general British population of single women.[173] Fat consumption has increased in both Iceland and Japan, and in the former it has been associated with a marked increase in incidence of breast cancer.[12] In Japan the increase in incidence has been much less marked.[174] Enig et al. have attempted to relate consumption of different types of fats to the apparent increase in incidence of breast and other cancers in the United States.[175] They have reported that the strongest association is that with the consumption of *trans*-fatty acids, which are fatty acids created in processes that convert liquid vegetable oils to margarine and solid vegetable shortening. However, it is not clear whether the U.S. incidence of breast cancer has actually been increasing beyond what would be expected on the basis of a trend toward later and fewer pregnancies. Within the United States, regional consumption of milk, an important fat source, is positively associated with rates of breast cancer, although consumption of eggs, a major cholesterol determinant, is inversely related to breast-cancer rates.[176]

There are few reported epidemiologic studies that address the relation between the fat intake of individual women and the occurrence of breast cancer. In one Canadian case–control study, total fat consumption was slightly higher among women in whom breast cancer developed than among control women, but this association was not statistically significant.[177] Although it was based on a small number of cases, a case–control study in Japan found a higher risk of breast cancer among women who consumed more high-fat foods,[178] and a preliminary report from Israel suggests the existence of an association between fat intake and breast cancer.[179] Using a very limited method of dietary assessment, a case–control study conducted in Alberta, Canada, found a strong positive association between breast cancer and the consump-

tion of beef and pork, the use of butter at the table, and the use of butter and margarine for frying.[180] However, in addition to the usual difficulty of obtaining dietary data in retrospect, the findings of this study are limited by the fact that data were collected in noncomparable ways from cases and controls and by a high nonparticipation rate among control subjects. Although not specifically designed to measure fat intake, a large case–control study by Graham et al.[40] found no association between fat consumption and breast-cancer incidence.

Some support for the hypothesis that high levels of dietary fat increase the rate of breast cancer is derived from studies that have related dietary factors to estrogen fractions, which are in turn likely to be related to breast-cancer risk.[181] Among postmenopausal women, omnivores, who generally consume substantial amounts of dietary fat, had higher urinary excretion of estriol and total estrogens[182] and higher plasma levels of estrone and estradiol[183] than vegetarian women. The relatively low plasma levels of estrogen among postmenopausal vegetarians in the last-cited study were shown to be at least partly the result of greatly enhanced fecal excretion of estrogens. Feeding a high-fat, Western diet to black South African women who typically consumed a low-fat vegetarian diet caused an apparent decrease in levels of luteinizing hormone, follicle-stimulating hormone, and prolactin.[184] In this study only a small increase in estradiol level was observed, and other estrogen fractions were apparently not measured.

Among premenopausal women, inconsistent associations of diet and sex hormones have been observed. Studies among vegetarian and nonvegetarian Seventh-Day Adventist teenagers[185] and among teenage girls in four countries with large differences in breast-cancer rates[186] found no meaningful associations between plasma or urinary estrogen levels and dietary factors. Although premenopausal American women who were omnivores were found to have higher levels of plasma estrone and estradiol than vegetarians,[17] an apparent decrease in estradiol level was caused by feeding a high-fat, Western diet to premenopausal South African women.[184] Each of these studies had limitations, including inadequate contrast in dietary intake,[185] the limitation of hormonal measurement to one portion of the menstrual cycle,[186] small numbers of subjects,[17] and lack of a concurrent control group.[184] Hence, the relation between dietary factors and hormonal levels among premenopausal women remains incompletely defined.

Although data on human beings are limited, the relation between various types of fat and breast cancer has been studied extensively in animal models.[1,187-190] In general, these studies show that higher levels of fat intake lead to an increased incidence of mammary tumors. Recent work suggests that the incidence of mammary tumors in rats is related to total fat intake but that at least a small amount of polyunsaturated fat is necessary for this effect to be manifested.[191,192]

Several mechanisms have been proposed by which dietary fat may increase the risk of breast cancer. Hill et al.[158] observed that estrogens are synthesized by gut flora and that this synthesis may be increased by adding fat to the diet. Alternatively, changes in colonic flora mediated by diet may increase the deconjugation and reabsorption of estrogens excreted by the biliary system.[17] Wynder et al. have suggested that fat may affect breast-cancer risk by altering prolactin secretion.[193] The existence of such a mechanism is supported by some animal studies,[194] although it has not been established that prolactin secretion is related to breast cancer in human beings. Adipose tissue can convert androstenedione to estrone,[195] and it makes an important contribution to circulating levels of estrogen in postmenopausal women. It is thus possible that dietary fat, through its high caloric content, may increase the risk of breast cancer by contributing to the development of excess fat stores. However, obesity may increase the risk of breast cancer only in older women[196]; several recent case–control studies suggest that obesity is associated with a lower rate of breast cancer among premenopausal women.[197,198] Another potential mechanism relates to the intake of polyunsaturated fatty acids that are subject to in vivo peroxidation.[83] This peroxidation, which may result in damage to macromolecules, can be reduced by vitamin E or selenium,[199] suggesting that an interaction between the type of dietary fat and antioxidant consumption may be related to the risk of breast cancer as well as other cancers.[200]

Although the hypothesis that at least some types of dietary fat cause breast cancer in human beings is reasonable, it is far from proved. Since it seems unlikely that the hypothesis can be tested in human beings experimentally, we must depend on observational studies of this relation. Unfortunately, this may also be one of the most difficult relations to study epidemiologically, for several reasons. First of all, the observations that the changes in rate of breast cancer among some immigrants do not occur until the second generation and that many hormone-related risk factors for breast cancer are operative before age 20 suggest that dietary variables may be most important relatively early in life. Secondly, within populations such as that of the United States there is considerably less variation in fat intake than in the intake of many other nutrients. Thirdly, dietary fat is obtained from a large number of foods with a highly variable fat composition, making it difficult to estimate intake. Finally, dietary fat, like fiber, is an extremely heterogeneous collection of nutrients.

It is to be hoped that several ongoing prospective studies of diet and cancer among women will provide a clearer characterization of the relation between fat intake and breast cancer. In these studies it will be important to address potential differences in the health effects of various types of fat.

Caloric Excess

Although our discussion has focused on specific nutrients, excess caloric intake relative to physical activity, as manifested by obesity, is associated with an increased risk of cancer at some specific sites.[201] The strongest association is with endometrial cancer. Carcinoma of the gallbladder likewise occurs more commonly in obese persons — a fact that is perhaps related to the more frequent occurrence of cholelithiasis in such persons.[202]

De Waard has reported that both greater weight and greater height are associated with breast cancer, so that postmenopausal women with large body-surface area have a fourfold excess risk of breast cancer as compared with women with small body-surface area.[203] However, these observations could result in part from incomplete control for the confounding effect of age, which is associated with a propensity to gain weight. If overweight is related to breast-cancer risk, this association is probably limited to breast cancer that occurs among postmenopausal women,[196] and the direction of the association may actually be reversed among premenopausal women.[197,204] Although further prospective data are required to define these relations more precisely, the excess risk of breast cancer due to general overnutrition is likely to be less than is suggested by the data of de Waard.[200]

A number of experiments in animals support a relation between excess caloric intake and cancer incidence,[205] as well as a nonspecific shortening of lifespan.[187] Caloric restriction, whether early or late in life, appears to decrease the incidence of tumors at multiple sites.[206,207] A number of mechanisms for the role of overfeeding in cancer have been suggested, including the stimulation of mitotic activity in young animals,[208] the alteration of hormonal levels at older ages,[209] or the reduction of immune competence.[210]

The study of caloric intake and cancer involves several special problems. First of all, persons with higher caloric intake tend to consume more of all the major nutrients. Thus, it will always be important to separate the effects of specific nutrients from the effects of total intake. In addition, the physiologic meaning of caloric intake remains somewhat obscure. To a considerable extent it represents a person's level of physical activity and size. However, it also probably reflects absorptive capacity and metabolic efficiency[211] in ways that are not well established or easily measurable.

Conclusion

Evidence from international studies, experiments in animals, and observational studies among individual subjects suggests that dietary factors have important causative and protective roles in carcinogenesis. However, information about specific dietary factors is generally inconsistent or incomplete. It is our own belief that available data are not sufficient to serve as a basis for strong specific dietary recommendations. The preliminary recommendations of the National Research Council[2] that people should generally eat less fat and more fruits, vegetables, and whole-grain products (in addition to moderating alcohol intake and minimizing the consumption of certain processed foods) seem sensible, not so much because of the firmness of any expectation that cancer rates will be lowered by such actions, but because the changes are unlikely to be harmful and may well be beneficial in the context of other diseases.

We are indebted to Dr. Meir Stampfer, Marilyn Bell, and Trudie Crowley for helpful comments and assistance in the preparation of this manuscript.

REFERENCES

85. Chow CK. Nutritional influence on cellular antioxidant defense systems. Am J Clin Nutr 1979; 32:1066-81.
86. Shamberger RJ, Tytko SA, Willis CE. Antioxidants and cancer. VI. Selenium and age-adjusted human cancer mortality. Arch Environ Health 1976; 31:231-5.
87. Shamberger RJ, Rukovena E, Longfield AK, Tytko SA, Deodhar S, Willis CE. Antioxidants and cancer. I. Selenium in the blood of normals and cancer patients. JNCI 1973; 50:863-70.
88. McConnell KP, Broghamer WL Jr, Blotcky AJ, Hurt OJ. Selenium levels in human blood and tissues in health and in disease. J Nutr 1975; 105:1026-31.
89. Broghamer WL Jr, McConnell KP, Blotcky AJ. Relationship between serum selenium levels and patients with carcinoma. Cancer 1976; 37:1384-8.
90. McConnell KP, Jager RM, Bland KI, Blotcky AJ. The relationship of dietary selenium and breast cancer. J Surg Oncol 1980; 15:67-70
91. Robinson MF, Godfrey PJ, Thomson CD, Rea HM, van Rij AM. Blood selenium and glutathione peroxidase activity in normal subjects and in surgical patients with and without cancer in New Zealand. Am J Clin Nutr 1979; 32:1477-85.
92. Willett WC, Polk BF, Morris JS, et al. Prediagnostic serum selenium and risk of cancer. Lancet 1983; 2:130-4.
93. Thomson CD, Robinson MF, Campbell DR, Rea HM. Effect of prolonged supplementation with daily supplements of selenomethionine and sodium selenite on glutathione peroxidase activity in blood of New Zealand residents. Am J Clin Nutr 1982; 36:24-31.
94. Levander OA, Alfthan G, Arvilommi H, et al. Bioavailability of selenium to Finnish men as assessed by platelet glutathione peroxidase activity and other blood parameters. Am J Clin Nutr 1983; 37:887-97.
95. Maugh TH II. Hair: a diagnostic tool to complement blood, serum, and urine. Science 1978; 202:1271-3.
96. Laker M. On determining trace element levels in man: the uses of blood and hair. Lancet 1982; 2:260-2.
97. Morris JS, Stampfer MJ, Willett W. Toenails as an indicator of dietary selenium. Biol Trace Element Res 1983; 5:529-37.
98. Jacobs MM, Matney TS, Griffin AC. Inhibitory effects of selenium on the mutagenicity of 2-acetylaminofluorine (AAF) and AAF derivatives. Cancer Lett 1977; 2:319-22.
99. Shamberger RJ, Beaman KD, Corlett CL, Kasten BL. Effect of selenium and other antioxidants on the mutagenicity of malonaldehyde. Fed Proc 1978; 37:261. abstract.
100. Marshall MV, Arnott MA, Jacobs MM, Griffin AC. Selenium effects on the carcinogenicity and metabolism of 2-acetylaminofluorine. Cancer Lett 1979; 7:331-8.
101. Clayton CC, Baumann CA. Diet and azo dye tumors: effect of diet during a period when dye is not fed. Cancer Res 1949; 9:575-82.
102. Shamberger RJ. Relationship of selenium to cancer. I. Inhibitory effect of selenium on carcinogenesis. JNCI 1970; 44:931-6.
103. Griffin AC, Jacobs MM. Effects of selenium on azo dye hepatocarcinogenesis. Cancer Lett 1977; 3:177-81.
104. Daoud AH, Griffin AC. Effects of selenium and retinoic acid on the metabolism of N-acetylaminofluorene and N-hydroxyacetylaminofluorene. Cancer Lett 1978; 5:231-7.
105. Greeder GA, Milner JA. Factors influencing the inhibitory effect of selenium on mice inoculated with Ehrlich ascites tumor cells. Science 1980; 209:825-7.
106. Thompson HJ, Becci PJ. Selenium inhibition of N-methyl-N-nitrosourea-induced mammary carcinogenesis in the rat. JNCI 1980; 65:1299-301.
107. Schrauzer GN, Ishmael D. Effects of selenium and of arsenic on the genesis of spontaneous mammary tumors in inbred C₃H mice. Ann Clin Lab Sci 1974; 4:441-7.
108. Medina D. Selenium and murine mammary tumorigenesis. Cancer Bull 1982; 34:162-5.
109. Burk RF, Lawrence RA, Lane JM. Liver necrosis and lipid peroxidation in the rat as the result of paraquat and diquat administration: effect of selenium deficiency. J Clin Invest 1980; 65:1024-31.
110. Ip C, Sinha DK. Enhancement of mammary tumorigenesis by dietary selenium deficiency in rats with a high polyunsaturated fat intake. Cancer Res 1981; 41:31-4.
111. Tappel AL. Vitamin E and selenium protection from in vivo lipid peroxidation. Ann NY Acad Sci 1980; 355:18-29.
112. Thompson HJ, Becci PJ. Effect of graded dietary levels of selenium on tracheal carcinomas induced by 1-methyl-1-nitrosourea. Cancer Lett 1979; 7:215-9.
113. Spallholz JE. Selenium: what role in immunity and immune cytotoxicity? In: Spallholz JE, Martin JL, Ganther HE, eds. Selenium in biology and medicine. Westport, Conn.: AVI Publishing, 1981:103-17.
114. Lemley RE. Selenium poisoning in the human: a preliminary report. The Journal–Lancet 1940; 60:528-31.
115. Burkitt DP. Epidemiology of cancer of the colon and rectum. Cancer 1971; 28:3-13.
116. Sherlock P, Lipkin M, Winawer SJ. Predisposing factors in carcinoma of the colon. Adv Intern Med 1975; 20:121-50.
117. Liu K, Stamler J, Moss D, Garside D, Persky V, Soltero I. Dietary cholesterol, fat, and fibre, and colon-cancer mortality: an analysis of international data. Lancet 1979; 2:782-5.
118. Bingham S, Williams DRR, Cole TJ, James WPT. Dietary fibre and regional large-bowel cancer mortality in Britain. Br J Cancer 1979; 40:456-63.
119. Bjelke E. Epidemiologic studies of cancer of the stomach, colon and rectum, with special emphasis on the role of diet. Vol. 3. Ann Arbor, Mich.: University Microfilm, 1973:273-343.
120. Graham S, Dayal H, Swanson M, Mittelman A, Wilkinson G. Diet in the epidemiology of cancer of the colon and rectum. JNCI 1978; 61:709-14.
121. Manousos O, Day NE, Trichopoulos D, Gerovassilis F, Tzonou A, Polychronopoulou A. Diet and colorectal cancer: a case-control study in Greece. Int J Cancer 1983; 32:1-5.
122. Modan B, Barell V, Lubin F, Modan M, Greenberg RA, Graham S. Low-fiber intake as an etiologic factor in cancer of the colon. JNCI 1975; 55:15-8.
123. Dales LG, Friedman GD, Ury HK, Grossman S, Williams SR. A case-control study of relationships of diet and other traits to colorectal cancer in American blacks. Am J Epidemiol 1978; 109:132-44.
124. Martinez I, Torres R, Frias Z, Colon JR, Fernandez N. Factors associated with adenocarcinomas of the large bowel in Puerto Rico. In: Birch JM, ed. Advances in medical oncology, research and education. Vol. 3. New York: Pergamon Press, 1979:45-52.
125. Southgate DAT. The definition and analysis of dietary fibre. Nutr Rev 1977; 35:31-7.
126. Glober GA, Nomura A, Kamiyama S, Shimada A, Abba BC. Bowel transit-time and stool weight in populations with different colon-cancer risks. Lancet 1977; 2:110-1.
127. Reddy BS, Hedges AR, Laakso K, Wynder EL. Metabolic epidemiology of large bowel cancer: fecal bulk and constituents of high-risk North American and low-risk Finnish population. Cancer 1978; 42:2832-8.
128. Story JA, Kritchevsky D. Comparison of the binding of various bile acids and bile salts in vitro by several types of fiber. J Nutr 1976; 106:1292-4.
129. Reddy BS, Wynder EL. Large-bowel carcinogenesis: fecal constituents of populations with diverse incidence rates of colon cancer. JNCI 1973; 50:1437-42.
130. Wilson RB, Hutcheson DP, Wideman L. Dimethylhydrazine-induced colon tumors in rats fed diets containing beef fat or corn oil with and without wheat bran. Am J Clin Nutr 1977; 30:176-81.
131. Freeman HJ, Spiller GA, Kim YS. A double-blind study on the effect of purified cellulose dietary fiber on 1,2-dimethylhydrazine-induced rat colonic neoplasia. Cancer Res 1978; 38:2912-7.
132. Asp NG, Bauer H, Dahlqvist A, Fredlund P, Öste R. Dietary fiber and experimental colon cancer in the rat. Nutr Cancer 1979; 1(2):70-3.
133. Reddy BS, Mori H, Nicolais M. Effect of dietary wheat bran and dehy-

drated citrus fiber on azoxymethane-induced intestinal carcinogenesis in Fischer 344 rats. JNCI 1981; 66:553-7.

134. Karlin DA, O'Donnell RT, Jensen WE. Effect of dioctyl sodium sulfosuccinate feeding on rat colorectal 1,2-dimethylhydrazine carcinogenesis. JNCI 1980; 64:791-3.

135. Wattenberg LW, Loub WD. Inhibition of polycyclic aromatic hydrocarbon-induced neoplasia by naturally occurring indoles. Cancer Res 1978; 38:1410-3.

136. Walker ARP. Colon cancer and diet, with special reference to intakes of fat and fiber. Am J Clin Nutr 1976; 29:1417-26.

137. Hirayama T. Epidemiology of cancer of the stomach with special reference to its recent decrease in Japan. Cancer Res 1975; 35:3460-3.

138. Lee JAH. Recent trends of large bowel cancer in Japan compared to United States and England and Wales. Int J Epidemiol 1976; 5:187-94.

139. Haenszel W, Berg JW, Segi M, Kurihara M, Locke FB. Large-bowel cancer in Hawaiian Japanese. JNCI 1973; 51:1765-79.

140. Haenszel W, Locke FB, Segi M. A case-control study of large bowel cancer in Japan. JNCI 1980; 64:17-22.

141. A co-operative trial in the primary prevention of ischemic heart disease using clofibrate: report from the Committee of Principal Investigators. Br Heart J 1978; 40:1069-118.

142. Kark JD, Smith AH, Hames CG. The relationship of serum cholesterol to the incidence of cancer in Evans County, Georgia. J Chronic Dis 1980; 33:311-22.

143. Garcia-Palmieri MR, Sorlie PD, Costas R Jr, Havlik RJ. An apparent inverse relationship between serum cholesterol and cancer mortality in Puerto Rico. Am J Epidemiol 1981; 114:29-40.

144. Kagan A, McGee DL, Yano K, Rhoads GG, Nomura A. Serum cholesterol and mortality in a Japanese-American population: the Honolulu Heart Program. Am J Epidemiol 1981; 114:11-20.

145. Linos DA, Beard CM, O'Fallon WM, Dockerty MB, Beart RW Jr, Kurland LT. Cholecystectomy and carcinoma of the colon. Lancet 1981; 2:379-81.

146. Vernick LJ, Kuller LH. Cholecystectomy and right-sided colon cancer: an epidemiological study. Lancet 1981; 2:381-3.

147. Nigro ND, Singh DV, Campbell RL, Pak MS. Effect of dietary fat on intestinal tumor formation by azoxymethane in rats. JNCI 1975; 54:439-42.

148. Reddy BS, Narisawa T, Vukusich D, Weisburger JH, Wynder EL. Effect of quality and quantity of dietary fat and dimethylhydrazine in colon carcinogenesis in rats. Proc Soc Exp Biol Med 1976; 151:237-9.

149. Broitman SA, Vitale JJ, Vavrousek-Jakuba E, Gottlieb LS. Polyunsaturated fat, cholesterol, and large bowel tumorigenesis. Cancer 1977; 40:2455-63.

150. Cruse JP, Lewin MR, Ferulano GP, Clark CG. Co-carcinogenic effects of dietary cholesterol in experimental colon cancer. Nature 1978; 276:822-5.

151. Bull AW, Soullier BK, Wilson PS, Hayden MT, Nigro ND. Promotion of azoxymethane-induced intestinal cancer by high-fat diet in rats. Cancer Res 1979; 39:4956-9.

152. Reddy BS, Weisburger JH, Wynder EL. Effects of high risk and low risk diets for colon carcinogenesis on fecal microflora and steroids in man. J Nutr 1975; 105:878-84.

153. Hill MJ. The role of unsaturated bile acids in the etiology of large bowel cancer. In: Hiatt HH, Watson JD, Winsten JA, eds. Origins of human cancer. Cold Spring Harbor, N.Y.: Cold Spring Harbor Laboratories, 1977:1627-40.

154. Reddy BS. Diet and excretion of bile acids. Cancer Res 1981; 41:3766-8.

155. Reddy BS, Mangat S, Sheinfil A, Weisburger JH, Wynder EL. Effect of type and amount of dietary fat, and 1,2-dimethylhydrazine on biliary bile acids, fecal bile acids, and neutral sterols in rats. Cancer Res 1977; 37:2132-7.

156. Quintão ESR, Brumer S, Stechhahn K. Tissue storage and control of cholesterol metabolism in man on high cholesterol diets. Atherosclerosis 1977; 26:297-310.

157. Lin DS, Conner WE. The long term effects of dietary cholesterol upon the plasma lipids, lipoproteins, cholesterol absorption, and the sterol balance in man: the demonstration of feedback inhibition of cholesterol biosynthesis and increased bile acid secretion. J Lipid Res 1980; 21:1042-52.

158. Hill MJ, Crowther JS, Drasar BS, Hawksworth GB, Aries V, Williams REO. Bacteria and aetiology of cancer of large bowel. Lancet 1971; 1:95-100.

159. Hill MJ, Drasar BS, Williams REO, et al. Fecal bile-acids and clostridia in patients with cancer of the large bowel. Lancet 1975; 1:535-9.

160. Reddy BS, Mastromarino A, Wynder EL. Further leads on metabolic epidemiology of large bowel cancer. Cancer Res 1975; 35:3403-6.

161. Reddy BS, Wynder EL. Metabolic epidemiology of colon cancer: fecal bile acids and neutral sterols in colon cancer patients and patients with adenomatous polyps. Cancer 1977; 39:2533-9.

162. Dietary fibre, transit time, faecal bacteria, steroids, and colon cancer in two Scandinavian populations: report from the International Agency for Research on Cancer Intestinal Microecology Group. Lancet 1977; 2:207-11.

163. Mudd DG, McKelvey STD, Norwood W, Elmore DT, Roy AD. Faecal bile acid concentrations of patients with carcinoma or increased risk of carcinoma in the large bowel. Gut 1980; 21:587-90.

164. Chomchai C, Bhadrachari N, Nigro ND. The effect of bile on the induction of experimental intestinal tumors in rats. Dis Colon Rectum 1974; 17:310-2.

165. Narisawa T, Magadia NE, Weisburger JH, Wynder EL. Promoting effect of bile acids on colon carcinogenesis after intrarectal installation of N-methyl-N'-nitro-N-nitrosoguanidine in rats. JNCI 1974; 53:1093-7.

166. Ranken R, Wilson R, Bealmear PM. Increased turnover of intestinal mucosal cells of germfree mice induced by cholic acid. Proc Soc Exp Biol Med 1971; 138:270-2.

167. Reddy BS, Watanabe K, Weisburger JH, Wynder EL. Promoting effect of bile acids in colon carcinogenesis in germ-free and conventional F344 rats. Cancer Res 1977; 37:3238-42.

168. Goldin BR, Swenson L, Dwyer J, Sexton M, Gorbach SL. Effect of diet and Lactobacillus acidophilus supplements on human bacterial enzymes. JNCI 1980; 64:255-61.

169. Waterhouse J, Muir C, Correa P, et al., eds. Cancer incidence in five continents. Vol. 3. Lyon: International Agency for Research on Cancer, 1976.

170. Stocks P. Breast cancer anomalies. Br J Cancer 1970; 24:633-43.

171. Phillips RL. Role of life-style and dietary habits in risk of cancer among Seventh-Day Adventists. Cancer Res 1975; 35:3513-22.

172. Phillips RL, Garfinkel L, Kuzma JW, Beeson WL, Lotz T, Brin B. Mortality among California Seventh-Day Adventists for selected cancer sites. JNCI 1980; 65:1097-107.

173. Kinlen LJ. Meat and fat consumption and cancer mortality: a study of strict religious orders in Britain. Lancet 1982; 1:946-9.

174. MacMahon B. Incidence trends in North America, Japan, and Hawaii. In: Magnus K, ed. Trends in cancer incidence. New York: McGraw-Hill, 1982:249-62.

175. Enig MG, Munn RJ, Keeney M. Dietary fat and cancer trends — a critique. Fed Proc 1978; 37:2215-20.

176. Gaskill SP, McGuire WL, Osborne CK, Stern MP. Breast cancer mortality and diet in the United States. Cancer Res 1979; 39:3628-37.

177. Miller AB, Kelly A, Choi NW, et al. A study of diet and breast cancer. Am J Epidemiol 1978; 107:499-509.

178. Hirayama T. Epidemiology of breast cancer with special reference to the role of diet. Prev Med 1978; 7:173-95.

179. Lubin F, Modan B. Correlations between dietary factors and pre- and postmenopausal breast cancer. Presented at the 12th International Congress of Nutrition, San Diego, August 1981.

180. Lubin JH, Burns PE, Blot WJ, Ziegler RG, Lees AW, Fraumeni JF Jr. Dietary factors and breast cancer risk. Int J Cancer 1981; 28:685-9.

181. MacMahon B, Cole P, Brown J. Etiology of human breast cancer: a review. JNCI 1973; 50:21-42.

182. Armstrong BK, Brown JB, Clarke HT, et al. Diet and reproductive hormones: a study of vegetarian and nonvegetarian postmenopausal women. JNCI 1981; 67:761-7.

183. Goldin BR, Adlercreutz H, Dwyer JT, Swenson L, Warram JH, Gorbach SL. Effect of diet on excretion of estrogens in pre- and postmenopausal women. Cancer Res 1981; 41:3771-3.

184. Hill P, Garbaczewski L, Helman P, Huskisson J, Sporangisa E, Wynder EL. Diet, lifestyle, and menstrual activity. Am J Clin Nutr 1980; 33:1192-8.

185. Gray GE, Williams P, Gerkins V, et al. Diet and hormone levels in Seventh-Day Adventist teenage girls. Prev Med 1982; 11:103-7.

186. Gray GE, Pike MC, Hirayama T, et al. Diet and hormone profiles in teenage girls in four countries at different risk for breast cancer. Prev Med 1982; 11:108-13.

187. Dunning WF, Curtis MR, Maun ME. The effect of dietary fat and carbohydrate on diethylstilbestrol-induced mammary cancer in rats. Cancer Res 1949; 9:354-61.

188. Benson J, Lev M, Grand CG. Enhancement of mammary fibroadenomas in the female rat by a high fat diet. Cancer Res 1956; 16:135-7.

189. Carroll KK, Khor HT. Effects of level and type of dietary fat on incidence of mammary tumors induced in female Sprague–Dawley rats by 7,12-dimethylbenz(α)anthracene. Lipids 1971; 6:415-20.

190. Chan P-C, Head JF, Cohen LA, Wynder EL. Influence of dietary fat on the induction of mammary tumors by N-nitrosomethylurea: associated hormone changes and differences between Sprague–Dawley and F344 rats. JNCI 1977; 59:1279-83.

191. Carroll KK, Hopkins GJ. Dietary polyunsaturated fat *versus* saturated fat in relation to mammary carcinogenesis. Lipids 1979; 14:155-8.

192. Hopkins GJ, Carroll KK. Relationship between amount and type of dietary fat in promotion of mammary carcinogenesis induced by 7,12-dimethylbenz[a]anthracene. JNCI 1979; 62:1009-12.

193. Wynder EL, MacCornack F, Hill P, Cohen LA, Chan PC, Weisburger JH. Nutrition and etiology and prevention of breast cancer. Cancer Detect Prev 1976; 1:293-310.

194. Chan P-C, Cohen LA. Effect of dietary fat, antiestrogen, and antiprolactin on the development of mammary tumors in rats. JNCI 1974; 52:25-30.

195. Grodin JM, Siiteri PK, MacDonald PC. Source of estrogen production in postmenopausal women. J Clin Endocrinol Metab 1973; 36:207-14.

196. de Waard F, Baanders-van Halewijn EA, Huizinga J. The bimodal age distribution of patients with mammary carcinoma: evidence for the existence of 2 types of human breast cancer. Cancer 1964; 17:141-51.

197. Helmrich SP, Shapiro S, Rosenberg L, et al. Risk factors for breast cancer. Am J Epidemiol 1983; 117:35-45.

198. Fasal E, Paffenbarger RS Jr. Oral contraceptives as related to cancer and benign lesions of the breast. JNCI 1975; 55:767-73.

199. Tappel AL. Vitamin E and selenium protection from *in vivo* lipid peroxidation. Ann NY Acad Sci 1980; 355:18-31.

200. Ames BN. Dietary carcinogens and anticarcinogens. Science 1983; 221:1256-66.

201. Lew EA, Garfinkel L. Variations in mortality by weight among 750,000 men and women. J Chronic Dis 1979; 32:563-76.

202. Zahor Z, Sternby NH, Kagan A, Uemura K, Vanecek R, Vichert AM. Frequency of cholelithiasis in Prague and Malmö: an autopsy study. Scand J Gastroenterol 1974; 9:3-7.

203. de Waard F. Breast cancer incidence and nutritional status with particular reference to body weight and height. Cancer Res 1975; 35:3351-6.

204. Choi NW, Howe GR, Miller AB, et al. An epidemiologic study of breast cancer. Am J Epidemiol 1978; 107:510-21.

205. Tannenbaum A. Relationship of body weight to cancer incidence. Arch Pathol 1940; 30:509-17.

206. Ross MH, Bras G. Lasting influence of early caloric restriction on prevalence of neoplasms in the rat. JNCI 1971; 47:1095-113.

207. Weindruch JR, Walford RL. Dietary restriction in mice beginning at 1 year of age: effect on life-span and spontaneous cancer incidence. Science 1982; 215:1415-8.

208. Stini WA. Early nutrition, growth, disease, and human longevity. Nutr Cancer 1978; 1(1):31-9.

209. Wynder EL, Mabuchi K. Etiological and preventive aspects of human cancer. Prev Med 1972; 1:300-34.

210. Jose DG, Good RA. Quantitative effects of nutritional protein and calorie deficiency upon immune responses to tumors in mice. Cancer Res 1973; 33:807-12.

211. De Luise M, Blackburn GL, Flier JS. Reduced activity of the red-cell sodium-potassium pump in human obesity. N Engl J Med 1980; 303:1017-22.

Mutagens, Carcinogens, and Tumor Promoters in our Daily Food

by Takashi Sugimura, M.D.

THE IDEA that cancer cells arise from normal cells through somatic mutation has a long history, and was suggested as early as 1928 by Bauer.[7] This idea is supported by the irreversibility of some cellular changes during carcinogenesis and the stability of most cancer phenotypes.

In 1957, Nakahara, Fukuoka and I[86] showed that 4-nitroquinoline 1-oxide (4NQO) was carcinogenic when painted on mouse skin. 4NQO was reported to be mutagenic towards *Aspergillus* in 1956.[150] Moreover, treatment of lysogenized *Escherichia coli* with this compound resulted in phage induction.[24] 4NQO is reduced to 4-hydroxyaminoquinoline 1-oxide (4HAQO) by enzymes in bacterial and mammalian cells with concomitant oxidation of reduced pyridine nucleotides.[119] 4HAQO has mutagenic activity[25] and phage-inducing activity on lysogenic bacteria[24] and can produce DNA strand scission *in vitro*.[120] Later Tada and Tada[124] showed that 4HAQO can form an adducts with DNA bases in the presence of serine, ATP and seryl-tRNA synthetase. The seryl-4HAQO thus formed is thought to be an ultimate mutagen and carcinogen, and so 4HAQO can be regarded as a proximate carcinogen. Further metabolic reduction of 4HAQO yields biologically much less active 4-aminoquinoline 1-oxide.[119] The metabolic pathway of 4NQO is shown in Figure 1.

These findings in our laboratory and other laboratories in Japan prompted us to study the carcinogenicity of mutagens, the interaction of carcinogens with DNA, and the metabolism of carcinogens. In 1960, the strong mutagenicity of N-methyl-N'-nitro-N-nitrosoguanidine (MNNG) was reported by Mandell and Greenberg.[63] In 1966, we reported that on subcutaneous injection, MNNG induced transplantable fibrosarcomas in rats.[117] In the same year, Schoenthal[101] and Druckrey and colleagues[22] also independently reported the carcinogenicity of this mutagen. After this discovery, a solution of MNNG was given to rats in their drinking water in our laboratory and found to produce adenocarcinomas of the glandular stomach (Fig. 2).[109,110] On the basis of this finding, we realized that gastric cancer, the most common cancer in Japanese, might be induced by carcinogens contained in traditional Japanese food, and that these carcinogens could be detected as mutagens.

In 1975, Ames and associates[5] reported a mutation test using *Salmonella typhimurium* to detect carcinogens in the environment. Many typical carcinogens have been demonstrated as mutagens by the *Salmonella* test, which is currently very widely used in research laboratories, industries, and regulatory agencies.[67,68,94-96] The *S. typhimurium* strains used in the Ames test have advantages in that they lack UV damage-repair capacity (*uvr*B) and most of the lipopolysaccharides of the cell wall (deep rough); these two characteristics make the bacteria very sensitive to mutagens. In the Ames test, S9 mix from the liver of rats previously treated with Aroclor 1254 (Analabs, North Haven, Conn.) is

From the National Cancer Center Research Institute, Tsukiji, Chuo-ku, Tokyo, Japan.

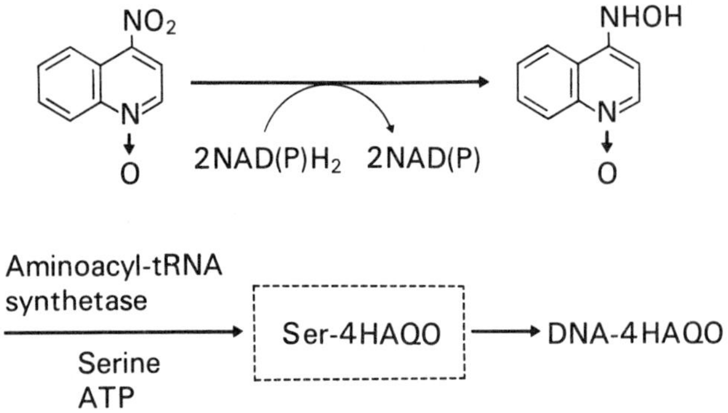

FIG. 1. Metabolism of 4NQO.

used to convert promutagens/procarcinogens to ultimate mutagens/ultimate carcinogens. In our laboratory, we demonstrated the marked overlap of mutagens revealed by the Ames test and carcinogens.[121] This finding prompted us to search for carcinogens through mutagens in the environment, especially in human food.

The Food Additive, AF-2

After World War II, food, especially food rich in protein, was limited in Japan. Since the sources of protein such as fish and meat were important, a series of nitrofuryl derivatives were developed as food preservatives. In 1965, the Ministry of Health and Welfare of Japan approved the use of AF-2, 2-(2-furyl)-3-(5-nitrofuryl)acrylamide, a nitrofuran derivative as a food preservative. The structure of AF-2 is shown in Figure 2. AF-2 was commonly added to fish and meat sausages at 20 ppm, to fish cake at 20 ppm, to soy bean curd at 10 ppm, and to red bean paste at 5 ppm. It was an extremely effective preservative. However, in 1973, AF-2 was found to induce chromosome aberrations in cultured human lymphoblasts,[135] and later its potent mutagenicity in *E. coli* WP2 mutant was reported.[49,57] AF-2 also gave a positive result in the mutation test using *S. typhimurium* TA100 and TA98.[148]

The approval of use of AF-2 by the Ministry of Health and Welfare had been based on a previous report of the noncarcinogenicity of AF-2 in rats. But the find-

FIG. 2. Structure of AF-2.

ing that AF-2 was mutagenic produced a controversy among academic people, consumers, and regulatory agencies who debated the safety of its use and whether or not it should be banned as a food additive. At that time, although the mutagenicity of typical carcinogens and the carcinogenicity of typical mutagens were being demonstrated in many laboratories,[68,95,121] proof of mutagenicity alone was not sufficient grounds for banning a substance. It was difficult to decide how to adjust laws which were becoming outdated by scientific advances.

During this period of controversy about AF-2, a bioassay in mice showed that AF-2 induced squamous cell carcinomas of the forestomach, and that the effect of AF-2 depended on its concentration in the diet.[46] These positive results on the carcinogenicity of AF-2 in mice were obtained in 1974 and its use as a food additive was immediately banned by the Ministry of Health and Welfare. Later, the carcinogenicity of AF-2 was further confirmed in mice,[129] rats,[20,129] and hamsters.[56]

The case of AF-2 provided several suggestions on the issue of mutagens and carcinogens in food. First, if any compound in food shows mutagenicity, its carcinogenicity should be seriously considered. Second, data reporting noncarcinogenicity, published before 1960, can not be considered conclusive. Furthermore, it became evident, in studies on AF-2, that *S. typhimurium* strains TA1535, TA1537 and TA1538, which were used as tester strains in Ames' original method,[4] could not be used to detect the mutagenicity of AF-2.[148] However, the TA100 and TA98 strains which contained plasmids and were introduced later by Ames and his associates,[69] were found to be very sensitive to the mutagenicity of AF-2.[147]

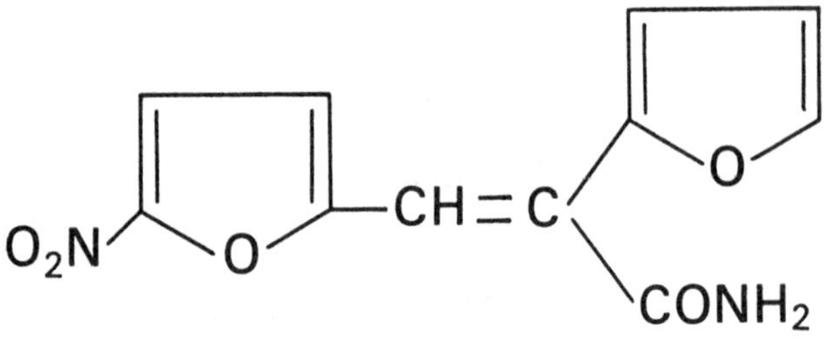

Improvement and Adoption of the Ames Test for Screening for Carcinogens in Food

During investigations into the mutagenicities of carcinogens, we noticed that several known carcinogens did not demonstrate mutagenicity. Therefore, we improved the Ames test to allow detection of the mutagenicities of carcinogens. Examples are provided in Figure 3. *N,N*-dimethylnitrosamine (DMN) is known to be carcinogenic to many animals. By adding a step of preincubation of the test chemical with bacteria and S9 mix, the mutagenicity of DMN was clearly demonstrated, whereas there was little mutagenicity without this step,[149] as shown in Figure 3a. Similarly, the mutagenicity of pyrolizidine alkaloids, known carcinogens which are present in some edible plants, could be demonstrated by the Ames test only with the preincubation procedure[156] (Fig. 3b). These findings led us to adopt the preincubation method in mutagenicity tests for all compounds, including those described below. Certain carcinogenic azo dyes, such as trypan blue and ponceau R, were demonstrated to be mutagenic only in the presence of riboflavin in S9 mix[66] (Fig. 3c). Riboflavin accelerates the reduction of the azo bond in forming the promutagen. On the other hand, the mutagenicity of *o*-aminoazotoluene was reduced by including riboflavin in S9 mix. The mutagenicities of carcinogenic yellow OB and *N*,*N*-diphenylnitrosamine were detected when norharman (β-carboline) was added to S9 mix[122] (Figure 3d). Norharman is produced by pyrolysis of tryptophan or proteins and is not mutagenic itself. The mutagenicities of aniline and *o*-toluidine were also demonstrated only in the presence of norharman[83] and the weak mutagenicity of 4-dimethylaminoazobenzene was tremendously enhanced by this chemical.[82] Norharman could thus be called a 'co-mutagen.'[83] Many naturally occurring mutagens exist as glycosides, and incubation with glycosidase is essential for demonstrating their mutagenicity. Examples are cycasin, demonstrated to be mutagenic with almond β-glucosidase,[66] and rutin, demonstrated to be mutagenic with hesperidinase from *Aspergillus niger*[78] (Figs. 3e and 3f).

With these modified incubation conditions and cofactors added as appropriate, many compounds were tested in our laboratory. The degree of overlapping of mutagenicity and carcinogenicity of chemicals depends very much on the types of compounds tested. With al-

kylating agent-type carcinogens, the overlap is nearly 100%, whereas with carcinogens such as chloroform or chlorinated aromatic compounds, the overlap is nearly zero. In this laboratory, we have not attempted to evaluate the usefulness of microbial mutation tests as screening methods for environmental carcinogens. Instead, we have used the microbial mutation test to find new mutagens, which we test later by long-term *in vivo* assay. The microbial test is recognized as a very useful method for obtaining preliminary, but crucial information on unknown carcinogenic compounds in foods. However, we have been reluctant to make any strong statements to regulatory agencies on the value of the microbial test in obtaining decisive information. Here I would like only to emphasize how useful the microbial mutation test has been in identifying new carcinogens in food. When a compound in our food is shown to be mutagenic, we definitely need further investigation into it.

Data from carcinogenicity tests found in the literature do not always provide a sufficient basis for evaluating the potency of carcinogenicity, which varies in a range of 10^6.[79] The potency of mutagenicity also varies in the same range. Thus, a discussion of overlap which does not mention the potencies of mutagenicity and carcinogenicity probably does not make much sense. Our results on more than 1000 compounds tested, showed that the overlap between the detection of mutagenicity and carcinogenicity was 70–80%.

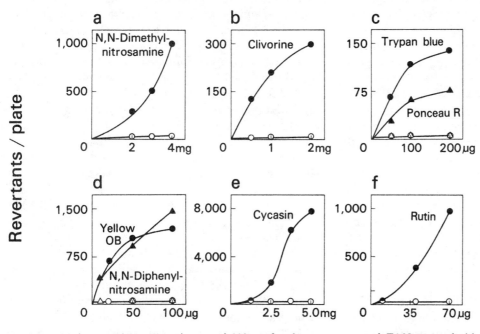

FIG. 3. Improvement of Ames *Salmonella* test. (a) Preincubation: Mutagenicity of *N*,*N*-dimethylnitrosamine was tested with (●——●) or without (○——○) preincubation at 25°C for 20 min. TA100 was used with S9 mix. (b) Preincubation: Mutagenicity of clivorine was tested with (●——●) or without (○——○) preincubation at 37°C for 20 min. TA100 was used with S9 mix. (c) Addition of riboflavin for the test of diazocompound: Mutagenicity of trypan blue was assayed with (●——●) or without (○——○) 0.1 μmol of riboflavin in the presence of S9 mix, and that of ponceau R was also tested with (▲——▲) or without (△——△) 1.0 μmol of riboflavin in the presence of S9 mix. TA98 and TA100 were used for trypan blue and ponceau R, respectively. (d) Addition of norharman: Yellow OB with (●——●) or without (○——○) 200 μg of norharman, and *N*,*N*-diphenylni-

trosamine with (▲——▲) or without (△——△) 200 μg of norharman were tested. TA98 was used with S9 mix. (e) Addition of β-glucosidase for the test of glucoside: *HisG46* and cycasin with (●——●) or without (○——○) β-glucosidase (30 units) were preincubated at 30°C, pH 6.5, for 90 min. (f) Addition of hesperidinase for the test of flavonol glycoside: Rutin was pretreated with (●——●) or without (○——○) 1 mg of hesperidinase, and then incubated with TA98 and S9 mix.

Carcinogenesis can be divided into two stages: initiation and promotion. Initiation is principally related to changes in DNA structure, whereas promotion is not necessarily related. If animal cells have been initiated by endogeneously formed mutagens or by mutagens in the environment, application of only a promoter will increase the incidence of tumors. Thus, compounds with tumor-promoting activity that do not have any mutagenic activity can also be termed 'carcinogens.' In many respects, discussion on the overlap of mutagens and carcinogens and on the value of the microbial assay for screening for environmental carcinogens is not fruitful if the significance of tumor promoters is not considered. It should be emphasized that the microbial tests currently available are useful only for identification of mutagens which might also be carcinogens. Further investigations, including carcinogenicity tests sometimes using tumor promoters, are necessary for identifying compounds as carcinogens.

Isolation and Identification of New Heterocyclic Amines from Pyrolysates of Amino Acids, Proteins and Proteinous Foods

It is well known that Japanese immigrants to Hawaii and California show much lower incidences of stomach cancer than Japanese in Japan;[105] in contrast, they show higher incidences of colon cancer.[39] Further, it is known that stomach cancer was also common in the early Meiji era in Japan, a century ago, prior to the development of modern technology. This suggests that the high incidence of stomach cancer in Japan may be due to the traditional food and life style in Japan, rather than to modern food, scientific technology and industry.[106] Screening for carcinogens with rodents has disadvantages in that it is time consuming and expensive, and requires much space and equipment. Moreover, it is not suitable for screening mutagens/carcinogens in food. For this purpose, short-term microbial tests are much more practical. Therefore, various foods, beverages and spices were subjected to mutation tests.

The presence of fairly strong mutagenicity in charred parts of beefsteak and grilled fish was observed first,[77,115] as shown in Figure 4. Heated beef or beef extract was also found to be mutagenic.[21] Later, the production of potent mutagens was found to be due to pyrolysis of amino acids and proteinous foods.[76,84] Food with a low water content and high protein content yields higher mutagenicity.[138]

By monitoring mutagenic activity, we purified mutagenic principles from pyrolysates of amino acids and determined their structures. These compounds have also been chemically synthesized. The compounds identified are listed in Figure 5. 3-amino-1,4-dimethyl-5*H*-pyrido[4,3-*b*]indole (Trp-P-1) and 3-amino-1-methyl-5*H*-

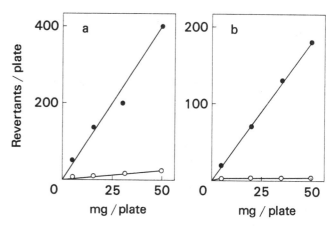

FIG. 4. Mutagenicities of the charred parts of beefsteak (a) and grilled sardine (b). TA98 was used with (●——●) or without (○——○) S9 mix.

pyrido[4,3-*b*]indole (Trp-P-2) were isolated from a tryptophan pyrolysate.[2,58,111,130] 2-amino-6-methyldipyrido[1,2-*a*:3′,2′-*d*]imidazole(Glu-P-1) and 2-aminodipyrido[1,2-*a*:3′,2′-*d*]imidazole (Glu-P-2) were isolated from a pyrolysate of glutamic acid.[131,155] 2-amino-5-phenylpyridine (Phe-P-1) was isolated from a phenylalanine pyrolysate.[58,111] Although not a heterocyclic amine, 3,4-cyclopentenopyrido[3,2-*a*]carbazole (Lys-P-1) was also isolated from a pyrolysate of lysine.[141] Yoshida *et al.*[159] isolated 2-amino-α-carboline (AαC) and 2-amino-3-methyl-α-carboline (MeAαC) from soybean globulin pyrolysate. More recently, 2-amino-3-methylimidazo[4,5-*f*]quinoline (IQ) and 2-amino-3,4-dimethylimidazo[4,5-*f*]quinoline (MeIQ) were isolated from broiled dried sardines by us.[51,53,54] Furthermore, 2-amino-3,8-dimethylimidazo[4,5-*f*]quinoxaline (MeIQx) was purified from fried beef.[52] Among these compounds, Trp-P-1, Trp-P-2, Glu-P-1, Glu-P-2, Lys-P-1, IQ, MeIQ, and MeIQx are newly registered compounds.[118]

The specific mutagenic activities of Trp-P-1, Trp-P-2, Glu-P-1, Glu-P-2, IQ, MeIQ, and MeIQx are extremely high, some being higher than that of aflatoxin B₁[114]. For comparison, their specific mutagenic activities are given in Table 1 with those of the typical carcinogens, AF-2 aflatoxin B₁, benzo(a)pyrene (B(a)P), *N,N*-diethylnitrosamine(DEN), DMN, MNNG and 4NQO.[106]

These newly identified compounds require metabolic activation to exert their mutagenic activities. S9 mix prepared from the liver of rats treated with polychlorinated biphenyls was most efficient for activation. S9 from the liver of rats treated with 3-methylcholanthrene (MC) was also effective for activating these compounds metabolically, but S9 from the liver of rats treated with phenobarbital (PB) was not as effective.[48] Consistent with these findings, a system reconstituted with cyto-

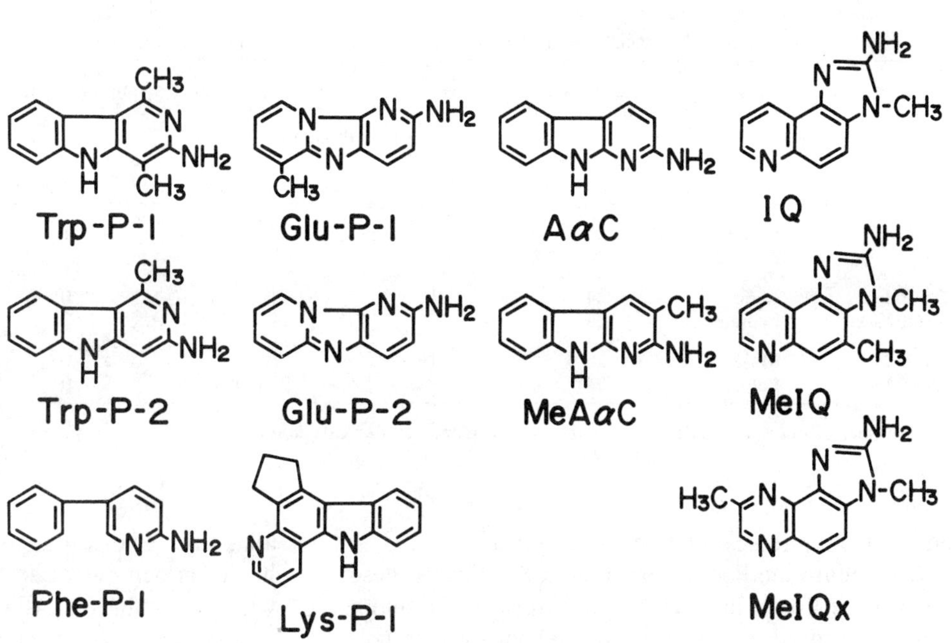

FIG. 5. Mutagens isolated from pyrolysates of amino acids, protein and proteinous foods.

chrome P-448 from the liver of rats treated with MC was much more active in metabolic activation of Trp-P-1 and Trp-P-2 than cytochrome P-450 purified from the liver of rats treated with PB.[47] Results obtained by using a specific antibody each against cytochrome P-448 (MC) and cytochrome P-450 (PB) also support the idea that P-448 (MC) is principally involved in the metabolic activation.[142]

Since Trp-P-1 and Trp-P-2 were the first of this series of compounds to be reported their pathway of metabolic activation and biological activity have been most inten-

TABLE 1. Specific Mutagenic Activities of the Compounds Isolated from Pyrolysates and Well Known Carcinogens

	Revertants/μg		
S. typhimurium TA98		*S. typhimurium* TA100	
MeIQ	661,000†	AF-2	42,000*
IQ	433,000†	MeIQ	30,000†
MeIQx	145,000†	Aflatoxin B$_1$	28,000†
Trp-P-2	104,200†	MeIQx	14,000†
Glu-P-1	49,000‡	4NQO	9,900*
Trp-P-1	39,000†	IQ	7,000†
AF-2	6,500*	Glu-P-1	3,200‡
Aflatoxin B$_1$	6,000†	Trp-P-2	1,800†
Glu-P-2	1,900‡	Trp-P-1	1,700†
4NQO	970*	Glu-P-2	1,200‡
B(a)P	320†	MNNG	870*
AαC	300§	B(a)P	660†
MeAαC	200§	MeAαC	120§
Lys-P-1	86§	Lys-P-1	99§
Phe-P-1	41§	Phe-P-1	23§
DEN	0.02§	AαC	20§
DMN	0.00§	DMN	0.23§
MNNG	0.00*	DEN	0.15§

* Without S9 mix; †10 μl; ‡30 μl; §150 μl S9/plate.

sively studied.[112] Conversion to the hydroxylamine derivative has been well established.[35,157] It has been suggested that acylation of the hydroxyamino group makes the compound more reactive, judging from the results of the interaction of the synthetic compound with DNA.[35] It is also suggested that seryl-tRNA synthetase and serine are involved in forming activated form of Trp-P-2[158] as in the case of 4HAQO.[124] The structures of the adducts of Trp-P-1 and Glu-P-1 with guanine base of DNA were elucidated.[33,34] All of these newly found mutagens were more mutagenic toward TA98 than TA100, and much less mutagenic toward TA1535 and TA1538 which do not have plasmids. Trp-P-1 and Trp-P-2 induced chromosome aberrations and sister chromatid exchanges in cultured human cells.[99,134] They produced transformed foci of cryopreserved Chinese hamster embryonal cells,[127,128] and cells from these foci were transplantable into the cheek pouches of hamsters.[127]

Experiments on the effects of feeding mice on diet containing either Trp-P-1 or Trp-P-2 demonstrated the hepatocarcinogenicity of these compounds[65] as shown in Table 2. Female mice were more susceptible than males. This is a specific characteristic of Trp-P-1 and Trp-P-2, not seen with most other hepatocarcinogens. Experiments now in progress on Glu-P-1, Glu-P-2 and MeAαC have already shown that these three chemicals are also hepatocarcinogens. In addition to malignant hepatomas, Glu-P-1 and Glu-P-2 induced hemangioendotheliosarcomas on the back between the scapulae.[64] It is interesting in this connection to recall that *o*-aminoazotoluene, which was the first compound reported to be hepatocarcinogenic in mice, also produces sar-

TABLE 2. Incidence of Hepatic Tumors in CDF$_1$ Mice Fed Diets Containing Trp-P-1 or Trp-P-2

| Treatment | Sex | Effective number | Number of mice with hepatic tumors | | | | |
| | | | Hepatocellular tumor | | | | |
			Adenoma	Carcinoma	Hemangioma	Total (%)	*P*
None	Male	25	0	0	1	1 (4)	
	Female	24	0	0	0	0	
Trp-P-1	Male	24	1	4	0	5 (21)	<0.179
(0.02%)	Female	26	2	14	0	16 (62)	<0.001
Trp-P-2	Male	25	1	3	0	4 (16)	<0.348
(0.02%)	Female	24	0	22 (2)*	0	22 (92)	<0.001

* Number of mice with pulmonary metastases of hepatocellular carcinomas.

comas in the interscapular region of mice.[6]

No standard method for exact quantification of these chemicals in foods has yet been established, although sequential procedures including partial purification, column chromatography, HPLC and gas chromatography-mass-spectrometry have been recommended.[118,151-154] By using these methods, we found 13.3 ng of Trp-P-1 and 13.1 ng of Trp-P-2 in one gram of broiled sardine[154] and 53 ng of Trp-P-1 in one gram of beef which had been broiled.[152] When one gram of dried squid was broiled, 280 ng of Glu-P-2 were found[151] and 158 ng of IQ and 72 g of MeIQ were detected in one gram of broiled dried sardine.[118]

Mutagens and Carcinogens in Edible Plants, Vegetables and Fruits

Cycad nuts have been found to be carcinogenic, the carcinogenic principle being cycasin, a glycoside of methylmethanol. Methyl azoxymethanol is mutagenic and carcinogenic.[59,103] Cycasin was found to be carcinogenic *in vivo* and mutagenic in the presence of glycosidase *in vitro*[59,66] as shown in Figure 3e.

Coltsfoots and comfrey have been reported to produce cancers in rats fed diets containing these plants.[40] The active principles in these plants are pyrrolizidine alkaloids. The mutagenicity of pyrrolizidine alkaloid has been demonstrated by the Ames method modified with preincubation. (Fig. 3b)[113,156]

The carcinogenicity of bracken is well established. Cows who graze in fields where bracken grows show a high incidence of urinary-bladder papillomas.[97] Rats fed diets containing bracken developed malignant tumors of the urinary bladder and ileocecal region.[26,91] The carcinogenic principle in bracken however, has not been fully identified. By monitoring the mutagenicity of the various fractions with the microbial test, during purification of the carcinogens from bracken, it was demonstrated that fractions containing flavonoids possess mutagenic activity.[30] Among various flavonoids, quercetin and kaempferol and their glycosides, rutin and astragalin, have been found most frequently in edible plants. Their structures are given in Figure 6. The mutagenicity of flavonoids has been reported independently by several groups,[9,13-15,32,62,78,116] and the specific mutagenic activity of quercetin is in the same order as that of B(a)P. Moreover, quercetin was found to be mutagenic not only to microbes, but also to cultured mammalian cells.[3,72,87] The content of flavonoids is very high in certain foods of plant origin. If flavonoids are carcinogenic, human beings must have been continuously and unavoidably exposed to carcinogens for

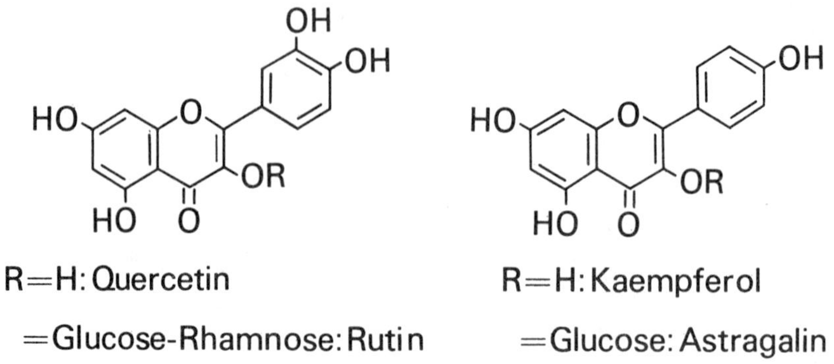

FIG. 6. Structures of quercetin, rutin, kaempferol and astragalin.

R=H: Quercetin
=Glucose-Rhamnose: Rutin

R=H: Kaempferol
=Glucose: Astragalin

many generations. But if flavonoids are not carcinogenic, what is the significance of their mutagenicity in *in vitro* tests?

As a result of the above findings, the Ministry of Health and Welfare of Japan organized a research group to test the carcinogenicities of flavonoids. Under this program, we carried out feeding experiments using ACI rats,[41] ddY mice[98] and Chinese hamsters.[74] The incidence of tumors in various organs of animals fed on quercetin or rutin diets were not different from those in the corresponding control groups. In contrast, in America, Pamukcu *et al.*[92] reported that quercetin feeding produced many tumors in the urinary bladder and ileocecal region of rats. The concentration of quercetin in their experiment was 0.1%, whereas in ours it was higher (0.2–10%); the duration of feeding was also longer in our experiments. The reason for this discrepancy between results in Japan and America is unknown. Recently, the National Toxicology Program in the United States included quercetin among compounds to be tested and results are being awaited with great concern. It is known, however, that flavonoids suppress the carcinogenic potency of $B(a)P$[144] and azo dye.[85]

It should be mentioned here that bracken is still being eaten by Japanese people, although its carcinogenicity has been well publicized. The carcinogenic potential of chemicals was expressed as the TD_{50} value by Hooper *et al.*[42] The TD_{50} values calculated for the notorious food additive AF-2 and for bracken were 60 mg/kg/day and 7000 mg/kg/day, respectively.[55] The total annual production of AF-2 in 1972 was three tons, and the total annual sale of bracken in 1974 was 2000 tons in Japan. The average human intake of AF-2 and bracken were thus calculated as 0.012 mg/kg/day and 1.1 mg/kg/day, respectively. The ratios of the average human intakes expressed as TD_{50} values to those of animals in carcinogenicity experiments were 1/5000

and 1/6400 for AF-2 and bracken, respectively. In other words, the risks from AF-2 and bracken were roughly of the same magnitude. Of course, many assumptions were made in these calculations. It is interesting to note that the general public paid more attention to a synthetic chemical than to a naturally occurring substance.

As seen with the cases of stomach cancer in Japan, the incidence of most common cancers depends on so-called life style. There seems to be a stronger possibility that the integration of the effects of many known and unknown carcinogens, rather than the effect of any one of them, which alone could be only a minor factor, is important in the development of human cancer.

Mutagens in Alcoholic Spirits, Spices, and Beverages

It should be emphasized that the presence of mutagens in food does not necessarily indicate the presence of carcinogens, as demonstrated clearly in the case of flavonoids.

Mutagens have been found in alcoholic spirits[60,61,80] such as wine, whiskey and brandy. Some of the mutagenicity of red wine was accounted for by flavonoids[8,11] and their glycosides,[132] but the nature of the mutagens in other alcoholic beverages has not been fully studied. Coffee shows mutagenicity toward TA100 without metabolic activation,[1,81] and the report by MacMahon *et al.*[70] of a correlation between coffee drinking and pancreatic cancer indicated the necessity for further studies of the mutagenic principles in coffee. We found almost equal mutagenic potential in brewed and instant coffee, whether regular or decaffeinated.[81] The mutagen in coffee was found to be inactivated by sulfite[123] (Fig. 7). If mutagens in coffee are confirmed to be hazardous, the use of sulfite as a coffee additive should be considered a practical possibility, since sulfite has been approved as a food additive and is already

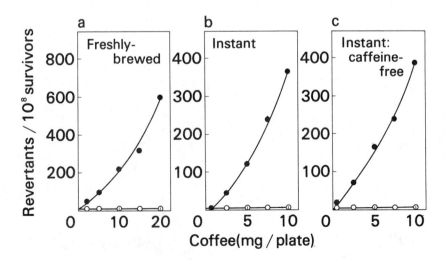

FIG. 7. Inactivation of mutagenic activity of coffee by sulfite. Freshly-brewed (a), instant (b) and caffeine free instant (c) coffee were incubated with (O —— O) or without (● —— ●) 300 μg of sulfite at room temperature for 30 min, and then assayed for mutagenicity by preincubation method using TA100 without S9 mix.

added to wine. Mutagenic activity was also found in spices such as sumac and dill weed. The mutagenic activity in sumac was due to quercetin,[102] and that in dill weed to sulfate esters of quercetin and isorhamnetin.[31] Mutagenic activity found in Japanese pickles was accounted for by flavonoids.[125] The mutagenic activities in both green and black tea were partially accounted for by flavonoids and their glycosides,[81,139] again indicating the necessity for determining the carcinogenicity of flavonoids.

Tumor Promoters and Life Style

As described above, there are many mutagens in the normal environment that cause DNA damage. In addition, exposure to cosmic rays and background radiation caused by naturally occurring radioactive isotopes, such as potassium-40, are continuously producing DNA damage. The oxygen radical, the organic peroxide radical and superoxide also cause DNA damage.[16] It is generally accepted that patients with heritable diseases involving DNA-repair deficiency tend to age easily and to suffer from cancer at a higher rate than normal subjects. It seems likely that there are many tumor initiators in our environment. Meanwhile, the concept of two-step carcinogenesis has been widely accepted by experimental oncologists, as well as by clinical oncologists and epidemiologists.[8,11] The crucial step in the development of human cancer may be the second stage of carcinogenesis, that of tumor promotion, not the first, tumor initiation stage.

Phorbol esters isolated from croton oil from the seeds of *Euphorbiaceae, Croton tiglium L.* have been most intensively studied as tumor promoters.[36,140] Their mode of action, especially their effect on the cell membrane of cultured mammalian cells, has been the subject of many investigations.[90,145] Phorbol esters are very effective promoters. Repeated paintings of initiated mouse skin with only a few μg of these compounds are sufficient to produce skin tumors in two-step carcinogenesis experiments. Phorbol esters also exert various biological activities *in vitro* at a concentration of 10^{-9}–10^{-8} M.[45]

For a long time, the phorbol ester 12-O-tetradecanoyl-phorbol-13-acetate (TPA) has been used in research as a typical tumor promoter.[36,37,140]

In our laboratory, a survey was made to detect other tumor promoters that were as effective as TPA. Induction of ornithine decarboxylase (ODC) activity in mouse skin after application of test compounds was used as a screening method. Various foodstuffs and extracts of plants and fungi were tested in this way. As a result, dihydroteleocidin B, teleocidin, and lyngbyatoxin A were found to induce ODC and exert various biological activities *in vitro*.[27,108] Their effective concentrations were about the same as that of TPA.

Teleocidin is a product of *Streptomyces* and dihydroteleocidin B is a catalytically hydrogenated derivative of teleocidin B,[126] and lyngbyatoxin is produced by the blue-green alga *Lyngbya majuscula*.[18] The structures of these compounds reported[18,126] are given in Figure 8. Teleocidin and lyngbyatoxin A are indole alkaloids, and structural isomers of these compounds have been found. The *in vivo* activity of these indole alkaloids has been demonstrated in two-step carcinogenesis experiment with mouse skin.[28,29] Figure 9 shows the results of the induction of skin tumors by applications of 7,12-dimethylbenz[a]anthracene (DMBA), TPA, dihydroteleocidin B, DMBA plus TPA, and DMBA plus dihydroteleocidin B. It is clear that dihydroteleocidin B is as potent as TPA. Table 3 summarizes the data on the histological findings from this experiment.

Dihydroteleocidin B, teleocidin, and lyngbyatoxin A have the same biological activity as TPA, as shown in Table 4.[27,28,43,44,50,88,108,137] More recently, aplysiatoxin, which was also isolated from another variety of the blue-green alga *Lyngbya majuscula* was found to have a similar potency for ODC induction in mouse skin and the same biological effects on cultured mammalian cells as TPA and indole alkaloids.[28,29] The biological activities of aplysiatoxin and its debromo-derivative, debromoaplysiatoxin, are summarized in Table 5. Interestingly, debromoaplysiatoxin is about 1/100 as effective on cultured cells as aplysiatoxin, but has activity almost

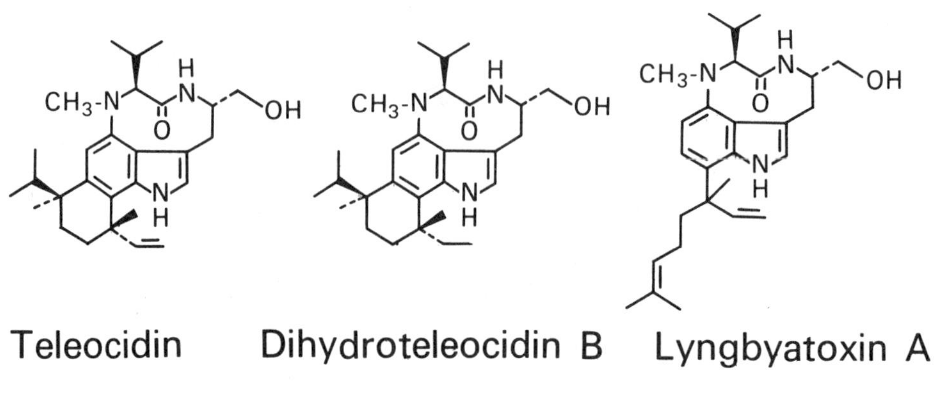

FIG. 8. Structures of teleocidin, dihydroteleocidin B and lyngbyatoxin A.

Teleocidin　　Dihydroteleocidin B　　Lyngbyatoxin A

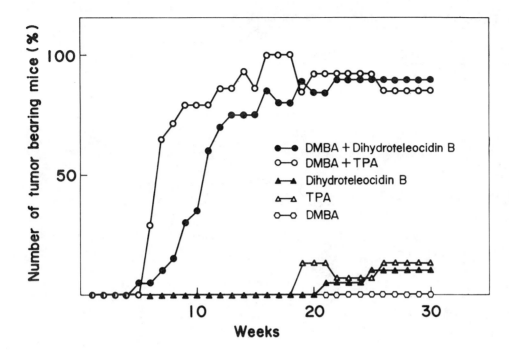

FIG. 9. Effect of dihydroteleocidin B on the formation of skin tumor. Female CD-1 mice were painted once with 100 μg of DMBA. After one week, painting with either 2.5 μg of dihydroteleocidin B or 2.5 μg of TPA was begun and continued twice a week until the end of experiment.

identical to the latter for ODC induction. The structures of aplysiatoxin and debromoaplysiatoxin both polyacetate compounds[75] are given in Figure 10. Since indole alkaloids are thought to be present in tropical seaweeds, the possibility that these compounds, as well as polyacetates and phorbol esters, are present in other foods should be investigated. Their possible significance as promoters of human cancer should also be studied. Other types of chemicals should also be tested as promoters.

In addition to the three above-mentioned classes of very potent tumor promoters, less strictly defined substances which are nevertheless considered tumor promoters may also be important in the development of human cancers. Chemicals that cause chronic damage of tissues and evoke chronic proliferation could be tumor promoters. Inhalation of tobacco smoke produces a condition of the bronchus that is favorable for tumor promotion; it has been reported that cigarette smoke condensate shows tumor promoter activity.[10] Food with a high content of sodium chloride causes chronic gastritis, which results in proliferation of the gastric epithelium.[100,133] PB is known to be a tumor promoter in the liver of rats previously treated with an initiator.[93]

Tryptophan[19] and saccharin[19,38] are tumor promoters in the urinary bladder of rats and bile acid derivatives might be promoters in carcinogenesis of the colon.[89] Estrogenic hormones may be involved in the promotion of breast cancer[71] and alcohol might be a tumor promoter in the esophagus when tumor initiation has occurred.[136] The mode of action of these tumor promoters may or may not be similar to that of TPA. More detailed experiments are required on the effects of the administration of carcinogens found in the normal environment in combination with various types of tumor promoters.

Concluding Comments

Although many new types of carcinogens are now being found and an appreciable amount of information is available on aromatic hydrocarbons, nitrosoamine compounds, aflatoxins and other mycotoxins, studies are still required on the endogenous formation of carcinogens and tumor promoters. Life style, and especially diet, may greatly influence conditions in the body such as in the endocrine and immunosurveillance systems in ways which affect the steps of carcinogenesis.

TABLE 3.   Histological Types of Skin Tumors

Promoter	Number of skin tumors examined	Number of squamous cell carcinoma	Number of papilloma	Number of hyperplasia
Dihydroteleocidin B	73	15 (21)*	56 (77)	2 (3)
TPA	132	11 (8)	117 (89)	4 (3)

* Figures in parenthesis are percentages.

TABLE 4. Biological Effects of TPA, Teleocidin, Dihydroteleocidin B and Lyngbyatoxin A

	TPA	Teleocidin	Dihydro-teleocidin B	Lyngbyatoxin A
ODC induction				
nmoles CO_2/5.0 μg compound	1.45	1.89	1.55	2.05
Inhibition (%) by retinoic acid	81.9	70.6	78.7	65.5
Irritancy				
ID_{50}^{24} nmole/ear	0.016	0.008	0.017	0.011
Hyperplasia	strong	strong	strong	strong
Induction of dark keratinocytes	strong	strong	strong	strong
Cell adhesion of HL-60				
ED_{50} ng/ml	1.5	4.0	0.3	7.0
Differentiation of HL-60				
ED_{30} ng/ml	2.5	3.6	1.4	2.5
Aggregation of NL-3 cells				
ED_{50} ng/ml	11.2	3.1	6.5	2.4
Differentiation of Friend erythroleukemia cells				
ED_{50} ng/ml	1.0	2.0	0.2	0.4
Inhibition of specific binding of ^{3}H-PDBu				
ED_{50} ng/ml	8.7	2.5	—	10.0
Incorporation of $^{32}PO_4$ into cellular phospholipid				
ED_{50} ng/ml	12	10	18	17

On the other hand, there are also many substances which are known to suppress various steps of carcinogenic process. For instance, vitamin C inhibits the formation of nitrosoamine compounds from nitrite and amines.[73] Some naturally occurring flavonoids inhibit the metabolic activation of various procarcinogens.[17,146] Vitamin E and sulfhydryl compounds inactivate many reactants derived from procarcinogens/promutagens[23,143]

TABLE 5. Biological Activities of Aplysiatoxin and Debromoaplysiatoxin

	Aplysiatoxin	Debromoaply-siatoxin
ODC induction		
nmoles CO_2/2.5 μg compound	3.62	2.97
Inhibition (%) by retinoic acid	89.7	74.1
Irritancy		
ID_{50}^{24} nmole/ear	0.005	0.005
Hyperplasia	strong	weak
Cell adhesion of HL-60		
ED_{50} ng/ml	2.0	180
Differentiation of HL-60		
ED_{30} ng/ml	1.7	100
Aggregation of NL-3 cells		
ED_{50} ng/ml	2.1	180

and vitamin A, as well as its related retinoic acid derivatives, can block a certain step of tumor promotion.[104]

Breslow and Enstrom[12] have recommended seven health habits to reduce cancer mortality: never smoke cigarettes, take regular physical exercise, drink little or no alcohol, sleep 7–8 hr, maintain a proper weight, eat breakfast, and do not eat between meals. People who had 6–7 of these habits were found to be much less likely to die of cancer than those with only 0–3 of these habits.

On the basis of all the information available, we tentatively propose the following 12 points for cancer prevention in a form easily understandable by the general public:[107]

1. Keep your diet well balanced, in terms of both taste and nutrition.
2. Do not eat the same foods repeatedly and exclusively. Also exercise caution in taking the same medication over long periods.
3. Avoid excessive eating.
4. Avoid drinking too much alcohol.
5. Refrain from excessive smoking.
6. Take optimal daily doses of vitamins A, C and E. Include a moderate amount of fibrous food ("roughage") in your diet.
7. Avoid excessive intake of salty food and do not

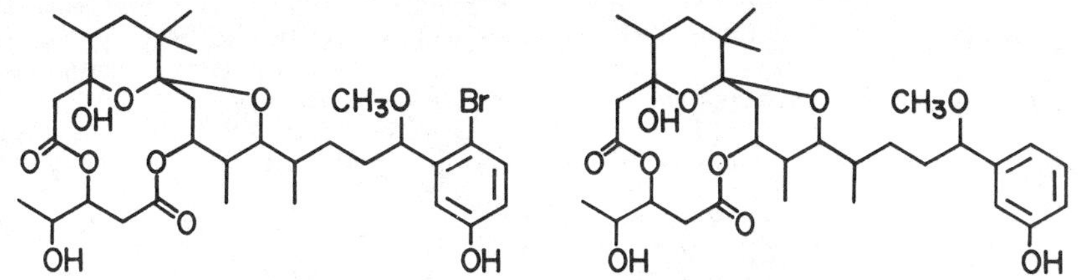

FIG. 10. Structures of aplysiatoxin and debromoaplysiatoxin.

drink too hot water, tea or coffee.

8. Avoid eating too many burnt parts of food, such as you find in charcoal-grilled meat and fish.
9. Avoid moldy food which is not intentionally moldy, such as cheese.
10. Avoid excessive exposure to the sun.
11. Avoid overwork so that you do not lower your resistance to disease.
12. Bathe or shower frequently.

These are, at best, very tentative recommendations for reducing exposure to carcinogens to prevent cancer, but currently this is the best advice we can give.

In the past 20 years, much progress has been made in the early detection and treatment of cancer. However, the high cost of treating patients has become a large social burden. Thus, even a 5 or 10% decrease in the number of cancer patients would greatly lighten the economic load. Therefore, the most urgent problem facing researchers today is preventing cancer.

REFERENCES

1. Aeschbacher HU, Würzner HP. An evaluation of instant and regular coffee in the Ames mutagenicity test. *Toxicol Lett* 1980; 5:139–145.
2. Akimoto H, Kawai A, Nomura H, Nagao M, Kawachi T, Sugimura T. Syntheses of potent mutagens in tryptophan pyrolysates. *Chem Lett* 1977; 1060–1064.
3. Amacher DE, Paillet SC, Turner GN, Ray VA, Salsburg DS. Point mutations at the thymidine kinase locus in L5178Y mouse lymphoma cells. II. Test validation and interpretation. *Mutation Res* 1980; 72:447–474.
4. Ames BN, Lee FD, Durston WE. An improved bacterial test system for the detection and classification of mutagens and carcinogens. *Proc Natl Acad Sci USA* 1973; 70:782–786.
5. Ames BN, McCann J, Yamasaki E. Methods for detecting carcinogens and mutagens with Salmonella/mammalian-microsome mutagenicity test. *Mutation Res* 1975; 31:347–364.
6. Andervont HB, Edward JE. Carcinogenic action of two azo compounds in mice. *J Natl Cancer Inst* 1943; 3:349–358.
7. Bauer KH. Mutationstheorie der Geschwulst-Entstehung, Übergang von Körperzellen in Geschwulst-Zellen durch Gen-Änderung. Berlin, Springer-Verlag, 1928.
8. Berenblum I. The mechanism of carcinogenesis. *Cancer Res* 1941; 1:807–814.
9. Bjeldanes LF, Chang GW. Mutagenic activity of quercetin and related compounds. *Science* 1977; 197:577–578.
10. Bock FG, Swain AP, Stedman RL. Composition studies on tobacco XLIV: Tumor-promoting activity of subfractions of the weak acid fraction of cigarette smoke condensate. *J Natl Cancer Inst* 1971; 47:425–426.

11. Boutwell RK. The role of the induction of ornithine decarboxylase in tumor promotion. In Book B, Hiatt HH, Watson JD, Winsten JA (eds): Origins of Human Cancer. New York, Cold Spring Harbor Laboratory, 1977; 773–783.
12. Breslow L, Enstrom E. Persistence of health habits and their relationship to mortality. *Preventive Med* 1980; 9:469–483.
13. Brown JP. A review of the genetic effects of naturally occurring flavonoids, anthraquinones and related compounds. *Mutation Res* 1980; 75:243–277.
14. Brown JP, Brown RJ, Roehm GW. The application of short-term microbial mutagenicity tests in the identification and development of non-toxic, non-absorbable food additives. In Scott D, Bridges BA, Sobels FH (eds): Progress in Genetic Toxicology. Amsterdam, Elsevier/North-Holland Biomedical Press, 1977; 185–190.
15. Brown JP, Dietrich PS. Mutagenicity of plant flavonols in the Salmonella/mammalian microsome test: Activation of flavonol glycosides by mixed glycosidases from rat cecal bacteria and other sources. *Mutation Res* 1979; 66:223–230.
16. Bruynincky WJ, Mason HS, Morse SA. Are physiological oxygen concentrations mutagenic? *Nature* 1978; 274:606–607.
17. Buening MK, Chang RL, Huang, M-T, Fortner JG, Wood AW, Conney AH. Activation and inhibition of benzo(a)pyrene and aflatoxin B_1 metabolism in human liver microsomes by naturally occurring flavonoids. *Cancer Res* 1981; 41:67–72.
18. Cardellina JH II, Marner F-J, Moore RE. Seaweed dermatitis: structure of lyngbyatoxin A. *Science* 1979; 204:193–195.
19. Cohen SM, Arai M, Jacobs JB, Friedell GH. Promoting effect of saccharin and DL-tryptophan in urinary bladder carcinogenesis. *Cancer Res* 1979; 39:1207–1217.
20. Cohen SM, Ichikawa M, Bryan GT. Carcinogenicity of 2-(2-furyl)-3-(5-nitro-2-furyl)acrylamide (AF-2) fed to female Sprague-Dawley rats. *Gann* 1977; 63:473–476.
21. Commoner B, Vithayathil AJ, Dolora P, Nair S, Madyastha P, Cuca GC. Formation of mutagens in beef and beef extract during cooking. *Science* 1978; 201:913–916.
22. Druckrey H, Preussmann R, Ivankovic S, So BT, Schmidt CH, Bücheler J. Zur Erzeugung subcutaner Sarkome an Ratten. Carcinogene Wirkung von Hydrazodicarbonsäure-bis-(methyl-nitrosamid), N-Nitroso-N-*n*-butylharnstoff, N-Methyl-N-nitroso-nitrosoguanidin und N-Nitroso-imidazolidon. *Z Krebsfrosch* 1966; 68:87–102.
23. Ellison NM, Londer H. Vitamins E and C and their relationship to cancer. In Newell GR, Ellison NM (eds): Nutrition and Cancer: Etiology and Treatment. New York, Raven Press, 1981; 233–241.
24. Endo H, Ishizawa M, Kamiya T. Induction of bacteriophage formation in lysogenic bacteria by a potent carcinogen, 4-nitroquinoline 1-oxide, and its derivatives. *Nature* 1963; 198:195–196.
25. Epstein SS, St. Pierre JA. Mutagenicity in yeast of nitroquinolines and related compounds. *Toxicol Appl Pharmacol* 1969; 15:451–460.
26. Evans IA, Mason J. Carcinogenic activity of bracken. *Nature* 1965; 208:913–914.
27. Fujiki H, Mori M, Nakayasu M, Terada M, Sugimura T. A possible naturally occurring tumor promoter; teleocidin B from Streptomyces. *Biochem Biophys Res Commun* 1979; 90:976–983.
28. Fujiki H, Mori M, Nakayasu M, Terada M, Sugimura T, Moore RE. Indole alkaloids; dihydroteleocidin B, teleocidin and lyngbyatoxin A, as a new class of tumor promoters. *Proc Natl Acad Sci*

USA 1980; 78:3872–3876.

29. Fujiki H, Sugimura T, Moore RE. New classes of environmental tumor promoters: Indole alkaloids and polyacetates. Abstracts of International Symposium on Health Effects of Tumor Promotion Cincinnati, 1981; 14.

30. Fukuoka M, Kuroyanagi M, Yoshihira K, Natori S, Nagao M, Takahashi Y, Sugimura T. Chemical and toxicological studies on bracken fern, *Pteridium aquilinum var. latuisculum*. IV. Surveys on bracken constituents by mutagen test. *J Pharm Dyn* 1978; 1:324–331.

31. Fukuoka M, Yoshihira K, Natori S, Sakamoto K, Iwahara S, Hosaka S, Hirono I. Characterization of mutagenic principles and carcinogenicity of dill weed and seed. *J Pharm Dyn* 1980; 3:236–244.

32. Hardigree AA, Epler JL. Comparative mutagenesis of plant flavonoids in microbial system. *Mutation Res* 1978; 58:231–239.

33. Hashimoto Y, Shudo K, Okamoto T. Structural identification of a modified base in DNA covalently bound with mutagenic 3-amino-1-methyl-5H-pyrido[4,3-b]indole. *Chem Pharm Bull* 1979; 27:1058–1060.

34. Hashimoto Y, Shudo K, Okamoto T. Metabolic activation of a mutagen, 2-amino-6-methyldipyrido[1,2-a:3',2'-d]imidazole. Identification of 2-hydroxyamino-6-methyldipyrido[1,2-a:3',2'-d]imidazole and its reaction with DNA. *Biochem Biophys Res Commun* 1980; 92:971–976.

35. Hashimoto Y, Shudo K, Okamoto T. Activation of a mutagen, 3-amino-1-methyl-5H-pyrido[4,3-b]indole. Identification of 3-hydroxyamino-1-methyl-5H-pyrido[4,3-b]indole and its reaction with DNA. *Biochem Biophys Res Commun* 1980; 96:355–362.

36. Hecker E. Phorbol esters from croton oil, chemical nature and biological activities. *Naturwissenschaften* 1967; 54:282–284.

37. Hecker E. Structure-activity relationships in diterpene esters irritant and cocarcinogenic to mouse skin. In Slaga TJ, Sivak A, Boutwell RK (eds): Carcinogenesis Vol 2, Mechanisms of Tumor Promotion and Cocarcinogenesis. New York, Raven Press, 1978; 11–48.

38. Hicks RM, Wakefield JStJ, Chowaniec J. Evaluation of a new model to detect bladder carcinogens or cocarcinogens: Results obtained with saccharin, cyclamate and cyclophosphamide. *Chem Biol Interact* 1975; 11:225–233.

39. Hirohata T. Shift in cancer mortality from 1920 to 1970 among various ethnic groups in Hawaii. In Gelboin HV, MacMahon B, Matsushima T, Sugimura T, Takayama S, Takebe H (eds): Genetic and Environmental Factors in Experimental and Human Cancer. Tokyo, Japan Scientific Societies Press, 1979; 341–350.

40. Hirono I, Mori H, Haga M, Fujii M, Yamada K, Hirata Y, Takanashi H, Uchida E, Hosaka S, Ueno I, Matsushima T, Umezawa K, Shirai A. Edible plants containing carcinogenic pyrrolizidine alkaloids in Japan. In Miller EC, Miller JA, Hirono I, Sugimura T, Takayama S (eds): Naturally Occurring Carcinogens-Mutagens and Modulators of Carcinogenesis. Tokyo, Japan Scientific Press, 1979; 79–87.

41. Hirono I, Ueno I, Hosaka S, Takanashi H, Matsushima T, Sugimura T, Natori S. Carcinogenicity examination of quercetin and rutin in ACI rats. *Cancer Lett* 1981; 13:15–21.

42. Hooper NK, Friedman AD, Sawyer CB, Ames BN. Carcinogenic potency: Analysis, utility for human risk assessment, and relation to mutagenic potency in Salmonella. Progress Report for IARC/WHO Meeting, Lyon, October 3–7, 1977.

43. Hoshino H, Miwa M, Fujiki H, Sugimura T. Aggregation of human lymphoblastoid cells by tumor-promoting phorbol esters and dihydroteleocidin B. *Biochem Biophys Res Commun* 1980; 95:842–848.

44. Hoshino H, Miwa M, Fujiki H, Sugimura T, Yamamoto H, Katsuki T, Hinuma Y. Enhancement of Epstein-Barr virus-induced transformation of human lymphocytes by teleocidin. *Cancer Lett* 1981; 13:275–280.

45. Huberman E, Callaham MF. Induction of terminal differentiation in human promyelocytic leukemia cells by tumor-promoting agents. *Proc Natl Acad Sci USA* 1978; 76:1293–1297.

46. Ikeda Y, Horiuchi S, Furuya T, Uchida O, Suzuki K, Azegami J. Induction of gastric tumors in mice by feeding of furylfuramide. Food Sanitation Study Council, Ministry of Health and Welfare, Japan, 1974.

47. Ishii K, Ando M, Kamataki T, Kato R, Nagao M. Metabolic activation of mutagenic tryptophan pyrolysis products (Trp-P-1 and Trp-P-2) by a purified cytochrome P-450-dependent monooxygenase system. *Cancer Lett* 1980; 9:271–276.

48. Ishii K, Yamazoe Y, Kamataki T, Kato R. Metabolic activation of mutagenic tryptophan pyrolysis products by rat liver microsomes. *Cancer Res* 1980; 40:2596–2600.

49. Kada T. *Escherichia coli* mutagenicity of furylfuramide. *Jpn J Genet* 1973; 48:301–305.

50. Kakunaga T, Hirakawa T, Fujiki H, Sugimura T. Extraordinary enhancement of chemically induced malignant transformation by a new chemical class of tumor promoter, dihydroteleocidin B. Proceedings of AACR and ASCO, Washington, D. C., 1981; 72.

51. Kasai H, Nishimura S, Wakabayashi K, Nagao M, Sugimura T. Chemical synthesis of 2-amino-3-methylimidazo[4,5-f]quinoline (IQ), a potent mutagen isolated from broiled fish. *Proc Jpn Acad* 1980; 56B:382–384.

52. Kasai H, Yamaizumi Z, Shiomi T, Yokoyama S, Miyazawa T, Wakabayashi K, Nagao M, Sugimura T, Nishimura S. Structure of a potent mutagen isolated from fried beef. *Chem Lett* 1981; 485–488.

53. Kasai H, Yamaizumi Z, Wakabayashi K, Nagao M, Sugimura T, Yokoyama S, Miyazawa T, Nishimura S. Structure and chemical synthesis of Me-IQ, a potent mutagen isolated from broiled fish. *Chem Lett* 1980; 1391–1394.

54. Kasai H, Yamaizumi Z, Wakabayashi K, Nagao M, Sugimura T, Yokoyama S, Miyazawa T, Spingarn NE, Weisburger JH, Nishimura S. Potent novel mutagens produced by broling fish under normal conditions. *Proc Jpn Acad* 1980; 56B:278–283.

55. Kawachi T. Personal communication. 1981.

56. Kinebuchi M, Kawachi T, Matsukura N, Sugimura T. Further studies on the carcinogenicity of a food additive, AF-2, in hamsters. *Food Cosmet Toxicol* 1979; 17:339–341.

57. Kondo S, Ichikawa-Ryo H. Testing and classification of mutagenicity of furylfuramide in *Escherichia coli*. *Jpn J Genet* 1973; 48:295–300.

58. Kosuge T, Tsuji K, Wakabayashi K, Okamoto T, Shudo K, Iitaka Y, Itai A, Sugimura T, Kawachi T, Nagao M, Yahagi T, Seino Y. Isolation and structure studies of mutagenic principles in amino acid pyrolysates. *Chem Pharm Bull* 1978; 26:611–619.

59. Laqueur GL. The induction of intestinal neoplasms in rats with the glycoside cycasin and its aglycone. *Virchows Arch Pathol Anat Physiol* 1965; 340:151–163.

60. Lee JSK, Fong LYY. Mutagenicity of Chinese alcoholic spirits. *Food Cosmet Toxicol* 1979; 17:575–578.

61. Loquet C, Toussaint G, LeTalaer JY. Studies on mutagenic constituents of apple brandy and various alcoholic beverages collected in western France, a high incidence area for oesophageal cancer. *Mutation Res* 1981; 88:155–164.

62. MacGregor JT, Jurd L. Mutagenicity of plant flavonoids: Structural requirements for mutagenic activity in *Salmonella typhimurium*. *Mutation Res* 1978; 54:297–309.

63. Mandell JD, Greenberg J. A new chemical mutagen for bacteria, 1-methyl-3-nitro-1-nitrosoguanidine. *Biochem Biophys Res Commun* 1960; 3:575–577.

64. Matsukura N. Personal communication. 1981.

65. Matsukura N, Kawachi T, Morino K, Ohgaki H, Sugimura T, Takayama S. Carcinogenicity in mice of mutagenic compounds from a tryptophan pyrolysate. *Science* 1981; 213:346–347.

66. Matsushima T, Sugimura T, Nagao M, Yahagi T, Shirai A, Sawamura M. Factors modulating mutagenicity in microbial tests. In Norpoth K, Garner RC (eds): Short-Term Mutagenicity Test Systems for Detecting Carcinogens. Berlin, Springer-Verlag, 1980; 271–285.

67. McCann J, Ames BN. Detection of carcinogens as mutagens in the Salmonella/microsome test: Assay of 300 chemicals: Discussion. *Proc Natl Acad Sci USA* 1976; 73:950–954.

68. McCann J, Choi E, Yamasaki E, Ames BN. Detection of carcinogens as mutagens in the Salmonella/microsome test: Assay of 300 chemicals. *Proc Natl Acad Sci USA* 1975; 72:5135–5139.

69. McCann J, Spingarn NE, Kobori J, Ames BN. Detection of carcinogens as mutagens: Bacterial tester strains with R factor plasmids. *Proc Natl Acad Sci USA* 1975; 72:979–983.

70. McMahon B, Yen S, Trichopoulos D, Warren K, Nardi G. Coffee and cancer of the pancreas. *N Engl J Med* 1981; 304:630–633.

71. Medina D. Mammary tumorigenesis in chemical carcinogen-treated mice. II. Dependence on hormone stimulation for tumorigenesis. *J Natl Cancer Inst* 1974; 53:223–226.

72. Meltz ML, MacGregor JT. Activity of the plant flavonol quercetin in the mouse lymphoma L5178Y TK$^{+/-}$ mutation, DNA single-strand break, and Balb/c 3T3 chemical transformation assays. *Mutation Res* 1981; 88:317–324.

73. Mirvish SS, Wallcave L. Ascorbate-nitrite reaction: Possible means of blocking the formation of carcinogenic N-nitroso compounds. *Science* 1972; 177:65–68.

74. Morino K, Matsukura N, Ohgaki H, Kawachi T, Sugimura T, Hirono I. Carcinogenicity test of quercetin and rutin in golden hamsters by oral administration. *Carcinogenesis* 1982 (in press).

75. Mynderes JS, Moore RE, Kashiwagi M, Norton TR. Antileukaemia activity in the oscillatoriaceae: Isolation of debromoaplysiatoxin from *Lyngbya*. *Science* 1977; 196:538–539.

76. Nagao M, Honda M, Seino Y, Yahagi T, Kawachi T, Sugimura T. Mutagenicities of protein pyrolysates. *Cancer Lett* 1977; 2:335–340.

77. Nagao M, Honda M, Seino Y, Yahagi T, Sugimura T. Mutagenicities of smoke condensates and the charred surface of fish and meat. *Cancer Lett* 1977; 2:221–226.

78. Nagao M, Morita N, Yahagi T, Shimizu M, Kuroyanagi M, Fukuoka M, Yoshihira K, Natori S, Fujino T, Sugimura T. Mutagenicities of 61 flavonoids and 11 related compounds. *Environ Mutagenesis* 1981; 3:401–419.

79. Nagao M, Sugimura T, Matsushima T. Environmental mutagens and carcinogens. *Ann Rev Genet* 1978; 12:117–159.

80. Nagao M, Takahashi Y, Wakabayashi K, Sugimura T. Mutagenicity of alcoholic beverages. *Mutation Res* 1981; 88:147–154.

81. Nagao M, Takahashi Y, Yamanaka H, Sugimura T. Mutagens in coffee and tea. *Mutation Res* 1979; 68:101–106.

82. Nagao M, Yahagi T, Honda M, Seino Y, Kawachi T, Sugimura T, Wakabayashi K, Tsuji K, Kosuge T. Comutagenic actions of norharman derivatives with dimethylaminoazobenzene and related compounds. *Cancer Lett* 1977; 3:339–346.

83. Nagao M, Yahagi T, Honda M, Seino Y, Matsushima T, Sugimura T. Demonstration of mutagenicity of aniline and *o*-toluidine by norharman. *Proc Jpn Acad* 1977; 53B:34–37.

84. Nagao M, Yahagi T, Kawachi T, Seino Y, Honda M, Matsukura N, Sugimura T, Wakabayashi K, Tsuji K, Kosuge T. Mutagens in foods, and especially pyrolysis products of protein. In Scott D, Bridges BA, Sobels FH (eds): Progress in Genetic Toxicology. Amsterdam, Elsevier/North Holland, 1977; 259–264.

85. Nagase S, Fujimaki C, Isaka H. Effect of administration of quercetin on the production of experimental liver cancers in rats fed 4-dimethylaminoazobenzene. *Proc Jpn Cancer Assoc*, 1964; 26–27..

86. Nakahara W, Fukuoka F, Sugimura T. Carcinogenic action of 4-nitroquinoline 1-oxide. *Gann* 1957; 48:129–137.

87. Nakayasu M. Unpublished data. 1981.

88. Nakayasu M, Fujiki H, Mori M, Sugimura T, Moore RE. Teleocidin, lyngbyatoxin A and their hydrogenated derivatives, possible tumor promoters, induce terminal differentiation in HL-60 cells. *Cancer Lett* 1981; 12:271–277.

89. Narisawa T, Magadia NE, Weisburger JH, Wynder EL. Promoting effect of bile acids on colon carcinogenesis after intrarectal instillation of N-methyl-N'-nitro-N-nitrosoguanidine in rats. *J Natl Cancer Inst* 1974; 53:1093–1097.

90. O'Brien TG, Diamond L. Ornithine decarboxylase, polyamines and tumor promoters. In Slaga TJ, Sivak A, Boutwell RK (eds): Carcinogenesis Vol 2, Mechanisms of Tumor Promotion and Cocarcinogenesis. New York, Raven Press, 1978; 273–287.

91. Pamukcu AM, Price JM. Induction of intestinal and urinary bladder neoplasms induced by feeding bracken fern (*Pteris aquilina*). *J Natl Cancer Inst* 1969; 43:275–281.

92. Pamukcu AM, Yalciner S, Hatcher JF, Bryan GT. Quercetin, an intestinal and bladder carcinogen present in bracken fern (*Pteridium aquilinum*). *Cancer Res* 1980; 40:3468–3472.

93. Peraino C, Fry RJM, Staffeldt E. Reduction and enhancement by phenobarbital of hepatocarcinogenesis induced in the rat by 2-acetylaminofluorene. *Cancer Res* 1971; 31:1506–1512.

94. Poirier LA, Weisburger EK. Selection of carcinogens and related compounds tested for mutagenic activity. *J Natl Cancer Inst* 1979; 62:833–840.

95. Purchase IFH, Longstaff E, Ashby J, Styles JA, Anderson D, Lefevre PA, Westwood FR. Evaluation of six short-term tests for detecting organic chemical carcinogens and recommendations for their use. *Nature* 1976; 264:624–627.

96. Rinkus SJ, Legator MS. Chemical characterization of 465 known or suspected carcinogens and their correlation with mutagenic activity in the *Salmonella typhimurium* system. *Cancer Res* 1979; 39:3289–3318.

97. Rosenberger G, Helschen W. Adlerfarn (*Pteris aquilina*)-die Ursache des sog. Stallrotes der Rinder (Haematuria vesicalis bovis chronica). *Dtsch Tieraerztl Wochenschr* 1960; 67:201–208.

98. Saito D, Shirai A, Matsushima T, Sugimura T, Hirono I. Test of carcinogenicity of quercetin, a widely distributed mutagen in food. *Teratog Carcinog Mutagen* 1980; 1:213–221.

99. Sasaki M, Sugimura K, Yoshida M, Kawachi T. Chromosome aberrations and sister chromatid exchanges induced by tryptophan pyrolysates, Trp-P-1 and Trp-P-2, in cultured human and Chinese hamster cells. *Proc Jpn Acad* 1980; 56B:332–337.

100. Sato T, Fukuyama T, Suzuki T, Takayanagi J, Murakami T, Shiotsuki N, Tanaka R, Tsuji R. Studies of the causation of gastric cancer. 2. The relation between gastric cancer mortality rate and salted food intake in general places in Japan. *Bull Inst Public Health* 1959; 8:187–198.

101. Schoental R. Carcinogenic activity of N-methyl-N-nitroso-N'-nitroguanidine. *Nature* 1966; 209:726–727.

102. Seino Y, Nagao M, Yahagi T, Sugimura T, Yasuda T, Nishimura S. Identification of a mutagenic substance in a spice, sumac, as quercetin. *Mutation Res* 1978; 58:225–229.

103. Smith DWE. Mutagenicity of cycasin aglycone (methyl-azoxymethanol), a naturally occurring carcinogen. *Science* 1966; 152:1273–1274.

104. Sporn MB, Dunlop NM, Newton DL, Smith JM. Prevention of chemical carcinogenesis by vitamin A and its synthetic analogs (retinoids). *Fed Proc* 1976; 35:1332–1338.

105. Stemmermann GN, Haenszel W, Locke F. Epidemiologic pathology of gastric ulcer and gastric carcinoma among Japanese in Hawaii. *J Natl Cancer Inst* 1977; 58:13–20.

106. Sugimura T. Naturally occurring genotoxic carcinogens. In Miller EC, Miller JA, Hirono I, Sugimura T, Takayama S (eds): Naturally Occurring Carcinogens-Mutagens and Modulators of Carcinogenesis. Tokyo, Japan Scientific Societies Press, 1979; 241–261.

107. Sugimura T. Tumor initiators and promoters associated with ordinary foods. In Arnott MS, van Eys J (eds): Molecular Interrelations of Nutrition and Cancer, New York, Raven Press, 1982 (in press).

108. Sugimura T, Fujiki H, Mori M, Nakayasu M, Terada M, Umezawa K, Moore RE. Teleocidin: new naturally occurring tumor promoter. In Hecker E, Fusenig N, Marks F, Kunz W (eds): Carcinogenesis, vol 7. New York, Raven Press, 1982; 69–73.

109. Sugimura T, Fujimura S. Tumor production in glandular stomach of rat by N-methyl-N'-nitro-N-nitrosoguanidine. *Nature* 1967; 216:943–944.

110. Sugimura T, Fujimura S, Baba T. Tumor production in the glandular stomach and alimentary tract of the rat by N-methyl-N'-nitro-N-nitrosoguanidine. *Cancer Res* 1970; 30:455–465.

111. Sugimura T, Kawachi T, Nagao M, Yahagi T, Seino Y, Okamoto T, Shudo K, Kosuge T, Tsuji K, Wakabayashi K, Iitaka Y, Itai A. Mutagenic principle(s) in tryptophan and phenylalanine pyrolysis products. *Proc Jpn Acad* 1977; 53:58–61.

112. Sugimura T, Kawachi T, Nagao M, Yamada M, Takayama S, Matsukura N, Wakabayashi K. Genotoxic carcinogens and comutagens in tryptophan pyrolysate. In Hayaishi O, Ishimura T, Kido R (eds): Biochemical and Medical Aspects of Tryptophan Metabolism. Amsterdam, Elsevier/North-Holland Biomedical Press, 1980; 297–310.

113. Sugimura T, Nagao M. Modification of mutagenic activity. In de Serres FJ, Hollaender A (eds): Chemical Mutagens, vol. 6. New York, Plenum Publishing Corporation, 1980; 41–60.

114. Sugimura T, Nagao M. The use of mutagenicity to evaluate carcinogenic hazards in our daily lives. In Heddle JA (ed): Muta-

genicity: New Horizons in Genetic Toxicology. New York, Academic Press, 1982; 73–88.

115. Sugimura T, Nagao M, Kawachi T, Honda M, Yahagi T, Seino Y, Sato S, Matsukura N, Matsushima T, Shirai A, Sawamura M, Matsumoto H. Mutagen-carcinogens in food, with special reference to highly mutagenic pyrolytic products in broiled foods. In Book C, Hiatt HH, Watson JD, Winsten JA (eds): Origins of Human Cancer. New York, Cold Spring Harbor Laboratory, 1977; 1561–1576.

116. Sugimura T, Nagao M, Matsushima T, Yahagi T, Seino Y, Shirai A, Sawamura M, Natori S, Yoshihira K, Fukuoka M, Kuroyanagi M. Mutagenicity of flavone derivatives. *Proc Jpn Acad* 1977; 53:194–197.

117. Sugimura T, Nagao M, Okada Y. Carcinogenic action of N-methyl-N'-nitro-N-nitrosoguanidine. *Nature* 1966; 210:962–963.

118. Sugimura T, Nagao M, Wakabayashi K. Mutagenic heterocyclic amines in cooked foods. In Egan H, Fishbein L, Castegnaro M, O'Neill IK, Bartsch H, Davis W (eds): Environmental Carcinogens-Selected Methods of Analysis Vol 4, Some Aromatic Amines and Azo Dyes in the General and Industrial Environmental. IARC Scientific Publications No 40, Lyon, International Agency for Research on Cancer, 1981; 251–267.

119. Sugimura T, Okabe K, Nagao M. The metabolism of 4-nitroquinoline 1-oxide, a carcinogen. III: An enzyme catalyzing the conversion of 4-nitroquinoline 1-oxide to 4-hydroxyaminoquinoline 1-oxide in rat liver and hepatomas. *Cancer Res* 1966; 26:1717–1721.

120. Sugimura T, Otake H, Matsushima T. Single strand scissions of DNA caused by a carcinogen, 4-hydroxyaminoquinoline 1-oxide. *Nature* 1968; 218:392.

121. Sugimura T, Sato S, Nagao M, Yahagi T, Matsushima T, Seino Y, Takeuchi M, Kawachi T. Overlapping of carcinogens and mutagens. In Magee PN, Takayama S, Sugimura T, Matsushima T (eds): Fundamentals in Cancer Prevention. Tokyo, Japan Scientific Societies Press, 1976; 191–215.

122. Sugimura T, Wakabayashi K, Yamada M, Nagao M, Fujino T. Activation of chemicals to proximal carcinogens. In Holmstedt B, Lauwerys R, Mercier M, Roberfroid M (eds): Mechanisms of Toxicity and Hazard Evaluation. Elsevier/North-Holland Biomedical Press, 1980; 205–217.

123. Suwa Y, Nagao M, Wakabayashi K, Kosugi A, Sugimura T. Abstracts of 3rd International Conference on Environmental Mutagens, Tokyo, 1981; 83.

124. Tada M, Tada M. Seryl-tRNA synthetase and activation of the carcinogen 4-nitroquinoline 1-oxide. *Nature* 1975; 255:510–512.

125. Takahashi Y, Nagao M, Fujino T, Yamaizumi Z, Sugimura T. Mutagens in Japanese pickle identified as flavonoids. *Mutation Res* 1979; 68:117–123.

126. Takashima M, Sakai H. A new toxic substance, teleocidin, produced by *Streptomyces*. *Bull Agr Chem Soc Japan* 1960; 24:647–651.

127. Takayama S, Hirakawa T, Sugimura T. Malignant transformation *in vitro* by tryptophan pyrolysis products. *Proc Jpn Acad* 1978; 54B:418–422.

128. Takayama S, Katoh Y, Tanaka M, Nagao M, Wakabayashi K, Sugimura T. *In vitro* transformation of hamster embryo cells with tryptophan pyrolysis products. *Proc Jpn Acad* 1977; 53B:126–129.

129. Takayama S, Kuwabara N. Carcinogenic activity of 2-(2-furyl)-3-(5-nitro-2-furyl)acrylamide, a food additive, in mice and rats. *Cancer Lett* 1977; 3:115–120.

130. Takeda K, Ohta T, Shudo K, Okamoto T, Tsuji K, Kosuge T. Synthesis of a mutagenic principle isolated from tryptophan pyrolysate. *Chem Pharm Bull* 1977; 25:2145–2146.

131. Takeda K, Shudo K, Okamoto T, Kosuge T. Synthesis of mutagenic principles isolated from L-glutamic acid pyrolysate. *Chem Pharm Bull* 1978; 26:2924–2925.

132. Tamura G, Gold C, Ferro-Luzzi A, Ames BN. Fecalase: A model for activation of dietary glycosides to mutagens by intestinal flora. *Proc Natl Acad Sci USA* 1980; 77:4961–4965.

133. Tatematsu M, Takahashi M, Fukushima S, Hananouchi M, Shirai T. Effects in rats of sodium chloride on experimental gastric cancers induced by N-methyl-N'-nitro-N-nitrosoguanidine or 4-nitroquinoline 1-oxide. *J Natl Cancer Inst* 1975; 55:101–105.

134. Tohda H, Oikawa A, Kawachi T, Sugimura T. Induction of

sister-chromatid exchanges by mutagens from amino acid and protein pyrolysates. *Mutation Res* 1980; 77:65–69.

135. Tonomura A, Sasaki MS. Chromosome aberrations and DNA repair synthesis in cultured human cells exposed to nitrofurans. *Jpn J Genet* 1973; 48:291–294.

136. Tuyns AJ. Epidemiology of alcohol and cancer. *Cancer Res* 1979; 39:2840–2843.

137. Umezawa K, Weinstein IB, Horowitz A, Fujiki H, Matsushima T, Sugimura T. Similarity of teleocidin B and phorbol ester tumor promoters in effects on membrane receptors. *Nature* 1981; 290:411–412.

138. Uyeta M, Kanada T, Mazaki M, Taue S, Takahashi S. Assaying mutagenicity of food pyrolysis products using the Ames test. In Miller EC, Miller JA, Hirono I, Sugimura T, Takayama S (eds): Naturally Occurring Carcinogen-Mutagens and Modulators of Carcinogenesis. Tokyo, Japan Scientific Societies Press, 1979; 169–176.

139. Uyeta M, Taue S, Mazaki M. Mutagenicity of hydrolysates of tea infusions. *Mutation Res* 1981; 88:233–240.

140. Van Duuren BL. Tumor-promoting agents in two-stage carcinogenesis. *Prog Exp Tumor Res* 1969; 11:31–68.

141. Wakabayashi K, Tsuji K, Kosuge T, Takeda K, Yamaguchi K, Shudo K, Iitaka Y, Okamoto T, Yahagi T, Nagao M, Sugimura T. Isolation and structure determination of a mutagenic substance in L-lysine pyrolysate. *Proc Jpn Acad* 1978; 54:569–571.

142. Watanabe J, Kawajiri K, Yonekawa H, Nagao M, Tagashira Y. Immunological analysis of the roles of two major types of cytochrome P-450 in mutagenesis of compounds isolated from pyrolysates. *Biochem Biophys Res Commun* 1982; 104:193–199.

143. Wattenberg LW. Inhibition of chemical carcinogenesis by antioxidants. In Slaga TJ (ed): Carcinogenesis Vol 5, Modifiers of Chemical Carcinogenesis. New York, Raven Press, 1980; 85–98.

144. Wattenberg LW, Leong JL. Inhibition of the carcinogenic action of benzo(a)pyrene by flavones. *Cancer Res* 1970; 30:1922–1925.

145. Weinstein IB, Mufson RA, Lee LS, Fisher PB, Laskin J, Horowitz A, Ivanovic V. Membrane and other biochemical effects of the phorbol esters and their relevance to tumor promotion. In Pullman B, Ts'o POP, Gelboin H (eds): Carcinogenesis, Fundamental Mechanisms and Environmental Effects. Amsterdam, R Reidel Pub. Co, 1980; 543–563.

146. Wiebel FJ, Gelboin HV, Bun-Hoi NP, Stont MG, Burnham WS. Flavones and polycyclic hydrocarbons as modulators of arylhydrocarbon [benzo(a)pyrene] hydroxylase. In Ts'o POP, Di Paolo JA (eds): Chemical Carcinogenesis. New York, Dekker, 1974; 249–270.

147. Yahagi T, Matsushima T, Nagao M, Seino Y, Sugimura T, Bryan GT. Mutagenicity of nitrofuran derivatives on a bacterial tester strain with an R factor plasmid. *Mutation Res* 1976; 40:9–14.

148. Yahagi T, Nagao M, Hara K, Matsushima T, Sugimura T, Bryan GT. Relationships between the carcinogenic and mutagenic or DNA-modifying effects of nitrofuran derivatives, including 2-(2-furyl)-3-(5-nitro-2-furyl)acrylamide, a food additive. *Cancer Res* 1974; 34:2266–2273.

149. Yahagi T, Nagao M, Seino Y, Matsushima T, Sugimura T, Okada M. Mutagenicities of N-nitrosamines on Salmonella. *Mutation Res* 1977; 48:121–130.

150. Yamagata K, Oda M, Ando T. Mutagenesis in Aspergillus(x): Chemical induction of mutations. Hakko Kogaku Zasshi 1956; 34:378–381 (in Japanese).

151. Yamaguchi K, Shudo K, Okamoto T, Sugimura T, Kosuge T. Presence of 2-aminodipyrido[1,2-a:3',2'-d]imidazole in broiled cuttlefish. *Gann* 1980; 71:743–744.

152. Yamaguchi K, Shudo K, Okamoto T, Sugimura T, Kosuge T. Presence of 3-amino-1,4-dimethyl-5H-pyrido[4,3-b]indole in broiled beef. *Gann* 1980; 71:745–746.

153. Yamaguchi K, Zenda H, Shudo K, Kosuge T, Okamoto T, Sugimura T. Presence of 2-aminodipyrido[1,2-a:3',2'-d]imidazole in casein pyrolysate. *Gann* 1979; 70:849–850.

154. Yamaizumi Z, Shiomi T, Kasai H, Nishimura S, Takahashi Y, Nagao M, Sugimura T. Detection of potent mutagens, Trp-P-1 and Trp-P-2, in broiled fish. *Cancer Lett* 1980; 9:75–83.

155. Yamamoto T, Tsuji K, Kosuge T, Okamoto T, Shudo K, Takeda K, Iitaka Y, Yamaguchi K, Seino Y, Yahagi T, Nagao M,

Sugimura T. Isolation and structure determination of mutagenic substances in L-glutamic acid pyrolysate. *Proc Jpn Acad* 1978; 54B:248–250.

156. Yamanaka H, Nagao M, Sugimura T, Furuya T, Shirai A, Matsushima T. Mutagenicity of pyrrolizidine alkaloids in the Salmonella/mammalian-microsome test. *Mutation Res* 1979; 68:211–216.

157. Yamazoe Y, Ishii K, Kamataki T, Kato R, Sugimura T. Isolation and characterization of active metabolites of tryptophan pyroly-sate mutagen, Trp-P-2, formed by rat liver microsomes. *Chem Biol Interact* 1980; 30:125–138.

158. Yamazoe Y, Tada M, Kamataki T, Kato R. Enhancement of binding of N-hydroxy-Trp-P-2 to DNA by seryl tRNA synthetase. *Biochem Biophys Res Commun* 1981; 102:432–439.

159. Yoshida D, Matsumoto T, Yoshimura R, Matsuzaki T. Mutagenicity of amino-α-carbolines in pyrolysis products of soybean globulin. *Biochem Biophys Res Commun* 1978; 83:915–920.

Dietary Carcinogens and Anticarcinogens: Oxygen Radicals and Degenerative Diseases

by Bruce N. Ames

Summary. The human diet contains a great variety of natural mutagens and carcinogens, as well as many natural antimutagens and anticarcinogens. Many of these mutagens and carcinogens may act through the generation of oxygen radicals. Oxygen radicals may also play a major role as endogenous initiators of degenerative processes, such as DNA damage and mutation (and promotion), that may be related to cancer, heart disease, and aging. Dietary intake of natural antioxidants could be an important aspect of the body's defense mechanism against these agents. Many antioxidants are being identified as anticarcinogens. Characterizing and optimizing such defense systems may be an important part of a strategy of minimizing cancer and other age-related diseases.

Comparison of data from different countries reveals wide differences in the rates of many types of cancer. This leads to hope that each major type of cancer may be largely avoidable, as is the case for cancers due to tobacco, which constitute 30 percent of the cancer deaths in the United States and the United Kingdom (*1*). Despite numerous suggestions to the contrary, there is no convincing evidence of any generalized increase in U.S. (or U.K.) cancer rates other than what could plausibly be ascribed to the delayed effects of previous increases in tobacco usage (*1–3*). Thus, whether or not any recent changes in life-style or pollution in industrialized countries will substantially affect future cancer risks, some important determinants of current risks remain to be discovered among

Bruce N. Ames is chairman of the Department of Biochemistry, University of California at Berkeley, 94720.

long-established aspects of our way of life. Epidemiologic studies have indicated that dietary practices are the most promising area to explore (*1, 4*). These studies suggest that a general increase in consumption of fiber-rich cereals, vegetables, and fruits and decrease in consumption of fat-rich products and excessive alcohol would be prudent (*1, 4*). There is still a lack of definitive evidence about the dietary components that are critical for humans and about their mechanisms of action. Laboratory studies of natural foodstuffs and cooked food are beginning to uncover an extraordinary variety of mutagens and possible carcinogens and anticarcinogens. In this article I discuss dietary mutagens and carcinogens and anticarcinogens that seem of importance and speculate on relevant biochemical mechanisms, particularly the role of oxygen radicals and their inhibitors in the fat-cancer relationship,

promotion, anticarcinogenesis, and aging.

Natural Mutagens and Carcinogens in Food

Plant material. Plants in nature synthesize toxic chemicals in large amounts, apparently as a primary defense against the hordes of bacterial, fungal, and insect and other animal predators (*5–40*). Plants in the human diet are no exception. The variety of these toxic chemicals is so great that organic chemists have been characterizing them for over 100 years, and new plant chemicals are still being discovered (*12, 24, 25*). However, toxicological studies have been completed for only a very small percentage of them. Recent widespread use of short-term tests for detecting mutagens (*41, 42*) and the increased number of animal cancer tests on plant substances (*6*) have contributed to the identification of many natural mutagens, teratogens, and carcinogens in the human diet (*5–40*). Sixteen examples are discussed below.

1) *Safrole, estragole, methyleugenol,* and related compounds are present in many edible plants (*5*). Safrole, estragole, and methyleugenol are carcinogens in rodents, and several of their metabolites are mutagens (*5*). Oil of sassafras, which had been used in "natural" sarsaparilla root beer, is about 75 percent safrole. Black pepper contains small

amounts of safrole and large amounts (close to 10 percent by weight) of the closely related compound *piperine* (26). Extracts of black pepper cause tumors in mice at a variety of sites at a dose of extract equivalent to 4 mg of dried pepper per day (about 160 mg/kg per day) for 3 months; an estimate of the average human intake of black pepper is over 140 mg per day (about 2 mg/kg per day) for life (26).

2) Most *hydrazines* that have been tested are carcinogens and mutagens, and large amounts of carcinogenic hydrazines are present in edible mushrooms. The widely eaten false morel (*Gyromitra esculenta*) contains 11 hydrazines, three of which are known carcinogens (28). One of these, *N*-methyl-*N*-formylhydrazine, is present at a concentration of 50 mg per 100 g and causes lung tumors in mice at the extremely low dietary level of 20 µg per mouse per day (28). The most common commercial mushroom, *Agaricus bisporus*, contains about 300 mg of *agaritine*, the δ-glutamyl derivative of the mutagen 4-hydroxy-methylphenylhydrazine, per 100 g of mushrooms, as well as smaller amounts of the closely related carcinogen *N*-acetyl - 4 - hydroxymethylphenylhydrazine (28). Some agaritine is metabolized by the mushroom to a diazonium derivative which is a very potent carcinogen (a single dose of 400 ng/g gave 30 percent of mice stomach tumors) and which is also present in the mushroom in smaller amounts (28). Many hydrazine carcinogens may act by producing oxygen radicals (43).

3) Linear *furocoumarins* such as *psoralen derivatives* are potent light-activated carcinogens and mutagens and are widespread in plants of the Umbelliferae family, such as celery, parsnips, figs, and parsley (for instance, 4 mg per 100 g of parsnip) (17, 19, 44). The level in celery (about 100 µg per 100 g) can increase about 100-fold if the celery is stressed or diseased (19). Celery pickers and handlers commonly develop skin rashes on their arms when exposed to diseased celery (19). Oil of bergamot, a citrus oil, is very rich in a psoralen and was used in the leading suntan lotion in France (17). Psoralens, when activated by sunlight, damage DNA and induce tanning more rapidly than the ultraviolet component of sunlight, which is also a carcinogen (17). Psoralens (plus light) are also effective in producing oxygen radicals (18).

4) The potato glycoalkaloids *solanine* and *chaconine* are strong cholinesterase inhibitors and possible teratogens and are present at about 15 mg per 200 g of potato (12, 13). When potatoes are diseased, bruised, or exposed to light, these and other (24) glycoalkaloids reach levels that can be lethal to humans (12). Plants typically respond to damage by making more (and often different) toxic chemicals as a defense against insects and fungi (19, 24, 25). The different cultivars of potatoes vary in the concentration of these toxic glycoalkaloids (the concentration is a major determinant of insect and disease resistance); one cultivar bred for insect resistance had to be withdrawn from use because of its toxicity to humans (> 40 mg of glycoalkaloids in a 200-g potato is considered to be a toxic level) (12).

5) *Quercetin* and several similar flavonoids are mutagens in a number of short-term test systems. Flavonoids are extremely widespread (daily levels close to 1 g) in the human diet (8, 16, 20, 21). There is evidence for the carcinogenicity of quercetin in two strains of rats (8), although it was negative in other experiments (21).

6) *Quinones* and their phenol precursors (9, 14, 16, 23, 45) are widespread in the human diet. Quinones are quite toxic as they can act as electrophiles or accept a single electron to yield the semiquinone radical, which can either react directly with DNA (14, 46) or participate in a redox cycle of superoxide radical generation by transferring the electron to O_2 (47). The superoxide radical and its metabolic product H_2O_2 can, in turn, lead to the oxidation of fat in cellular membranes by a lipid peroxidation chain reaction, thus generating mutagens and carcinogens, as discussed below. A number of quinones and dietary phenols have been shown to be mutagens (7, 9, 16, 23, 44). Mutagenic anthraquinone derivatives are found in plants such as rhubarb and in mold toxins (7, 16, 48). Many dietary phenols can spontaneously autoxidize to quinones, generating hydrogen peroxide at the same time [examples are catechol derivatives such as the caffeic acid component of chlorogenic acid (9), which is present at about 250 mg per

cup of coffee]. The amounts of these phenols in human urine (and in the diet) are appreciable (45). Catechol, for example, is excreted in urine at about 10 mg per day and appears to be mainly derived from metabolism of plant substances (45). Catechol is a potent promoter of carcinogenesis (45), an inducer of DNA damage, a likely active metabolite of the carcinogen benzene (46), and a toxic agent in cigarette smoke (45). Catecholamine induction of cardiomyopathy is thought to occur through generation of oxygen radicals (49).

7) *Theobromine*, a relative of caffeine, has been shown to be genotoxic in a variety of tests, to potentiate (as does caffeine) DNA damage by various carcinogens in human cells, and to cause testicular atrophy and spermatogenic cell abnormalities in rats (27). Cocoa powder is about 2 percent theobromine, and therefore humans may consume hundreds of milligrams of theobromine a day from chocolate. Theobromine is also present in tea.

8) *Pyrrolizidine* alkaloids are carcinogenic, mutagenic, and teratogenic and are present in thousands of plant species (often at > 1 percent by weight), some of which are ingested by humans, particularly in herbs and herbal teas and occasionally in honey (7, 29). Pyrrolizidine alkaloid poisonings in humans (as well as in other mammals) cause lung and liver lesions and are commonly misdiagnosed (29).

9) The broad (fava) bean (*Vicia faba*), a common food of the Mediterranean region, contains the toxins *vicine* and *convicine* at a level of about 2 percent of the dry weight (30). Pythagoras forbade his followers to eat the beans, presumably because he was one of the millions of Mediterranean people with a deficiency of glucose-6-phosphate dehydrogenase. This deficiency results in a low glutathione concentration in blood cells, which causes increased resistance to the malarial parasite, probably accounting for the widespread occurrence of the mutant gene in malarial regions. However, the low glutathione concentration also results in a marked sensitivity to agents that cause oxidative damage, such as the fava bean toxins and a variety of drugs and viruses. Sensitive individuals who ingest fava beans develop a severe hemolytic anemia caused by the

enzymatic hydrolysis of vicine to its aglycone, *divicine*, which forms a quinone that generates oxygen radicals (*30*).

10) *Allyl isothiocyanate*, a major flavor ingredient in oil of mustard and horseradish, is one of the main toxins of the mustard seed and has been shown to cause chromosome aberrations in hamster cells at low concentration (*50*) and to be a carcinogen in rats (*31*).

11) *Gossypol* is a major toxin in cottonseed and accounts for about 1 percent of its dry weight (*32*). Gossypol causes pathological changes in rat and human testes, abnormal sperm, and male sterility (*32, 33*). Genetic damage has been observed in embryos sired by gossypol-treated male rats: dominant lethal mutations in embryos were measured after males were taken off gossypol treatment and allowed to mate (*33*). Gossypol appears to be a carcinogen as well: it has been reported to be a potent initiator and also a promoter of carcinogenesis in skin painting studies with mice (*34*). Crude, unrefined cottonseed oil contains considerable amounts of gossypol (100 to 750 mg per 100 ml). Thus human consumption may be appreciable in countries, such as Egypt, where fairly crude cottonseed oil is commonly used in cooking. Gossypol is being tested as a male contraceptive in over 10,000 people in China (at an oral dose of about 10 mg per person per day), as it is inexpensive and causes sterility during use (*33*). Gossypol's mode of action as a spermicide may be through the production of oxygen radicals (*35*).

Plant breeders have developed "glandless cotton," a new strain with low levels of gossypol, but seeds from this strain are much more susceptible to attack by the fungus *Aspergillus flavus*, which produces the potent carcinogen aflatoxin (*36*).

12) *Sterculic acid* and *malvalic acid* are widespread in the human diet. They are toxic cyclopropenoid fatty acids present in cottonseed oil and other oils from seeds of plants in the family Malvaceal (for instance, cotton, kapok, okra, and durian) (*51*). Another possible source of human exposure is consumption of fish, poultry, eggs, and milk from animals fed on cottonseed (*51*). Cyclopropenoid fatty acids are carcinogens in trout, markedly potentiate the carcinogenicity of aflatoxin in trout, cause athero-

sclerosis in rabbits, are mitogenic in rats, and have a variety of toxic effects in farm animals (*51*). The toxicity of these fatty acids could be due to their ease of oxidation to form peroxides and radicals (*51*).

13) Leguminous plants such as lupine contain very potent teratogens (*22*). When cows and goats forage on these plants, their offspring may have severe teratogenic abnormalities; an example is the characteristic "crooked calf" abnormality due to the ingestion of *anagyrine* from lupine (*22*). In addition, significant amounts of these teratogens are transferred to the animals' milk, so that drinking the milk during pregnancy is a serious teratogenic hazard (*22*). In one rural California family, a baby boy, a litter of puppies, and goat kids all had "crooked" bone birth-defect abnormalities. The pregnant mother and the dog had both been drinking milk obtained from the family goats, which had been foraging on lupine (the main forage in winter) (*22*). It was at first mistakenly thought that the birth defects were caused by spraying of 2,4-D.

14) *Sesquiterpene lactones* are widespread in many plants (*37*), although because they are bitter they are not eaten in large amounts. Some have been shown to be mutagenic (*37*). They are a major toxin in the white sap of *Lactuca virosa* (poison lettuce), which has been used as a folk remedy. Plant breeders are now transferring genes from this species to commercial lettuce to increase insect resistance (*38*).

15) The *phorbol esters* present in the Euphorbiacea, some of which are used as folk remedies or herb teas, are potent promoters of carcinogenesis and may have been a cause of nasopharyngeal cancer in China and esophageal cancer in Curaçao (*39*).

16) Alfalfa sprouts contain *canavanine*, a highly toxic arginine analog that is incorporated into protein in place of arginine. Canavanine, which occurs in alfalfa sprouts at about 1.5 percent of their dry weight (*40*), appears to be the active agent in causing the severe lupus erythematosus–like syndrome seen when monkeys are fed alfalfa sprouts (*40*). Lupus in man is characterized by a defect in the immune system which is associated with autoimmunity, antinuclear antibodies, chromosome breaks, and various types of pathology (*40*). The chromosome

breaks appear to be due to oxygen radicals as they are prevented by superoxide dismutase (*52*). The canavanine–alfalfa sprout pathology could be due in part to the production of oxygen radicals during phagocytization of antibody complexes with canavanine-containing protein.

The 16 examples above, plus coffee (discussed below), illustrate that the human dietary intake of "nature's pesticides" is likely to be several grams per day—probably at least 10,000 times higher than the dietary intake of man-made pesticides (*53*).

Levels of plant toxins that confer insect and fungal resistance are being increased or decreased by plant breeders (*38*). There are health costs for the use of these natural pesticides, just as there are for man-made pesticides (*41, 54*), and these must be balanced against the costs of producing food. However, little information is available about the toxicology of most of the natural plant toxins in our diet, despite the large doses we are exposed to. Many, if not most, of these plant toxins may be "new" to humans in the sense that the human diet has changed drastically with historic times. By comparison, our knowledge of the toxicological effects of new man-made pesticides is extensive, and general exposure is exceedingly low (*53*).

Plants also contain a variety of anticarcinogens (*55*), which are discussed below.

Alcohol. Alcohol has long been associated with cancer of the mouth, esophagus, pharynx, larynx, and, to a lesser extent, liver (*1, 56*), and it appears to be an important human teratogen, causing a variety of physical and mental defects in babies of mothers who drink (*57*). Alcohol drinking causes abnormalities in mice (*57a*) and is a synergist for chromosome damage in humans (*58*). Alcohol metabolism generates acetaldehyde, which is a mutagen and teratogen (*59*), a cocarcinogen, and possibly a carcinogen (*60*), and also radicals that produce lipid hydroperoxides (*61*) and other mutagens and carcinogens (*62*; see below). In some epidemiologic studies on alcohol (*56*), it has been suggested that dietary green vegetables are a modifying factor in the reduction of cancer risk.

Mold carcinogens. A variety of mold carcinogens and mutagens are present in mold-contaminated food such as corn, grain, nuts, peanut butter, bread, cheese, fruit, and apple juice (*15, 63*). Some of these, such as sterigmatocystin and aflatoxin, are among the most potent carcinogens and mutagens known (*15, 63*). Dietary glutathione has been reported to counteract aflatoxin carcinogenicity.

Nitrite, nitrate, and nitrosamines. A number of human cancers, such as stomach and esophageal cancer, may be related to nitrosamines and other nitroso compounds formed from nitrate and nitrite in the diet (*64, 65*). Beets, celery, lettuce, spinach, radishes, and rhubarb all contain about 200 mg of nitrate per 100-g portion (*65*). Anticarcinogens in the diet may be important in this context as well (*66*).

Fat and cancer: possible oxidative mechanisms. Epidemiologic studies of cancer in humans suggest, but do not prove, that high fat intake is associated with colon and breast cancer (*1, 4, 67*). A number of animal studies have shown that high dietary fat is a promoter and a presumptive carcinogen (*4, 67, 68*). Colon and breast cancer and lung cancer (which is almost entirely due to cigarette smoking) account for about half of all U.S. cancer deaths. In addition to the cyclopropenoid fatty acids already discussed, two other plausible mechanisms involving oxidative processes could account for the relation (*69*) between high fat and both cancer and heart disease.

1) *Rancid fat.* Fat accounts for over 40 percent of the calories in the U.S. diet (*67*), and the amount of ingested oxidized fat may be appreciable (*70, 71*). Unsaturated fatty acids and cholesterol in fat are easily oxidized, particularly during cooking (*70, 71*). The lipid peroxidation chain reaction (rancidity) yields a variety (*71–73*) of mutagens, promoters, and carcinogens such as fatty acid hydroperoxides (*62*), cholesterol hydroperoxide (*74*), endoperoxides, cholesterol and fatty acid epoxides (*74–77*), enals and other aldehydes (*44, 59, 78*), and alkoxy and hydroperoxy radicals (*44, 72*). Thus the colon and digestive tract are exposed to a variety of fat-derived carcinogens. Human breast fluid can contain enormous levels (up to 780 μM) (*75*) of cholesterol epoxide (an oxidation product of cholesterol), which could originate from either ingested oxidized fat or oxidative processes in body lipids. Rodent feeding studies with oxidized fat (*79*) have not yielded definitive results.

2) *Peroxisomes* oxidize an appreciable percentage of dietary fatty acids, and removal of each two-carbon unit generates one molecule of hydrogen peroxide (a mutagen, promoter, and carcinogen) (*80, 81*). Some hydrogen peroxide escapes the catalase in the peroxisome (*80, 82, 83*), thus contributing to the supply of oxygen radicals, which also come from other metabolic sources (*72, 83–85*). Hydroperoxides generate oxygen radicals in the presence of iron-containing compounds in the cell (*72*). Oxygen radicals, in turn, can damage DNA and can start the rancidity chain reaction which leads to the production of the mutagens and carcinogens listed above (*72*). Drugs such as clofibrate, which cause lowering of serum lipids and proliferation of peroxisomes in rodents, result in age pigment (lipofuscin) accumulation (a sign of lipid peroxidation in tissues) and liver tumors in animals (*80*). Some fatty acids, such as $C_{22:1}$ and certain *trans* fatty acids, appear to cause peroxisomal proliferation because they are poorly oxidized in mitochondria and are preferentially oxidized in the peroxisomes, although they may be selective for heart or liver (*86*). There has been controversy about the role of *trans* fatty acids in cancer and heart disease, and recent evidence suggests that *trans* fatty acids might not be a risk factor for atherosclerosis in experimental animals (*87*). Americans consume about 12 g of *trans* fatty acids a day (*87*) and a similar amount of unnatural *cis* isomers [which need further study (*88*)], mainly from hydrogenated vegetable fats. Dietary $C_{22:1}$ fatty acids are also obtained from rapeseed oil and fish oils (*86*). Thus oxidation of certain fatty acids might generate grams of hydrogen peroxide per day within the peroxisome (*86*). Another source of fat toxicity could be perturbations in the mitochondrial or peroxisomal membranes caused by abnormal fatty acids, yielding an increased flux of superoxide and hydrogen peroxide. Mitochondrial structure is altered when rats are fed some abnormal fatty acids from partially hydrogenated fish oil (*89*). Dietary $C_{22:1}$ fatty acids and clofibrate also induce ornithine decarboxylase (*86*), a common attribute of promoters.

A recent National Academy of Sciences committee report suggests that a reduction of fat consumption in the American diet would be prudent (*4*), although other scientists argue that, until we know more about the mechanism of the fat-cancer relation and about which types of fat are dangerous, it is premature to recommend dietary changes (*90*).

Cooked Food as a Source of Ingested Burnt and Browned Material

Work of Sugimura and others has indicated that the burnt and browned material from heating protein during cooking is highly mutagenic (*21, 91*). Several chemicals isolated on the basis of their mutagenicity from heated protein or pyrolyzed amino acids were found to be carcinogenic when fed to rodents (*21*). In addition, the browning reaction products from the caramelization of sugars or the reaction of amino acids and sugars during cooking (for instance, the brown material on bread crusts and toasted bread) contain a large variety of DNA-damaging agents and presumptive carcinogens (*23, 38, 92*). The amount of burnt and browned material in the human diet may be several grams per day. By comparison about 500 mg of burnt material is inhaled each day by a smoker using two packs of cigarettes (at 20 mg of tar per cigarette) a day. Smokers have more easily detectable levels of mutagens in their urine than nonsmokers (*93*), but so do people who have consumed a meal of fried pork or bacon (*94*). In the evaluation of risk from burnt material it may be useful (in addition to carrying out epidemiologic studies) to compare the activity of cigarette tar to that of the burnt material from cooked food (or polluted air) in short-term tests and animal carcinogenicity tests involving relevant routes of exposure. Route of exposure and composition of the burnt material are critical variables. The risk from inhaled cigarette smoke can be one reference standard: an average life shortening of about 8 years for a two-pack-a-day smoker. The amount of burnt material inhaled from severely polluted city air, on the other hand, is relatively small: it would be necessary to breathe smoggy Los Angeles air (111 $\mu g/m^3$ total particulates; 31 $\mu g/m^3$ soluble organic matter) for 1 to 2 weeks to equal the soluble organic matter of the particulates or the mutagenicity from one cigarette (20 mg of tar) (*95*). Epidemiologic studies have not shown significant risks from city air pollution alone (*1, 96*). Air in the houses of smokers is considerably more polluted than city air outside (*97*).

Coffee, which contains a considerable amount of burnt material, including the mutagenic pyrolysis product methylglyoxal, is mutagenic (*21, 98*). However, one cup of coffee also contains about 250 mg of the natural mutagen chlorogenic acid (*9*) [which is also an antinitrosating agent (*66*)], highly toxic atractylosides (*10*), the glutathione transferase inducers kahweal palmitate and cafestol palmitate (*11*), and about 100 mg of caffeine [which inhibits a DNA-repair system and can increase tumor yield (*99*) and cause birth defects at high levels in several experimental species (*100*)]. There is preliminary, but not conclusive, epidemiologic evidence that heavy coffee drinking is associated with cancer of the ovary, bladder, pancreas, and large bowel (*101*).

Cooking also accelerates the rancidity reaction of cooking oils and fat in meat (*70, 71*), thus increasing consumption of mutagens and carcinogens.

Anticarcinogens

We have many defense mechanisms to protect ourselves against mutagens and carcinogens, including continuous shedding of the surface layer of our skin, stomach, cornea, intestines, and colon (*102*). Understanding these mechanisms should be a major goal of cancer, heart, and aging research. Among the most important defenses may be those against oxygen radicals and lipid peroxidation if, as discussed here, these agents are major contributors to DNA damage (*103*). Major sources of endogenous oxygen radicals are hydrogen peroxide (*83*) and superoxide (*72, 104*) generated as side products of metabolism, and the oxygen radical burst from phagocytosis after viral or bacterial infection or the inflammatory reaction (*105*). A variety of environmental agents could also contribute to the oxygen radical load, as discussed here and in recent reviews (*72, 106*). Many enzymes protect cells from oxidative damage; examples are superoxide dismutase (*104*), glutathione peroxidase

(*107*), DT-diaphorase (*108*), and the glutathione transferases (*109*). In addition, a variety of small molecules in our diet are required for antioxidative mechanisms and appear to be anticarcinogens; some of these are discussed below.

1) *Vitamin E* (tocopherol) is the major radical trap in lipid membranes (*72*) and has been used clinically in a variety of oxidation-related diseases (*110*). Vitamin E ameliorates both the cardiac damage and carcinogenicity of the quinones adriamycin and daunomycin, which are mutagenic, carcinogenic, cause cardiac damage, and appear to be toxic because of free radical generation (*111*). Protective effects of tocopherols against radiation-induced DNA damage and mutation and dimethylhydrazine-induced carcinogenesis have also been observed (*112*). Vitamin E markedly increases the endurance of rats during heavy exercise, which causes extensive oxygen radical damage to tissues (*113*).

2) β-*Carotene* is another antioxidant in the diet that could be important in protecting body fat and lipid membranes against oxidation. Carotenoids are free-radical traps and remarkably efficient quenchers of singlet oxygen (*114*). Singlet oxygen is a very reactive form of oxygen which is mutagenic and particularly effective at causing lipid peroxidation (*114*). It can be generated by pigment-mediated transfer of the energy of light to oxygen, or by lipid peroxidation, although the latter is somewhat controversial. β-Carotene and similar polyprenes are present in carrots and in all food that contains chlorophyll, and they appear to be the plants' main defense against singlet oxygen generated as a byproduct from the interaction of light and chlorophyll (*115*). Carotenoids have been shown to be anticarcinogens in rats and mice (*116*). Carotenoids (in green and yellow vegetables) may be anticarcinogens in humans (*1, 56, 117*). Their protective effects in smokers might be related to the high level of oxidants in both cigarette smoke and tar (*45, 118*). Carotenoids have been used medically in the treatment for some genetic diseases, such as porphyrias, where a marked photosensitivity is presumably due to singlet oxygen formation (*119*).

3) *Selenium* is another important dietary anticarcinogen. Dietary selenium (usually selenite) significantly inhibits

the induction of skin, liver, colon, and mammary tumors in experimental animals by a number of different carcinogens, as well as the induction of mammary tumors by viruses (*120*). It also inhibits transformation of mouse mammary cells (*121*). Low selenium concentrations may be a risk factor in human cancer (*122*). A particular type of heart disease in young people in the Keshan area of China has been traced to a selenium deficiency, and low selenium has been associated with cardiovascular death in Finland (*123*). Selenium is in the active site of glutathione peroxidase, an enzyme essential for destroying lipid hydroperoxides and endogenous hydrogen peroxide and thus helping to prevent oxygen radical–induced lipid peroxidation (*107*), although not all of the effects of selenium may be accounted for by this enzyme (*120*). Several heavy-metal toxins, such as Cd^{2+} (a known carcinogen) and Hg^{2+}, lower glutathione peroxidase activity by interacting with selenium (*107*). Selenite (and vitamin E) has been shown to counter the oxidative toxicity of mercuric salts (*124*).

4) *Glutathione* is present in food and is one of the major antioxidants and antimutagens in the soluble fraction of cells. The glutathione transferases (some of which have peroxidase activity) are major defenses against oxidative and alkylating carcinogens (*109*). The concentration of glutathione may be influenced by dietary sulfur amino acids (*125, 126*). N-Acetylcysteine, a source of cysteine, raises glutathione concentrations and reduces the oxidative cardiotoxicity of adriamycin and the skin reaction to radiation (*127*). Glutathione concentrations are raised even more efficiently by L-2-oxothiazolidine-4-carboxylate, which is an effective antagonist of acetaminophen-caused liver damage (*126*). Acetaminophen is thought to be toxic through radical and quinone oxidizing metabolites (*128*). Dietary glutathione may be an effective anticarcinogen against aflatoxin (*129*).

5) Dietary *ascorbic acid* is also important as an antioxidant. It was shown to be anticarcinogenic in rodents treated with ultraviolet radiation, benzo[*a*]pyrene, and nitrite (forming nitroso carcinogens) (*64, 65, 130*), and it may be inversely associated with human uterine cervical dysplasia (although this is not

proof of a cause-effect relationship) (*131*). It was recently hypothesized that ascorbic acid may have been supplemented and perhaps partially replaced in humans by uric acid during primate evolution (*132*).

6) *Uric acid* is a strong antioxidant present in high concentrations in the blood of humans (*132*). The concentration of uric acid in the blood can be increased by dietary purines; however, too much causes gout. Uric acid is also present in high concentrations in human saliva (*132*) and may play a role in defense there as well, in conjunction with lactoperoxidase. A low uric acid level in blood may possibly be a risk factor in cigarette-caused lung cancer in humans (*133*).

7) Edible plants and a variety of substances in them, such as phenols, have been reported to inhibit (cabbage) or to enhance (beets) carcinogenesis (*11, 55, 134*) or mutagenesis (*23, 66, 92, 135*) in experimental animals. Some of these substances appear to inhibit by inducing cytochrome P-450 and other metabolic enzymes [(*134*); see also (*11*)], although on balance it is not completely clear whether it is generally helpful or harmful for humans to ingest these inducing substances.

The hypothesis that as much as 80 percent of cancer could be due to environmental factors was based on geographic differences in cancer rates and studies of migrants (*136*). These differences in cancer rates were thought to be mainly due to life-style factors, such as smoking and dietary carcinogens and promoters (*136*), but they also may be due in good part [see also (*1*)] to less than optimum amounts of anticarcinogens and protective factors in the diet.

The optimum levels of dietary antioxidants, which may vary among individuals, remain to be determined; however, at least for selenium (*120*), it is important to emphasize the possibility of deleterious side effects at high doses.

Oxygen Radicals and Degenerative Diseases Associated with Aging

Aging. A plausible theory of aging holds that the major cause is damage to DNA (*102, 137*) and other macromolecules and that a major source of this damage is oxygen radicals and lipid peroxidation (*43, 84, 103, 138–141*). Cancer and other degenerative diseases, such as heart disease (*102*), are likely to be due in good part to this same fundamental destructive process. Age pigment (lipofuscin) accumulates aging in all mammalian species and has been associated with lipid peroxidation (*73, 84, 138, 139*). The fluorescent products in age pigment are thought to be formed by malondialdehyde (a mutagen and carcinogen and a major end product of rancidity) cross-linking protein and lipids (*138*). Metabolic rate is directly correlated with the rate of lipofuscin formation (and inversely correlated with longevity) (*139*).

Cancer increases with about the fourth power of age, both in short-lived species such as rats and mice (about 30 percent of rodents have cancer by the end of their 2- to 3-year life-span) and in long-lived species such as humans (about 30 percent of people have cancer by the end of their 85-year life-span) (*142*). Thus, the marked increase in life-span that has occurred in 60 million years of primate evolution has been accompanied by a marked decrease in age-specific cancer rates; that is, in contrast to rodents, 30 percent of humans do not have cancer by the age of 3 (*142*). One important factor in longevity appears to be basal metabolic rate (*139, 141*), which is much lower in man than in rodents and could markedly affect the level of endogenous oxygen radicals.

Animals have many antioxidant defenses against oxygen radicals. Increased levels of these antioxidants, as well as new antioxidants, may also be a factor in the evolution of man from short-lived prosimians (*143*). It has been suggested that an increase in superoxide dismutase is correlated (after the basal metabolic rate is taken into account) with increased longevity during primate evolution, although this has been disputed (*141*). Ames *et al.* proposed (*132*) that as uric acid was an antioxidant and was present in much higher concentrations in the blood of humans than in other mammals, it may have been one of the innovations enabling the marked increase in life span and consequent marked decrease in age-specific cancer rates which occurred during primate evolution. The ability to synthesize ascorbic acid may have been lost at about the same time in primate evolution as uric acid levels began to increase (*144*).

Cancer and promotion. Both DNA-damaging agents (initiating mutagens) (*21, 41, 42*) and promoters (*145*) appear to play an important role in carcinogenesis (*21, 146*). It has been postulated that certain promoters of carcinogenesis act by generation of oxygen radicals and resultant lipid peroxidation (*73, 146–149*). Lipid peroxidation cross-links proteins (*43, 150*) and affects all aspects of cell organization (*72*), including membrane and surface structure, and the mitotic apparatus. A common property of promoters may be their ability to produce oxygen radicals. Some examples are fat and hydrogen peroxide (which may be among the most important promoters) (*67, 68, 81*), TCDD (*151*), lead and cadmium (*152*), phorbol esters (*147, 149, 153*), wounding of tissues (*154*), asbestos (*155*), peroxides (*156*), catechol (*45*) (see quinones above), mezerein and teleocidin B (*147*), phenobarbital (*157*), and radiation (*72, 158*). Inflammatory reactions involve the production of oxygen radicals by phagocytes (*105*), and this could be the basis of promotion for asbestos (*155*) or wounding (*154*). Some of the antioxidant anticarcinogens (discussed above) are also antipromoters (*73, 121, 146, 159, 160*), and phorbol ester–induced chromosome damage (*149*) or promotion of transformation (*159*) is suppressed by superoxide dismutase, as would be expected if promoters were working through oxidative mechanisms. Many ''complete'' carcinogens cause the production of oxygen radicals (*73, 161*); examples are nitroso compounds, hydrazines, quinones, polycyclic hydrocarbons (through quinones), cadmium and lead salts, nitro compounds, and radiation. A good part of the toxic effects of ionizing radiation damage to DNA and cells is thought to be due to generation of oxygen radicals (*103, 162*), although only a tiny part of the oxygen radical load in humans is likely to be from this source.

Recent studies give some clues as to how promoters might act. Promoters disrupt the mitotic apparatus, causing hemizygosity and expression of recessive genes (*163*). Phorbol esters generate oxygen radicals, which cause chromosome breaks (*164*) and increase gene copy number (*165*). Promoters also cause formation of the peroxide hormones of the prostaglandin and leukotriene family by oxidation of arachidonic acid and other C_{20} polyenoic fatty acids, and inhibitors of this process appear to be antipromoters (*160*). These hormones are intimately involved in cell division, differentiation, and tumor growth (*166*) and could have arisen in evolution as signal molecules warning the cell of oxidative damage. Effects on the cell membrane have also been suggested as the important factor in promotion, causing inhibition of intercellular communication (*167*) or protein kinase activation (*167a*).

Heart disease. It has been postulated that atherosclerotic lesions, which are derived from single cells, are similar to benign tumors and are of somatic mutational origin (*102, 168*). Fat appears to be one major risk factor for heart disease as well as for colon and breast cancer (*69*). In agreement with this, a strong correlation has been observed between the frequency of atherosclerotic lesions and adenomatous polyps of the colon (*69*). Thus, the same oxidative processes involving fat may contribute to both diseases. Oxidized forms of cholesterol have been implicated in heart disease (*169*), and atherosclerotic-like lesions have been produced by injecting rabbits with lipid hydroperoxide or oxidized cholesterol (*169*). The anticarcinogens discussed above could be anti–heart disease agents as well. As pointed out in the preceding section, vitamin E ameliorates both the cardiac damage and carcinogenicity of the free-radical-generating quinones adriamycin and daunomycin; *N*-acetylcysteine reduces the cardiotoxicity of adriamycin; and selenium is an antirisk factor for one type of heart disease.

Other diseases. The brain uses 20 percent of the oxygen consumed by man and contains an appreciable amount of unsaturated fat. Lipid peroxidation (with consequent age pigment) is known to occur readily in the brain (*72*), and possible consequences could be senile dementia or other brain abnormalities (*84*). Several inherited progressive diseases of the central nervous system, such as Batten's disease, are associated with lipofuscin accumulation and may be due to a lipid peroxidation caused by a high concentration of unbound iron (*170*). Mental retardation is one consequence of an inherit-

ed defective DNA repair system (XP complementation group D) for depurinated sites in DNA (*171*).

Senile cataracts have been associated with light-induced oxidative damage (*172*). The retina and an associated layer of cells, the pigment epithelium, are extremely sensitive to degeneration in vitamin E and selenium deficiency (*173*). The pigment epithelium accumulates massive amounts of lipofuscin in aging and dietary antioxidant deficiency (*173*). The eye is well known to be particularly rich in antioxidants.

The testes are quite prone to lipid peroxidation and to the accumulation of age pigment. A number of agents, such as gossypol, which cause genetic birth defects (dominant lethals) may be active by this mechanism. The various agents known to cause cancer by oxidative mechanisms are prospective mutagenic agents for the germ line. Thus, vitamin E, which was discovered 60 years ago as a fertility factor (*72*), and other antioxidants such as selenium (*174*), may help both to engender and to protect the next generation.

Risks

There are large numbers of mutagens and carcinogens in every meal, all perfectly natural and traditional [see also (*21, 23*)]. Nature is not benign. It should be emphasized that no human diet can be entirely free of mutagens and carcinogens and that the foods mentioned are only representative examples. To identify a substance, whether natural or man-made, as a mutagen or a carcinogen, is just a first step. Beyond this, it is necessary to consider the risks for alternative courses of action and to quantitate the approximate magnitude of the risk, although the quantification of risk poses a major challenge. Carcinogens differ in their potency in rodents by more than a millionfold (*175*), and the levels of particular carcinogens to which humans are exposed can vary more than a billionfold. Extrapolation of risk from rodents to humans is difficult for many reasons, including the longevity difference, antioxidant factors, and the probable multicausal nature of most human cancer.

Tobacco smoking is, without doubt, a major and well-understood risk, causing about 30 percent of cancer deaths and 25

percent of fatal heart attacks (as well as other degenerative diseases) in the United States (*1*). These percentages may increase even more in the near future as the health effects of the large increase in women smokers become apparent (*1*). Diet, which provides both carcinogens and anticarcinogens, is extremely likely to be another major risk factor. Excessive alcohol consumption is another risk, although it does not seem to be of the same general importance as smoking and diet. Certain other high-dose exposures might also turn out to be important for particular groups of people—for instance, certain drugs, where consumption can reach hundreds of milligrams per day; particular cosmetics; and certain occupational exposures (*2*), where workers inhale dusts or solvents at high concentration. We must also be prudent about environmental pollution (*41, 54*). Despite all of these risks, it should be emphasized that the overall trend in life expectancy in the United States is continuing steadily upward (*176*).

The understanding of cancer and degenerative disease mechanisms is being aided by the rapid progress of science and technology, and this should help to dispel confusion about how important health risks can be identified among the vast number of minor risks. We have many methods of attacking the problem of environmental carcinogens (and anticarcinogens), including human epidemiology (*1*), short-term tests (*41, 42, 177*), and animal cancer tests (*175*). Powerful new methods are being developed [for instance, see (*58, 177*)] for measuring DNA damage or other pertinent factors with great sensitivity in individuals. These methods, which are often noninvasive as they can be done on blood or urine (even after storage), can be combined with epidemiology to determine whether particular factors are predictive of disease. Thus, more powerful tools will be available for optimizing antioxidants and other dietary anti-risk factors, for identifying human genetic variants at high risk, and for identifying significant health risks.

References and Notes

1. R. Doll and R. Peto, *J. Natl. Cancer Inst.* **66**, 1192 (1981).
2. R. Peto and M. Schneiderman, Eds., *Banbury Report 9. Quantification of Occupational Cancer* (Cold Spring Harbor Laboratory, Cold Spring Harbor, N.Y., 1981).

3. *Cancer Facts and Figures, 1983* (American Cancer Society, New York, 1982).
4. National Research Council, *Diet, Nutrition and Cancer* (National Academy Press, Washington, D.C., 1982).
5. E. C. Miller, J. A. Miller, I. Hirono, T. Sugimura, S. Takayama, Eds., *Naturally Occurring Carcinogens-Mutagens and Modulators of Carcinogenesis* (Japan Scientific Societies Press and University Park Press, Tokyo and Baltimore, 1979); E. C. Miller *et al.*, *Cancer Res.* **43**, 1124 (1983); C. Ioannides, M. Delaforge, D. V. Parke, *Food Cosmet. Toxicol.* **19**, 657 (1981).
6. G. J. Kapadia, Ed., *Oncology Overview on Naturally Occuring Dietary Carcinogens of Plant Origin* (International Cancer Research Data Bank Program, National Cancer Institute, Bethesda, Maryland, 1982).
7. A. M. Clark, in *Environmental Mutagenesis, Carcinogenesis, and Plant Biology*, E. J. Klekowski, Jr., Ed. (Praeger, New York, 1982), vol. 1, pp. 97–132.
8. A. M. Pamukcu, S. Yalciner, J. F. Hatcher, G. T. Bryan, *Cancer Res.* **40**, 3468 (1980); J. F. Hatcher, A. M. Pamukcu, E. Erturk, G. T. Bryan, *Fed. Proc. Fed. Am. Soc. Exp. Biol.* **42**, 786 (1983).
9. H. F. Stich, M. P. Rosin, C. H. Wu, W. D. Powrie, *Mutat. Res.* **90**, 201 (1981); A. A. Aver'yanov, *Biokhimiya* **46**, 256 (1981); A. F. Hanham, B. P. Dunn, H. F. Stich, *Mutat. Res.* **116**, 333 (1983).
10. K. H. Pegel, *Chem. Eng. News* **59**, 4 (20 July 1981).
11. L. K. T. Lam, V. L. Sparnins, L. W. Wattenberg, *Cancer Res.* **42**, 1193 (1982).
12. S. J. Jadhav, R. P. Sharma, D. K. Salunkhe, *CRC Crit. Rev. Toxicol.* **9**, 21 (1981).
13. R. L. Hall, *Nutr. Cancer* **1** (No. 2), 27 (1979).
14. H. W. Moore and R. Czerniak, *Med. Res. Rev.* **1**, 249 (1981).
15. I. Hirono, *CRC Crit. Rev. Toxicol.* **8**, 235 (1981).
16. J. P. Brown, *Mutat. Res.* **75**, 243 (1980).
17. M. J. Ashwood-Smith and G. A. Poulton, *ibid.* **85**, 389 (1981).
18. A. Ya. Potapenko, M. V. Moshnin, A. A. Krasnovsky, Jr., V. L. Sukhorukov, *Z. Naturforsch.* **37**, 70 (1982).
19. G. W. Ivie, D. L. Holt, M. C. Ivey, *Science* **213**, 909 (1981); R. C. Beier and E. H. Oertli, *Phytochemistry*, in press; R. C. Beier, G. W. Ivie, E. H. Oertli, in "Xenobiotics in Foods and Feeds," *ACS Symp. Ser.*, in press; _____, D. L. Holt, *Food Chem. Toxicol.* **21**, 163 (1983).
20. G. Tamura, C. Gold, A. Ferro-Luzzi, B. N. Ames, *Proc. Natl. Acad. Sci. U.S.A.* **77**, 4961 (1980).
21. T. Sugimura and S. Sato, *Cancer Res. (Suppl.)* **43**, 2415s (1983); T. Sugimura and M. Nagao, in *Mutagenicity: New Horizons in Genetic Toxicology*, J. A. Heddle, Ed. (Academic Press, New York, 1982), pp. 73–88.
22. W. W. Kilgore, D. G. Crosby, A. L. Craigmill, N. K. Poppen, *Calif. Agric.* **35** (No. 11) (November 1981); D. G. Crosby, *Chem. Eng. News* **61**, 37 (11 April 1983); C. D. Warren, *ibid.*, p. 3 (13 June 1983).
23. H. F. Stich, M. P. Rosin, C. H. Wu, W. D. Powrie, in *Mutagenicity: New Horizons in Genetic Toxicology*, J. A. Heddle, Ed. (Academic Press, New York, 1982), pp. 117–142; _____, W. D. Powrie, *Cancer Lett.* **14**, 251 (1981).
24. N. Katsui, F. Yagihashi, A. Murai, T. Masamune, *Bull. Chem. Soc. Jpn.* **55**, 2424 (1982); _____, *ibid.*, p. 2428; R. M. Bostock, R. A. Laine, J. A. Kuc, *Plant Physiol.* **70**, 1417 (1982).
25. H. Griesebach and J. Ebel, *Angew. Chem. Int. Ed. Engl.* **17**, 635 (1978).
26. J. M. Concon, D. S. Newburg, T. W. Swerczek, *Nutr. Cancer* **1** (No. 3), 22 (1979).
27. H. W. Renner and R. Munzner, *Mutat. Res.* **103**, 275 (1982); H. W. Renner, *Experientia* **38**, 600 (1982); D. Mourelatos, J. Dozi-Vassiliades, A. Granitsas, *Mutat. Res.* **104**, 243 (1982); J. H. Gans, *Toxicol. Appl. Pharmacol.* **63**, 312 (1982).
28. B. Toth, in *Naturally Occurring Carcinogens-Mutagens and Modulators of Carcinogenesis*,

E. C. Miller, J. A. Miller, I. Hirono, T. Sugimura, S. Takayama, Eds. (Japan Scientific Societies Press and University Park Press, Tokyo and Baltimore, 1979), pp. 57–65; A. E. Ross, D. L. Nagel, B. Toth, *J. Agric. Food Chem.* **30**, 521 (1982); B. Toth and K. Patil, *Mycopathologia* **78**, 11 (1982); B. Toth, D. Nagel, A. Ross, *Br. J. Cancer* **46**, 417 (1982).
29. R. Schoental, *Toxicol. Lett.* **10**, 323 (1982); R. J. Huxtable, *Perspect. Biol. Med.* **24**, 1 (1980); H. Niwa, H. Ishiwata, K. Yamada, *J. Chromatogr.* **257**, 146 (1983).
30. M. Chevion and T. Navok, *Anal. Biochem.* **128**, 152 (1983); V. Lattanzio, V. V. Bianco, D. Lafiandra, *Experientia* **38**, 789 (1982); V. L. Flohe, G. Niebch, H. Reiber, *Z. Klin. Chem. Klin. Biochem.* **9**, 431 (1971); J. Mager, M. Chevion, G. Glaser, in *Toxic Constituents of Plant Foodstuffs*, I. E. Liener, Ed. (Academic Press, New York, 1980), pp. 265–294.
31. J. K. Dunnick *et al.*, *Fundam. Appl. Toxicol.* **2**, 114 (1982).
32. L. C. Berardi and L. A. Goldblatt, in *Toxic Constituents of Plant Foodstuffs*, I. E. Liener, Ed. (Academic Press, ed. 2, New York, 1980), pp. 183–237.
33. S. P. Xue, in *Proceedings, Symposium on Recent Advances in Fertility Regulation* (Beijing, 2 to 5 September, 1980), p. 122.
34. R. K. Haroz and J. Thomasson, *Toxicol. Lett. Suppl.* **6**, 72 (1980).
35. M. Coburn, P. Sinsheimer, S. Segal, M. Burgos, W. Troll, *Biol. Bull. (Woods Hole, Mass.)* **159**, 468 (1980).
36. C. Campbell, personal communication.
37. G. D. Manners, G. W. Ivie, J. T. MacGregor, *Toxicol. Appl. Pharmacol.* **45**, 629 (1978); G. W. Ivie and D. A. Witzel, in *Plant Toxins*, vol. 1, *Encyclopedic Handbook of Natural Toxins*, A. T. Tu and R. F. Keeler, Eds. (Dekker, New York, in press).
38. J. C. M. Van der Hoeven *et al.*, in *Mutagens in Our Environment*, M. Sorsa and H. Vainio, Eds. (Liss, New York, 1982), pp. 327–338; J. C. M. van der Hoeven, W. J. Lagerweij, I. M. Bruggeman, F. G. Voragen, J. H. Koeman, *J. Agric. Food Chem.*, in press.
39. T. Hirayama and Y. Ito, *Prev. Med.* **10**, 614 (1981); E. Hecker, *J. Cancer Res. Clin. Oncol.* **99**, 103 (1981).
40. M. R. Malinow, E. J. Bardana, Jr., B. Pirofsky, S. Craig, P. McLaughlin, *Science* **216**, 415 (1982).
41. B. N. Ames, *ibid.* **204**, 587 (1979). "Mutagen" will be used in its broad sense to include clastogens and other DNA-damaging agents.
42. H. F. Stich and R. H. C. San, Eds., *Short-Term Tests for Chemical Carcinogens* (Springer-Verlag, New York, 1981).
43. P. Hochstein and S. K. Jain, *Fed. Proc. Fed. Am. Soc. Exp. Biol.* **40**, 183 (1981).
44. D. E. Levin, M. Hollstein, M. F. Christman, E. Schwiers, B. N. Ames, *Proc. Natl. Acad. Sci. U.S.A.* **79**, 7445 (1982). Many additional quinones and aldehydes have now been shown to be mutagenic.
45. S. G. Carmella, E. J. LaVoie, S. S. Hecht, *Food Chem. Toxicol.* **20**, 587 (1982).
46. K. Morimoto, S. Wolff, A. Koizumi, *Mutat. Res. Lett.* **119**, 355 (1983); T. Sawahata and R. A. Neal, *Mol. Pharmacol.* **23**, 453 (1983).
47. H. Kappus and H. Sies, *Experientia* **37**, 1233 (1981).
48. L. Tikkanen, T. Matsushima, S. Natori, *Mutat. Res.* **116**, 297 (1983).
49. P. K. Singal, N. Kapur, K. S. Dhillon, R. E. Beamish, N. S. Dhalla, *Can. J. Physiol. Pharmacol.* **60**, 1390 (1982).
50. A. Kasamaki *et al.*, *Mutat. Res.* **105**, 387 (1982).
51. J. D. Hendricks, R. O. Sinnhuber, P. M. Loveland, N. E. Pawlowski, J. E. Nixon, *Science* **208**, 309 (1980); R. A. Phelps, F. S. Shenstone, A. R. Kemmerer, R. J. Evans, *Poult. Sci.* **44**, 358 (1964); N. E. Pawlowski, personal communication.
52. I. Emerit, A. M. Michelson, A. Levy, J. P. Camus, J. Emerit, *Hum. Genet.* **55**, 341 (1980).
53. FDA Compliance Program Report of Findings. FY79 Total Diet Studies—Adult (No. 7305.002); available from National Technical Information Service, Springfield, Va.). It is

estimated that the daily dietary intake of synthetic organic pesticides and herbicides is about 60 μg, with chlorpropham, malathion, and DDE accounting for about three-fourths of this. An estimate of 150 μg of daily exposure in Finland to pesticide residues has been made by K. Hemminki, H. Vainio, M. Sorsa, S. Salminen [*J. Environ. Sci. Health* C1 (No. 1), 55 (1983)].
54. N. K. Hooper, B. N. Ames, M. A. Saleh, J. E. Casida, *Science* **205**, 591 (1979).
55. L. W. Wattenberg, *Cancer Res. (Suppl.)* **43**, 2448s (1983).
56. J. Hoey, C. Montvernay, R. Lambert, *Am. J. Epidemiol.* **113**, 668 (1981); A. J. Tuyns, G. Pequignot, M. Gignoux, A. Valla, *Int. J. Cancer* **30**, 9 (1982); A. Tuyns, in *Cancer Epidemiology and Prevention*, D. Schottenfeld and J. F. Fraumeni, Jr., Eds. (Saunders, Philadelphia, 1982), pp. 293–303; R. G. Ziegler *et al.*, *J. Natl. Cancer Inst.* **67**, 1199 (1981); W. D. Flanders and K. J. Rothman, *Am. J. Epidemiol.* **115**, 371 (1982).
57. E. L. Abel, *Hum. Biol.* **54**, 421 (1982); H. L. Rosset, L. Weiner, A. Lee, B. Zuckerman, E. Dooling, E. Oppenheimer, *Obstet. Gynecol.* **61**, 539 (1983).
57a. R. A. Anderson, Jr., B. R. Willis, C. Oswald, L. J. D. Zaneveld, *J. Pharmacol. Exp. Ther.* **225**, 479 (1983).
58. H. F. Stich and M. P. Rosin, *Int. J. Cancer* **31**, 305 (1983).
59. R. P. Bird, H. H. Draper, P. K. Basrur, *Mutat. Res.* **101**, 237 (1982); M. A. Campbell and A. G. Fantel, *Life Sci.* **32**, 2641 (1983).
60. V. J. Feron, A. Kruysse, R. A. Woutersen, *Eur. J. Cancer Clin. Oncol.* **18**, 13 (1982).
61. T. Suematsu *et al.*, *Alcoholism: Clin. Exp. Res.* **5**, 427 (1981); G. W. Winston and A. I. Cederbaum, *Biochem. Pharmacol.* **31**, 2301 (1982); L. A. Videla, V. Fernandez, A. de Marinis, N. Fernandez, A. Valenzuela, *Biochem. Biophys. Res. Commun.* **104**, 965 (1982); T. E. Stege, *Res. Commun. Chem. Pathol. Pharmacol.* **36**, 287 (1982).
62. M. G. Cutler and R. Schneider, *Food Cosmet. Toxicol.* **12**, 451 (1974).
63. Y. Tazima, in *Environmental Mutagenesis, Carcinogenesis and Plant Biology*, E. J. Klekowski, Jr., Ed. (Praeger, New York, 1982), vol. 1, pp. 68–95.
64. P. N. Magee, Ed., *Banbury Report 12. Nitrosamines and Human Cancer* (Cold Spring Harbor Laboratory, Cold Spring Harbor, N.Y., 1982); P. E. Hartman, in *Chemical Mutagens*, F. J. de Serres and A. Hollaender, Eds. (Plenum, New York, 1982), vol. 7, pp. 211–294; P. E. Hartman, *Environ. Mutagen.* **5**, 111 (1983).
65. Committee on Nitrite and Alternative Curing Agents in Food, Assembly of Life Sciences, National Academy of Sciences, *The Health Effects of Nitrate, Nitrite, and N-Nitroso Compounds* (National Academy Press, Washington, D.C., 1981).
66. H. F. Stich, P. K. L. Chan, M. P. Rosin, *Int. J. Cancer* **30**, 719 (1982); H. F. Stich and M. P. Rosin, in *Nutritional and Metabolic Aspects of Food Safety*, M. Friedman, Ed. (Plenum, New York, in press).
67. L. J. Kinlen, *Br. Med. J.* **286**, 1081 (1983); D. J. Fink and D. Kritchevsky, *Cancer Res.* **41**, 3677 (1981).
68. C. W. Welsch and C. F. Aylsworth, *J. Natl. Cancer Inst.* **70**, 215 (1983).
69. P. Correa, J. P. Strong, W. D. Johnson, P. Pizzolato, W. Haenszel, *J. Chronic Dis.* **35**, 313 (1982).
70. F. B. Shorland *et al.*, *J. Agric. Food Chem.* **29**, 863 (1981).
71. M. G. Simic and M. Karel, Eds., *Autoxidation in Food and Biological Systems* (Plenum, New York, 1980).
72. W. A. Pryor, Ed., *Free Radicals in Biology* (Academic Press, New York, 1976 to 1982), vols. 1 to 5.
73. H. B. Demopoulos, D. D. Pietronigro, E. S. Flamm, M. L. Seligman, *J. Environ. Pathol. Toxicol.* **3**, 273 (1980).
74. F. Bischoff, *Adv. Lipid Res.* **7**, 165 (1969).
75. N. L. Petrakis, L. D. Gruenke, J. C. Craig, *Cancer Res.* **41**, 2563 (1981).
76. H. S. Black and D. R. Douglas, *ibid.* **32**, 2630

77. H. Imai, N. T. Werthessen, V. Subramanyam, P. W. LeQuesne, A. H. Soloway, M. Kanisawa, *Science* 207, 651 (1980).
78. M. Ferrali, R. Fulceri, A. Benedetti, M. Comporti, *Res. Commun. Chem. Pathol. Pharmacol.* 30, 99 (1980).
79. N. R. Artman, *Adv. Lipid Res.* 7, 245 (1969).
80. J. K. Reddy, J. R. Warren, M. K. Reddy, N. D. Lalwani, *Ann. N.Y. Acad. Sci.* 386, 81 (1982); J. K. Reddy and N. D. Lalwani, *CRC Crit. Rev. Toxicol.*, in press.
81. H. L. Plaine, *Genetics* 40, 268 (1955); A. Ito, M. Naito, Y. Naito, H. Watanabe, *Gann* 73, 315 (1982); G. Speit, W. Vogel, M. Wolf, *Environ. Mutagen.* 4, 135 (1982); H. Tsuda, *Jpn. J. Genet.* 56, 1 (1981); N. Hirota and T. Yokoyama, *Gann* 72, 811 (1981).
82. S. Horie, H. Ishii, T. Suga, *J. Biochem. (Tokyo)* 90, 1691 (1981); D. P. Jones, H. Eklow, H. Thor, S. Orrenius, *Arch. Biochem. Biophys.* 210, 505 (1981).
83. B. Chance, H. Sies, A. Boveris, *Physiol. Rev.* 59, 527 (1979).
84. D. Harman, *Proc. Natl. Acad. Sci. U.S.A.* 78, 7124 (1981); in *Free Radicals in Biology*, W. A. Pryor, Ed. (Academic Press, New York, 1982), vol. 5, pp. 255–275.
85. I. Emerit, M. Keck, A. Levy, J. Feingold, A. M. Michelson, *Mutat. Res.* 103, 165 (1982).
86. C. E. Neat, M. S. Thomassen, H. Osmundsen, *Biochem. J.* 196, 149 (1981); J. Bremer and K. R. Norum, *J. Lipid Res.* 23, 243 (1982); M. S. Thomassen, E. N. Christiansen, K. R. Norum, *Biochem. J.* 206, 195 (1982); H. Osmundsen, *Int. J. Biochem.* 14, 905 (1982); J. Norseth and M. S. Thomassen, *Biochim. Biophys. Acta*, in press.
87. M. G. Enig, R. J. Munn, M. Keeney, *Fed. Proc. Fed. Am. Soc. Exp. Biol.* 37, 2215 (1978); J. E. Hunter, *J. Natl. Cancer Inst.* 69, 319 (1982); A. B. Awad, *ibid.*, p. 320; H. Ruttenberg, L. M. Davidson, N. A. Little, D. M. Klurfeld, D. Kritchevsky, *J. Nutr.* 113, 835 (1983).
88. R. Wood, *Lipids* 14, 975 (1979).
89. E. N. Christiansen, T. Flatmark, H. Kryvi, *Eur. J. Cell Biol.* 26, 11 (1981).
90. Council for Agricultural Science and Technology, *Diet, Nutrition, and Cancer: A Critique* (Special Publication 13, Council for Agricultural Science and Technology, Ames, Iowa, 1982).
91. L. F. Bjeldanes *et al.*, *Food Chem. Toxicol.* 20, 357 (1982); M. W. Pariza, L. J. Loretz, J. M. Storkson, N. C. Holland, *Cancer Res. (Suppl.)* 43, 2444s (1983).
92. H. F. Stich, W. Stich, M. P. Rosin, W. D. Powrie, *Mutat. Res.* 91, 129 (1981); M. P. Rosin, H. F. Stich, W. D. Powrie, F. W. Wu, *ibid.* 101, 189 (1982); C.-I. Wei, K. Kitamura, T. Shibamoto, *Food Cosmet. Toxicol.* 19, 749 (1981).
93. E. Yamasaki and B. N. Ames, *Proc. Natl. Acad. Sci. U.S.A.* 74, 3555 (1977).
94. R. Baker, A. Arlauskas, A. Bonin, D. Angus, *Cancer Lett.* 16, 81 (1982).
95. D. Schuetzle, D. Cronn, A. L. Crittenden, R. J. Charlson, *Environ. Sci. Technol.* 9, 838 (1975); G. Gartrell and S. K. Friedlander, *Atmos. Environ.* 9, 279 (1975); L. D. Kier, E. Yamasaki, B. N. Ames, *Proc. Natl. Acad. Sci. U.S.A.* 71, 4159 (1974); J. N. Pitts, Jr., *Environ. Health Perspect.* 47, 115 (1983).
96. J. E. Vena, *Am. J. Epidemiol.* 116, 42 (1982); R. Cederlof, R. Doll, B. Fowler, *Environ. Health Perspect.* 22, 1 (1978); F. E. Speizer, *ibid.* 47, 33 (1983).
97. B. Brunekreef and J. S. M. Boleij, *Int. Arch. Occup. Environ. Health* 50, 299 (1982).
98. H. Kasai *et al.*, *Gann* 73, 681 (1982).
99. V. Armuth and I. Berenblum, *Carcinogenesis* 2, 977 (1981).
100. S. Fabro, *Reprod. Toxicol.* 1, 2 (1982).
101. D. Trichopoulos, M. Papapostolou, A. Polychronopoulou, *Int. J. Cancer* 28, 691 (1981); P. Hartge, L. P. Lesher, L. McGowan, R. Hoover, *ibid.* 30, 531 (1982); B. MacMahon, *Cancer (Brussels)* 50, 2676 (1982); H. S. Cuckle and L. J. Kinlen, *Br. J. Cancer* 44, 760 (1981); R. L. Phillips and D. A. Snowdon, *Cancer Res. (Suppl.)* 43, 2403s (1983); L. D. Marrett, S. D. Walter, J. W. Meigs, *Am. J. Epidemiol.* 117,

113 (1983); D. M. Weinberg, R. K. Ross, T. M. Mack, A. Paganini-Hill, B. E. Henderson, *Cancer (Brussels)* 51, 675 (1983).
102. P. E. Hartman, *Environ. Mutagen.*, in press.
103. J. R. Totter, *Proc. Natl. Acad. Sci. U.S.A.* 77, 1763 (1980).
104. I. Fridovich, in *Pathology of Oxygen*, A. Autor, Ed. (Academic Press, New York, 1982), pp. 1–19; L. W. Oberley, T. D. Oberley, G. R. Buettner, *Med. Hypotheses* 6, 249 (1980).
105. B. Halliwell, *Cell Biol. Int. Rep.* 6, 529 (1982); A. I. Tauber, *Trends Biochem. Sci.* 7, 411 (1982); A. B. Weitberg, S. A. Weitzman, M. Destrempes, S. A. Latt, T. P. Stossel, *N. Engl. J. Med.* 308, 26 (1983). Neutrophils also produce HOCl, which is both a chlorinating and oxidizing agent.
106. M. A. Trush, E. G. Mimnaugh, T. E. Gram, *Biochem. Pharmacol.* 31, 3335 (1982).
107. L. Flohe, in *Free Radicals in Biology*, W. A. Pryor, Ed. (Academic Press, New York, 1982), vol. 5, pp. 223–254.
108. C. Lind, P. Hochstein, L. Ernster, *Arch. Biochem. Biophys.* 216, 178 (1982).
109. M. Warholm, C. Guthenberg, B. Mannervik, C. von Bahr, *Biochem. Biophys. Res. Commun.* 98, 512 (1981).
110. J. G. Bieri, L. Corash, V. S. Hubbard, *N. Engl. J. Med.* 308, 1063 (1983).
111. Y. M. Wang *et al.*, in *Molecular Interrelations of Nutrition and Cancer*, M. S. Arnott, J. van Eys, Y.-M. Wang, Eds. (Raven, New York, 1982), pp. 369–379.
112. C. Beckman, R. M. Roy, A. Sproule, *Mutat. Res.* 105, 73 (1982); M. G. Cook and P. McNamara, *Cancer Res.* 40, 1329 (1980).
113. K. J. A. Davies, A. T. Quintanilha, G. A. Brooks, L. Packer, *Biochem. Biophys. Res. Commun.* 107, 1198 (1982).
114. C. S. Foote, in *Pathology of Oxygen*, A. Autor, Ed. (Academic Press, New York, 1982), pp. 21–44; J. E. Packer, J. S. Mahood, V. O. Mora-Arellano, T. F. Slater, R. L. Willson, B. S. Wolfenden, *Biochem. Biophys. Res. Commun.* 98, 901 (1981); W. Bors, C. Michel, M. Saran, *Bull. Eur. Physiopathol. Resp.* 17 (Suppl.), 13 (1981).
115. N. I. Krinsky and S. M. Deneke, *J. Natl. Cancer Inst.* 69, 205 (1982); J. A. Turner and J. N. Prebble, *J. Gen. Microbiol.* 119, 133 (1980); K. L. Simpson and C. O. Chichester, *Annu. Rev. Nutr.* 1, 351 (1981).
116. G. Rettura, C. Dattagupta, P. Listowsky, S. M. Levenson, E. Seifter, *Fed. Proc. Fed. Am. Soc. Exp. Biol.* 42, 786 (1983); M. M. Mathews-Roth, *Oncology* 39, 33 (1982).
117. R. Peto, R. Doll, J. D. Buckley, M. B. Sporn, *Nature (London)* 290, 201 (1981); R. B. Shekelle *et al.*, *Lancet* 1981-II, 1185 (1981); T. Hirayama, *Nutr. Cancer* 1, 67 (1979); G. Kvale, E. Bjelke, J. J. Gart, *Int. J. Cancer* 31, 397 (1983).
118. W. A. Pryor, M. Tamura, M. M. Dooley, P. I. Premovic, D. F. Church, in *Oxy-Radicals and Their Scavenger Systems: Cellular and Medical Aspects*, G. Cohen and R. Greenwald, Eds. (Elsevier, Amsterdam, 1983), vol. 2, pp. 185–192; W. A. Pryor, B. J. Hales, P. I. Premovic, D. F. Church, *Science* 220, 425 (1983).
119. M. M. Mathews-Roth, *J. Natl. Cancer Inst.* 69, 279 (1982).
120. A. C. Griffin, in *Molecular Interrelations of Nutrition and Cancer*, M. S. Arnott, J. Van-eys, Y. M. Wang, Eds. (Raven, New York, 1982), pp. 401–408; D. Medina, H. W. Lane, C. M. Tracey, *Cancer Res. (Suppl.)* 43, 2460s (1983); M. M. Jacobs, *Cancer Res.* 43, 1646 (1983); H. J. Thompson, L. D. Meeker, P. J. Becci, S. Kokoska, *ibid.* 42, 4954 (1982); D. F. Birt, T. A. Lawson, A. D. Julius, C. E. Runice, S. Salmasi, *ibid.*, p. 4455; C. Witting, U. Witting, V. Krieg, *J. Cancer Res. Clin. Oncol.* 104, 109 (1982).
121. M. Chatterjee and M. R. Banerjee, *Cancer Lett.* 17, 187 (1982).
122. W. C. Willett *et al.*, *Lancet*, in press.
123. J. T. Salonen, G. Alfthan, J. Pikkarainen, J. K. Huttunen, P. Puska, *ibid.* 1982-II, 175 (1982).
124. M. Yonaha, E. Itoh, Y. Ohbayashi, M. Uchiyama, *Res. Commun. Chem. Pathol. Pharmacol.* 28, 105 (1980); L. J. Kling and J. H. Soares, Jr., *Nutr. Rep. Int.* 24, 39 (1981).

125. N. Tateishi, T. Higashi, A. Naruse, K. Hikita, Y. Sakamoto, *J. Biochem. (Tokyo)* 90, 1603 (1981).
126. J. M. Williamson, B. Boettcher, A. Meister, *Proc. Natl. Acad. Sci. U.S.A.* 79, 6246 (1982).
127. CME Symposium on "*N*-Acetylcysteine (NAC): A Significant Chemoprotective Adjunct," *Sem. Oncol.* 10 (Suppl. 1), 1 (1983).
128. J. A. Hinson, L. R. Pohl, T. J. Monks, J. R. Gillette, *Life Sci.* 29, 107 (1981).
129. A. M. Novi, *Science* 212, 541 (1981).
130. W. B. Dunham *et al.*, *Proc. Natl. Acad. Sci. U.S.A.* 79, 7532 (1982); G. Kallistratos and E. Fasske, *J. Cancer Res. Clin. Oncol.* 97, 91 (1980).
131. S. Wassertheil-Smoller *et al.*, *Am. J. Epidemiol.* 114, 714 (1981).
132. B. N. Ames, R. Cathcart, E. Schwiers, P. Hochstein, *Proc. Natl. Acad. Sci. U.S.A.* 78, 6858 (1981).
133. A. Nomura, L. K. Heilbrun, G. N. Stemmermann, in preparation.
134. J. N. Boyd, J. G. Babish, G. S. Stoewsand, *Food Chem. Toxicol.* 20, 47 (1982).
135. A. W. Wood, *et al.*, *Proc. Natl. Acad. Sci. U.S.A.* 79, 5513 (1982).
136. T. H. Maugh II, *Science* 205, 1363 (1979) (interview with John Higginson).
137. H. L. Gensler and H. Bernstein, *Q. Rev. Biol.* 6, 279 (1981).
138. A. L. Tappel, in *Free Radicals in Biology*, W. A. Pryor, Ed. (Academic Press, New York, 1980), vol. 4, pp. 1–47.
139. R. S. Sohal, in *Age Pigments*, R. S. Sohal, Ed. (Elsevier/North-Holland, Amsterdam, 1981), pp. 303–316.
140. J. E. Fleming, J. Miquel, S. F. Cottrell, L. S. Yengoyan, A. C. Economos, *Gerontology* 28, 44 (1982).
141. J. M. Tolmasoff, T. Ono, R. G. Cutler, *Proc. Natl. Acad. Sci. U.S.A.* 77, 2777 (1980); R. G. Cutler, *Gerontology*, in press; J. L. Sullivan, *ibid.* 28, 242 (1982).
142. R. Peto, *Proc. R. Soc. London Ser. B* 205, 111 (1979); D. Dix, P. Cohen, J. Flannery, *J. Theor. Biol.* 83, 163 (1980).
143. R. G. Cutler, in *Testing the Theories of Aging*, R. Adelman and G. Roth, Eds. (CRC Press, Boca Raton, Fla., in press).
144. D. Hersh, R. G. Cutler, B. N. Ames, in preparation.
145. E. Boyland, in *Health Risk Analysis* (Franklin Institute Press, Philadelphia, 1980), pp. 181–193; E. Boyland, in *Cancer Campaign*, vol. 6, *Cancer Epidemiology*, E. Grundmann, Ed. (Fischer, Stuttgart, 1982), pp. 125–128.
146. J. L. Marx, *Science* 219, 158 (1983).
147. B. D. Goldstein, G. Witz, M. Amoruso, D. S. Stone, W. Troll, *Cancer Lett.* 11, 257 (1981); W. Troll, in *Environmental Mutagens and Carcinogens*, T. Sugimura, S. Kondo, H. Takebe, Eds. (Univ. of Tokyo Press, Tokyo, and Liss, New York, 1982), pp. 217–222.
148. B. N. Ames, M. C. Hollstein, R. Cathcart, in *Lipid Peroxide in Biology and Medicine*, K. Yagi, Ed. (Academic Press, New York, 1982), pp. 339–351.
149. I. Emerit and P. A. Cerutti, *Proc. Natl. Acad. Sci. U.S.A.* 79, 7509 (1982); *Nature (London)* 293, 144 (1981); P. A. Cerutti, I. Emerit, P. Amstad, in *Genes and Proteins in Oncogenesis*, I. B. Weinstein and H. Vogel, Eds. (Academic Press, New York, in press); I. Emerit, A. Levy, P. Cerutti, *Mutat. Res.* 110, 327 (1983).
150. J. Funes and M. Karel, *Lipids* 16, 347 (1981).
151. S. J. Stohs, M. Q. Hassan, W. J. Murray, *Biochem. Biophys. Res. Commun.* 111, 854 (1983).
152. C. C. Reddy, R. W. Scholz, E. J. Massaro, *Toxicol. Appl. Pharmacol.* 61, 460 (1981).
153. H. Nagasawa and J. B. Little, *Carcinogenesis* 2, 601 (1981); V. Solanki, R. S. Rana, T. J. Slaga, *ibid.*, p. 1141; T. W. Kensler and M. A. Trush, *Cancer Res.* 41, 216 (1981).
154. H. W. Simon, C. H. Scoggin, D. Patterson, *J. Biol. Chem.* 256, 7181 (1981); T. S. Argyris and T. J. Slaga, *Cancer Res.* 41, 5193 (1981).
155. G. E. Hatch, D. E. Gardner, D. B. Menzel, *Environ. Res.* 23, 121 (1980).
156. A. J. P. Klein-Szanto and T. J. Slaga, *J. Invest. Dermatol.* 79, 30 (1982).

157. C. C. Weddle, K. R. Hornbrook, P. B. McCay, *J. Biol. Chem.* **251**, 4973 (1976).

158. A. G. Lurie and L. S. Cutler, *J. Natl. Cancer Inst.* **63**, 147 (1979).

159. C. Borek and W. Troll, *Proc. Natl. Acad. Sci. U.S.A.* **80**, 1304 (1983); C. Borek, in *Molecular Interrelations of Nutrition and Cancer*, M. S. Arnott, J. van Eys, Y.-M. Wang, Eds. (Raven, New York, 1982), pp. 337–350.

160. T. J. Slaga *et al.*, in *Carcinogenesis: A Comprehensive Treatise* (Raven, New York, 1982), vol. 7, pp. 19–34; K. Ohuchi and L. Levine, *Biochim. Biophys. Acta* **619**, 11 (1980); S. M. Fischer, G. D. Mills, T. J. Slaga, *Carcinogenesis* **3**, 1243 (1982).

161. R. P. Mason, in *Free Radicals in Biology*, W. A. Pryor, Ed. (Academic Press, New York, 1982), vol. 5, pp. 161–222.

162. G. McLennan, L. W. Oberley, A. P. Autor, *Radiat. Res.* **84**, 122 (1980).

163. J. M. Parry, E. M. Parry, J. C. Barrett, *Nature (London)* **294**, 263 (1981); A. R. Kinsella, *Carcinogenesis* **3**, 499 (1982).

164. H. C. Birnboim, *Can. J. Physiol. Pharmacol.* **60**, 1359 (1982).

165. A. Varshavsky, *Cell* **25**, 561 (1981).

166. T. J. Powles *et al.*, Eds. *Prostaglandins and Cancer: First International Conference* (Liss, New York, 1982).

167. J. E. Trosko, C.-C. Chang, A. Medcalf, *Cancer Invest.*, in press.

167a. I. B. Weinstein, *Nature (London)* **302**, 750 (1983).

168. J. A. Bond, A. M. Gown, H. L. Yang, E. P. Benditt, M. R. Juchau, *J. Toxicol. Environ. Health* **7**, 327 (1981).

169. Editorial, *Lancet* **1980-I**, 964, (1980); K. Yagi, H. Ohkawa, N. Ohishi, M. Yamashita, T. Nakashima, *J. Appl. Biochem.* **3**, 58 (1981).

170. J. M. C. Gutteridge, B. Halliwell, D. A. Rowley, T. Westermarck, *Lancet* **1982-II**, 459 (1982).

171. J. E. Cleaver, in *Metabolic Basis of Inherited Disease*, J. B. Stanbury, J. B. Wyngaarden, D. S. Fredrickson, J. L. Goldstein, Eds. (McGraw-Hill, ed. 5, New York, 1983), pp. 1227–1250.

172. K. C. Bhuyan, D. K. Bhuyan, S. M. Podos, *IRCS Med. Sci.* **9**, 126 (1981); A. Spector, R. Scotto, H. Weissbach, N. Brot, *Biochem. Biophys. Res. Commun.* **108**, 429 (1982); S. D. Varma, N. A. Beachy, R. D. Richards, *Photochem. Photobiol.* **36**, 623 (1982).

173. M. L. Katz, K. R. Parker, G. J. Handelman, T. L. Bramel, E. A. Dratz, *Exp. Eye Res.* **34**, 339 (1982).

174. D. Behne, T. Hofer, R. von Berswordt-Wallrabe, W. Elger, *J. Nutr.* **112**, 1682 (1982).

175. B. N. Ames, L. S. Gold, C. B. Sawyer, W. Havender, in *Environmental Mutagens and Carcinogens*, T. Sugimura, S. Kondo, H. Takebe, Eds. (Univ. of Tokyo Press, Tokyo, and Liss, New York, 1982), pp. 663–670.

176. National Center for Health Statistics, Advance Report, Final Mortality Statistics, 1979, *Monthly Vital Statistics Report* **31**, No. 6, suppl. [DHHS publication (PHS) 82-1120, (Public Health Service, Hyattsville, Md., 1982]; Metropolitan Life Insurance Company Actuarial Tables, April 1983.

177. B. A. Bridges, B. E. Butterworth, I. B. Weinstein, Eds., *Banbury Report 13. Indicators of Genotoxic Exposure* (Cold Spring Harbor Laboratory, Cold Spring Harbor, N.Y., 1982); R. Montesano, M. F. Rajewsky, A. E. Pegg, E. Miller, *Cancer Res.* **42**, 5236 (1982); H. F. Stich, R. H. C. San, M. P. Rosin, *Ann. N.Y. Acad. Sci.*, in press; I. B. Weinstein, *Annu. Rev. Public Health* **4**, 409 (1983).

178. I am indebted to G. Ferro-Luzzi Ames, A. Blum, L. Gold, P. Hartman, W. Havender, N. K. Hooper, G. W. Ivie, J. McCann, J. Mead, R. Olson, R. Peto, A. Tappel, and numerous other colleagues for their criticisms. This work was supported by DOE contract DE-AT03-76EV70156 to B.N.A. and by National Institute of Environmental Health Sciences Center Grant ES01896. This article has been expanded from a talk presented at the 12th European Environmental Mutagen Society Conference, Espoo, Finland, June 1982 [in *Mutagens in Our Environment*, M. Sorsa and H. Vainio, Eds. (Liss, New York, 1982)]. I wish to dedicate this article to the memory of Philip Handler, pioneer in the field of oxygen radicals.

Diet and Breast Cancer

by Ernst L. Wynder and David P. Rose

Epidemiologic and experimental data strongly implicate high dietary fat as a major factor in the etiology of breast cancer, particularly after menopause. Evidence of interactions between fat intake and hormone status is reviewed. Although the association is not open-and-shut, there is a good case for reduction of dietary fat to 30% of total calories.

Human breast cancer—in common with the vast majority of other human cancers—has a largely environmental etiology. This view is supported by epidemiologic data demonstrating widely differing international breast cancer rates. Specifically, the breast is the leading site for cancer in women of most Western countries, but it does not rank nearly as high in the rest of the world's female population, especially in Asia and Africa. That environmental, rather than racial or genetic, factors best account for these differences is further supported by studies of migrant populations. The risk of breast cancer increases in descendants of groups who move from a non-Western to a Western country, and within only a few generations it approximates the risk prevailing in the host country (see J. Higginson, "The Face of Cancer Worldwide," HP, November 1983).

Another significant epidemiologic finding is that worldwide differences in breast cancer incidence and mortality are more pronounced in older age groups, with the rates in low-risk countries leveling off or declining after menopause and those in high-risk countries continuing to rise. This international pattern is paralleled within the high-risk population of the United States, where county-by-county breast cancer mortality has been reported to be almost uniform among premenopausal women but high among postmenopausal women living in northeastern states. Such pat-

terns imply that some etiologic factors in postmenopausal disease are distinct from those in premenopausal disease. In addition to menstrual status, however, it should be noted that other hormone-based factors have been variously incriminated in both pre- and postmenopausal breast cancer risk (see J. F. Fraumeni, Jr., "The Face of Cancer in the United States," HP, December 1983).

Although epidemiologic assessment of the role played by dietary factors in modulating cancer risk is fraught with well-recognized difficulties, and although the relevance of animal models to human disease is always open to question, a large body of evidence points to high fat intake as a causative factor in breast cancer. Furthermore, the worldwide distribution of breast cancer is very similar to that of colorectal cancer; in both cases, tumor risk has been shown to increase with an increasing proportion of fat in the diet (see D. P. Burkitt, "Etiology and Prevention of Colorectal Cancer," HP, February).

In this article, we will take a closer look at the age- and diet-related aspects. An important part of our discussion will be a consideration of mechanisms by which hormone status and excessive dietary fat may interact in the development of postmenopausal breast cancer. As we will see, key questions remain to be answered. But with increasing use of metabolic epidemiology and other multidisciplinary approaches, we finally may be asking the *right* questions about breast carcinogenesis.

Dr. Wynder is President and Dr. Rose is Chief of Nutrition and Endocrinology, American Health Foundation. Dr. Rose is also Acting Director, Mahoney Institute, New York.

First, we should note that there are exceptions, inconsistencies, and ambiguities in the evidence regarding the etiology of breast cancer, particularly in the epidemiologic data. In the main, however, these problems are more apparent than real; rather than challenging the view that diet and hormone status are major factors in the development of breast cancer, they simply illustrate the concept that the etiology of cancer is nearly always multifactorial.

For example, one well-recognized risk factor for breast cancer is a positive family history of the tumor (see Table 1). Numerous pedigrees describing a familial variant of human breast cancer have been reported, and the risk involved has been shown to increase with closer genetic relationship to the affected family member. Like other genetically influenced cancers, moreover, familial breast cancer tends to occur at a much younger age than its sporadic counterpart and tends to involve more than one site (i.e., both breasts). This indicates that nonenvironmental factors are sometimes important in breast cancer's etiology. But by all accounts, familial disease represents no more than a tiny fraction of human breast cancer; in the vast majority of cases, nongenetic factors are involved.

In this regard, increased breast cancer risk has also been associated with high socioeconomic status in the United States and northern Europe. Most investigators view this finding as a reflection of dietary practices among the more affluent subgroups of these populations—those who, often quite literally, live on the "fat" of the land. But the possibility that the increased risk derives from some other, nondietary and as

Table 1. Risk Factors for Breast Cancer

Characteristic	Risk Group	
	High	Low
Race	Caucasian	Oriental
Family history	Yes	No
Socioeconomic status	High	Low
Marital status	Single	Married
Parity	Nulliparous	Parous
Age at first completed pregnancy	Late	Early
Menarche	Early	Late
Natural menopause	Late	Early
Artificial menopause	No	Yes
Weight	?Obese	?Thin

yet unidentified environmental factor(s) still cannot be excluded; for example, low-income groups in industrial countries may also have high fat intake. In addition, the results of several epidemiologic studies show that isolation of fat as the crucial dietary determinant of human breast cancer risk is often extremely difficult.

To illustrate, in a 1968 study of data from 22 countries, K. K. Carroll and associates reported that there were significant positive correlations between age-adjusted breast cancer mortality and per capita intake of both fats and total calories. Similarly, in 1970 and again in 1978, G. Hems found that breast cancer incidence in 41 countries was positively correlated with estimated per capita fat, animal protein, and total calorie consumption and that each dietary factor was so closely linked with the others that it was impossible to determine which was the most important in breast cancer risk. In a somewhat different form, this theme was echoed in a more recent study by

Carroll, who in 1977 reviewed data from 37 countries with high, low, or intermediate breast cancer mortality. In this study, the death rates rose with increasing animal fat and animal protein intake, and the two dietary factors could not be analyzed separately (see Figure 1).

Some experimental findings support epidemiologic correlations between increased breast cancer risk and high total calorie or animal protein intake. As far back as the 1940s and 1950s, for example, studies by A. Tannenbaum, H. Silverstone, and others showed that reduced calorie intake in laboratory animals inhibited carcinogenesis, including the spontaneous development of mammary neoplasms and their induction by exogenous estrogens. These results were largely achieved, however, by feeding the animals a low-fat diet.

Regarding protein intake, recent clinical studies indicate that specific amino acid components of protein can stimulate release of growth hormone. Whether the hormone plays a role in human breast cancer is unknown, but it has been shown to be lactogenic and to compete effectively with prolactin for prolactin receptors in normal tissues and mammary cancers. Prolactin is clearly important in rodent models of breast carcinogenesis; in numerous studies, it has promoted the growth (or regrowth) of chemically induced mammary tumors. In a recent study by J. J. Noonan and one of us (DPR), however, growth hormone obtained from sheep was found to act synergistically with prolactin in promoting such growth.

Finally, although the epidemiologic evidence for breast cancer's hormonal basis is very strong, there is some disagreement about how this relationship is manifested. In studies over the years, increased risk for the tumor has been variously associated with nulliparity, late age at first completed pregnancy, early age at menarche, late age at natural menopause, the absence of surgically induced menopause up to about age 40, and obesity. That not all studies agree on each of these putative risk factors is shown in the results of a 1978 study reported by F. A. MacCornack, S. D. Steilman, and one of us (ELW). In that study, data from 785 breast cancer patients in the United States were compared with those from matched controls. The risk factors identified in this study were largely limited to late age at first completed pregnancy (for pre- and perimenopausal but not postmenopausal breast cancer) and a family history of breast cancer. Slightly more cases than controls also reported such premenstrual symptoms as breast swelling or tenderness, but there was no difference found for age at menarche, number of births,

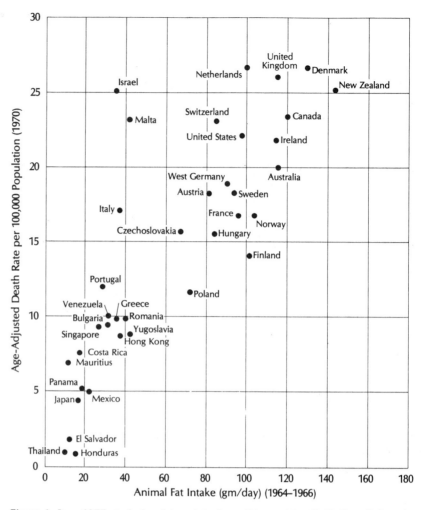

Figure 1. *In a 1977 study involving data from 37 countries, K. K. Carroll found that breast cancer mortality was positively correlated with estimated per capita*

weight change, or use of exogenous estrogens or oral contraceptives. In addition, there was very little difference between cases and controls regarding nulliparity or late menopause.

In our view, such findings do not undermine the argument that endogenous hormones are etiologic factors in breast cancer. Rather, they serve to underscore the concept that dietary fat best accounts for breast cancer rates that differ from group to group or country to country. They also suggest that the overall evidence regarding a role for hormone status in breast cancer is more important than specific evidence regarding aspects of hormone status. In short, the

case for dietary fat and endogenous hormones as major etiologic factors for the tumor is impressive. Essentially, it holds that hormonal factors act as a pathogenetic bridge between fat intake and tumor development, especially in the postmenopausal years. Whatever may be said about deficiencies in the supporting evidence, the view makes sense—logically and biologically.

To present the case, let us begin with some familiar observations. In the worldwide epidemiology of breast cancer, contrasts between the high-risk population of the United States and the low-risk population of Japan are often cited. Thus, for the period between 1968 and

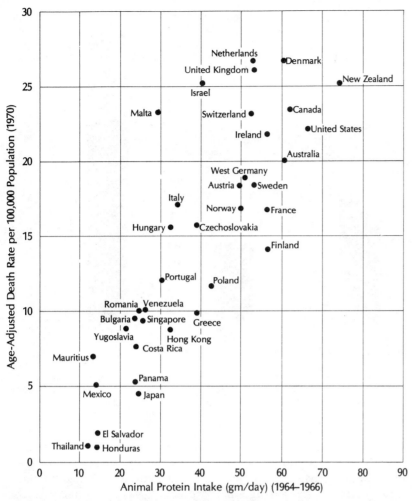

animal fat (left) and animal protein (right) intake. In terms of biologic plausibility, dietary fat appears to be more crucial determinant of breast cancer risk.

1972, the annual age-adjusted incidence of breast cancer among women living in Miyagi, Japan, was 13/100,000, whereas the corresponding figure reported for Connecticut women during that period was about 5.5 times greater (71.4/100,000). In addition, if similar data on nationwide breast cancer rates in the United States and Japan are broken down according to age or menstrual status, the difference between the two populations in the incidence of premenopausal disease is about threefold, and that in the incidence of postmenopausal disease about eightfold.

Among the results of various correlation studies designed to account for international differences, data from national dietary surveys often stand out. In particular, two such surveys, reported in 1968 and 1969, showed that Americans consumed three times the amount of fat consumed by the Japanese. Although protein intake by Americans was also significantly higher, excessive fat intake was the principal source of the difference of 1000 calories per day between the American and Japanese diets (see Figure 2).

Although breast cancer is still relatively uncommon in Japan, it may not be widely appreciated that the disease has recently gained importance as a public health problem there. In a 1978

review, for example, T. Hirayama noted that the annual number of deaths from breast cancer in Japan had doubled in the 20-year period from 1955 to 1975. That trend was most pronounced in postmenopausal women, especially those living in urban areas. Using 1970 data, Hirayama showed that age-adjusted breast cancer mortality in various districts of Japan correlated closely with daily per capita fat intake; the same was true regarding pork intake. As might be expected, urban residents tended to have the highest fat intake and the highest breast cancer death rates.

In another 1978 study, Y. Kagawa pointed out that the period from the 1950s through the 1970s was marked by an increasing westernization of the Japanese diet. Occurring primarily among the younger, more affluent, and urban segments of the Japanese population, the trend was characterized by dramatic increases in the consumption of fats—principally animal fats. Kagawa found also that at age 12, Japanese girls showed steady increases in height and weight from 1950 to 1974, a period in which the age of menarche in Japan steadily declined. By 1974, 12-year-old Japanese girls had almost the same average height and weight (148.5 cm and 41 kg) as their Caucasian United States counterparts (149.1 cm and 40.9 kg); in addition, the age of menarche in Japanese and American subjects in 1974 was virtually identical (12.2 and 12.5 years, respectively), with the Japanese value representing a three-year reduction compared with that seen in 1950 (see Figure 3).

These post-World War II Japanese trends recapitulate the experience of much of the Western world over the past hundred

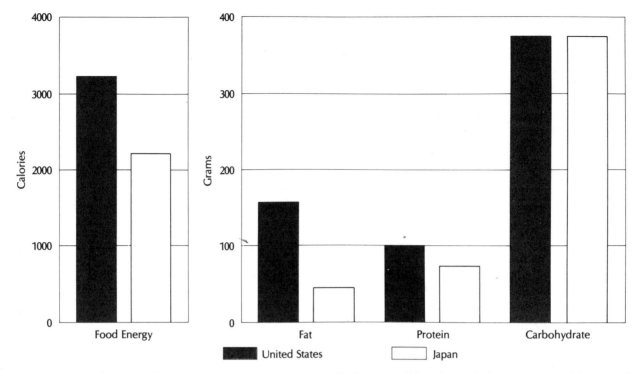

Figure 2. *In 1968 and 1969, dietary surveys in the United States and Japan showed that, per capita, Americans consumed approximately 1000 calories per day more than did the Japanese. Although protein intake accounted for part of this difference, the principal reason was that fat intake in the American diet was three times greater.*

years or so. In many Western countries menarche now occurs, on average, several years earlier than previously, and early menarche in these populations is associated with increased breast cancer risk. It is also recognized that nutritional factors influence weight and height, which in turn can affect menstrual status. Statistically, there is a critical weight-for-height that must be achieved in order for menarche to occur. This is reflected in two observations— 1) that girls whose menses have begun are taller and heavier than girls of the same age who have not yet reached menarche, and 2) that the mean weight of girls at onset of menarche is the same, whether that event is early or late.

In a series of studies, R. E. Frisch, R. Revelle, and co-workers suggested that attainment of the critical weight involves an increase in stored fat that is needed to trigger altered metabolic activity. That alteration reduces the sensitivity of hypothalamic centers to estrogens, which in turn resets feedback mechanisms controlling blood gonadotropin and sex steroid levels. The end result is that the levels are raised enough to induce uterine and ovarian maturation, and thus menarche.

Once menarche is achieved, diet continues to influence menstrual function; its influence may be seen directly or discerned in hormonal changes related to body weight. An extreme example of weight-related hormonal changes is the development of amenorrhea and hirsutism in young women with anorexia nervosa. Less dramatically, the relationship between diet and hormones is exemplified in the results of a 1977 study performed by Peter Hill and others at our center. The study showed that the duration of the menstrual cycle (interval between cycles) was shortened in women who changed from a diet high in animal fat and animal protein to one devoid of meat and meat products. They also found that the altered menstrual activity was accompanied by reductions in plasma prolactin (see Figure 4)' and testosterone concentrations.

More recently, B. Sherman and co-workers reviewed the relationship of the Quetelet index (metric body weight/height[2]) to menstrual patterns in American women. Their retrospective study showed that the subjects who were most obese at age 18 had experienced menarche at a mean age of 12.4 years, compared with 13 years for the least obese 18-year-olds. In addition, those who were heavier at age 18 and who later also gained at least five more pounds had longer and more irregular menstrual cycles in the first seven years after menarche. Finally, there was a positive correlation between body mass at 18 years and subsequent menopausal age, with the heavier subjects undergoing a later menopause.

Additional evidence that body weight—and hence diet—affects the timing of menopause can be found in data from the Framingham study of cardiovascular disease. In a 1976 report, M. C. Hjortland, P. M. McNamara, and W. B. Kannel noted that at every age level, women who had undergone menopause had a lower body weight than those who remained premenopausal. Similar findings—but with more relevance to concepts of dietary composition and tumor risk—were reported in 1977 by B. K. Armstrong. In Australia, Seventh-Day Adventists (who tend to follow an ovo-lacto-vegetarian diet) had lower mean body weights and menopause at an earlier age than did omnivorous controls. Seventh-Day Adventists have significantly lower rates of breast (and large-bowel) cancer than are seen in most other subgroups of Western populations.

The indications that diet directly or indirectly influences age at menarche, age at menopause, and menstrual function are suggestive, particularly in light of previously noted associations between increased breast cancer risk and early menarche, late menopause, or obesity. But what hormonal mechanisms account for the associations? Equally important, what accounts for the failure of some studies to confirm that they are indeed determinants of breast cancer risk?

Definitive answers to these and other key questions about breast carcinogenesis are still lacking. In a number of respects, however, animal models

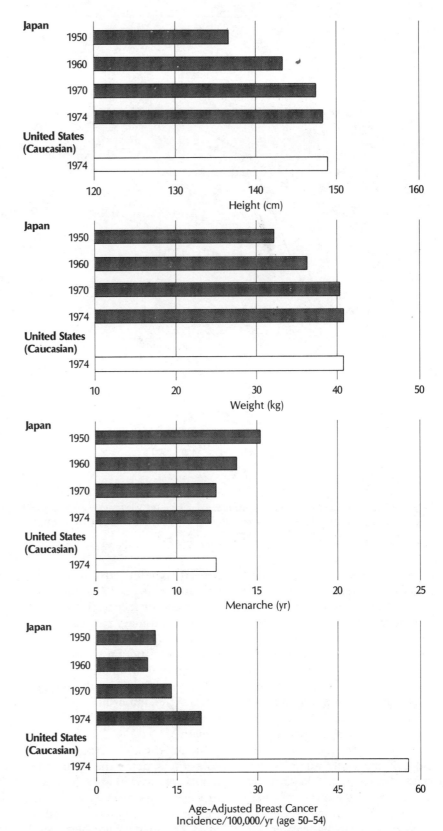

Figure 3. *Population study by Y. Kagawa noted that between 1950 and 1974 the height and weight of 12-year-old Japanese girls rose to values seen in U.S. counterparts and that the age of menarche in Japanese girls fell to the U.S. level. During the same period Japanese breast cancer rates also began to rise.*

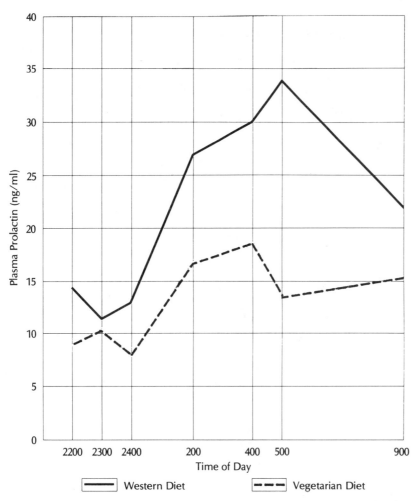

Figure 4. *In four healthy subjects alternately fed a high-fat Western and a low-fat vegetarian diet, P. Hill found that the high-fat diet significantly increased mean prolactin output, particularly during early-morning hours.*

of the disease have provided some good clues.

The literature on experimental mammary carcinogenesis is extensive. It stretches back to the 1940s, when Tannenbaum and Silverstone showed that a high-fat diet enhanced chemically induced and spontaneous mammary cancer in rodents and that protein, carbohydrate, or other macronutrient intake did not markedly affect tumor yield. Subsequent studies by other investigators confirmed those early findings of dietary fat's role in breast cancer. Of many models designed to elucidate the tumor's etiologic mechanisms, one that has

proved particularly revealing over the years uses 7,12-dimethylbenz(*a*)anthracene (DMBA) to induce mammary cancer in the rat. The DMBA model not only permits distinction between initiating and promoting events in carcinogenesis but demonstrates the importance of hormonal factors in breast tumor growth.

During the 1970s, Carroll and co-workers, using the DMBA rat model, showed that a high-fat diet exerts its primary effect on the promotion phase of mammary carcinogenesis, that diets rich in polyunsaturated fatty acids tend to be more effective tumor promoters than diets rich

in saturated fatty acids, and that the effect of fat intake on the development of mammary tumors is separate and distinct from that of calorie intake or obesity. Other investigators showed that approximately 70% of DMBA-induced tumors regress after ovariectomy, with as many as 75% regrowing at the original site at varying intervals after regression. The model's potential relevance to human disease is apparent when one considers that breast cancer in the Western world predominantly affects women without periodic ovarian activity and that human breast cancers often recur after endocrine ablative surgery.

Recently, L. A. Cohen, P. C. Chan, and one of us (ELW) took the DMBA rat model one step further—using it to demonstrate the tumor-enhancing effect of a high-fat diet after ovariectomy. Fifty Sprague-Dawley female rats were given a single dose of DMBA at 50 days of age. Eighty days later (when six of the animals already had detectable mammary tumors), each rat underwent bilateral ovariectomy. After another seven days, the animals were divided into two groups of 25, with three tumor-bearing animals in each group. For the next 40 weeks, one group was maintained on a diet containing 0.5% lard, the other on one containing 20% lard.

When the surviving animals were then killed and autopsied, 13 of 23 rats in the high-fat-diet group had mammary tumors, compared with only five of 20 rats in the low-fat-diet group. The high-fat-diet group was also more severely affected by multiple tumors: 0.78 tumors per rat at risk, compared with only 0.25 in the low-fat-diet group. All six of the previously established tumors regressed within a week of ovariectomy, and three of these (two in high-fat-diet animals) regrew at their original sites during the study period.

It is noteworthy that the high-fat diet supplied 40% to 50% of total calories as fat and thus was equivalent to the average per capita fat intake of the high-risk United States population. In contrast, the low-fat diet contained about 1% of calories as fat—well below the average value seen in such low-risk countries as Japan. Additionally, although both diets were fed ad libitum, weight gain was similar in the two groups. The calculated energy density of the high-fat diet (4.45 kcal/gm) was greater than that of the low-fat diet (3.52 kcal/gm), and the high-fat-diet animals consumed less food per day than the low-fat-diet animals (16 to 18 gm versus 20 to 22 gm, respectively). The similar weight gains indicated that tumor development was neither positively related to obesity (in the high-fat-diet group) nor negatively related to undernutrition (in the low-fat-diet group). Rather, differences in tumor yields in the two groups appeared to be due to dietary fat content per se.

As noted, most animals in the study lacked palpable mammary tumors at the time of ovariectomy, suggesting that dietary fat stimulated the early stages of DMBA-induced tumor development. A 1977 study by J. Russo and co-workers provides pertinent reference points: In female Sprague-Dawley rats given DMBA at age 50 days, ductal hypertrophy at day 70 was the first discernible evidence of cell transformation; intraductal proliferation of altered epithelial cells occurred between days 80 and 90, and the first intraductal carcinomas appeared at day 95. Since our animals were ovariectomized at age 130 days, 80 days after DMBA administration, it is therefore likely that most of their intraductal lesions were already present at the time of surgery. Assuming that both groups had roughly equal numbers of such lesions upon ovariectomy, one may conclude that high fat intake in the absence of normal periodic ovarian steroid secretion increased the rate of progression to overt carcinomas.

Before we consider hormonal mechanisms that may be responsible for the tumor-enhancing effect of a high-fat diet, a word about obesity and experimental mammary carcinogenesis. Several animal studies have demonstrated that overnutrition significantly increases the frequency of spontaneous and chemically induced tumors, including those of the mammary glands. In mice, spontaneous mammary tumors have been shown to occur far more frequently in obese than in nonobese subjects. More to the point, the same has been shown for ovariectomized obese as compared with ovariectomized nonobese mice. In 1966, S. H. Waxler and M. F. Leef reported that ovariectomized C3H mice that were injected with gold thioglucose to induce obesity had significantly more spontaneous mammary tumors than nonobese ovariectomized controls. Since the two groups in the study were fed similar diets, obesity per se appeared able to overcome the inhibitory effect of ovariectomy on mammary tumor development. A more recent study by Waxler and others reported a higher frequency of spontaneous mammary tumors in intact obese mice fed a high-fat diet than in intact obese mice fed a low-fat diet. Altogether, these results suggest that both obesity and high dietary fat intake increase mammary tumor frequency, but they probably do so by independent mechanisms.

In the rat at least, one prominent mechanism for dietary fat's tumor-enhancing effect is mediated by the pituitary hormone prolactin. That has been shown in various ways in our laboratory and elsewhere, most often with DMBA as the initiating agent. Thus, drug-induced hyperprolactinemia has been linked with augmented mammary tumor growth in rats exposed to DMBA, and exogenous prolactin has caused tumor regrowth after hypophysectomy had induced tumor regression. In addition, drug-induced stimulation of prolactin secretion has reversed the therapeutic effects of antiestrogens, luteinizing hormone releasing factor analogues, and ovariectomy in the DMBA rat model.

Our studies have shown that high-fat diets in the rat induce increases in serum prolactin but not estrogen concentrations. That effect was most pronounced during the proestrus and estrus stages of the rat's estrus cycle and resulted in chronic periodic increases in the prolactin:estrogen ratio. Additionally, our investigators have reported that ovariectomized rats fed a high-fat diet had a higher incidence of mammary tumors than ovariectomized rats fed a low-fat diet and that the high-fat-diet animals also had higher serum prolactin levels. In contrast, rats given an antiprolactin drug showed no increase in tumor yield. We obtained similar results by using *N*-nitrosomethylurea as the initiating agent—more mammary tumors in rats on a high-fat than on a low-fat diet, with the high-fat-diet group showing increases in serum prolactin levels and in the serum prolactin:estrogen ratio.

We noted earlier that tumor regression following ovariectomy is common in rats treated with DMBA but that the regression is transient and often followed by regrowth at the original tumor site. The results of a 1977 study performed in our laboratory suggest a possible explanation. Although serum prolactin concentrations in the rat fell abruptly, they began to rise within 12 to 16 weeks after ovariectomy. The magnitude of the postovariectomy increases was significantly greater in rats fed a high-fat diet than in those fed a low-fat diet.

Along those lines, C. F. Aylsworth and co-workers recently reported an elegant variation on the hormone-dependent DMBA tumor model. Animals were ovariectomized five days after DMBA exposure and shortly thereafter were placed on a high-fat or low-fat diet. Some rats were also given an estrogen replacement dose, daily haloperidol injections to raise serum prolactin, or both. The results: 1) Intact control animals on the high-fat diet showed pronounced enhancement of tumor development, but no tumor excess was seen in ovariectomized animals on either diet; 2) in ovariectomized rats fed the high-fat diet and given either estrogen replacement or haloperidol, tumor incidence did not differ significantly from that in similarly treated rats fed the low-fat diet; and 3) when ovariectomized rats were given estrogen replacement *and* made hyperprolactinemic by haloperidol *and* fed the high-fat diet, their tumor incidence equaled that in the intact controls fed the high-fat diet. Those results indicated that dietary fat's promotion of mammary tumor development in the rat may require interactions involving both prolactin and estro-

gens. The investigators observed that their findings implied a direct role for dietary fat in breast carcinogenesis, possibly by sensitizing DMBA-initiated mammary cells to hormone promoters.

Before considering mechanisms by which obesity may promote breast cancer development, we should first point out that the epidemiologic evidence linking obesity to breast cancer is scanty. Indeed, studies in U.S. populations have generally failed to confirm that obesity is a risk factor for the tumor, possibly because critical differences in the nutritional basis of obesity may affect the composition of adipose tissue. Specifically, it may be speculated that obesity induced by a high-fat diet may increase the risk of breast cancer, whereas obesity induced by a high-carbohydrate diet may not. These hypotheses, however, require study.

As we have seen, prolactin figures prominently—though not exclusively—in rat models of dietary fat's role in postmenopausal disease. According to many investigators, however, estrogens assume particular importance in current concepts of obesity's possible role in postmenopausal breast cancer. Somewhat paradoxically, those concepts center on an *androgen*—the C_{19} steroid androstenedione. They also lead to consideration of the thesis that breast cancer may share etiologic mechanisms with endometrial cancer.

In premenopausal women, androstenedione is secreted along with other androgens, progesterone, and estrogens from both the ovaries and the adrenals. Amounts of androstenedione secreted from each glandular source are about the same premenopausally, but after menopause the adrenal cortex be-

comes the major source of the steroid. The potential relevance of these observations to obesity-induced mechanisms of breast cancer development crystallized in 1973, when J. M. Grodin, P. K. Siiteri, and P. C. MacDonald showed that postmenopausal circulating estrogens are largely derived from the aromatization of androstenedione, which results in the formation of the estrogen estrone. They also showed that the principal site for this conversion is adipose tissue—and the character of adipose tissue depends in part on the composition of the diet.

In postmenopausal women, plasma estrone levels are similar to those in premenopausal women during the follicular phase of the menstrual cycle. With increasing age during adulthood, however, the rate at which androstenedione is converted into estrone has been shown to rise. This conversion rate has also been shown to be positively correlated with body weight. Thus, the older and heavier a woman is, the greater her peripheral estrogen formation.

Does the resulting increase in circulating estrogen influence breast cancer risk? Observations in endometrial cancer may be relevant: First, like breast cancer, endometrial cancer predominantly affects Western populations, correlates closely with dietary fat, and most often occurs after menopause. Among the recognized risk factors for endometrial cancer are obesity, late menopause, and treatment with exogenous estrogens to relieve menopausal symptoms (see Table 2). Less clearly, some epidemiologic data suggest that early menarche also increases the risk for this tumor. In addition, premenopausal endometrial cancer is sometimes associated with Stein-Leventhal syn-

---

Table 2. Risk Factors for Endometrial Cancer

Obesity
  Elevated estrone production from
  androstenedione

Impaired fertility and menstrual abnormalities
  ?Early menarche

  Late menopause

  Stein-Leventhal syndrome

Endometrial hyperplasia
  Adenomatous hyperplasia

  Granulosa-theca cell tumors

Exogenous estrogens (e.g., for menopausal symptoms)

---

drome or with granulosa-theca cell tumors; in both, ovarian dysfunction leads to excessive estrogen stimulation of the endometrium, endometrial hyperplasia, and a heightened risk of malignant transformation. Finally, some studies have shown that endometrial cancer patients exhibit increased aromatization of androstenedione and that their plasma estrone concentrations are elevated. Those findings are not specific to endometrial cancer but primarily reflect the excessive body weight that is common in women with the tumor. For example, plasma estrone levels have been found to be elevated by about the same extent in healthy controls matched for age and weight.

With regard to circulating steroid levels in breast cancer patients, the findings are mixed. Normal or elevated estrone concentrations and reduced, normal, or elevated androstenedione concentrations have been reported. In one of the larger studies, H-O. Adami and co-workers reported from Sweden in 1979 on 122 postmenopausal breast cancer patients and the same number of age-matched controls. Serum samples from the breast cancer group, obtained shortly after mastectomy, showed considerable elevations in estrone and androstenedione concentrations, plus a slight but statistically significant increase in testosterone. Although the higher serum estrone concentrations in the breast cancer patients may be interpreted as resulting from increased availability of androstenedione precursor, it is noteworthy that the cases and controls in this study did not differ significantly in weight, height, or Quetelet index. On its face, this observation is not consistent with the concept that increased conversion of androstenedione to estrone in excessive adipose tissue contributes to postmenopausal breast cancer risk. Other investigators have failed to demonstrate that androstenedione production or conversion rates are elevated in postmenopausal breast cancer patients. The same may be said for virtually any hormonal or dietary factor implicated in human breast cancer. The etiologic role of each of the major elements we have discussed—dietary fat, obesity, and endog-

enous hormones of the steroid and peptide varieties—still needs to be clarified.

Regarding dietary fat and obesity, one possible approach is to rethink our definitions of such crucial terms, especially obesity. Simply put, whether in the diet or in the body, fat is not necessarily the same from individual to individual. Distinctions among total fat intake, animal fat intake, and saturated versus poly-(or mono-)unsaturated fatty acid intake are beginning to be appreciated by most investigators. But important questions about the biologic effects of those and other variables remain to be explored. For example, does a high-fat diet per se increase breast cancer risk, or is this effect seen only in the presence of a certain degree or type of obesity? Among possible mechanisms by which dietary fat might promote tumor development in the absence of obesity is alteration of the lipid content of cell membranes, membrane-bound receptors, or both, in breast tissue. Alternatively, since prostaglandins are the biologically active derivatives of the essential fatty acids arachidonate and linolate, dietary fat's tumor-producing effect might involve alteration of prostaglandin synthesis. As for obesity, the failure of some epidemiologic studies to confirm its role as a risk factor in breast cancer could stem from differences in nutritional basis (high fat versus high carbohydrate consumption, high saturated versus high unsaturated fat consumption) that may affect the composition of adipose tissue. In addition, it is possible that differences in the degree of obesity or in the distribution of excessive adipose tissue, or both, may influence tumor risk.

Concerning the role of hormones in breast cancer, it is becoming clear that multifactorial interactions are probably involved and that a multidisciplinary approach is most likely to be fruitful. Metabolic epidemiology is already providing some insights. In recent years, for example, we have begun to measure hormone levels in breast secretions, acting on the thesis that the hormone-mediated effects of dietary components on the target tissue may not be reflected by hormone levels in the blood. In one such study involving healthy Finnish women, we noted a twofold increase in prolactin and a sixfold increase in estrogen in breast fluid as compared with serum concentra-

tions (see Figure 5 for findings in a similar study). In other studies that are still in progress, we found that the amount of free cholesterol in ductal aspirates from American women was more than twice as high as that found in aspirates from Japanese women. We have also found evidence that at least part of the lipid content in some ductal aspirates is made up of exfoliated mammary parenchyma cells that stain heavily for lipids. This finding raises the possibility that the cellular content of breast secretions may reflect the integrity of the ductal epithelium of the breast and that differences in this regard between Ameri-

can and Japanese women, if present, may in turn reflect the relative risk of breast cancer in these populations. More specifically, it may also be hypothesized that the lipid content of breast fluid or mammary cell membranes determines the interaction of water-soluble prolactin and fat-soluble estrogens with their respective receptors. Obviously, however, much more study is needed to define the relevance of such findings and hypotheses to breast cancer development. What is clear is that future research in the hormonal etiology of breast cancer will be based on analysis of hormone concentrations in the breast and not in the serum.

Finally, no discussion of the factors that appear to influence the development of human breast cancer would be complete without consideration of the factors that may affect the course of the disease after it is established. Data from numerous investigations suggest that the same factors are important in both situations. Thus, retrospective studies have variously correlated disease-free survival or overall survival with reproductive history, family history of breast cancer, or obesity. A recent National Cancer Institute case-control study involving breast cancer patients in California showed a two- to three-fold excess risk associated with long-term use of conjugated estrogens among women who had undergone bilateral ovariectomy. Clinically, about one third of premenopausal breast cancer patients experience at least a temporary remission of disease after bilateral ovariectomy. About two thirds of patients whose breast cancers contain significant amounts of estrogen receptors respond to treatment with an estrogen antagonist, such as

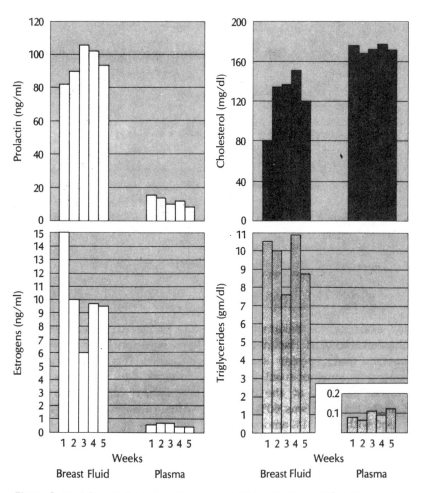

Figure 5. *In eight apparently healthy, nonlactating premenopausal women, mean cholesterol concentrations in breast fluid were comparable with those in plasma, but breast-fluid levels of other putative mediators of breast cancer risk—prolactin, estrogens, and triglycerides—were several times greater than those found in plasma.*

tamoxifen. Conversely, no more than 10% of patients with receptor-negative breast cancers respond to such treatment.

As in breast cancer induction, some human studies have found that obesity plays no role in disease-free or overall survival, whereas others have found that obese breast cancer patients have an increased risk of early recurrence and shorter survival compared with nonobese patients. It may be that methodologic variables of the type already noted—differing definitions of obesity and differences in the nutritional basis of obesity—also account for these inconsistencies.

That dietary fat may influence survival of breast cancer patients is another hypothesis requiring further study. As we have seen, the most dramatic difference in breast cancer incidence between the high-risk, high-fat-intake population of the United States and the low-risk, low-fat-intake population of Japan occurs in postmenopausal age groups. Similarly, postmenopausal breast cancer patients in Japan have markedly better survival rates after surgery than their U.S. counterparts. In 1979, for example, G. Sakamoto, H. Sugano, and W. H. Hartmann reported that 10-year survival among postmenopausal breast cancer patients at the Japan Cancer Institute was 60%, compared with only 31% among similar patients at Vanderbilt University Hospital. In both centers, however, premenopausal patients exhibited virtually the same 10-year survival—66% among the Japanese and 61% among the Americans.

The relevance of dietary fat to postmenopausal breast cancer survival is supported by recent studies in Hawaii reported by L. N. Kolonel and co-workers and by M. Ward-Hinds and co-workers. The first study found that the per capita fat intake of white Hawaiians was greater than that of Japanese Hawaiians and that this difference increased with advancing age. The second study found that, whereas the incidence of in situ breast carcinoma was about the same in white Hawaiians and Hawaiians of Japanese ancestry, the rate at which the lesions progressed to clinical disease was significantly greater in the whites, but only among postmenopausal patients.

These and other findings suggest that it may be appropriate to perform a randomized prospective clinical trial on the efficacy of a low-fat diet as adjuvant therapy in postmenopausal breast cancer. The diet used might be based on the Japanese model, consisting of 20% to 25% of calories as fat and having a polyunsaturated : saturated : monounsaturated (P/S/M) ratio of 1:1:1. For comparison, the control diet would be typically American, with 40% of calories as fat and a P/S/M ratio of 0.4:1:1. An important stipulation for such a trial is that it be limited to postmenopausal patients with lymph-node involvement (stage II disease); this subgroup is often most resistant to chemotherapy and is also most likely to respond to dietary adjuvant therapy. In fact, such trials are currently under consideration at the National Cancer Institute.

As for preventing human breast cancer and especially postmenopausal disease, we would endorse the recommendation that fat intake in the Western diet be reduced to about 25% of total calories, or even lower if possible. Burkitt and others have noted that the probable benefits of such a reduction are not likely to be limited to one disease but may lessen the frequency of several diseases common in modern Western societies. We agree. In the case of breast cancer, we feel that the evidence regarding the etiologic role of a high fat intake is sufficiently strong to justify recommending specific preventive or remedial actions. These actions should not have to wait until the precise role of dietary fat is elucidated.

Selected Reading

Wynder EL: Dietary factors related to breast cancer. Cancer 46:899, 1980

Rose DP: Diet, hormones, and breast cancer. *In* Endocrinology of Cancer, Rose DP (Ed), CRC Press, Boca Raton, Fla, 1982, pp 93–111

Cohen LA, Chan PC, Wynder EL: The role of a high-fat diet in enhancing the development of mammary tumors in ovariectomized rats. Cancer 47:66, 1981

Rose DP: Diet, hormones, and cancer. Food Technol, March 1983, p 58

Wynder EL: Reflections on diet, nutrition, and cancer. Cancer Res 43:3024, 1983

Wynder EL: Tumor enhancers: Underestimated factors in the epidemiology of lifestyle-associated cancers. Environ Health Perspect 50:15, 1983

Wynder EL, Cohen LA: A rationale for dietary intervention in the treatment of postmenopausal breast cancer patients. Nutr Cancer 3:195, 1982

Hill P et al: Breast cancer: Diet and hormone metabolism. *In* Banbury Report 8: Hormones and Breast Cancer, Cold Spring Harbor Laboratory, Cold Spring Harbor, NY, 1981, pp 257–277

Potential Risks From Low-Fat Diets

by Joseph T. Judd, June L. Kelsay, and Walter Mertz

THE DIETARY FAT INTAKE of different population groups ranges from less than 10% to more than 40% of the energy intake. Diets with this range of fat intake may be nutritionally adequate if the total energy intake is in proportion to the requirements and if the nonfat components of the diet furnish adequate amounts of the essential nutrients. If these conditions are not met, diets very low in fat (less than 10% of the energy intake) can become limiting in total energy intake and in fat-soluble essential nutrients, whereas diets very high in fat (more than 40% of the energy intake), because of their energy density, may predispose to obesity and may limit the intake of nonfat essential nutrients. This statement clearly indicates that fat must be considered as part of the total diet and that potential risks of low-fat diets must be examined in the context of all nutrients whose concentration may be affected. A reduction in the proportion of dietary fat must be compensated for by a corresponding increase in other nutrients, if the energy content of a diet is to be maintained. No responsible recommendations have advocated the replacement of fat by simple carbohydrates or protein, in view of the well-documented dangers arising from excessive intakes of these nutrients. On the other hand, almost all recommendations advocate the replacement of fat calories by sources of complex carbohydrates, including fiber, such as whole grain cereal products, fruits, and vegetables. For this reason, the following discussion will attempt to examine potential risks of low and moderate fat diets from two points of view: the potential risks that may be associated with low-fat intake per se, and those that may arise from a high consumption of dietary fiber. While the following discussion is based mainly on well-documented risks of extreme intakes, there is no evidence of deleterious effects of diets moderately low in fat (20% to 30% of the energy intake) and moderately high in fiber for most age groups. However, at the present state of knowledge it is not possible to define a diet of ideal fat and fiber content that would be optimal for all people in minimizing risk for disease.

ROLES OF FAT IN THE DIET

Source of energy. Fat is a very important energy source in the human diet. Among the major nutrients, it has the highest caloric density, averaging about 2.25 times that of carbohydrates or protein. Such a high-caloric density is important in situations where the bulk of food may become limiting to the energy intake. This applies to the elderly, the edentulous, children, and the sick. In severely cold temperatures, its ready digestibility together with its high-fuel value make fat an especially important dietary energy source.

Carrier of fat-soluble vitamins. Carotene and vitamin A and vitamins D, E, and K are

From the US Department of Agriculture, Agricultural Research Service, Beltsville Human Nutrition Research Center, Beltsville, Md.

Address reprint requests to Joseph T. Judd, US Department of Agriculture, Agricultural Research Service, Beltsville Human Nutrition Research Center, Beltsville, MD 20705.

associated with fat in the diet. While moderately low-fat diets should provide adquate amounts of these substances, severe restriction of fat may affect not only the amount of vitamins but also their absorption. Such severely restricted diets, if consumed for considerable periods of time, should be carefully evaluated to determine if supplementation with fat-soluble vitamins is needed.

Source of essential fatty acids. Dietary fat is the only source of the essential fatty acids required by man and other mammals. Of these substances, linoleic acid is by far the most important, as it cannot be synthesized by mammalian organisms. This fatty acid, and its derivatives, are functional components of cell membranes and precursors of the powerful biological regulators, the prostaglandins and thromboxanes. The vital role of these substances in the normal and abnormal functioning of many diverse body systems is only beginning to be understood.

Present estimates[1] of desirable dietary intakes of essential fatty acids are based on very general observations, primarily on amounts needed to prevent major deficiency symptoms. It is possible that continued investigations of relationships of the amount of dietary essential fatty acids to

specific effects in the body may well lead to establishment of optimal intakes above the presently recommended levels. An indication of an optimal level of essential fatty acid intake considerably above that of the very general Recommended Dietary Allowances (RDA) is seen in our own studies at the Beltsville Human Nutrition Research Center. In one of a series of investigations of the role of polyunsaturated fatty acids in the regulation of blood pressure, carefully formulated diets composed of foods commonly eaten by the US population were fed to adult volunteers.[2] All of the diets provided the RDA for all known essential nutrients. In addition, they were designed to provide moderate protein levels (about 16% of energy), a balance (1:1) between simple and complex carbohydrates, and either usual (about 43% of calories) or moderately reduced (25% of calories) energy from fat. The type of fat was controlled to provide a polyunsaturated:saturated (P/S) fatty acid ratio of either 0.3 or 1.0. A detailed analysis of some of these diets has been published.[3] Diets with the higher P/S ratio, with either usual (Fig. 1A, B) or moderately low (Fig. 1C, D) fat-energy levels, resulted in lowering of both systolic and diastolic blood pressures. The greatest effect,

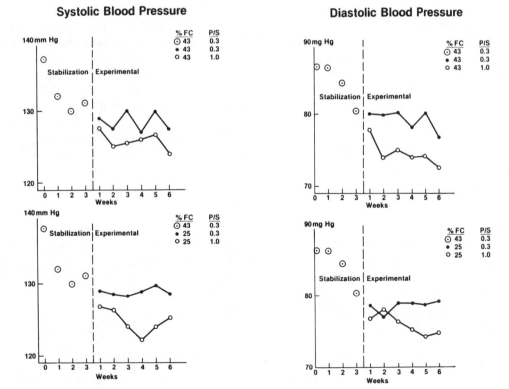

Fig. 1. Effect of varying the amount of polyunsaturated fatty acid (P/S ratio) on blood pressures in adult men fed normal (43% FC) and moderately low- (25% FC) fat diets.

however, appeared to be with the moderately low-fat diets (25% fat calories) and a P/S ratio of 1.0 (Fig. 1). The comparison between the two low-fat diets suggests that the optimal level of essential fatty acid (polyunsaturated fat) may be above the RDA. The diet with 25% fat and a P/S ratio of 0.3 slightly exceeds the RDA for essential fatty acids while the diet with 25% fat, P/S ratio 1.0, has a higher content of essential fatty acids. This study suggests that clinical trials of low-fat diets should have a P/S ratio near one.

Care should be taken by those consuming even moderately low-fat diets that sufficient essential fatty acid is provided. The latest edition of the Recommended Dietary Allowances[1] states that for those consuming relatively low amounts of fat (below 25% of calories), linoleic acid should provide 3% of the energy. In order to attain this essential fatty acid intake, it is critical that the low-fat diet contain a high level of polyunsaturated vegetable oil in amounts relatively great in comparison to the other sources of fat in the diet. We have attempted to illustrate this by the theoretical calculations shown in Table 1. From this example it may be estimated that polyunsaturated fats (such as the margarine in the example) must provide about 40% of the total fat intake. This leaves little room for consumption of many traditional foods in the US diet that are high in saturated fat and contain little or no polyunsaturated fatty acids.

Other roles of dietary fat. Fat increases the palatability of food, has a high satiety value, and affects gastrointestinal motility. Fat interacts with other nutrients or dietary components such as cholesterol, fiber, and calcium in their absorption and elimination from the digestive tract.

LOW-FAT DIETS FOR ADULTS

With the exception of the aged, the edentulous, and ill people, a moderate reduction of the dietary fat intake to 20% to 25% of the energy does not appear to constitute a health risk if an adequate ratio of polyunsaturated:saturated fatty acids is maintained. That level of intake would result in a reduction in the intake of fat-soluble vitamins, but such reduction is not believed to be consequential. The decreased intake of preformed vitamin A would be compensated for by an increase of the vitamin A precursors, the carotenes, present in many products of vegetable origin, if fatty foods are replaced by those rich in complex carbohydrates. The requirement for vitamin E is proportional to the dietary fat intake;[1] it decreases in proportion to decreases of dietary fat. The remaining fat-soluble vitamins, D and K, are synthesized in the healthy adult; the dietary intake is believed to be inconsequential.

LOW-FAT DIETS FOR CHILDREN

Recommendations of modified diets for the control of heart disease emphasize the desirability or even the necessity of life-long adoption by the whole population, including children,[4,5] to achieve the desired result. In our opinion, however, children constitute a special high-risk group with respect to their nutritional requirements, and any general recommendations for dietary changes that include them must be weighed very carefully. The American Heart Association committee report "Diet in the Healthy Child"[6] sets forth specific recommendations or guidelines for diets in healthy children, while recognizing that "some children in the United States are nutritionally deprived," and the "recommendations to them about diet might, through good intentions, lead to a compounding of nutritional deficiencies." Among their primary recommendations is that total fat should be approximately 30% of calories, with 10% from saturated fat, 10% from monounsaturated fat, and 10% or less from polyunsaturated fat. The question may well be raised as to whether this recommendation could create a

---

Table 1. Example of Fat Intake on Moderately Low-Fat Diet Providing RDA for Linoleic Acid

Calculations based on a daily energy intake of 2700 kcal with 25% of energy from fat and 3% of energy from linoleic acid (LoA):

kcal/d from fat = 2700 kcal/d × 0.25 = 675 kcal/d

kcal/d from LoA = 2700 kcal/d × 0.03 = 81 kcal/d

Assuming an average fuel value for fat and LoA of 9 kcal/g:

Fat intake/d = 675 kcal/d/9 kcal/g = 75 g/d

LoA intake/d = 81 kcal/d/9 kcal/g = 9 g/d

Typical source of fat in US diet that would meet this requirement:

Soft margarine made from partially hydrogenated and regular corn oil having approximately 30 g LoA/100 g fat.[36]

9 g LoA/d/0.3 g LoA/g fat = 30 g fat (margarine)/d

Of the total daily fat intake of 75 g, 40% or 30 g would need to be provided by a fat source(s) high in linoleic acid (about 30% LoA), with only 60% or 45 g remaining for all other fat sources, eg, meats, eggs, dairy products, and animal fats.

risk for a large segment of the children in the United States, those in the lower economic groups.

Celender, et al[7] in reviewing dietary trends in the United States pointed out that while most Americans have nutritionally adequate diets, notable exceptions occur in low-income populations, especially children. Support for this view cited by Celender was in the Ten-State Nutrition Survey,[8] which was biased by inclusion of an unproportionately high sample from lower economic groups; children under 6 years of age had low iron and vitamin A levels, and, in the same survey, growth retardation was generally found among low-income children, while in Mexican-Americans in low income areas there was a high prevalence of low-vitamin A levels. In addition, in the First Health and Nutritional Examination Survey (HANES), 1971 to 1972,[9] vitamin A intakes were below the RDA levels for low-income white females ages 18 to 44 and normal income black adolescents ages 12 to 17. In another survey cited by these workers, low-socioeconomic black children were reported to have lower intakes of calcium, vitamin A, and vitamin C than did white children.[10]

In view of these findings it appears prudent to ascertain the full adequacy for all nutrients of children's diets before recommending substantial modifications.

RISKS OF CONSUMING HIGH-FIBER DIETS

Among the beneficial effects claimed for high-fiber diets are the prevention and treatment of diverticular disease, cancer of the colon, ischemic heart disease, and diabetes mellitus. These possible benefits appear promising enough that a higher level of fiber intake is being widely recommended by physicians, nutritionists, and health scientists. The undisputed claim that fiber is beneficial in maintaining good bowel function and in preventing constipation is sufficient reason for making recommendations for consumption of a moderate level of fiber.

At the same time there is some evidence that high fiber intakes have adverse effects on the availability of nutrients to the body. Nutrients may be bound to the fiber as they occur in nature and, thus, may not be readily available. Some nutrients, particularly minerals, may become adsorbed to the fiber as its passes through the digestive tract, and may be rendered unavailable to the body.

Increased fecal excretion of energy, nitrogen,

and fat resulting in decreased apparent digestibility of these parameters have been reported in the literature by a number of investigators.[11–16] This effect of fiber is demonstrated in the results of a study carried out by Kelsay, et al., 1981.[17] Twelve adult men consumed each of four diets for 3 weeks in a 4 × 4 Latin square design. The four diets contained 2, 10, 19, and 26 g neutral detergent fiber (NDF—hemicellulose, cellulose, and lignin). Intake of energy, fat, and protein was similar on all four diets. The digestibility of energy, fat, and protein decreased as the fiber intake increased (Fig. 2). The difference in fecal calories on the lowest and highest fiber diets was 142 calories/d. A higher-fiber diet such as this might make a significant contribution to weight loss if consumed over a sufficient length of time. Probably the most important effect of fiber in the diet on energy intake is the decrease in high-energy food intake as a result of consuming satiating high-fiber foods. In developing countries this dilution of calories by the presence of large amounts of fiber in the diet may be of concern. It could be a problem particularly with children and with the elderly, whose caloric intakes are likely to be low. The decrease in fat absorption due to a high-fiber intake is probably of little physiological importance. However, the lower absorption of nitrogen may be of concern in countries where intakes of protein are low and intakes of fiber are high.

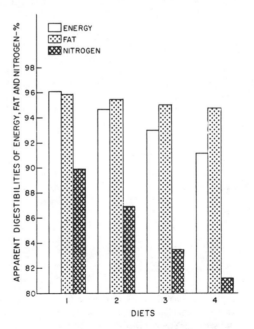

Fig. 2. Apparent digestibilities of energy, fat, and nitrogen (%) when levels of fiber were fed. Adapted from Kelsay, et al.[17]

There are reports of decreased or even negative mineral balances when the level of fiber in the diet is increased. These reports have been reviewed previously.[18,19] Iron and phosphorus balances did not seem to be generally affected by addition of fiber to the diet, possibly because of high intakes of these minerals in the studies reported. However, increased fiber in the diet was reported to decrease calcium and magnesium balances in most studies, and zinc and copper balances in some. Decreased absorption of minerals due to binding by fiber is not so important if mineral intakes are sufficiently high to maintain near zero or positive balances. Other dietary components, such as phytate and oxalate, can also bind minerals and reduce their availability.

Studies in which negative mineral balances with increased fiber intake were reported are listed in Table 2. Factors that may have a bearing on the negative mineral balances reported are listed: (1) Levels of mineral intake. In the first study by McCance and Widdowson,[20] the subjects were in more negative calcium balance with intakes of 500 mg/d of calcium on the brown high-fiber bread diet than with intakes of 1200 mg/d on the brown bread diet. In their second study[21] the subjects had intakes of 500 mg calcium per day and were again in negative calcium balance. Two of three subjects studied by Walker, et al[22] had calcium intakes of about 500 mg/d during the experimental period of the study but were consuming approximately 1100 mg/d on their usual diets consumed before the experiment. The change in level of intake of calcium may partially account for the negative calcium balances during the first 4 weeks on the experimental diet containing brown bread. (2) Presence of phytate. The presence of phytate may be partially responsible for negative mineral balances observed on brown bread intakes, since unrefined cereals are high in phytate content. In the second study by McCance and Widdowson[21] values for absorption of calcium, magnesium, and phosphorus on dephytinized brown bread intakes were between the values obtained for brown bread and white bread diets. The studies

Table 2. Level of Fiber Intake and Negative Mineral Balances

Investigators	Fiber Source*	Fiber Intake (g/d)	Negative Balances
McCance and Widdowson[20]	Brown bread	20–33†	Ca
	White bread	7–12†	
McCance and Widdowson[21]	Brown bread	25–43†	Ca
	Dephytinized brown bread	25–43†	Ca
	White bread	7–12†	
Walker, et al[22]	Brown bread	39†	Ca, Mg
	White bread	12†	
Reinhold, et al[23]	Wholemeal bread	30†	Ca, Zn
	White bread	9†	
Reinhold, et al[24]	Wholemeal bread	32‡	Ca, Mg, P, Zn
	White bread	22‡	
Ismail-Beigi, et al[34]	Cellulose in apple compote	35‡	Ca, Mg, An
	Control diet	19‡	
Cummings, et al[25]	Wheat fiber	53§	Ca
	Control diet	22§	
Drews, et al[32]	Hemicellulose	21‖	Mg, Zn, Cu
	Control diet	7‖	
Kies, et al[33]	Hemicellulose	32‖	Zn
	Control diet	12‖	
Slavin and Marlett[26]	Cellulose	24¶	Ca, Mg
	Control diet	10¶	
Kelsay, et al[28,29]	Fruits and vegetables	24¶	Ca, Mg, Zn, Cu
	Control diet	5¶	
Kelsay and Prather[30]	Fruits and vegetables	24¶	Ca, Mg, Zn
	Control diet	5¶	

*In all of these studies, fiber sources were added to a basal diet of mixed foods.

†Estimated from McCance and Widdowson's food tables. Values include fiber from bread only.

‡Analyzed acid detergent fiber values, which do not include hemicellulose.

§Calculated from McCance and Widdowson's food tables by Cummings, et al.[25]

‖Values from respective publications by Drews, et al[32] and Kies, et al.[33]

¶Analyzed neutral detergent fiber values, which include hemicellulose, cellulose, and lignin.

of Walker, et al,[22] Reinhold, et al,[23,24] and Cummings, et al[25] were also complicated by the presence of phytate in the diet. Reinhold, et al[23] first attributed the decreased mineral balances to the presence of phytate. However, in the second study[24] they fed leavened wholemeal bread and obtained negative mineral balances even though the phytate had been destroyed. (3) Level of protein intake. The high-protein diets fed by Cummings, et al[25] and by Slavin and Marlett[26]

Table 3. Menu and Work Sheet for Lipid Study 3, Day 5, 25% Fat Calories, P/S = 0.3

Name _____ Date _____

	Measure	g	Calories 2400	2800	3200	3600	4000
Breakfast							
Grapefruit sect, cn	1 C	254	½ C	1 C	1 C	1 C	1 C
Wheaties	1 C	25	25	50	50	50	50
Banana	—	—	0	0	0	0	175
Corn muffin	1 ea av	40	2 ea	2 ea	2 ea	2 ea	2 ea
Milk, 2%	1 C	246	1 C	1 C	1 C	1 C	1 C
Milk, skim	1 C	245	0	0	0	0	0
Coffee, tea							
Lunch							
Broiled cubed steak	1 oz	30	90	90	90	90	90
French fries, Z	10 pc	57	57	57	57	171	171
Wax beans, canned	1 C	125	125	125	125	125	125
Salad							
Sliced tomato	—	—	200	200	200	200	200
Lettuce leaf	—	—	25	25	25	25	25
Mayonnaise	1 Tb	15	0	0	0	0	0
Hamburger roll	1 ea av	49	1 ea	1 ea	1 ea	1 ea	1 ea
Brownie	1 pc	20	20	20	20	20	20
Pears, canned	1 C	255	150	255	345	218	435
Pears, diet, canned	1 C	255	0	0	0	0	0
Catsup	1 pkg	11	2 pkg	1 pkg	1 pkg	3 pkg	3 pkg
Coffee, tea							
Dinner							
Baked Haddock	1 oz	30	90	120	150	150	150
Corn oil	1 tsp	5	0	5	5	5	0
Bread crumbs	—	25	5	5	5	5	5
Lemon wedge	1 pc	20	20	20	20	20	20
Catsup	1 pkg	11	1 pkg	1 pkg	1 pkg	1 pkg	1 pkg
Noodles	½ C	80	80	80	160	120	80
Asparagus, Z	—	—	60	60	60	60	60
Salad							
Apple	—	—	75	75	75	75	185
Orange	—	—	90	90	180	180	180
Lemon juice	1 tsp	5	1 tsp	1 tsp	0	0	0
Lettuce leaf	—	—	25	25	25	25	25
French dressing	1 Tb	15	0	0	8	0	0
Roll, soft	1 ea av	28	2 ea	2 ea	2 ea	3 ea	3 ea
Jello, strawberry	1 C	240	65	130	130	130	130
Royal Anne cherries, cn	—	—	150	150	150	150	200
RA cherries, diet, cn	—	—	0	0	0	0	0
Coconut, dry, sw			0	0	0	25	0
Pineapple, sl, jc, pk, cn			0	0	0	200	186
Milk, 2%	1 C	246	0	0	⅓ C	1 C	1 C
Milk, skim	1 C	245	0	0	0	0	0
Coffee, tea							
Butter	1 pat	5	6 pat	7 pat	8 pat	5 pat	8 pat
Jelly	1 pkg	11	3 pkg	3 pkg	3 pkg	5 pkg	5 pkg
Sugar	1 pkg	5	4 pkg	3 pkg	3 pkg	3 pkg	4 pkg
Salt							

Z = frozen.

may have had an effect on the negative mineral balances reported in these studies. High-protein diets have been reported to decrease calcium balance.[27] (4) Presence of oxalic acid. The oxalic acid present in spinach in the diets fed by Kelsay, et al[28-30] was shown to contribute to results originally believed to be effects of fiber alone. In the second study, Kelsay, et al[29] compared a low-fiber diet containing spinach with the higher-fiber diet with and without spinach. Only the higher-fiber diet containing spinach resulted in negative mineral balances. (5) Kind of fiber. It has been shown in vitro that different fibers have different affinities for binding materials.[31] Drews, et al[32] found significant decreases in magnesium, zinc, and copper balances when hemicellulose, but not cellulose or pectin, was fed; this effect of hemicellulose was verified by Kies, et al.[33] However, Slavin and Marlett[26] and Ismail-Beigi, et al[34] reported negative balances of minerals when cellulose was added to the diet. (6) Level of fiber intake. Most investigators who reported negative mineral balances had fed levels of fiber greater than 25 g/d.[20-25,33,34] In four studies listed above, fiber intakes in the breads were calculated by us using values from McCance and Widdowson's food tables[35] and do not include fiber in the basal diet. The basal diet probably included another 10 g fiber. Slavin and Marlett[26] reported negative calcium and magnesium balances on 24 g NDF/d. The NDF values would be lower than the McCance and Widdowson values, because the latter include soluble fibers, whereas NDF values include only insoluble hemicellulose, cellulose, and lignin. (7) Length of study period. In the study by Walker, et al[22] the subjects with negative calcium and magnesium balances for the first 4 weeks had positive balances during the week 8. This indicates that subjects may be able to adjust to a lower mineral availability due to increased fiber if they are given sufficient time. The study by

Drews, et al[32] was short term, and the time may not have been sufficient to allow for adaptation to changes in diet. However, the study by Kies, et al[33] was for two 7-day periods, and no difference was seen between zinc balances for the two periods.

Further studies are needed on high levels of fiber intake in which other complicating factors have been eliminated in order to give a satisfactory answer to the question of effect of fiber on mineral balances. Studies could be conducted for a sufficient length of time to assure adjustment to changes in level of mineral intakes.

A moderately low-fat experimental menu containing 25% fat calories and having a P/S ratio of 0.3 is presented in Table 3. This diet was fed in studies conducted by Iacono, et al and Marshall et al.[2,3] The fiber content of this menu was calculated using McCance and Widdowson's fiber values[35] and was found to contain 32 g fiber at the 2800 kcal level.

CONCLUSION

The data presented above lead to the following conclusions: (1) Diets extremely low in fat (less than 10% of kcal) consumed over extended periods of time present quantifiable health risks because of low-energy density and reduced intake of fat-soluble vitamins and essential fatty acids. The substitution of the required high amounts of fiber-rich foods can result in a significant decrease in the utilization of nutrients, especially the mineral elements. Infants, children, the aged, sick, and edentulous are especially at risk from such diets.

There is no evidence to indicate a health risk to the healthy adult of diets moderately low in fat and moderately high in fiber. Although an ideal composition cannot be stated, diets containing fat at 20% or more of the total energy and less than 25 g of neutral detergent fiber can be considered safe.

REFERENCES

1. Recommended Dietary Allowances. Washington, DC, National Academy of Sciences, 1980

2. Iacono JM, Judd JT, Marshall MW, et al: Role of dietary polyunsaturated fatty acids and prostaglandins in reducing blood pressure and improving thrombogenic indices, in Beitz DC, Gaurth Hansen R (eds): Animal Products in Human Nutrition. New York, Academic Press, 1982

3. Marshall MW, Judd JT: Calculated vs. analyzed com

position of four modified fat diets. J Amer Dietetic Assoc. 80:537–549, 1982

4. Senate Select Committee on Nutrition and Human Needs: Dietary Goals for the United States. Washington, DC, US Govt Print Office, 1977

5. American Heart Association, Nutrition Committee: Rationale of the diet-heart statement of the american heart association. Verbatim transcript of AHA Committee Report.

Nutrition Today. 1982

6. American Heart Association: Diet in the healthy child. Circulation 67:1411A, 1983

7. Celender IM, Shapero M, Sloan AE: Dietary trends and nutritional status in the United States. Food Technology. 1978

8. Department of Health, Education, and Welfare: Ten-State Nutrition Survey 1968–1970. Washington, DC, HEW, 1972

9. Department of Health, Education, and Welfare: First Health and Nutrition Examination Survey, United States 1971–1972. Washington, DC, HEW, 1972

10. Owen GM, Kram KM, Gurry PJ, et al: A study of nutritional status of preschool children in the United States, 1968–1970. Pediatrics 53:597, 1974

11. McCance RA, Widdowson EM: The digestibility of English and Canadian wheats with special reference to the digestibility of protein by Man. J Hyg 45:59–64, 1947

12. Southgate DAT, Durnin JVGA: Calorie conversion factors. An experimental reassessment of the factors used in the calculation of energy value on human diets. Brit J Nutr 24:517–535, 1970

13. Beyer PL, Flynn MA: Effects of high- and low-fiber diets on human feces. J Am Dietet Assoc 72:271–277, 1978

14. Calloway DH, Kretsch MJ: Protein and energy utilization in men given a rural Guatemalan diet and egg formulas with and without added oat bran. Am J Clin Nutr 31:1118–1126, 1978

15. Southgate DAT, Branch WJ, Hill MJ, et al: Metabolic responses to dietary supplements of bran. Metabolism 25:1129–1135, 1976

16. Kelsay JL, Behall KM, Prather ES: Effect of fiber from fruits and vegetables on metabolic responses of human subjects. I. Bowel transit time, number of defecations, fecal weight, urinary excretions of energy and nitrogen and apparent digestibilities of energy, nitrogen, and fat. Am J Clin Nutr 31:1149–1153, 1978

17. Kelsay JL, Clark WM, Herbst BJ, et al: Nutrient utilization by human subjects consuming fruits and vegetables as sources of fiber. J Agri Food Chem 29:461–465, 1981

18. Kelsay JL: Effect of diet fiber level on bowel function and trace mineral balances of human subjects. Cereal Chem 54:2–5, 1981

19. Kelsay JL: Effects of fiber on mineral and vitamin bioavailability, in Vahouny GV, Kritchevsky D (eds): Dietary Fiber in Health and Disease. New York, Plenum Publishing Corporation, 1982, pp 91–103

20. McCance RA, Widdowson EM: Mineral metabolism of healthy adults on white and brown bread dietaries. J Physiol 101:44–85, 1942

21. McCance RA, Widdowson EM: Mineral metabolism on dephytinized bread. J Physiol 101:304–313, 1942

22. Walker ARP, Fox FW, Irving JT: Studies in human mineral metabolism. I. The effect of bread rich in phytate phosphorus on the metabolism of certain mineral salts with special reference to calcium. Biochem J 42:452–462, 1948

23. Reinhold JG, Nasr K, Lahimgarzadeh A, et al: Effects of purified phytate and phytate-rich bread upon metabolism of zinc, calcium, phosphorus and nitrogen in man. Lancet 1:283–288, 1973

24. Reinhold JG, Faradji B, Abadi P, et al: Decreased absorption of calcium, magnesium, zinc and phosphorus by humans due to increased fiber and phosphorus consumption as wheat bread. J Nutr 106:493–503, 1976

25. Cummings JH, Hill MJ, Jivraj T, et al: The effect of meat protein and dietary fiber on colonic function and metabolism. I. Changes in bowel habit, bile acid excretion, and calcium absorption. Am J Clin Nutr 32:2086–2093, 1979

26. Slavin JL, Marlett JA: Influence of refined cellulose on human bowel function and calcium and magnesium balance. Am J Clin Nutr 33:1932–1939, 1980

27. Hegsted M, Linkswiler HM: Long-term effects of level of protein intake on calcium metabolism in young adult women. J Nutr 111:244–251, 1981

28. Kelsay JL, Behall KM, Prather ES: Effect of fiber from fruits and vegetables on metabolic responses of human subjects. II. Calcium, magnesium, iron, and silicon balances. Am J Clin Nutr 32:1876–1880, 1979

29. Kelsay JL, Jacob RA, Prather ES: Effect of fiber from fruits and vegetables on metabolic responses of human subjects. III. Zinc, copper, and phosphorus balances. Am J Clin Nutr 32:2307–2311, 1979

30. Kelsay JL, Prather ES: Effect of fiber and oxalic acid on mineral balances of adult human subjects. Fed Proc 40:854, 1981

31. Camire AL, Clydesdale FM: Effect of pH and heat treatment on the binding of calcium, magnesium, zinc, and iron to wheat bran and fractions of dietary fiber. J Food Science 46:548–551, 1981

32. Drews LM, Kies C, Fox HM: Effect of dietary fiber on copper, zinc, and magnesium urilization by adolescent boys. Am J Clin Nutr 32:1893–1897, 1979

33. Kies C, Fox HM, Beshgetoor D: Effect of various levels of dietary hemicellulose on zinc nutritional status of men. Cereal Chem 56:133–136, 1979

34. Ismail-Beigi F, Reinhold JG, Faradji B, et al: Effects of cellulose added to diets of low and high fiber content upon the metabolism of calcium, magnesium, zinc, and phosphorus by man. J Nutr 107:510–518, 1977

35. Paul AA, Southgate DAT: McCance and Widdowson's The Composition of Foods. London, HMSO, 1978

36. Agricultural Handbook No. 8–4. Washington, DC, 1979

Vitamins and Cancer Prevention: Issues and Dilemmas

by Vernon R. Young and Paul M. Newberne

Vitamins are a class of organic compounds that are essential components of an adequate diet. They or their derivatives function as coenzymes, cellular antioxidants, and/or regulators of gene expression. Fourteen vitamins are recognized in human nutrition (Vitamins A, D, E, K, B_1, B_2, B_6, B_{12}, C, niacin, folacin, pantothenic acid, biotin, choline), with deficiencies or excesses in intake leading to changes in protein, nucleic acid, carbohydrate, fat and/or mineral metabolism. Thus, the integrity of physiological systems, including those associated with detoxification, cellular repair, immune processes, and neural and endocrine function, depends upon the nutritional and vitamin status of the host. For these reasons, it may be anticipated that the adequacy of the vitamin supply to cells and tissues would affect the development, progress, and outcome of cancers. In this review, the definition and functions of and requirements and recommended allowances for vitamins are discussed briefly before exploring the evidence, largely from studies in experimental animals, that indicates the nature of the link between vitamins and cancer. Although evidence based on studies in animal systems reveals that vitamin intake and status can modulate the outcome of experimental carcinogenesis, the findings are often conflicting and difficult to interpret. Furthermore, it is not yet possible to develop a suitable prediction of the role of the individual vitamins in tumor development. The significance of these observations for human nutrition and cancer *prevention*, particularly in reference to ascorbic acid (vitamin C), vitamin E, and B-complex vitamins is considered. Vitamin A and retinoid compounds are discussed elsewhere in the symposium. The many popular misconceptions and unsound advice concerning vitamins and health, including "fake" vitamins-pangamic acid ("vitamin B_{15}") and laetrile ("vitamin B_{17}")-are also discussed. On the basis of current evidence, it would be inappropriate to recommend either substantial changes in habitual vitamin intakes, as provided by an adequate, well-balanced diet, or promotion of megavitamin intakes, as a means of reducing risk from cancers in the human population. However, a prudent approach toward diet and food habits, as a means of better optimizing the health consequences of our complex lifestyle is to be recommended.

Cancer 47:1226–1240, 1981.

A HIGH PROPORTION OF human cancers is attributable to environmental factors.[17,25] Evidence obtained from studies with experimental animals and from human populations implicates nutritional factors and dietary constituents in the causation of cancers at different sites in the body.[6] Previously, we have discussed some facts and fallacies concerning nutrients, vitamins and minerals in human cancer prevention.[77] Hence, in this paper we consider more specifically, in reference to the final session on Issues and Dilemmas on this Conference, the relationship between vitamins and incidence and development of various cancers. Our purpose is not to review in detail this aspect of the diet–cancer axis, because this has been done previously by us and others.[46,48,72,73] Furthermore, the specific issues of vitamin A and

Presented at the American Cancer Society National Conference on Cancer Prevention and Detection, Chicago, Illinois, April 17–19, 1980.

From the Department of Nutrition and Food Science, Massachusetts Institute of Technology, Cambridge, Massachusetts.

Address for reprints: Dr. Vernon R. Young, Department of Food and Nutrition, 56-333, Massachusetts Institute of Technology, 77 Massachusetts Avenue, Cambridge, MA 02139.

retinoids have been discussed by Sporn[63] and elsewhere in this Conference. Rather, we hope to provide the health professional with an overview of current knowledge, and based on this, to offer our opinion about the appropriate advice to be given to the general public.

Before turning to the vitamins *per se*, however, it is worth emphasizing that a number of dietary variables may contribute to the development of human cancers[72]; these are summarized in Table 1.[25] The thrust of our discussion will be with respect to item 3 in this table, because the essential nutrients (protein, essential fatty acids, energy sources, minerals, vitamins, water, and oxygen) regulate cell and organ metabolism. Thus, it is rational to consider that these nutrients and the nutritional state of the host could play a role in promoting or inhibiting the development of cancers at certain sites. Furthermore, there is an increased interest by health professionals concerning the relation between diet and the major degenerative diseases in our population, and this is paralleled by the attention of the consumer to diet and food purchases, for reasons that include attempts to improve personal health. The frequency with which nutrition and diet form the basis of a headline feature in popular newspapers attests to the interest by the public in nutrition issues, as does the proliferation of books with incorrect or even extravagant claims concerning the role of diet and essential nutrients in health maintenance. These sources of information frequently may be misleading, inappropriate, or even detrimental to health. The subtle interweaving of articles about news from laboratory investigations concerned with vitamins in health and disease, between advertisements for vitamin supplements in popular magazines, leads to a false interpretation of the value of buying these supplements.

Indeed, dietary regimens are among the cruel and deceptive practices used by "quacks" in attracting healthy people as well as cancer patients to follow their approaches and dangerous philosophy. These regimens may include the "grape cure," a carrot juice diet, or coffee enemas.[26] Because of the broad acceptance, by those without a scientific understanding of nutrition, that vitamins play an important role in health maintenance, there is great opportunity to misinform and misguide the consumer about the role of vitamins in health and in cancer prevention particularly. Hence, we will begin our paper with a definition of vitamins and a discussion of their role in human physiology and then consider current estimates of requirements for the vitamins. This will be followed by a brief review of the findings that

TABLE 1. Dietary Variables of Relevance in Cancer Causation and Prevention*

1. Preformed potential carcinogens (aflatoxin, pyrolysates).
2. Carcinogen precursers (secondary amines, nitrites).
3. Type and relative proportion of nutrients.
4. Non-nutrients (fibers, biologically active compounds).
5. Nonspecific effects (energy intakes)

* Based on Higginson and Muir: *J Natl Cancer Inst* 1979; 63: 1291–1298.

indicate the nature of the association between vitamin intake and vitamin status and development of cancers. The relevance of these findings to considerations of human nutrition and cancer prevention then will be assessed before we offer, based on present knowledge, our advice and draw our summary conclusions. We must emphasize that the thrust of our discussion is concerned with nutrition in relation to cancer *prevention*, and we are not concerned here with the nutritional therapy of the patient already diagnosed with cancer. This latter aspect of cancer treatment and therapeutic nutrition is a separate and quite different topic that is beyond the scope of our mandate at this Conference.

The Vitamins

Definition

Vitamins are organic compounds the body requires for the growth and maintenance of normal cell and organ functions (Table 2). Because they cannot be made in sufficient quantities, they are required in small amounts in the diet. For some vitamins, such as biotin, the intestinal microflora might synthesize amounts that are significant in meeting the requirement of the host.

These compounds are essential constituents of an adequate diet because the cells lack the enzymatic machinery necessary to accomplish their synthesis at rates required to meet the needs of the body. Two examples may be given to emphasize the fact that a deletion of enzymes has created a dietary requirement for vitamins in human nutrition.

TABLE 2. Definition of a Vitamin

(a) An organic compound required in small amounts for complete health and well-being of the organism.
(b) Not utilized primarily to supply energy or as a source of structural tissue components.
(c) Function to promote physiologic processes vital to continued existence.
(d) Cannot be synthesized by the organism and must be supplied *de novo*.
(e) Deficiency causes a well-defined disease that is prevented or cured by the appropriate vitamin.

First, in addition to primates, guinea pigs, fishes, and flying mammals, humans are dependent on dietary sources of ascorbic acid. This is due to the loss of the enzyme L-gulonolactone oxidase that catalyzes the last step in the conversion of glucose to ascorbic acid (Fig. 1). In this sense, therefore, scurvy might be regarded as a "hereditary metabolic disease," but one of an unusual type since the inborn error is carried as a dominant trait by all members of the human population.[51]

The second example is derived from a recent report of a case of atypical phenylketonuria. Of significance is that the coenzyme for the enzymes phenylalanine hydroxylase, tryrosine-3-hydroxylase, and tryptophan-5-hydroxylase is L-erythro-5,6,7,8-tetrahydrobiopterin (THB), the latter being derived normally from guanosine triphosphate (GTP) by a series of reactions (Fig. 1).[9] However, Niederweisser *et al.*[50] found that a six-month-old female infant with mental retardation and elevated serum phenylalanine lacked the capacity to convert dihydroneopterin to sepiapterin. Oral administration of this latter intermediate reduced serum phenylalanine and so was required by this infant for formation of the cofactor (THB). Hence, because of this enzymatic block, sepiapterin became a vitamin for this child. Although this is a rather unusual case, it further underscores the metabolic basis for the vitamin requirement and illustrates that the need for essential nutrients, including vitamins, is determined ultimately by our genetic background.

From the above definition, 14 vitamins have been identified in human nutrition. The trivial names and generic descriptors for these vitamins and their related compounds are listed in Table 3.[28]

These are the only compounds currently recognized by the nutrition profession as vitamins and, in this context, as essential constituents of the human diet. Consideration will be given to the "fake" vitamins, including laetrile and B-15, when we discuss the topic of vitamins and human cancers.

Functions

Vitamins participate in a wide variety of biochemical and physiological processes. Because of the availability of numerous reviews of the metabolic functions of the individual vitamins, it is appropriate, therefore, to summarize only briefly the major functions of the 14 vitamins (Table 4). This will provide a rationale for further exploring the role that these nutrients may play in cancer causation and prevention.

An important function, shared by the B vitamins, is as precursors of coenzymes which are required for the activity of specific enzymes.[61] Each of the coenzymes participates in the catalysis of specific types of reactions which are associated with the metabolism of carbohydrates, lipids proteins, and nucleic acids. Thus, the utilization of energy, formation of cellular constituents, and the integrity of the repair and defense mechanisms involve the vitamins. Furthermore, a single metabolic pathway, such as the catabolism of a single amino acid, may require

A COMMON AND AN UNUSUAL VITAMIN

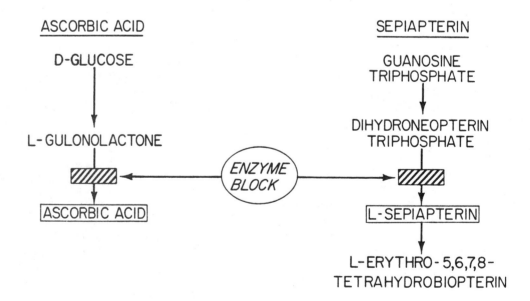

FIG. 1. Deletion of an enzyme, as a result of genetic factors, in a metabolic pathway leads to the evolution of a vitamin requirement.

TABLE 3. Generic Descriptions and Trivial Names for Vitamins and Related Compounds in Human Nutrition*

Vitamin term	Generic use
	(compounds with qualitatively the biological activity of:)
Fat-soluble vitamins and related compounds	
Vitamin A	β-ionone derivatives with retinol activity
Provitamin A carotenoids	Carotenoids with β-carotene-activity
Vitamin D	Steroids with cholecalciferol activity
Vitamin E	Tocol and tocotrienol derivatives with activity of α-tocopherol
Vitamin K	2-methyl-1,4,naphthoquinone and derivatives with phylloquinone activity
Water-soluble vitamins and related compounds	
Folacin	Folic acid and compounds with folic acid activity (e.g., THFA)
Niacin	Pyridine 3-carboxylic acid and derivatives with nicotinamide activity
Riboflavin (B_2) Thiamine (B_1) Vitamin B_6	2-methylpyridine and derivatives with pyridoxine activity
Vitamin B_{12}	Corrinoids exhibiting cyanocobalamin activity
Vitamin C	Compounds with ascorbic acid activity
Pantothenic Acid	
Biotin	
Choline	

* Summarized from IUNS Committee on Nomenclature: *Nutr Abs. Rev.* 1970; 40:395–400.

TABLE 4. Functions of Vitamins

Function	Vitamin
1. *Precursor of coenzyme*	Biotin Nicotinic acid Pantothenic acid Vitamin B_6
2. *Transmission of genetic information* (Transcription, translation, post-translation)	Vitamin A Vitamin K Vitamin D
3. *Antioxidant and electron transport*	Vitamin E Vitamin C
4. *Specialized"* Photosensitive reactions Neural transmission Macromolecular structure	Vitamin A Thiamin? B_6?

simultaneously many of the vitamins in their active coenzyme form.[61]

A second function met by some vitamins is related to the expression of genetic information. Therefore, vitamins might influence this process via (1) the synthesis of mRNA and/or its transport to the cytoplasm (*transcription*); (2) the formation of proteins at the *translation* stage, including involvement of ribosomes, protein factors, and amino-acyl-tRNA; (3) the addition of a prosthetic group to a newly made protein (*post-translation*); or (4) by affecting a cell surface constituent which might regulate cell function, division, or differentiation. Thus, the differentiation of epithelial cells is determined, in part, by vitamin A.[76] Vitamin D, via its conversion to 1,25 dihydrocholesterol vitamin D_3, possibly induces the transcription of mRNA of a specific gene(s) which codes for proteins responsible for intestinal calcium transport.[16] In the case of vitamin K, it participates in the post-translational modification of prothrombin precursors, involving carboxylation of glutamate residues, with the formation of active prothrombin.[52]

An antioxidant or electron transport function is served importantly by two vitamins, namely vitamins E and C.[29] Thus, vitamin E acts as an *in vivo* antioxidant.[29] These vitamins are reducing substances that keep the redox potential of tissues at a low level. Vitamin E protects cellular lipids from free-radical attack and stops the chain reactions by which these reactive species are multiplied.[29] It should be noted that vitamin E constitutes only a part of the cell's defense against oxygen-containing radicals, since glutathione peroxidase, a selenium-containing enzyme, is intimately involved in this system.[13] Vitamin C (ascorbic acid) is also known to possess antioxidant activity and its function in human metabolism may, in part, relate to this property. However, in relation to normal physiology, the main electron transfer role of vitamin C appears to be that of reducing metals so that the associated enzyme systems can act in the transport of molecular oxygen, as in hydroxylation of proline during collagen synthesis and in the formation of noradrenaline.[29]

Finally, some of the vitamins exhibit specialized functions not easily included in the above three major categories. An example of this is vitamin A, which is associated with the formation of rhodopsin, the light-sensitive pigment of the retina.[76] In addition, a nonmetabolic role for thiamin triphosphate in nerve excitation has been proposed.[3] It is also possible that pyridoxal phosphate might serve to modulate the binding to receptor-steroid complexes with nucleii and their removal from nucleii.[2]

In view of the foregoing, it should be obvious that

vitamins play a key role in cellular metabolism and in the maintenance of various physiologic processes. In addition, there is ample evidence that vitamin deficiencies or excesses lead to changes in the efficiency and status of the immune, detoxification, protective, repair, growth, and differentiation systems of body cells and organs.

Hence, in theory, it is possible that individual vitamins can contribute to the promotion or alleviation of cancers by acting as cocarcinogens, or by affecting the cellular mechanisms that lead to the formation of carcinomas. In addition to these physiologic functions it is, of course, possible that some vitamins may act as pharmacologic or pharmaceutical agents on processes that are of significance in cancer causation and prevention. We will consider this possibility later, but before doing so, it is appropriate to review, briefly, estimates of vitamin intakes that are considered to be sufficient to maintain adequate health in human populations.

Requirements and Allowances

Estimates of the human requirement for the individual vitamins has been based largely on the results of metabolic studies in relatively small populations of experimental subjects of various ages.[19] Data obtained from such studies are extended by findings obtained in animal systems and from epidemiologic and dietary surveys. When combined, these data provide the rationale for arriving at recommended daily dietary allowances for each of the vitamins. In addition to estimates of the mean requirement for a vitamin in a given population group, knowledge is also required of the extent of variation in requirements among apparently similar individuals within that population. From this information, dietary allowances are proposed and are judged to be intake levels sufficient to meet the needs of nearly all healthy subjects within the population.[19,45] Therefore, the actual requirement for most members of the population will be less than the allowance because the latter is set at an intake level necessary to meet the needs of individuals with the highest requirement.

Table 5 gives the most recent daily dietary allowances for vitamins for adult men, as recommended by the U. S. Food and Nutrition Board.[19] The reader may wish to consult this report[19] for further details concerning the philosophy on which these allowances have been made, and of the way in which they are to be interpreted and used in the evaluation of dietary survey data. However, it is important to emphasize that the dietary allowances are to be applied in reference to healthy populations

TABLE 5. Recommended Daily Dietary Intakes of the Vitamins

Vitamin	Name	Recommended intake* (adult male)
A	Retinol	100 μg
D	Calciferol	5 μg
E	Tocopherol	10 mg
K	Menaquinone	70–140 μg†
C	Ascorbic acid	60 mg
—	Biotin	100–200 μg†
B₁	Thiamin	104 mg
—	Niacin	18 mg
B₂	Riboflavin	1.6 mg
—	Folic acid	400 μg
B₆	Pyridoxine	2.2 mg
B₁₂	Cyanocobalamin	3 μg
—	Pantothenic acid	4–7 μmg†
—	Choline	Not determined

* From Recommended Dietary Allowances (1980).
† Estimated safe and adequate intake.

and are not intended to represent therapeutic intakes for treatment of disease conditions. Thus, they represent intakes which should prevent the development of nutritional deficiency disease and maintain the long-term health in most individuals. Furthermore, a diet based on a wide selection of foods will assure vitamin intakes that equal or exceed the allowances. Also, there is no evidence that inadequate vitamin status represents a major nutritional or health problem in our society. Vitamin supplements supplying amounts approaching the recommended daily allowances may be considered an "insurance" against the development of deficiencies arising from a poorly selected diet.[30] However, vitamin intakes that are considerably in excess of these allowances are not to be recommended as a broad public health policy. The specific issues of vitamin supplements and cancers will be considered in a later section of this paper.

Vitamins and Cancers

Nature of Evidence for Role in Cancer Causation

The availability of many popular articles and books concerned, in part, at least, with vitamins and cancers makes it imperative to assess the present state of knowledge in this area. particularly since in many of these popular publications, the issues have not been examined critically. Such literature often presents a picture that we consider to be unsound and may give poor advice or offer false hopes. Thus, for example, in the book by Berkley[7], advice is given to take extra amounts of vitamins, particularly B vitamins, A, C and E, and to make extensive use of food supplements. The author also states that he takes 4000 units (presumably 4 g) of vitamin C daily. We have pointed out previously, in reference to other popular publications, the falacious advice concerning recommendations given to consumers about vitamin supplements and cancer prevention.[77]

Hence, what is the relationship between vitamins and cancers? Because this topic has been reviewed by us and others,[46,48,49,59,73] we will summarize here the major points that can be drawn from the available literature.

Basically, there are no valid grounds to believe that there is any unique relationship between these nutrients and cancer prevention, except in specific cases, as described below. Certainly cancer cells require the nutrients for growth and proliferation, and they are susceptible to nutritional deficiencies as in the case of normal cells. This fact is made clear by use of vitamin analogs which interfere with the normal utilization of vitamins. Thus, methotrexate, which interferes with the normal cellular function of folic acid, has been found useful as a basis for cancer treatment. To date, however, other vitamin analogs such as isoriboflavin, pyrithiamin, and desoxypryidoxine, all antagonists of riboflavin, thiamin, and pyridoxine, respectively, have not found use in therapy of neoplastic disease. It does appear important, however, to further examine the possible therapeutic role of these and other vitamin antagonists in the control of tumor growth and metastasis.

Numerous animal studies (Table 6) have shown that the dietary intake of many of the vitamins may alter the outcome of experimental carcinogenesis. Thus, vitamin deficiencies or excesses may either enhance or inhibit cancer development, depending upon the specific vitamin and experimental condition examined. Some studies examining the effects of alterations in the entire vitamin B complex in relation to carcinogenesis have not demonstrated appreciable evidence for an inhibitory effect on tumor induction. In addition, diets low in B-complex vitamins had no significant effect on the induction of skin tumors in mice.[8] Furthermore, variations in the level of vitamin B-complex ranging as high as nine times the normal dietary level had no influence on mammary tumor incidence in DBA mice or on the induction of skin tumors in C_3H or DBA mice.[64]

Thiamin (vitamin B_1) has not been shown to have any influence on induction of intestinal tumors by Bracken fern.[53] However, more than 50% of the animals given thiamin supplement developed bladder tumors. Thus, it appears that thiamin, a vitamin that can be destroyed by some enzymes (thiaminases) in the diet, promoted bladder carcinogenesis in rats fed Bracken fern. To date these observations have not been confirmed.

Riboflavin affects liver tumor inductions by azo dyes. Kensler et al.[32] showed that riboflavin inhibited formation of dimethylaminoazobenzene (DAB)-induced liver tumors. Miller and Miller[40] proposed that this inhibition was a result of the role of riboflavin in the detoxification of the azo dye. In diets low in riboflavin, the enzyme responsible for detoxifying the azo dye was not sufficiently active to prevent carcinogenesis. Some riboflavin analogs are even more effective against azo dye carcinogenesis than the parent compound.[34] Thus, riboflavin may have anticarcinogenic effects through its action as a cofactor in enzyme systems that deactivate carcinogens. Pyridoxine (vitamin B_6) may have an indirect effect through its influence on tryptophan metabolism, and it perhaps permits animals to live

TABLE 6. A Selective Survey of Studies, in Experimental Animals, Concerned with the Effects of Vitamin Intake and Status on Carcinogenesis

Vitamin	Dietary condition	Observation	Author
Riboflavin	High riboflavin intake	Reduced hepatoma induction by azo dyes	Miller *et al.* (1941)
	Riboflavin deficiency	Increased aflatoxin sensitivity in chickens	Hamilton *et al.* (1974)
	Riboflavin supplementation	No effect on aflatoxin B_1 induction of liver carcinoma	Newberne *et al.* (1974)
	Riboflavin deficiency	Retards growth of tumors	Rivlin (1973)
Folic acid B_{12} Choline	Deficiency	Enhance chemical induction of liver, colon and esophageal tumors	Rogers (1975)
B_6	Deficiency	Reduced growth sarcoma 180 in mice	Littman *et al.* (1964)
B-complex	High intakes	No influence on mammary tumor induction in DBA mice	Tannenbaum and Silverstone (1952)
Thiamin	Deficiency	Protects chicks from aflatoxin B_1	Hamilton *et al.* (1974)
Vitamin A	Supplementation	Prevents epithelial tumors	Newberne and McConnel (1980)

longer so that they develop bladder tumors from acetyl-aminofluorene (AAF).[37]

In view of the role played by vitamin E in lipid peroxidation reactions *in vivo* and because free radicals might be important in tumor development,[70,75] the effects of vitamin E intake on experimental carcinogenesis have also been examined. Again, however, the results obtained in these various animal studies are not consistent.[73] It is apparent that additional investigation will be required before any definitive conclusions can be made about the relationship between vitamin E intake and cancer induction in animal model systems.

The problem is however also indicated in the listing given in Table 6, that the findings reported in literature are often conflicting and/or results difficult to evaluate. Thus, vitamin deficiencies affect overall food intake in animals; this alone might influence the utilization and metabolism of carcinogens or the metabolic status of cells. Also, interpretation of animal studies is further complicated as a result of (1) interdependent metabolic interactions among vitamins at the cellular level, as in the case of vitamin B_6, riboflavin, and niacin[60]; (2) variations in the composition of the experimental diets; (3) sex and strain of animal species; and (4) specific type of carcinogen. Rogers and Newberne[59] have pointed out these complicating factors in a recent review of the effects of lipotrope deficiency (choline, methionine, folate, B_{12}) on chemically induced hepatocarcinogenesis; however in this experimental situation of lipotrope deficiency, there is a consistent increased development of liver tumors. Nevertheless, the application to human disease of results obtained in model systems, including cell cultures and tumor-bearing animals, is difficult and uncertain. There are, however, a number of clinical findings that require mention, particularly in relation to vitamins C (ascorbic acid) and E.

Is Ascorbic Acid a General Anticancer Vitamin?

Ascorbic acid has attracted considerable attention. Two books, one dealing with the common cold and the other with cancers, have given the public, as well as professionals, much to think about. Furthermore, megadoses of vitamin C are being taken by thousands of patients with cancer, and it is pertinent to give particular emphasis here to this vitamin.

The possible role of vitamin C in the occurrence and treatment of malignant disease may be deduced from various lines of evidence; these have been discussed by Cameron *et al.*[12] in a recent review of this subject. As summarized in Table 7, ascorbic acid plays a key role in the maintenance of the intercellular matrix, whose integrity is important in the growth

TABLE 7. The Vitamin C—Cancer Connection

Theoretical aspects
   Vitamin C deficiency alters intercellular matrix
   Intercellular matrix dissolution aids tumor cell invasion and growth
   Guinea pig tumors; concentration of Vitamin C
   Vitamin C may be required for synthesis of hyaluronidose inhibitor
   Cancer patients low ascorbate reserves
   High Vitamin C intakes change immunocompetence
   Vitamin C required for phagocytosis
   Vitamin C has *in vitro* antiviral activity
Animal studies
   Conflicting results
Human studies
   Epidemiologic evidence limited
Clinical studies
   Need controlled studies

and proliferation of tumors. Ascorbic acid inhibits hyaluronidase, and it influences humoral and cellular immune function[1,54] and the metabolic processes associated with cell repair. For these reasons, it is reasonable to propose that the vitamin C status of the host would influence the development and/or outcome of human cancers. Although a reasoning similar to that given by Cameron *et al.*[12] for vitamin C could be offered for a number of the vitamins, it is important to examine whether vitamin C intakes in considerable excess of those[19] considered to be sufficient to maintain long-term health would offer a major protection from the development of human cancers. Furthermore, the following conclusion drawn by Cameron and Pauling[11] requires comment, in view of its implications for public health policy.

> We believe that the officially recommended dietary intake of about 45 mg of vitamin C intake per day is so much less than the optimum as to constitute in itself a significant cause of cancer. It is our opinion that to keep the age-specific incidence of cancer and of other diseases low it is necessary that the daily intake be at least 250 mg, and for most people a daily intake between 1g and 10g per day may lead to the best of health. · · ·

In their review of the associations between ascorbic acid and cancer, Cameron *et al.*[12] point to the equivocal nature of *in vivo* studies of the effects of ascorbic acid on tumors in experimental animals.[62] Furthermore, these investigators also considered the results of epidemiologic studies and of clinical trials in the management of human cancer. In the former instance, evidence is limited.[36] In the latter, a number of uncontrolled experiments, including those of De Cosse *et al.*,[15] where a daily supplement of ascorbic acid, 3g, was given to patients with familial polyposis, have suggested that an increasing ascorbic acid intake *might* have beneficial effects in the treatment of cancers. A quite recent, controlled study by Cregan *et al.*[14] has failed to confirm a therapeutic benefit from 10 g vitamin C per day in patients with advanced cancer (see Table 8). Although Pauling[55] considers that the earlier work of Cameron[11] was not adequately reinvestigated by Cregan *et al.*[14] in their study, and that the prior chemotherapy of the patients included in this experiment might have negated the possible benefits of vitamin C, we are forced to the conclusion that adequate, direct evidence to support the above proposition by Cameron and Pauling[11] is still lacking. In agreement with the view of Moertel and Cregan,[44] claims for benefit from high-dose vitamin C at *any* stage of malignant disease remain to be established by properly designed, prospective, randomized, and concurrently controlled studies. If positive results are obtained in such studies, it would also be important to examine dose responses since Migliozzi[39] found that, in the methylcholanthrene-induced guinea pig system, tumor regression was noted in 55% of animals receiving a low vitamin C intake (0.3 mg/kg/day), whereas tumor growth was stimulated by massive doses (10g/kg/day), of ascorbic acid in this model system.

This does not mean that vitamin supplementation, including ascorbic acid, should not be part of the treatment of cancer patients, who often show low vitamin C status[12]; and drug therapy can also interfere with the utilization of individual vitamins.[22] Thus, it must be recognized that systemic and infectious diseases often lead to increased losses of vitamins, including ascorbic acid[69] from the body; under these circumstances, the need for them, as well as for other essential nutrients, is raised.[5] The specific problem, however, is that there is no evidence to suggest that this catabolic response is specific for neoplastic disease or for vitamin C, in particular. It is important that adequate nutrition constitutes an essential component of comprehensive treatment in *all* hospitalized patients. In our judgment, therefore, recommendations for megadose intakes of vitamin C as a means of preventing human cancers is premature and unsupported on the basis of present evidence. Nevertheless, the proponents of this approach have developed a rationale that merits further critical investigation in human studies.

Vitamin C and E in Relation to Formation of Nitrosamine and Fecal Mutagens

Since the early 1960s, published reports have shown that nitrite can react with other chemicals (amines or amides) to form a family of compounds called nitrosamines.[27] Nitrite formation occurs within the body.[66,68]

TABLE 8. Summary of Results of Double-Blind Study on High-dose Vitamin C in Cancer Patients*

	Vitamin C group	Placebo
No. of patients	60	63
Tumor characteristics		
Colorectal	24	26
Pancreas	12	12
Lung	6	6
Stomach	5	5
Other	12	16
Previous treatment		
None	5	4
Radiation	17	18
Chemotherapy	52	56
Results		
Survival	—No difference—	
Symptoms	—No difference—	

* Cregan *et al.* (*N Engl J Med 1979*; 301:687–691).

Furthermore, this nitrite can then be converted to a nitrosating agent. Via interaction with a suitable secondary or tertiary nitrogen compound, it gives rise to potentially carcinogenic N-nitroso compounds. This process occurs extensively throughout the digestive tract and this may contribute significantly to the body burden of carcinogens.[66,71] Of particular relevance to the present topic is the discovery that ascorbic acid can block these nitrosation reactions, *in vitro* and *in vivo*, with consequent reductions in formation of nitrosamine[43,43] and nitrosamide.[56,72] In addition, vitamin E also inhibits these reactions.[31,38] Furthermore, as summarized in Table 9, the combined actions of ascorbic acid and vitamin E may serve to enhance inhibition of these reactions.[67] Because nitrosation can take place in both the aqueous and lipid phases of the intestinal tract contents, and since ascorbate occurs in the aqueous phase and of tocopherol in the non-aqueous phase, a possible synergistic effect on the inhibition of formation N-nitroso compounds may be obtained when both vitamins are given together. However, it should be pointed out that these blocking functions of ascorbic acid and tocopherol are unrelated to their physiologic functions as vitamins.

TABLE 9. Effect of Vitamins C and E on Formation of N-Nitroso Compounds

1. N-nitroso compounds: From interaction of nitrosating agent with secondary or tertiary N compound
2. N-nitroso compounds: many carcinogenic
3. Nitrite converted to nitrosating agent
4. Vitamin C blocks nitrosation
5. Vitamin E blocks nitrosation
6. These vitamins may act in concert (*i.e.*, in aqueous and lipid phases)
7. Blocking action unrelated to vitamin function

Finally, Bruce and coworkers[10] have found that the amount of mutagen in the feces of normal humans can be reduced by administering vitamin C, and that high oral doses of vitamin E acetate result in increased fecal levels of vitamin E in healthy adults.[67]

These various observations offer an exciting opportunity for further research, but there is still a great deal to be learned before these aspects of the chemistry of vitamins C and E can be translated into safe and rational food and public health policy.

The "Fake" Vitamins

As stated earlier, cancer quackery includes dietary regimens, and this encompasses promotion of substances that are stated to be vitamins in human nutrition and alleged to provide a "cure" for cancers. Among these compounds are laetrile and pangamic acid. These have been the topic of two popular but not-to-be-recommended books that we purchased recently at a major bookstore that serves the private and university community in the Cambridge area. Neither substance is a vitamin, according to the accepted definition discussed earlier; nor are they effective in the prevention or treatment of cancers or any other condition.[18,20,23,24]

Briefly, laetrile, sometimes called vitamin B_{17} by its proponents, is a cyanogenic glucoside, consisting of glucose, benzaldehyde, and cyanide. It is present in the pits of peaches, apricots, bitter almonds, and in other plant material. This substance has caused death in a number of recently documented cases,[23] and the laetriles have long been known to be poisonous. Claims of its efficacy as a cancer "cure" are based on anecdotal evidence that lacks scientific support. The rationale for its use, namely, the selective release of lethal amounts of hydrocyanic acid in tumor cells, is spurious.[20] Furthermore, Herbert[23] has presented evidence that laetriles may actually *cause* cancer. *In vitro* and *in vivo* testing in animal tumor systems have shown that amygdalin is entirely devoid of anticancer activity.[23]

Another substance, termed "B_{15}" or pangamic acid, currently appears in advertisements for vitamin supplements. The substance consists of a variable mixture that includes calcium gluconate, calcium chloride, dimethylglycine, D-gluconic acid-6-bis(1-methylethyl)amino acetate, glycine, and diisopropylamine dichloracetate. However, as Herbert[24] has pointed out, there is no standard of identity for the product, the term "pangamic acid" apparently is used indiscriminately regardless of which of the various adducts are on the ester linkage. There is no proof that it is safe for human use, nor has any therapeutic benefit been demonstrated in scientifically acceptable studies, despite allegations that it has value in the treatment of various diseases, including schizophrenia, hepatitis, and cancer. Indeed, Herbert[24] states that the product may be mutagenic. Finally, in reference to the food additive regulations by the U. S. Food and Drug Administration, it is illegal to promote pangamic acid as a dietary supplement.

In summary, the promotion and selling of laetrile and pangamic acid are among the worst of "remedies." Indeed, Dorr and Paxinos[18] have concluded that studies in humans with laetrile would appear to be contraindicated from the data available in animal studies and observed human toxicities to this substance.

Recommendations

Research

Based on the foregoing, there is little doubt that there are many experimental circumstances in which the level of intake of individual vitamins and/or the vitamin status of the host organism can influence the development of cancers. However, the present state of knowledge does not provide a clear picture of the role of vitamins, either individually or in combination with others, in cancer causation. Thus, there is little basis at present for drawing definitive conclusions or predictive value and significance for sound public health and nutrition policy. In order to achieve this goal, it is essential to explore further and better understand the mechanisms by which nutritional factors in general and vitamin deficiencies or excesses in particular modulate the response of animals to carcinogens. This will require testing of additional model systems and further exploration and refinement of those that have already been described. Nevertheless, it is evident that use of nutritional factors adds to the tools available for investigation of the mechanisms of carcinogenesis. In this context, the study of vitamin intakes in animals provides an immediate contribution to the challenge of reducing cancer incidence and risk in human populations.

The evidence that the intakes of vitamins and vitamin nutritional status in apparently healthy individuals in our population, or any other for that matter, play a causative role in the major cancer types is fragmentary and largely circumstantial. However, for some cancers and vitamins there have been some important research developments that justify intensification of efforts to identify and unravel the possible relationships between vitamins and human cancers. This is particularly relevant in the case of vitamin A or its analog and cancers of epithelial tissues, as well as for Vitamins C and E in relation to their nonvitamin or pharmaceutical role in blocking formation of putative carcinogenic N-nitroso compounds. Furthermore, a metabolic rationale has been offered that vitamin C may be a general anticancer agent,[12] and this deserves further study. However, it should be recognized that from a knowledge of the metabolic functions played by many of the individual vitamins, an equally strong argument for further investigation of the possible involvement of these vitamins in the development of human carcinomas can be made.

It is also desirable to explore, in epidemiologic studies, the role of vitamins in cancer prevention, but this will not be easily accomplished.

(1) First, there are close associations between the various dietary factors that complicate study of the possible importance of vitamins, *per se*.[33]

(2) Second, the assessment of vitamin nutritional status is not readily achieved, either because of the limited applicability of the most precise methods for determination of vitamin nutriture in extensive field surveys of populations involving subjects of all ages, or because current methods may not be adequate for evaluating the role of vitamin nutrition and status in populations with differing cancer type and incidence.

(3) Third, the prolonged lag time between initiation of a carcinogenic insult and the development of a carcinoma, and in view of the fact that clinical cancer is the end result of multiple influences at the cellular level,[25] makes the epidemiologic study of the role of vitamins in cancer causation and prevention an even more difficult task. However, in spite of these problems, careful attention should be given to the possibility that inappropriate intakes of some of the vitamins may enhance human susceptibility to some of the major cancers. The possibility of improving treatment of established cancers through selective use of vitamins, or their analogs and their antagonists deserves increased research attention. This, of course, concerns therapy rather than prevention.

Consumers

What recommendations are appropriate for the consumer or the patient who requests the advice of a health professional about vitamins and cancer, considering the nature of the available evidence discussed above? Should generous supplements of vitamins C and E be recommended when we eat our meals, especially those including pickled and highly salted foods, and broiled or fried meats? Is there a place for multivitamin supplements as a general and effective means of reducing cancer risk? Should we buy pills of vitamin A, C, E and/or other vitamins each

time we purchase a processed food at the local supermarket? Our answer is that present evidence *does not* support the promotion of *any* vitamin supplement as an effective or rational approach to reducing risk of cancer in humans at any stage of their lives, providing the diet is based on a wide selection of foods that are commonly available and at reasonable cost for the majority of people. Although Williams,[74] who has made important contributions to the further understanding of the basis and extent of the variability in nutrient requirements among individuals, might regard our conclusions as representative of a "waiting" philosophy, or, as he states, "wait until cancer growth becomes apparent then try to cut it out or burn it out with suitable radiation," we maintain that our view is the best that can be offered and there is no evidence to the contrary, in relation to vitamins and cancer causation and prevention in our population.

Indeed, the consumer should also be made aware of the fact that vitamins can be toxic and they cannot be used indiscriminately. For example, high doses of vitamin C are not without untoward effects[4] and some of these are listed in Table 10, as an example. Most of the unfavorable responses that have been described are more troublesome than they are a threat to health, but in some cases, they may have serious consequences. Indeed, from the above, we cannot subscribe to the notion that "high potency" vitamin supplements or the continued intakes of "megadoses" of vitamins provide an important and effective approach to protection from degenerative diseases, including cancer. Prescription of specific vitamins in therapeutic or pharmacological amounts should be made only where there is evidence of vitamin deficiencies or increased requirements to support maintenance of normal physiologic and behavioral states. Vitamin supplements to meet recommended daily dietary allowances, as we have already stated, may be taken as an "insurance" against poor dietary habits, but, in this case, the more adequate nutritional advice would be to improve overall dietary habits. Furthermore, it is easy to choose a diet based on common foods that will meet the energy requirements of individuals and, at the same time, supply the 14 vitamins in excess of the recommended daily allowances.[19] This diet, therefore, would meet the needs of some individuals with vitamin requirements

TABLE 10. Some Reported Untoward Effects of Ascorbic Acid

Acidosis	Fatigue
Oxaluria	Sterility
Renal stones	B_{12} destruction
GI disturbances	
Conditioned need	

that are considerably higher than those for most other members of the population. Nevertheless, we do recognize that in view of the growing evidence concerning the possible causative interrelationships between nitrosamines and ascorbic acid in the incidence of gastric cancer, a case might be made for recommending a moderate level of ascorbic acid supplementation in individuals at high risk, such as those with atrophic gastritis, partial gastrectomy, or whenever gastric acid secretion is significantly compromised. In addition, individuals with high risk of cancers of the lower bowel, for example, such as those with polyposis or ulcerative colitis, may also benefit from a supplement of ascorbic acid. This is speculative and an optimum supplementation schedule cannot be defined, at this stage, if indeed there is one. We anticipate with continued research progress in this area of vitamins and cancer prevention that a more specific recommendation should be possible within the next few years.

The above does not mean, of course, that particular attention should not be given to diet and nutritional factors as a means of reducing risk of developing cancer. Present evidence suggests that prudence in dietary choices and food habits offers the most reasonable approach to modifying the nutritional component of our increasingly complex environment and pattern of lifestyle. However, drastic changes in dietary habits or exclusion of individual foods are probably not necessary for the vast majority of individuals.

This advice is based on our informed reasoning and it is consistent with the discharge of the responsibilities that we, as nutrition professionals, must be prepared to make in translating the fruits of nutrition research to the health and welfare of the society. It would be irresponsible to recommend otherwise.

REFERENCES

1. Anderson R, Oasthuizen R, Maritz R, Theron A, Van Rensburg AJ. The effects of increasing weekly doses of ascorbate on certain cellular and humoral immune functions in normal volunteers. *Am J Chem Nutr* 1980; 33:71–76.
2. Anon. Does pyridoxal phosphate have a non-coenzymatic role in steroid-hormone action? *Nutr Rev* 1980; 38:93–95.
3. Barchi RL. In: Gubler CJ, Fujiwara M, Dreyfus PM, eds. Thiamin. New York: John Wiley and Sons, 1975:283–305.
4. Barness LA. Some toxic effects of vitamin C. In: Hauck A, Ritzel G, eds. Re-evaluation of vitamin C. Bern, Switzerland: Verlag Hans Huber, 1977:23–29.
5. Beisel WR. Nutrient wastage during infection. In: McKigney JI, Munro HN, eds. Nutrient requirements in adolescence. Cambridge, Mass.: M.I.T. Press, 1975:257–278.
6. Berg JW. Can nutrition explain the pattern of international epidemiology of hormone-dependent cancers? *Cancer Res* 1975; 35:3345–3350.
7. Berkley GE. Cancer: How to prevent it and how to help your doctor fight it. Englewood Cliff: Prentice Hall, Inc., 1978:242.
8. Boutwell RK, Brush MK, Rusch HP. The influence of vitamins of the B complex on the induction of epithelial tumors in mice. *Cancer Res* 1949; 9:747–752.
9. Brown GM. The biosynthesis of pteridines. *Adv Enzymol* 1971; 35:35–77.
10. Bruce WR, Varghesa AJ, Furner R, Land PC. A mutagen in the feces of normal humans. In: Origins of human cancer. New York: Cold Spring Harbor Laboratory, 1977:1641–1642.
11. Cameron E, Pauling L. Cancer and vitamin C. Menlo Park, Cal.: Linus Pauling Institute of Science and Medicine 1979:238.
12. Cameron E, Pauling L, Leibowitz B. Ascorbic acid and cancer: A review. *Cancer Res* 1979; 39:663–681.
13. Chow CK. Nutritional influence on cellular antioxidant defense systems. *Am J Clin Nutr* 1979; 32:1066–1081.
14. Cregan ET, Moertel CG, O'Fallon JR, et al. Failure of high-dose vitamin C (ascorbic acid) therapy to benefit patients with advanced cancer: A controlled trial. *N Eng J Med* 1979; 301:68–691.
15. De Cosse JJ, Adams MB, Kuzma JF, LoGerfo P, Condon RE. Effect of ascorbic acid on rectal polyps of patients with familial polyposis. *Surgery* 1975; 78:608–612.
16. De Luca H. Vitamin D. In: Alfin-Slater RB, Kritchevsky D, eds. Nutrition and the adult: Micronutrients. New York: Plenum Press, 1980:205–244.
17. Doll R. Strategy for detection of cancer hazards to man. *Nature* 1977; 265:589–596.
18. Dorr RT, Paxinos J. The current status of laetrile. *Ann Int Med* 1978; 89:389–397.
19. Food and Nutrition Board. Recommended Dietary Allowances, 9th rev ed. Washington, DC: National Academy Sciences, 1979.
20. Greenberg DM. The vitamin found in cancer quackery. *West J Med* 1975; 122:354–358.
21. Hamilton PB, Tung HT, Wyatt RD, Donaldson WE. Interaction of dietary aflatoxin with some vitamin deficiencies. *Poult Sci* 1974; 53:871–877.
22. Hathcock JN, Coon J eds. Nutrition and drug interrelationships. New York: Academic Press, 1978:927.
23. Herbert V. Laetrile: The cult of cyanide. Promoting poison for profit. *Am J Clin Nutr* 1979; 32:1121–1158.
24. Herbert V. Pangamic acid ("Vitamin B$_{15}$") *Am J Clin Nutr* 1979; 32:1534–1540.
25. Higginson J, Muir CS. Environmental carcinogens: Misconceptions and limitations to cancer control. *J Natl Cancer Inst* 1979; 63:1291–1298.
26. Isler C. The fatal choice: Cancer quackery. *RN* 1974; 37:55–59.
27. Issenberg P. Nitrite, nitrosamines and cancer. *Fed Proc* 1976; 35:1322–1326.
28. IUNS—International Union of Nutritional Sciences, Committee on Nomenclature. Tentative rules for generic descriptors and trivial names of vitamins and related compounds. *Nutr Abstr Rev* 1970; 40:395–400.
29. Johnson FC. The antioxidant vitamins. CRC *Crit Rev Food Sci Nutr* 1979; 11:217–310.
30. Jukes TH. Megavitamins and food fads. In: Hodges RE, ed. Nutrition metabolic and clinical applications New York: Plenum Press, 1979; 257–292.
31. Kamm JJ, Dashman T, Newmark H. Inhibition of aminonitrate hepatotoxicity by α-tocopherol. *Toxicol Appl Pharmacol* 1977; 41:575–583.
32. Kensler CJ. Sugiuira K, Young MF, Halter CR, Rhoads, CP. Partial protection of rats by riboflavin with casein against liver cancer caused by dimethylamino azobenzene. *Science* 1941; 93:308–310.
33. Knox EG. Foods and diseases. *Br J Prev Soc Med* 1977; 31:71–80.
34. Lambooy JP. Riboflavin protection against azo hepatoma induction in the rat. *Proc Soc Exp Biol Med* 1970; 134:192–194.
35. Littman ML, Taguchi T, Shimizu Y. Retarding effect of vitamin deficient and cholesterol free diets on growth and sarcoma. *Proc Soc Exp Biol Med* 1964; 116:95–101.

36. Marquardt H, Rufino F, Weisberger JH. On the aetiology of gastric cancer: Mutagenicity of food extracts after incubation with nitrite. *Food Cosmet Toxicol* 1977; 15:97–100.

37. Melicow MM, Uson AC, Price ID. Bladder tumor induction in rats fed 2-AAF and a pyridoxine deficient diet. *J Urol* 1964; 91:520–529.

38. Mergens WJ, Kamm JJ, Newmark HL. Alpha-tocopherol: Uses in preventing nitrosamine formation. In: Environmental aspects of N-nitroso compounds. *IARC Sci Publ* 1978; 19: 199–212.

39. Migliozzi JA. Effect of ascorbic acid on tumor growth. *Br J Cancer* 1977; 35:448–543.

40. Miller JA, Miller EC. The carcinogenic amino azo dyes. *Adv Cancer Res* 1953; 1:339–396.

41. Miller JA, Minor DL, Rusch HP, Baumann CA. Diet and hepatic tumor formation. *Cancer Res* 1941; 1:699.

42. Mirvish SS. Blocking the formation of N-nitroso compounds with ascorbic acid *in vitro* and *in vivo*. *Am NY Acad Sci* 1975; 258:175–180.

43. Mirvish SS. N-nitroso compounds: Their chemical and *in vivo* formation and possible importance as environmental carcinogens. *J Toxicol Environ Health* 1977; 2:1267–1277.

44. Moertel CG, Cregan ET. Letter to editor. *N Engl J Med* 1980; 302:694–695.

45. Munro HN. Nutritional requirements in health. *Crit Care Med* 1979; 8:2–8.

46. Newberne PM. Environmental modifiers of susceptibility to carcinogenesis. *Cancer Detection and Prevention* 1976; 1: 129–173.

47. Newberne PM, Chan WM, Rogers AE. Influence of light, riboflavin and carotene on the response of rats to acute toxicity of aflaxtoxin and monocrotaline. *Toxicol Appl Pharmacol* 1974; 28:200–208.

48. Newberne PM, McConnell RG. Nutrient deficiencies in cancer causation. *J Environ Pathol Toxicol* 1980; 3:323–356.

49. Newberne PM, Rogers AE, Gross RL. Nutritional modulation of carcinogenesis. In: Nieburgs HE, ed. Prevention and detection of cancer, Part 1. Prevention. Volume 1. Etiology. New York: Marcel Dekker, Inc., 1977:665–691.

50. Niederwieser A, Curtius H-Ch, Betloni O, *et al.* Atypical phenylketonuria caused by 7,8-dihydrobiopterin synthetase deficiency. *Lancet* 1979; 1:131–133.

51. Nishikimi M, Uderfriend S. Scurvy as an inborn error of ascorbic acid biosynthesis. *TIBS* May 1980; 111–113.

52. Olson RE. Vitamin K. In: Alfin-Slater RB, Kritchev D, eds. Nutrition and the adult: Micronutrients. New York: Plenum Press, 1980:267–286.

53. Pamucka AM, Walciner S, Price JM, Bryan GT. Effects of the co-administration of thiamine on the incidence of urinary bladder carcinomas in rats fed Bracken fern. *Cancer Res* 1970; 30:2671–2674.

54. Panush RS, Delafuente JC. Modulation of certain immunological responses by vitamin C. In: Hanck A, Ritzel G, eds. Vitamin C. Bern, Switzerland: Hans Huber Publishers, 1979: 179–199.

55. Pauling L. Vitamin C therapy of advanced cancer. *N Eng J Med* 1980; 302:694.

56. Raineri R, Weisberger JH. Reduction of gastric carcinogens with ascorbic acid. *Ann NY Acad Sci* 1975; 258:181–189.

57. Rivlin RS. Riboflavin and cancer: A review. *Cancer Res* 1975; 33:1977.

58. Rogers AE. Variable effects of a lipotrope-deficient, high-fat diet on chemical carcinogenesis in rats. *Cancer Res* 1975; 35:2469–2474.

59. Rogers AE, Newberne PM. Lipotrope deficiency in experimental carcinogenesis. *Nutrition and Cancer* 2:2 1980:104–112.

60. Sauberlich HE. Biosynthesis of vitamin B_6. In: Sebell WH Jr, Harris RS, eds. The vitamins, Vol. II. New York: Academic Press, 1968:31–33.

61. Shive W, Lansbord EM, Jr. Roles of vitamins as coenzymes. In: Alfin-Slater RB, Kritchevsky D, eds. Nutrition and the Adult: Micronutrients. New York: Plenum Press, 1980:1–71.

62. Siegel BW, Leibovitz DP. Vitamin C in aging and cancer. In: Hanck A, Ritzel G, eds. Vitamin C. Bern, Switzerland: Hans Huber Publishers, 1970:9–24.

63. Sporn MB, Dunlop NM, Newlon DL, Smith JM. Prevention of chemical carcinogenesis by vitamin A and its synthetic analogs (retinoids). *Fed Proc* 1976; 35:1332–1338.

64. Tannenbaum A, Silverstone H. The genesis and growth of tumors. V. Effects of varying the level of B. vitamins in the diet. *Cancer Res* 1952; 12:744–749.

65. Tannenbaum A, Silverstone H. Nutrition and the genesis of tumors. In: Raven RW, ed. Cancer. London: Butterworth and Company, 1957:306–334.

66. Tannenbaum SR. Endogeneous formation of nitrite and N-nitroso compounds. In: Miller EC, *et al.*, eds. Naturally occurring carcinogens—mutagens and modulators of carcinogenesis. Baltimore: University Park Press, 1979:211–220.

67. Tannenbaum SR, Mergens W. Reaction of nitrite with vitamins C and E. In: Proc Conf on Micronutrient interactions: Vitamins, minerals and hazardous elements. New York Acad. Sci. Feb. 20, 1980 (in press).

68. Tannenbaum SR, Young VR. Endogenous nitrate formation in man. *J Environ Pathol Toxicol* 1980; 3:357–368.

69. Tolbert BM. Ascorbic and metabolism and physiological function. In: Hanck A, Ritzel G, eds. Vitamin C. Bern, Switzerland: Hans Huber Publishers, 1979:127–142.

70. Ts'o POP, Caspary WJ, Lorentzen RJ. The involvement of free radicals in chemical carcinogenesis. In: Pryor WA, ed. Free radicals in biology. Vol. III, Chpt 7. New York: Academic Press, 1977:251–303.

71. Weisberger JH, Raineri R. Dietary factors and the etiology of gastric cancer. *Cancer Res* 1975; 35:3469–3474.

72. Weisberger HJ. Mechanism of action of diet as a carcinogen. *Nutrition and Cancer* 1979; 1:74–81.

73. Wells P, Alfin-Slater RB. The relationship of diet and nutritional status to cancer. In: Hodges RE, ed. Nutrition metabolic and clinical applications. New York: Plenum Press, 1979; 183–214.

74. Williams RJ. Nutrition against disease. New York: Pitman Publ. Corp., 1971:370.

75. Wilson RL, Hydroxyl radicals and biological damage *in vitro*: What relevance *in vivo*? In: Oxygen free radicals and tissue damage. CIBA Foundation Symposium 65 (new series) Amsterdam: Excerpta Medica, 1980:19–35.

76. Wolf G. Vitamin A. In: Alfin-Slater RB, Kritchevsky D, eds. Nutrition and the adult: Micronutrients. New York: Plenum Press, 1980:97–203.

77. Young VR, Richardson DP. Nutrients, vitamins and minerals in cancer prevention. Facts and fallacies. *Cancer* 1979; 43: 2125–2136.

Manipulation of Nutrients to Prevent Cancer

by Peter Greenwald

Laboratory and epidemiologic data strongly suggest that changes in diet can influence human cancer risk. To develop more definitive information, the National Cancer Institute has two research programs: one to investigate the safety and efficacy of specific chemicals and micronutrients; the other to study the effects of macronutrients such as fat on cancer incidence.

It is generally agreed that environmental factors are involved in most human cancers, and two factors, tobacco and diet, have a particularly large impact. According to some estimates, each of the two may account for 30% or more of all cancers in the U.S. and similar populations. (Tobacco will be discussed by C. Everett Koop in the next article in this series.)

Admittedly, the influence of diet on the development of human cancer is currently not as clearly defined as that of tobacco, and the proportion of cancers in which diet may play an etiologic role cannot yet be estimated with precision. Those deficiencies reflect the complexities inherent in the study of both nutrition and tumor development. As is well known, diet is a multifaceted entity; it is made up of broad food groups, or macronutrients, with a host of individual constituents, or micronutrients. Since overt human cancers may take many years to develop, and since experimental models of carcinogenesis show that tumors evolve through a multistage process in which more than one etiologic factor may participate, it is easy to appreciate the difficulties in establishing links between dietary factors and cancer.

Nevertheless, such links exist, however imperfectly understood they may be. Data from a large

Dr. Greenwald is Director, Division of Cancer Prevention and Control, National Cancer Institute, National Institutes of Health, Bethesda.

body of epidemiologic and laboratory studies conducted during the past few decades converge to support the hypothesis that some diets can increase cancer risk, whereas others offer some protection. Those data also provide us with specific leads, some of which have already been mentioned or discussed in this series. For example, among macronutrients implicated as modifiers of tumor development, high fat intake looms prominently as a likely cause of large-bowel and breast cancers and may also be involved in cancers of the prostate, endometrium, and other sites; conversely, high dietary fiber intake is postulated to protect against large-bowel cancer (see D. P. Burkitt, "Etiology and Prevention of Colorectal Cancer," HP, February; and E. L. Wynder and D. P. Rose, "Diet and Breast Cancer," HP, April). As for micronutrients that may influence carcinogenesis, much attention has been focused on the possibly protective effects of vitamins C, E, and A—the last including both naturally occurring (e.g., the vitamin A precursor β-carotene) and synthetic retinoids; in addition, a similar role has been suggested for some minerals, of which perhaps the foremost is selenium.

Now that we have such leads, what will we do with them, and how will we find and develop other leads?

To answer that question, the National Cancer Institute charged its Division of Cancer Prevention and Control with planning and administering two closely related programs: the Diet, Nutrition, and Cancer Program, which was established in 1975 and is now receiving increased emphasis, and the recently established Chemoprevention Program. The former deals chiefly with macronutrients; its studies will examine the effects of rough percentage changes—additions or subtractions—in food classes or nutrient content that may lower cancer incidence. The Chemoprevention Program focuses on micronutrients; it entails the introduction into the diet of vitamins, synthetic analogues, and other defined chemicals—again, with a view toward reducing cancer incidence.

The two programs, of course, are a good deal more complex than those thumbnail descriptions suggest. Both programs will address questions about the bioavailability of possibly helpful food constituents and chemopreventive agents along with those concerning safety, metabolic, and other host factors and their interactions with environmental factors. Moreover, both programs rely on an integration of basic epidemiologic and laboratory data as a prerequisite to devising human intervention studies in high-risk or general populations.

Of the two largely dietary approaches to cancer control, it is readily apparent that chemoprevention has two major theoretical advantages. First, it examines the effects of discrete, relatively well-defined substances, and the findings may therefore be easier to analyze. The second can be stated in the proposition that, from a public health point of view, it is often easier to prescribe rather than to proscribe. The prevention of cancer in the general population may be easier to achieve by adding relatively small amounts of some constituent(s) to the diet than by attempting major modifications in dietary habits and life-styles.

With or without inherent advantages, any effective program must define its agenda and organize its activities. For that purpose, both the Chemoprevention Program and the Diet, Nutrition, and Cancer Program follow a planning model developed by Louis Carrese and his colleagues at the National Cancer Institute. Based on a method known as the convergence technique, the model is essentially an outline of a process in which four major components interact: research, methods development, operations, and resources. In turn, each of the components is organized around three activities: laboratory, epidemiologic, and human intervention studies.

Each component is made up of stages, with decision points along the way controlling movement from stage to stage. The first, or research, component requires a description of research judged necessary to reach program objectives plus the formulation of sequentially ordered stages for that research to follow. The second component involves identification of the methods available or in need of development that are required to conduct the research described in each of the stages for laboratory, epidemiologic, and human intervention studies. The managerial, administrative, and informational supports necessary for the program are described in the third component; and finally, the personnel, facilities, materials, and funds that are needed for each stage are identified in the fourth.

As noted, all working components of the model consist of laboratory, epidemiologic, and human intervention research. The flow of that research logic is envisioned as beginning with one sequence of stages in laboratory research and another in epidemiologic research and leading from the application of either source in human intervention studies (Figure 1).

To illustrate, the Chemoprevention Program's first stage in laboratory research is a review of available information on potential cancer inhibitors. If further laboratory evaluation of a given substance is judged appropriate, stage II studies are performed to clarify its efficacy, pharmacology, and toxicity in animals. If the agent is still promising, stage III animal studies are performed: comparison with other agents, its effects in combination with other agents, and additional toxicity studies—particularly, long-term studies—which are prerequisites to possible human use. The results are then evaluated for advancement to human intervention studies.

Running parallel with this sequence is a series of epidemiologic studies. It, too, begins with a review of the literature and current research in order to identify agents for further investigation. But its first stage includes two other activities as well: identifying suitable populations for epidemiologic and human intervention studies and monitoring ongoing "natural experiments" (e.g., changes in a population's life-style, especially with respect to dietary or environmental factors). Stage II studies will be more rigorous and critically focused. If a lead is already strong enough not to require such confirmatory studies, the data may be reviewed

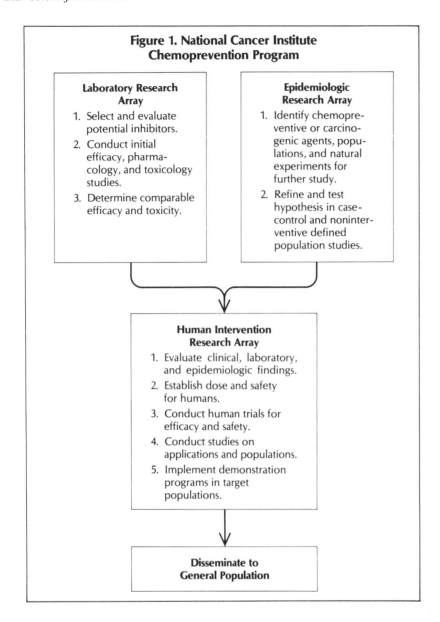

Figure 1. National Cancer Institute Chemoprevention Program

Laboratory Research Array

1. Select and evaluate potential inhibitors.
2. Conduct initial efficacy, pharmacology, and toxicology studies.
3. Determine comparable efficacy and toxicity.

Epidemiologic Research Array

1. Identify chemopreventive or carcinogenic agents, populations, and natural experiments for further study.
2. Refine and test hypothesis in case-control and noninterventive defined population studies.

Human Intervention Research Array

1. Evaluate clinical, laboratory, and epidemiologic findings.
2. Establish dose and safety for humans.
3. Conduct human trials for efficacy and safety.
4. Conduct studies on applications and populations.
5. Implement demonstration programs in target populations.

Disseminate to General Population

against the next set of decision criteria for possible direct advancement to human intervention studies.

Finally, there are five stages in the human intervention sequence. The first is an evaluation of all information gathered thus far. At that decision point, a lead may progress to human studies for either of two reasons: The laboratory or the epidemiologic data are very strong, or the laboratory and the epidemiologic data together are moderately

strong. For agents meeting either criterion, the next stage involves small-scale trials in order to establish dosage and safety levels for humans. In stage III, the data base on the agent's efficacy and safety is expanded, with a risk-benefit analysis figuring heavily in the evaluation of findings. If the results are promising, the fourth stage, in which research on applications and populations is performed, may be begun. That stage addresses questions concerning

the various ways in which an agent may be used (e.g., in capsule form or added to the diet) and the types of populations that might benefit most from such applications. After all criteria are met, the fifth, and final, stage is a demonstration program in larger target populations, followed by an evaluation point at which ongoing monitoring of the populations must document that the anticipated effect actually occurred.

The same process is followed in the Diet, Nutrition, and Cancer Program. Where the two programs differ lies largely in the methods used to answer some specific questions along the way; the methods are dictated by obvious differences in the nature of the factors under study. In the Chemoprevention Program, for example, stage II laboratory studies may involve identifying, acquiring, or producing a given agent. In addition, the agent's pharmacology and toxicology at levels required to inhibit carcinogenesis in animals are investigated. In contrast, stage II laboratory studies in the Diet, Nutrition, and Cancer Program use experimental and control diets to accomplish its goals, which include determining whether the intake of those diets and their biochemical end points can be monitored adequately. Similarly, the Chemoprevention Program's stage II human intervention studies involve pharmacologic end points to help establish initial intake and safety levels for humans, whereas the equivalent studies in the Diet, Nutrition, and Cancer Program emphasize biochemical end points.

With both programs organized according to that planning model, we now have a systematic strategy for pursuing new and future research on cancer prevention through dietary means. That is clearly better than having no strategy at all, since it shortens the time for achievement of broad public benefit from current research. For the first time, human cancer prevention trials are being emphasized. But investigation of the influence of macronutrients and micronutrients (and related substances) on tumor development is hardly new. It stretches back many years, and there are a number of projects in the field that already have a long history in laboratory and epidemiologic research.

How well does the strategy deal with investigator-initiated research? For large-scale, collaborative trials, the answer is still being worked out, particularly in the Diet, Nutrition, and Cancer Program, whose activities are not yet as developed as those in the Chemoprevention Program. Progress made in the latter program, however, suggests that the overall planning model is indeed flexible enough to accommodate previously established as well as new research projects. To illustrate, our Chemoprevention Program is currently sponsoring about 20 human intervention trials. Most of them were investigator-initiated, but many were also stimulated by advisory-group and workshop efforts that went into planning the program. Some developed in response to a request for applications that our division formulated and announced as "The Role of Natural Inhibitors in the Prevention of Cancer."

No fewer than 15 of the trials relate, at least in part, to retinoids. There are already considerable data on the influence of retinoids—vitamin A, provitamin A (mainly β-carotene), and synthetic analogues of vitamin A—on the development of cancer (see M. B. Sporn, "Retinoids and Suppression of Carcinogenesis," HP, October 1983). Altogether, the existing laboratory research on the subject certainly makes a strong case for further studies of retinoids and cancer, especially with respect to synthetic retinoids. But what about the complementary data from epidemiologic research?

Over the years, at least 24 studies have examined human cancer risk in relation to dietary intake of vitamin A or β-carotene; nearly all found an inverse correlation. To be sure, there are weaknesses in the evidence. In order to estimate vitamin A intake, for example, data on the consumption of such foods as milk, cheese, butter, eggs, and liver are needed; for β-carotene intake, consumption of dark-green leafy vegetables, carrots, and certain yellow or red fruits and vegetables must be analyzed. But it is often extremely difficult to determine with any precision what people eat, especially in retrospective studies. It also is widely recognized that an epidemiologic association between a given dietary component and cancer protection may be incidental, thus reflecting unrecognized ingestion of truly protective components or avoidance of harmful components. For example, someone whose vegetable consumption is above average may get high levels of β-carotene but also gets other micronutrients and usually has a lower than average intake of fat.

One strong argument against the influence of those and other potential flaws is that the available epidemiologic data on dietary retinoid intake and cancer risk are consistent with related findings in the laboratory. Another is that the epidemiologic data are internally consistent; that is, the results of studies of and by different groups and involving various protocols generally agree.

To illustrate the second point, I will briefly review some salient studies in the literature. In 1975, E. Bjelke reported on 8,278 Norwegian men who had responded to mailed questionnaires about smoking and diet and were then followed for five years, with the development of cancer monitored by a linkup with Norway's cancer registry. At the end of the study period, 36 bronchus or lung cancers had developed in the group. Using the dietary information, Bjelke devised a vitamin A index that was based chiefly on consumption levels of carrots, milk, and eggs. When the cancer and dietary data were stratified according to smoking status, it was found that, with respect to the vitamin A index, men in the bottom third of the study group had about three times the risk of lung cancer as those in the top two thirds (Table 1). Bjelke recently updated that study, which now includes more than 100 cases of cancer and further supports a negative association between lung cancer incidence and vitamin A intake.

In 1979, T. Hirayama reported the results of a similar prospective study in Japan. It involved 265,118 people, who completed an extensive dietary questionnaire in 1965 and were then followed for 10 years. Among that group, 807 died of lung cancer during the study period. When the data were standardized for age, sex, and smoking status, Hirayama found that the relative risk of lung cancer was a statis-

Table 1. Lung Cancer Risk Related to Cigarette Smoking and Dietary Vitamin A

Cigarette-Smoking Status	Vitamin A Index*		
	A. < 5	B. > 5	B ÷ A
	5-Year Lung Ca Incidence/1,000		
≥ 20 per day	21.0	7.4	0.35
1–19 per day	12.8	5.7	0.45
Ex-smoker	6.1	1.5	0.25
Nonsmoker	1.1	1.2	1.10
All subjects	7.3	2.8	0.38

*Index is based chiefly on carrots, milk, and eggs.
Adapted from E. Bjelke

tically significant 1.4 for those in the group who ate yellow-green vegetables containing in excess of 1000 IU of β-carotene per 100 grams less often than daily, compared with others in the group who did eat those vegetables daily. Hirayama also reported statistically significant negative associations between daily consumption of vegetables containing β-carotene and incidence of stomach and prostate cancers.

In the United States, two large-scale epidemiologic studies examined whether dietary vitamin A or β-carotene intake protects against cancer. One, reported by R. B. Shekelle and co-workers in 1981, involved 1,954 middle-aged men whose dietary practices were determined at the outset in personal interviews and questionnaire responses; all subjects, who worked in a Chicago-area Western Electric plant, were then followed for 19 years. Shekelle and co-workers found that intake of preformed vitamin A or other micronutrients was not significantly related to lung cancer risk and that the same was generally true of carotene intake and the risk of a variety of nonlung carcinomas.

They did find, however, a statistically significant inverse relationship between carotene intake and lung cancer incidence. Specifically, the relative risks of lung cancer in the lowest to the highest quartiles of carotene intake distribution among all men in the Western Electric study were 7, 5.5, 3, and 1, respectively; for those in the study who had smoked cigarettes for 30 years or more, the corresponding values were 8.1, 5.6, 3.9, and 1 (Figure 2).

The second U.S. study, reported in installments in recent years by S. Graham, C. Mettlin, and others at Roswell Park Memorial Institute, Buffalo, N.Y., is retrospective. It involves a few thousand cancer patients and a similar number of noncancer controls, all of whom were admitted to that center and completed dietary questionnaires during the late 1950s and early 1960s. Like Bjelke and Hirayama, the Roswell Park investigators found that an estimate of increasing vitamin A intake was associated with a decreasing incidence of lung cancer, after adjustment for smoking status. Specifically, estimated vitamin A intake was lower in 292 male

lung cancer patients than in 801 hospitalized controls, and comparison of the two groups showed a dose-response gradient in which the relative risk of the tumor among lung cancer patients with the lowest vitamin A intakes was 2.4. In other analyses, the investigators found similar trends for vitamin A intake and the risks of bladder (Table 2), esophageal, and laryngeal cancers.

Except for the study by Shekelle and colleagues, it is difficult to distinguish between vitamin A protection and that of β-carotene; yet there may be an important distinction. In a recent review, R. Peto and co-workers pointed out that the term "vitamin A" in nutritional studies commonly embraces both preformed retinol and its carotenoid precursors. They also commented that the total amount of vitamin A in human diets that is derived from β-carotene and related substances often exceeds that derived from preformed retinol itself. More specifically, the investigators noted that both Bjelke's vitamin A index and that used by Graham, Mettlin, and co-workers were based in part on consumption levels of carrots and other carotene-containing vegetables. The implication was that at least some of the protective effects attributed to vitamin A might actually have been from β-carotene.

That point, among others, is still moot. As Peto and co-workers also pointed out, the literature contains two recent prospective studies of stored blood samples in which low total serum retinol levels were associated with an increased risk of cancer. One study, reported in 1980 by N. Wald and associates from the United Kingdom, involved sera from approximately

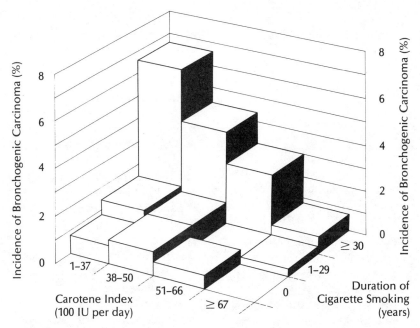

Figure 2. *In R. B. Shekelle and co-workers' 19-year prospective study of 1,954 men, the development of lung cancer in 33 subjects was inversely associated with daily carotene intake and directly associated with duration of cigarette smoking.*

was found to be 2.2 times greater for those in the lowest than in the highest quintile of the serum retinol distribution. The other study, reported in 1981 by J. D. Kark and co-workers, involved serum samples from 3,102 apparently healthy residents of Evans County, Ga. After a 12- to 14-year follow-up, 85 members of the group had developed cancer. Fluorometric measurement of retinol concentrations in stored serum samples from those persons and from 174 matched controls showed that the relative risk of cancer for people in the lowest retinol quintile was 5.3 times greater than that for those in the highest quintile (Table 3).

Unfortunately, the significance of those findings is obscured because relatively few cancers were observed in each study. In addition, although Kark and associates reported that serum retinol appeared to be stable in terms of light exposure, thawing, and refreezing, the effects of

16,000 apparently healthy men. After one to four years, samples from 86 men who developed cancer were retrieved from storage, thawed, and analyzed by high-pressure liquid chromatography to determine retinol levels; for comparison, sera from 172 controls were also analyzed. After adjustment for age, smoking status, and serum cholesterol, the relative risk of cancer

Table 2. Bladder Cancer Risk Correlated with Dietary Vitamin A

Vitamin A Level (1000 IU per month)	Females			Males		
	Cases (N=112)	Controls (N=256)	Relative Risk	Cases (N=377)	Controls (N=645)	Relative Risk
≤25	8	10	3.08	32	42	1.87
26–50	31	46	2.59	82	120	1.67
51–75	32	57	2.16	92	143	1.58
76–100	11	39	1.08	57	109	1.28
101–125	13	32	1.56	43	79	1.33
126–150	4	22	0.70	31	54	1.41
≥151	13	50	1.00	40	98	1.00

Food items included in the index and their vitamin A content in international units per 100-gm edible portion are beef (50), beets (20), broccoli (2500), brussels sprouts (520), cabbage (130), carrots (11,000), cauliflower (60), chicken (200), coleslaw (130), cucumber (100), fish (280), fruit (517), kale (8000), kohlrabi (20), lettuce (330), milk (340/cup), parsnips (30), pickles (100), red cabbage (40), rutabaga (550), and sauerkraut (50).

Adapted from C. Mettlin, S. Graham, and M. Swanson

Table 3. Cancer Risk and Total Blood Retinol in Stored Blood

Country	Blood Retinol Quintile Lowest → Highest					Number of Cancers (all sites)
United States (Georgia)	5.3	2.9	3.8	3.0	1.0*	85
United Kingdom	2.2	1.7	1.6	1.1	1.0	86
United States (Boston, Mass.)	1.0	1.0	0.9	0.7	1.1	111

*Top quintile is based on only seven cancers and, therefore, is unreliable.

long-term storage on serum retinol are not fully known. The retinol levels reported in both studies fell within the broad normal range. Finally, homeostatic mechanisms in the liver may keep retinol (but not β-carotene) blood levels constant over a wide range of dietary intake.

Overall, the available epidemiologic evidence about the relative importance of dietary vitamin A or β-carotene intake is inconclusive. The evidence does permit us to conclude, however, that since either factor may be an important determinant of cancer risk, both deserve further study. It remains to be seen whether β-carotene's apparent anticancer effects are related to its provitamin A activity, directly or indirectly, or to conversion to retinol in the human intestine. For example, some investigators postulate that β-carotene may exert anticancer effects by quenching the excitation energy of singlet oxygen or by trapping certain organic free radicals—properties that might prevent oxidative damage caused by such chemical species. On the other side of the issue, it remains to be seen whether vitamin A's role as a possible cancer inhibitor is limited to total, unbound, or carrier-bound blood retinol or involves extrinsic factors (e.g., hormones) that may influence retinol concentration. For example, blood retinol levels may be elevated in women who use oral contraceptives.

Practically speaking, of course, questions of mechanism(s) of action are less pressing than determining whether the micronutrients actually protect against human cancer. Toward that end, a number of human intervention trials are already under way, with each scheduled for completion before the end of this decade. What follows are examples of the β-carotene and vitamin A (or synthetic retinoid) studies that are in progress. They have been selected to represent the four major categories into which the Chemoprevention Program's human intervention trials tend to fall: general-population studies, studies of high-risk groups, studies of patients with precancerous lesions, and studies of the prevention of new primaries in cancer patients.

Perhaps the best known of all is the five-year general-population study being conducted by Charles Hennekens at Harvard. That randomized double-blind trial, which involves 22,000 U.S. physicians, is testing the efficacy of alternate-day aspirin (325 mg) and β-carotene (50 mg) in the prevention of coronary heart disease and cancer, re-

spectively. Since Hennekens's study population is not exactly typical of the general U.S. population (e.g., in terms of smoking), we also are collaborating with Finnish health authorities on a similar study involving a more broadly based and presumably less health-conscious population.

In the high-risk category, Irving Selikoff, at the Mount Sinai School of Medicine, New York, is prospectively studying five-year lung cancer mortality in relation to previously determined serum retinol and β-carotene levels in approximately 2,500 asbestos workers.

With regard to precancerous lesions, both Frank Meyskens, at the University of Arizona, and Seymour Romney, at the Albert Einstein College of Medicine, New York, are performing stage I clinical trials of a topically administered retinoid in women with mild-to-moderate cervical dysplasia. At West Virginia University, John Durham is studying the effects of 13-*cis*-retinoic acid in patients with familial polyposis coli. In addition to determining whether such treatment reduces the risk of colon cancer in such patients, the trial will examine specific biochemical effects of retinoid treatment on colonic polyps and skin fibroblasts. A related study by Phyllis Bowen is under way at the University of Illinois. Its subjects are persons with adenomatous colonic polyps. One phase is a clinical trial using β-carotene; another will examine the relationship between low vitamin A consumption or marginal vitamin A status and the development of colonic adenomatous polyps, colonic adenocarcinoma, or both.

The principal focus of current human intervention trials of chemoprevention for new primary tumors is non-melanoma skin cancer. Robert Greenberg, at Dartmouth College, will study the efficacy of orally administered β-carotene. At Memorial Hospital for Cancer and Allied Diseases, New York, Bijan Safai, will study oral β-carotene in combination with ascorbic acid and α-tocopherol. At the University of Arizona, Thomas Moon will examine the efficacy of 13-*cis*-retinoic acid or vitamin A in reducing skin cancer risk. A study conducted by Joseph Tangrea and Earl Gross at the National Cancer Institute, involving Veterans Administration hospitals throughout the United States, focuses on 13-*cis*-retinoic acid as a chemopreventive agent for basal cell skin carcinoma.

What about other chemopreventive approaches? As noted earlier, the major micronutrients that have been proposed as possible cancer inhibitors include vitamin C, vitamin E, and the trace metal selenium. Each is also currently under study in human intervention trials or related clinical projects sponsored by the Chemoprevention Program.

At Memorial Hospital, New York, for example, Jerome De Cosse is assessing the effects of dietary ascorbic acid and α-tocopherol, with or without wheat fiber, on rectal adenomas in patients with polyposis coli who have undergone colectomy and ileorectal anastomosis. Roy Shore, at the New York University Medical Center, will use a case-control protocol to assess the influence of dietary vitamin C, vitamin E, and selenium (plus dietary vitamin A, β-carotene, protease inhibitors, and fat and fiber) on the development of colorectal cancer. The relationship between dietary selenium and the risk of breast,

lung, or large-bowel cancer will be investigated in a case-control study by Walter Willett at the Harvard School of Public Health. Finally, Frank Polk, at The Johns Hopkins University, is performing a prospective study of the development of cancer in relation to previously determined serum concentrations of vitamins A, C, and E; selenium; hormones, and antibodies to cytomegalovirus and Epstein-Barr virus.

As with vitamin A and β-carotene, the mechanisms by which vitamin C, vitamin E, and selenium may exert anticancer effects are unknown. For all three of the latter micronutrients, however, protection against free radical damage has been suggested as one possibility. Many recognized carcinogens are themselves free radicals; that is, they possess an unpaired electron, such as that of singlet

oxygen, in an outer orbital. In addition, some are either directly converted in the body into free radicals or stimulate free radical production.

Selenium is a functional component of glutathione peroxidase, which destroys hydroperoxidases and lipoperoxidases and thereby protects cell constituents against damage caused by free radical reactions. But the relevance of glutathione peroxidase activity to selenium's apparent anticancer effects is still unclear. Moreover, little is known about the relative importance, if any, of the various forms of selenium to which human beings may be exposed; they include both organic (e.g., selenomethionine) and inorganic (e.g., sodium selenite) compounds. (Positive experimental findings with selenium are shown in Figure 3.)

Both water-soluble vitamin C

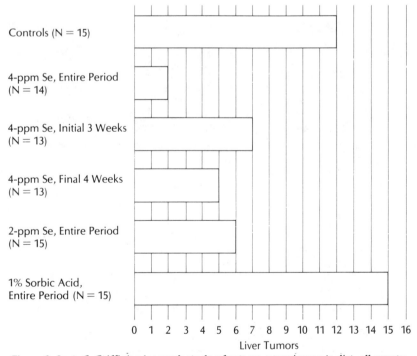

Figure 3. *In A. C. Griffin's nine-week study of rats on a carcinogenic diet, all groups given selenium had fewer liver tumors than the controls or those given sorbic acid. Selenium's apparent antitumor effect was greatest at the highest dosage and longest duration of exposure that was used. A group given 0.5% butylated hydroxytoluene and neither selenium nor sorbic acid had no tumors at end of study period.*

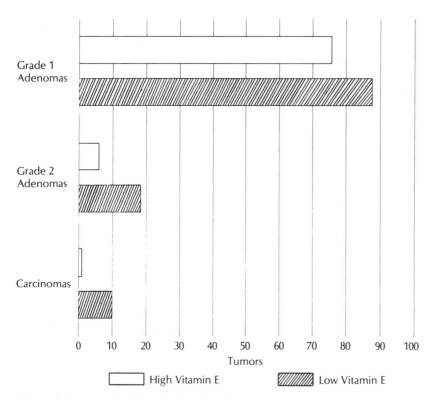

Figure 4. *In a study of chemically induced colorectal tumors, M. G. Cook and P. McNamara found that the number of neoplasms was significantly reduced in mice fed high vitamin E, compared with those fed low vitamin E. Data were restricted to animals who survived 23 weeks of carcinogen injections. Low group had high mortality and higher percentage of survivors with one or more tumors.*

Selected Reading

Greenwald P: Cancer control research: Directions and opportunities. *In* Progress in Cancer Control III: A Regional Approach, Mettlin C, Murphy G (Eds). Alan R Liss, New York, 1983, pp 21–29

Carrese LM, Baker CG: The convergence technique: A method for the planning and programming of research efforts. Management Science 13(8):B420, 1967 (US Department of Health, Education and Welfare)

Greenwald P, DeWys WD: Nutritional status and chemoprevention in relation to lung cancer. *In* Lung Cancer: Causes and Prevention, Mizell M, Correa P (Eds). Verlag Chemie, Deerfield Beach, Fla (in press)

Peto R et al: Can dietary beta-carotene materially reduce human cancer rates? Nature 290:201, 1981

Bjelke E: Dietary vitamin A and human lung cancer. Int J Cancer 15:561, 1975

Hirayama T: Diet and cancer. Nutr Cancer 1:67, 1979

Shekelle RB et al: Dietary vitamin A and risk of cancer in the Western Electric study. Lancet 2:1185, 1981

Mettlin C, Graham S, Swanson M: Vitamin A and lung cancer. J Natl Cancer Inst 62:1435, 1979

Wald N et al: Low serum-vitamin-A and subsequent risk of cancer: Preliminary results of a prospective study. Lancet 2:813, 1980

Kark JD et al: Serum vitamin A (retinol) and cancer incidence in Evans County, Georgia. J Natl Cancer Inst 66:7, 1981

Willett WC et al: Relation of serum vitamins A and E and carotenoids to the risk of cancer. N Engl J Med 310:430, 1984

and fat-soluble vitamin E also may inhibit carcinogenesis by interfering with free radical reactions in target tissues. Additionally, those micronutrients may alter the metabolism of carcinogens or procarcinogens by decreasing the formation of activated products or increasing the formation of detoxified products. A salient example is the demonstrated ability of vitamins C and E to inhibit endogenous formation of nitrosamines and nitrosamides. (For an example of experimental findings with vitamin E, see Figure 4.)

For the Diet, Nutrition, and Cancer Program, much more work remains to be done. The two major leads for further investigation are the roles played by dietary fat and fiber in human cancer. In particular, we think that the efficacy of low-fat diets in protecting against female breast cancer deserves examination in human intervention trials. Studies of the efficacy of high-fiber diets are also attractive. However, more information is needed about the possible relationships between different aspects of dietary fiber—cellulose, hemicellulose, pectins, etc—and cancer risk; initially, those questions may best be addressed in laboratory studies.

Two of the major recommendations in a recent report on diet and cancer by the National Academy of Sciences were for Americans to reduce fat intake from 40% to 30% of total calories and to eat more whole-grain cereals, fruits, and vegetables. Those three food groups contain fiber and other nutrients. If widely adopted, those changes would probably reduce the cancer burden in the United States significantly. The need to reduce that burden is obvious: In 1983, there were 850,000 estimated new cases of cancer and nearly

450,000 cancer deaths in the United States.

Adopted or not, however, prudent public health practices do not replace the underlying need for definitive research answers on cancer prevention and control through dietary means. Although it will take time to obtain such answers and to realize their benefits, the National Cancer Institute's plans in that area aim for a major impact on cancer incidence and mortality by the year 2000.

Role of Retinoids in Differentiation and Carcinogenesis

by Michael B. Sporn and Anita B. Roberts

It has been known for more than 50 years that retinoids, the family of molecules comprising both the natural and synthetic analogues of retinol, are potent agents for control of both cellular differentiation and cellular proliferation (70). In their original classic paper describing the cellular effects of vitamin A deficiency in the rat, Wolbach and Howe clearly noted that there were distinct effects on both differentiation and proliferation of epithelial cells. During vitamin A deficiency, it was found that proper differentiation of stem cells into mature epithelial cells failed to occur and that abnormal cellular differentiation, characterized in particular by excessive accumulation of keratin, was a frequent event. Furthermore, it was noted that there was excessive cellular proliferation in many of the deficient epithelia. Although the conclusion that an adequate level of retinoid was necessary for control of normal cellular differentiation and proliferation was clearly stated in the original paper by Wolbach and Howe, a satisfactory explanation of the molecular mechanisms underlying these effects on both differentiation and proliferation still eludes us more than 50 years later.

It was inevitable that the basic role of retinoids in control of cell differentiation and proliferation would eventually find practical application in the cancer field, and there have been great advances in this area, particularly for prevention of cancer. Many studies have shown that retinoids can suppress the process of carcinogenesis *in vivo* in experimental animals (for reviews, see Refs. 7, 33, 51, 54, 56, and 57), and these results are now the basis of current attempts to use retinoids for cancer prevention in humans. Furthermore, there is now an extensive literature on the ability of retinoids to suppress the development of the malignant phenotype *in vitro* (for reviews, see Refs. 6, 8, 30, and 31), and these studies corroborate the use of retinoids for cancer prevention. Finally, most recently, it has been shown that reti-

noids can exert effects on certain fully transformed, invasive, neoplastic cells, leading in certain instances to a suppression of proliferation (30) and in other instances to terminal differentiation of these cells, resulting in a more benign, nonneoplastic phenotype (10, 11, 60, 62). Even though there are many types of tumor cells for which this is not the case (33, 52) (indeed, at present there are only a limited number of instances in which such profound effects of retinoids on differentiation and proliferation of invasive tumor cells have been shown), this finding nevertheless has highly significant implications for the problem of cancer treatment. It emphasizes that in many respects cancer is fundamentally a disease of abnormal cell differentiation (36, 44), and it raises the possibility that even invasive disease may eventually be controlled by agents which control cell differentiation rather than kill cells. Since carcinogenesis is essentially a disorder of cell differentiation, the overall scientific problem of the role of retinoids in either differentiation or carcinogenesis is essentially the same problem and will be considered as a single problem in this brief review.

Major Problems Relating to Retinoids and Cancer

In the broadest sense, there are 2 major domains relating to retinoids and the cancer problem: (*a*) the practical development and use of retinoids for either cancer prevention or treatment; and (*b*) the elucidation of the cellular and molecular mechanisms underlying the first domain. The first domain has attracted a great deal of attention in the past 5 years and requires the coordinated efforts of synthetic organic chemists, cell biologists, investigators in experimental carcinogenesis and chemotherapy, pharmacologists, toxicologists, and clinical investigators in order to synthesize new retinoids, test them both *in vitro* and *in vivo* for useful biological activity, establish their pharmacokinetic and toxicological properties, and then bring the best new retinoids to clinical trial for either prevention or treatment of specific types of cancer. This is a problem of immense scope, complexity, and

Michael B. Sporn and Anita B. Roberts are with the Laboratory of Chemoprevention, Division of Cancer Cause and Prevention, National Cancer Institute, Bethesda, MD 20205.

expense, which is currently being pursued with vigorous interest throughout the world. We have reviewed some of the key issues in this first domain in previous articles (54, 56, 57) and will not discuss them further at this point. Instead, we will focus the rest of this short review on the problem of cellular and molecular mechanisms. Studies in this area are not only of great theoretical interest but should also facilitate the practical development and use of retinoids for prevention and treatment of cancer. Elucidation of the mechanism of action of retinoids may also lead to new applications for their use. It is reasonable to suggest that retinoids may find applications in the prevention or treatment of diseases other than cancer, the pathogenesis of which involves abnormalities of cell differentiation and/or proliferation (55). In terms of the scientific challenge, it is again worth emphasizing that the problem of cellular and molecular mechanism is still unsolved more than 50 years after the initial description of the overall biological activity of the retinoids. The problem of the mechanism of action of retinoids may be studied at 3 levels, namely, in the whole animal, at the cellular level, and finally at the molecular level, which we shall now consider in turn, using effects on both differentiation and carcinogenesis as markers.

Mechanism of Action of Retinoids in Differentiation and Carcinogenesis Studied in the Whole Animal

Although the earliest studies on retinoid deficiency in the whole animal emphasized its effects on epithelial cell differentiation and proliferation, the possibility that retinoid deficiency caused abnormalities in nonepithelial cells derived from mesenchymal elements was also noted by several careful investigators. Indeed, in the 1920s, it was reported that there was a reduction in hematopoietic cells in the bone marrow of vitamin A-deficient animals (21, 70). In the 1930s and 1940s, many studies were performed on the need for retinoids for proper bone formation (34, 39), and there was detailed investigation of the control of osteoblasts and osteoclasts (cells derived from mesenchyme) by retinoids (34). However, in the ensuing years, there was a much greater emphasis on studies on the role of retinoids in control of epithelial cell differentiation and proliferation, and the dogma that retinoids were selectively involved in the control of epithelial cells and were of relatively minor importance with respect to cells of mesenchymal origin became scientific folklore.

In contrast, in the area of experimental embryology and teratology, there accumulated an impressive body of information which indicated that retinoids had significant, selective teratogenic action on cells of mesenchymal origin in rat, mouse, hamster, and chick embryos; we have reviewed these data elsewhere (58). Particularly striking were the effects of either retinol deficiency or retinoic acid excess on the development of the very early vascular system of either the chick or the rat embryo. In the 1-day-old chick embryo, retinol deficiency causes failure of mesenchymal cells to proliferate and differentiate to form the early vascular system (Refs. 66, 67; Fig. 1); treatment of rat or chick embryos with excess retinol or retinoic acid has similar effects (40).[1] Furthermore, in the retinoid-deficient chick embryo, normal development of the vascular system can be restored by injection of appropriate amounts of various retinoids, including esters of retinoic acid (66, 67). These results indicate a very stringent requirement for retinoids, with either deficiency or excess leading to abnormal development of tissues derived from primitive mesenchyme. The effects of retinoids on the

---

[1] M. B. Sporn and D. L. Newton, unpublished results.

developing vascular system of the early embryo appear to be quite selective, since many other cell types do not appear to be affected to anywhere near the same extent (58, 66, 67). In the early embryo, a common stem cell type has long been believed to be a precursor to both blood cells themselves and those cells which will form the walls of the earliest blood vessels (50). The preceding observations, made with only the simplest of morphological techniques, suggest that retinoids play a role in controlling the proliferation and differentiation of these mesenchymal precursor cells or their early progeny; more recent work, using sophisticated cell culture and recombinant DNA techniques, has added important further information, as will be discussed later.

Mechanistic studies in the whole animal on the role of retinoids in prevention of carcinogenesis have dealt largely with the prevention of epithelial carcinogenesis. There are especially convincing data on the efficacy of many different retinoids in prevention of skin, breast, and bladder cancer in experimental animals (5, 7, 33, 37, 38, 57, 59, 65). Overall, these studies suggest that retinoids exert a hormone-like control of either cell proliferation or cell differentiation. However, in the whole animal, it is extremely difficult to separate these 2 parameters; they are intimately linked with each other. Some investigators have stressed the role of retinoids as antiproliferative agents (38), while others have emphasized that the role of retinoids in control of differentiation, rather than proliferation, may be more important (4). Whole-animal studies do not easily lend themselves to separate analysis of these 2 parameters. Indeed, the problem of the separation of the effects of retinoids on cell proliferation, as contrasted to effects on cell differentiation, may turn out to be more semantic than real, once a complete genetic analysis, using recombinant DNA methods, is available. The key problem is not to deal with the semantics of whether retinoids preferentially affect cell proliferation or cell differentiation but to identify the specific genes, the function of which is ultimately controlled by retinoids, either directly or indirectly. This problem cannot be solved in the whole animal; it requires isolated cellular systems and modern methods of molecular analysis. We will now discuss the application of studies in these areas to understanding the role of retinoids in differentiation and carcinogenesis.

Cellular Mechanism of Action of Retinoids in Differentiation and Carcinogenesis

Significant advances in understanding the mechanism of action of retinoids did not occur until *in vitro* systems were used as experimental tools. The development of methods for organ culture of tissues, such as the skin and the prostate, in which retinoids are particularly active, was a major advance. In the 1950s, the classic studies of Fell and Mellanby (20) showed that the differentiated phenotype of chick epidermis in organ culture could be changed from keratinized to mucus producing by treatment with retinol or retinyl acetate. In cultures treated with retinoids, the keratinizing cells of the epidermis disappeared and were replaced by mucus-producing cells, and in some instances even by ciliated cells, which are not found in normal skin (20). These organ culture experiments were essentially the reverse of those performed by Wolbach and Howe in the 1920s in the whole animal. In the Wolbach-Howe studies, retinoid *deficiency* caused disappearance of normal mucociliary epithelium, with replacement by keratinizing cells (keratinizing squamous metaplasia); in the Fell-Mellanby experiments, retinoid *excess* caused disappearance of normal keratinizing epithelium, with replacement by mucus and ciliated cells (mucus metaplasia).

The next significant advance in this area also used organ culture methodology. Lasnitzki (26), working in the same laboratory as Fell and Mellanby, was able to show that the premalignant phenotype of mouse prostate glands that had been treated with the carcinogen, 3-methylcholanthrene, could be altered by retinoids. The atypical epithelial cells that were induced by the carcinogen disappeared upon retinoid treatment of the organ cultures, and they were replaced by cells with more normal morphology (26). The effects of the retinoids were to suppress abnormal cellular differentiation that had been induced by the carcinogen in the epithelium of the prostate gland and to restore a more normal pattern of epithelial differentiation. In other organ culture studies, Lasnitzki (27) also made the important observation that there were significant morphological similarities between vitamin A-deficient prostatic epithelium and prostatic epithelium in cultures that had been treated with methylcholanthrene; these studies provide further evidence for the concept that the mechanisms of action of retinoids in both differentiation and carcinogenesis are closely linked.

In spite of the advances that were made in the above experiments, organ culture methods have definite liabilities for analysis of mechanism; they use mixed-cell populations, from which it is very difficult, if not impossible, to obtain replicate samples of homogeneous cells. The introduction of cell culture methodology to studies of retinoid mechanism was therefore of great importance and now is allowing molecular investigation of the role of retinoids in differentiation and carcinogenesis. In contrast to the organ culture studies, in which the emphasis was on the role of retinoids in control of epithelial differentiation, cell culture studies have emphasized the role of retinoids in cells of mesenchymal origin, if only because such cells are grown more easily in culture. One may suppose that, as better systems are developed for epithelial cell culture, there will be increasing investigation of retinoids in many different types of epithelium using these methods; this has already happened with epidermal cell culture (72).

Continuous cell lines of mesenchymal origin have been widely used to study the effects of retinoids on both differentiation and carcinogenesis; the cell lines which have been used are both neoplastic and nonneoplastic. The experiments which opened up this area of investigation were those of Merriman and Bertram (35) and Harisiadis *et al.* (24), which showed that retinoids can act directly on nonneoplastic cells to suppress the process of malignant transformation induced by either chemicals or radiation. In the case of the experiments done with suppression of chemical carcinogenesis, it was clearly shown that retinoids were effective in suppressing transformation even when they were applied to cells a full week after original exposure of the cells to carcinogen. Whatever the genetic damage caused by the carcinogen, it had already occurred. The role of the retinoids in these experiments was thus clearly shown to be a suppressor of the expression of the malignant phenotype in cells that had been previously initiated by a carcinogen (35). Furthermore, in these experiments, continuous presence of the retinoids was required to suppress the malignant phenotype; removal of the retinoids from the culture allowed expression of the transformed state.

Retinoids can also change the differentiation of invasive neoplastic cells growing in either monolayer or suspension culture. The most striking example of this phenomenon is the induction of terminal differentiation in murine F9 teratocarcinoma cells (60, 62) or human promyelocytic leukemia cells (Refs. 10 and 11; Fig. 2); in these cases, the differentiated phenotype is drastically changed from neoplastic to nonneoplastic, and proliferation of the induced cells is permanently suppressed. In the F9 system,

retinoids induce terminal differentiation of teratocarcinoma stem cells to cells which resemble parietal endoderm; a variety of new proteins is induced in the differentiated cells (62, 63). In the human promyelocytic leukemia system, retinoids can induce terminal differentiation of malignant leukemia cells, leading to formation of morphologically mature granulocytes, which have functional markers of the mature neutrophil (10, 11); these results have been obtained with the established HL60 cell line (11), as well as with primary cultures of other promyelocytic leukemia cells (10). These studies with neoplastic leukemia cells in turn have had a major influence on studies on possible effects of retinoids on normal myeloid differentiation. Since some of the leukemias may be viewed as diseases in which there is a block or arrest in normal myeloid differentiation and maturation (14, 23) and since retinoids can apparently overcome this block in certain leukemia cells, it has been suggested that retinoids may also be involved in normal hematopoiesis (11, 18).

The mechanism of all of these effects of retinoids, whether they be to alter the differentiated phenotype in nonneoplastic or preneoplastic epithelial cells in organ culture, to suppress the appearance of the neoplastic phenotype in nonneoplastic mesenchymal cells in monolayer culture, or to induce the terminally differentiated phenotype in fully neoplastic cells in monolayer culture, is not known. It is tempting to believe that there is a common mechanism (or limited number of mechanisms), which underlies all of these phenomena. In cell culture studies, as we noted before in the studies on whole animals, various investigators again have chosen to emphasize the role of retinoids in control of either cell proliferation (30) or cell differentiation (72). It would appear that retinoids control both processes and that any dispute over which is more important is relatively fruitless at present. Rather, it would seem more productive to focus on the specific molecular processes involved, to which we shall now turn.

Molecular Mechanism of Action of Retinoids in Differentiation and Carcinogenesis

Over the years, numerous hypotheses on the molecular mechanism of action of retinoids in control of differentiation have been proposed, but none has stood up to the experimental data. In particular, any hypothesis relating to molecular mechanism of action must take into account the evidence, now overwhelming, that retinoic acid will support growth in the whole animal as effectively as retinol (74), that retinoic acid is more active than retinol or retinal in numerous *in vitro* test systems (11, 30, 57, 62), and that there is no evidence that the mammalian organism can convert retinoic acid to retinol (19). In many test systems, retinoic acid is at least 100 to 1000 times more active than is retinol (11, 57, 62), and biological activity can be measured at levels as low as 10^{-11} M (57). Thus, the hypothesis, proposed in the 1960s, that retinol directly modifies membrane structure (16) to exert its biological effects is now of only historical interest.

More recently, it has been suggested that a primary biological role of the retinoids is to participate in sugar transfer reactions by means of the intermediate retinyl phosphate mannose, which is a metabolite of retinol (1, 15, 71). This hypothesis cannot be rationalized with the experimental data on retinoic acid, summarized above. Neither is there any convincing evidence at present for a metabolite of retinoic acid which is involved in sugar transfer reactions. The recent synthesis of a new series of retinoids (29), which may be viewed as retinoidal benzoic acid derivatives (Chart 1) and which are even more potent than

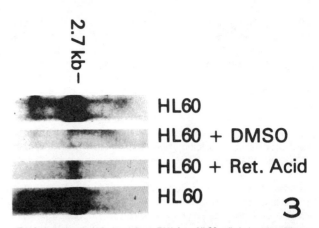

Chart 1. Structure of a new retinoidal benzoic acid derivative, which is 1000 times more active than is retinol or retinyl acetate in several test systems, both *in vitro* and *in vivo*.

retinoic acid in many test systems both *in vivo* and *in vitro*, provides even further experimental evidence against any essential role for retinyl phosphate mannose in control of differentiation or carcinogenesis. The new analogue shown in Chart 1 (or its derivatives) will support growth in the whole animal fed a vitamin A-deficient diet (29), is at least 1000 times more active than retinol in suppressing skin carcinogenesis in the mouse (29), is more than 100 times as active as retinol in the hamster tracheal organ culture system (57), and is more than 1000 times as active as retinol or retinyl acetate in the F9 teratocarcinoma or HL60 promyelocytic leukemia test systems (61). With data such as these at hand, it is unreasonable to believe that retinyl phosphate mannose plays any universally critical role in the control of differentiation or carcinogenesis. Although one cannot exclude the possibility that there may be some situations in which retinyl phosphate mannose may play some role, currently available information would relegate this metabolite to a minor role in control of differentiation and carcinogenesis.

If one wishes to develop a molecular hypothesis of retinoid mechanism that is compatible with the broadest range of experimental data, then the simplest one that can be proposed at present is to suggest that retinoids modify gene expression. This, of course, is not a new idea. If one takes this as a general proposition, then 2 important questions follow: (*a*) *which* genes are controlled by retinoids; and (*b*) *how* are these genes controlled by retinoids? (is the mechanism one of direct or indirect control?). We will provide only an outline of what is known regarding these 2 questions.

With respect to which genes are known to be controlled by retinoids, one is impressed by the number of recent reports which indicate that retinoids control the expression of many proteins which either are direct constituents of the cytoskeleton and extracellular matrix or participate in the formation of cytoskeleton and matrix. These proteins include keratins (22), collagen (62, 63), collagenase (12), transglutaminase (53, 73), and laminin (63). Determination of the specific types of cytoskeletal or matrix proteins which are produced in cells is now being used as a specific marker for cell differentiation, and it would appear that retinoids are intimately involved in this process. Other proteins the expression of which is known to be controlled by retinoids include plasminogen activator (62, 63), alkaline phosphatase (48, 63), and the receptor for epidermal growth factor (25, 47). Furthermore, the important observation has recently been made in the HL60 system that retinoic acid controls the expression of the *myc* oncogene. Using a specific molecular probe for the *myc* gene, it has been shown that physiological levels of all-*trans*-retinoic acid suppress *myc* gene expression in HL60 cells (Ref. 68; Fig. 3). Although the specific molecular function for the *myc* gene product has not yet been elucidated, it is presumed that in some way the excessive expression of this gene and its product is correlated with the excessive proliferation (and perhaps with the arrested differentiation) of the HL60 cell. However, the possibility must be considered that an oncogene

2.7 kb—

HL60
HL60 + DMSO
HL60 + Ret. Acid
HL60

3

Fig. 3. Hybridization of *myc* probe to RNA from HL60 cells induced to differentiate. Degree of differentiation was judged by the percentage of cells able to reduce nitroblue tetrazolium, as well as morphological criteria (see Fig. 2). *Left* to *right*: *Lane 1*, RNA from uninduced HL60 (less than 2% of cells nitroblue tetrazolium positive); *Lane 2*, RNA from HL60 induced to differentiate with dimethyl sulfoxide (*DMSO*) (87% of cells nitroblue tetrazolium positive); *Lane 3*, RNA from HL60 induced to differentiate with retinoic (*Ret.*) acid (40% of cells nitroblue tetrazolium positive); *Lane 4*, a second isolate of RNA from uninduced HL60 (less than 2% of cells nitroblue tetrazolium positive). On a molar basis, retinoic acid is approximately 1 million times more active than is dimethyl sulfoxide in inducing differentiation in HL60 (11). Reprinted with permission from Ref. 68.

other than *myc* may also contribute to the neoplastic behavior of the HL60 cell[2] and that retinoic acid may have significant interactions with this gene as well. Furthermore, as of the present, the kinetics of the interaction of retinoic acid with *myc* in HL60 has not been determined, and it is not yet clear whether retinoic acid controls *myc* expression directly or indirectly.

Thus, at the gene level, it appears that retinoids affect the expression of genes or gene products involved with both differentiation and proliferation. The remaining, and most difficult, question is, "How do they do it?" The overall problem of the control of gene expression is beyond the scope of this article; one may conceive of both direct and indirect mechanisms that involve either regulation of gene transcription itself, regulation of processing of primary gene transcripts, or regulation of translation of processed message. Little is known about retinoids in any of these areas. Recent experiments have demonstrated effects of retinoids on genomic expression in retinoid-deficient rat tissues (43); however, the complexity of the experimental system precludes analysis of the molecular mechanisms involved. By analogy with the steroids, it has been suggested that the effects of retinoids in controlling gene expression are mediated by specific intracellular binding proteins (13). However, retinoids have significant effects in control of both differentiation and carcinogenesis in 2 important cell systems, namely HL60 and 10T½ fibroblasts, in which no retinoid-binding protein (analogous to steroid-binding proteins) can be detected (17, 28).[3]

The alternative to a steroid-like mechanism for retinoids is to suggest that they control gene expression via interactions with protein kinases, both cyclic AMP[4] dependent and cyclic AMP independent. Retinoids have been shown to increase cyclic AMP-dependent protein kinase activity in B16 melanoma cells (32), which are highly sensitive to their antiproliferative effects (30), as well as in F9 teratocarcinoma cells which are induced to

---

[2] R. A. Weinberg, personal communication.
[3] T. R. Breitman, personal communication.
[4] The abbreviation used is: cyclic AMP, cyclic adenosine 3':5'-monophosphate.

differentiate by retinoic acid (45). Furthermore, $N^6,O^{2'}$-dibutyryl cyclic adenosine 3':5'-monophosphate markedly potentiates the differentiating effects of retinoic acid in both F9 teratocarcinoma cells (63) and HL60 leukemia cells (42). Very recent work has also suggested that a secondary effect of retinoic acid may be the induction in the F9 system of a calcium- and phospholipid-dependent, cyclic AMP-independent protein kinase activity (2, 41, 64) and that some of the interactions between retinoids and phorbol esters may be mediated through this system (2). These latest studies on a calcium-dependent protein kinase system provide an important link between retinoids and calcium, which is now assuming an increasing importance in control of cell proliferation and differentiation (46, 69). Thus, although studies on the interactions between retinoids and the various protein kinase systems of the cell have only recently begun, they have already yielded significant new data which will need to be integrated into an overall hypothesis of mechanism of action.

Ultimately, it would appear that the problem of the molecular mechanism of action of retinoids in control of differentiation and carcinogenesis is converging on one of the central problems in all of biology, namely, the control of gene expression. There may be new mechanisms, yet to be discovered, that may be critically involved in this process. For example, yet another question that awaits further experimentation is the functional relationship between retinoids and polypeptide growth factors that control cell proliferation and differentiation (58). The role of peptide growth factors in controlling these processes is of fundamental importance (for a review, see Ref. 9); for example, there is evidence that a new family of transforming growth factors (type α and type β), which we have recently described (3, 49), may play a key role in the processes of carcinogenesis and differentiation. Clearly, any future hypothesis dealing with mechanism of action of retinoids will need to integrate the role of retinoids, peptide growth factors, and specific genes controlling differentiation and proliferation. In particular, it must define the precise relationship between retinoids, transforming growth factors, and cellular oncogenes. The breadth, potency, and specificity of retinoids in the control of cell function all suggest that retinoids will be valuable tools for the experimental scientist to unravel molecular mechanisms, in addition to their practical usefulness in controlling differentiation and carcinogenesis.

Acknowledgments

We thank Ruth Morsillo for expert assistance with the preparation of the manuscript.

References

1. Adamo, S., De Luca, L. M., Silverman-Jones, C. S., and Yuspa, S. H. Mode of action of retinol. Involvement in glycosylation reactions of cultured mouse epidermal cells. J. Biol. Chem., *254:* 3279–3287, 1979.
2. Anderson, W. B., Kraft, A. S., and Evain-Brion, D. Effect of retinoic acid and phorbol ester treatment of embryonal carcinoma cells on calcium, phospholipid-dependent protein kinase activity. Cold Spring Harbor Conf. Cell Proliferation, *10:* in press, 1983.
3. Anzano, M. A., Roberts, A. B., Meyers, C. A., Komoriya, A., Lamb, L. C., Smith, J. M., and Sporn, M. B. Synergistic interaction of two classes of transforming growth factors from murine sarcoma cells. Cancer Res., *42:* 4776–4778, 1982.
4. Astrup, E. G., and Paulsen, J. E. Effect of retinoic acid pretreatment on 12-O-tetradecanoylphorbol-13-acetate-induced cell population kinetics and polyamine biosynthesis in hairless mouse epidermis. Carcinogenesis (Lond.), *3:* 313–320, 1982.
5. Becci, P. J., Thompson, H. J., Grubbs, C. J., Squire, R. A., Brown, C. C., Sporn, M. B., and Moon, R. C. Inhibitory effect of 13-cis-retinoic acid on urinary bladder carcinogenesis induced in C57BL/6 mice by N-butyl-N-(4-hydroxybutyl)nitrosamine. Cancer Res., *38:* 4463–4466, 1978.
6. Bertram, J. S., Mordan, L. J., Domanska-Janik, K., and Bernacki, R. J. Inhibition of in vitro neoplastic transformation by retinoids. In: M. S. Arnott, J. van Eys, and Y. M. Wang (eds.), Molecular Interrelations of Nutrition and Cancer, pp. 315–335. New York: Raven Press, 1982.
7. Bollag, W. Retinoids and cancer. Cancer Chemother. Pharmacol., *3:* 207–215, 1979.
8. Borek, C. Vitamins and micronutrients modify carcinogenesis and tumor promotion in vitro. In: M. S. Arnott, J. van Eys, and Y. M. Wang (eds.), Molecular Interrelations of Nutrition and Cancer, pp. 337–350. New York: Raven Press, 1982.
9. Bradshaw, R. A., and Sporn, M. B. (eds.). Symposium: Polypeptide growth factors and the regulation of cell growth and differentiation. Fed. Proc., *42:* 2590–2634, 1983.
10. Breitman, T. R., Collins, S. J., and Keene, B. R. Terminal differentiation of human promyelocytic leukemia cells in primary culture in response to retinoic acid. Blood, *57:* 1000–1004, 1981.
11. Breitman, T. R., Selonick, S. E., and Collins, S. J. Induction of differentiation of the human promyelocytic leukemia cell line (HL-60) by retinoic acid. Proc. Natl. Acad. Sci. U. S. A., *77:* 2936–2940, 1980.
12. Brinckerhoff, C. E., and Harris, E. D., Jr. Modulation by retinoic acid and corticosteroids of collagenase production by rabbit synovial fibroblasts treated with phorbol myristate acetate or poly(ethylene glycol). Biochim. Biophys. Acta, *677:* 424–432, 1981.
13. Chytil, F., and Ong, D. E. Cellular retinol- and retinoic acid-binding proteins in vitamin A action. Fed. Proc., *38:* 2510–2514, 1979.
14. Clarkson, B. C. Acute myelocytic leukemia in adults. Cancer (Phila.), *30:* 1572–1582, 1972.
15. De Luca, L. M., Bhat, P. V., Sasak, W., and Adamo, S. Biosynthesis of phosphoryl and glycosyl phosphoryl derivatives of vitamin A in biological membranes. Fed. Proc., *38:* 2535–2539, 1979.
16. Dingle, J. T., and Lucy, J. A. Vitamin A, carotenoids, and cell function. Biol. Rev., *40:* 422–461, 1965.
17. Douer, D., and Koeffler, H. P. Retinoic acid—inhibition of the clonal growth of human myeloid leukemia cells. J. Clin. Invest., *69:* 277–283, 1982.
18. Douer, D., and Koeffler, H. P. Retinoic acid enhances growth of human early erythroid progenitor cells in vitro. J. Clin. Invest., *69:* 1039–1041, 1982.
19. Dowling, J. E., and Wald, G. The biological function of vitamin A acid. Proc. Natl. Acad. Sci. U. S. A., *46:* 587–608, 1960.
20. Fell, H. B., and Mellanby, E. Metaplasia produced in cultures of chick ectoderm by high vitamin A. J. Physiol., *119:* 470–488, 1953.
21. Findlay, G. M., and McKenzie, R. D. The bone marrow in deficiency diseases. J. Pathol. Bacteriol., *25:* 402–403, 1922.
22. Fuchs, E., and Green, H. Regulation of terminal differentiation of cultured human keratinocytes by vitamin A. Cell, *25:* 617–625, 1981.
23. Gallo, R. C. On the origin of human acute myeloblastic leukemia: virus-"hot spot" hypothesis. In: R. Neth, R. C. Gallo, S. Spiegelman, and F. Stohlman (eds.), Modern Trends in Human Leukemia, pp. 227–236. Munich: J. F. Lehmanns Verlag, 1974.
24. Harisiadis, L., Miller, R. C., Hall, E. J., and Borek, C. A vitamin A analogue inhibits radiation-induced oncogenic transformation. Nature (Lond.), *274:* 486–487, 1978.
25. Jetten, A. M. Retinoids specifically enhance the number of epidermal growth factor receptors. Nature (Lond.), *284:* 626–629, 1980.
26. Lasnitzki, I. The influence of A hypervitaminosis on the effect of 20-methylcholanthrene on mouse prostate glands grown in vitro. Br. J. Cancer, *9:* 434–441, 1955.
27. Lasnitzki, I. Hypovitaminosis-A in the mouse prostate gland cultured in chemically defined medium. Exp. Cell Res., *28:* 40–51, 1962.
28. Libby, P. R., and Bertram, J. S. Lack of intracellular retinoid-binding proteins in a retinol-sensitive cell line. Carcinogenesis (Lond.), *3:* 481–484, 1982.
29. Loeliger, P., Bollag, W., and Mayer, H. Arotinoids, a new class of highly active retinoids. Eur. J. Med. Chem., *15:* 9–15, 1980.
30. Lotan, R. Effects of vitamin A and its analogs (retinoids) on normal and neoplastic cells. Biochim. Biophys. Acta, *605:* 33–91, 1980.
31. Lotan, R., Thein, R., and Lotan, D. Suppression of the transformed cell phenotype expression by retinoids. In: F. L. Meyskens and K. Prasad (eds.), The Modulation and Mediation of Cancer by Retinoids. Basel: S. Karger AG, in press, 1983.
32. Ludwig, K. W., Lowey, B., and Niles, R. M. Retinoic acid increases cyclic AMP-dependent protein kinase activity in murine melanoma cells. J. Biol. Chem., *255:* 5999–6002, 1980.
33. Mayer, H., Bollag, W., Hänni, R., and Rüegg, R. Retinoids, a new class of compounds with prophylactic and therapeutic activities in oncology and dermatology. Experientia (Basel), *34:* 1105–1119, 1978.
34. Mellanby, E. Vitamin A and bone growth: the reversibility of vitamin A deficiency changes. J. Physiol., *105:* 382–399, 1947.
35. Merriman, R. L., and Bertram, J. S. Reversible inhibition by retinoids of 3-methylcholanthrene-induced neoplastic transformation in C3H/10T½ CL8 cells. Cancer Res., *39:* 1661–1666, 1979.
36. Mintz, B., and Fleischman, R. A. Teratocarcinomas and other neoplasms as developmental defects in gene expression. Adv. Cancer Res., *34:* 211–278, 1981.
37. Moon, R. C., Grubbs, C. J., Sporn, M. B., and Goodman, D. G. Retinyl acetate inhibits mammary carcinogenesis induced by N-methyl-N-nitrosourea. Nature (Lond.), *267:* 620–621, 1977.
38. Moon, R. C., Thompson, H. J., Becci, P. J., Grubbs, C. J., Gander, R. J., Newton, D. L., Smith, J. M., Phillips, S. L., Henderson, W. R., Mullen, L. T., Brown, C. C., and Sporn, M. B. N-(4-Hydroxyphenyl)retinamide, a new retinoid for prevention of breast cancer in the rat. Cancer Res., *39:* 1339–1346, 1979.

39. Moore, L. A. Relationship between carotene, blindness due to constriction of the optic nerve, papillary edema, and nyctalopia in calves. J. Nutr., *17:* 443–459, 1939.

40. Morriss, G. M., and Steele, C. E. Comparison of the effects of retinol and retinoic acid on postimplantation rat embryos in vitro. Teratology, *15:* 109–119, 1977.

41. Nishizuka, Y., and Takai, Y. Calcium and phospholipid turnover in a new receptor function for protein phosphorylation. Cold Spring Harbor Conf. Cell Proliferation, *8:* 237–249, 1981.

42. Olsson, I. L., Breitman, T. R., and Gallo, R. C. Priming of human myeloid leukemic cell lines HL-60 and U-937 with retinoic acid for differentiation effects of cyclic adenosine 3′:5′-monophosphate-inducing agents and a T-lymphocyte-derived differentiation factor. Cancer Res., *42:* 3928–3933, 1982.

43. Omori, M., and Chytil, F. Mechanism of vitamin A action: gene expression in retinol deficient rats. J. Biol. Chem., *257:* 14370–14374, 1982.

44. Pierce, G. B., Shikes, R., and Fink, L. M. Cancer—A Problem of Developmental Biology, Englewood Cliffs, N. J.: Prentice Hall, 1978.

45. Plet, A., Evain, D., and Anderson, W. B. Effect of retinoic acid treatment of F9 embryonal carcinoma cells on the activity and distribution of cyclic AMP-dependent protein kinase. J. Biol. Chem., *257:* 889–893, 1982.

46. Rasmussen, H. Calcium and cAMP as Synarchic Messengers. New York: John Wiley & Sons, Inc., 1981.

47. Rees, A. R., Adamson, E. D., and Graham, C. F. Epidermal growth factor receptors increase during the differentiation of embryonal carcinoma cells. Nature (Lond.), *281:* 309–311, 1979.

48. Reese, D. H., Fiorentino, G. J., Claflin, A. J., Malinin, T. I., and Politano, V. A. Rapid induction of alkaline phosphatase activity by retinoic acid. Biochem. Biophys. Res. Commun., *102:* 315–321, 1981.

49. Roberts, A. B., Frolik, C. A., Anzano, M. A., and Sporn, M. B. Transforming growth factors from neoplastic and non-neoplastic tissues. Fed. Proc., *42:* 2621–2626, 1983.

50. Romanoff, A. L. The Avian Embryo. New York: The Macmillan Co., 1960.

51. Saffiotti, U., Montesano, R., Sellakumar, A. R., and Borg, S. A. Experimental cancer of the lung. Inhibition by vitamin A of the induction of tracheobronchial squamous metaplasia and squamous cell tumors. Cancer (Phila.), *20:* 857–864, 1967.

52. Schroder, E. W., Rapaport, E., and Black, P. H. Retinoids and cell proliferation. Cancer Surv., in press, 1983.

53. Scott, K. F. F., Meyskens, F. L., and Russell, D. H. Retinoids increase transglutaminase activity and inhibit ornithine decarboxylase activity in Chinese hamster ovary cells and in melanoma cells stimulated to differentiate. Proc. Natl. Acad. Sci. U. S. A., *79:* 4093–4097, 1982.

54. Sporn, M. B., Dunlop, N. M., Newton, D. L., and Smith, J. M. Prevention of chemical carcinogenesis by vitamin A and its synthetic analogs (retinoids). Fed. Proc., *35:* 1332–1338, 1976.

55. Sporn, M. B., and Harris, E. D., Jr. Proliferative diseases. Am. J. Med., *70:* 1231–1236, 1981.

56. Sporn, M. B., and Newton, D. L. Chemoprevention of cancer with retinoids. Fed. Proc., *38:* 2528–2534, 1979.

57. Sporn, M. B., and Newton, D. L. Retinoids and chemoprevention of cancer. In: M. S. Zedeck and M. Lipkin (eds.), Inhibition of Tumor Induction and Development, pp. 71–100. New York: Plenum Publishing Corp., 1981.

58. Sporn, M. B., Newton, D. L., Roberts, A. B., De Larco, J. E., and Todaro, G. J. Retinoids and suppression of the effects of polypeptide transforming fac-
tors—a new molecular approach to chemoprevention of cancer. In: A. C. Sartorelli, J. S. Lazo, and J. R. Bertino (eds.), Molecular Actions and Targets for Cancer Chemotherapeutic Agents, pp. 541–554. New York: Academic Press, Inc., 1981.

59. Sporn, M. B., Squire, R. A., Brown, C. C., Smith, J. M., Wenk, M. L., and Springer, S. 13-cis-Retinoic acid: inhibition of bladder carcinogenesis in the rat. Science (Wash. D. C.), *195:* 487–489, 1977.

60. Strickland, S. Mouse teratocarcinoma cells: prospects for the study of embryogenesis and neoplasia. Cell, *24:* 277–278, 1981.

61. Strickland, S., Breitman, T. R., Frickel, F., Nürrenbach, A., Hädicke, E., and Sporn, M. B. Structure-activity relationships of a new series of retinoidal benzoic acid derivatives as measured by induction of differentiation of murine F9 teratocarcinoma cells and human HL-60 promyelocytic leukemia cells. Cancer Res., in press, 1983.

62. Strickland, S., and Mahdavi, V. The induction of differentiation in teratocarcinoma stem cells by retinoic acid. Cell, *15:* 393–403, 1978.

63. Strickland, S., Smith, K. K., and Marotti, K. R. Hormonal induction of differentiation in teratocarcinoma stem cells: generation of parietal endoderm by retinoic acid and dibutyryl cAMP. Cell, *21:* 347–355, 1980.

64. Takai, Y., Kishimoto, A., Kawahara, Y., Minakuchi, R., Sano, K., Kikkawa, U., Mori, T., Yu, B., Kaibuchi, K., and Nishizuka, Y. Calcium and phosphatidylinositol turnover as signalling for trans-membrane control of protein phosphorylation. Adv. Cyclic Nucleotide Res., *14:* 301–308, 1981.

65. Thompson, H. J., Becci, P. J., Brown, C. C., and Moon, R. C. Effect of the duration of retinyl acetate feeding on inhibition of 1-methyl-1-nitrosourea-induced mammary carcinogenesis in the rat. Cancer Res., *39:* 3977–3980, 1979.

66. Thompson, J. N. The role of vitamin A in reproduction. In: H. F. DeLuca and J. W. Suttie (eds.), The Fat-Soluble Vitamins, pp. 267–281. Madison, Wis.: The University of Wisconsin Press, 1969.

67. Thompson, J. N., Howell, J. M., Pitt, G. A. J., and McLaughlin, C. I. The biological activity of retinoic acid in the domestic fowl and the effects of vitamin A deficiency on the chick embryo. Br. J. Nutr., *23:* 471–490, 1969.

68. Westin, E. H., Wong-Staal, F., Gelmann, E. P., Dalla Favera, R., Papas, T. S., Lautenberger, J. A., Eva, A., Reddy, E. P., Tronick, S. R., Aaronson, S. A., and Gallo, R. C. Expression of cellular homologues of retroviral onc genes in human hematopoietic cells. Proc. Natl. Acad. Sci. U. S. A., *79:* 2490–2494, 1982.

69. Whitfield, J. F., Boynton, A. L., MacManus, J. P., Rixon, R. H., Sikorska, M., Tsang, B., and Walker, P. R. The roles of calcium and cyclic AMP in cell proliferation. Ann. N. Y. Acad. Sci., *339:* 216–240, 1980.

70. Wolbach, S. B., and Howe, P. R. Tissue changes following deprivation of fat soluble A vitamin. J. Exp. Med., *42:* 753–777, 1925.

71. Wolf, G., Kiorpes, T. C., Masushige, S., Schreiber, J. B., Smith, M. J., and Anderson, R. S. Recent evidence for the participation of vitamin A in glycoprotein synthesis. Fed. Proc., *38:* 2540–2543, 1979.

72. Yuspa, S. H. Retinoids and tumor promotion. In: D. A. Roe (ed.), Diet and Cancer: From Basic Research to Policy Implications. New York: Alan R. Liss, in press, 1983.

73. Yuspa, S. H., Ben, T., and Steinert, P. Retinoic acid induces transglutaminase activity but inhibits cornification of cultured epidermal cells. J. Biol. Chem., *257:* 9906–9908, 1982.

74. Zile, M., and DeLuca, H. F. Retinoic acid: some aspects of growth-promoting activity in the albino rat. J. Nutr., *94:* 302–308, 1968.

Blocking the Formation of *N*-Nitroso Compounds with Ascorbic Acid *in Vitro* and *in Vivo*

by Sidney S. Mirvish

N-Nitroso compounds (NO-compounds), such as nitrosamines and nitrosamides, are produced by the reaction of nitrite with nitrogen compounds. The formation of these compounds *in vitro* and *in vivo* was recently reviewed.[1] Kinetic studies showed that differences of up to 200,000 × occur in the ease of nitrosation of various nitrogen compounds, as measured by the kinetic rate constants. The most readily nitrosated classes of compounds are the weakly basic secondary amines (e.g. morpholine, piperazine, and *N*-methylaniline), tertiary enamines (e.g. aminopyrine), *N*-alkylureas, and *N*-alkylcarbamates. Nitrite occurs in nitrite–preserved meat and fish, spoiled foods (where nitrate is reduced by bacterial action), and human saliva (which has about 10 mg $NaNO_2$/liter). Amines, ureas, and carbamates occur widely as food constituents, food additives, drugs, and/or pesticides. More than 100 NO-compounds have been found to induce tumors in rodents, in the stomach, liver, esophagus, lungs, nervous system and pancreas. Many of these tumors are similar to tumors in man, where they show wide geographic and temporal variations in incidence, suggesting that they are induced by chemical agents. Hence the possibility arises that these tumors are induced in man by NO-compounds. These could reach the body from external sources, food and cigarette smoke, for example, or be formed *in vivo*, especially, since nitrosation is acid-catalyzed, in the stomach. The latter situation has been produced in rats and mice, where feeding nitrite together with amines or ureas has given rise to acute liver damage and tumors of various organs.

The concentration of NO-compounds so far determined in food is usually small, <0.1 mg/kg, and it remains to be established whether NO-compounds present a significant risk to human populations. However, populations exposed to high levels of nitrate (which could be reduced to nitrite) appear to show raised incidences of gastric and liver cancer.[1, 2] In conclusion, the points briefly reviewed here indicate that involvement of NO-compounds in the etiology of human cancer is a real possibility.

* Supported by contract PH-43-68-959 from the National Cancer Institute and grant BC-39B from the American Cancer Society.

Sidney S. Mirvish is with the Eppley Institute for Research in Cancer, University of Nebraska Medical Center, Omaha, Nebraska 68105.

Therefore, it would be useful to be able to prevent the formation of NO-compounds in food and *in vivo*. Since a number of readily nitrosated drugs are administered orally in large doses, their possible nitrosation *in vivo* is particularly disturbing. Among such drugs are piperazine, phenmetrazine, aminopyrine, ethambutol, and (possibly) oxytetracycline (OTC) and disulfiram. Many other drugs have yielded NO-derivatives, but often only under extreme conditions. The present paper reviews evidence indicating that ascorbic acid (ASC) could be used to block *in vivo* nitrosation of such drugs.

Chemical Experiments

In 1972 we tried to repeat a published experiment showing that nitrosation of the tertiary amine OTC gave rise to dimethylnitrosamine (DMN). Our sample of OTC failed to yield DMN, but we later confirmed that the pure drug did yield DMN. Since pharmaceutical OTC contains 80% ASC (added as an antioxidant), it struck us that ASC might be used to block the formation of NO-compounds. As an experimental model, we showed that ASC blocked the *in vitro* formation of NO-compounds by the reaction of nitrite with dimethylamine, morpholine, piperazine, methylurea, N-methylaniline, and OTC.[3] Under suitable conditions, blockages of 98–100% could be obtained, except for N-methylaniline, where the blockage was 45–60%. In these studies, a solution of nitrite at a given pH was added to a solution containing both the amine (or urea) and ASC at the same pH, and NO-compound formation was compared to that when ASC was omitted. The basis for the effect was clearly the well-known reaction of ASC with nitrite to give dehydro-ASC and nitric oxide, so that ASC competed with the nitrogen compound for the nitrite.

The kinetics of the ASC-nitrite reaction[4] indicates that ascorbate anion reacts with nitrite 230 $\times$ faster than ascorbic acid (pK_a 4.3). Since the formation of most nitrosamines shows a pH optimum of 3.4, and nitrosamide formation proceeds most rapidly at an even lower pH, ASC should act more efficiently at pH 3–5 (when ascorbate anion is present) than at pH 1–3. Our results[3] supported this view. We therefore proposed[3] that drugs that are readily nitrosated should be formulated with sufficient ASC to block their intragastric nitrosation by nitrite arising from food and saliva. This suggestion seemed particularly promising, since the pH of gastric contents after a meal is gradually lowered from 5 to 1, so that ASC might react with nitrite before it could produce NO-compounds.

Because of the reaction between nitrite and ASC, ASC is often added to nitrite-preserved meat. It serves to increase the formation of nitric oxide, which is responsible for the pink color of nitrosomyoglobin.[5] In this connection, Fiddler et al.[6] reported that ASC inhibited DMN production in frankfurters cured with high levels of nitrite.

In later studies by us,[7] the nitrosation of aminopyrine, which very readily produces DMN, was nevertheless successfully blocked by ASC: 20 mM AP and 25 mM nitrite were reacted at 0° C and pH 2 for 30 seconds to give 2.3 mM DMN. Inclusion of 6.2 mM ASC in the reaction mixture completely blocked DMN production. Aminopyrine is no longer used as an analgesic in this country, because it occasionally induced fatal agranulocytosis. One wonders whether this side reaction was due to *in vivo* production of DMN. The drug is still widely used in Europe and should be a prime candidate there for formulation with ASC or replacement by safer drugs.

We compared the action of ASC with that of other compounds that react with nitrite. Urea was relatively ineffective.[3] Ammonium sulfamate was a good blocker of morpholine and piperazine nitrosation at pH 1 and 2, but was less effective at pH 3 and 4.[3] We also examined the action of gallic acid, tannin, cysteine, and sulfite.[1] Some of these compounds were as effective as ASC in blocking morpholine nitrosation, but ASC remained the most effective compound for blocking piperazine nitrosation. The reaction of 10 mM piperazine and 10 mM nitrite at pH 3 and 25° C for 10 minutes gave 5.7 mM mononitrosopiperazine. On addition of 10 mM blocking agent, ASC gave 96% blocking while the other agents gave 26–63% blocking. Piperazine nitrosation offers a more critical test than morpholine nitrosation, because piperazine is nitrosated more rapidly than morpholine and hence competes more effectively with blocking agent for the nitrite.

Fan and Tannenbaum [8] studied the effect of ASC on morpholine nitrosation. When the ASC:morpholine ratio exceeded 2:1, nitrosomorpholine formation was completely blocked. When the ratio was less than 2:1, nitrosomorpholine formation was partly blocked. Under the latter conditions, nitrite concentration was up to 40% greater when measured by the Griess reaction than when calculated from the rate of morpholine nitrosation. Possibly ASC and nitrite reacted to form a nitrite compound determined by Griess reagent but not available for morpholine nitrosation.

Sen and Donaldson [9] studied the nitrosation of piperazine adipate, the form of piperazine usually used in treating intestinal worms. ASC blocked the formation of the relatively weak carcinogen mononitrosopiperazine by up to 80%. However, small amounts of the strong carcinogen dinitrosopiperazine were detected in the presence, but not the absence, of ASC. This is apparently connected with the use of adipate, since piperazine free base did not produce the dinitroso derivative, even in the presence of ASC.[25] Glutathione was an alternative blocking agent that did not lead to production of dinitroso compound.

In Vivo Experiments

Kamm et al.,[10] Greenblatt,[11] and Cardesa et al.[12] showed that ASC could completely prevent the acute hepatotoxic effects produced by gavage (administration by stomach tube) of rats and mice with nitrite + dimethylamine or AP. In these experiments, two solutions were gavaged, one containing nitrite and the other amine and ASC. For both dimethylamine and AP, the toxic effect was attributed to DMN formation. These studies are discussed by Kamm elsewhere in this monograph.[13]

ASC was also reported not to affect the acute toxic action of DMN.[11, 12] Unfortunately, a preliminary statement [10] that ASC did inhibit the toxic action of DMN, which was later withdrawn,[13] was extended by Edgar [14] to the suggestion that ASC might inhibit carcinogenesis by nitrosamines and, indeed, all alkylating carcinogens. As pointed out by Mirvish and Shubik,[15] Edgar's suggestion has no experimental basis.

The historical origin of Edgar's suggestion could be the report by Harman [16] that antioxidants increased the life span and decreased the spontaneous tumor incidence in some mouse strains, though Harman found no effect for ASC. In this connection, Black [17] reported that a mixture of ASC, glutathione, and butylated hydroxytoluene, added to the diet, appeared to inhibit the induction by ultraviolet light of skin tumors in hairless mice (tumor incidence was reduced from 5 of 21 to 0 of 13). The effect was attributed to a reduction of the light–induced formation of cholesterol-α-oxide (a carcinogenic epoxide) in the skin.

Oral administration of ASC inhibited tumor induction in rats and mice by nitrite + amines and ureas. Thus, nervous-system tumors and hydrocephalus were induced in the offspring of pregnant rats gavaged with ethylurea + nitrite. These effects were completely prevented by simultaneous gavage of ASC.[18] ASC did not affect induction of these tumors by ethylnitrosourea gavaged to pregnant rats.

In studies from our institute, the induction of lung adenomas in strain A mice was used to examine the amine/urea + nitrite system. Lung adenomas were induced by treatment with nitrite + (among other compounds) morpholine, piperazine, and methylurea. Nitrite was administered in the drinking water and the amines, ureas, and ASC in powdered food. Treatment was continued for 20 weeks. The mice were then left for 10 weeks, killed, and surface lung adenomas were counted.[19] We reported [20] that piperazine (6.25 g/kg food) + $NaNO_2$ (1.0 g/liter water) induced 8.6 adenomas/mouse, and that inclusion of 23 g sodium ASC/kg food reduced the tumor incidence to 1.0 adenomas/mouse. This approaches the level for untreated controls of 0.3 adenomas/mouse and represents a 91% inhibition of tumor induction. However, the inhibition was only 37% for 5.75 g ASC/kg.

Our latest experiments [21] will now be summarized. ASC alone (23 g/kg food) did not induce lung adenomas, in agreement with previous reports on the noncarcinogenicity of ASC.[22, 23] The effect of ASC was examined on the morpholine (6.33 g/kg) + $NaNO_2$ (1.0 g/liter) system, which induced 9.9 adenomas/mouse in the absence of ASC. With 23 g ASC/kg, the inhibition was 89%, and with 5.75 g ASC/kg, the inhibition was 72%. Thus at lower ASC levels the morpholine system was blocked more effectively than the piperazine system. When methylurea (2.68 g/kg) + $NaNO_2$ (1.0 g/liter) was given, 4.7 adenomas/mouse were induced. Inclusion of Na ASC (11.6 g/kg food) reduced the tumor yield to 0.1 adenomas/mouse more than the untreated controls (98% inhibition). Thus, high ASC levels effectively blocked the nitrite + amine/urea system, but at low ASC levels the blockage depended on the individual amine or urea.

We also tested whether ASC affected lung adenoma induction by preformed nitrosamines. In a preliminary experiment, ASC (23 g/kg) given with mono-nitrosopiperazine (34.5 mg/liter) increased the adenoma yield by 59%, from 12.9 (for nitrosamine alone) to 20.4 adenomas/mouse. Measurement of the consumption of nitrosamine–containing water suggested that ASC increased the nitrosamine dose by causing the mice to drink more water. Six repetitions of this experiment were carried out, 3 with mononitrosopiperazine and 3 with nitrosomorpholine. In all 6 groups, adenoma yield was greater (by 15–41%) than in controls treated with nitrosamine alone. The increases were statistically significant in 4 groups. Measurement of water consumption (done only 2–4 $\times$ during the experiment) showed no significant differences. We concluded that ASC produced a slight increase in adenoma induction by the nitrosamines, but the possibility that the effect was due merely to increased water consumption was not excluded, especially since ASC had no effect on the acute toxic action of DMN. If real, the effect could be due to an increase in the microsomal metabolic activation of nitrosamines, via α-oxidation, to give carcinogenic alkylating agents. This is plausible because the microsomal metabolism of some drugs is increased in guinea pigs receiving high doses of ASC.[24] We are now testing the effect of ASC, given in the food, on adenoma induction by nitrosamines, given by i.p. injection (so that the dose is known).

In conclusion, the present evidence supports the suggestion that ASC should be administered with readily nitrosatable drugs to block *in vivo* nitrosation. A slight potentiation by ASC of the tumorigenic action of nitrosamines, if confirmed, may not be too important. However, some caution should possibly be exercised before recommending high doses of ASC for general use.

References

1. MIRVISH, S. S. Formation of *N*-nitroso compounds: Chemistry, kinetics, and *in vivo* occurrence. Toxicol. Appl. Pharmacol. In press.
2. HILL, M. J., G. HAWKSWORTH & G. TATTERSALL. 1973. Bacteria, nitrosamines and cancer of the stomach. Brit. J. Cancer **28:** 562–567.
3. MIRVISH, S. S., L. WALLCAVE, M. EAGEN & P. SHUBIK. 1972. Ascorbate-nitrite reaction: possible means of blocking the formation of carcinogenic *N*-nitroso compounds. Science **177:** 65–68.
4. DAHN, H., L. LOEWE & C. A. BUNTON. 1960. Über die Oxydation von Ascorbinsäure durch salpetrige Säure. VI. Übersicht und Diskussion der Ergebnisse. Helvet. Chim. Acta **43:** 320–333.
5. WATTS, B. M. & B. T. LEHMANN. 1952. The effect of ascorbic acid on the oxidation of hemoglobin and the formation of nitric oxide hemoglobin. Food Res. **17:** 100–108.
6. FIDDLER, W., J. W. PENSABENE, E. G. PIOTROWSKI, R. C. DOERR & A. E. WASSERMAN. 1973. Use of sodium ascorbate or erythorbate to inhibit formation of *N*-nitrosodimethylamine in frankfurters. J. Food Sci. **38:** 1084.
7. MIRVISH, S. S., B. GOLD, M. EAGEN & S. ARNOLD. 1974. Kinetics of the nitrosation of aminopyrine to give dimethylnitrosamine. Z. Krebsforsch. **82:** 259–268.
8. FAN, T. Y. & S. R. TANNENBAUM. 1973. Natural inhibitors of nitrosation reactions: The concept of available nitrite. J. Food Sci. **38:** 1067–1069.
9. SEN, N. P. & B. DONALDSON. The effect of ascorbic acid and glutathione on the formation of nitrosopiperazines from piperazine adipate and nitrite. *In N*-Nitroso Compounds in the Environment. P. Bogovski, E. A. Walker & W. Davis, Eds. International Agency for Research on Cancer, Lyon, France. In press.

10. KAMM, J. J., T. DASHMAN, A. H. CONNEY & J. J. BURNS. 1973. Protective effects of ascorbic acid on hepatotoxicity caused by sodium nitrite plus aminopyrine. Proc. Nat. Acad. Sci. U.S.A. **70**: 747–749.
11. GREENBLATT, M. 1973. Ascorbic acid blocking of aminopyrine nitrosation in NZO/Bl mice. J. Nat. Cancer Inst. **50**: 1055–1056.
12. CARDESA, A., S. S. MIRVISH, G. T. HAVEN & P. SHUBIK. 1974. Inhibitory effect of ascorbic acid on the acute toxicity of dimethylamine plus nitrite in the rat. Proc. Soc. Exp. Biol. Med. **145**: 124–128.
13. KAMM, J. J. Effect of ascorbic acid on amine-nitrite toxicity. This monograph.
14. EDGAR, J. A. 1974. Ascorbic acid and biological alkylating agents. Nature **248**: 136–137.
15. MIRVISH, S. S. & P. SHUBIK. 1974. Ascorbic acid and nitrosamines. Nature (London) **250**: 684.
16. HARMAN, D. 1962. Role of free radicals in mutation, cancer, aging, and the maintenance of life. Radiat. Res. **16**: 753–763.
17. BLACK, H. S. 1974. Effects of dietary antioxidants on actinic tumor induction. Res. Commun. Chem. Path. Pharmacol. **7**: 783–786.
18. IVANKOVIC, S., W. J. ZELLER, D. SCHMÄHL & R. PREUSSMANN. 1973. Verhinderung der pränatal carcinogenen Wirkung von Äthylharnstoff und Nitrit durch Äscorbinsaure. Naturwissenschaften. **60**: 525.
19. GREENBLATT, M. & S. S. MIRVISH. 1973. Dose–response studies with concurrent administration of piperazine and sodium nitrite to strain A mice. J. Nat. Cancer Inst. **50**: 119–124.
20. MIRVISH, S. S., A. CARDESA, L. WALLCAVE & P. SHUBIK. 1973. Effect of sodium ascorbate on lung adenoma induction by amines plus nitrite. Proc. Amer. Assoc. Cancer Res. **14**: 102.
21. MIRVISH, S. S., A. CARDESA, L. WALLCAVE & P. SHUBIK. Induction of mouse lung adenomas by amines and ureas plus nitrite and by *N*-nitroso compounds: Effect of nitrite dose and of ascorbate, gallate, thiocyanate, and caffeine. Submitted for publication.
22. PIPKIN, G. E., J. U. SCHLEGEL, R. NISHIMURA & G. N. SHULTZ. 1969. Inhibitory effect of L-ascorbate on tumor formation in urinary bladders implanted with 3-hydroxyanthranilic acid. Proc. Soc. Exp. Biol. Med. **131**: 522–524.
23. SCHLEGEL, J. U., G. E. PIPKIN, R. NISHIMURA & G. N. SHULTZ. 1969. The role of ascorbic acid in the prevention of bladder tumor formation. Trans. Amer. Ass. Genitourin. Surg. **61**: 85–89.
24. ZANNONI, V. & P. H. SATO. Effects of ascorbic acid on microsomal drug metabolism. This monograph.
25. SEN, N. P. 1974. Personal communication.

Cancer Prevention as a Realizable Goal

by Isaac Berenblum

IT IS, I suppose permissible, on a rare occasion like this, to deal with some broader issues than those conventionally included in scientific reviews, and to try to project the resulting image onto a wider screen. Assuming that one is more or less familiar with what has so far been achieved in a particular field, the question then arises: "Where do we go from here?"

In science, as in many other spheres of human endeavor, sophistication enables one to cope with problems which would otherwise remain insoluble. But there is, of course, a price to pay for this. It not only involves the use of complicated techniques and the need for ample budgets, manpower, etc.; it also creates difficulties at the *interpretative* level—to decide how to make best use of the information for practical, beneficial purposes.

I should like to deal briefly with the latter aspect —more specifically, with trying to extrapolate existing knowledge of the etiology and pathogenesis of tumors *as a guide to cancer prevention in man.*

Thirty or forty years ago, this problem seemed simple enough: All that had to be done was to identify the carcinogens in our environment and eliminate them, or at least, prevent us from being exposed to them. Since no more than 5–10% of all human cancers were then thought to be of environmental origin, and the remainder assumed to be of spontaneous origin, the scope for cancer prevention seemed, at that time, rather limited.

Presented on receipt of the Alfred P. Sloan Award of the General Motors Cancer Research Foundation, Washington, DC, June 18, 1980.

From the Weizmann Institute of Science, Rehovot, Israel.

Address for reprints: Isaac Berenblum, The Weizmann Institute of Science, Rehovot, Israel.

Accepted for publication December 30 , 1980.

How one's views have changed since then!

First of all, it is now fairly clear that the low estimate of human cancers attributable to environmental factors is widely off the mark—that *70–90 percent of human cancers* are, in one way or another, determined by environmental influences.[9,10,19] On the other hand, one now realizes that in only a small proportion of cases do such environmental factors operate as "complete" carcinogens.[3,9,10]

To speak of "complete" carcinogens implies that there are also "incomplete" carcinogens, or expressed differently, that there are all kinds of "associated factors"—cocarcinogens, promoting agents, etc.— which are able to determine whether a carcinogen will, or will not, cause a tumor to develop.

This information, initially derived from extensive series of animal experiments,[2,3,4,5,17] has in recent years been found also to be true for human cancer.[9,10,20] This has brought about a radical change in outlook among cancer epidemiologists, who are now more and more preoccupied with "associated factors" of this kind. It is also likely, in time, to bring about comparable changes in attitude with regard to laboratory testing for incriminating agents, putting greater emphasis on "precipitating factors," as a guide to cancer prevention.

From the practical viewpoint, it really matters very little whether one is dealing with "complete" or "incomplete" carcinogens, so long as their elimination can prevent the disease from developing.

But prevention *by eliminating "complete" or "incomplete" causative agents* represents only one means of reducing the cancer incidence. There is also the alternative method of interfering with the carcinogenic process. This could offer even brighter prospects of eradicating the disease, or at least, serve as a valuable supplement to cancer prevention based on *elimination* of causative agents.

Prevention *by methods of interference* can operate at three different levels: (1) during the pre-carcinogenic stage; (2) during the course of carcinogenic action; and (3) during the post-carcinogenic stage.

I should like to give a few examples of each, to serve as a sort of blueprint of cancer prevention for the future.

One example of interference at the precarcinogenic level has to do with the production of carcinogenic nitrosamines in the stomach, through chemical interaction between nitrites and secondary amines.[15] We now know that this can be strongly inhibited by the simultaneous presence of vitamin C in the stomach.[13] Here, then, is an opportunity of preventing cancer development *before carcinogenesis even begins to operate.*

Another example relates to the fact that most carcinogens have first to be ''activated'' in the body, by enzymic conversion into ''ultimate'' carcinogens, before they can react with cells to transform them into tumor cells.[12] But carcinogens tend also to be enzymically detoxicated in the body.[12] Actually, the potency of a carcinogenic compound largely depends on which of the two competing processes gains the upper hand. In time, it will almost certainly be possible to manipulate these two enzymic processes, and to shift the balance in favor of detoxication—thereby providing another method or prevention *by interference at the pre-carcinogenic stage.*

A third example is by lowering *the responsiveness of a tissue* to carcinogenic action. Responsiveness is known to vary during different phases of development; *e.g.*, in breast tissue, in which the functional changes are determined by an interplay of different hormones.[14] By artificially changing the hormonal pattern, it should become possible, in time, to render that organ less responsive to whatever carcinogenic agent that might be present.

Interference *during the course of carcinogenic action* is an altogether different proposition, which might be figuratively described as ''putting a spoke in the wheel,'' thereby preventing *the completion* of the carcinogenic process. The methods will naturally differ according to the particular phase of the multistage process of carcinogenesis which is being blocked or reversed.

The primary, rapid, *initiating* phase of carcinogenesis is now generally accepted as being brought about by a gene mutation, providing the cell with new ''tumor-type'' information,[6,7] thus converting it into a potential or ''dormant tumor cell.''

While a gene mutation may, in a sense, be looked upon as an irreversible change, both in genetic makeup and potential function, mutated genes can, in fact, be repaired in the body by specific enzymes, the cell reverting to normal.[8] This probably occurs more commonly than is generally supposed.

Once the enzymes responsible for the repair are identified, it might become possible to stimulate their action artificially and encourage the repair process to function more effectively, *thereby blocking any further stages of carcinogenic action.*

Interference with the *promoting* phase of carcinogenesis would seem to offer the best prospects for cancer prevention,[3] if only because the promoting phase covers most of the latent period of carcinogenesis (which, in man, may be 30 years or more), during which there is considerable scope for interfering action.

''Anticarcinogens'' have been known for a very long time. It was actually my good fortune (back in 1929) to discover, by pure chance, the first example of such agents—sulfur mustard, which inhibited tar carcinogenesis in mouse skin.[1] It is still the most potent anticarcinogen known; but is highly toxic and, therefore, altogether unsuitable for human use.

Many other anticarcinogenic agents and influences have since been discovered in various laboratories[18] some being specific for certain organs or tissues, others (such as caloric restriction of the diet) apparently acting in a more general way. Toxicity is still the major stumbling block in attempting to apply anticarcinogenic agents for human use. Much attention is nowadays directed to examining chemical analogues of known inhibitors, in the hope that some of these will be relatively free from toxic side-effects while still exerting inhibitory action on carcinogenesis. Among the more recent examples are the ''retinoids,'' related to vitamin A, which seem to possess fairly pronounced anticarcinogenic action.[16] While the earlier members of the group did have undesirable toxicity, some of the later ones seem to have less harmful side-effects. There are also other types of anticarcinogenic agents, discovered in recent years, which might have similar useful applications.[18]

One of the interesting features of such anticarcinogenic agents is that so many of them seem to be effective in inhibiting carcinogenesis in animals when administered at quite an advanced stage during the long latent period.

But all this is trying to interfere with the promoting phase of carcinogenesis *by trial and error.* How much more logical it would be to discover how promoting action operates, and then design *specific* methods of blocking the process. This is, in fact, one of the major preoccupations of present-day research workers in the field of carcinogenesis.

We already have a good idea about how *initiating*

action operates—by inducing a gene mutation (as I have already intimated). The mechanism of *promoting* action is still something of a mystery. Once the mystery is solved—and we seem to be getting closer and closer to the solution of the problem[11]—one would be in a position to devise *specific* methods of blocking the process, *and thereby introduce rational methods of cancer prevention.*

There is finally interference during the post-carcinogenic stage—which might seem, at first sight, a contradiction in terms. For how can one interfere with something that is already finished? The answer is that there is a large gap, or transition phase, between the completion of carcinogenesis and the earliest clinical evidence of a growing tumor.

The most obvious example is "carcinoma *in situ*" in the cervix of the uterus, consisting of committed cancer cells which are still confined to their site of origin, but identifiable by the Papanicolaou Smear Test. Surgical removal of the lesion can thus be described as "preventive" *therapy* at the post-carcinogenic stage."

The other well-known example refers to a cancer which is already at the growing stage, yet barely detectable—as in early breast cancer, unsuspected but recognized during a routine check-up at a Cancer Detection Center. Whether this may justifiably be included under "cancer prevention" is a matter of semantics. But the fact remains that *early* detection of an established cancer may lead to a successful cure, and the term "prevention" may be used here in the sense of avoiding the danger of the disease reaching a stage no longer curable.

The picture I have tried to present seems promising enough, even if somewhat speculative in parts, As an optimist, I naturally believe that the virtual eradication of the disease is, in the long run, a realizable goal. Others might take a less optimistic view. The distinction between extrapolating existing knowledge and sheer fanciful speculation is, after all, not well defined.

In any case, success will not only have to depend on translating theory into practice; it will also have to rely on the public being ready to cooperate, when such methods of prevention become available.

There is a story, relating to the time when my country was militarily in a precarious state, about an old man being heard to say: "Stop relying on miracles and start reading the Psalms instead." Perhaps I am guilty of offering the same kind of advice—in a secular sense.

REFERENCES

1. Berenblum I. The modifying influence of dichloro-ethyl sulphide on the induction of tumours in mice by tar. *J Pathol Bacteriol* 1929; 32:425–434.
2. Berenblum I. A re-evaluation of the concept of cocarcinogenesis. *Prog Exp Tumor Res* 1969; 11:21–30.
3. Berenblum I. Carcinogenesis as a biological problem. In: Frontiers of biology, Amsterdam: North-Holland Publ. Co., and New York: Elsevier, vol. 34, 1974.
4. Berenblum I. Some basic problems in assessing carcinogenic risks. *Br J Cancer* 1980; 41:490–493.
5. Boutwell RK. The function and mechanism of promoters of carcinogenesis. *CRC Crit Rev Toxicol* 1974; 2:419–444.
6. Brookes P. Mini review: Covalent interaction of carcinogens with DNA. *Life Sciences* 1975; 16:331–344.
7. Chu EHY, Trosko JE, Chang C-C. Mutational approaches to the study of carcinogenesis. *J Toxicol Environ Health* 1977; 2: 1317–1334.
8. Cleaver JE. DNA repair with purines and pyrimidines in radiation- and carcinogen-damaged normal and Xeroderma pigmentosum human cells. *Cancer Res* 1973; 33:362–369.
9. Doll R. Strategy for detection of cancer hazards to man. *Nature* 1977; 265:589–596.
10. Higginson J, Muir CS. Guest Editorial: Environmental carcinogenesis: Misconceptions and limitations to cancer control. *J Natl Cancer Inst* 1979; 63:1291–1298.
11. Mechanisms of tumor promotion and cocarcinogenesis. In: Carcinogenesis: A comprehensive survey. Slaga TJ, Sivak A, Boutwell RK, eds. New York: Raven Press, 1978.
12. Miller EC. Some current perspectives on chemical carcinogenesis in humans and experimental animals: Presidential address. *Cancer Res* 1978; 38:1479–1496.
13. Mirvish SS. Formation of N-nitroso compounds: Chemistry, kinetics and *in vivo* occurrence. *Toxicol Appl Pharmacol* 1975; 31:325–351.
14. Nandi S. Hormonal carcinogenesis: A novel hypothesis for the role of hormones. *J Environ Pathol & Toxicol* 1978; 2:13–20.
15. Sander S, Bürkle G. Induktion maligner Tumoren bei Ratten durch gleichzeitige Verfütterung von Nitrit und sekundären Aminen. *Z Krebsforsch* 1969; 73:54–66.
16. Sporn MB, Dunlop NM, Newton DL, Smith JM. Prevention of chemical carcinogenesis by vitamin A and its synthetic analogs (retinoids). *Fed Proc* 1976; 35:1332–1338.
17. Van Duuren BL. Tumor-promoting and co-carcinogenic agents in chemical carcinogenesis. In: Searle CE, ed. Chemical Carcinogens. ACS Monograph 173. Washington, DC: American Chemical Society 1976; 24–51.
18. Wattenberg LW. Inhibitors of chemical carcinogenesis. *Adv Cancer Res* 1977; 26:197–226.
19. WHO Technical Rep. Series, Geneva: 1964; 276.
20. Wynder EL, Gori GB. Guest editorial: Contribution of the environment to cancer incidence: An epidemiological exercise. *J Natl Cancer Inst* 1977; 58:825–832.

Clinical Trials: A Recent Emphasis in the Prevention Program of the National Cancer Institute

by William D. DeWys and Peter Greenwald

RESEARCH on the etiology and prevention of cancer has been a major emphasis of the National Cancer Institute (NCI) since its beginning and has included epidemiologic research, research with animal models, and basic research. Recently, NCI has increased its emphasis on clinical trials in prevention.

The relationship between diet and cancer incidence has not yet been precisely defined, but data increasingly point to a role of dietary factors in determining cancer incidence.[1] Published estimates of the percentage reduction in cancer deaths that could be accomplished by dietary changes have ranged as high as 60% to 70%,[2,3] but 30% seems a reasonable, conservative estimate. These estimates are based on several assumptions and can only be validated by the results of controlled clinical trials. Nonetheless, these estimates are valuable for setting research priorities, estimating the feasibility of clinical trials, and designing clinical trials.

Interest in the effect of diet on cancer incidence dates from the classic animal studies of Tannenbaum reported in the 1940s;[4] however, the possible relevance of these studies to humans is based on epidemiologic studies published dur-

From the Division of Resources, Centers, and Community Activities, National Cancer Institute, Bethesda, Md.

Address reprint requests to William D. DeWys, National Institutes of Health, National Cancer Institute, Blair Bldg, Rm 6A07, 9000 Rockville Pike, Bethesda, MD 20205.

ing the 1970s. Using these studies as a basis, in 1979 the NCI developed and published a set of dietary principles that included a reduction of dietary fat, an increase in dietary fiber, and moderation in alcohol consumption.[5] In 1980, NCI commissioned the National Academy of Sciences to study all available information on diet and cancer incidence, to summarize the state of knowledge in this area,[1] and to make recommendations about future research directions.[6] Concurrently, NCI staff and its advisory boards reviewed the status of research on diet and cancer and planned for the development of future research.[7] The early implementation phases of these plans are discussed in this paper.

THE NEED FOR CLINICAL TRIALS

The development of clinical trials is an integral part of NCI research plans in diet and cancer prevention. The rationale for doing clinical trials includes theoretical and practical considerations. At a theoretical level, it is important to test an attractive theory rigorously to reveal any flaws in the theory.[8] At the practical level, clinical trials must address issues of specificity not resolved in epidemiologic studies, uncertainty about the clinical relevance of animal models, questions about participant acceptance of the intervention, and the cost/benefit ratio.

As noted in several of the reviews in this issue, although epidemiologic studies may suggest a correlation between a specific nutrient and the incidence of cancer, they often lack specificity and are not free from confounding effects. For example, diets that are low in vitamin A are likely to be low in vitamin C and folate as well. Also, diets that are high in β carotene will also be high in several nonnutritive factors that may have anticarcinogenic effects. While improvements in epidemiologic research methods and improvements in the data base on food composition may partially remedy the specificity issue, clinical trials are the most direct approach to resolving questions of specificity. In a clinical trial, intake of a single nutrient, such as β carotene, can be manipulated while all other aspects of the diet are left unchanged. The technique of randomization should result in two groups that differ only in the specific nutrient being studied.

Studies in animal models can be used to address issues of specificity, but we are presently uncertain about which animal models are most relevant to human disease. In cancer treatment, animal models have been found to differ considerably in their predictability of the activity of chemotherapy agents in humans. We envision a strategy in which numerous animal models will be studied for each intervention that is to be studied in humans. Retrospective analyses will then be used to select a smaller number of animal models for determining which cancer preventive agents and diets to study in humans.

Behavioral research will be an important component of clinical trials, especially to elucidate issues of participant acceptance and adherence to specific intervention strategies, such as drug therapy or change of diet. Much of the current knowledge about behavior is based on treatment of persons with illnesses or unwanted conditions, such as obesity. Participants in cancer prevention trials will, for the most part, be free of illnesses; however, they may be at an increased risk for developing cancer and thus may be motivated to accept the intervention. Symptoms caused by minor intercurrent illnesses may be falsely attributed to cancer prevention interventions and could result in noncompliance and dropping out.

Finally, clinical trials will provide the basis for determining the risk/benefit ratio for each intervention. The trials will introduce relatively nontoxic levels of the intervention agent; however, description of the complete pattern and degree of toxicity requires a large clinical trial. Phase 1 studies will provide preliminary information about toxicity and will be the basis for selecting the dose level for phase 3 trials. Selection of doses for phase 3 trials must consider the tradeoff issues. The degree of toxicity that is acceptable to prevent lung cancer may be higher than for prevention of skin cancer. On the benefit side, studies may have a spectrum of endpoints, such as reversal of precursor lesions, reduction in the incidence of cancer, reduction in deaths from cancer, reduction in overall death rate, and improvement in overall survival. Careful delineation of toxicity and accurate assessment of the study endpoints will determine the risk/benefit ratio.

The clinical trials program has been divided into two subject areas — chemoprevention, and diet and cancer prevention. The areas overlap partially, but each has unique emphasis.

THE DIET AND CANCER PREVENTION ACTIVITIES

NCI will fund clinical trials of diets and other research that will strengthen the clinical trials. The initial clinical trials will study the effects of a 20% fat diet as the intervention compared to the typical American diet in which approximately 40% of calories are derived from fat. Two separate trials will be conducted among different target populations.

One trial will be of women at high risk for developing breast cancer; the endpoint will be a reduced incidence of breast cancer. Of these women, one group will have a first-degree relative with a history of breast cancer and will have had a first pregnancy at 30 years or more of age, or will have had two or more breast biopsies for benign disease. A second group will be women who have two or more first-degree relatives with a history of breast cancer. We estimate that these selection criteria will result in a population with an annual incidence of breast cancer of 1%. The rationale for this trial is that the level of dietary fat correlates positively in epidemiologic studies with the incidence of breast cancer. In studies of migrants, the increases in the incidence of breast cancer coincides with increases in dietary fat. Major economic events such as war have been associated with changes in dietary fat and changes in breast cancer incidence. Studies in laboratory animals indicate that dietary fat affects cancer incidence when the diet is changed during the promotion phase of carcinogenesis; reduced dietary fat, even if late in the promotion phase, has resulted in a reduced incidence of breast cancer. The clinical trial will test whether reducing dietary fat will slow or halt the promotion phase of carcinogenesis and reduce the incidence of breast cancer in the study population. This clinical trial will evaluate the specificity of the epidemiologic studies and will test whether the impact of a low-fat diet intervention in humans duplicates animal model results. This trial will also provide insights into strategies for influencing eating behavior and will document the safety of the study diet.

The second trial involving a 20% fat diet will study women with stage 2 breast cancer, the endpoint being a reduction or delay of the development of metastases. The rationale for this trial is that the prognosis for patients with breast cancer differs among countries. Japanese patients have better survival rates than US patients[9,10] for all stages and extent of disease.[11] The differences in survival cannot be explained by difference in histology[10] or by differences in medical care since similar differences were observed in Hawaii where Japanese and white patients receive similar medical care.[12] Rather, differences in dietary fat consumption may underlie these differences in survival.[13–17] The differences in survival are greater for postmenopausal women than for premenopausal women[18] possibly because the differences in fat consumption between white and Japanese women increases with age. Older Japanese women are less likely to be westernized than younger Japanese women.[12]

The mechanism by which dietary fat or obesity might influence prognosis is not understood, but hormonal changes might be involved, such as abnormalities in the pattern of prolactin secretion,[19] decreased levels of gonadotropins,[20] increased conversion of androstenedione to estrone,[21] or altered sex hormone-binding globulin, free androgen and free estrogen.[22]

A challenge in diet research is obtaining and maintaining adherence to the diet. Boyd and colleagues documented a 1-year period of adherence to a 20% fat diet by women with radiographic evidence of breast dysplasia.[23] Their approach included intensive personalized contact between the research staff and the study participants, an approach that may not be feasible in large-scale trials. The endurance of the adhering behavior is uncertain and reinforcing strategies will be important. NCI will be supporting research to develop and test various strategies for modifications of eating behavior that are highly efficacious, cost effective, and lasting.

We also anticipate conducting clinical trials in the near future to change the fiber, carotene, or vitamin A contents of the diets. First, however, a more complete data base will be necessary on the fiber components in the diet because the various fiber components may have different potential for cancer prevention. Also the carotenes (which are precursors of vitamin A) and the various forms of vitamin A may have different cancer prevention potentials, antioxidant properties, and potential for toxicity. NCI will support studies to determine the fiber, vitamin A, and carotene content of foods.

CHEMOPREVENTION ACTIVITIES

Chemoprevention research differs from diet research in that well-defined chemicals in precise doses are administered as the intervention. In chemoprevention, as in diet, we will aim for a balance between investigator-initiated research and research that follows a preconceived strategy. An example of a RFA (request for application) for investigator-initiated research is in the area of natural and synthetic inhibitors of carcinogenesis. The purpose of these studies will be to identify new naturally occurring inhibitors of the carcinogenic process, to develop methods for isolating specific constituents, and to describe the mechanisms of action of the inhibitors.

Other studies are being developed to implement a preconceived strategy.[7] These studies will include preclinical screening, studies in a battery of animal models (different species, different tumor sites, and different carcinogens), and preclinical toxicology. All of these studies will provide leads and background information for selection of agents and doses for initial human studies. Initial human studies will be phase 1 studies to define patterns of toxicity and establish tolerable doses for humans. These studies will differ from phase 1 studies of cancer chemotherapy drugs in duration of treatment and the need to discover toxic events that may occur infrequently. Because chemoprevention agents will be administered for long periods of time, phase 1 studies must be designed to detect delayed or chronic toxicity. Also, chemoprevention agents will be administered to large numbers of well people, thus necessitating knowledge of infrequently occurring side effects.

In addition to phase 1 studies, biologic studies in humans may assist in formulating phase 3 protocols. For example, current selenium studies are evaluating physiologic parameters of selenium administration (blood levels and platelet

Table 1. NCI-Supported Chemoprevention Clinical Trials

Study Population	Institution	Agent(s)
Healthy population		
Physicians	Harvard	β caroten
		aspirin
Dentists	Harvard	Vit E
		Vit A
		Vit B_6
		Na Selenite
Lung		
Dysplasia	U Alabama	Vit B_{12} and folic acid
Asbestos workers	U Washington	13-cis retinoc acid
Male smokers	U Washington	13-cis retinoc acid
Large bowel		
Familial polyposis	MSKCC	Vit C, Vit E, Bran
	W Va U	13-cis retinoic acid
Polyposis	U Illinois	β carotene
Skin (basal/squamous)	MSKCC	Vit C, vit E,
		β carotene
	Dartmouth	β carotene
	U Arizona	13-cis retinoic acid
	NCI, VA, Army, Navy	13-cis Retinoic acid
	Africa (albinos)	β carotene and canthaxanthin
Cervic		
Dysplasia, topical	U Arizona	All trans retinoic acid
	A Einstein	Retinyl acetate
Dysplasis, systemic	U of Washington	Folic acid

glutathione peroxidase) for different forms of selenium (selenite and selenomethionine). Also under study is the effect of concommitant ingestion of food on selenium pharmacokinetics.

The keystone of chemoprevention research is the phase 3 clinical trial. At present, NCI is supporting 16 clinical trials that are either in progress or about to be initiated (Table 1). Target sites for which we are encouraging studies are shown in Table 2; patients who have been treated successfully for certain cancers are at increased risk for developing a second cancer.

An overall plan has been developed and implemented for reviewing and monitoring NCI-sponsored prevention trials. All projects undergo study section peer review. We encourage investigators developing phase 3 protocols to use a standardized format to facilitate review, exchange of information between investigators, and implementation of the protocol (Table 3). Protocols are then reviewed by a DRCCA staff committee to assure: (1) that all potential adverse effects have been considered and addressed in the protocol, (2) adequacy of monitoring for toxicity, (3) adequacy of monitoring for participant adherence to the protocol, and (4) completeness and clarity of the informed consent process. All investigators will be asked to submit semiannual progress reports to NCI. Site visits may be made

to NCI staff when the protocol is initiated depending on investigator experience and protocol complexity. Site visits generally will be conducted annually thereafter. A meeting of all funded investigators will be held annually for sharing of experiences. For many of these trials NCI will file an Investigational New Drug Application (IND) with the Food and Drug Administration (FDA) and will file an annual report with the FDA.

APPLICATION TO THE POPULATION AT LARGE

When positive results are obtained from any of the trials discussed above, we will be interested in

Table 2. Target Groups for Future Chemoprevention Trials

Prevention of primary or second primary
in the following sites:
    bladder
    breast
    head and neck
    lung

Reduction in incidence of second primaries of various sites
in patients successfully treated for:
    acute leukemia
    Hodgkins disease
    Lymphoma
    Ovarian cancer

Table 3. Protocol Format.

Face Sheet
Table of Contents
Schema of Study
1. Introduction and background
2. Objectives
3. Participant selection:
    eligibility
    exclusions
4. Prestudy requirements
5. Intervention assignments
6. Intervention plan
7. Toxicity
8. Compliance
9. Measurement of efficacy
10. Duration of treatment
11. Methods of analysis and statistical considerations
12. Forms and records
13. Pathology review
14. Drug requirements
15. Informed consent
16. Adverse effects reporting

applying these results to the population at large. This will bring new challenges such as disseminating information, stimulating and maintaining acceptance of the new behavior (diet, pill taking, etc), monitoring the population for adherence to the new behavior, and monitoring the impact in terms of adverse effects and changes in cancer incidence. These applications may require new types of research (cancer control phases 4 and 5) and new uses for existing monitoring systems. Specifically, we plan to use the Health and Nutrition Examinations Survey (HANES) of the National Center for Health Statistics to monitor acceptance of preventive behaviors by population.[5] The Surveillance, Epidemiology, and End Results (SEER) program of NCI will monitor changes in cancer incidence. Linkage between these two data systems will be useful for monitoring cause and effect relationships.

REFERENCES

1. National Academy of Sciences, Committee on Diet, Nutrition and Cancer: Diet, Nutrition and Cancer. Washington, DC, National Academy Press, 1982, pp 496

2. Wynder EL, Gori GB: Contribution of the environment to cancer incidence: An epidemiologic exercise. J Natl Can Inst 58:825–832, 1977

3. Doll R, Peto R: The causes of cancer: Quantitative estimates of available risks of cancer in the United States today. J Natl Can Inst 66:1192–1308, 1981

4. Tannenbaum A: The genesis and growth of tumors. III. Effects of a high fat diet. Cancer Res 2:468–475, 1942

5. Upton AC: Statement on diet, nutrition and cancer. Hearings of the Subcommittee on Nutrition, Senate Committee on Agriculture, Nutrition and Forestry. 1979

6. National Academy of Sciences, Committee on Diet, Nutrition and Cancer: Diet, Nutrition and Cancer: Directions for Research. Washington, DC, National Academy Press, 1983, pp 74

7. DeWys WD, Greenwald P: The diet, nutrition and cancer prevention plan of the National Cancer Institute (in press)

8. Popper KR: The logic of scientific discovery. London, Hutchinson, 1959

9. Wynder EL, Kajatani T, Kumo J, et al: A comparison of survival rates between American and Japanese patients with breast cancer. Surg Gynecol Obstet 117:196–200, 1963

10. Morrison AS, Lowe CR, MacMahon B, et al: Some international differences in treatment and survival in breast cancer. Int J Cancer 18:269–273, 1976

11. Nemoto T, Tominaga T, Chamberlain A, et al: Differences in breast cancer between Japan and the United States. J Natl Cancer Inst 58:193, 1977

12. Ward-Hinds M, Kolonel LN, Nomura AMY, et al: Stage specific breast cancer incidence rates by age among Japanese and Caucasian women in Hawaii. Brit J Cancer 45:118–123, 1982

13. Armstrong B, Doll R: Environmental factors and cancer incidence and mortality in different countries with special reference to dietary practice. Brit J Cancer 15:617–631, 1975

14. Carroll KK, Gammal EB, Plunkett ER: Dietary fat and mammary cancer. Cancer Med Assoc J 93:590–594, 1968

15. Wynder EL, MacCormick F, Hill P, et al: Nutrition and the etiology and prevention of breast cancer. Cancer Detection and Prevention 1:293–310, 1976

16. Donegan WL, Marty AJ, Rimm AA: The association of body weight and recurrent cancer of the breast. Cancer 41:1590–1594, 1978

17. Kolonel LN, Hankin JH, Lee J, et al: Nutrient intakes in relation to cancer incidence in Hawaii. Brit J Cancer 44:332, 1981

18. Sakamoto G, Sugano H, Hartman WH: Comparative clinicopathological study of breast cancer among Japanese and American females. Jpn J Clin Oncol 25:161, 1979

19. Kwa HG, Bulbrook RD, Cleton F, et al: An abnormal early evening peak of plasma prolactin in nulliparous and obese post-menopausal women. Int J Cancer 22:691–693, 1978

20. deWaard F, Baanders-Van Halewijn EA: A prospective study in general practice on breast cancer risks in postmenopausal women. Int J Cancer 14:153–160, 1974

21. McDonald R, Grodin J, Sitteri P: The utilization of plasma androstendione for estrone production in women in endocrimology. Excerpta Med Int Congr Sem 184:770–776, 1969

22. O'Dea J, Wieland R, Hallberg M, et al: Effect of dietary weight loss on sex steroid binding, sex steroids and gonadotropins on obese postmenopausal women. J Lab Clin Med 93:1004–1008, 1979

23. Boyd NF, Cousins ML, Bayliss SE, et al: Diet modification in clinical trials: Behavioral issues in the prevention of cancer, in Burish TG, Levy SM, Meyerowitz BE (eds): Nutrition, Taste Aversion and Cancer: A Biobehavioral Perspective (in press)

Epidemiology: A Step Forward in the Scientific Approach to Preventing Cancer Through Chemoprevention

by Peter Greenwald

At the National Cancer Institute (NCI) in the Division of Cancer Prevention and Control, we have recently taken a long, hard look at the concepts of prevention and control as they have been historically understood and applied. We found an important lesson for future cancer research in two examples, one negative and one positive.

The negative example is our short progress on the route to preventing lung cancer caused by cigarette smoking. Although research has established for at least two decades that the most effective means of preventing lung cancer is to eliminate cigarette smoking, only recently has a concentrated effort been made to develop policies to achieve that goal. We still lack knowledge about how to influence smoking behavior, especially among youths. Had we developed a strategy 20 years ago for ascertaining when a research base is adequate to support policymaking and information dissemination, and acted more forcefully on that strategy, we might have fewer deaths from lung cancer today.

The positive example is the clinical progress made in cancer therapy since the 1950s. A research strategy evolved, based on clinical trials as a means of evaluating the efficacy of treatments. Then, in 1955, the National Cooperative Chemotherapy Program was organized, ensuring participation of the best researchers in the nation, high standards, and compatibility of studies. As results became available, they were quickly communicated and adopted. New leads for further advances were systematically brought into the process. Advanced tests led into well-defined phases of human clinical trials.

Until quite recently, the rigor and systematic approach applied to clinical research had never been applied to cancer prevention research. During 1982–83, however, the NCI carefully reviewed the needs and potentials in cancer prevention and control and developed a new policy for prevention research, guided by three basic assumptions:

- that the scientific method of inquiry is an essential part of cancer control;
- that the pursuit of excellence in science and the potential for reducing incidence, morbidity, and mortality in numerically important ways are prime considerations in setting priorities for action;
- that the planning and conduct of activities are built on existing strengths of the National Cancer Program.

The policy is also based on a clear, consistent definition of cancer prevention. Cancer prevention has as a major foundation etiologic research. Cancer prevention is defined as *applied research* to *systematically* test or introduce a specific *intervention* aimed at having a *mea-*

Dr. Greenwald is Director of the Division of Cancer Prevention and Control, National Cancer Institute. The article is based on his presentation at the Second Binational Symposium: United States–Israel, held at Bethesda, Md., October 17–19, 1983.

Tearsheet requests to Dr. Peter Greenwald, Director, DCPC, National Cancer Institute, National Institutes of Health, Bldg. 31, Rm. 4A–32, Bethesda, Md. 20205.

Reprinted with permission from *Public Health Reports,* Vol. 99, No. 3, May-June 1984, pp. 259-264.

surable impact on an important cancer problem. The purpose of the intervention is to reduce cancer incidence (and, thus, also morbidity and mortality) rates in populations.

Prevention Research: Strategy

The outcome of this planning effort was a major strategy for prevention research. The Division of Cancer Prevention and Control (DCPC) now requires that development of cancer interventions follow an orderly sequence of research phases (fig. 1). The phases are designed to enable DCPC to assess the rigor of proposed interventions in a systematic manner. Each phase carefully, incrementally advances the research concept, thus allowing only those interventions evaluated and proven to be effective to be brought to widespread implementation.

In Phase I, *Hypothesis Development*, research leads are derived from a synthesis of available scientific evidence, from basic laboratory, epidemiologic, and clinical studies, about a cancer problem and possible interventions. A testable hypothesis is formulated about the effectiveness of the intervention in reducing incidence, morbidity, or mortality rates in populations. Phase I develops the hypothesis; Phases II–V test the hypothesis in comparative or controlled studies.

In Phase II, *Methods Development*, the accuracy and validity of procedures are ensured before the study is begun, to test the hypothesis. Phase II might include the following types of studies: pilot tests to investigate the feasibility or acceptance of using a proposed intervention in a specific population subgroup; studies to assess potential participation (compliance) in future intervention studies; development, pilot testing, and validation of data-collection forms, instruments, or questionnaires; testing of translations of materials from other languages; comparative pilot tests of alternative forms or approaches to performing the intervention; and tests of the applicability of methods used with other diseases or disciplines. Often an intervention must be assessed in terms of sensitivity and specificity, cost-effectiveness, and minimal subject risks.

In Phase III, *Controlled Intervention Trials*, the hypothesis developed in Phase I is tested, using the methods validated in Phase II. A Phase III study tests the efficacy of the preventive intervention in a group of individuals. Rather than being a representative sample, the group may be more homogeneous than the actual target population, and may be chosen in a setting that facilitates research management. In controlled intervention trials, the study group is compared with a group that does not receive an intervention, or different interventions are compared with one another, and/or with a control group.

In Phase IV, *Defined Population Studies*, an intervention proven to be efficacious in Phase III is applied in a carefully controlled study of a defined population. The study population is a large, distinct, and well-characterized population or is a representative sample of such a population. Results from a well-designed population study can be generalized to the entire target population. For example, estimates can be derived for rates of exposure, incidence, morbidity, mortality, and survival, and for predicting changes in these as a result of the intervention under study. Thus, the studies provide the evidence of potential benefit that warrants proceeding to demonstration and implementation studies on a broader scale.

Figure 1. Cancer control phases

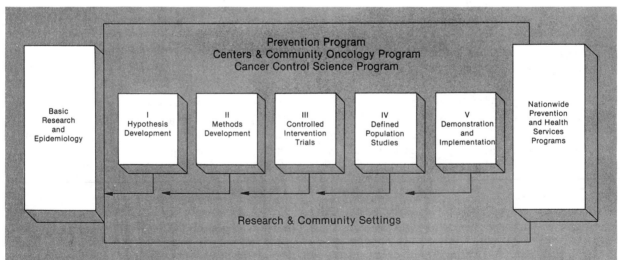

In Phase V, *Demonstration and Implementation*, the research process culminates in studies that apply a proven intervention to a community at large. An evaluation component is built into Phase V studies to provide the final assessment of costs and benefits of implementing the cancer prevention intervention on a nationwide scale. Thus, at the end of Phase V, a proven intervention with public health effectiveness in reducing cancer incidence, morbidity, or mortality would have been introduced in a population with known characteristics, and a process for monitoring the impact of the program would be in place.

Role of Epidemiology in Research Plans

The DCPC's prevention program was reorganized and expanded in 1983; it now has five content priorities: smoking, tobacco, and cancer; chemoprevention; diet and cancer; occupational cancer; and cancer detection. For all these prevention areas, we use a research flow design that includes epidemiologic research.

All prevention research and methods development derive from three research categories: laboratory research, epidemiologic research, and human intervention studies. The flow of this research logic is shown in figure 2 in terms of the chemoprevention program. We envision an

array of stages in laboratory research, an array of stages in epidemiologic research, and leads from either of these to be brought into human intervention studies that may lead to broad preventive application. A decision point ("DP" in the figure) is established at the end of each array and also at the end of each stage. The decision points require establishment of criteria for evaluating the leads at that array or stage.

The epidemiologic research array (fig. 2) begins with a review of available literature and current research. In addition to identifying potential agents for further study, the objective is to identify populations for epidemiologic studies and for human intervention studies. The third activity in this initial stage is a monitoring function: identifying and evaluating naturally occurring experiments. For example, populations may unexpectedly change an aspect of their lifestyles, such as diet. We must be prepared to monitor the relationships between such changes and subsequent cancer incidence and mortality.

At the Stage I decision point, there are two possible directions. One possibility is to bring the lead forward by additional epidemiologic studies that are more focused than the initial leads. The second possibility is that the lead so strongly fulfills the decision criteria that it may be reviewed against the next set of decision criteria without

Figure 2. NCI Chemoprevention Program

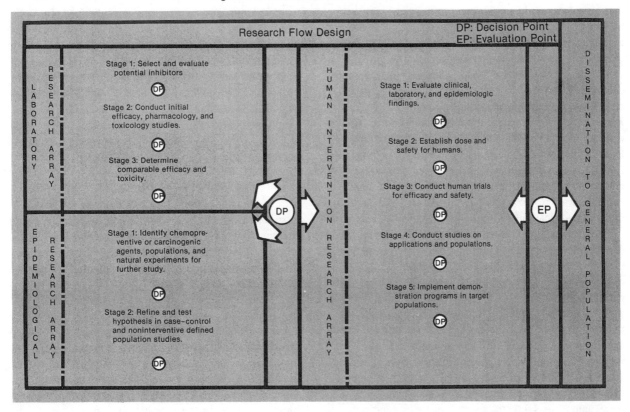

additional studies. The lead, then, could move to human intervention studies. Thus, Stage II studies refine and test hypotheses about agents in target populations in case-control and nonintervention defined population studies. Analytical epidemiologic methods are used to determine preventive effects in selected populations and perhaps in the population at large. Again, criteria are specified, and leads fulfilling these criteria are then brought into human trials.

The human intervention array involves five stages. In the initial stage, combined information from laboratory and epidemiologic arrays is evaluated. A lead may enter clinical studies if it is very strong in terms of laboratory data or epidemiologic data, or moderately strong in both. After all criteria are met in the first four stages, the final stage is a demonstration program in larger target populations, followed by an evaluation point that requires ongoing monitoring of the population to document the anticipated effect of the intervention.

The Chemoprevention Research Plan

Chemoprevention is the introduction into the diet of specific chemicals, such as vitamins, synthetic analogs, or other substances, for the purpose of reducing cancer incidence. The agents to be used are chemically defined and can be admininstered in precisely specified dosages. An advantage of the chemoprevention approach is that it may be easier to add a constituent to the diet for preventive purposes than to achieve acceptance of a major modification of dietary patterns.

In contrast to the chemoprevention research program, which deals with micronutrients, the related diet and cancer research program focuses on macronutrients that may be either added to or subtracted from the diet. Rather than examining precise dosages of one or a few defined agents, the dietary studies will examine the effects of dietary changes in classes of foods or nutrient content in roughly estimated percentages. For both programs, the ultimate aim is to develop effective and acceptable ways to lower cancer incidence by means of dietary modifications.

The growing and converging bodies of basic and epidemiologic evidence on the inhibition of cancer suggest that chemoprevention merits an aggressive research effort. Potential chemopreventive agents include several naturally occurring substances found in many foods, such as vitamin A and its precursor, beta-carotene; vitamins C and E; and the trace metal selenium. Other agents now being studied in the laboratory include phenolic antioxidants, protease inhibitors, prostaglandin synthesis inhibitors, indoles, and uric acid. The goal of the chemoprevention program is to determine whether these natural or synthetic agents can lower cancer inci-

dence. The objectives of the chemoprevention research plan are to:

• identify and characterize agents with proven activity in preventing carcinogenesis in animals,
• identify agents from epidemiologic studies,
• test the efficacy and toxicological effects of such agents to select the most promising,
• conduct Stage III human trials of potential chemoprevention agents, and
• apply research results to the general population.

As an outcome of our planning procedures, which considered existing research data to determine the most promising avenues of chemoprevention research, we have funded 20 chemoprevention trials, all of which were in progress by the end of 1983.

Research on vitamin A and cancer. Many of the chemoprevention trials we have funded are testing the relationship between cancer and dietary vitamin A, beta-carotene, and synthetic retinoids (analogs of vitamin A). Beta-carotene is present in leafy green and yellow vegetables; it is converted to vitamin A in the digestive tract. Laboratory and human studies have led to the hypothesis that ingestion of these agents is inversely related to cancer. A historically important study in chemoprevention was done by Lasnitzki (*1*), who developed a method for growing mouse prostate cells on a watch glass, for transforming these cells into cancer cells by adding a carcinogen, and for inhibiting the transformation by adding vitamin A. She also inhibited a later stage of cancer cell development by adding vitamin A. Subsequently, other researchers showed that retinoic acid inhibits and reduces cancer (*2,3*).

Epidemiologic data also support the vitamin A hypothesis. About 20 studies in various parts of the world suggest an inverse association between eating foods containing vitamin A or beta-carotene and various types of human cancer; risk is thereby reduced by 30–50 percent. For example, several case-control epidemiologic studies show lower vegetable consumption or lower estimates of vitamin A intake among cancer patients than among controls. This relationship is supported by three cohort studies in which a negative association between lung cancer and an index of vitamin A was observed. The first of these studies, by Bjelke (*4*), involved 8,278 Norwegian men. Hirayama (*5*) made a similar observation in a study of 265,118 Japanese adults and suggested that ex-smokers might particularly benefit from daily vegetable consumption. Shekelle and associates (*6*) found dietary carotene to be inversely related to lung cancer in 2,107 American men. Three studies of serum or plasma vitamin A in lung cancer patients, as compared with controls, showed mixed results, but two prospective studies were consistent in demonstrating an inverse relationship between retinol in stored sera and subsequent occurrence of lung cancer (7,8).

In the only intervention trial reported to date, Gouveia and associates (9) examined the effect of the synthetic retinoid Etretinate on 34 heavy smokers with bronchial metaplasia. The index of metaplasia scores dropped significantly in the 12 study subjects who completed 6 months of treatment. This preliminary study will need confirmation because the number of cases is small and the precision of the metaplasia score is uncertain.

The combined strength of these and other research leads is being tested in a number of the 20 human trials supported by the National Cancer Institute in its chemoprevention program. These trials comprise studies of prevention in general populations and high-risk groups, studies aimed at preventing precancerous lesions from becoming malignant, and studies of ways to prevent new primary cancers. Examples of NCI-funded research in each of these four categories follow.

General population study. In a general population intervention study, researchers are currently testing whether cancer can be reduced in study subjects as compared with matched controls. The subjects of this study, being conducted by Dr. Charles Hennekens and colleagues at Harvard University, are about 22,000 physicians in the United States. The 5-year, randomized human trial will examine whether or not beta-carotene contributes to a decrease in total cancer incidence in this population and whether aspirin reduces cardiovascular mortality.

High-risk groups. In another human trial, Dr. Gilbert Omenn and his associates at the University of Washington are investigating the relationship between lung cancers and mesotheliomas in asbestos workers and these workers' intake of vitamin A and retinoids. The study population consists of 2,500 men, 45 years of age or older, who are at risk for bronchogenic carcinoma or malignant mesothelioma, as defined by diagnostic signs of asbestosis. The specific aims of the trial are (a) to determine the efficacy of chemoprevention of these malignancies with daily, oral administration of 13-cis retinol, and (b) to assess toxicity and safety of such a chemoprevention regimen. This is one of the first studies aimed at seeing if cancer risk can be reduced *after* exposure to carcinogens has occurred.

Another study, by Dr. Gary Goodman at the same institution, is testing the efficacy of vitamin A and a synthetic retinoid in reducing lung cancer risk among a population of smokers. This may be especially useful for ex-smokers.

Precancerous lesions. Other human trials are studying the potential of chemopreventive measures for preventing conditions that may be precancerous from developing into cancer. One of these conditions is cervical dysplasia, an abnormal cell formation in the cervix of the uterus. NCI has funded two Stage I trials of a retinoid to study the prevention of cervical dysplasia and to determine if any topical or systemic toxicity occurs with increased dosages of the retinoid.

Dr. Frank Meyskens, at the University of Arizona, is using retinyl acetate in gel form. It is embedded in a collagen sponge, within a cervical cap, and is applied by a physician. In Dr. Seymour Romney's study at the Albert Einstein School of Medicine in New York, the patient applies the retinyl acetate gel to her cervix with a vaginal applicator. These Stage I trials will be followed by double-blind studies to compare the preventive effects of the retinoid with those of a placebo.

Prevention of new primary cancers. Nearly 400,000 new cases of basal cell carcinoma, one type of skin cancer, are diagnosed each year. Although surgery yields a cure rate of at least 95 percent, the development of new tumors in these patients ranges from 20 percent in patients with one or more previous basal cell carcinomas to nearly 100 percent in patients with eight or more.

The subject of four chemoprevention trials is the prevention of new primary skin cancers in patients previously treated for basal cell carcinoma. Two studies use beta-carotene and two use the synthetic retinoid 13-cis retinoic acid (isotretinoin). For example, Drs. Joseph Tangrea and Earl Gross of the National Cancer Institute are conducting a 5-year study of 1,800 white men and women, ages 45–70 years, who have had two or more basal cell carcinomas. This study will evaluate the effectiveness of low-dosage levels of 13-cis retinoic acid in reducing new incidence of basal cell carcinomas and will examine possible side effects associated with long-term administration of this agent. The knowledge from these trials will also provide insights useful in the design of studies aimed at preventing more aggressive types of cancer.

The relationship between diet and cancer has not yet been precisely defined. Published estimates of the percentage of cancer deaths attributable to diet range as high as 60–70 percent (10,11), but 30 percent seems a reasonable, conservative estimate. Although we hope chemoprevention initiatives will be useful against many types of cancer, including lung cancer, the best thing we can all do about lung cancer is to encourage people not to smoke. Chemoprevention and diet-and-cancer research are promising areas that will receive increasing emphasis.

References ································

1. Lasnitzki, I.: The influence of a hyper-vitaminosis on the effect of 20-methylcholanthrene on mouse prostate glands grown in vitro. Br J Cancer 9: 438–439 (1955).

2. Becci, P. J.: Inhibitory effect of 13-cis retinoic acid on urinary bladder carcinogenesis induced in C57BL/6 mice by N-Butyl-N-(4-hydroxybutyl) nitrosamine. Cancer Res 38: 4464 (1978).

3. Thompson, J. H., et al.: Inhibition of 1-Methyl-1-nitrosourea-induced mammary carcinogenesis in the rat by the retinoid axerophthene. Arneim.-Forsch./Drug Res 30–2: 1128 (1980).

4. Bjelke, E.: Dietary vitamin A and human lung cancer. Int J Cancer 15: 561–565 (1975).

5. Hirayama, T.: Diet and cancer. Nutr Cancer 1: 67–81 (1979).

6. Shekelle, R. B., et al.: Dietary vitamin A and risk of cancer in the Western Electric study. Lancet 28: 1185–1190, November 1981.

7. Wald, N., et al.: Low serum-vitamin A and subsequent risk of lung cancer; preliminary results of a prospective study. Lancet 18: 813–815, October 1980.

8. Kark, J. D., et al.: Serum vitamin A (retinol) and cancer incidence in Evans County, Georgia. JNCI 66: 7–16 (1981).

9. Gouveia, J., et al.: Degree of bronchial metaplasia in heavy smokers and its regression after treatment with a retinoid. Lancet 27: 710–712, March 1982.

10. Wynder, E. L., and Gori, G. B.: Contribution of the environment to cancer incidence: an epidemiologic exercise. JNCI 58: 825–832 (1977).

11. Doll, R., and Peto, R.: The causes of cancer: quantitative estimates of available risks of cancer in the United States today. JNCI 66: 1192–1308 (1981).

Carcinogens Occurring Naturally in Foods

by James A. Miller, Ph.D., and Elizabeth C. Miller, Ph.D.

ABSTRACT

Humans are susceptible to the carcinogenic action of a small group of organic and inorganic chemicals in certain industrial, medical, and social habit exposures. A larger number and wider variety of chemical carcinogens, primarily organic compounds, are known for experimental animals. Chemical carcinogens are also found among the metabolites of living cells. No common structure is evident among chemical carcinogens, and a majority of these agents are precarcinogens that require metabolic activation into reactive electrophilic ultimate carcinogens. These strong electrophiles combine covalently with nucleophilic sites in DNAs, RNAs, and proteins in target tissues. One or more of these adducts appear to initiate carcinogenesis. About 20 naturally occurring organic chemical carcinogens, primarily metabolites of green plants and fungi, are known; some occur in some human foods. Many other naturally occurring chemical carcinogens doubtless exist among the vast number of uncharacterized nonnutritive minor components of living systems, some of which are sources of human foods. The electrophilic forms of chemical carcinogens are mutagenic, and mammalian tissue-mediated mutagenicity assays appear promising in the detection of potential chemical carcinogens. These assays should serve at least as a prescreen for conventional lifetime tests in rodents for the carcinogenic activity of food components and contaminants. Epidemiological approaches appear necessary to evaluate the importance of the naturally occurring chemical carcinogens in the occurrence of human cancer.—**Miller, J. A., and E. C. Miller.** Carcinogens occurring naturally in foods. *Federation Proc.* 35: 1316–1321, 1976.

From the Wendell H. Griffith Memorial Symposium on *Nutrition and Cancer* presented by the American Institute of Nutrition at the 59th Annual Meeting of the Federation of American Societies for Experimental Biology, Atlantic City, NJ, April 15, 1975.

The work of the authors and their collaborators in chemical carcinogenesis has been supported by funds from grants CA 07175, CA-15785, and CRTY-5002 of the National Cancer Institute, Public Health Service.

James A. Miller and Elizabeth C. Miller are with the McArdle Laboratory for Cancer Research, University of Wisconsin Medical Center, Madison, Wisconsin 53706.

It has been known for over 2 centuries that humans are susceptible to the carcinogenic action of certain chemicals, and today over a dozen such chemicals and chemical mixtures are known (Table 1) (14, 19, 20, 35). Most of these human carcinogens were discovered from observations on small population groups that were exposed to large amounts of specific agents for many years. In most cases these exposures occurred in industrial situations, but some resulted from the use of carcinogenic drugs or from social habits (e.g., cigarette smoking and betel nut chewing). More recently it has become apparent that carcinogens are also found among the metabolites of living cells and that at least two classes (nitrosamines and nitrosamides) may also be formed nonenzymatically during storage of foods or in gastric contents. Thus, there is considerable concern at this time for the detection of naturally occurring carcinogens in foods, the elucidation of their chemical natures, the determination of their carcinogenic properties, and an assessment of the possible importance in the development of human cancer of those carcinogens that may occur in foods. An important reason for this concern is that studies in cancer epidemiology in the past 2 decades have provided strong evidence for the importance of environmental factors in the etiology of many human cancers (21, 22). The high potency in experimental animals of some of the carcinogens that can occur naturally in certain food products makes such compounds suspect as causative agents for some human cancers.

Extensive discussion and documentation on the naturally occurring chemical carcinogens are not possible in the confines required of this review. Some of the less studied or apparently less important naturally

TABLE 1. Chemicals recognized as carcinogens in the human as well as in experimental animals[a]

Carcinogen	Targets in the human
2-Naphthylamine, benzidine, 4-aminobiphenyl, 4-nitrobiphenyl	Urinary bladder
N,N-bis(2-Chloroethyl-2-naphthylamine	Urinary bladder
bis(2-Chloroethyl) sulfide	Respiratory tract
Diethylstilbestrol	Vagina
Chloromethyl methyl ether, bis(chloromethyl)ether	Lungs
Vinyl chloride	Liver
Certain soots, tars, oils	Skin, lungs
Cigarette smoke	Lungs, other tissues
Betel nuts	Buccal mucosa
Chromium compounds	Lungs
Nickel compounds	Lungs, nasal sinuses
Asbestos	Lungs, pleura
Arsenic compounds[b]	Skin, lungs

[a] See references 14, 19, 20, and 35. [b] Inactive in rodents.

occurring chemical carcinogens are mentioned only briefly or not at all. Furthermore, some of the compounds described below occur in what may appear to be nonfood sources. However, they are included since it appears impossible to categorize a naturally occurring compound as one that is not now or will not at some time be contained in a human food source. More comprehensive reviews of the naturally occurring carcinogens have been published elsewhere (36, 58), and reviews on specific aspects are referenced below. The reader is likewise referred to recent reviews on chemical carcinogenesis for more detailed accounts of knowledge in this field (3, 34, 35).

BIOCHEMICAL REACTIVITY OF CHEMICAL CARCINOGENS AND THEIR METABOLITES

Although only a small percentage of the known chemicals appear to be carcinogenic, this class of compounds includes a wide range of structures; in the forms administered, the carcinogens show no overall structural similarity. The carcinogenic chemicals include a few inorganic compounds (such as certain Ni^{2+}, Be^{2+}, Cd^{2+} and Co^{2+} compounds, chro-

mates, and certain silicates), some relatively simple organic molecules (e.g., carbon tetrachloride, ethyl carbamate, and thioacetamide), a wide variety of alkylating agents, some acylating agents, a large number of polycyclic aromatic hydrocarbons, a number of aromatic amines and their derivatives, a large group of aliphatic nitrosamines and nitrosamides, and a variety of other organic structures (including the naturally occurring carcinogens discussed in this review).

The majority of the classes of synthetic chemical carcinogens and the naturally occurring chemical carcinogens that have been investigated appear not to initiate neoplasia in the forms administered. These compounds are thus precarcinogens, and are metabolized, sometimes through intermediate proximate carcinogens, to ultimate carcinogens that initiate the carcinogenic reaction (Fig. 1). Metabolism of chemical carcinogens to inactive derivatives can usually occur at each stage of activation, and the balance between the metabolism to ultimate carcinogens and to noncarcinogenic derivatives is an important factor in determining the potency of an administered compound.

It is axiomatic that, in the same manner as other pharmacologic agents, ultimate chemical carcinogens must induce tumors through some interaction(s), direct or indirect, with critical cellular components. Further, the heritable and at least quasipermanent nature of the conversion of normal cells to malignant cells suggests that the critical cellular

targets must include informational molecules, such as the nucleic acids or proteins, or both, that are involved in the control of growth. Covalent binding in vivo of chemical carcinogens to proteins, RNA, and DNA of target tissues has been well documented in all cases that have been carefully examined and with a wide variety of carcinogen structures. Inactive related compounds generally do not exhibit similar levels of covalent macromolecular binding.

The levels of covalent bindings observed in vivo for chemical carcinogens range from 1 carcinogen residue per 10^4 to 1 residue per 10^7 nucleotide or amino acid residues in the total crude nucleic acids and proteins of the target tissues. In several cases, but not all, fairly good correlations exist between the gross amounts of macromolecular binding and the carcinogenicities of closely related structures. Detailed studies have shown that there are numerous sites of covalent binding of carcinogen residues in the macromolecules, and some of the more complex chemical carcinogens form more than one reactive metabolite in vivo. It now seems likely that the probability of initiating a carcinogenic event may differ markedly depending on the form of the carcinogen that reacts, the monomer residue that is substituted, and the particular DNA, RNA, or protein molecule or portion thereof that is altered.

With the elucidation of the natures of the covalent interactions in vivo it has become evident that the ultimate reactive forms of most, if not all,

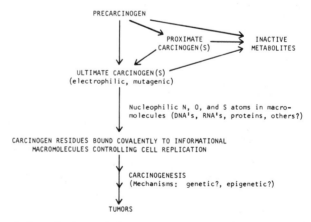

Figure 1. General scheme for the metabolism of carcinogens to inactive and active forms and for the reactions of ultimate carcinogens with cellular constituents in the initiation of carcinogenesis.

chemical carcinogens are strong electrophilic reactants (34, 35, 37). That is, the precarcinogens, despite their wide structural variety, are all metabolized to an electronic form in which there is a relatively electron-deficient carbon or nitrogen atom. These electrophilic species then react with electron-rich (nucleophilic) sites in cellular molecules to yield covalently bound carcinogen residues. It has further become evident that, whenever it has been possible to bring these strongly electrophilic forms of chemical carcinogens into contact with DNA in mutagenicity tests, these reactive derivatives have exhibited mutagenic activity (33). While this strong formal relationship between carcinogenic and mutagenic activity does not have any necessary mechanistic implications for mechanisms of carcinogenesis, it provides a powerful tool for detection of potential carcinogens in foods.

CARCINOGENS FROM GREEN PLANTS

Cycasin

One of the more potent plant carcinogens is cycasin (methylazoxymethanol-β-glucoside) (Fig. 2), which occurs in the palm-like cycad trees (*Cycas circinalis* and other species of the family Cycadaceae) (55). These trees have provided food for natives of tropical and subtropical regions. Though the sliced cycad nuts are extracted with water prior to use, acute poisonings have occurred. No

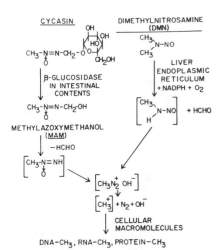

Figure 2. The conversion of cycasin and dimethylnitrosamine into methylating species.

evidence has been presented for the carcinogenicity of cycasin in humans.

When administered orally, cycasin is highly carcinogenic for the liver and kidney of rats and also induces tumors in other species (27). Rat tissues generally do not contain detectable levels of β-glucosidase, but cycasin is hydrolyzed by β-glucosidase from the intestinal bacteria. The product, methylazoxymethanol, decomposes at neutral pH to an electrophilic intermediate that methylates nucleic acids and proteins both in vitro and in vivo (30). These findings and the carcinogenicity of methylazoxymethanol (27) have implicated it as a proximate carcinogenic metabolite of cycasin. The metabolic activation of cycasin appears to yield a methylating species similar to or identical with that formed in the metabolic activation of the much studied synthetic carcinogen dimethylnitrosamine (Fig. 2) which has carcinogenic properties similar to those of cycasin.

Nitrosamines and nitrosamides

Nitrosamines and nitrosamides present a potential carcinogenic hazard either as natural constituents of food or, probably more frequently, as the result of reactions between nitrite and amines or amides in the food, especially at acid pH in the stomach. Nitrosamines may also result from bacterial action. These important problems are not discussed in this review, since they are considered in detail by Issenberg (25) in this symposium, and in other reviews (4, 28).

Pyrrolizidine alkaloids

The pyrrolizidine alkaloids from the *Senecio*, *Crotalaria*, and *Heliotropium* genera have long been known to include a number of highly hepatotoxic members (8, 32) (Fig. 3). These plants may contaminate forages and food grains, and the alkaloids they contain have caused acute and chronic poisoning of livestock in many parts of the world. Some of the alkaloids appear to be highly hepatocarcinogenic for experimental animals if the experimental protocol permits long-term survival. Acute poisoning of humans with hepatic damage has occurred, but critical evidence that these compounds are carcinogenic in the

Figure 3. The metabolic activation of pyrrolizidine alkaloids by the mixed function oxidases.

human is not available.

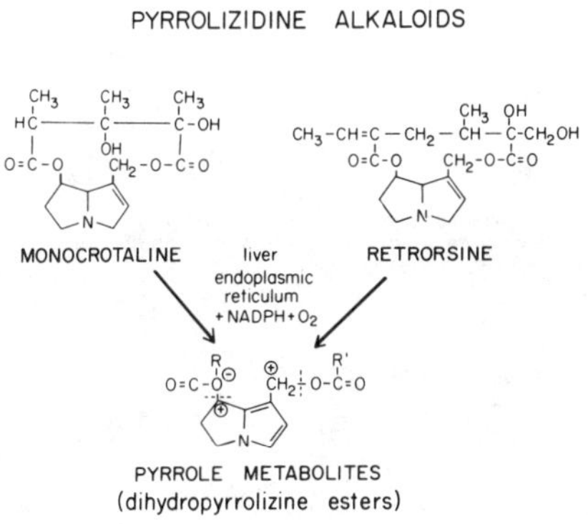

An allylic ester structure appears to be required for both the hepatotoxicity and hepatocarcinogenicity of the pyrrolizidine alkaloids, and usually the naturally occurring alkaloids with branched chain allylic esters are more hepatotoxic than those with less complex ester functions. While the pyrrolizidine alkaloids are electrophilic at high pH, their reactivity at neutrality is very low. However, the alkaloids are converted in vitro to much stronger electrophilic reactants by dehydrogenation by a mixed function oxidase system in liver and lung (Fig. 3) (31, 54). These pyrrole metabolites are acutely toxic, readily alkylate cellular constituents, and become bound to cellular macromolecules. In the pyrrole metabolites with two ester functions both are allylic, and thus in these cases there is a potential for bifunctional alkylation (54). The evidence, including the formation of pyrrolic derivatives of the alkaloids in vivo, strongly points to the pyrrolic ester metabolites as the major toxic metabolites of the pyrrolizidine alkaloids and suggests that they are also ultimate carcinogenic metabolites.

Allyl and propenyl benzene derivatives

Safrole (1-allyl-3,4-methylenedioxybenzene) (Fig. 4) is a minor constituent of several spices and a major component of some essential oils such as oil of sassafras. It was used as a flavoring agent in the U.S. prior to the report in 1960 that it caused liver tumors when fed as 0.5%

Figure 4. The metabolism of safrole to electrophilic metabolites and the products of the reactions of 1'-acetoxysafrole with guanylic acid and methionine.

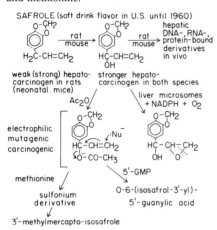

of the diet to adult rats. Safrole is a moderately strong hepatocarcinogen when administered to mice prior to weaning. Safrole is hydroxlyated in vivo to 1'-hydroxysafrole, and the latter metabolite is a stronger hepatocarcinogen than is the parent carcinogen (5, 6). Further metabolic activation can occur by at least two routes (Fig. 4) (5, 6, 44, 56, 57). The synthetic ester 1'-acetoxysafrole is a stronger carcinogen at sites of application than is 1'-hydroxysafrole. 1'-Acetoxysafrole is also a moderately strong electrophilic reactant, as evidenced by its reactions at neutrality with methionine to yield 3'-methylmercaptoisosafrole and with guanylic acid to yield O^6-(isosafrol-3'-yl)-guanylic acid. 1'-Hydroxysafrole yields a reactive metabolite (presumably the sulfuric acid ester) in a 3'-phosphoadenosine-5'-phosphosulfate-dependent reaction catalyzed by liver cytosol (56). Degradation of a small fraction of the hepatic protein-bound derivatives formed from 1'-hydroxysafrole in vivo to 3'-methylmercaptoisosafrole has provided tentative evidence for the formation of some ester of 1'-hydroxysafrole in vivo (57). Liver microsomes convert 1'-hydroxysafrole to the 2',3'-oxide, an electrophilic reactant with a relatively long half-life and with a capacity for initiating papilloma formation in the skin of mice (56).

A variety of allyl and propenyl benzene derivatives related to safrole occur in many essential oils and spices. These compounds have re-

ceived only limited, if any, tests for carcinogenic activity. Estragole (1-allyl-4-methoxybenzene) induced hepatomas when administered to mice prior to weaning; its 1'-hydroxy metabolite is a stronger carcinogen than the parent compound (J. A. Miller, N. Drinkwater and E. C. Miller, unpublished data). Oil of calamus, which contains β-asarone (*cis*-1-propenyl-2,4,5-trimethoxybenzene) as a major component, induced mesenchymal tumors of the small intestine when fed to rats at high levels for long periods (18, 51).

Bracken fern

Ingestion of bracken fern as several percent of the diet induces urinary bladder carcinomas in cattle, urinary bladder carcinomas and intestinal adenocarcinomas in rats, pulmonary adenomas in mice, and intestinal adenocarcinomas in Japanese quail (12, 39). Bracken fern is used in human dietaries in several parts of the world, but its role, if any, in the causation of cancers in human populations is not known. Although intensively investigated, the component(s) responsible for the carcinogenicity of bracken fern have not been identified.

Other plant carcinogens

The occurrence of trace amounts of polycyclic aromatic hydrocarbons in land plants and marine flora and fauna is well known. These hydrocarbons may come from contamination with pyrolysis products or, at low levels, from synthesis by plants (7, 17). The amounts of polycyclic aromatic hydrocarbons in foods can be increased in broiling where pyrolysis products from burning fat are deposited on the food (29). Thiourea, which is found in seeds of certain plants of the genus *Laburnum*, caused tumors of the thyroid, liver, eyelid, and ear duct gland on administration as 0.1–1% of the diet of rats for long periods (26, 40, 42).

CARCINOGENS ELABORATED BY FUNGI

Aflatoxins

Aflatoxin B_1 (Fig. 5), the most potent known hepatocarcinogen for experi-

Figure 5. The structures of several carcinogenic mold metabolites.

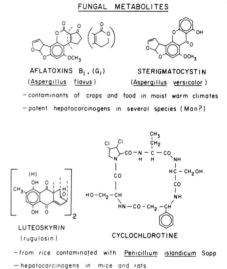

mental animals, is elaborated by certain strains of *Aspergillus flavus*. This compound, which is carcinogenic in a wide range of species, induces moderate to high incidences of hepatocellular carcinomas in rats fed only 15 ppb in the diet over long periods of time (9, 23). These *Aspergillus* strains also produce aflatoxin G_1 (Fig. 5), which is less hepatocarcinogenic. Aflatoxins B_2 and G_2, in which the 2,3-bond is saturated, are much less carcinogenic. Infection of crops such as peanuts and grains with *Aspergillus flavus* can occur during improper harvesting and storage conditions. Aflatoxins have been found in human foods, especially in certain tropical and subtropical areas, and appreciable quantities of aflatoxin M_1, the 4-hydroxy metabolite of aflatoxin B_1, have been detected in the urine of some individuals. The results of epidemiological studies are consistent with a possible role for aflatoxins B_1 and/or G_1 in the high incidences of hepatocellular carcinoma found in human populations in certain parts of Africa and Asia (9, 23, 38, 53).

About 10% of a dose of aflatoxin B_1 is converted to protein- and nucleic acid-bound forms in rat liver (Fig. 6) (48). Macromolecule-bound aflatoxin B_1 derivatives are also obtained on incubation of aflatoxin B_1 with reduced pyridine nucleotide-fortified liver microsomes (16). These data, together with the much lower

Figure 6. The metabolism of aflatoxin B_1 to the putative ultimate carcinogen aflatoxin B_1-2,3-oxide and the reactivities of the latter compound and its synthetic analog, aflatoxin B_1-2,3-dichloride.

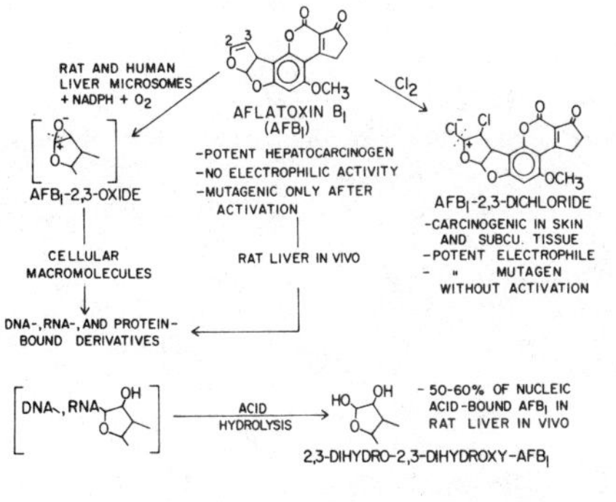

level of binding and carcinogenicity of aflatoxin B_2, implicated aflatoxin B_1-2,3-oxide as a possible ultimate carcinogenic metabolite. The release by mild acid hydrolysis from nucleic acid-aflatoxin B_1 adducts of 2,3-dihydro-2,3-dihydroxyaflatoxin B_1 has provided strong evidence for the metabolic formation of the epoxide (48, 49). Although it has not been possible to isolate aflatoxin B_1-2,3-oxide for study, the reactivity and carcinogenicity of aflatoxin B_1-2,3-dichloride, a synthetic electronic model for the epoxide, are consistent with the proposed role of the 2,3-oxide as an ultimate carcinogenic metabolite (50).

Sterigmatocystin

Sterigmatocystin (Fig. 5), a product of several *Aspergillus* species, has approximately one-tenth the hepatocarcinogenic activity of aflatoxin B_1 (52). Since it lacks the strong characteristic fluorescence of the aflatoxins, data on its occurrence are incomplete. However, the conditions that favor the formation of aflatoxins also favor the formation of sterigmatocystin, and this mycotoxin must be considered as a possible carcinogen for certain native human populations. The 2,3-unsaturated furanofuran structure of sterigmatocystin suggests that its 2,3-oxide may be an ultimate carcinogenic derivative.

Yellow rice toxins

Much attention has been devoted to the characterization of the hepato-toxic and hepatocarcinogenic metab-

olites produced by the growth of *Penicillium islandicum* Sopp on rice (11). A metabolite designated (−) luteoskyrin (Fig. 5) caused liver adenomas and hepatomas in mice fed a few tenths of a milligram daily for 2 years. Another component, cyclochlorotine (Fig. 5), is a more potent acute hepatotoxin, but chronic administration resulted in only low tumor yields.

Griseofulvin

Griseofulvin (Fig. 7) and several of its ring-substituted derivatives are produced by certain *Penicillium* species. Administration of this antibiotic in the diet for long periods to mice resulted in liver damage and hepatomas and in cocarcinogenic effects on the development of s___ tumors (36). Griseofulvin has be__ administered in repeated large o__ doses for prolonged periods in th__ ___ of several serious huma__ ____ mycoses; no data appe__ ___ able on its possible __ __ foods or on the pos__ ___ fects of griseofulv__ therapeutically.

CARCINOGENS PRODUCED BY ACTINOMYCET___ ___ BACTERIA

Streptomyces products

Since the carcinogens produc__ __ *Streptomyces* strains have received lit-tle or no testing by the ___ ___ their importance as possible carcino-gens in foods remains to be ___ These compounds include actino-mycin D and mitomycin C, both of which induce sarcomas on repeated subcutaneous injections of microgram doses (24, 46). Streptozotocin (2-deoxy-2-(3-methyl-3-nitrosoureido)-glucopyranose (2, 41) and elaiomycin (D-*threo*-4-methoxy-3-(1-octenylazoxy)-2-butanol (43) are potential alkylating agents. Single intravenous injections in rats of streptozotocin have induced high incidences

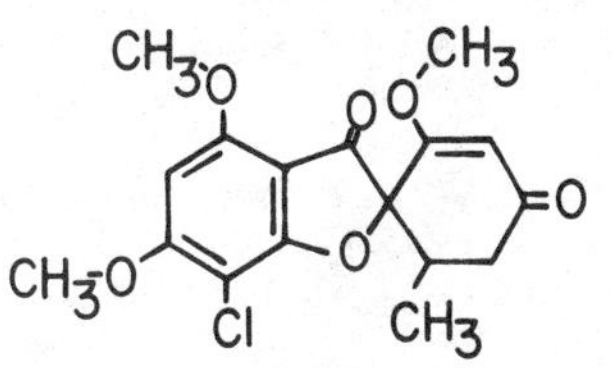

Figure 7. The structure of griseofulvin.

of tumors of the kidney cortex or, with concurrent administration of nicotinamide, of the pancreas.

Ethionine

Ethionine, the S-ethyl analog of methionine, is a metabolite of several bacteria, including *Escherichia coli* (15). Chronic administration of about 0.25% in the diet of rats results in high incidences of hepatocellular carcinomas (13). Administration of ethionine results in the ethylation of hepatic nucleic acids (13, 47), and it seems likely that the ethylation occurs via S-adenosylethionine. The latter compound, the formation of which has been documented in vivo, is a candidate ultimate carcinogen; transfer of the ethyl group occurs enzymatically. Whether or not mammals ___ ___osed to ethionine formed by ____ __ ___ lower gastrointestinal ____ ___ ___ studied.

_____ __ __ ___ _an be formed by ____ __ ___, and this important ____ ___ ___ ___ wed elsewhere in this __ _).

FUTURE APPROACHES

The great complexity of natural foods, the known toxicities of some of their components (10), and the very limited testing for carcinogenic activity that the numerous, mostly uncharacterized, natural components of foods have received make it virtually certain that the number of carcinogens known to occur naturally in foods will continue to increase. This high probability, together with the large role that cancers play as causes of human morbidity and mortality and the apparent importance of environmental factors as causes of human cancers, makes further studies on carcinogens that occur naturally in foods of great importance.

The laboratory approaches to screening for chemical carcinogens have undergone considerable evolution in the past few years (45). Thus, the fact that the mutagenic activity of a chemical implies that it or a metabolite is probably an electrophilic reactant and hence has a considerable probability of being carcinogenic (33) has led to the development of mutagenicity assays as prescreens for chemicals with carcinogenic activity. Of particular importance are those systems that utilize mammalian tissue systems for metabolism of the test chemical, so that metabolism characteristic of mammalian tissues can be coupled with the great sensitivity of mutagenicity assays. These tests are rapid and relatively inexpensive. The data currently available from the assays devised by Ames and his collaborators (1), which depend on the reversion of specially designed histidineless mutants of *Salmonella typhimurium*, are very encouraging for the development of a predictive screen with considerable utility. Assays for mammalian tissue-mediated malignant transformation of mammalian cell cultures by chemicals are currently under development. These tests would have the advantage that the product scored would be essentially similar to that scored in tumor development in vivo.

For the present it seems necessary to continue to test naturally occurring compounds suspected of being carcinogenic, especially if they prove to be mutagenic, in the conventional long-term feeding tests with rodents. These animal tests have as their major advantage the fact that the endpoint is cancer production in an intact animal. However, they have the major disadvantages of being relatively insensitive (a function of the number of animals that can be put under test), very time-consuming, and very expensive. The use of mutagenicity and/or cell transformation assays as prescreens should permit the necessarily limited facilities for whole animal screening to be used to best advantage.

Finally, further epidemiologic studies on human populations that have been inadvertently exposed to foodstuffs suspected of being carcinogenic will be important tools in the assessment of the hazard to humans of such materials and to an understanding of the basic causes of human cancer. The above studies, together with a greater awareness of the carcinogenic chemicals that may occur naturally in foods, and improved techniques for their detection, characterization, and study in animal systems should help us to deal rapidly and satisfactorily with problems as they arise. Reduction of the amounts of carcinogenic natural products in human dietaries may eventually constitute a useful weapon in the prevention of important human cancers.

Addendum (1984):
Reinvestigation showed that N^2-(*trans*-isosafrol-3'-yl)guanylic acid is the major product formed on reaction of guanylic acid with 1'-acetoxysafrole; no O^6-(isosafrol-3'-yl)guanylic acid was detected (Phillips, D. H., Miller, J. A., Miller, E. C., and Adams, B. *Cancer Res. 41:* 2664-2671, 1981).

REFERENCES

1. **Ames, B. N., J. McCann and E. Yamasaki.** *Mutation Res.* 31: 347, 1975.
2. **Arison, R. N., and E. L. Feudale.** *Nature London* 214: 1254, 1967.
3. **Becker, F. F.** *Cancer, a Comprehensive Treatise.* Vol. 1. *Etiology: Chemical and Physical Carcinogenesis.* New York/London: Plenum, 1975.
4. **Bogovski, P., R. Preussmann, E. A. Walker and W. Davis.** *N-Nitroso Compounds—Analysis and Formation.* IARC Scientific Publications No. 3. Lyon: International Agency for Research on Cancer, 1972.
5. **Borchert, P., J. A. Miller, E. C. Miller and T. K. Shires.** *Cancer Res.* 33: 590, 1973.
6. **Borchert, P., P. G. Wislocki, J. A. Miller and E. C. Miller.** *Cancer Res.* 33: 575, 1973.
7. **Borneff, J., F. Selenka, H. Kunte and A. Maximos.** *Environ. Res.* 2: 22, 1968.
8. **Bull, L. B., C. C. J. Culvenor and A. T. Dick.** *The Pyrrolizidine Alkaloids.* Amsterdam: North-Holland, 1968.
9. **Butler, W. H.** In: *Mycotoxins*, edited by I. F. H. Purchase. Amsterdam/Oxford/New York: Elsevier, 1974, p. 1.
10. **Committee on Food Protection.** *Toxicants Occurring Naturally in Foods.* Washington, D.C.: Natl. Acad. Sci. 1973, 2nd ed.
11. **Enomoto, M., and I. Ueno.** In: *Mycotoxins*, edited by I. F. H. Purchase. Amsterdam/Oxford/New York: Elsevier, 1974, p. 303.
12. **Evans, I. A.** *Cancer Res.* 28: 2252, 1968.
13. **Farber, E.** *Adv. Cancer Res.* 7: 383, 1963.
14. **Figueroa, W. G., R. Raszkowski and W. Weiss.** *New Engl. J. Med.* 288: 1096, 1973.
15. **Fisher, J. F., and M. F. Mallette.** *J. Gen. Physiol.* 45: 1, 1961.
16. **Garner, R. C., E. C. Miller and J. A. Miller.** *Cancer Res.* 32: 2058, 1972.
17. **Graf, W., and W. Nowak.** *Arch. Hyg. Bakteriol.* 150: 513, 1966.
18. **Gross, M. A., W. I. Jones, E. L. Cook and C. C. Boone.** *Proc. Am. Assoc. Cancer Res.* 8: 24, 1967.
19. **Heath, C. W., Jr., H. Falk, and J. L. Creech.** *Ann. N.Y. Acad. Sci.* 246: 231, 1975.
20. **Herbst, A. L., H. Ulfelder and D. C. Poskanzer.** *New Engl. J. Med.* 284: 878, 1971.
21. **Higginson, J.** *Can. Cancer Conf.* 8: 40, 1969.
22. **Higginson, J., and C. Muir.** In: *Cancer Medicine*, edited by J. F. Holland and E. Frei, III. Philadelphia: Lea & Febiger, 1973, p. 241.
23. *IARC Monographs on the Evaluation of the Carcinogenic Risk of Chemicals to Man. Natural Products.* Lyon: International Agency for Research on Cancer, 1972, Vol. 1, p. 145.
24. **Ikegami, R., Y. Akamatsu and M. Haruta.** *Acta Pathol. Jpn.* 17: 495, 1967.
25. **Issenberg, P.** *Federation Proc.* 35: 1322, 1976.
26. **Klein, G., and E. Farkass.** *Oester. Bot. Z.* 79: 107, 1930.
27. **Laqueur, G. L., and M. Spatz.** *Cancer Res.* 28: 2262, 1968.
28. **Lijinsky, W., and S. S. Epstein.** *Nature, London* 225: 21, 1970.
29. **Lijinsky, W., and P. Shubik.** *Science* 145: 53, 1964.
30. **Matsumoto, H., and H. H. Higa.** *Biochem. J.* 98: 20C, 1966.
31. **Mattocks, A. R.** *Nature, London* 217: 723, 1968.
32. **McLean, E. K.** *Pharmacol. Rev.* 22: 429, 1970.
33. **Miller, E. C., and J. A. Miller.** In: *Chemical Mutagens—Principles and Methods for their Detection.* New York/London: Plenum, 1971, vol. 1, p. 83.
34. **Miller, E. C., and J. A. Miller.** In: *Molecular Biology of Cancer*, edited by H. Busch. New York/London: Academic, 1974, p. 377.
35. **Miller, J. A.** *Cancer Res.* 30: 559, 1970.
36. **Miller, J. A.** In: *Toxicants Occurring Naturally in Foods.* Washington, D. C.: Natl. Acad. Sci., 1973, 2nd. ed., p. 508.
37. **Miller, J. A., and E. C. Miller.** In: *The Jerusalem Symposia on Quantum Chemistry and Biochemistry, Vol. 1, Physicochemical Mechanisms of Carcinogenesis.* Jerusalem: The Israel Academy of Sciences and Humanities, 1969, p. 237.
38. **Peers, F. G., and C. A. Linsell.** *Br. J. Cancer* 27: 473, 1973.
39. **Price, J. M., and A. M. Pamukcu.** *Cancer Res.* 28: 2247, 1968.
40. **Purves, H. D., and W. E. Griesbach.** *Br. J. Exp. Pathol.* 28: 46, 1947.
41. **Rakieton, N., B. S. Gordon, A. Beaty, D. A. Conney, R. H. Davis and P. S. Schein.** *Proc. Soc. Exp. Biol. Med.* 137: 280, 1971.
42. **Rosin, A., and H. Ungar.** *Cancer Res.* 17: 302, 1957.
43. **Schoental, R.** *Nature, London* 221: 765, 1969.
44. **Stillwell, W. G., M. J. Carman, L. Bell and M. G. Horning.** *Drug Metab. Dispos.* 2: 489, 1974.
45. **Stoltz, D. R., L. A. Poirier, C. C. Irving, H. F. Stich, J. H. Weisburger and H. C. Grice.** *Toxicol. Appl. Pharmacol.* 29: 157, 1974.
46. **Svoboda, D., J. Reddy and C. Harris.** *Cancer Res.* 30: 2271, 1970.
47. **Swann, P. F., A. E. Pegg, A. Hawks, E. Farber, and P. N. Magee.** *Biochem. J.* 123: 175, 1971.
48. **Swenson, D. H., E. C. Miller and J. A. Miller.** *Biochem. Biophys. Res. Commun.*

60: 1036, 1974.

49. **Swenson, D. H., J. A. Miller and E. C. Miller.** *Biochem. Biophys. Res. Commun.* 53: 1260, 1973.

50. **Swenson, D. H., J. A. Miller and E. C. Miller.** *Cancer Res.* 35: 3811, 1975.

51. **Taylor, J. M., W. I. Jones, E. C. Hagan, M. A. Gross, D. A. Davis and E. L. Cook.** *Toxicol. Appl. Pharmacol.* 10: 405, 1967.

52. **Van der Watt, J. J.** In: *Mycotoxins,* edited by I. F. H. Purchase. Amsterdam/Oxford/New York: Elsevier, 1974, p. 369.

53. **Van Rensburg, S. J., J. J. Van Der Watt, I. F. H. Purchase, L. Pereira Coutinho and R. Markham.** *S. Afr. Med. J.* 48: 2508a, 1974.

54. **White, I. N. H., and A. R. Mattocks.** *Biochem. J.* 128: 291, 1972.

55. **Whitting, M. G.** *Econ. Bot.* 17: 271, 1963.

56. **Wislocki, P. G.** *On the Proximate and Ultimate Carcinogenic Metabolites of Precarcinogens: Safrole and Certain Aminoazo Dyes.* (Ph.D. Thesis) Madison, WI: Univ. of Wisconsin, 1974.

57. **Wislocki, P. G., P. Borchert, E. C. Miller and J. A. Miller.** *Proc. Am. Assoc. Cancer Res.* 14: 19, 1973.

58. **Wogan, G. N.** In: *The Physiopathology of Cancer.* Vol. 1. *Biology and Biochemistry* edited by F. Homburger. Basel: Karger, 1974, p. 64.

Large-Bowel Carcinogenesis: Fecal Constituents of Populations with Diverse Incidence Rates of Colon Cancer

by Bandaru S. Reddy and Ernst L. Wynder

Bandaru S. Reddy and Ernest L. Wynder, *Division of Nutrition and Division of Epidemiology of Naylor Dana Institute for Disease Prevention, The American Health Foundation, New York, New York 10021*

SUMMARY—We studied the quantitative and qualitative aspects of fecal neutral sterols and bile acids and fecal β-glucuronidase activity from populations with various dietary patterns to elucidate the etiologic role of these compounds on colon cancer. The fecal microflora of Americans consuming a mixed Western diet were more able to hydrolyze glucuronide conjugates than were those of American vegetarians and Seventh-Day Adventists, and Japanese and Chinese. The daily fecal excretion of coprostanol, coprostanone, and total neutral sterols was higher in Americans than in other groups. Americans who ate a Western-type diet excreted high levels of bile acids and more microbially degraded bile acids than did others. Our data showed a strong association between the incidence of colon cancer and the fecal bile acid and neutral sterol excretion.—J Natl Cancer Inst 50: 1437–1442, 1973.

THE INCIDENCE of colon cancer varies with geographic area and socioeconomic level. It is high in Northwest Europe, North America, and other Anglo-Saxon areas, and low in South America, Africa, and Asia (*1–5*). A number of epidemiologic

Received November 17, 1972; accepted February 5, 1973.

Supported by Public Health Service contract NIH-NCI-71-2310 from the National Cancer Institute.

We thank Dr. Nobuhiro Maruchi of the Division of Epidemiology for the collection of fecal samples, and Mrs. Laurice Gorbran and Mr. David Vukusich for excellent technical assistance.

studies indicate that colon cancer is associated mainly with environmental factors (*1–6*). Related observations (*1, 4, 5, 7*) suggest that dietary factors may affect the risk of colon cancer. Populations in high risk areas consume diets high in animal protein and fat; people in low risk areas eat food low in such components but high in vegetable protein and fiber.

The key question is what diet-dependent compounds in the lumen are carcinogenic. Hill et al. (*8*) established a strong correlation between high concentrations of neutral sterols and bile acid derivatives in the feces and incidence of colon cancer.

Reprinted with permission from *Journal of the National Cancer Institute*, Vol. 50, No. 6, June 1973, pp. 1437-1442.

Other investigators (*9–12*) found that several bile acids could induce sarcomas at the site of injection. Deoxycholic acid can be converted chemically to 3-methylcholanthrene, and some species of intestinal microflora might transform a bile acid into a carcinogen (*12, 13*). A similar conversion might be possible for cholesterol (*8*). Furthermore, the intestinal microflora in a given population is generally diet dependent (*14–17*).

Dietary factors thus both determine fecal composition and influence the type and number of intestinal microflora. Also, the metabolism of bile acids and/or cholesterol into known carcinogens by diverse intestinal microflora may be another factor in the etiology of colon cancer.

We investigated the qualitative and quantitative aspects of bile acids and neutral sterols in the feces of various groups who eat different foods; our aim was to determine high and low risk populations for colon cancer. We also determined the microbial β-glucuronidase (E.C. 3.2.1.31) activity in the feces to assess the degree of microbial capacity for the enzymic hydrolysis of various complex conjugates in the large bowel.

MATERIALS AND METHODS

Subjects studied and fecal sample collection.—Daily 2-day fecal samples were collected from adults: American volunteers on a typical mixed Western diet; Seventh-Day Adventists on a mixed Western diet without meat, but with vegetable protein; Japanese who migrated from Japan in the 6 months to 3 years before they became volunteers and who were still on a Japanese diet; Chinese-Americans on a Chinese diet; strict vegetarians on a diet of vegetables, milk, and eggs (table 1). Fecal samples were collected into a special plastic bag attached to toilets, gased with CO_2, frozen in dry ice in an air-tight container, and stored at −40° C.

Biochemical determinations.—For the determination of β-glucuronidase activity, a sample of well-mixed stool specimen was diluted with prereduced anaerobic media (Robbin Labs., Fiskeville, R.I.) and centrifuged at $100 \times g$ in an International model PR-6 centrifuge at 4° C for 30 minutes to remove undigested food particles and other coarse materials. The supernatant fraction which contained bacteria was spun for 30 minutes at $15,000 \times g$ in a Sorvall RC 2-B centrifuge at 4° C (Ivan Sorvall Inc., Newtown, Conn.). The pellet was washed 3 times with 10 ml sterile normal saline by resuspension and centrifugation at $15,000 \times g$ for 30 minutes. The supernatant from all washings was pooled. The final sediment was suspended in 10 ml ice-cold normal saline and disrupted in a Sonic Dismembrator (Artek Systems Corp., Farmingdale, N.Y.) for 15 minutes at 4° C.

β-Glucuronidase activity in the bacterial pellet and the supernatant fraction was assayed as described by Fishman (*18*). The reaction mixture, containing 0.1 ml 0.01m phenolphthalein glucuronide, pH 5.5, 0.8 ml 0.1m acetate buffer, pH 5.8, and 0.1 ml enzyme source (bacterial pellet fraction and supernatant fraction) was incubated for 5 hours at 37° C in a water bath. The reaction was terminated by adding 2.5 ml 0.1m glycine solution and 1 ml 5% trichloroacetic acid. Phenolphthalein freed was measured at 540 mμ in a Beckman DB-GT spectrophotometer. The β-glucuronidase activity was expressed as μg substrate hydrolyzed per hour at 37° C.

To determine neutral sterols and bile acids, whole feces samples were homogenized in an equal volume of normal saline, and 1-g fractions were transferred to 250-ml centrifuge bottles. The techniques of Grundy et al. (*19*) for the analysis of neutral sterols and the methods of Miettinen et al. (*20*), with slight modifications (*21*), for analysis of bile acids were used. As internal recovery standards, cholesterol-4-^{14}C and cholic acid-24-^{14}C of high specific activity were added to correct at the end of the procedure for incomplete recoveries during extraction and thin-layer chromatography (TLC) (*19, 20*).

To determine neutral sterols, 1 g homogenized sample was saponified with 20 ml 1N NaOH in 90% ethanol by refluxing over steam for 1 hour. The nonsaponifiable fraction containing neutral sterols was extracted 5 times with 50 ml redistilled hexane and concentrated in a Flash-Evaporator (Buchler Instruments, Fort Lee, N.J.). The

TABLE 1.—*Dietary habits of various population groups*

Population groups	Age	Origin	Dietary habits
Americans (17)*	28–60	Staff members of The American Health Foundation and other volunteers from New York City.	Normal Western diet containing high fat and animal protein.
American vegetarians (12)	30–62	New York City	Vegetable protein, lentils, little butter, milk, and wheat or rice.
American Seventh-Day Adventists (11).	30–75	New York City area	Soybeans and vegetable protein, rice or wheat products, milk, eggs, and little butter.
Japanese (21)	35–45	Migrants to New York City area from Japan within 3 years.	Typical Japanese food containing vegetables, fish, little beef, eggs, milk, and little butter.
Chinese (11)	28–45	Migrants to New York City area from Taiwan and Hong Kong within 5 years.	Typical Chinese food containing vegetables, little beef, eggs, milk, and little butter.

*Number of subjects shown in parentheses.

individual components of neutral sterols were separated by TLC on Silica Gel GF plates (Analtech Inc., Newark, Del.) developed in a bath of diethyl ether and heptane (55:45). The individual bands were eluted with redistilled chloroform, evaporated to dryness, dissolved in 2 ml ethyl acetate with a known amount of 5α-cholestane as internal standard for gas chromatographic analysis, and divided into 2 segments; one was intended for radioactive counting and the other for gas-liquid chromatography (GLC). The portion intended for GLC was silylated with 0.3 ml 9:3:1 dry pyridine, hexamethyldisilazane, and trimethylchlorosilane (Pierce Chemical Co., Rockford, Ill.) and analyzed quantitatively with a Hewlett-Packard, Model 7610A, Gas Chromatograph Instrument on a column packed with 1% SE-30 on 100–120 mesh Gas-Chrom Q (prepacked from Applied Science Laboratories, State College, Pa.). Column temperature was 220° C; the temperature of the flash heater was about 250° C and that of the detector about 260° C. Nitrogen was used as carrier gas. Radioactivity was measured with an Intertechnique model SL-36 scintillation counter (Intertechnique, Dover, N.J.).

To analyze bile acids, the aqueous phase (free of neutral sterols) from the converted sample was further saponified rigorously under pressure at 15 psi for 3 hours with 2 ml 10N NaOH, then acidified to pH 2.0 with HCl and methanol. The bile acids were extracted 3 times with about 150 ml chloroform, evaporated to dryness, and methylated overnight with 10 ml of 3% wt/wt HCl in methanol. The methylating solution was prepared by slow addition of 5 ml acetyl chloride to 100 ml methanol; it was held at least for 15 minutes. After evaporation of the methylated bile acid solution, the residue was dissolved in about 0.4 ml chloroform-methanol (2:1), subjected to TLC on Silica Gel GF plates developed in chloroform-benzene (1:1) and isooctane-isopropanol-acetic acid (120:4:01). The plates were sprayed with 8-hydroxy-1,3,6-pyrenetrisulfonic acid in ethanol (*22*). The individual bands were eluted with acetone, evaporated to dryness, and dissolved in 2 ml ethyl acetate with a known amount of 5α-cholestone as internal standard for GLC. A fraction was treated with silylating reagents and then analyzed quantitatively by gas-liquid chromatography with 1% SE-30 and QF-1 columns as described. Bile acids were identified by comparison with TLC and GLC behavior of standard reference

bile acids. Radioactive measurements were performed as described.

The data were analyzed statistically by Student's *t* test.

RESULTS

The data for various age groups and males and females indicate no significant difference between males and females or between young adults and old people in the fecal β-glucuronidase activity or in bile acid and neutral sterol excretion. The weight of stools passed per day was (mean dry wt in g): Americans, 28.7; American vegetarians, 22.4; Seventh-Day Adventists, 26.5; Japanese, 23.5; Chinese, 20.8.

Table 2 shows the bacterial pellet and total β-glucuronidase activity in feces from Americans, American vegetarians and Seventh-Day Adventists, Japanese, and Chinese. Total activity included that from the bacterial pellet as well as the activity released into the supernatant fraction by bacteria. Bacterial and supernatant β-glucuronidase activity was optimal at pH 5.8, and the optimum pH values in the groups studied were comparable. Bacterial and total β-glucuronidase activity per mg protein and total units excreted per day were significantly higher in Americans on a Western diet than in other groups of populations. This indicates that the intestinal microflora of Americans on a mixed Western diet is more able to hydrolyze glucuronide conjugates than is that of other groups.

Table 3 summarizes daily neutral sterol excretion in feces of different populations. The fecal neutral sterols reported here include cholesterol and its microbial conversion products, coprostanol and coprostanone. The daily fecal excretion of coprostanol, coprostanone, and total neutral sterols was

TABLE 2.—*Fecal β-glucuronidase activity in different populations**

Population groups	Bacterial		Total	
	U/mg protein	Total U/day/10^{-3}	U/mg protein	Total U/day/10^{-3}
Americans (17)†	246±31‡	350±74	134±18	425±80
American vegetarians (10)	100±25§	52±12§	55±13§	73±15§
American Seventh-Day Adventists (11)	114±21§	93±26‖	89±20‖	180±40‖
Japanese (21)	52±7¶	40±6‖	32±5¶	61±9¶
Chinese (11)	102±30§	56±18§	54±15§	66±19§

*Unit of activity expressed as µg phenolphthalein formed/hr at 37° C.
†Number of subjects shown in parentheses.
‡Mean±SE.
§Significantly different from Americans at $P<0.01$.
‖Significantly different from Americans at $P<0.05$.
¶Significantly different from Americans at $P<0.001$.

Table 3.—*Daily fecal neutral sterol excretion in different populations*

Population groups	Cholesterol (mg/day)	Coprostanol (mg/day)	Coprostanone (mg/day)	Total sterols (mg/day)
Americans (17)*_____	30. 3±8. 8†	571±98	217±84	817±115
American vegetarians (12)_____	66. 5±16. 5‡	231±49§	20. 0±6. 0‡	318±53‡
American Seventh-Day Adventists (11)_____	74. 0±21. 7‡	178±43‖	13. 6±4. 3‡	266±42‡
Japanese (17)_____	145±28§	109±26§	12. 4±3. 0‡	266±29§
Chinese (11)_____	74. 9±20‡	102±26§	17. 9±7. 5‡	195±38§

*Number of subjects shown in parentheses.
†Mean ±SE.
‡Significantly different from Americans at $P<0.05$.
§Significantly different from Americans at $P<0.001$.
‖Significantly different from Americans at $P<0.01$.

significantly higher in Americans than in the other groups. The magnitude of difference among American vegetarians and Seventh-Day Adventists, Japanese, and Chinese was relatively small. The pattern of cholesterol excretion was unique. American subjects showed the lowest daily fecal cholesterol excretion. This observation, with the data on coprostanol and coprostanone excretion, suggests an increased microbial activity in Americans on a Western diet. The fact that the ratio of coprostanol and coprostanone to cholesterol and percent of cholesterol degraded were elevated considerably in Americans (table 4) is a further indication of increased microbial degradation of cholesterol.

Table 5 summarizes the daily excretion of fecal bile acids which comprise cholic acid, deoxycholic acid, lithocholic acid, and other microbially modified bile acids. A significant increase in the excretion of lithocholic acid (4- to 5-fold), deoxycholic acid (2.5- to 4-fold), and total bile acids (2- to 5-fold) was observed in Americans eating Western food. However, there was no significant difference in cholic acid excretion between American subjects and other groups. Initially, cholesterol (table 3) and cholic acid (table 5) might be higher in the American subjects, but were lower in fecal samples because of microbial degradation.

DISCUSSION

The results of our study indicate that the Americans on a Western-type diet excrete high levels of total neutral sterols and bile acids in feces compared to American vegetarians and Seventh-Day Adventists, Japanese, and Chinese. The data are in line with the observations of Hill et al. (8). One explanation for this difference in neutral sterol and bile acid excretion obviously relates to dietary habits. A change in the composition of food in terms of fats, proteins, and carbohydrates produced a marked change in pool size and production of bile acids secreted into bile and in the excretion of fecal bile acids and neutral sterols in man and animals (23–26).

Our data also indicate that fecal cholesterol and bile acids were much more extensively degraded in Americans on a Western-type diet than in other groups. Our preliminary observations and data from other investigators (8) show that the feces of Americans eating Western food contained more anaerobic bacteria (which metabolize cholesterol and bile acids more actively than do aerobes). This suggests that the quantitative aspects of intestinal microflora are affected by the composition of the diet, and the effects of diet on the extent to which cholesterol and bile acids are transformed into these microbial metabolites depend on the changes in the composition of intestinal microflora. Also relatively high levels of microbial

Table 4.—*Degree of microbial activity as indicated by degradation of cholesterol into coprostanol and coprostanone**

Population groups	Ratio of degradation†	Percent of cholesterol degraded‡
Americans(17) §_____	26. 0	96. 4
American vegetarians (12)_____	3. 8	78. 9
American Seventh-Day Adventists(11)_	2. 6	72. 0
Japanese(17)_____	0. 8	46. 6
Chinese(11)_____	1. 6	61. 5

*Calculated from table 3.
†Ratio of coprostanol and coprostanone (microbial degradation products) to cholesterol.
‡ $\dfrac{Coprostanol+coprostanone}{Total\ neutral\ sterols}$
§Number of subjects shown in parentheses.

TABLE 5.—*Daily fecal bile acid excretion in different populations*

Population groups	Cholic acid (mg/day)	Deoxycholic acid (mg/day)	Lithocholic acid (mg/day)	Total bile acids* (mg/day)
Americans (17)†	8. 48 ± 5. 80‡	106 ± 19	81. 1 ± 12. 9	256 ± 34
American vegetarians (12)	6. 84 ± 5. 76	32. 3 ± 5. 8§	23. 4 ± 4. 7‖	133 ± 15§
American Seventh-Day Adventists (11)	1. 14 ± 0. 83	24. 7 ± 5. 2§	15. 0 ± 4. 1‖	54 ± 16‖
Japanese (18)	5. 27 ± 2. 80	40. 0 ± 5. 6§	22. 8 ± 3. 3‖	83 ± 8‖
Chinese (11)	2. 98 ± 1. 46	22. 1 ± 6. 4§	20. 0 ± 5. 7§	54 ± 13‖

*Total bile acids include cholic, deoxycholic, lithocholic, and other bile acids.
†Number of subjects are shown in parentheses.
‡Mean±SE.
§Significantly different from Americans at $P<0.01$.
‖Significantly different from Americans at $P<0.001$.

β-glucuronidase activity are excreted in the feces of Americans on a Western diet (table 2). β-Glucuronidase activity is further correlated with a relative increase in fecal microbial activity (*8, 14*). We do not believe that β-glucuronidase activity per se has a function in large-bowel carcinogenesis, but rather it indicates the degree of microbial activity which could amplify the biologic activity of many exogenous and endogenous compounds.

From an epidemiologic study of colon cancer in American and Japanese populations, we suggested that dietary fat and cholesterol were closely associated with colon cancer (*4, 5*). Burkitt (*1, 27*) proposed a similar correlation for the intake of simple carbohydrates as well as low-fiber foods. The data from the present study support further an etiologic function for animal fat and/or animal proteins which in turn exert significant effects on the composition of fecal constituents (bile acids and neutral sterols), including microflora. The incidence of colon cancer among American vegetarians is not known. Seventh-Day Adventists are reported to have 20% less large-bowel cancer than control American whites (*28*). To produce more meaningful data, the rate of colon cancer incidence among the Seventh-Day Adventists should be verified, including subjects who were Seventh-Day Adventists from birth or who were converted Seventh-Day Adventists with a varied early history of their strict adherence to a non-meat diet. This biochemical study, in line with our epidemiologic studies (*4, 5*), suggests that, in a given population, the risk of colon cancer may be determined by the composition of diet.

REFERENCES

(*1*) BURKITT DP: Epidemiology of cancer of the colon and rectum. Cancer 28:3–13, 1971

(*2*) BREMNER CG, ACKERMAN LV: Polyps and carcinoma of the large bowel in the South African Bantu. Cancer 26:991–999, 1970

(*3*) DOLL R: The geographical distribution of cancer. Br J Cancer 23:1–8, 1969

(*4*) WYNDER EL, SHIGAMATSU T: Environmental factors of cancer of the colon and rectum. Cancer 20:1520–1561, 1967

(*5*) WYNDER EL, KAJITANI T, ISHIKAWA S, et al: Environmental factors of cancer of the colon and rectum. II. Japanese epidemiological data. Cancer 23:1210–1220, 1969

(*6*) STEMMERMANN GN: Patterns of disease among Japanese living in Hawaii. Arch Environ Health 20:266–273, 1970

(*7*) GREGOR O, TOMAN R, PRUSOVA F: Gastrointestinal cancer and nutrition. Gut 10:1031–1034, 1969

(*8*) HILL MJ, DRASER BS, ARIES V, et al: Bacteria and etiology of cancer of large bowel. Lancet 1:95–99, 1970

(*9*) LACASSAGNE A, BUU-HOI NP, ZAJDELA F: Carcinogenic activity of apocholic acid. Nature (Lond) 190:1007–1008, 1961

(*10*) ———: Carcinogenic activity in situ of further steroid compounds. Nature (Lond) 209:1026–1027, 1966

(*11*) COOK JW, KENNAWAY EL, KENNAWAY NM: Production of tumours in mice by deoxycholic acid. Nature (Lond) 145:627, 1940

(*12*) HADDOW A: Chemical carcinogens and their modes of action. Br Med Bull 14:79–92, 1958

(*13*) ———: The possible causes of cancer—our present knowledge. *In* Abbottempo, Bk. 4. Abbot Universal Lts., 1970, pp 8–11

(*14*) ARIES V, CROWTHER JS, DRASER BS, et al: Bacteria and the etiology of cancer of large bowel. Gut 10:334, 1969

(*15*) HOFFMAN K: Untersuchungen uber die Zusammensetsung der Stuhlflora wahrend eines langdauernden

Ernahrungsversuches mit Kohlenhydratreicher, mit fettreicher und mit eiweissreicher Kost. Zbl Bkt 1 Abt Orig 192:500–508, 1964

(*16*) Smith HW: Observations on the flora of the alimentary tract of animals and factors affecting its composition. J Pathol Bacteriol 89:95–122, 1965

(*17*) Smith HW, Crabb WE: The fecal flora of animals and men: Its development in the young. J Pathol Bacteriol 82:53–66, 1961

(*18*) Fishman WH: β-Glucuronidase. *In* Methods of Enzymatic Analysis (Bergmeyer HU, ed.). New York and London, Academic Press, Inc., 1965, pp 869–874

(*19*) Grundy SM, Ahrens EH, Miettinen TA: Quantitative isolation and gas-liquid chromatographic analysis of total fecal bile acids. J Lipid Res 6:397–410, 1965

(*20*) Miettinen TA, Ahrens EH, Grundy SM: Quantitative isolation and gas-liquid chromatographic analysis of total dietary and fecal neutral steroids. J Lipid Res 6:411–424, 1965

(*21*) Eneroth P, Sjovall J: Extraction, purification, and chromatographic analysis of bile acids in biological materials. *In* The Bile Acids (Nair PP, Kirtchevsky D, eds.), vol 1. New York, Plenum Press, 1971, pp 121–171

(*22*) Kellogg T: An improved spray reagent for detection of bile acids on thin-layer chromatogplates. J Lipid Res 11:498–499, 1970

(*23*) Danielsson H: Present status of research on catabolism and rexcetion of cholesterol. Adv Lipid Res 1:335–385, 1963

(*24*) Avigan J, Steinber GD: Steroid and bile acid excretion in man and the effect of dietary fat. J Clin Invest 44:1845–1856, 1965

(*25*) Portman OW, Murphy P: Excretion of bile acids and β-hydroxysterols by rats. Arch Biochem Biophys 76:367–376, 1958

(*26*) Portman OW, Stare FJ: Dietary regulation of serum cholesterol levels. Physiol Rev 39:407–442, 1959

(*27*) Burkitt DP, Walker AR, Painter NS: Effect of dietary fiber on stools and transit-times and its role in the causation of disease. Lancet ii: 1408–1412, 1972

(*28*) Lemon FR, Walden RT, Woods RW: Cancer of the lung and mouth in Seventh-Day Adventists. Preliminary report on population study. Cancer 17:486–497, 1964

A Mutagen in the Feces of Normal Humans

by W. R. Bruce, A. J. Varghese, R. Furrer, and P. C. Land

Cancer of the colon is a major cause of cancer mortality in Western countries, and the incidence of the disease appears to be associated with diet (Armstrong and Doll 1975). When considering etiology, it is thus tempting to ask: Do the feces of individuals from Western countries contain carcinogens derived from their food? Heretofore, this has been almost an unanswerable question. The feces contain many thousands of compounds, and assays for carcinogens are slow and expensive. However, the recent success of using *Salmonella* tester strains to identify carcinogens as mutagens (McCann and Ames 1976) makes it meaningful to ask instead: Do feces contain mutagens? We report here our early findings which show that some feces from individuals on Western diets do indeed contain high levels of mutagens.

The feces we have studied were collected from normal males, 25 to 45 years of age, who were on no medication or vitamin supplements and were on full Western diets containing meats, potatoes, desserts, etc. We examined feces from normal individuals on this type of diet because the epidemiologic findings cited above indicated that tumors might develop after prolonged exposure of normal individuals to carcinogens in, or produced from, these foods. The feces were quickly frozen to −70°C and were then freeze-dried and extracted according to the scheme shown in Figure 1. Each fraction was reconstituted to a concentration corresponding to 1 g dry weight starting material per milliliter of dimethylsulfoxide (DMSO).

The assay we used was that described by McCann et al. (1975) based on the measurement of the induction of back mutations in *Salmonella* strains which permit these cells to grow in the absence of histidine. McCann and Ames have shown that the *Salmonella* tester strains, under appropriate conditions, detect as mutagens 90% of a sample of known carcinogens. We thus applied the DMSO-reconstituted feces samples to their tester strains TA98, TA100, TA1535, and TA1537 at four or more concentrations with and without liver microsomes (S-9 Mix) according to the method described by Ames et al. (1975).

The authors are with The Ontario Cancer Institute, Toronto, M4X 1K9, Ontario, Canada.

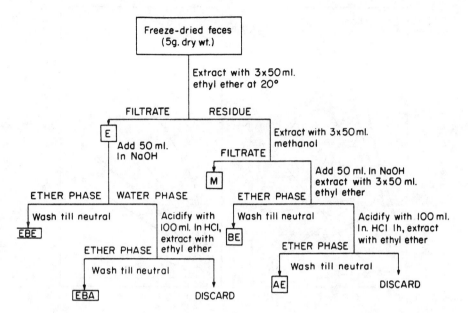

Figure 1

The extraction and early fractionation used in the study of feces. Peroxide-free ethyl ether, methanol, and other reagents were free of mutagenic activity. The fractions E, EBE, EBA, M, BE, and AE were dried and resuspended in dimethyl-sulfoxide at a concentration of 1 g dry starting material per ml and assayed at a concentration corresponding to 0.05 to 0.5 ml/dish using the method of Ames et al. (1975). The samples were processed and assayed in subdued or yellow light.

The results of preliminary studies soon showed that there was an agent in the ether extract, E, of many feces that was directly active on strain TA100. These samples were also active on TA1535 and to a lesser degree on TA98. However, the highest activities were usually seen in fraction EBE, a sample derived from E by washing with a basic aqueous solution. The results of assays of eight consecutive stool samples from one donor are shown in Figure 2. The dose–response curves obtained with many of the EBE samples are linear and, in the case of several of such fractions (right panel), extend to a level of 1000 mutations at a dose corresponding to 200 mg of dried stool. The corresponding mutations induced by fractions from the ether samples, E, are also shown (left panel). The levels of revertants observed for the ether fraction were usually much lower than those observed for the EBE fraction. The results shown in Figure 2 were higher than those encountered frequently. Table 1 gives data for four individuals for samples of all stools passed over a period of 8 days. The levels obtained with these donors are generally lower, but for at least one sample from each donor the levels appear to be above background. Again, we noted differences between the E and EBE fractions.

The apparently greater activity of EBE as compared to fraction E suggested that the water-soluble fraction, EBA of E, might inhibit the mutagenesis of the fraction EBE. If this were indeed the case, the procedure for assaying samples in the future could not assume that the total activity of a sample was equal to the sum of the activities of the fractionated components, as had been found to be the case by Kier et al. (1974) in their study of cigarette condensates. To test this possibility, a simple reconstruction test was performed both with a known mutagen, *N*-methyl-*N*′-nitro-*N*-nitrosoguanidine, and with EBE together with fraction E and fraction EBA. The results of one such comparison (Table 2) demonstrate that there are factors in feces which

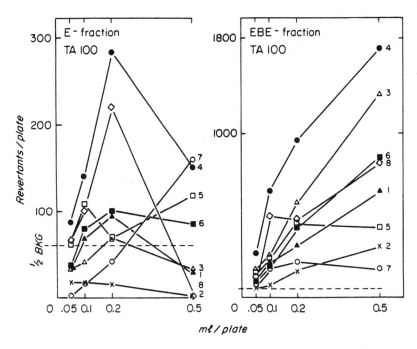

Figure 2
The mutagenic activity, in revertants/plate, of fractions E (*left*) and EBE (*right*) from a normal donor. Dose–response curves for eight consecutive feces samples are shown. Background counts (BKG), averaging 150 per plate, have been subtracted from the data.

inhibit the expression of mutations by known mutagens and by the factor EBE in feces. This means that the actual mutagenicity of a sample in feces can only be determined after chemical separation of the active material from the inhibitor in the feces.

Preliminary steps toward purification of the mutagen were made using pooled active samples from the donor described in Figure 2. Fraction EBE was applied in benzene to a 1 × 20-cm silica gel column and was then eluted with benzene and ether. Seven major fractions were recovered and assayed for their activity on TA100. The sixth fraction contained most of the activity, as shown in Figure 3, and yielded a linear dose–effect curve through 1000 mutations per plate. Although the major constituent of the active fraction was a neutral steroid, extensive purification of this steroid yielded a product which was inactive on the bacterial assay. Further studies are in progress to determine the chemical nature of the active material.

Our results show that the mutagenic factor in the feces of normal individuals may represent a hazard as a carcinogen and may indeed be responsible for cancer of the colon. Since many other tumors display the same epidemiologic pattern shown by cancer of the colon (Armstrong and Doll 1975), it is possible that a mutagen in the feces is responsible for all these conditions. Experiments are under way to (1) determine which particular items in the diet are responsible for the marked swings in the mutagen levels in feces, (2) compare the levels of the mutagen in cancer and noncancer patients, (3) compare the levels in low- and high-risk populations, and (4) characterize further the structure of the active material so that it may be tested directly for carcinogenic activity.

Table 1

The Mutagenic Activity, in Revertants/Plate, of Feces Obtained from Four Donors over a Period of 8 Days

Donor	Day	TA100, EBE no. of revertants	
		0.2 ml	0.5 ml
1	1	5	26
1	2	38	66[a]
1	4	0	0
2	1	0	0
2	2	0	0
2	3	19	42
2	4	12	1
2	5	0	0
2	6	107[a]	189[a]
2	8	0	0
3	1	56	84[a]
3	2	66[a]	39
3	3	35	0
3	4	62	30
3	8	44	61
4	1	26	18
4	2	21	48
4	4	57	34
4	5	75[a]	74[a]
4	8	16	24

[a] These results are considered to be unequivocally positive.

Table 2

Observed Mutagenic Activity of Known Mutagen, MNNG, and Fecal Mutagen, EBE, by Themselves and after the Addition of Relatively Inactive Fecal Fractions EBA and E

Conditions	TA100 no. of revertants	Percent reduction
MNNG (1 μg)	603	
EBA (0.2 ml)	31	
MNNG + EBA	378	37.3
EBE (0.5 ml)	240	
E (0.2 ml)	104	
EBE + E	158	34.2

A reduction of measured mutagenicity is noted.

Note Added in Proof

The mutagen has been further purified by high-pressure liquid chromatography and identified as an *N*-nitroso compound. The purified mutagen gave a positive response on an *N*-nitroso-compound-specific Thermal Energy

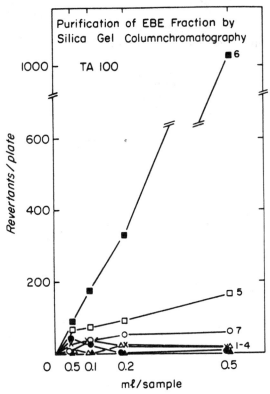

Figure 3

The mutagenic activity, in revertants/plate, of seven fractions recovered from a silica gel chromatographic separation of fraction EBE from a normal donor.

Analyser interfaced to a high-pressure liquid chromatograph. Chemical properties, such as the liberation of nitrite in acidic aqueous solution and the ability to alkylate *p*-(4-nitrobenzyl)-pyridine, provided additional evidence that the mutagen is an *N*-nitroso compound. Furthermore, it has been found that the levels of nitroso compounds, as well as the levels of mutagen, are reduced by over 60% in the feces of all four donors when their normal diets were supplemented with ascorbic acid.

Acknowledgments

We thank Dr. C. R. Fuerst for help in implementing the test system and Dr. L. Siminovitch for reviewing the manuscript. This investigation was supported by the National Cancer Institute of Canada. P. L. was supported by a National Institutes of Health National Research Service Award #1 F32 GM 05658-01 from the National Institute of General Medical Sciences.

REFERENCES

Ames, B.N., J. McCann and E. Yamasaki. 1975. Methods for detecting carcinogens and mutagens with the *Salmonella*/mammalian microsome mutagenicity test. *Mutat. Res.* **31**:347.

Armstrong, B. and R. Doll. 1975. Environmental factors and cancer incidence and mortality in different countries, with special reference to dietary practices. *Int. J. Cancer* **15:**617.

Kier, L.D., E. Yamasaki and B.N. Ames. 1974. Detection of mutagenic activity in cigarette smoke condensate. *Proc. Natl. Acad. Sci.* **71:**4159.

McCann, J. and B.N. Ames. 1976. Detection of carcinogens as mutagens in the *Salmonella*/microsome test: Assay of 300 chemicals. Discussion. *Proc. Natl. Acad. Sci.* **73:**950.

McCann, J., N.E. Spingarn, J. Kobori and B.N. Ames. 1975. Detection of carcinogens as mutagens: Bacterial tester strains with R factor plasmids. *Proc. Natl. Acad. Sci.* **72:**979.

Mutagens in the Feces of 3 South-African Populations at Different Levels of Risk for Colon Cancer

by Marion Ehrich, James E. Aswell, Roger L. Van Tassell, Tracy D. Wilkins, Alexander R. P. Walker, and Neville J. Richardson

Summary

The incidence of mutagens in the feces of 3 South-African populations at different risk levels for colon cancer has been determined. Lyophilized fecal samples were extracted with ether and the mutagenicity of the extracts determined using the Salmonella/mammalian microsome mutagenicity test. 19% of the samples from urban white South-Africans, a population at a high risk for colon cancer, were mutagenic using *Salmonella typhimurium* strain TA100. This incidence was significantly greater ($p < 0.001$) than the incidence of mutagen excretion in the low-risk populations of urban blacks (2%) and rural blacks (0%). This pattern was also obtained using *Salmonella typhimurium* strain TA98. The incidence of mutagen excretion for urban whites was 10%, as compared to 5% and 2% for urban and rural blacks, respectively.

The incidence of colon cancer varies geographically throughout the world. This disease occurs with greater frequency in economically developed nations, and, therefore, North-Americans are considered a high-risk population for colon cancer. Over 99 000 new cases of colon cancer are diagnosed each year in the United States alone, but the incidence rate does not seem to follow a sexual or racial pattern [2,15,30,35]. Unfortunately, positive diagnosis is generally made late in the course of the disease and the mortality rate is about 50% [20, 30].

Marion Ehrich, James E. Aswell, Roger L. Van Tassell, and Tracy D. Wilkins are with the Anaerobe Laboratory, Virginia Polytechnic Institute and State University, Blacksburg, Virginia 24061.

Alexander R. P. Walker and Neville J. Richardson are with The South African Institute for Medical Research, Johannesburg, South Africa.

Environmental factors, especially diet, have been implicated as an explanation for the variation in the occurrence of this type of cancer [3,5,13,16,28, 34]. A diet high in animal fat and low in fiber is generally consumed by populations considered to be at increased risk for colon cancer. It has been observed [14,33] that African blacks, whether in a primitive rural environment or living in large urban centers, rarely developed colon cancer. The diet consumed by these population groups was adequate in protein, but low in fat and high in crude fiber [29,34]. Although high dietary fat can promote colon carcinogenesis in some animal models [3,22,25,26], these data are not sufficient to prove that fat is a causative agent in cancer of the colon.

Although it is possible to identify a small percentage of individuals who are genetically predisposed to this disease, specific agents responsible for the development of colon cancer in humans have not been identified. Recently, Bruce et al. [4,33] detected ether-extractable mutagens in certain human fecal specimens by use of the Salmonella/mammalian microsome mutagenicity test of Ames [1]. We have also demonstrated the presence of mutagens in ether extracts of feces from our local Virginia residents. Since 85—90% of known carcinogens tested are mutagenic using the Ames test [19,23], the presence of mutagenic substances·in feces might increase the risk of colon cancer for individuals excreting these substances.

If fecal mutagens are in fact implicated in colon carcinogenesis, excretion of these compounds may be more prevalent in populations at high risk for colon cancer. Therefore, we examined the feces of 3 populations at different risk levels to determine whether mutagen excretion varied among these groups.

Materials and methods

Fecal samples

We examined fecal samples from members of 3 South-African populations. Urban whites living in Johannesburg consume a "western-type" diet and the incidence of colon cancer is similar to North-Americans, a high-risk population. Black South-Africans living in Johannesburg and rural blacks of Ruskinburg were considered as representative of two low-risk populations [34]. The diet of rural blacks was adequate in protein, but low in fat and high in crude fiber [29, 34]. The diet of urban blacks was similar to that of their rural counterparts, but would be expected to contain slightly more meat and fat.

Fecal samples from all populations were collected within the same 4-month period. Donors of these samples were individuals of either sex, aged 30 or older, and had no history of colonic diseases. For the urban white population, 23 of the 42 samples were from males and 19 were from females. Each individual donated a single sample. The average age of urban white donors was 46 ± 8 (mean ± standard deviation). The sex of the rural black donors was evenly divided, with samples obtained from 54 males and 54 females. The average age was 51 ± 15. For the urban black population, 50 of the 82 samples were from males, and the average age of this group was 47 ± 9.

All fecal samples were collected under similar conditions. Samples were frozen within 15 min of passage and stored frozen at $-15°C$ for a maximum of one week prior to freeze-drying. Water content and pH of the fecal samples were determined. The pH was determined potentiometrically using a slurry of wet feces and saline. The freeze-dried samples were coded in South Africa and shipped together by air to the United States. Samples were analyzed for the presence of fecal mutagens within 12 days of arrival.

Mutagenicity testing

Samples were prepared for mutagenicity testing in the following manner: lyophilized feces were extracted twice with cold ether (20 then 10 ml per gram dry feces) and the solvent was vacuum-filtered through Whatman No. 1 filter paper. The ether extracts were combined, evaporated to dryness, and the residue resuspended in 1 ml dimethyl sulfoxide (DMSO) per gram dry feces. The DMSO suspensions were mixed by vortexing and then centrifuged for 2 min at 10 000 × g in a Brinkman Eppendorf centrifuge. Aliquots (0.2 ml equivalent to 200 mg dry feces) of the supernatant were added to the molten agar overlay used in the Salmonella mutagenicity test of Ames et al. [1]. Plates were incubated at 37°C for 48 h, and then the revertant colonies were counted by hand.

For analysis of fecal extracts we used histidine-requiring *Salmonella typhimurium* test strains obtained from B.N. Ames. The test strains used were TA98 and TA100, which detect frame-shift mutations and base-pair substitutions, respectively. All samples were assayed with and without the liver microsomal enzymes (S9 mix described by Ames [1]) which are necessary for activation of some mutagens. Each sample was tested, in duplicate, in 2—4 different assays, and the results were averaged. The number of revertant colonies on experimental plates varied less than 15% from assay to assay. Each assay had a minimum of 14 control plates. The average control values over the entire test period for spontaneous revertants of TA98 and TA100 without the S9 mix were 15 ± 2 and 117 ± 7 (mean ± S.D.), respectively. The number of spontaneous revertants was slightly higher for TA98 and slightly lower for TA100 when the mammalian enzyme system was included in the assay system. These values were very stable over the time period in which these fecal extracts were tested for mutagenicity. The Salmonella cells were tested for histidine requirements and ampicillin resistance prior to every mutagenicity assay. Representative colonies from experimental plates were tested for true reversion using a radial streak technique. Isolated colonies were streaked from the edge to the center of a minimal agar plate which contained 20 μl of 0.01 M histidine on a paper disk. All colonies tested were true revertants and grew equally well along the entire streak.

We expressed results as mutagenic ratios. The mutagenic ratio is the number of *his*$^+$ revertant colonies on the test plates divided by the number of *his*$^+$ spontaneous revertant colonies on control plates for the assay in which the sample was run. Thus, the higher the mutagenic ratio, the more mutagenic the sample. Following the recommendation of Ames et al. [1], we considered samples positive for the presence of mutagens only if the mutagenic ratio was equal to or greater than 2.0. Tester strain TA98 has a low spontaneous reversion rate, and previous experience had demonstrated that a mutagenic ratio of 2.0 was needed to assure the selection of samples with reproducible mutagenic activity.

Results

Fig. 1 shows the distribution of mutagenic ratios obtained for ether extracts assayed with *Salmonella typhimurium* TA100. The mutagenic ratios are the average value for 2—4 assays. More urban whites had mutagenic ratios greater than 2.0 than did the rural or urban blacks.

Samples that were mutagenic for either TA100 or TA98 were examined for a dose-response by varying the amount of extract included in the assay. As shown by representative samples in Fig. 2, mutagenic ratios increased in relation to the amount of fecal extract added. For nonmutagenic samples, increasing or decreasing the amount of fecal extract did not change mutagenic ratios.

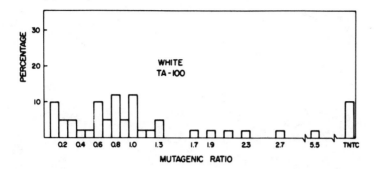

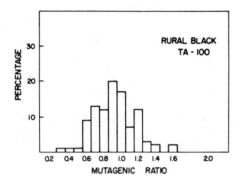

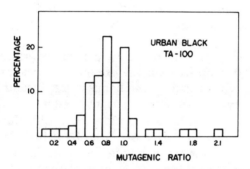

Fig. 1. Distribution of mutagenic ratios of fecal extracts with *Salmonella typhimurium* TA100. The percentage of the samples from urban whites (Fig. 1a), rural blacks (Fig. 1b), and urban blacks (Fig. 1c) was plotted against the average mutagenic ratio from 2—4 assays on each sample. Mutagenic ratios were calculated by dividing the number of revertant colonies on experimental plates by the average number of spontaneous revertant colonies. The number of samples was 42, 108 and 82 for urban whites, rural blacks and urban blacks, respectively.

Samples which produced mutagenic ratios less than 1.0 under the standard assay conditions were diluted. Upon dilution these fecal extracts were no longer inhibitory for the growth of *Salmonella typhimurium*. Some fecal extracts from urban white donors produced more revertant colonies per plate than we could count accurately. These samples were also diluted and dilution brought the number of revertant colonies within the countable range. Results in Fig. 1 were, however, tabulated using standard conditions for all samples.

The distribution of mutagenic ratios obtained with *Salmonella typhimurium* TA98 is shown in Fig. 3. Again, more of the urban whites excreted substances mutagenic on TA98 that the urban or rural blacks.

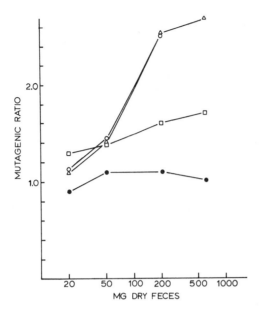

Fig. 2. Dose—response data for representative fecal samples. The mutagenic ratios were plotted against the equivalent weight of lyophilized feces suspended in DMSO. Open triangles, mutagenic sample TA100; open circles, mutagenic sample TA98. Open square, nonmutagenic samples TA98; closed circle, nonmutagenic sample TA100.

The mutagenic ratios shown in Figs. 1 and 3 were obtained in the absence of the mammalian enzyme (S9) mixture. The fecal mutagens acted directly on *Salmonella typhimurium*. The S9 mix actually inactivated the mutagenic fecal extracts, bringing them back to control levels.

To simplify the results shown in Figs. 1 and 2, we considered samples with mutagenic ratios greater than 2.0 as positive for the presence of fecal mutagens. Of the 42 fecal extracts from whites living in Johannesburg, 9 samples were mutagenic with the *Salmonella typhimurium* test strains used in this study. Of these samples, 3 were mutagenic both with TA100 and with TA98. None of the samples from 108 rural blacks and only 2 of those from 82 urban blacks were positive with *S. typhimurium* TA100. A Chi-square test used in conjunction with a contingency table showed that these differences between the black and white populations with TA100 were significant ($p < 0.001$). Excretion of mutagens acting on *Salmonella typhimurium* test strain TA98 was also higher in the urban white population than in the urban blacks and rural blacks, being 10%, 5% and 2% respectively. The difference between urban whites and rural blacks with TA98 was also statistically significant ($p < 0.01$). The differences

TABLE 1

MUTAGENIC RESPONSE OF *Salmonella typhimurium* TO FECAL EXTRACTS

Population group	Number of samples	% samples with MR > 2.0			
		TA98	TA100	TA 98 and TA 100	Total % of mutagenic samples
Urban whites	42	10	19	7	21
Urban blacks	82	5 [a]	2 [b]	1 [b]	6 [a]
Rural blacks	108	0 [a]	2 [b]	0 [b]	2 [a]

[a] Comparison with urban whites, $p < 0.01$, Chi-square test used in conjunction with a contingency table.
[b] Comparison with urban whites, $p < 0.001$.

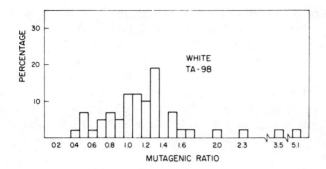

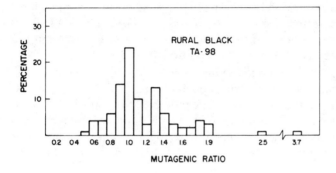

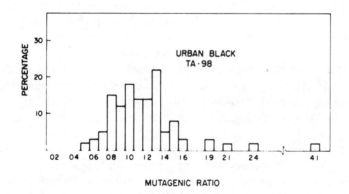

Fig. 3. Distribution of mutagenic ratios of fecal extracts with *Salmonella typhimurium* TA98. See legend for Fig. 1.

between rural and urban blacks, however, was not.

We also analyzed data relative to the age and sex of the donors of fecal samples. The ages of the donors of mutagenic samples did not differ statistically from the average age of the groups as a whole. Sex was also not correlated with excretion of fecal mutagens; the ratio of males : females with mutagenic samples corresponded to the ratio of males : females in each population group. For the urban whites, fecal samples from 5 males and 4 females were mutagenic. For the rural blacks, positive samples were obtained from 2 males and for the urban blacks, 3 males and 2 females. Samples from 4 individuals (3 from the urban white group and 1 urban black) were mutagenic both with TA100 and TA98.

The water content of the feces also did not vary among the 3 populations tested and did not differ between mutagenic and nonmutagenic samples within the same population. Percent water was 72 ± 5, 75 ± 7, and 76 ± 7 for urban whites, rural blacks, and urban blacks, respectively.

There was however, a pH difference among fecal samples from the 3 South-African populations. For urban whites, fecal pH was 7.1 ± 0.6. For rural and urban blacks, fecal pHs were 6.5 ± 0.4 and 6.5 ± 0.6, respectively. The difference in pH values between urban whites and rural blacks was statistically significant using the student's *t* test ($p < 0.01$). The difference between urban whites and urban blacks was not. There were no significant differences in pH between mutagenic and nonmutagenic fecal specimens from the same populations. Mutagenic fecal samples had pH values of 7.2 ± 0.9, 6.3 ± 0.5, and 6.6 ± 0.7 for urban whites, rural blacks, and urban blacks, respectively.

Discussion

We have confirmed the report of Bruce et al. [4] that certain human fecal samples contain mutagens which act on *Salmonella typhimurium* TA100. In their studies and ours, the presence of mammalian enzymes was not required for expression of mutagenicity. We have also demonstrated that human fecal extracts can be mutagenic for *Salmonella typhimurium* TA98. Since the presence of mutagens in human feces was not reported until 1977 [4], it is too soon to assess whether they are carcinogens and whether they are involved in colon cancer. Many mutagens are carcinogens, however, and we have demonstrated that the incidence of mutagen excretion is higher in a population at relatively high risk for colon cancer than in two populations with lower risk levels.

Our study also shows a trend towards higher excretion of mutagens in urban blacks as compared to rural blacks. Composite diet studies have not yet been done with the urban blacks of South Africa, but these individuals are likely to have a slightly increased exposure to animal fat as well as increased exposure to industrial pollutants than their rural counterparts. Although the rates for colon cancer are at present similar between rural and urban blacks, this incidence may change relative to the exposure to a more industrialized society, as it has with rural Japanese who have immigrated to Hawaii [35].

Factors responsible for the excretion of fecal mutagens have not yet been defined. Differences in fecal flora between populations at low and high risk for colon cancer have been described [8,9], but these differences are not consistent from population to population. It seems more likely, therefore, that differences in bacterial metabolism as affected by diet, are more important than differences in bacterial species between populations at different risk levels for colon cancer [7,10,11,21,25,27,28]. Studies on more populations are needed to determine whether these factors are important in excretion of fecal mutagens.

Mutagens can be produced from foods such as fish [17,18], hamburger [6], and broiled foods [32] under certain conditions. Whether or not these mutagens are subsequently excreted in the feces remains to be determined. Recent studies by W.R. Bruce (personal communication) have indicated that ether extracts from certain human fecal samples contain an *N*-nitroso oleamide which is mutagenic. He believes that this substance is produced in the body rather than ingested in the diet. We have not yet determined whether *N*-nitroso oleamides are present in the mutagenic ether extracts of feces from our South-African donors. Sperry et al. [31], however, showed that concentrations of oleic acid were lower in the feces of South-African rural blacks than in the feces of North-Americans, a population at high risk for colon cancer.

The detection of mutagens in feces and urine [36] indicates that potential carcinogens are present in the human body. It is too soon, however, to determine whether they are the agents responsible for cancer. Fecal mutagens, for instance, are excreted at a relatively low level. Since the average age of onset of colon cancer is over 50 years, a long exposure period may be required for the development of this disease. Therefore, absolute correlation between excretion of fecal mutagens and risk for colon cancer will be difficult to establish. We are, however, examining the frequency at which mutagens are found in fecal samples from certain individuals. We are also currently investigating the incidence of mutagen excretion in other populations at different risk levels for colon cancer. If a positive correlation between fecal mutagen excretion and increased risk for cancer of the colon could be established, it would greatly facilitate the identification and early diagnosis of this disease.

Comment on obtaining human-fecal samples

Colon cancer is a disease which occurs only in humans and for which no completely satisfactory animal models have been developed. Consequently, epidemiological studies, such as are presented in the manuscript we have submitted, are the only real lead available on the etiology of the disease. Unfortunately, populations at low risk for colon cancer, such as the rural African blacks we have studied, are isolated from centers of medical and biological research. Collections of samples from these populations has certain difficulties which were mentioned by some of the reviewers. We feel that we had to sample this population in its own environment while consuming their normal diet. To do otherwise would have introduced variables difficult to ascertain or to describe. We feel we must point out that it is impossible to control experimental conditions in an isolated village 100 miles from Johannesburg in the way one can in a hospital situation. Collection of the samples required the use of a specially equipped Land-Rover and it is doubtful that we could have obtained any samples if we had required that they be collected at a prescribed time. To determine if donors were blood relatives, as one reviewer suggested, would have required in depth interviews in the village. This is more appropriate to an anthropological study than to a biological one, as the participants in the study have only first names.

Even with the urban white population we experienced difficulty in obtaining the fecal samples we included in the study. It is not easy to get 100 volunteers for a project of this type.

With appropriate caution in interpretation of the data from the low-risk population in accordance with the reviewers comments and our awareness of their limitations, our epidemiological study should be of value in determining the etiology of colon cancer.

Acknowledgements

This work was supported by a grant from the Abercrombie Foundation and by NCI Contract No. NO1-CP-55685.

References

1 Ames, B.N., J. McCann and E. Yamasaki, Method for detecting carcinogens and mutagens with the Salmonella/mammalian-microsome mutagenicity test, Mutation Res., 31 (1975) 347—364.

2 Blot, W.J., J.F. Fraumeni Jr., B.J. Stone and F.W. McKay, Geographic patterns of large bowel cancer in the United States, J. Natl. Cancer Inst., 57 (1976) 1225—1231.

3 Broitman, S.A., J.J. Vitale, E. Vavrousek-Jukuba and L.S. Gottlieb, Polyunsaturated fat, cholesterol, and large bowel tumorigenesis, Cancer, 40 (1977) 2455—2463.

4 Bruce, W.R., A.J. Varghese, R. Furrer and P.C. Land, A mutagen in the feces of normal humans, in: H.H. Hiatt, J.P. Watson and J.A. Winsten (Eds.), Origins of Human Cancer, Cold Spring Harbor Laboratory, Cold Spring Harbor, N.Y., (1977) pp. 1641—1646.

5 Burkitt, D.P., Colonic-rectal cancer: fiber and other dietary factors, Am. J. Clin. Nutr., 31 (1978) S58—S64.

6 Commoner, B., A.J. Vithayathil, P. Dolara, S. Nair, P. Madyastha and G.C. Cuca, Formation of mutagens in beef and beef extract during cooking, Science, 201 (1978) 913—916.

7 Drasar, B.S., and D.J.A. Jenkins, Bacteria, diet, and large bowel cancer, Am. J. Clin. Nutr., 29 (1976) 1410—1416.

8 Finegold, S.M., and V.L. Sutter, Fecal flora in different populations, with special reference to diet, Am. J. Clin. Nutr., 31 (1978) S112—116.

9 Fuchs, H.M., S. Dorfman and M.H. Floch, The effect of dietary fiber supplementation in man, II. Alteration in fecal physiology and bacterial flora, Am. J. Clin. Nutr., 29 (1976) 1443—1447.

10 Goldin, B., and S.L. Gorbach, Alteration in fecal microflora enzymes related to diet, age, Lactobacillus supplement and dimethylhydrazine, Cancer, 40 (1977) 2421—2426.

11 Hill, M.J., The role of colon anaerobes in the metabolism of bile acids and steroids and its relation to colon cancer, Cancer, 36 (1975) 2387—2400.

12 Hentges, D.J., Fecal flora of volunteers on controlled diets, Am. J. Clin. Nutr., 31 (1978) S123—S124.

13 Huang, C.T., G.S. Gopalakrishna and B.L. Nichols, Fiber, intestinal sterols, and colon cancer, Am. J. Clin. Nutr., 31 (1978) 516—526.

14 Kenda, J.F.N., Cancer of the large bowel in the African: a 15-year survey at Kinshusa University Hospital, Zaire, Br. J. Surg., (1976) 966—968.

15 Lowenfels, A.B., Etiological aspects of cancer of the gastro-intestinal tract, Surg. Gynecol. Obstet., 137 (1973) 291—298.

16 MacLannan, R., et al., Report from the International Agency for Research on Cancer Intestinal Micro-ecology Group, Dietary fibre, transit-time, faecal bacteria, steroids, and colon cancer in two Scandinavian populations, Lancet, 2 (1977) 207—211.

17 Marquardt, H., F. Rugino and J.H. Weisburger, Mutagenic activity of nitrite-treated foods, Human stomach cancer may be related to dietary factors, Science, 196 (1977) 1000—1001.

18 Marquardt, H., F. Rugino and J.H. Weisburger, On the aetiology of gastric cancer: Mutagenicity of food extracts after incubation with nitrite, Fd. Cosmet. Toxicol., 15 (1977) 97—100.

19 McCann, J., and B.N. Ames, Detection of carcinogens as mutagens in the Salmonella/microsome test: Assay of 300 chemicals, Proc. Natl. Acad. Sci. (U.S.A.), 72 (1975) 5135—5139.

20 Miller, S.F., and A.R. Knight, The early detection of colorectal cancer, Cancer, 40 (1977) 945—959.

21 Moore, W.E.C., E.P. Cato and L.V. Holdeman, Some current concepts in intestinal bacteriology, Am. J. Clin. Nutr., 31 (1978) S33—S42.

22 Nigro, N.D., R.L. Campbell, D.V. Singh and Y.N. Lin, Effect of diet high in beef fat on the composition of fecal bile acids during intestinal carcinogenesis in the rat, J. Natl. Cancer Inst., 57 (1976) 833—888.

23 Poirier, L.A., and V.F. Simmon, Mutagenic—carcinogenic relationships and the role of mutagenic screening tests for carcinogenicity, Clin. Pharmacol. Toxicol., 9 (1976) 761—771.

24 Reddy, B.S., and E.L. Wynder, Large-bowel carcinogenesis: Fecal constituents of populations with diverse incidence rates of colon cancer, J. Natl. Cancer Inst., 50 (1973) 1437—1442.

25 Reddy, B.S., S. Mangat, J.H. Weisburger and E.L. Wynder, Effect of high-risk diets for colon carcinogenesis on intestinal mucosal and bacterial β-glucuronidase activity in F344 rats, Cancer Res., 37 (1977) 3533—3536.

26 Reddy, B.S., T. Narisawa and J.H. Weisburger, Effect of a diet with high levels of protein and fat on colon carcinogenesis in F344 rats treated with 1,2-dimethylhydrazine, J. Natl. Cancer Inst., 57 (1976) 567—569.

27 Reddy, B.S., J.H. Weisburger and E.L. Wynder, Fecal β-glucuronidase: Control by diet, Science, 183 (1974) 416—417.

28 Reddy, B.S., and E.L. Wynder, Large bowel carcinogenesis: Fecal constituents of populations with diverse incidence rates of colon cancer, J. Natl. Cancer Inst., 50 (1973) 1437—1442.

29 Salyers, A.A., J.F. Sperry, T.D. Wilkins, A.R.P. Walker and N.J. Richardson, Neutral steroid concentrations in the feces of North American white and South African black populations at different risks for cancer of the colon, S.A. Med. J., 51 (1977) 823—827.

30 Seidman, H., E. Silverberg and A.I. Holleb, Cancer statistics, A comparison of white and black populations, CA, 26 (1976) 1—7.

31 Sperry, J.F., A.A. Salyers and T.D. Wilkins, Fecal long chain fatty acids and colon cancer risk, Lipids, 11 (1976) 637—639.

32 Sugimura, T., M. Nagao, T. Kawachi, M. Honda, T. Yahagi, Y. Seino, S. Sato, N. Matsukura, T. Matsushima, A. Shirai, M. Sawamura and H. Matsumoto, Mutagen—carcinogens in food, with special reference to highly mutagenic pyrolytic products in broiled foods, in: H.H. Hiatt, J.P. Watson and J.A. Winsten (Eds.), Origins of Human Cancer, Cold Spring Harbor Laboratory, Cold Spring Harbor, N.Y., 1977, pp. 1561—1577.

33 Varghese, A.J., P. Land, R. Furrer and W.R. Bruce, N-Nitroso compounds in the human body, Proc. Am. Ass. Cancer Res., 18 (1977) 80.

34 Walker, A.R.P., and D.P. Burkitt, Colon cancer — hypotheses of causation, dietary prophylaxis, and future research, Am. J. Dig. Dis., 21 (1976) 910—917.

35 Wynder, E.L., and T. Hirayama, Comparative epidemiology of cancers of the United States and Japan, Prevent. Med., 6 (1977) 567—594.

36 Yamasaki, E., and B.N. Ames, Concentration of mutagens from urine by adsorption with the nonpolar resin XAD-2: Cigarette smokers have mutagenic urine, Proc. Natl. Acad. Sci. (U.S.A.), 74 (1977) 3555—3559.

Metabolic Epidemiology of Large Bowel Cancer: Fecal Mutagens in High- and Low-Risk Population for Colon Cancer, a Preliminary Report

by Bandaru S. Reddy, Chand Sharma, Loretta Darby, Kristina Laakso and Ernst L. Wynder

Naylor Dana Institute for Disease Prevention, American Health Foundation, Dana Road, Valhalla, NY 10595 (U.S.A.)

Summary

Because of potential significance of fecal mutagens in the pathogenesis of colon cancer, the dietary pattern and fecal mutagens of 3 populations with distinct risk for the development of colon cancer, a high-risk population in New York Metropolitan area (non-Seventh-Day Adventists), a low-risk population of vegetarian Seventh-Day Adventists in New York Metropolitan area and a low-risk population in rural Kuopio, Finland were studied. The average daily intake of protein was the same in the 3 groups, but the sources were different, a greater portion coming from meat in the New York non-Seventh-Day Adventists and from vegetables in Seventh-Day Adventists. The intake of fat was lower in Seventh-Day Adventists and higher in Kuopio and in New York non-Seventh-Day Adventists. The intake of dietary fiber was high in Kuopio compared to other groups.

Fecal samples collected for 2 days were freeze-dried extracted with peroxide-free diethyl ether, partially purified on a silica-gel column and assayed for mutagenicity using the Salmonella/mammalian microsome mutagenicity test. The mutagenic activity was observed with *Salmonella typhimurium* tester strain TA98 without microsomal activation and with TA100 with and without microsomal activation in high-risk subjects from New York consuming a high-fat, high-meat diet. The incidence of fecal mutagen activity was higher in volunteers from New York consuming a high-fat, high-meat diet compared to low-risk rural Kuopio population. None of the vegetarian Seventh-Day Adventists showed any mutagenic activity.

Epidemiologic studies suggest that colon-cancer incidence is associated with dietary factors, particularly high intake of total dietary fat and meat and relative lack of dietary fiber and certain vegetables [3,6,14,15,36]. The role of dietary fat and certain fibers in colon cancer has received support from studies in animal models [5,25,27,34]. It has also been shown that the effect of dietary fat in the rat is at the level of promotion, but not the initiation phase of colon carcinogenesis [5]. The suspected effect of dietary factors may be related to changes in the metabolic activity of gut microflora and in the concentration of secondary bile acids in colon contents [2,16,25,27,28,29]. These secondary bile acids — deoxycholic acid and lithocholic acid — have been shown to act as colon-tumor promoters, but not complete carcinogens [31]. Recently studies have shown that certain dietary fibers increase the stool bulk, which dilutes the above tumorigenic compounds, as well as modify the metabolism of those suspected tumorigenic compounds [28,29].

Until recently the nature of the carcinogens responsible for colon cancer not only were obscure, but there were no real leads. Recently, Bruce et al. [4] have reported the presence of mutagenic substances positive to *Salmonella typhimurium*, strains TA100 and TA98 without S9 activation in the stools of certain individuals consuming a high-fat, mixed-Western diet. Ehrich et al. [11] have demonstrated that the stools of South-African urban whites were higher in mutagenic activity with TA98 and TA100 without microsomal activation compared to South-African urban and rural blacks who are at low risk for the development of colon cancer. If the fecal mutagens are involved in the genesis of colon cancer, it would be of interest to extend these studies to various populations at varied risk for colon-cancer development.

The incidence of colon cancer in Finland is one of the lowest in the developed countries [10,18]. The age-adjusted colon-cancer incidence rates for white males in the United States and in rural Finland (Kuopio) are 28.5 and 5.6 per 100 000 respectively [8,17]. There are no sexual and racial differences in incidence and mortality rates. Comparative studies of religious groups have been motivated by the search for leads for factors that would link the lifestyle of individual groups within a small geographical area and their site-specific cancer risks. Active Mormons (Church of Jesus Christ of Latter-Day Saints) in Utah and California have colon-cancer mortality rates lower than United States white population [12]. The Mormon church not only advises against the use of tobacco, alcohol, coffee and tea, but recommends a well-balanced diet, particularly the use of whole grains, fruits and fresh vegetables and moderation of meat [12]. The North-American Seventh-Day Adventists who consume little or no meat are reported to have about 60% of the rate for a comparable general population [26]. A case-control study of colon cancer among Seventh-Day Adventists show statistically significant relative risks for colon cancer of 2.8 for past use of meat, and for current food use a relative rate of 2.3 for beef, 2.7 for lamb and 2.1 for highly saturated fat foods [26].

The study reported here was designed to investigate whether the differences in colon-cancer risk in 3 populations, namely North-American non-Seventh-Day Adventists, North-American Seventh-Day Adventists and Finnish population are associated with their fecal mutagenic activity.

Materials and methods

Chemicals, media and bacterial strains

All chemicals used in this study were of highest grade purity. 2-Acetylaminofluorine (2-AAF), *N*-methyl-*N'*-nitro-*N*-nitrosoguanidine (MNNG), Picrolonic acid, dimethyl sulfoxide (DMSO) were obtained from Aldrich Chemical Company, Milwaukee, WI, Aroclor 1254 from Monsanto Chemical Co., St. Louis, MI, and silical gel from Mallinckrodt, St. Louis, MI.

Salmonella typhimurium strains TA100 (for detection of base-pair substitution) and TA98 (for detection of frame-shift mutations) were provided by the laboratory of Dr. Bruce N. Ames, University of California, Berkeley, CA, and checked for histidine requirement, crystal-violet sensitivity, ampicillin-resistant R factor, UV sensitivity and spontaneous reversions. All media were prepared as described [1,22].

Study population

3 groups of volunteers from Kuopio (Finland), and from the New York metropolitan area were studied. In the first group were 15 middle-aged healthy males from Kuopio; in the second group there were 11 healthy male Seventh-Day Adventists consuming a vegetarian diet from the New York metropolitan area; and in the third group there were 18 healthy males from the New York metropolitan area (non-Seventh-Day Adventists) consuming a high-fat, high-meat, low-fiber diet. All volunteers were matched for age. The average age of all volunteers was 49 ± 5 years.

Subjects were excluded if they had a history of regular use of antibiotics within 4 weeks of the study, any gastrointestinal disease, surgical resection of partial or total stomach or intestine, or if they were on a special diet other than their normal diet. All volunteers were life-long residents of that particular country. The subjects were interviewed by a nutritional epidemiologist and diet histories recorded. The diet questionnaire contained the information on any major change in their dietary pattern over the past 25 years, and on food items normally eaten from childhood. In order to obtain accurate information on what was eaten during and just before stool collection, a 5—14 day diet recall was obtained from each participant.

Collection of stool specimens

Methods for the collection of stool specimens have been developed in our laboratory and described [28]. All fecal samples were collected under similar conditions and treated similarly. Individual 24-h specimens were collected from each volunteer for 2 days. Stool samples were collected into a special plastic bag attached to the toilet, frozen immediately after defecation in dry ice supplied to each participant in an air-tight container. All samples were stored in dry ice until they were shipped. Samples from Finland were air-shipped in a dry-ice container within 1 week of collection and the samples from the New York area stored in dry ice were brought to the laboratory. All samples were stored in a cold room (−20°C) in our laboratory before they were processed.

Sample preparation for mutagenesis

Fecal samples collected for 2 days from each individual were pooled and homogenized in a cold room (4°C) and then freeze-dried. During freeze-drying, it is possible that an unknown amount of volatile mutagens could have been lost. Standard experimental procedures for the extraction of fecal specimens have been described by Bruce et al. [4] and Varghese et al. [33]. Briefly, 10—20 g freeze-dried sample from each volunteer was extracted 3 times with peroxide-free diethyl ether (10 ml/g sample). The extract was filtered through Whatman No. 1 filter paper. The filtrate was evaporated to dryness in a flash evaporator under vacuum, reconstituted in about 5 ml diethyl ether and applied on a silica gel (Silic AR, CC-7) column (50 × 4 cm) for purification. The column was first eluted with about 500 ml benzene and subsequently with 500 ml diethyl ether to recover the mutagenic fraction. Benzene fraction did not show any significant activity in both TA98 and TA100 tester systems. The ether eluate was concentrated to a small volume in a flash evaporator, passed through a Millipore filter, 0.5 mμ (HAWG 04700 from Millipore Corp., Bedford, MA), dried under nitrogen and resuspended in DMSO for mutagenic assay.

Preparation of S9

Liver S9 mix was prepared as described by Ames et al. [1] Male Sprague—Dawley rats (200—300 g) received a single intraperitoneal injection of Aroclor 1254 (500 mg/kg body wt.) 6 days before sacrifice. Rats were decapitated and their livers homogenized in 3 vol. of sterile, cold KCl (150 mM, buffered with 10 mM sodium phosphate, pH 7.4). The homogenate was centrifuged at 9000 g for 10 min and stored at —80°C, filter sterilized. 1 vol. of the resulting supernatant was mixed with 1 vol. of 25 mM MgCl$_2$—100 mM KCl and 1 vol. 12 mM MgCl$_2$—100 mM KCl and 1 vol. 12 mM NADP—15 mM glucose 6-phosphate—150 mM sodium phosphate, pH 7.4.

Mutagenesis assay

Standard experimental procedures have been described by Ames et al. [1, 22]. Sample was completely dissolved in DMSO by shaking the tubes in water bath at 45°C for a few seconds at a time. The test compound (0.025—0.1 ml aliquots of DMSO solution equivalent to approx. 50—250 mg of dry feces) and 0.1 ml of over-night nutrient broth culture of bacteria were added to 2 ml top agar and overlayed on the Vogel—Bonner E-medium plates. 0.5 ml of S9 preparation was added for screening the fecal metabolites requiring activation. Each sample was plated using TA98 and TA100 with and without S9 mix. Plates were incubated for 40—48 h and colonies counted. Each sample was tested, in duplicate, in 3—4 different doses and the results were averaged. Remaining portions of fecal samples that gave positive results were subjected to entire extraction and testing procedure and found to be positive.

Every experiment contained positive controls for checking the activity of the metabolizing system and mutability of the bacteria as well as negative controls in the form of sterility controls and incubation without test compound. The revertant colonies were checked for true reversion by streaking the isolated colonies on a minimal agar plate which contained histidine on a paper disk and found to be true revertants.

Toxicity effects were evaluated by examination of the back-ground lawn, size and appearance of colonies. There was no evidence of toxicity of the fecal extracts that showed positive mutagenic activity. Fecal extracts that gave mutation ratio of less than 1 at the lowest concentration under standard mutagenesis assay, were diluted and tested again for mutagenic activity. Our results indicate that most of the samples retested after further dilution were not inhibitory to TA98 and TA100. The data presented here for all samples include the results obtained with standard assay procedure.

Results

The diet analyses from a 5—14 day dietary recall from each volunteer indicate that the total calorie consumption in the 3 groups was comparable (Table 1). The dietary intake of fat was higher in New York non-Seventh-Day Adventists and in Finland, compared to Seventh-Day Adventists; the protein content was similar in all groups. The dietary intake of fiber was higher in volunteers from Kuopio compared to Seventh-Day Adventists and non-Seventh-Day Adventists; however, Seventh-Day Adventists consumed more fiber than non-Seventh-Day Adventists from New York. The consumption of meat was greater in the non-Seventh-Day Adventists, whereas the consumption of milk and other

TABLE 1

DAILY NUTRIENT INTAKE OF HEALTHY VOLUNTEERS FROM KUOPIO (FINLAND) AND NEW YORK METROPOLITAN AREA [a]

Nutrient (g/day)	Kuopio [15]	Metropolitan New York	
		Seventh-Day [b] Adventists [11]	Non-Seventh Day [c] Adventists [18]
Protein	95 ± 4 [d]	86 ± 8	92 ± 6
Fat	97 ± 2	72 ± 5	98 ± 2
Carbohydrate	318 ± 4	340 ± 10	276 ± 8
Fiber	32 ± 3	20 ± 2	12 ± 1

[a] The data were calculated from 5—14 day diet recall.
[b] Vegetarians consuming a vegetarian diet for more than 10 years and included milk but not fish, poultry and meat.
[c] Normal population consuming a high-fat, high-meat, western diet.
[d] Averages ±S.E.M.

dairy products was higher in Finland. The sources of fat were different, a greater portion coming from meat in New York non-Seventh-Day Adventist population and from milk and other dairy products from Kuopio and Seventh-Day Adventists. The volunteers from Kuopio consumed more whole grain rye bread and cereals and less green vegetables and fruits than New York population, whereas Seventh-Day Adventists consumed more fresh vegetables and fruits than New York non-Seventh-Day Adventists and Kuopio population.

All the data of mutagenic response are expressed as mutagenic ratios which are the number of his^+ revertant colonies on the test plates divided by the number of his^+ spontaneous revertant colonies on control plates for each dose tested in each assay. Samples were considered positive for the presence of mutagenic ratio was equal to or greater than 3.0. Ames et al. [1] and Ehrich et al. [11] considered samples positive for the presence of mutagenic activity if the mutagenic ratio was equal to or greater than 2. However, in our experience, a mutagenic ratio of 3 was needed to assure the selection of samples with reproducible mutagenic activity.

Fig. 1 illustrates the dose-dependent relationship of representative fecal extracts from New York non-Seventh-Day Adventists using *Salmonella typhimurium* TA98 and TA100, with or without S9 activation. The assays were performed by varying the amount of extract included in the test system. As shown in Fig. 1, the mutagenic response to the fecal extracts was dose-related. For those samples which did not show any mutagenic response, increasing or decreasing the dose of fecal extract did not alter mutagenic ratios. The dose—response curves of certain samples exhibited a decrease in mutagenic activity at higher concentrations as shown in Fig. 1 (TA98 without S9 and TA100 with S9 activation). The decrease in mutagenic activity at higher dose levels may be attributed to toxicity and/or competition for the activation enzymes.

Figs. 2—4 and Table 2 summarize the distribution of mutation ratios for the fecal samples of 3 population groups who are at varied risk for the development of colon cancer. Samples collected from non-Seventh-Day Adventists of New York were highly mutagenic (mutagenic ratio greater than 3) in TA98 without S9, followed by TA100 without S9 and TA100 with S9 (Fig. 2). In the case of Seventh-Day Adventists, none of the samples tested showed mutagenic activity in any of the tester systems (Fig. 3), whereas Kuopio samples exhibited activity only in TA98 with S9 (Fig. 4). In New York non-Seventh-Day Adventists, 2 samples were mutagenic both with TA98 and TA100 (Table 2). All the samples

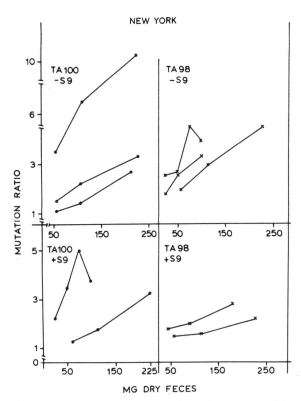

Fig. 1. Dose—response curves for the mutagen extracted from fecal samples of New York non-Seventh-Day Adventists consuming a high-fat, high-meat, low-fiber diet. The data were from representative fecal specimens and expressed as mutation ratio. The ether extract equivalent of 45—225 mg dry feces was suspended in DMSO and assayed for mutagenicity using *Salmonella typhimurium* TA98 and TA100 with and without S9 mix.

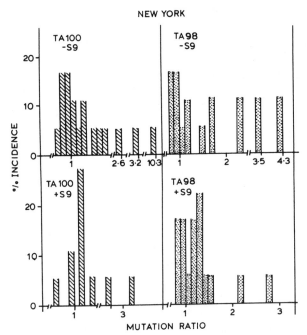

Fig. 2. Distribution of mutagenic activity of fecal extracts from New York non-Seventh-Day Adventists consuming a high-fat, high-meat, low-fiber diet. Fecal samples were extracted with ether, suspended in DMSO and assayed for mutagenicity using *Salmonella typhimurium* TA98 and TA100 with and without S9 mix. A dose—response curve was obtained for each sample using 3—4 different doses of ether extract. The percentage of the samples (% incidence) showing mutagenic activity was plotted against mutation ratio. A mutation ratio of 3 or more was considered positive.

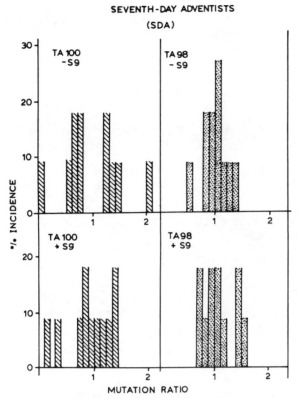

Fig. 3. Distribution of miutagenic activity of fecal extracts from New York Seventh-Day Adventists consuming vegetarian diet. Fecal samples were extracted with ether, suspended in DMSO and assayed for mutagenicity using *Salmonella typhimurium* TA98 and TA100 with and without S9 mix. Refer Fig. 2 for additional legend.

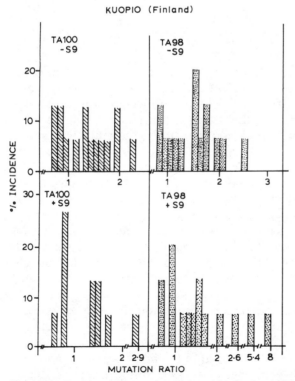

Fig. 4. Distribution of mutagenic activity of fecal extracts from Kuopio population consuming a high-fat, low-meat, high-fiber diet. Fecal samples were extracted with ether, suspended in DMSO and assayed for mutagenicity using *Salmonella typhimurium* TA98 and TA100, with and without S9 mix. Refer Fig. 2 for additional legend.

TABLE 2

MUTAGENIC ACTIVITY OF FECAL SAMPLES COLLECTED FROM HEALTHY MALE SUBJECTS FROM KUOPIO (FINLAND) AND NEW YORK METROPOLITAN AREA

Population group	% samples with mutagenic ratio greater than 3 [a]					
	TA98		TA100		TA98 and TA100 [c]	% samples showing mutagenic activity in at least one test system
	+S9	−S9	+S9	−S9		
New York non-Seventh-Day Adventists [18] [b]	0	22	6	11	11	22
Kuopio [15]	13	0	0	0	0	13
New York Seventh-Day Adventists [11]	0	0	0	0	0	0

[a] Mutagenic ratio is the number of his^+ revertant colonies on the test plate divided by the number of his^+ spontaneous revertant colonies on control plates.

[b] Number of samples tested is shown in parenthesis.

[c] Samples showing activity both in TA98 and TA100 tester systems.

that were active in TA100 without S9 also were active in TA98 without S9 (Table 2 and Fig. 2). In general, the fecal extracts of the non-Seventh-Day Adventists from New York consuming a high-fat, high-meat, low-fiber diet showed a higher mutagenic activity than did volunteers from Kuopio consuming a high-fat/high-fiber diet.

Table 3 presents the means of revertants per plate and standard deviation for TA98 and TA100 with or without microsomal activation, as recommended by De Serres and Shelby [9]. Fecal samples which gave a mutagenic ratio of 3 or more (Table 2) and all the samples which gave a mutagenic ratio 3 (Figs. 2—4) are included in the table.

Discussion

Previous studies have demonstrated that the fecal excretion of mutagens positive to *Salmonella typhimurium* TA100 and TA98 without S9 activation were higher in South-African urban whites who are at high risk for the development of colon cancer than in the South-African urban and rural blacks, a low-risk population for colon cancer [11]. In another study, the mutagenic activity was observed without microsomal activation on TA100 in volunteers consuming a Western diet and reduced when the diet was supplemented with ascorbic acid or α-tocopherol [4,33]. In the present study, the concentration of mutagens as well as the percentage of fecal samples showing mutagenic activity were higher in New York people consuming a high-fat, high-meat, low-fiber diet, compared with people in Kuopio, Finland; none of the Seventh-Day Adventists tested showed any mutagenic activity. The differences in mutagenic activity among the non-Seventh-Day Adventists and Seventh-Day Adventists from New York area and Finnish population from Kuopio might very well be related to their dietary habits.

The question may be asked as to factors responsible for the excretion of fecal mutagens. Bruce et al. [4,33] have reported the presence of mutagenic substances in the stools of some individuals that they identified as *N*-nitroso compounds and believed them to be produced in the body rather than ingested in the diet. Nagao et al. [23], Commoner et al. [7], Spingarn and Weisburger [32] and Weisburger et al. [35] demonstrated the presence of mutagens in fried fish and meat, fried hamburgers and broiled foods. Since most of the mutagens

TABLE 3

MUTAGENICITY OF FECAL EXTRACTS FROM HEALTHY MALE SUBJECTS FROM KUOPIO (FINLAND) AND NEW YORK METROPOLITAN AREA WITH SALMONELLA/MICROSOME TEST [a]

Samples and control	Amount of sample tested	Number of his^+ revertants/plate			
		TA98		TA100	
		−S9	+S9	−S9	+S9
Controls [44] [b]		18 ± 3 [c]	34 ± 3	126 ± 10	135 ± 10
Positive controls					
2-AAF [25]	1 μg		73 ± 16		159 ± 29
	5 μg		437 ± 27		364 ± 35
	10 μg		868 ± 62		515 ± 54
MNNG [25]	1 μg			248 ± 37	
	5 μg			619 ± 40	
	10 μg			1683 ± 230	
Picrolonic acid [25]	250 μg	691 ± 37			
Fecal extracts, [d] all samples					
Non-Seventh-Day Adventists [18]	50 mg [e]	26 ± 16	36 ± 12	155 ± 53	144 ± 30
	150 mg	28 ± 18	37 ± 14	181 ± 57	163 ± 34
	250 mg	38 ± 27	38 ± 11	226 ± 157	241 ± 172
Kuopio [15]	50 mg	20 ± 9	40 ± 16	145 ± 38	139 ± 45
	150 mg	22 ± 7	57 ± 23	162 ± 56	150 ± 58
	250 mg	21 ± 6	68 ± 30	158 ± 38	139 ± 45
Seventh-Day Adventists [11]	50 mg	17 ± 6	37 ± 8	109 ± 45	126 ± 49
	150 mg	16 ± 6	38 ± 12	110 ± 53	119 ± 60
	250 mg	16 ± 4	32 ± 14	110 ± 50	120 ± 62
Fecal extracts showing [f] mutagenic ratio more than 3					
Non-Seventh-Day Adventists	50 mg	50 ± 18 (4) [b]		337 ± 94 (2)	172 (1)
	150 mg	71 ± 11	none	538 ± 206	230
	250 mg	84 ± 10		804 ± 248	439
Kuopio	50 mg		90 ± 30 (2)		
	150 mg	none	155 ± 1	none	none
	250 mg		228 ± 74		
Seventh-Day Adventists		none	none	none	none

[a] Summary of the data presented in Table 2 and Figs. 2—4.
[b] Number of assays are shown in parenthesis. Each assay was done in duplicate.
[c] Mean ± standard deviation.
[d] Values represent all samples tested (Figs. 2—4).
[e] Amount of sample tested equal to 50, 150 and 250 mg of dry feces, except 50, 150 and 225 mg in case of TA100 with S9.
[f] Values represent samples which showed a mutagenic ratio of more than 3 (see Table 2 and Figs 2—4).

formed by the cooking process require S9 activation [7,23,32] and the fecal mutagens thus far tested are active, for the most part, without S9 [4,11], the source of fecal mutagens is not completely understood and remains to be determined. In addition, analysis of fecal specimens from other population groups could lead to the detection of different types of mutagens.

The present study and those of others [4,11] demonstrated the presence of mutagens in the feces of various populations. However, the procedures used in all these studies do not estimate the total mutagenic load of fecal samples. There are reports that certain compounds are not mutagenic when tested alone, but enhance the mutagenic properties of carcinogens and are termed co-mutagens [21,24]. It is possible that the fecal samples may contain co-mutagens and anti-mutagens which contribute to overall mutagenic potential of the feces. Isolation and identification of these compounds could lead to a better understanding of the mutagenic load in the colon.

It also remains to be determined whether the fecal mutagenic activity along with fecal bacterial enzymes such as β-glucuronidase, 7α-dehydroxylase and 7α-hydroxysteroid dehydrogenase [13,19,20,28,30] could be used as key indicators or markers which distinguish low- and high-risk population groups or individuals for large bowel cancer. Studies should be expanded to large number of populations to permit a more extensive evaluation of these discriminants for the large bowel cancer.

Acknowledgments

This work was supported by the National Cancer Institute, Grant CA-16382, through the National Large Bowel Project and Grants CA-12376 and CA-24217 from the National Cancer Institute.

References

1 Ames, B.N., J. McCann and E. Yamasaki, Methods for detecting carcinogens and mutagens with the Salmonella/mammalian-microsome mutagenicity test, Mutation Res., 31 (1975) 347—364.

2 Aries, V.C., J.S. Crowther, B.S. Drasar, M.J. Hill and R.E.O. Williams, Bacteria and the etiology of cancer of the large bowel, Gut, 10 (1969) 334—335.

3 Armstrong, B., and R. Doll, Environmental factors and cancer incidence and mortality in different countries with special reference of dietary practices, Int. J. Cancer, 15 (1975) 617—631.

4 Bruce, W.R., A.J. Varghese, R. Furrer and P.C. Land, A mutagen in the feces of normal humans, in: H.H. Hiatt, J.P. Watson and J.A. Winsten (Eds.), Origins of Human Cancer, Vol. 4, Cell Proliferation Series, Cold Spring Harbor Symposium, Cold Spring Harbor, NY, 1977, pp. 1641—1646.

5 Bull, A.W., B.K. Soullier, P.S. Wilson, M.T. Hayden and N.D. Nigro, Promotion of azoxymethane-induced intestinal cancer by high fat diet in rats, Cancer Res., 39 (1979) 4956—4959.

6 Burkitt, D.P., Large bowel carcinogenesis: An epidemiologic jigsaw puzzle, J. Natl. Cancer Inst., 54 (1975) 3—6.

7 Commoner, B., A.J. Vithayathil, P. Dolara, S. Nair, P. Madyastha and G.C. Cuca, Formation of mutagens in beef and beef extract during cooking, Science, 201 (1978) 913—916.

8 Cutler, S.J., and J.L. Young, Demographic patterns of cancer incidence in the United States, in J.F. Fraumeni Jr. (Ed.), Persons at High Risk of Cancer, Academic Press, New York, 1975, pp. 307—342.

9 de Serres, F.J., and M.D. Shelby, Recommendations on data production and analysis using the Salmonella/microsome mutagenicity assay, Mutation Res., 64 (1979) 159—165.

10 Doll, R., The geographical distribution of cancer, Br. J. Cancer, 23 (1969) 1—8.

11 Ehrich, M., J.E. Ashell, R.L. Van Tassell, T.D. Wilkins, A.R.P. Walker and N.J. Richardson, Mutagens in the feces of 3 South African populations at different levels of risk for colon cancer, Mutation Res., 64 (1979) 231—240.

12 Enstrom, J.E., Cancer and total mortality among active Mormons, Cancer, 42 (1978) 1943—1951.

13 Goldin, B.R., and S.L. Gorbach, The relationship between diet and rat fecal bacterial enzymes implicated in colon cancer, J. Natl. Cancer Inst., 57 (1976) 371—375.

14 Graham, S., H. Dayal, M. Swanson, H. Mittelman and G. Wilkinson, Diet in the epidemiology of cancer of the colon and rectum, J. Natl. Cancer Inst., 61 (1978) 709—714.

15 Haenszel, W., J.W. Berg, M. Segi, M. Kurihara and F.B. Locke, Large bowel cancer in Hawaiian Japanese, J. Natl. Cancer Inst., 51 (1973) 1765—1769.

16 Hill, M.J., B.S. Drasar, V. Aries, J.S. Crowther, G.M. Hawksworth and R.E.O. Williams, Bacteria and etiology of cancer of the large bowel, Lancet, 1 (1971) 90—100.

17 I.A.R.C. Microecology Group, Dietary fiber, transit the fecal bacteria, steroids and colon cancer in two Scandinavian populations, Lancet, 2 (1977) 207—211.

18 Jensen, O.M., J. Mosbech, M. Salaspuro and T. Jhamaki, A comparative study of the diagnostic basis for cancer of the colon and cancer of the rectum in Denmark and Finland, Int. J. Epidemiol., 3 (1974) 183—186.

19 MacDonald, I.A., G.R. Webb and D.E. Mahony, Fecal hydroxysteroid dehydrogenase activities in vegetarian Seventh-Day Adventists control subjects and bowel cancer patients, Am. J. Clin. Nutr., 31 (1978) S233—238.

20 Mastromarino, A., B.S. Reddy and E.L. Wynder, Metabolic epidemiology and colon cancer: Enzymic activity of fecal flora, Am. J. Clin. Nutr., 29 (1976) 1455—1460.

21 Matsumoto, T., D. Yoshida and S. Mizusaki, Enhancing effect of harman on mutagenicity in Salmonella, Mutation Res., 56 (1977) 85—88.

22 McCann, J., N.E. Spingarn, J. Kobori and B.N. Ames, Detection of carcinogens as mutagens: bacterial tester with R. Factor plasmids, Proc. Natl. Acad. Sci. (U.S.A.), 72 (1975) 979—983.

23 Nagao, M., M. Honda, Y. Seino, T. Yahagi and T. Sugimura, Mutagenicities of smoke condensates and the charred surface of fish and meat, Cancer Lett., 2 (1977) 221—226.

24 Nagao, M., T. Yahagi, T. Kawachi, T. Kosuge, K. Tsuji, K. Wakabayashi, S. Mizusaki and T. Matsumoto, Co-mutagenic action of norharman and harman, Proc. Jpn. Acad., 53 (1977) 95—98.

25 Nigro, N.D., D.V. Singh, R.L. Campbell and M.S. Pak, Effect of dietary beef fat on intestinal tumor formation by azoxymethane in rats, J. Natl. Cancer Inst., 54 (1975) 439—442.

26 Phillips, R.L., Role of lifestyle and dietary habits in risk of cancer among Seventh-Day Adventists, Cancer Res., 35 (1975) 3513—3522

27 Reddy, B.S., Nutrition and colon cancer, Adv. Nutrit. Res., 2 (1979) 199—218.

28 Reddy, B.S., A.R. Hedges, K. Laakso and E.L. Wynder, Metabolic epidemiology of large bowel cancer: Fecal bulk and constituents of high-risk North American and low-risk Finnish population, Cancer, 42 (1978) 2832—2838.

29 Reddy, B.S., K. Watanabe and A. Sheinfil, Effect of dietary wheat bran, alfalfa, pectin and carrageenan on plasma cholesterol and fecal bile acid and neutral sterol excretion in rats, J. Nutr. (in press).

30 Reddy, B.S., J.H. Weisburger and E.L. Wynder, Fecal bacterial β-glucuronidase: Control by diet, Science, 183 (1974) 416—417.

31 Reddy, B.S., J.H. Weisburger and E.L. Wynder, Colon cancer: Bile salts as tumor promoters, in: T.J. Slaga, A. Sivak and R.K. Boutwell (Eds.), Carcinogenesis, Vol. 2, Raven, New York, 1978, pp. 453—464.

32 Spingarn, N.E., and J.H. Weisburger, Formation of mutagens in cooked foods, I. Beef, Cancer Lett., 7 (1979) 259—264.

33 Varghese, A.J., P. Land, R. Furrer and W.R. Bruce, N-Nitroso compounds in the human body, Proc. Am. Ass. Cancer Res., 18 (1977) 80.

34 Watanabe, K., B.S. Reddy, J.H. Weisburger and D. Kritchevsky, Effect of dietary alfalfa, pectin and wheat bran on azoxymethane- or methylnitrosourea-induced colon carcinogenesis in F344 rats, J. Natl. Cancer Inst., 63 (1979) 141—145.

35 Weisburger, J.H., B.S. Reddy, N.E. Spingarn and E.L. Wynder, Current views on the mechanisms involved in the etiology of colorectal cancer, in: S.J. Winawer, P. Sherlock and D. Schottenfeld (Eds.), Progress in Cancer Research, Raven, New York (in press).

36 Wynder, E.L., T. Kajitani, S. Ishikawa, H. Dodo and A. Takano, Environmental factors of cancer of the colon and rectum, II. Japanese epidemiological data, Cancer, 23 (1969) 1210—1220.

Benzo(a)pyrene and Other Polynuclear Hydrocarbons in Charcoal-Broiled Meat

by W. Lijinsky and P. Shubik

Abstract. *The possible production of carcinogenic polynuclear hydrocarbons in the charcoal broiling of food has been investigated. Fifteen steaks were cooked and the polynuclear compounds were extracted, separated by chromatography, and identified spectrometrically. Many polynuclear hydrocarbons were identified, but no nitrogen heterocyclic compounds were detected. The carcinogen benzo(a)-pyrene was present in the average amount of 8 micrograms per kilogram of steak.*

It has been suggested many times that high-temperature cooking of food might give rise to carcinogenic hydrocarbons of the polynuclear aromatic group. Indeed, there has been one report of the finding of dibenz(a,h)anthracene in charcoal-broiled meat (*1*). Five years ago an analysis of charcoal-broiled steak was carried out in this laboratory and several polynuclear hydrocarbons were separated and identified, including pyrene, fluoranthene, chrysene, benz(a)anthracene, and benzo(g,h,i)perylene. The analytical method used was cumbersome and lengthy, involving alkaline and acid hydrolyses occupying several weeks, and undoubtedly introduced serious losses, particularly of any unstable hydrocarbons present. The experiment has been re-

At the time this article was written, the authors were with the Division of Oncology, Chicago Medical School, Chicago, Illinois. W. Lijinsky is currently Laboratory Director, Frederick Cancer Research Facility, Frederick, Maryland 21701.

peated with a simpler and more sensitive method now available (*2*).

Fifteen steaks were charcoal broiled, the outer layers were removed and extracted, the polynuclear material was extracted from the lipids, and the polynuclear aromatic hydrocarbons were separated by column and paper chromatography. Identification and measurement were made by ultraviolet absorption and by fluorescence spectrometry.

The results of the analysis (Table 1) show that the mixture of hydrocarbons extracted from the broiled meat is similar qualitatively to that obtained in the pyrolysis of other organic materials, such as cigarettes and coal. Most notable is the presence of benzo(a)pyrene to the extent of 9 μg steak (8 μg/kg). This is the quantity of benzo(a)pyrene in the smoke of approximately 600 cigarettes (*3*). Meat protein is apparently not pyrolyzed.

The most likely source of the polynuclear hydrocarbons is the melted fat which drips on the hot coals and is

pyrolyzed at the prevailing high temperature. The polynuclear hydrocarbons in the smoke are then deposited on the meat as the smoke rises. The significant absence of pyrolysis of protein indicates that other methods of cooking meat such as oven broiling or roasting would be unlikely to produce carcinogenic hydrocarbons.

The analysis was performed by broiling 15 large steaks (1.1 kg each), with a total surface area of approximately 1 m², to "well-done" on a standard charcoal broiler. Wood charcoal was ignited with purified isooctane and allowed to reach a uniform glowing red heat before the meat was placed over the fire. The distance of the meat from the coals was about 6 inches (15 cm). Both sides of each steak were cooked. The outer half centimeter of each side was cut off and extracted with acetone in a Soxhlet apparatus for several hours. Acetone and water were removed by distillation in a vacuum. The bones and fat were washed with 1 liter of acetone and 2 liters of benzene, and the solution was evaporated under nitrogen until only fat remained. The two residues were combined; the total weight was approximately 500 g.

The polynuclear compounds were separated from the bulk of the aliphatic material by solvent partition. The lipid

Table 1. Polynuclear hydrocarbons in charcoal-broiled steaks.

Compound	Total (μg)	Concentration in μg		
		Per steak	Per kilogram	Per 100 cm²
Anthanthrene	29	2	2	0.3
Anthracene	71	5	4.5	0.7
Benz(*a*)anthracene	76	5	4.5	0.8
Alkyl-benzanthracene	40	2.7	2.4	0.4
Benzo(*b*)chrysene	7.5	0.5	0.5	0.08
Benzo(*g,h,i*)perylene	76	5	4.5	0.8
Benzo(*a*)pyrene	133	9	8	1.3
Benzo(*e*)pyrene	97	6.5	6	1.0
Chrysene	21	1.5	1.4	0.2
Coronene	37	2.5	2.3	0.4
Dibenz(*a,h*)anthracene	3.5	0.2	0.2	0.04
Fluoranthene	321	21	20	3.2
Phenanthrene	180	12	11	1.8
Pyrene	286	19	18	2.9
Perylene	34	2	2	0.3

residue was dissolved in 500 ml of hexane [this and all other solvents were freed of polynuclear aromatic material by appropriate procedures (*4*)] and shaken with two 500-ml portions of nitromethane, the total extract being then distilled to dryness under nitrogen in a vacuum. The extraction of polynuclear aromatic material from the hexane solution was completed with three 200-ml portions of dimethylsulfoxide. To this extract were added 750 ml of hexane and 1.4 liters of water; the hexane layer was distilled to dryness and the oily residue was added to that from the nitromethane extract to give 8.8 g of oil. This was dissolved in 40 ml of isooctane and chromatographed on a 20- by 3.5-cm column of silica gel (100 to 200 mesh). Filtration of a further 200 ml of isooctane through the adsorbent eluted much dark brown material, after which the eluate was almost colorless. The adsorbed aromatic material was finally eluted with 250 ml of benzene, and the solvent was distilled under nitrogen. The residue (490 mg) was diluted to 2.5 ml with benzene, and 250 μl of solution was chromatographed on each of ten 15- by 50-cm strips of Whatman No. 1 paper that had been impregnated with *N,N*-dimethylformamide. The chromatograms were developed by the descending technique, with isooctane as mobile phase (*5*) and the analogous fluorescent

zones on all of the papers were combined, ultraviolet absorption spectra taken and fractions were rechromatographed as necessary in the same system until spectra were obtained which could be identified with those of known polynuclear compounds. The identifications were confirmed, where possible, by the fluorescence emission spectra.

Although many polynuclear hydrocarbons were identified in the steaks (Table 1), some hydrocarbons were present which could not be adequately identified or estimated because of their low concentration; among these are possibly picene, benzo(*j*)fluoranthene, benzo(*b*)fluoranthene, benzo(*k*)fluoranthene, dibenzo(*a,l*)pyrene, and dibenzo-(*a,i*)pyrene. The concentration of any of these compounds, if present, is certainly below 0.5 μg per steak. At least two compounds were present in concentrations comparable with those of the identified compounds, but they could not be identified spectroscopically with any known polycyclic aromatic compound. One of these was compound "Y," which has been found previously in solvents, waxes, and so forth (*4*); the other is a compound of low R_F in the dimethylformamide/isooctane system and having absorption maxima at 405, 400, 383, 362, 340, and 325 mμ.

The concentrations given for the various hydrocarbons are, of course, minimum values. The losses that occur

during repeated chromatography set an effective limit to the obtainable purification of some of the rarer components of the mixture. The identification of dibenz(*a,h*)anthracene and benzo(*b*)-chrysene is consequently not quite definite. That of benzo(*a*)pyrene, on the other hand, is unequivocal. In addition to benz(*a*)anthracene, a compound with a very similar spectrum but quite sharply separated from the former (and with higher R_F) was present. This is probably an alkylbenz(*a*)anthracene, which might or might not be a carcinogen. More of this material is needed for positive identification.

Several conclusions may be drawn tentatively from this preliminary experiment. The profile of polynuclear hydrocarbons present on the meat as a result of charcoal broiling is very similar to that present in other pyrolysis products, with one notable difference. Since no nitrogen-containing polynuclear compounds were detected, it can be inferred that pyrolysis of only carbon-, hydrogen-, and oxygen-containing compounds is involved. Carbazoles and acridines are very evident in the pyrolysates of nitrogen-containing materials, such as coal, vegetable matter (tobacco), and liquid smoke (produced by dry distillation of wood) (*6*). Reports of the analysis of the pyrolysates of cigarette paper (C, H, and O only) have given no evidence of the presence of nitrogen heterocycles (*7*).

References and Notes

1. A. Seppilli and S. G. Scassellati, *Boll. Soc. Ital. Biol. Sper.* **39**, 110 (1963).
2. I. I. Domsky, W. Lijinsky, K. Spencer, P. Shubik, *Proc. Soc. Exptl. Biol. Med.* **113**, 110 (1963).
3. *Smoking and Health*, Report of the Advisory Committee to the Surgeon General of the Public Health Service, Publ. No. 1103 (Govt. Printing Office, Washington, D.C., 1964).
4. W. Lijinsky and C. R. Raha, *Toxicol. Appl. Pharmacol.* **3**, 469 (1961).
5. W. Lijinsky, *Anal. Chem.* **32**, 684 (1960).
6. ———, I. Domsky, G. Mason, H. Ramahi, T. Safavi, *Anal. Chem.* **35**, 952 (1963); B. L. Van Duuren, J. A. Bilbao, C. A. Joseph, *J. Natl. Cancer Inst.* **25**, 53 (1960); W. Lijinsky and P. Shubik, unpublished observations.
7. R. L. Cooper and A. J. Lindsey, *Chem. Ind. London* **1954**, 1260 (1954); R. L. Cooper, J. A. S. Gilbert, A. J. Lindsey, *Brit. J. Cancer* **9**, 442 (1955).
8. Supported by NIH grant CS-9212.

9 April 1964

Artificial Sweeteners and Human Bladder Cancer: Preliminary Results

by Robert N. Hoover and Patricia Hartge Strasser

Summary   3010 patients with cancer of the urinary bladder and 5783 controls drawn from the general population of ten geographic areas of the U.S.A. were interviewed. Subjects who reported ever having used artificial sweeteners or artificially sweetened foods or beverages showed no elevation in risk. However, positive associations between various measures of use of artificial sweeteners and risk of bladder cancer were seen in several subgroups. Inconsistencies in the data suggest that the positive associations may be due to chance, but it is noteworthy that the subgroups were those chosen, a priori, to test hypotheses derived from laboratory experiments.

Introduction

In 1977 a case-control interview study[1] revealed that men who used artificial sweeteners (AS) had a 60% increase in their risk of bladder cancer, with evidence of a dose-response relationship. However, women had a non-significant decrease in risk. A subsequent unpublished report from an ongoing case-control study also disclosed an excess risk of bladder cancer among male users of AS but not among female users,[2] but a later report from the same study found no excess.[3] Other case-control studies have not revealed an association for either sex.[4-7] Experimental evidence has shown that saccharin, a combination of cyclamate and saccharin, and a metabolite of cyclamate can each cause bladder tumours in rats if the animals are given high doses.[8-11] The results for saccharin were most obvious if the exposure began in utero. Laboratory studies have also shown that saccharin promotes the carcinogenic effects of other agents.[12,13]

We conducted a large, population-based case-control interview study for two purposes: to resolve some of the apparent conflicts in the findings of the epidemiological studies and to look for evidence of either of the two biological mechanisms suggested for saccharin by laboratory data—weak carcinogenesis when given by itself, and potentiation of carcinogenesis when given with other carcinogens. We concluded that a large study was needed in order to provide adequate numbers of subjects in separate subgroups where these two mechanisms might be manifest. In particular, we wished to examine the subjects who were at the highest level of exposure. We also wished to examine the subjects at low background risk of bladder cancer among whom a small addition to risk might be most discernible. Third, we wished to examine the subjects exposed to known bladder carcinogens before they were exposed to AS, among whom evidence of promotion might be detectable.

Methods

Cases comprised all residents of designated counties in the metropolitan areas of Atlanta, Detroit, New Orleans, San Francisco, and Seattle and in the states of Connecticut, Iowa, New Jersey, New Mexico, and Utah, aged 21–84, who were newly diagnosed with a histologically confirmed carcinoma of the urinary bladder (or papilloma not specified as benign) during a one-year period beginning in December, 1977. Cases with previous lower-urinary-tract cancers were excluded. The

Robert N. Hoover and Patricia Hartge Strasser are with the Environmental Epidemiology Branch, National Cancer Institute, Bethesda, Maryland 20205.

The following sixteen co-authors took part in this collaborative study: MARGARET CHILD, Atlanta Surveillance Center; THOMAS J. MASON, MAX MYERS, and DEBRA SILVERMAN, National Cancer Institute; DONALD AUSTIN, California State Department of Health; RONALD ALTMAN and ANNETTE STEMHAGEN, New Jersey State Department of Health; KENNETH CANTOR, Environmental Protection Agency; AMBATI NARAYANA, University of Iowa; DAVID THOMAS, Fred Hutchinson Cancer Research Center, Seattle, Washington; CHARLES KEY, University of New Mexico; J. W. SULLIVAN, Louisiana State University Medical Center; DEE WEST, University of Utah; MARIE W. SWANSON, Michigan Cancer Foundation; J. WISTER MEIGS and LARAINE D. MARRETT, Yale University.

cases were found through the Surveillance, Epidemiology and End Results Network and the New Jersey Cancer Registry. Controls were an age and sex stratified random sample of the general populations of the ten geographic areas, frequency-matched at a 2:1 ratio of controls to cases.

Controls aged 65–84 were randomly sampled from the files of the Health Care Financing Administration, which enumerated an estimated 98% of individuals over age 65 in the U.S.A. Controls aged 21–64 were selected in a three-stage process: telephone numbers were chosen at random from all residential telephones in the ten geographic areas;[14] an interviewer called each number and recorded the age and sex of each household member aged 21–64; a stratified random sample was selected from the household censuses.

Personal interviews were conducted in the subjects' homes. Questionnaire items included detailed histories of use of AS in three forms (as a table-top sweetener, in diet drinks, in diet foods) as well as tobacco use, occupation, residence, source of water, coffee use, hair-dye use, and illnesses.

In the analysis, the unexposed groups included only subjects who were never exposed to any form of AS. In tables referring to only one form of AS, the exposed groups included only those who used that form (whether or not exposed to other forms). Since only 1% of the subjects used diet food but not diet drinks or table-top AS, data are not presented for diet foods in detail.

The measure of strength of association used is the maximum likelihood estimate of relative risk (RR) derived from the odds ratio.[15] Where noted, analyses were controlled for other potentially confounding variables by multiple contingency table analysis[16] or logistic regression.[17] One-tailed tests for statistical significance were used—the Mantel-Haenszel summary chi-squared[18] and the Mantel extension of the Mantel-Haenszel test, a test for linear trend.[19]

During the study, 4045 eligible cases were identified, of whom 1% had papillomas and 99% had carcinomas. From the files of the Health Care Financing Administration, we drew 4058 controls aged 65–84. Of the 25 826 residential telephone numbers we chose at random, 88% yielded household censuses. We could not attempt to interview subjects from households that gave no census. Nor could we interview those who had died (7% of cases, 1% of controls) or those severely disabled (7% of cases, 3% of controls). Among those approached for an interview, cooperation rates were 87% for all cases, 85% for controls aged 21–64, 87% for controls aged 65–84, 86% for subjects overall. If the numbers of identified cases and controls are combined with the estimated number of controls that would have been eligible had telephone censuses been obtained, the total is 11 430, of whom we interviewed 8793.

Results

75% of the cases (and controls) were male and the median age was 67. Compared with the control series, the case series included more White subjects, more cigarette-smokers, and more workers exposed to dye, rubber, leather, ink, or paint. These patterns replicated those of previous studies.[20]

Men who had ever used AS showed a relative risk of 0·99 and the corresponding women showed a relative risk of 1·07, after adjustment for the identified risk factors in the total group—race, cigarette-smoking, coffee-drinking, and chemical exposures at work (table I). Relative risks for use of each major form of AS did not differ appreciably from 1·00. Additional control (for age, sex, history of diabetes, geographic area, and education) did not alter the estimates of relative risk.

Users of table-top AS or diet drink were classified according to their usual level of intake (table II).

TABLE I—HISTORY OF USE OF ARTIFICIAL SWEETENERS, BY SEX

	Cases	Controls	R R*	95% Confidence limits
Males				
Never used AS	1349	2554	1·00	
Ever used diet drink	607	1204	0·95	(0·84, 1·07)
Ever used table-top	592	1066	1·04	(0·92, 1·18)
Ever used diet food	240	442	1·02	(0·85, 1·22)
Ever used any form	909	1723	0·99	(0·89, 1·10)
Females				
Never used AS	358	767	1·00	
Ever used diet drink	262	504	1·02	(0·83, 1·25)
Ever used table-top	236	474	1·04	(0·84, 1·28)
Ever used diet food	130	239	1·13	(0·87, 1·47)
Ever used any form	384	732	1·07	(0·89, 1·29)
Both sexes				
Never used AS	1707	3321	1·00	
Ever used diet drink	869	1708	0·97	(0·87, 1·07)
Ever used table-top	828	1540	1·04	(0·93, 1·16)
Ever used diet food	370	681	1·05	(0·91, 1·22)
Ever used any form	1293	2455	1·01	(0·92, 1·11)

* Relative risk adjusted for race, cigarette smoking, coffee drinking, and occupational exposure.

TABLE II—AVERAGE DAILY USE OF TABLE-TOP SWEETENERS, AND OF DIET DRINK

—	Males			Females		
	Cases	Controls	R R*	Cases	Controls	R R*
Never used AS	1349	2554	1·00	358	767	1·00
<1 use table-top	109	190	1·09	39	113	0·73
1–1·9 uses table-top	105	229	0·88	56	96	1·28
2–3·9 uses table-top	164	299	1·08	72	110	1·42
4–5·9 uses table-top	62	118	0·97	22	45	0·99
⩾6 uses table-top	39	59	1·05	16	20	1·36
	($\chi^2=0·181; p=0·43$)			($\chi^2=1·938; p=0·03$)		
<1 serving diet drink	349	723	0·93	146	294	1·01
1–1·9 servings diet drink	107	207	0·93	44	108	0·83
2–2·9 servings diet drink	48	63	1·44	24	29	1·72
⩾3 servings diet drink	25	41	1·01	15	20	1·37
($\chi^2=0·352; p=0·36$)	($\chi^2=0·352; p=0·36$)			($\chi^2=0·942; p=0·17$)		

* Relative risk adjusted for age, race, and cigarette smoking. p values are based on one-tailed tests.

Although males with heavier usual consumption of diet drinks showed elevated risks, there was no consistent gradation of risk with increased use of diet drinks or table-top AS. Among females, the risks were elevated with heavier use, and the trend for table-top AS was statistically significant. However, the relative risks were below 1·0 in some categories and the patterns were variable. Combined consumption of diet drinks and table-top AS was also considered, with categories defined to reflect the fact that one average serving of diet drink contains 2–3

TABLE III—AVERAGE NUMBER OF DAILY USES OF TABLE-TOP
SWEETENERS BY AVERAGE NUMBER OF DAILY SERVINGS OF DIET
DRINK: MALES AND FEMALES COMBINED

Uses of table-top AS daily:	Diet drinks daily:		
	None	<2	≥2
None	1.00* (1707, 3321)†	0.94 (314, 638)	1.21 (38, 60)
<3	1.02 (189, 367)	0.98 (212, 417)	1.26 (35, 54)
3–5	1.15 (80, 136)	0.76 (59, 146)	1.56 (20, 25)
≥6	0.99 (18, 34)	1.53 (28, 34)	1.64 (7, 8)

* Relative risk of bladder cancer adjusted for age, race, sex
† (Number of cases, number of controls)

TABLE IV—AVERAGE DAILY USE OF ARTIFICIAL SWEETENERS
AMONG LOW-RISK* WHITE FEMALES

—	Table-top sweeteners			Diet drinks		
	Cases	Controls	RR†	Cases	Controls	RR†
Never used AS	130	402	1.0	130	402	1.0
Ever used table-top /diet drink	82	210	1.2 ($\chi^2=1.163$; p=0.12)	71	219	1.1 ($\chi^2=0.387$; p=0.35)
<1 use/serving	15	53	0.9	36	132	0.9
1–1.9 uses/servings	17	43	1.2	16	43	1.2
2–2.9 uses/servings	21	36	1.8	7	14	1.6
≥3 uses/servings	22	38	1.8 ($\chi^2=2.630$; p<0.01)	3	6	1.6 ($\chi^2=1.075$; p=0.14)
≥2 uses/servings for 5 yr	14	34	1.3	1	6	0.5
≥2 uses/servings for 5–9 yr	13	22	1.8	3	7	1.4
≥2 uses/servings for ≥10 yr	16	18	2.7 ($\chi^2=3.240$; p<0.01)	6	7	3.0 ($\chi^2=1.654$; p<0.05)

* Never smoked cigarettes and never handled dye, rubber, leather, ink, or paint on any job; † adjusted for age. p values are based on one-tailed tests.

TABLE V—AVERAGE DAILY CONSUMPTION OF TABLE-TOP AS AND
DIET DRINKS AMONG WHITE MALES WHO SMOKED MORE THAN 40
CIGARETTES DAILY

—	Cases	Controls	R R*
Never used AS	104	167	1.00
Table-top AS:			
<1 use	12	15	1.28
1–1.9 uses	19	14	2.07
2–3.9 uses	16	13	1.96
4–5.9 uses	8	10	1.33
≥6 uses	7	7 ($\chi^2=2.220$; p=0.01)	1.86
Diet drinks:			
<1 serving	39	53	1.20
1–1.9 servings	14	19	1.20
2–2.9 servings	10	5	3.33
≥3 servings	6	4 ($\chi^2=2.339$; p=0.01)	2.62

* Adjusted for age. p values are based on one-tailed tests

times as much AS as one average use of table-top AS (table III). Subjects who used both forms, at least one of them heavily, showed an increased risk. Logistic regression analysis controlling for sex, age, race, smoking, occupational exposures, region, and education yielded a relative risk of 1.45 for those who used at least three servings of table-top AS and at least two diet drinks daily or who used at least some diet drinks and at least six servings of table-top AS (the three categories of greatest use in table III). (The 95% confidence interval was from 1.00 to 2.10.) For males, the relative risk was 1.47; for females, 1.41.

When subjects were categorised according to the duration of exposure or according to the years since the first exposure, no consistent patterns emerged for either sex. In fact, for males and females, the lowest risk was seen in the subjects with longest use. An analysis of estimated lifetime consumption (average daily dose multiplied by duration) showed no trends for males but a statistically significant, although erratic, positive trend for table-top AS among females.

In addition to the total study group, several subgroups of the study population were examined. First, we searched for effects detectable only in the absence of major bladder-cancer risk factors. Since males had three times the risk of females, and smokers had twice the risk of non-smokers, and those exposed to dye, leather, rubber, ink, or paint had 1.3 times the risk of those unexposed, we examined a group of female non-smokers unexposed to dye, rubber, leather, ink, or paint. Because we had few non-White women in this group, we further restricted the group to White women. These low-risk subjects had a crude risk of about 5 cases per 100 000 per year. Among these low-risk White women, we found a pattern of increased risk with increased levels of intake of AS (table IV). These findings were unaffected by adjustment for coffee-drinking, history of diabetes, geographic region, education, obesity, use of hair dyes, or history of urinary infections. A relation of risk to duration was not apparent in the total subgroup. However the low-risk women who consumed diet drinks or table-top sweeteners at least twice daily showed increased relative risk with longer duration of use. Low-risk White females who consumed table-top AS at least twice daily for ten years or more had 2.7 times the risk of non-users; those who drank at least two diet drinks daily for ten years or more had 3.0 times the risk.

To search for potentiation of known bladder carcinogens, we examined a high-risk group composed of White men who smoked cigarettes most heavily (more than 40 per day) (table v). Within this group, consumers of diet drinks or table-top AS were at higher risk than those who never used AS. There were gradations in risk suggestive of dose-response for diet drinks, but not for table-top AS.

These findings were restricted to the heavy smokers; non-smoking men and those who smoked 40 or fewer cigarettes per day showed no significant trends in relative risk with increased use of either table-top AS or diet drinks. In fact, the non-smoking males showed a non-significant decreasing trend with increased daily use of diet drinks. Among the heaviest-smoking females (more than 20 cigarettes daily) the heavier users of table-top AS and diet drinks (≥ 2 servings per day) also showed higher relative risks than those who never used AS. The trend in relative risk was significant for diet drinks. No consistent trends were seen for either form of AS among women who smoked 20 or fewer cigarettes daily.

Discussion

The data from this study do not provide support for earlier reports of a relative risk as high as 1·6 for men who used table-top AS. Thus, this study rules out a strong or moderate carcinogenic effect on the human bladder of artificial sweeteners as these have been used in the U.S.A. in the past. In the total study group, there was no evidence of increased risk to long-term users or to those first exposed decades ago.

However, an excess risk was seen among subjects who reported use of both table-top AS and diet drinks and heavy use of one of the forms (six or more daily uses of table-top AS, or two or more daily servings of diet drinks). The relative risks were small by epidemiological standards, and did not show a consistent dose-response relationship. Further, the estimates for the heaviest users were based on small numbers of subjects.

Because of inconsistencies in the patterns observed, the elevations in risk require cautious interpretation and further analyses. Nonetheless, the findings give some cause for concern. First, it is not implausible that a carcinogenic effect might be seen only among the few subjects who were heavily exposed. Second, to the extent that levels of AS consumption have been rising, the future overall association between AS use and bladder cancer may be better approximated by the associations seen at higher doses than by the average past experience of the total group of subjects.

We examined a subgroup of women at low risk of bladder cancer because experiments with laboratory animals suggested that saccharin and cyclamates are weak carcinogens, whose effects may be more easily identified in persons unexposed to potent risk factors. Indeed, in the low-risk group there was evidence of an association with heavier consumption of diet drinks and table-top AS. It is noteworthy that a very recently reported study revealed no overall association between bladder cancer and artificial sweeteners, but did show an association among non-smoking females.[21] We were unable to determine whether the lack of association among low-risk males reflected their higher background risk compared with females or the role of chance in the positive association among females.

When we classified subjects according to their usual level of cigarette smoking, we found some associations between bladder cancer and AS among the heavier smokers. These elevated risks may reflect potentiation by AS of the carcinogenic effect of cigarette smoking, but further analyses of duration, total dose, and other factors are needed before an interpretation can be offered confidently.

While the positive associations observed in this study may reflect biological reality, other explanations are possible. Cases were identified and interviewed promptly, but 14% were too ill or had died. If these cases had histories of AS use greatly different from those of healthier cases, our estimates of relative risk would be biased. This would also happen if the cases or the controls who refused or were unlocated had histories greatly different from those of respondents. However, our response rates were high and were similar for cases and controls. Other biases could arise—for instance, if publicity had caused bladder-cancer patients to recall their AS use to a greater or lesser extent than other people, or if physicians were more likely to diagnose bladder cancer in an AS user. We think it unlikely that biases would have produced either the patterns of positive associations observed in various subgroups, which vary by extent of exposure and by other factors, or the overall lack of association with average AS use in the total study population. It is harder to exclude the possibility of chance. By chance alone, we could have missed a small but real elevation in risk associated with average past levels of use; and, by chance alone, we could have observed positive associations in subgroups of a study which, overall, showed no association between bladder cancer and AS use. On the basis of the confidence intervals, we doubt that chance played an important role in producing the overall lack of association.

The study did not assess the effects of exposure to AS in utero. Nor could it assess the long-term effects of certain newly established patterns of AS use, such as relatively heavy exposure begun in childhood. The analyses presented do not separate cyclamates (in use in the 1960s) from saccharin, but none of the associations seen were derived solely from exposures in the 1960s.

We conclude that past AS use has had a minimal effect, if any, on bladder cancer rates. We also conclude that the positive associations in this study do not by themselves establish a causal link between AS use and bladder cancer. However, we think it noteworthy that the pattern of positive associations is consistent with experimental data that suggest that artificial sweeteners are weakly carcinogenic when given alone and potentiating when given with other carcinogens.

This study was sponsored by the U.S. Food and Drug Administration, National Cancer Institute, and Environmental Protection Agency. We wish to thank especially the patients, their physicians, and the members of the general population whose cooperation made this study possible.

Requests for reprints should be addressed to R. N. H.

REFERENCES

1. Howe GR, Burch JD, Miller AB, et al. Artificial sweeteners and human bladder cancer. *Lancet* 1977; ii: 578–81.
2. Wynder EL, Stellman SK, Austin H. Saccharin usage and bladder cancer. Annual Report to NCI and Subcontract SHP-74-106C under NO1-CP-55666.
3. Wynder EL, Stellman SK. Saccharin usage and bladder cancer. *Science* 1980; **207**: 1214–16.
4. Jain MG, Morgan RW. Bladder cancer: smoking, beverages, and artificial sweeteners. *Can Med Assoc J* 1974; **111**: 1067–70.
5. Wynder EK, Goldsmith R. The epidemiology of bladder cancer: a second look. *Cancer* 1977; **40**: 1246–68.
6. Simon D, Yen S, Cole P. Coffee drinking and cancer of the lower urinary tract. *J Nat Cancer Inst* 1975; **54**: 587–91.
7. Kessler II, Clark JP. Saccharin, cyclamate and human bladder cancer. *JAMA* 1978; **240**: 349–55.
8. Arnold DL, Moodie CA, Grice HC, et al. Long-term toxicity of ortho-toluene sulfonamide and sodium saccharin in the rat: an interim report. Ottawa, Canada: National Health & Welfare Ministry, Health Protection Branch, Toxicology Research Division, 1977: 37.
9. U.S. Department of Health, Education and Welfare Food and Drug Administration. Histopathologic evaluation of tissues from rats following continuous dietary intake of sodium saccharin and calcium cyclamate for a maximum period of two years. Final Report (Project P-169-170). Wash-

ington, DC: U.S. Dept Health, Education, Welfare, Public Health Service, Food and Drug Administration, 1973.

10. Wisconsin Alumni Research Foundation. Long term saccharin feeding in rats: final report. Madison, Wisconsin: WARF, 1973.

11. Price JM, Biava CG, et al. Bladder tumors in rats fed cyclohexylamine or high doses of a mixture of cyclamate and saccharin. *Science* 1970; **167**: 1131–32.

12. Hicks RM, Chowaniec J. The importance of synergy between weak carcinogens in the induction of bladder cancer in experimental animals and human. *Cancer Res* 1977; **37**: 2943–49.

13. Cohen SM, Arai M, Jacobs JB, and Friedell GH. Promoting effect of saccharin and DL-tryptophan in urinary bladder carcinogenesis. *Cancer Res* 1979; **39**: 1207–17.

14. Waksberg J. Sampling methods for random digit dialing. *J Am Stat Assoc* 1978; **73**: 40–46.

15. MacMahon B, Pugh TF. Epidemiology principles and methods. Boston: Little, Brown, 1970.

16. Gart JJ. Point and interval estimation of the common odds ratio in the combination of 2×2 tables with fixed marginals. *Biometrika* 1970; **57**: 471–75.

17. Prentice R. Use of the logistic model in retrospective studies. *Biometrics* 1976; **32**: 599–606.

18. Mantel N, Haenszel W. Statistical aspects of the analysis of data from retrospective studies of disease. *J Nat Cancer Inst* 1959; **22**: 719–48.

19. Mantel N. Chi-square tests with one degree of freedom; extension of the Mantel-Haenszel procedure. *J Am Stat Assoc* 1963; **58**: 690–700.

20. Morrison AS, Cole P. Epidemiology of bladder cancer. *Urol Clin N Am* 1976; **3**: 13–29.

21. Morrison AS, Buring JE. Artificial sweeteners and cancer of the lower urinary tract. *N Engl J Med* 1980; **302**: 537–41.

Dietary Constituents Altering the Responses to Chemical Carcinogens[1,2]

by Lee W. Wattenberg, William D. Loub, Luke K. Lam and Jennine L. Speier

ABSTRACT

This paper deals with two categories of compounds having the capacity to inhibit the neoplastic effects of chemical carcinogens on the host. The first are inducers of increased microsomal mixed function oxidase activity. An increasing number of these inducers are being found in natural products. Cruciferous vegetables including brussels sprouts, cabbage, and cauliflower contain such compounds. Recently indole-3-acetonitrile, indole-3-carbinol and 3,3′-diindolylmethane have been identified as inducers in these three plants. Other naturally occurring inducers include flavones, safrole, isosafrole, β-ionone, and oxidized sterols. Since previous work has shown that synthetic inducers may protect against chemical carcinogens, the composition of the diet could play a role in inhibiting the neoplastic response to these carcinogenic agents. The second category of inhibitors comprises the antioxidants. Several of these compounds have been found to inhibit the carcinogenic effects of a variety of chemical carcinogens. Considerable work of this nature has been done with butylated hydroxyanisole and butylated hydroxytoluene, two antioxidants extensively used as food additives. Other antioxidants having carcinogen inhibiting capacities include ethoxyquin, disulfiram, and dimethyldithiocarbamate.— **Wattenberg, L. W., W. D. Loub, L. K. Lam and J. L. Speier.** Dietary constituents altering the responses to chemical carcinogens. *Federation Proc.* 35: 1327–1331, 1976.

E̲pidemiological studies have shown diversities in the incidence of a substantial number of neoplasms in different geographical areas. Likewise, changes occur in the incidence of particular neoplasms in the same region over a period of time, for example, the decrease in cancer of the stomach in the USA. In both instances, the differences that are found may be due to either alterations in levels of exposure to carcinogenic agents, or alternately, to changes in factors protecting the host against the effect of the carcinogenic agent involved. This presentation deals with the latter possibility. Two classes of compounds potentially protecting against chemical carcinogenesis will be discussed. The first compounds are inducers of increased microsomal mixed function oxidase activity; the second are a group of antioxidants, some of which are extensively employed as food additives.

INDUCTION OF INCREASED MIXED FUNCTION OXIDASE ACTIVITY BY DIETARY CONSTITUENTS

The microsomal mixed function oxidase system is a complicated biochemical entity that metabolizes a wide variety of xenobiotic compounds including many chemical carcinogens (6, 21). The activity of this system can be increased by administration of various inducers. These can differ in the number and type of substrates that they cause to be metabolized at an increased rate (5, 20). The nature of the metabolites formed can also be altered (20, 33). The inducing compounds may or may not bear a chemical relationship to the substrates for which activity is increased (6). The induction process entails new protein synthesis (13).

Since induction of increased microsomal mixed function oxidase activity could change the host response to compounds metabolized by this system, including chemical carcinogens, there has been considerable interest in the characteristics of inducers (6). In particular, substantial work has

[1] From the Wendell H. Griffith Memorial Symposium on *Nutrition and Cancer* presented by the American Institute of Nutrition at the 59th Annual Meeting of the Federation of American Societies for Experimental Biology, Atlantic City, NJ, April 15, 1975.

[2] Supported by Public Health Service grants CA-09599 and CA-14146, and Contract N01-33364 from the National Cancer Institute.

Abbreviations: AHH, aryl hydrocarbon hydroxylase; BHA, butylated hydroxyanisole; BHT, butylated hydroxytoluene; BP, benzo(a)pyrene; DMBA, 7,12-dimethylbenz(a)anthracene.

been reported on inducers of increased microsomal hydroxylation of aromatic polycyclic hydrocarbons, a class of compounds that includes a large number of carcinogens found widely dispersed in the environment. This particular group of mixed function oxidase reactions has been termed aryl hydrocarbon hydroxylase (AHH). Polycyclic hydrocarbons, phenothiazines, flavones, and 2-phenylbenzothiazoles have all been shown to induce increased AHH activity. Some data on the relationship of chemical structure to inducing activity have been obtained (8, 54, 58, 59).

In early studies of AHH activity, it had been assumed that normal levels of activity of substantial magnitude exist. The assumption is true for the liver but is incorrect for the small intestine and lung. Most if not all of the AHH activity in these two organs, which are major portals of entry, results from exposure to exogenous inducers present in crude diets (46–48). The first evidence for this came from studies of starved female Sprague-Dawley rats. The animals showed almost total loss of AHH activity in the small intestine and lung. Subsequently, studies were carried out employing a balanced purified diet, i.e., vitamin-free casein 27%, starch 59%, corn oil 10%, salt mix 4%, plus a complete vitamin supplement (Normal Protein Test Diet, Nutritional Laboratories, Cleveland). Again, there was almost a total loss of AHH activity in the small intestine and lung. Determination of the effects of starvation and feeding a purified diet were also carried out on 3-methyl-4-methylaminoazobenzene N-demethylase activity of the small intestine. Both of these regimens result in a profound decrease in the activity of this reaction as compared to the level of activity in animals fed Purina Rat Chow (3).

Efforts were begun to identify the inducers of increased AHH activity present in the crude diets using Purina Rat Chow as a prototype. Various constituents of the diet were tested. Inducing activity was found in the vegetable component which consists of alfalfa meal. Experiments with alfalfa meal showed that this material has inducing activity. Subsequently, the plant itself was obtained from a farm in which no chemical treatment

of the soil or plant had been employed. This alfalfa also had inducing activity when added to purified diets fed to rats (48).

Because of the results obtained with alfalfa, investigations of the inducing activity of other vegetables were carried out. Many vegetables induce increased AHH activity, some do not. The most potent studied thus far are members of the Brassicaceae family including brussels sprouts, cabbage, turnips, broccoli, and cauliflower. Addition of brussels sprouts or cabbage to the diet has also been found to induce increased O-dealkylation of phenacetin and 7-ethoxycoumarin by the small intestine of the rat (17). Further studies with brussels sprouts and cabbage showed quite marked differences in AHH-inducing activity with different varieties of the vegetable, more so for cabbages than brussels sprouts.

Work was initiated to characterize the inducers in cruciferous plants using brussels sprouts, cabbages, and cauliflower as starting materials. The inducing activity was found in a fraction containing indoles. From this fraction, three indoles having inducing capacity were identified. These are indole-3-acetonitrile, indole-3-carbinol, and 3,3′-diindolylmethane (19). These indoles result from the hydrolysis of a parent compound, indolylmethyl glucosinolate (Fig. 1) (44). The parent compound along with the enzyme myrosinase that hydrolyzes it occurs in plant cells in their viable state.

Figure 1. The enzymatic degradation of indolylmethyl glucosinolate.

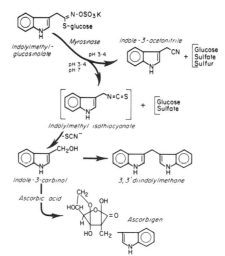

With cellular disruption the enzyme and substrate are brought together and hydrolysis occurs. As can be seen from Fig. 1, the relative amounts of the various hydrolysis products are dependent on the conditions of the reaction.

Other compounds found in plants also have inducing activity. A number of flavones induce increased AHH activity (59). Flavone, which is a naturally occurring compound, is an inducer. Polyhydroxylation of this compound results in loss of inducing activity. Since the vast majority of naturally occurring flavones are polyhydroxylated, they are ineffective as inducers. A few flavones such as 5,6,7,8,4′-pentamethoxyflavone (tangeretin) and 5,6,7,8,3′,4′-hexamethoxyflavone (nobiletin) contain methoxy rather than hydroxy groups. These compounds which occur in citrus fruits do have inducing activity. Additional naturally occurring inducers include safrole, isosafrole and β-ionone (31, 32). Oxidation of a variety of sterols including cholesterol results in their having inducing activity (4). A number of insecticides and polychlorinated biphenyls are inducers so that contamination of the diet with these compounds could enhance mixed function oxidase activity (2, 15, 35).

EFFECTS OF INDUCTION OF INCREASED MIXED FUNCTION OXIDASE ACTIVITY ON THE RESPONSE TO CHEMICAL CARCINOGENS

The microsomal mixed function oxidase system has the capacity to both detoxify chemical carcinogens and also to activate them to proximate or ultimate carcinogenic forms (27–29, 45). A substantial number of in vivo studies have shown that induction of increased mixed function oxidase activity protects against challenge by chemical carcinogens (Table 1). Because of the existence of activation reactions, the possibility that induction of increased mixed function oxidase activity might increase the carcinogenic response to a chemical carcinogen also exists. However, data clearly showing such an increased carcinogenic response in vivo have not been published. This may be due to the fact that rapid activation of carcinogens simply does not enhance

TABLE 1. Inhibition of carcinogenesis by induction of increased microsomal enzyme activity

Carcinogen	Inducer	Species	Organ	Ref
3'-Methyl-4-dimethyl-aminoazobenzene	Polycyclic hydrocarbons, α-benzene hexachloride, polychlorinated biphenyls	Rat	Liver	22,26,34,41
2-Acetylaminofluorene	Polycyclic hydrocarbons, polychlorinated biphenyls	Rat	Liver, breast, small intestine	22,26
Diethylnitrosamine	Polychlorinated biphenyls	Rat	Liver	22
4-Dimethylaminostilbene	Polycyclic hydrocarbons	Rat	Ear duct	40
Urethane	Pentobarbital	Mouse	Lung	1,38
Urethane	β-Naphthoflavone, chlordane, phenobarbital	Mouse	Lung	61
Benzo(a)pyrene	β-Naphthoflavone	Mouse	Lung, skin	57
7,12-Dimethylbenz(a)anthracene	Polycyclic hydrocarbons	Rat	Breast	18,60
7,12-Dimethylbenz(a)anthracene	Phenothiazines	Rat	Breast	55
7,12-Dimethylbenz(a)anthracene	β-Naphthoflavone	Rat	Breast	56
7,12-Dimethylbenz(a)anthracene	β-Naphthoflavone	Mouse	Lung	56
Aflatoxin	Phenobarbital	Rat	Breast	25
Bracken fern carcinogen	Phenothiazine	Rat	Small intestine, bladder	30

carcinogenicity. Chemical carcinogenesis is a low threshold (or perhaps even a no threshold) phenomenon (10). Thus, rapid activation could result in loss of activated carcinogen species due to nonavailability of critical binding sites or due to secondary reactions. In contrast, induction of increased activity of microsomal mixed function oxidase reactions detoxifying carcinogens would have a protective effect. Thus there is the expectation, which is in fact supported by the results of animal experimentation, that enhanced microsomal mixed function oxidase activity would inhibit chemical carcinogenesis if it has any effect at all. This latter qualification is added since in some experiments no effect on carcinogenesis is obtained. Presumably this is due to the fact that in some tissues the mixed function oxidase activity is very low. Accordingly, if doses of carcinogen substantially beyond the metabolic capacities of the system are employed, no difference in tumor incidence may be observed.

In the previous discussion, implications of in vivo alterations in mixed function oxidase activity have been presented. Considerable in vitro work has been done. Because of the nature of the enzyme system involved, there is potential hazard in assuming that the results of alteration of this system in cell cultures and those for the intact organism will parallel one another. The mixed function oxidase system is a highly integrated mechanism for rendering compounds more polar so that they can be further metabolized, frequently by conjugation, and excreted. In cell cultures, instead of being excreted, metabolites remain within the culture medium and may cause a variety of changes that would not have occurred had they been removed in comparable fashion to that existing in vivo. Thus while increased transformation can be produced in cell cultures by induction of increased mixed function oxidase activity, no such in vivo counterpart has been reported (23). In contrast, as is seen in Table 1, protection has been obtained in many instances.

INHIBITION OF CHEMICAL CARCINOGENESIS BY ANTIOXIDANTS

During the past several years, studies have been carried out which have shown that several antioxidants will inhibit the carcinogenic effects of a substantial variety of chemical carcinogens (Table 2) (49–53). The most extensive work of this type has been done with phenolic antioxidants; in particular, butylated hydroxyanisole (BHA) and butylated hydroxytoluene (BHT). Inhibition occurs under a number of experimental conditions. It has been found in situations where the route of administration results in direct contact of carcinogen with the target tissue, i.e., neoplasia of the forestomach in mice fed benzo(a)-pyrene (BP) or 7,12-dimethylbenz-(a)anthracene (DMBA). Comparable suppression of neoplasia is also obtained in experiments in which the carcinogen is acting at a site remote from that of administration, i.e., inhibition of mammary tumor formation in rats given DMBA orally. Of interest with regard to gastrointestinal neoplasia are a number of experiments in which the BHA or BHT was added to diets containing polycyclic hydrocarbon carcinogens. In these studies the target tissue in which neoplasia occurred was the forestomach. Those animals receiving BHA or BHT in the diet along with the carcinogen showed pronounced suppression of neoplasia at this site. Butylated hydroxyanisole and BHT are extensively used as food additives. Of the two compounds, BHA is preferable in that it has a lower toxicity than BHT. However, both compounds can be employed at very high

TABLE 2. Inhibition of carcinogen-induced neoplasia by antioxidants

Carcinogen	Antioxidant	Species	Site of neoplasm inhibited	Ref
Benzo(*a*)pyrene	BHA, BHT, ethoxyquin	Mouse	Forestomach, lung	49,51
Benzo(*a*)pyrene	Disulfiram	Mouse	Forestomach	52
7,12-Dimethylbenz(*a*)anthracene	BHA, BHT, ethoxyquin	Mouse	Forestomach, lung	49,51
7,12-Dimethylbenz(*a*)anthracene	BHA, BHT, ethoxyquin	Rat	Breast	49
7,12-Dimethylbenz(*a*)anthracene	Disulfiram, dimethyl-dithiocarbamate	Rat	Breast	52
7,12-Dimethylbenz(*a*)anthracene	Cysteamine	Rat	Breast	24
7-Hydroxymethyl-12-methylbenz(*a*)-anthracene	BHA	Mouse	Lung	51
Dibenz(*a,h*)anthracene	BHA	Mouse	Lung	51
Diethylnitrosamine	BHA, ethoxyquin	Mouse	Lung	50
4-Nitroquinoline-*N*-oxide	BHA, ethoxyquin	Mouse	Lung	50
Uracil mustard	BHA	Mouse	Lung	51
Urethane	BHA	Mouse	Lung	51
N-2-Fluorenylacetamide	BHT	Rat	Liver	42
N-Hydroxy-*N*-2-fluorenylacetamide	BHT	Rat	Liver, breast	42
p-Dimethylaminoazobenzene	BHT	Rat	Liver	12
Dimethylhydrazine	Disulfiram	Rat	Large intestine	53

doses before evidence of toxicity appears.

In addition to BHA and BHT, inhibition of polycyclic hydrocarbon-induced carcinogenesis of the forestomach has been brought about by antioxidants with different chemical structures. One of these is ethoxyquin (6 - ethoxy - 1,2 - dihydro - 2,2,4 - trimethylquinoline), an antioxidant that is widely used as an additive in commercial animal diets, but not in food for human consumption (Table 2). More recently, studies have been carried out with several sulfur-containing antioxidants (52). Two of these compounds, disulfiram and dimethyl-dithiocarbamate, exert a strong inhibitory effect against neoplasia induced by polycyclic hydrocarbons. In addition, disulfiram inhibits neoplasia of the large bowel resulting from administration of dimethylhydrazine (53).

During the studies of the inhibitory properties of sulfur-containing antioxidants against chemical carcinogens, experiments were carried out in which benzylthiocyanate was employed as a possible inhibitor. This compound caused suppression of DMBA-induced mammary tumor formation in the rat. In subsequent work, it was found that benzylisothiocyanate will inhibit DMBA-induced mammary tumor formation and also BP-induced tumor formation of the mouse forestomach (unpublished observations). These data are of some interest because of the occurrence of thiocyanates and isothiocyanates in a number of edible vegetables (43).

Other antioxidants have been reported to inhibit neoplasia from chemical carcinogens. A contradictory literature, previously reviewed, exists with regard to α-tocopherol (49). Selenium has also been reported to inhibit chemical carcinogenesis in experimental animals and has been suggested as a possible environmental factor exerting an effect on tumor incidence in man (36, 37).

The actual mechanism or mechanisms by which the various antioxidants listed in Table 2 inhibit chemical carcinogenesis has not been determined. The compounds may be acting via an antioxidant function. However, they have other biological actions including the capacity to alter enzyme activity (9, 11, 14, 16). At present it is not clear which type of mechanism is involved. Several studies have been recently carried out on the mechanism of BHA inhibition of neoplasia in the mouse. It has been found that feeding BHA under conditions protecting against BP-induced neoplasia results in altered microsomal metabolism of the carcinogen (39). Incubation of BP and calf thymus DNA with liver microsomes from BHA-fed mice shows about one-half the binding of BP metabolites to DNA as compared to controls. The amount of cytochrome P450 is increased per unit weight of microsomal protein and liver in mice fed BHA. The ethyl isocyanide binding spectrum was measured to see if alterations of cytochrome P450 might be produced by BHA feeding. The maximum at 430 nm is the same in control and BHA-fed mice. However, the maximum at 455 nm is lower in BHA-fed mice than in the controls indicating some change has occurred due to BHA feeding. The data obtained show that

BHA feeding results in altered properties of liver microsomes including a decrease in BP metabolite binding to DNA. It is not known whether this is a unique situation or if it has a more universal occurrence. An intriguing possibility is that there is an altered form of cytochrome P450 which results in a carcinogen metabolite pattern having a diminished amount of the activated species causing neoplasia; but this remains to be established.

REFERENCES

1. Adenis, L., M. N. Vlaeminck and J. Driessens. *C. R. Soc. Biol.* 164: 560, 1970.
2. Bickers, D. R., L. C. Harber, A. Kappas and A. P. Alvares. *Res. Commun. Chem. Pathol. and Pharmacol.* 3: 505, 1972.
3. Billings, R., and L. W. Wattenberg. *Proc. Soc. Exp. Biol. Med.* 139: 865, 1972.
4. Brown, R. R., J. A. Miller and E. C. Miller. *J. Biol. Chem.* 209: 211, 1954.
5. Conney, A. H. *Pharmacol. Rev.* 19: 317, 1967.
6. Conney, A. H., and J. J. Burns. *Science* 178: 576, 1972.
7. Conney, A. H., C. Davison, R. Gastel and J. J. Burns. *J. Pharmacol. Exp. Therap.* 130: 1, 1960.
8. Conney, A. H., E. C. Miller and J. A. Miller. *J. Biol. Chem.* 228: 753, 1957.
9. Dietrich, R. A., and V. G. Erwin. *Mol. Pharmacol.* 301, 1971.
10. DiPaolo, J. A., P. J. Donovan and R. L. Nelson. *Nature, New Biol.* 230: 240, 1971.
11. DuBois, K. P., A. P. Raymond and B. E. Hietbrink. *Toxicol. Appl. Pharmacol.* 3: 236, 1961.
12. Frankfurt, O. S., L. P. Lipchina, T. V. Bunto, et al. *Bull. Exp. Biol. Med.* 8: 86, 1967.
13. Gelboin, H. V., and R. N. Blackburn. *Cancer Res.* 24: 356, 1964.
14. Grantham, P. H., J. H. Weisburger and E. K. Weisburger. *Food Cosmet. Toxicol.* 11: 209, 1973.
15. Hart, L. G., and J. R. Fouts. *Proc. Soc. Exp. Biol. Med.* 114: 388, 1963.
16. Hathaway, D. E. In: *Advances in Food Research*, edited by M. Mrak and G. F. Stewart, New York: Academic, 1966, p. 1–56.
17. Hsiao, K.-C., E. J. Pantuck, L. W. Wattenberg, R. Kuntzman, M. Jacobson and A. H. Conney. *Federation Proc.* 34: 742, 1975.
18. Huggins, C., G. Lorraine and R. Fukunishi. *Proc. Natl. Acad. Sci. USA* 51: 737, 1964.
19. Loub, W. D., L. W. Wattenberg and D. W. Davis. *J. Natl. Cancer Inst.* 54: 985, 1975.
20. Lu, A. Y., L. Luntzman, S. West, and A. H. Conney. *Biochem. Biophys. Res. Comm.* 42: 1200, 1971.
21. Lu, A. Y., R. Luntzman, S. West, M. Jacobson and A. H. Conney. *J. Biol. Chem.* 247: 1727, 1972.
22. Makiura, S., H. Aoe, S. Sugihara, K. Hirao, A. Masayuki and N. Ito. *J. Natl. Cancer Inst.* 53: 1253, 1974.
23. Marquardt, H., and C. Heidelberger. *Cancer Res.* 32: 721, 1972.
24. Marquardt H., M. D. Saponzink and M. S. Zedeck. *Cancer Res.* 34: 3387, 1974.
25. McLean, A. E., and A. Marshall. *Br. J. Exp. Pathol.* 52: 322, 1971.
26. Miller, E. C., J. A. Miller, R. R. Brown and J. C. MacDonald. *Cancer Res.* 18: 469, 1958.
27. Miller, J. A. *Cancer Res.* 30: 559, 1970.
28. Miller, J. A., and E. C. Miller. *Prog. Exp. Tumor Res.* 11: 273, 1969.
29. Miller, J. A., and E. C. Miller. *J. Natl. Cancer Inst.* 47: v–xiv, 1971.
30. Pamukcu, A. M., L. W. Wattenberg, J. M. Price and G. T. Bryan. *J. Natl. Cancer Inst.* 47: 155, 1971.
31. Parke, D. V., and H. Rahman. *Biochem. J.* 119: 53P, 1970.
32. Parke, D. V., and H. Rahman. *Biochem. J.* 113: 12P, 1969.
33. Rasmussen, R. E., and I. Y. Wang. *Cancer Res.* 34: 2290, 1974.
34. Richardson, H. L., A. R. Stein and E. Borson-Nacht-Nebel. *Cancer Res.* 12: 356, 1952.
35. Sell, J. L., and K. L. Davison. *Federation Proc.* 32: 2003, 1973.
36. Shamberger, R. J. *J. Natl. Cancer Inst.* 44: 931, 1970.
37. Shamberger, R. J., and C. E. Willis. *Clin. Lab. Sci.* 2: 211, 1971.
38. Silva, E. A. *Hospital, Rio de Janeiro* 71: 1483, 1966.
39. Speier, J. L., and L. W. Wattenberg. *J. Natl. Cancer Inst.* 55: 469, 1975.
40. Tawfic, H. N. *Acta Pathol. Jpn.* 15: 255, 1965.
41. Thamavit, W., Y. Hiasa, N. Ito and N. Phamarapravati. *Cancer Res.* 34: 337, 1974.
42. Ulland, B. M., J. H. Weisburger, R. S. Yammamoto and E. K. Weisburger. *Food Cosmet. Toxicol.* 11: 199, 1973.
43. Virtanen, A. I. *Angew. Chem. Int. Ed. Engl.* 1: 299, 1962.
44. Virtanen, A. I. *Phytochemistry* 4: 207, 1965.
45. Wattenberg, L. W. *Cancer Res.* 26: 1520, 1966.
46. Wattenberg, L. W. *Prog. Exp. Tumor Res.* 14: 89, 1970.
47. Wattenberg, L. W. *Cancer* 20: 99, 1971.
48. Wattenberg, L. W. In: *Twenty-fourth Annual Symposium on Fundamental Research, 1971, at the University of Texas M. D. Anderson Hospital and Tumor Institute.* Baltimore: Williams & Wilkins, 1972, p. 241–255.
49. Wattenberg, L. W. *J. Natl. Cancer Inst.* 48: 1425, 1972.
50. Wattenberg, L. W. *Federation Proc.* 31: 633, 1972.
51. Wattenberg, L. W. *J. Natl. Cancer Inst.* 40: 1541, 1973.
52. Wattenberg, L. W. *J. Natl. Cancer Inst.* 52: 1583, 1974.
53. Wattenberg, L. W. *J. Natl. Cancer Inst.* 54: 1005, 1975.
54. Wattenberg, L. W., and J. L. Leong. *Cancer Res.* 24: 365, 1965.
55. Wattenberg, L. W., and J. L. Leong. *Federation Proc.* 26: 692, 1967.
56. Wattenberg, L. W., and J. L. Leong. *Proc. Soc. Exp. Biol. Med.* 128: 940, 1968.
57. Wattenberg, L. W., and J. L. Leong. *Cancer Res.* 30: 1922, 1970.
58. Wattenberg, L. W., M. A. Page and J. L. Leong. *Cancer Res.* 28: 2539, 1968.
59. Wattenberg, L. W., M. A. Page and J. L. Leong. *Cancer Res.* 29: 934, 1968.
60. Wheatley, D. N. *Br. J. Cancer* 22: 787, 1968.
61. Yamamoto, R. S., J. H. Weisburger and E. K. Weisburger. *Cancer Res.* 31: 483, 1971.

Recommendations for Dietary Change

Dietary Guidelines for Americans

from a hearing before a subcommittee of the Committee on Appropriations, United States Senate

DEPARTMENT OF HEALTH AND HUMAN SERVICES

STATEMENT OF J. MICHAEL McGINNIS, M.D., DEPUTY ASSISTANT SECRETARY FOR HEALTH, DEPARTMENT OF HEALTH AND HUMAN SERVICES

ACCOMPANIED BY ROBERT I. LEVY, M.D., DIRECTOR, NATIONAL HEART, LUNG AND BLOOD INSTITUTE, DEPARTMENT OF HEALTH AND HUMAN SERVICES

INTRODUCTION OF ASSOCIATES

Senator EAGLETON. The committee will once again be in order.

We have the aforementioned people from the Department of Health and the Department of Agriculture.

Dr. McGinnis, you are first.

Dr. McGINNIS. Thank you very much, sir.

Mr. Chairman, we thank you for the opportunity to meet with you today to review a substantial number of issues related to appropriate dietary recommendations for Americans.

If I may, I would like to begin by introducing, obviously, Dr. Levy, who you have seen on several occasions before, and Dr. C. Wayne Callaway as well, who acts as Executive Secretary of the Department's Nutrition Coordinating Committee.

PREPARED STATEMENT

I would also like, with your permission, to submit my testimony for the record and speak less formally.

Senator EAGLETON. That is fine. The full testimony will appear in the record.

Dr. McGINNIS. Thank you.

[The statement follows:]

Reprinted from *Dietary Guidelines for Americans,* a hearing before a subcommittee of the Committee on Appropriations, United States Senate, Ninety-Sixth Congress, Second Session, U.S. Government Printing Office, Washington, 1980.

PREPARED STATEMENT OF J. MICHAEL MCGINNIS, M.D.

DEPUTY ASSISTANT SECRETARY FOR HEALTH
(DISEASE PREVENTION AND HEALTH PROMOTION)
DEPARTMENT OF HEALTH AND HUMAN SERVICES

Thank you for the opportunity to meet with you today to discuss our mutual concern with appropriate dietary recommendations for healthy Americans. With me is Dr. Robert I. Levy, whom you know well. As Director of the National Heart, Lung and Blood Institute and as one of the leaders in the effort to understand the relationships between diet, blood lipid levels, and atherosclerosis, Dr. Levy can speak with authority about the scientific evidence linking diet with heart disease and about current research efforts to elucidate these relationships.

Before you hear from Dr. Levy, however, I would like to focus our attention briefly on three separate questions that are implicit -- although not always clearly identified -- in the discussions that have occurred today. First is the question of scientific evidence: What are the facts? Second is the question of public health policy: Given the facts, what should be done from a public health standpoint in order to reduce the morbidity and mortality associated with the diseases and conditions to which the U.S. population is subject? Thirdly, apart from purely health issues, what are the other considerations that must be taken into account in determining over-all public policy?

I believe that some of the confusion that has followed pursuant to the report of the panel of the Food and Nutrition Board, "Toward Healthful Diets," has been due to our failure to distinguish these three levels of consideration. If we wish to emerge from these hearings with greater clarity and understanding, it is essential that we make such distinctions.

SCIENTIFIC BASIS FOR THE GUIDELINES

Few scientific ideas can claim abclute proof. However, it is possible to obtain some degree of consensus on many scientific questions, including questions concerning the links between diet and diseases. To be effective, dietary recommendation should not spring forth de novo, but should reflect the best scientific consensus available at the time.

One of the more successful attempts to express such consensus is the Report of the Task Force on the Evidence Relating Six Dietary Factors to the Nation's Health, published as a supplement to the December, 1979 issue of The American Journal of Clinical Nutrition. The Task Force was assembled by the American Society for Clinical Nutrition at the request of the Assistant Secretary for Health and Surgeon General, Dr. Julius B. Richmond. Its panels were representative of the broad range of scientific opinion on various questions regarding diet and health.

Perhaps most interesting was the method used to evaluate the strength and consistency of the evidence linking specific classes of nutrients with specific diseases.

Each position paper considered the relationship between a given dietary factor and a specific disease under three headings:

o   Kinds of evidence

o   Quality and strength of the evidence

o   Risks and benefits of changing the intake of the dietary factor.

The kinds of evidence were divided into three broad categories:

o   Epidemiologic or population studies

o   Animal experimental studies

o   Human experimentation, including clinical intervention trials.

The quality and strength of the evidence was assessed and the panel members were asked to assign a score of 0 to 20 for the strength of the evidence relating specific nutrient classes to ten major conditions, according to the following five categories:

o   Associations among various population groups

o   Associations among individuals within a population

o   Intervention studies

o   Animal models

o   Biological explanation.

Thus, a "perfect" score would be 100, indicating that the panel considered the evidence in all five categories to be overwhelmingly convincing.

The scores of the various panel members were then tallied, and expressed as a mean score, with standard deviations for each mean (as an indication of the degree of divergence of opinion among members of the panel).

The highest associations were recorded for:

o   Alcohol and liver disease

o   Carbohydrates and dental caries

o   Sodium and high blood pressure

o   Cholesterol <u>and</u> fat and atherosclerosis

The scores for cholesterol alone or for fat alone were somewhat lower than for the combination of cholesterol and fat taken together (Table 1).

TABLE 1

AMERICAN SOCIETY FOR CLINICAL NUTRITION TASK FORCE EVALUATION

Diet--Disease Issues	Mean Score	Standard Deviation
Alcohol--Liver Disease	88	8
Carbohydrates--Dental Caries	87	6
Salt--High Blood Pressure	74	9
Cholesterol and Fat--Atherosclerosis	73	15
Excess Calories--Health Hazard	68	18
Cholesterol--Atherosclerosis	62	20
Saturated Fat--Atherosclerosis	58	15
Carbohydrates--Diabetes	13	17
Alcohol--Atherosclerosis	13	15
Carbohydrates--Atherosclerosis	11	8

In assessing the scientific evidence, we relied heavily upon such consensus-type documents. In addition to the American Society for Clinical Nutrition report, we had the benefit of other authoritative documents, including:

o Background papers developed by the Institute of Medicine of the National Academy of Sciences for Healthy People, The Surgeon General's Report on Health Promotion and Disease Prevention, released last summer.

o "American Medical Association Concepts of Nutrition and Health," a statement from the AMA Council on Scientific Affairs (JAMA, 242: 2335-2338, November 23, 1979).

o "Breast Feeding." Nutrition Committee of the Canadian Pediatric Society and Committee on Nutrition of the American Academy of Pediatrics (Pediatrics, 62: 591-601, 1978).

o "Research Needs for Establishing Dietary Guidelines for the U.S. Population",Food and Nutrition Board, National Research Council, National Academy of Sciences, 1979.

o "Diet and Cancer Relationship" Statement of Dr. Arthur C. Upton, Director, National Cancer Institute, NIH, before the Subcommittee on Nutrition of the Committee on Agriculture, Nutrition, and Forestry, United States Senate, October 2, 1979.

Careful reading of all of these statements reveals an impressively high degree of agreement on the facts:

o Plasma cholesterol concentrations are clearly and unequivocally associated with risks of heart attacks.

o Other major risk factors amenable to treatment or behavioral change include cigarette smoking and high blood pressure.

o The determinants of plasma cholesterol concentrations are complex, but include most importantly heredity and diet. As with any phenomenon involving "nature and nurture," the more homogeneous the environment, the greater the relative role of heredity. Thus, within a population eating a similar diet, heredity will appear more important in determining plasma cholesterol levels than will diet. However, among populations eating dissimilar diets, dietary factors will be found to have more prominent significance.

o The dietary determinants of plasma cholesterol concentrations include saturated fats and cholesterol, both of which nearly always are to be found in the same food items.

About these facts there is little disagreement. Likewise, in regard to other dietary recommendations, there is widespread agreement that obesity is associated with a variety of diseases and chronic disorders; that sugars and sugar alcohols (along with inadequate fluoridation in the water supply and the presence of certain bacteria in the mouth) contribute to dental caries; that sodium plays a role in the development and maintenance of some types of high blood pressure; and that excessive alcohol is the major cause of cirrhosis of the liver and a contributing cause of several types of cancer. The roles of other dietary factors in various types of cancer are not well understood but there is at least suggestive evidence that obesity and diets high in fat may be of importance.

PUBLIC HEALTH POLICY

Given these facts, what should be public health policy?

Let me quote the recent report of the Food and Nutrition Board: ". . . in our present state of knowledge, sound medical and public health practice should aim at reducing the known risk factors to the extent possible." We are in full agreement with this conclusion.

The known risk factors for our major causes of death and disability are listed in Table 2; those that are underlined are thought to be diet-related. The dietary factors that can be identified are excess calories relative to energy expenditures; excess sodium; excess total fat, saturated fats and

TABLE 2

PROMINENT RISK FACTORS

Cause of Death	Risk Factors
Heart Disease	Smoking,* high blood pressure,* elevated blood cholesterol,* lack of exercise, diabetes, stress
Cancer	Smoking,* worksite carcinogens,* environmental carcinogens, alcohol, diet
Motor Vehicle Accidents	Alcohol,* no seat belts,* speed,* roadway design
Other Accidents	Alcohol,* drug abuse, smoking (fires), product design, handgun availability
Stroke	High blood pressure,* smoking,* elevated blood cholesterol,* stress
Homicide	Stress,* handgun availability,* alcohol
Suicide	Stress,* alcohol, drug abuse
Cirrhosis of Liver	Alcohol,* possible nutrient deficiencies
Influenza/Pneumonia	Smoking*
Diabetes	Obesity*
Cause of Morbidity	**Risk Factors**
Dental Caries	Fluoridation,* mouth bacteria,* diet*
Bowel Dysfunctions	Diet,* stress

*Major Risk Factor

cholesterol; excess alcohol; perhaps inadequate dietary fiber; and frequent ingestion of sugars and sugars alcohols in forms that stick to the teeth (Table 3).

Given this knowledge and given the principle of "sound medical and public health practice", we arrive at the seven dietary guidelines released last February by this Department and the U.S. Department of Agriculture (Table 4).

I would call your attention to several important caveats, expressed explicitly in the first two pages of that pamphlet.

o   We don't know enough about nutrition to identify an "ideal diet" for each individual.

o   People differ -- and their food needs vary depending on age, sex, family history, body size, physical activity, and other conditions such as pregnancy or illness.

o   In those chronic conditions where diet may be important -- heart attacks, high blood pressure, strokes, dental caries, diabetes and some forms of cancer -- the roles of specific nutrients have not been defined.

TABLE 3

DIET-RELATED RISK FACTORS

Risk Factor	Possible Dietary Factors
High Blood Pressure	Sodium, excess calories*
Elevated Blood Cholesterol	Total fat, saturated fats, cholesterol, excess calories
Diabetes	Excess calories
Alcohol Abuse	Alcohol
Dietary Factors in Cancer	Excess calories, total fat, polyunsaturated fats, fiber, alcohol
Dietary Factors in Dental Caries	Carbohydrates, including sugars and sugar alcohols; form and frequency of eating; fluoride in water supply
Dietary-Bowel Dysfunctions	Fiber

*Relative to energy expenditure. (Note: Dietary sources of calories include fats, oils, starches, sugars and alcohol, as well as protein.)

TABLE 4

DIETARY GUIDELINES FOR AMERICANS

- Eat a variety of foods

- Maintain ideal weight

- Avoid too much fat, saturated fat, and cholesterol

- Eat foods with adequate starch and fiber

- Avoid too much sugar

- Avoid too much sodium

- If you drink alcohol, do so in moderation

○ The guidelines are suggested for most Americans. They do not apply to people who need special diets because of diseases or conditions that interfere with normal nutrition.

○ No guidelines can guarantee health or well-being.

Please also note the discussion under the guideline regarding total **fat**, saturated fat and cholesterol:

o There are wide variations among people -- related to heredity and the way each person's body uses cholesterol.

o Some people can consume diets high in cholesterol and still keep normal blood cholesterol levels. Other people, unfortunately, have high blood cholesterol levels even if they eat low-fat, low-cholesterol diets.

o There is controversy about what recommendations are appropriate for healthy Americans.

o The recommendations are not meant to prohibit the use of any specific food item.

o Eggs . . . contain many essential vitamins and minerals as well as protein (and) can be eaten in moderation as long as your overall cholesterol intake is not excessive.

We believe these recommendations to be sound and sensible, given (1) the best consensus we could obtain regarding scientific knowledge, (2) current data on the health of Americans and the diseases and disorders that they are likely to experience, and (3) a realistic estimate as to what might be achieved by any type of dietary advice. The recommendations are carefully worded to limit their susceptibility for extreme or rigid interpretations.

Why, then, the apparent controversy? Apart from what are perhaps inevitable differences in interpretation, there is a fundamental distinction between the approach that might be appropriate for a physician to take in regard to an individual patient and the approaches that might be appropriate for broad public health policy. We can refer to these separate approaches as the "medical model" and the "public health model." The two approaches are complementary, not contradictory. Each can be valid when applied to its appropriate circumstances.

When specific diseases, disorders, or risk factors are identified in an individual patient, a health care provider should individualize the the dietary recommendations. This is the foundation of rational <u>medical</u> care.

For public health purposes, however, one must maintain a different perspective. For the most part, we are dealing with aggregate data, with the population as a whole or with major subgroups within that population. Programs or policies that may have a minimal effect on any single individual, nevertheless, may have major importance in terms of the entire population. Thus, dietary changes that reduce average cholesterol concentrations by only a small percentage, might result in significant reductions in total morbidity and rates of mortality due to heart attacks. As long as more than half the U.S. population have plasma cholesterol levels greater than optimal, sound public health policy would suggest dietary recommendations that might reduce average cholesterol levels.

OVERALL PUBLIC POLICY

Given the current scientific evidence and given what we consider to be sound public health policy, we are still faced with the question of over-all policy -- or, if you will, with implementation.

The policy of the Department of Health and Human Services has been to offer dietary recommendations for informational and educational purposes. The guidelines are suggestions for dietary behavior; they are not designed to impose any type of uniform diet on the American public. To the contrary, the guidelines stress that good eating habits are based on variety and moderation. The guidelines are not prescriptions for guaranteed health, nor are they proscriptions against any specific food items.

As a consequence of this reasonable and moderate approach, the guidelines have met with widespread acceptance and endorsement. Indeed, much of the promotion of the principles expressed in the guidelines has been undertaken at the initiative and the expense of industry and other private institutions. To cite but a few examples:

o General Foods, Inc., has published full-page newspaper advertisements, containing the introductory section and the discussions under each of the seven guidelines, along with informative commentary explaining significant points, in eight major newspapers representing General Foods' major market areas.

o ARA Services, the largest commercial supplier of cafeteria meals for government, corporate and private institutions, has developed a nutrition and physical fitness program based upon the dietary guidelines. The program will soon be introduced into selected cafeterias and ultimately may be offered as an alternative to standard dietary fare for up to 10 million daily customers.

o Food Marketing Institute, the major trade organization for grocery chains, has obtained plates for reprinting the Guidelines and distributing them to member companies.

o Nutrition Today, one of the more widely circulated nutrition magazines, has reproduced the Guidelines in their entirety as part of the March/April 1980 issue.

If our dietary recommendations are understood in this perspective, I believe that some of the concern that has been expressed, expecially by certain food producers, might be allayed.

CONCLUSION

"The health of the American people has never been better."* Why, then do we need dietary recommendations -- or any other preventive measures? The answer to such a question should be obvious. By the standards we use to measure health (e.g., death rates, life-expectancy, infant mortality), the health of the American people has continually improved during the 20th century. Such progress has come about because of persistant efforts to identify the major diseases and disorders that afflict our population, to study the multiple interrelated factors in their causation, and to translate such knowledge into intelligible and sensible programs. By continuing to do so, we can hope always to say, "The health of the American people has never been better." This is the basis of sound public health policy. Our dietary recommendations are one part of that effort.

PRINCIPAL QUESTIONS RELATING TO PUBLIC HEALTH

Dr. McGINNIS. What I am going to do in my testimony is address three principal questions. The first is from the perspective of public health policy, "what are the important dietary factors to address to reduce disease and disability of Americans overall?" The second is "what is the scientific basis for the level of agreement for recommendations for these factors?" And the third is "what is the level of public interest and demand for these kinds of recommendations?"

DIETARY FACTORS RELATING TO DISEASE OF AMERICANS

Turning first to the initial question from the perspective of health policy—what are the important dietary factors or habits to address to reduce the disease, disability of the Americans. I think that the report of the Food and Nutrition Board, which has been discussed in detail this morning, emphasizes the importance of reducing known risk factors to the extent possible, as sound medical and public health policy. The question we face is what are those risk factors?

The first chart, if I can ask Dr. Callaway to assist, presents those risk factors according to the leading causes of death. That is table II in the draft testimony. On the left-hand side of the chart are the 10 leading causes of death, and on the bottom are the two leading causes of morbidity. On the right-hand side are the risk factors prominently associated with each of those leading causes of mortality and morbidity.

Senator EAGLETON. I have a one-track mind. Yesterday's testimony was that Alzheimers disease and other related neurological disorders

---

* Healthy People, The Surgeon General's Report on Health Promotion and Disease Prevention.

were the fifth most prevalent cause of death. That came from the National Institutes of Health.

Dr. McGinnis. I cannot explain the data from the National Institute of Aging. This list of the 10 leading causes of death is in terms of potential of years lost, the aggregate numbers of years lost before the age of 65. So those causes of death which tend to hit people at younger ages are listed more prominently here because what we are talking about is dietary recommendations for the bulk of the population.

Again, the asterisks indicate the major risk factors and those underlined indicate diet related.

It is important to note that virtually all the leading causes of morbidity and mortality are associated with some diet-related risk factors. That point is brought out more prominently on the second chart, which is table III in the text.

DIET-RELATED FACTORS ASSOCIATED WITH RISK

The question that is addressed by this particular chart is of those dietary factors associated with the leading factors of death, what nutrients are involved? This chart elaborates on those diet-related factors and elaborates on the possible dietary factors associated with risk. On the left-hand side are the risk factors, taken from the underlined portions of the previous table, and the right-hand side of the chart are the possible dietary factors.

Let me just list them.

Sodium excess and calories are important factors related to high blood pressure. Total fat, saturated fat, and cholesterol are related to blood cholesterol. Excess calories are related to diabetes. Alcohol is related to alcohol abuse. Excess calories, total fat, polyunsaturated fats, fiber and alcohol are related to dietary factors in cancer—again, not proven, but suspect. Carbohydrates—including sugars and sugar alcohols—form and frequency of eating, and fluoride in the water supply relate to the dietary factors in dental caries. And fiber is related to dietary-bowel dysfunctions.

LESSONS LEARNED FROM INDIVIDUAL RISK PROFILES

It is important to note that for individual practitioners and health care providers it is important to assess the risk profiles of individual patients for these possible factors involved in disease. But for public health policy we have to address the profile of population as a whole as we make recommendations. The question we then face is what are the lessons for us as consumers, the public as a whole, included in this listing of possible dietary factors?

First, if we focus on the right-hand side of the chart, there are possible dietary factors, and we can note that different dietary factors carry different risks. The lesson here is we ought to eat a variety of food. Too much of any one factor may carry some risks for individuals.

The second lesson is we ought to eat or consume in balance. We see excess calories appear in a number of places on the chart, so it is important that we balance our caloric consumption with appropriate exercise patterns.

The third lesson that we can learn is that we have to avoid too much fat, saturated fat, and cholesterol, for a number of reasons. Not only do we see fat, saturated fat, and cholesterol together as contributors to increased blood cholesterol, but also noted as a possible dietary factor related to cancer and perhaps even more important as contributors to excess calories.

The fourth lesson we can obtain is we ought to avoid too much sodium intake.

The fifth is we ought to avoid too much sugar intake. Sugar is noted both with respect to dietary factors in dental caries and with respect to its role in yielding excess calories in the absence of other nutrients.

Sixth, we ought to consume alcohol only in moderation, obviously because of its relation to alcohol abuse, but also because of its possible relation to cancer and its contribution to excess calories in the absence of other nutrients.

Seventh is that we ought to insure that our diets contain adequate fiber and complex carbohydrates, both because of the relationship between lack of fiber in the diet and dietary-bowel dysfunction and the possible relationship between low-fiber diet and cancer.

The third chart lists those conclusions in the aggregate as the dietary guidelines which have emerged. I think it is fair to say that these are not earthshaking recommendations or guidelines, that they in fact are common sense. They are very reasonable statements, and they are general in their direction. They are the most reasonable statements we can make given the scientific base we have at hand.

GUIDELINE DEVELOPMENT

That brings me to the second question that I would like to address relatively briefly; what is the scientific basis or level of agreement for these recommendations? How were the guidelines developed?

Actually, the consensus, I think, is reasonably solid, much more so than the level of discussion around the guidelines seems to imply. That is the important point to bear in mind. Our guidelines clearly did not spring de novo into being, but were based on a number of recent consensus statements. Indeed, we might view 1979 as a banner year for consensus statements, because there were a number of consensus statements issued by a number of bodies. They are included in my prepared testimony. They include background papers to the Surgeon General report which were prepared by the Institute of Medicine of the National Academy of Sciences.

I would like to draw attention, in particular, to one of those statements of consensus that was involved last year, because I think it is particularly pioneering as an effort to quantify the level of consensus. It was one alluded to earlier in the hearing, namely, the effort of the American Society for Clinical Nutrition to assemble a group which could quantify the level of consensus about a number of dietary factors. Before getting into this, I have to emphasize that this was not an effort to decide scientific principles, but only to specify for the public the general level of consensus or disagreement that existed about diet-disease relationships so that the public could then make decisions on their own habits.

If I can have the next table please. It lists 10 proposed relationships that were considered by this task force of nine scientists that was alluded to earlier. Again, the process of assessing the proposed relationships is described in some detail in my written testimony, so I will not go through that to any great extent. However, I would like to note, if I can, the specific quantified results of that particular assessment.

The first three items on the chart—the relationship between alcohol and liver disease, the relationship between carbohydrates and dental caries, and the relationship between salt and high blood pressure—as you can see, yield very little disagreement in the consensus statement. This consensus is expressed not only as a mean score of agreement but with a standard deviation, which gives us some indication of the level of divergence of opinion among the scientists.

Senator EAGLETON. There were nine in the number?

Dr. McGINNIS. There were nine.

Senator EAGLETON. The National Academy of Sciences had 15. So they are ahead 15 to 9.

Dr. McGINNIS. One might view it in that way, although I think that we have to view the preponderance of the evidence in the aggregate.

Senator EAGLETON. Fifteen out of twenty-four.

Dr. McGINNIS. A number of scientists on the Food and Nutrition Board were participants in this exercise, and were in fact in full agreement on the concensus of the outcome.

The first three items on this consensus statement, if you will, obviously are items about which there is little disagreement, as noted in the standard deviation. Not only is there a high mean score for those items, but little standard deviation. Yet there is a wider spread of opinion for the next item, that is, of the relationship between cholesterol and fat together and atherosclerosis. There is, nonetheless, a substantial level of consensus, and a level which is even higher than that for excess calories and health hazard, a relationship fairly highly accepted among the professional and public communities. I think this represents an important statement. In summary, it does indicate there is an impressive consensus around the recommended dietary guidelines, including the recommendation on avoiding too much fat, saturated fat, and cholesterol.

PUBLIC INTEREST IN RECOMMENDATIONS

If I can, I would like to move on to the third question, which is what is the level of public interest in and demand for these kinds of recommendations? In a word, it is enormous. You may be aware of a survey reported by Yankelovich, Skelly and White which indicated that 76 percent of the public felt they were either poorly informed or simply uninformed on diet and nutrition. Because the public remains desirous of the nutrition information and because the public remains confused about——

Senator EAGLETON. That is not the only thing Yankelovich reported. You are correct, but that same Yankelovich report went on to say that it found that of those interviewed, only 25 percent had a lot of confidence in health warnings provided by their Government, and that only 1 percent of those surveyed believed that it was the Government's responsibility to see to it that their children are taught good health and nutrition habits. So if you look to Brother Yankelovich as having some weight for your particular point of view, you better look at his other points.

Dr. McGINNIS. With respect to the warnings point, 72 percent of the public in that same survey stated it was better to be safe than sorry, and they would prefer to see the Government issue warnings, if necessary, prior to definite proof.

FINDINGS IN YANKELOVICH REPORT

Senator EAGLETON. Do you challenge the findings in the Yankelovich report with respect to the two matters I have just stated?

Dr. McGINNIS. No; not at all.

Senator EAGLETON. For whatever weight they carry, and they may have no weight, may be ridiculous, frivolous, or innocuous, but you don't fault their methodology in arriving at the results they reflected in their report; do you?

Dr. McGINNIS. That is correct. The only points that I do think bear emphasis are the points——

Senator EAGLETON. You only want to emphasize the points supportive of your views, and you don't want to emphasize the points attacking your views.

Dr. McGINNIS. There are two points in support of our point of view.

Senator EAGLETON. "Don't bother me with the facts; my mind is already made up."

Dr. McGINNIS. Because of the fact the public clearly remains confused about nutrition in spite of the fact there is substantial consensus about overall dietary trends, publications such as Dietary Guidelines are important contributors to meeting a perceived public need in this respect.

I have to note, in addition, we are clearly by no means the only ones who sense this demand. You have heard it from others today. Because the guidelines are sensible and moderately stated, they have met with, I think, widespread acceptance and endorsement. Professional groups like the American College of Preventive Medicine, the American Heart Association, the American Public Health Association, and so forth and so on, have welcomed publicly the release of the guidelines. Industry has also been active in publicizing the guidelines. I think it might be worth noting just a few of these activities in brief.

RELEASE OF GUIDELINES BY PRIVATE SECTOR

General Foods ran a series of newspaper ads in major metropolitan newspapers reviewing each of the guidelines in detail as well as the summary, a very important involvement of the private sector in working with Government in this respect. The ARA Concessionary Co., which serves 10 million people in cafeterias, is developing a plan to focus on the guidelines for all of their clients in various cafeterias around the country. Again, I think this is an important manifestation of private support for this important interaction. The Food Marketing Institute, which is a trade association for markets, will also be distributing the guidelines to a number of their grocery stores, "Nutrition Today," which is a widely circulated nutrition magazine, has reproduced the guidelines in their entirety.

In sum, to quote from the Surgeon General's report, "The health of the American people has never been better." Dietary improvements have been important contributors to the gains we have made today, and the released guidelines are an important part of our effort to insure that health continues to improve.

Thank you, Mr. Chairman.

Public Health Considerations in Reducing Cancer Risk: Interim Dietary Guidelines

by Sushma Palmer and Kulbir Bakshi

RESEARCH into the etiology and prevention of cancer has occupied center stage for several decades. However, emphasis on dietary components as potential causative and protective agents and, therefore, modification of the diet in an attempt to reduce cancer risk is relatively recent. As described in the foregoing chapters, the last four decades have generated an abundance of epidemiological and laboratory data concerning cancer and its association with dietary patterns, food groups, foods, and individual food constituents that either occur naturally, are used as food additives, or inadvertently contaminate the food supply. At the request of the National Cancer Institute, this evidence was recently evaluated by a 14-member multidisciplinary panel—the Committee on Diet, Nutrition, and Cancer (the committee) of the National Research Council/National Academy of Sciences (NRC/NAS). In June 1982, the committee issued a comprehensive report critiquing the epidemiological and experimental evidence relating dietary factors to the etiology and pre-

From the National Academy of Sciences, Washington, DC.

This article is based on work conducted pursuant to contract number NO–1–CP–05603 with the National Cancer Institute.

Address reprint requests to Sushma Palmer, Project Director, National Academy of Sciences, 2101 Constitution Ave NW, Washington, DC 20418.

vention of cancer.[1] Overall, the committee concluded that "the differences in rates at which various cancers occur in different human populations are often correlated with differences in diet. The likelihood that some of these correlations reflect causality is strengthened by laboratory evidence that similar dietary patterns and components of food also affect the incidence of certain cancers in animals." However, unlike Wynder and Gori[2] who had estimated that ~40% of cancers in males and ~60% in females could be attributed to dietary factors and Doll and Peto[3] who had proposed that 10% to 70% of all deaths due to cancer could be reduced by practical dietary means, the committee was unable to quantitate the contribution of diet to the overall cancer risk or to determine the percent reduction in risk that might be achieved by dietary modifications. Nevertheless, in the judgment of the committee, cancers of most major sites appear to be influenced by diet, and the epidemiological and experimental evidence was sufficiently convincing to formulate the following interim dietary guidelines that are both consistent with sound nutritional practices and are likely to reduce the risk of certain diet-sensitive cancers (Table 1).[4]

These interim guidelines were based on concordance between epidemiological and laboratory evidence that served as a prerequisite to developing recommendations.

Table 1. Interim Dietary Guidelines to Lower Cancer Risk*

- Reduce intake of both saturated and unsaturated fats from ~40% to approximately 30% of total calories.
- Include fruits, vegetables, and whole-grain cereal products in daily diet; especially citrus fruits, dark green, and deep yellow vegetables, and carotene-rich and cruciferous vegetables. Avoid high doses of dietary supplements.
- Minimize consumption of cured, pickled, and smoked foods.
- Use alcohol only in moderation.

*Recommended by the NAS Committee on Diet, Nutrition, and Cancer,[1] and adapted from Palmer.[4]

SCIENTIFIC BASIS FOR, AND CONSIDERATIONS IN, THE APPLICATION OF INTERIM GUIDELINES

Table 2 summarizes the scientific basis for recommending a reduction in total fat intake. The average American diet contains ~40% of calories in the form of fats and three food groups, ie, fatty cuts of meat, whole milk dairy products, and oils and fats contribute the bulk of fat, each providing approximately one third of the total calories.[5] The 25% reduction in fat intake proposed by the committee applies to total dietary fat and not simply to saturated fats. The reduction may be achieved by frequently selecting leaner cuts of meat (eg, round steak, chuck steak,

Table 2. Fat Intake and Cancer: Basis for Recommendation

Epidemiological Evidence

Increased incidence of, or mortality from, cancers of the breast, colon, prostate, or other sites among populations or individuals consuming high fat diets.

Evidence derived from correlation studies (international and intranational), migrant studies, and case-control studies.

Laboratory Evidence

Increased incidence, reduced lifespan, and/or increased multiplicity of tumors of the mammary gland, intestine, pancreas, liver, or other organs in rats or mice fed high-fat diets.

There is some evidence of a dose response. Evidence derived mainly from spontaneous tumors or chemically-induced tumors using a variety of carcinogens (eg, DMBA or DMH),* but some evidence also from transplantable tumors.

Possible Mechanism

Tumor promotion.

*DMBA = dimethylbenzanthracene, DMH = dimethylhydrazine.

This table presents a summary of the epidemiological and laboratory evidence that formed the basis of the first recommendation in Table 1. The epidemiological evidence was judged to be good, though not entirely consistent. The inconsistencies are explained in the report. The laboratory data were found to be supportive of the epidemiological findings. The evidence concerning the proposed mechanisms for the action of fat was sparse, but indicative of a promotional effect.[1]

Adapted from Palmer.[4]

lamb shoulder or leg, pork center shank, chicken and turkey without skin, and fish, including tuna packed in water), trimming all visible fat from meats and removing skin from poultry, selecting low-fat or skim milk dairy products (eg, low-fat yoghurt, low-fat or skim milk, low-fat cheeses, and skimmed evaporated milk), and using smaller amounts of oils and fats in spreads, salads, and cooking.

Table 3 outlines the epidemiological and experimental basis for recommending inclusion of certain fruits, vegetables, and whole-grain cereal products in the daily diet. The epidemiological evidence pertains to both raw and cooked vegetables. Most of the epidemiological data provide indirect evidence for a protective role for vitamin C and carotene (which is enzymatically converted in vivo to vitamin A) in human cancer because they are based on the consumption of foods (especially citrus fruits, green and yellow vegetables, and cruciferous vegetables such as cabbage, cauliflower, broccoli, and brussels sprouts) rich in these nutrients, rather than on actual measurements of nutrient intake. Cruciferous vegetables also contain nonnutritive compounds (eg, indoles, flavonoids, phenols, and aromatic isothiocyanates) that inhibit chemically induced carcinogenesis in laboratory animals. Although several constituents of fruits and vegetables (nutritive and nonnutrive) appear to inhibit experimentally induced carcinogenesis, which of these agents are predominantly responsible for this protective effect observed in epidemiological studies is not yet known. For example, there is no conclusive evidence that total dietary fiber per se (of the kind present in fruits and vegetables) offers protection against colon cancer.[1] Thus, the committee has recommended the consumption of "foods" and suggested avoiding high-potency supplements that may not be the beneficial agents and that may in large doses have adverse or unpredictable effects.

Table 4 summarizes the scientific basis for the guideline to minimize the consumption of cured, pickled, and smoked foods. On the basis of some data, the degree of risk posed by the consumption of cured and smoked foods may be presumed to be determined by their content of polycyclic aromatic hydrocarbons (PAHs) and nitrite (that may be converted during cooking or in vivo to carcinogenic nitrosamines); however, the precise causative agents in these foods have not yet been clearly identified. In the United States, modifications in manufacturing practices (such as using liquid smoke instead of wood smoke and

Table 3. Fruit and Vegetable Consumption and Lower Cancer Risk: Basis for Recommendation*

Epidemiological Evidence

Index of Carotene and Vitamin A Intake

Frequent consumption of carotene-rich vegetables and vitamin A-rich foods and indirectly estimated carotene or vitamin A intake is inversely associated in case-control and cohort studies with cancers of the lung (in Norway, Singapore, and the United States) and larynx, bladder, esophagus, stomach, colon/rectum, and prostate (in various countries).

Serum vitamin A is inversely associated with total cancer incidence in three cohort studies in the United States and United Kingdom.

Index of Vitamin C Intake

Frequent consumption of vegetables and certain fruits and indirectly estimated vitamin C intake is inversely associated in case-control studies with cancers of the stomach and esophagus (mainland United States, Iran, Hawaii, Norway, and Japan).

Limited evidence also for laryngeal cancer.

Raw and Cruciferous Vegetables

Frequent consumption of raw or cruciferous vegetables is inversely associated in case-control and cohort studies with cancers of the stomach and colon (in different parts of the world including the United States).

Laboratory Evidence

Vitamin A and Related Compounds

Vitamin A deficiency increases incidence of chemically induced carcinogenesis in the lung, bladder, and colon (in rats mostly).

Vitamin A excess decreases incidence of chemically induced cancer of the lung, forestomach, cervix, and skin (in rats, mice, or hamsters), whereas exceedingly high doses enhanced tumor incidence in some studies.

Vitamin A may act via an effect on cell differentiation.

Retinoids (synthetic analogs of vitamin A) inhibit chemically induced neoplasia of the breast, bladder, skin, lung, and other organs in most studies, and cause regression of skin papillomas.

Data on the anticarcinogenic effect of β carotene are limited.

Vitamin C

Vitamin C inhibits nitrosation in vitro and in vivo and leads to regression and/or prevention of malignant transformation of cells in culture.

Data on inhibition of carcinogenesis in vivo are limited and inconclusive.

Nonnutritive Chemicals in Fruits and Cruciferous Vegetables

Indoles, phenols, flavones, aromatic isothiocyanates and β-sitosterol inhibit carcinogenesis in vivo, act as blocking agents, antiinitiators, or antipromoters.

Vegetables tested in animals and humans induce MFO and glutathione-S-transferase activity.

Some flavonoids (eg, quercetin in onions) are mutagenic, but extracts of most fruits and vegetables are antimutagenic.

*Based on National Academy of Sciences,[1] and adapted from Palmer.[4]

Table 4. Salt-Cured, Pickled, and Smoked Foods, and Increased Cancer Risk

Epidemiological Evidence

Frequent or greater consumption of cured, pickled, or smoked foods is directly associated in correlation, migrant, or case-control studies with the incidence of cancer of the esophagus (China), or stomach (Japan, U.S.S.R., Norway, Iceland, Hungary, and the United States [Hawaii, high-risk counties of Wisconsin, Minnesota, and Michigan]).

Experimental Evidence

Nitrate and nitrite (present in cured meats) are not directly carcinogenic, but nitrite is mutagenic in mammalian systems, and both nitrate and nitrite are converted to N-nitrosocompounds in vitro and in vivo.

N-nitrosocompounds: Over 90% of the ~300 compounds tested are carcinogenic in multiple animal species and mutagenic in various test systems.

Polycyclic aromatic hydrocarbons (BaP, DBA, BA)* (present in certain smoked foods, and found in charcoal broiled meats and fish, especially fatty meats) induce cancers of multiple sites in animals and are strongly mutagenic.

*BaP = benzo[a]pyrene, DBA = dibenzanthracene, BA = benzanthracene.

A summary of the epidemiological and experimental evidence that formed the basis for the third recommendation in Table 1. The epidemiological data on esophageal cancer are limited compared to those for stomach cancer. Laboratory experiments to test the carcinogenicity of some components of cured, pickled, or smoked foods support the epidemiological findings.[1]

Adapted from Palmer.[4]

report did not define moderation. Alcohol abusers often consume a substantial percentage of calories (10% to 50% or more) as alcohol and may suffer from malnutrition, which in turn may play a key role in development of cancers of the head and neck.[8] Factors such as age, general health and nutritional status, smoking habits, and prior history of alcohol consumption would need to be considered in determining an acceptable level of alcohol consumption for each individual. Similarly, no conclusions were reached about the relative degree of risk from different types of alcoholic beverages. However, because the types and levels of contaminants in alcohol may play a role in carcinogenesis,[9] beverages produced under uncontrolled or noncommercial conditions (eg, home distilled wine or beer) may pose a potentially greater risk.

Table 6 explains why no dietary guidelines were formulated concerning other dietary constituents such as total caloric intake, cholesterol, protein, fiber, and selenium.

The Committee on Diet, Nutrition, and Cancer was unable to reach firm conclusions about the role of food additives, contaminants, and naturally occurring toxicants. This is partly because most dietary microconstituents that are

reducing the level of residual nitrite in foods) have succeeded in making available a variety of cured foods with low levels of nitrite and smoked foods with a low PAH content.[6,7]

Table 5 explains the scientific basis for suggesting moderation in the use of alcohol. The

Table 5. Alcohol and Cancer: Basis for Recommendation*

Excessive beer drinking is directly associated with colorectal cancer among populations in some parts of the world including the United States.

Excessive alcohol consumption, especially combined with cigarette smoke appears to synergistically increase the risk of cancers of the mouth, larynx, esophagus and respiratory tract.

Postulated Mechanisms: Alcohol may act as a carcinogen, cocarcinogen, or promoter; or indirectly as a solvent facilitating intracellular transport of carcinogens; as an inducer of microsomal enzymes; as a source of putative carcinogens (contaminants); or through an effect on nutritional or immunological status.

*Based on National Academy of Sciences,[1] and adapted from Palmer.[4]

added to foods, and many others that are contaminants, have not yet been tested for carcinogenicity. Tentatively, the committee concluded that food additives, such as butylated hydroxytoluene, and naturally occurring or other contaminants such as molds or pesticide residues individually are unlikely to be major contributors to the risk of cancer in the United States. However, collectively these substances may pose significant risks, and no firm conclusions can be drawn until more evidence becomes available. In the interim, it was suggested that efforts be continued towards minimizing contamination of foods, establishing permissible levels for unavoidable contaminants, and monitoring the dietary levels of these contaminants.[1]

Similarly, only preliminary conclusions could be drawn about the role of mutagens in the diet. Mutagens occur naturally in foods and can be produced during cooking, especially high-temperature cooking, and other processing of foods. For example, smoking or charcoal broiling of foods leads to deposition of PAHs, many of which are mutagenic and carcinogenic.[10] Although mutagens are suspect carcinogens, carcinogenicity must be confirmed by long-term animal bioassays. Because most mutagens that have been detected in food have not been tested for carcinogenicity, the committee was unable to determine their contribution to the incidence of cancer in humans. In the interim, the committee recommended to regulatory agencies that dietary exposure to mutagens be reduced where feasible.[1]

COMPARISON WITH DIETARY RECOMMENDATIONS BY OTHER GROUPS

Table 7 compares seven dietary recommendations that have been issued to the public in the past decade. It demonstrates that with two exceptions[13,16] all other organizations listed above have proposed reduction in dietary fat intake.[1,11,12,14,15,17] Similar to the NAS committee, the American Heart Association (AHA)[17] and the Senate Select Subcommittee[11] suggested reduction in fat intake to ~30% of total calories. Reduction in saturated fat intake also appears to

Table 6. Basis for Lack of Dietary Guidelines*

Food Component	Epidemiological Evidence	Laboratory Evidence
Total calories	Epidemiological evidence indirect and limited	Reduction in total food intake decreases age-specific tumor incidence, effect of calories per se *v* macronutrients not clear
Cholesterol	Serum cholesterol inversely associated with colon cancer in males in some prospective cohort studies and intervention trials, but not in others; usually, no association observed in females; dietary cholesterol usually directly associated with colon cancer	Dietary cholesterol cocarcinogenic in the bowel in some studies but not in others
Dietary fiber	Data from international correlations good; from intranational correlations poor	Different fiber components inhibit or enhance carcinogenesis depending on experimental conditions
	Case-control data inconsistent for total dietary fiber; fat intake, possible confounding variable	Results inconsistent and difficult to equate with human studies
Protein	Epidemiological data limited and weaker compared to fat, especially case-control studies	Overall, low-protein diets inhibit and high-protein diets enhance tumorigenesis, but data inconsistent and limited compared to fat
Selenium	Epidemiological data limited to few geographic correlation studies	Exerts antitumorigenic effect but frequently at doses that may be toxic in humans

*Based on National Academy of Sciences,[1] and adapted from Palmer.[4]

Table 7. Dietary Recommendations to the American Public, 1977–1982*

	Limit or Reduce Total Fat (% Calories)	Reduce Saturated Fat (% Calories)	Increase Polyunsaturated Fat (% Calories)	Limit Cholesterol (mg/d)	Limit Simple Sugars
Dietary[11] goals, 1977; general	27% to 33%	Yes	Yes	250–350	Yes
Surgeon general,[12] 1979; general	Yes	Yes	NS†	Yes	Yes
AMA,[13] 1979; general	No	No	No	No	Yes
NCI,[14] 1979; cancer	Yes	NC	No	NC	NC
USDA-[15]DHEW, 1980; general	Yes	Yes	No	Yes	Yes
NAS/[16]FNB, 1980; general	For weight reduction only	No	No	No	For weight reduction only
AHA,[17] 1982; heart disease	~30%	To ~10%	To ~10%	~300	Yes
NAS/[1]DNC, 1982; cancer	~30%	As total fat only	No	NC	NC

*Adapted from McNutt,[18] and reprinted with permission from Palmer.[4]
†Not specifically.
‡No comment.

be consistently recommended by the same groups, but there is no consensus among scientists on the desirability of increasing polyunsaturated fats or of lowering cholesterol in the diet. This is partly because the recommendations were made with different objectives in mind. For polyunsaturated fats, although an increase to ~10% of calories has been proposed by the AHA to lower the risk of heart disease, it is not yet clear whether the same would be desirable for cancer.[1] Similarly, although limiting dietary cholesterol would seem desirable for reducing the risk of heart disease,[17] the role of cholesterol in carcinogenesis is not well understood.[1] Therefore, caution needs to be exercised in advising the public. However, there appears to be agreement among several groups that a lower intake of total fat is desirable for promoting health and reducing the risk of chronic diseases.[1,11,12,14,15,17] Other guidelines (ie, concerning the intake of carbohydrates [simple and complex], dietary fiber, sodium, and alcohol, and for limiting body weight),

while not identical for each disease, appear not to be inconsistent. Some of the seeming inconsistencies in dietary guidelines may be attributed to philosophical differences among scientists about the criteria for and the advisability of making recommendations to the general public rather than to subgroups that are at high risk, and these are discussed elsewhere.[4]

REFERENCES

1. National Academy of Sciences, Committee on Diet, Nutrition, and Cancer: Diet, Nutrition, and Cancer. Washington, DC, National Academy Press, 1982, 496 pp

2. Wynder EL, Gori GB: Contribution of the environment to cancer incidence: An epidemiologic exercise. J Natl Cancer Inst 58:825–832, 1977

3. Doll R, Peto R: The causes of cancer: Quantitative estimates of avoidable risks of cancer in the United States today. J Natl Cancer Inst 66:1192–1308, 1981

4. Palmer S: Diet, nutrition, and cancer: The future of dietary policy. Cancer Res 43(suppl):2509s–2514s, 1983

5. US Department of Agriculture, Human Nutrition Information Service: Nutrient Content of the National Food

Increase Complex Carbohydrates	Increase Fiber	Restrict Sodium Chloride (g/d)	Moderation in Alcohol	Maintain Ideal Body Weight, Exercise	Other Recommendations
Yes	Yes	<8	Yes	Yes	Reduce additives and processed foods
Yes	NS	Yes	Yes	Yes	More fish, poultry, and legumes; less red meat
NC‡	NC	12	Yes	Yes	Consider high-risk groups
NS	Yes	NC	Yes	Yes	Variety in diet
Yes	Yes	Yes	Yes	Yes	Variety in diet, consider high-risk groups
No	No	3–8	Yes	Yes	Variety in diet, consider high-risk groups
To ~50% calories	NS	Yes	NS	Yes	Public education
Through whole-grains, fruits, and vegetables	NS	Through salt-cured, pickled, smoked foods	Yes	NC	Emphasize fruits and vegetables; avoid high doses of supplements

Supply. A Table of Food Consumption Per Capita for 1947–49, 1957–59 Averages, and Annual 1967 and 1970–80. Hyattsville, Md, US Department of Agriculture, Science, and Education Administration, Human Nutrition Information Service, Consumer Nutrition Center, 8 pp

6. National Academy of Sciences, Committee on Nitrite and Alternative Curing Agents in Food: The Health Effects of Nitrate, Nitrite, and *N*-Nitroso Compounds. Washington, DC, National Academy Press, 1981, 529 pp

7. National Academy of Sciences, Committee on Pyrene and Selected Analogues: Polycyclic Aromatic Hydrocarbons: Evaluation of Source and Effects. Washington, DC, National Academy Press, 1983, 460 pp

8. Kissin B, Kaley MM: Alcohol and cancer, in Kissin B, Begleiter H (eds): The Biology of Alcoholism, Clinical Pathology, vol 3. New York and London, Plenum Press, 1974, pp 481–511

9. Goff EU, Fine DH: Analysis of volatile *N*-nitrosamines in alcoholic beverages. Food Cosmet Toxicol 17:569–573, 1979

10. Lijinsky W, Shubik P: Benzo(a)pyrene and other polynuclear hydrocarbons in charcoal-broiled meat. Science 145:53–55, 1964

11. Select Subcommittee on Nutrition and Human Needs, US Senate: Dietary Goals for the United States (ed 2). Washington, DC, US Government Printing Office, stock no. 052–070–94376–8, 1977

12. Department of Health, Education, and Welfare: Healthy People: The Surgeon General's Report on Health Promotion and Disease Prevention. Washington DC, DHEW (Public Health Service) publication no. 79–55071, 1979, 177 pp

13. American Medical Association, Council on Scientific Affairs: J Am Med Assoc 242:2335–2338, 1979

14. Upton AC: Statement on diet, nutrition, and cancer. Hearings of the Subcommittee on Nutrition, Senate Committee on Agriculture, Nutrition, and Forestry, October 2, 1979

15. US Department of Agriculture and Department of Health, Education, and Welfare: Nutrition and Your Health—Dietary Guidelines for Americans. Washington, DC, USDA-DHEW, 1980, 20 pp

16. National Academy of Sciences, Food, and Nutrition Board. Toward Healthful Diets. Washington, DC, National Academy of Sciences, 1980, 24 pp

17. American Heart Association, Committee on Nutrition: Rationale of the Diet — Heart Statement of the American Heart Association. Circulation 65(4):839A–854A, 1982

18. McNutt K: Dietary advice to the public. Nutr Rev 38(10):353–360, 1980

Nutrition and Cancer: Cause and Prevention

an American Cancer Society Special Report

In most instances exposure to cancer-causing agents (carcinogens) takes place 20 to 30 years before a statistically significant increase in cancer can be detected. Only then can it be adduced that the increase in cancer may have been caused by exposure to specific carcinogens.

There is now good reason to suspect that dietary habits contribute to human cancer, but it is important to understand that the interpretation of both human population (epidemiologic) and laboratory data is very complex, and as yet does not allow clear-cut conclusions. Although associations of dietary patterns with various forms of cancer have been found, association does not necessarily imply causation. Causation in cancer is extremely difficult to establish.

This report is based on a study by Sidney Weinhouse, Ph.D., Professor of Biochemistry of Fels Research Institute, Temple University School of Medicine in Philadelphia, Pennsylvania, and a Member of the Board of the American Cancer Society. He acknowledges with thanks the assistance of: David Kritchevsky, Ph.D., Associate Director of Wistar Institute in Philadelphia, Pennsylvania; Sushma Palmer, D.Sc., Project Director of the Committee on Diet, Nutrition and Cancer of the National Research Council, Commission on Life Sciences in Washington, D.C.; Michael J. Prival, Ph.D. of the Genetic Toxicology Branch of the Food and Drug Administration in Washington, D.C.; and Lee W. Wattenberg, M.D., of the Department of Pathology of the University of Minnesota School of Medicine in Minneapolis, Minnesota.

In recent years a considerable number of dietary constituents have been found to protect against the occurrence of cancers in experimental animals. The diversity and widespread occurrence of these compounds in food suggest that it may be virtually impossible to consume a diet that does not contain substances that can inhibit carcinogenesis. Recognition of the range of inhibitors in the diet has led to two major lines of investigation that are currently being pursued. The first is directed toward understanding the impact that these inhibitors now play in preventing cancer and the second, how protective effects might be enhanced. Foods may have constituents that cause or promote cancer on the one hand or protect against it on the other.

No concrete dietary advice can be given that will guarantee prevention of any specific human cancer. The American Cancer Society nonetheless believes that there is sufficient inferential information to make a series of interim recommendations about nutrition that, in the judgment of experts, are likely to provide some measure of reducing cancer risk. These dietary recommendations are consistent in general with the maintenance of good health. They are similar to and largely drawn from background statements previously issued by the American Cancer Society, the National Research Council of the National Academy of Sciences, and the National Cancer Institute. As new information is obtained from research, the Society's recommendations will be changed accordingly.

The first section of this report contains practical recommendations in areas where there are sufficient data. The second section includes comments on substances about which there is insufficient evidence to make specific recommendations at this time. Source materials are listed at the end.

Section I
Recommendations

1. Avoid obesity.

That obese people are at increased risk of certain cancers has been demonstrated by the massive prospective study, Cancer Prevention Study I (CPS I), conducted by the American Cancer Society. This study, conducted over a 12-year period (1960–1972), found a markedly increased incidence of cancers of the uterus, gallbladder, kidney, stomach, colon and breast, associated with obesity. In this study, when data for obese men and women 40 percent or more overweight were reviewed, the women were found to have a 55 percent greater risk, and the men, a 33 percent greater risk of cancer than those of normal weight. Experiments in animals had indicated much earlier that the incidence of cancer is reduced and the life span is lengthened by providing nutritionally adequate diets that maintained animals at close to an ideal weight. For people who are obese, weight reduction may be one way to lower cancer risk.

2. Cut down on total fat intake.

Accumulating evidence from both human population and laboratory studies implies that excessive fat intake increases the chance of developing cancers of the breast, colon and prostate. Excessive intake of both saturated and unsaturated fats, whether from plant or animal sources, has been found to enhance human cancer growth in some studies. Numerous experimental studies have shown that high fat diets increase the incidence of breast and colon cancer in rats exposed to chemical carcinogens. Americans consume about 40 percent of total calories as fat. A decrease in the amount of fat we consume to 30 percent of total calories, on the average, has been suggested in the report of the National Academy of Sciences. For most people, this should mean a simple change in food habits, readily achieved by moderation in the consumption of fats, oils, and foods rich in fats—an effective way to reduce total calories.

3. Eat more high fiber foods, such as whole grain cereals, fruits and vegetables.

Fiber is a term used to cover many food components that are not readily digested in the human intestinal tract. These substances, abundant in whole grains, fruits and vegetables, consist largely of complex carbohydrates of diverse chemical composition. Agreement on fiber's role in cancer prevention is not universal. Proponents cite a large body of epidemiologic evidence that colon cancer is low in populations who live on a diet of largely unrefined food high in fiber. Other scientists point to epidemiologic data that do not support a preventive role of dietary fiber. They suggest that since refined diets low in fiber are likely to be high in fat, the latter factor may play a more prominent role in elevating cancer risk than low fiber intake. Even if fiber itself may not prove to have a protective effect against cancer, high fiber-containing fruits, vegetables and cereals can be recommended as a wholesome substitute for fatty foods.

4. Include foods rich in vitamins A and C in the daily diet.

a. Dark green and deep yellow vegetables and certain fruits are rich in caro-

tene, a form of vitamin A. Many laboratory tests point to vitamin A (and certain synthetic chemicals related to vitamin A) as reducing the incidence of certain cancers in animals, and a number of human population studies indicate that foods rich in carotene or vitamin A may lower the risk of cancers of the larynx, esophagus and lung. Examples of foods rich in carotene are carrots, tomatoes, spinach, apricots, peaches and cantaloupes. Excessive vitamin A in the form of supplements (tablets or capsules) is not recommended because of possible toxicity.

b. Epidemiologic studies indicate that people whose diets are rich in ascorbic acid (vitamin C), i.e., those consuming diets high in fruits and vegetables, are less likely to get cancer, particularly of the stomach and esophagus. It is still uncertain whether it is vitamin C itself or other constituents of the vitamin C-containing fruits and vegetables that exert the protective effect. Vitamin C can inhibit the formation of carcinogenic nitrosamines in the stomach. The possible role of this inhibition of nitrosamine formation in modifying the incidence of human stomach and esophageal cancer is not known.

5. Include cruciferous vegetables, such as cabbage, broccoli, Brussels sprouts, kohlrabi and cauliflower in the diet.

Cruciferous vegetables belong to the mustard family, whose plants have flowers with four leaves in the pattern of a cross. Some epidemiologic studies have suggested that consumption of these vegetables may reduce the risk of cancer, particularly of the gastrointestinal and respiratory tracts. Tests in laboratory animals have revealed that the inclusion of cruciferous vegetables in the diet may be highly effective in the prevention of chemically induced cancer. A great deal of experimental work is in progress to determine what components of these foods are protective against cancer.

6. Be moderate in consumption of alcoholic beverages.

Heavy drinkers of alcohol, especially those who are also cigarette smokers, are at unusually high risk for cancers of the oral cavity, larynx and esophagus. Alcohol abuse can result in cirrhosis, which may sometimes lead to liver cancer. Epidemiologic studies in Africa, France and China have shown that the consumption of wine and other alcoholic beverages is associated with a high risk of esophageal cancer.

7. Be moderate in consumption of salt-cured, smoked and nitrite-cured foods.

Conventionally smoked foods such as hams, some varieties of sausage, fish and so forth, absorb some of the tars that arise from incomplete combustion. These tars contain numerous carcinogens that are similar chemically to the carcinogenic tars in tobacco smoke. The risks may apply primarily to conventionally smoked meats and fish. The food processing industry is now using a "liquid smoke" that is thought to be less hazardous.

There is limited inferential evidence that salt-cured or pickled foods may increase the risk of stomach and esophageal cancer. In parts of the world where nitrate and nitrite are prevalent in food and water, as in Colombia, or where cured and pickled foods are common in the diet, such as in Japan and China, stomach and esophageal cancers are common; and there is good chemical evidence that nitrate and nitrite can enhance nitrosamine formation, both in foods and in our digestive tracts. Many nitrosamines are potent carcinogens in animals and may be human carcinogens. Nitrite has been employed traditionally in meat preservation, where it acts as a preventive against botulism (food poisoning) and improves the color and flavor of meats. The U.S. Department of Agriculture and the American meat industry already have substantially decreased the amount of nitrite in prepared meats and are searching for improved methods of meat preservation.

Section II
Topics of General Interest with No Specific Recommendations

The following substances or dietary practices have received much attention and therefore are reviewed, but no recommendations are made at this time. All are under investigation.

Food Additives

Various chemicals are added to foods to improve color and flavor, and to prevent spoilage. Some have been found to cause cancer in animals and have been banned. Several others are thought to be protective against carcinogens. Knowledge about the possible cancer risks or benefits of food additives is insufficient to warrant a recommendation for or against their use.

Vitamin E

There is no evidence that vitamin E prevents cancer in humans. While vitamin E is an antioxidant, and antioxidants may prevent some cancers in animals, more research is needed before the role of vitamin E in human cancer prevention can be assessed.

Selenium

Although there is evidence that selenium, a trace element, may offer protection against some cancers, this evidence is much too limited to justify a recommendation that selenium intake be increased. Because of the potential hazard of selenium poisoning, the *medically unsupervised* use of selenium as a food supplement cannot be recommended.

Artificial Sweeteners

At high levels, saccharin has been shown to cause bladder cancer in rats. Epidemiologic studies offer no clear evidence for an increase in risk of bladder cancer among people who are moderate users of this artificial sweetener. Of possible concern is the consumption of saccharin by children and pregnant women. The long-term consequences of this possible risk cannot be predicted from current epidemiologic data. New non-caloric sweeteners are now entering the market. Their long-term effects have not yet been studied in humans.

Coffee

Evidence about coffee as a risk factor in human cancer is inconclusive. Although some epidemiologic studies implicate high intake of coffee in bladder and pancreas cancer, others fail to make such a connection. Available information does not suggest a recommendation against its moderate use. There is no indication that caffeine, which is a natural component of both coffee and tea, is a risk factor in human cancer.

Meat and Fish Cooked at High Temperatures, such as by Frying or Broiling

Recent studies have demonstrated that the cooking of meat and fish at high temperatures such as by frying or broiling gives rise to a number of potent mutagens (agents that cause genetic changes) in bacteria, and some of them have induced cancers in animal tests. This subject is now being investigated in several laboratories.

Cholesterol

Although cholesterol is considered to be a risk factor for heart or blood vessel disease, there is little evidence that a high cholesterol intake or a high cholesterol level in the blood also poses the risk of cancer. Evidence relating low blood cholesterol to human cancer is inconclusive.

Background

An optimal diet cannot yet be defined. If we knew what an optimal diet was, additional research in nutrition would not be necessary. There is abundant evidence, however, that the usual American diet is not optimal, and this is adequate reason to recommend modification. Current dietary recommendations were developed to prevent the occurrence of nutritional deficiency disease in the 1930s and 1940s. They have been largely successful. New information about diet and cancer, hypertension, obesity, diabetes, etc. leads to sensible and consistent dietary recommendations to moderate the dietary practices of most Americans.

D.M. Hegsted, Ph.D.
Professor of Nutrition
Harvard School of Public Health

Proceedings of the ACS and NCI National Conference on Nutrition and Cancer, 1979.

About 450,000 people now die of cancer in the United States each year. The deaths of about 135,000—30 percent —are due to cigarette smoking. Rough estimates indicate that genetic factors, radiation, air pollution and certain occupational exposures may together contribute to another 10 to 20 percent. An as yet unknown but probably small number of cancers may be due to viruses. This leaves the causes of the majority of all cancers in this country still unknown. Scientific evidence gathered from studies in the United States and other countries indicates that dietary habits may contribute to the development of a significant, though undetermined, proportion of the cancers whose origins are still not clearly understood.

A search for the causes of human cancer and methods of preventing it is being pursued by many scientists throughout the world. In this country, massive efforts are supported by the National Cancer Institute and the American Cancer Society.

Much of what has been learned about the role of the diet in the development of

cancer has come from three methods of investigation:

1. *Epidemiologic studies* relate cancer incidence and mortality in well-defined human populations to known dietary patterns and other environmental factors. Evidence of the importance of diet as a factor in cancer initially came from epidemiologic studies of migrant populations. More convincing evidence is now being obtained from investigations of cancer-diet relationships in *controlled studies* of individuals and groups.

2. *Laboratory studies* in which food intakes in rats or mice have been systematically designed to reveal effects of specific dietary components not only have provided a means of verifying inferences obtained from epidemiologic studies but also have given leads to additional epidemiologic studies and yielded valuable insights into the effects of cancer-inducing substances on cell machinery. Recently, experimental methods have been devised to detect carcinogens by their ability to cause cancer in cells cultured outside the body. This approach is still in the research stage and may offer promise for the future.

3. A third way of identifying cancer-causing chemicals is to determine their ability to cause mutations (genetic changes). There is evidence that substances that cause mutations in bacteria or in other types of cells or organisms are likely to be cancer-inducing. Mutagenicity testing provides a useful preliminary means of detecting substances suspected of carcinogenicity, but it does not establish that a substance is or is not carcinogenic.

Migrating Populations

Relationships between diet and human cancer have been deduced from studies of migrating populations. For example, the Japanese who migrated to Hawaii have developed a cancer pattern closer to other Hawaiian residents than to the Japanese in Japan as their diet gradually became similar to the Hawaiian diet. Other studies of migrating populations—eastern Europeans who migrated to the United States and Canada, Icelanders who migrated to Canada, and southern Europeans who migrated to Australia—have shown similar types of changes in cancer incidence.

There have been hundreds of studies of the relationship of diet, dietary changes and food components, yielding some evidence relating nutrition to the incidence of many types of cancers. Most have focused, however, on cancers of the gastrointestinal tract, and on the hormonally related cancers, such as those of the breast and prostate. There also have been studies of the influence of diet on respiratory tumors and those of the urinary bladder.

The relationships noted in human epidemiologic studies are, in many cases, supported by evidence from laboratory animal studies.

ACS Nutrition Research

The Society's extensive research program includes investigations into various aspects of nutrition. The effort has been greatly expanded in recent years, as research findings have indicated a possible protective role of some food substances against cancer. The ACS sponsored its first symposium on nutrition and cancer in 1974. The Society conducted another national conference on nutrition in 1979 and plans a third conference for 1985. A workshop conference on nutrition in cancer causation and prevention was held in 1982.

Currently, the Society is conducting in-house research and is supporting 24 grants in nutrition research, which together represent committed funds of more than $18 million.

The American Cancer Society's intramural research, a huge multi-year epidemiologic project known as Cancer Prevention Study II (CPS II), is examining the lives, habits, activities, work and environmental exposures of approximately 1.2 million Americans. Each participant has filled out a detailed personal questionnaire and will be followed by one of 75,000 American Cancer Society volunteer researchers for six years. The current study is patterned after CPS I, which started in 1959 and produced, among other important data, evidence of the link between cigarette smoking and lung cancer, heart attacks and other disease that led to the landmark Surgeon General's Report on Smoking and Health in 1964. CPS II asks a number of new questions about cancer and the environment. It is hoped that the new study will reveal new negative and positive links between diet, nutrition and cancer. For 1982–1983 its budget was $3.2 million, largely for information processing; its total budget is approximately $9 million.

Bibliography

1. Silverberg E: Cancer statistics, 1983. CA 33:9–25, 1983.

2. National Research Council Committee on Diet, Nutrition and Cancer. Washington, DC, National Academy Press, 1982.

3. Doll R, Peto R: The causes of cancer: quantitative estimates of avoidable risks of cancer in the United States today. JNCI 66:1191–1308, 1981.

4. Arnott MS, Van Eys J, Wang YM (eds): Molecular Interrelations of Nutrition and Cancer. New York, Raven Press, 1982.

5. Byers T, Graham S: The Epidemiology of Diet and Cancer, in Advances in Cancer Research, vol 41. New York, Academic Press, 1984, pp 1–69.

6. Nutrition in Cancer Causation and Prevention. Proceedings of a Workshop Conference under auspices of the American Cancer Society. Cancer Res (suppl) 43:2385s–2519s, 1983.

7. Nutrition and Your Health: Dietary Guidelines for Americans. Washington, DC, Government Printing Office.

Part 2: Epidemiologic Support for the Link Between Cancer and Diet

Epidemiology plays a crucial role in research undertaken to clarify the relationship between cancer and diet and nutrition. Indeed, the science of epidemiology is essential to investigations of cause and prevention of any disease that affects as large a percentage of the world population as does cancer. As discussed in Part 1, epidemiology may be considered a less-than-exact science, and it therefore is important to understand the nature and validity of epidemiologic studies before applying and manipulating the resultant data to formulate theories on causation and prevention. Readers should be sure to read the papers in the second section of Part 1 as background for the studies included in Part 2.

Epidemiologic studies must be used in concert with experimental laboratory studies employing animal models because only epidemiologic studies can tell us whether observations from laboratory experiments also hold true for humans. Conversely, many epidemiologic methods usually can provide only inferences, not proof, of causation and prevention and leave us only with working hypotheses as to the role of any causative factor, including diet and nutrition. Clinical trials and other types of interdisciplinary research, together with *in vitro* and *in vivo* laboratory experiments, therefore are necessary to confirm correlations found in large-scale epidemiologic studies. Investigators of cancer causation must confirm and reconfirm, test and retest, working hypotheses and must understand exactly how conclusive the various types of studies are, on their own and in conjunction with other research results.

For the most part, epidemiologic investigation of a problem progresses from large-scale correlation studies to smaller case-control studies and finally to clinical trials with humans. This sequence has been particularly useful in cancer-diet research because it has long been recognized, through broad-based correlation studies, that there are vast geographical variations in rates of cancer incidence and mortality, presumably caused by differences in environmental factors. Studies comparing such rates among Eastern and Western countries, among migrant populations, and among populations known for particular lifestyle characteristics (such as proscription of certain foods) have led to working theories on the role of various dietary factors in cancer causation and prevention.

While such epidemiologic studies have served to suggest research for the present and future, these studies do have significant limitations, which should be recognized. First, large-scale correlation studies often cannot account for factors besides diet that contribute to the differences in cancer incidence among various countries. Second, as discussed in Part 1, until recently dietary assessment methods rarely yielded accurate reflections of the subjects' actual diets, especially over a number of years in the past. Third, it is beyond the capability of many epidemiologic studies to identify the exact effect exerted by diet. It is here that experimental laboratory research can complement the results and inferences of cancer epidemiology and explore the biologic mechanisms whereby diet influences the development of cancer.

The papers in this second part of the *Sourcebook* are meant to serve as examples of the types of studies undertaken by cancer epidemiologists investigating the role of diet and to present significant trends in cancer incidence and cancer mortality and how diet affects those rates.

The first section, "Statistics and Trends by Population and Geographic Locale," presents current trends in both cancer incidence and mortality and nutrition. The papers included progress from a review of U.S. nutrition over 75 years to large-scale correlation studies that have been used widely by current investigators. Readers should note that certain geographic populations have been singled out for particular attention in the research because the accessibility and reliability of data gleaned from them may make a significant contribution to our future knowledge of the cancer-diet link. This section concludes with an example of a study done in a smaller geographic population that showed a low incidence of cancer, in an attempt to identify some chemopreventive factor(s).

The second section, "Statistics and Trends by Cancer Site with Population Correlatives," presents data collected for those cancer sites thought to have the strongest causal connection with diet. Researchers have found it easiest to make such a connection for cancer at gastrointestinal and hormone-influenced sites such as the colon, stomach, esophagus, breast, and prostate. While other cancer sites have been studied for possible dietary causality, the data in these cases are less cohesive and less indicative of true causality; therefore, cancer sites included here have been limited to those with the strongest connection to dietary factors.

Abby G. Ershow, Sc.D.
Staff Fellow
Division of Cancer Etiology
National Cancer Institute

Statistics and Trends by Population and Geographic Locale

Nutrition in the United States, 1900 to 1974

by Willis A. Gortner

Summary

Food and nutrient intakes are being examined for possible relationship to the occurrence or the progress of various types of cancer in man. This paper describes the state of our knowledge on the nutritional status of various population groups in the United States and on the food consumption patterns and their nutritional consequences during the 1900's. Only a few medical studies of nutritional status have been conducted on a national or even a regional basis. These extend back less than 2 decades. Dietary information is available back to the 1930's, and statistical data on use of food in the United States can be found beginning with 1909. Sources of information are suggested for the use of and detailed study by the epidemiologist.

Introduction

The past 4 decades have seen a dramatic turnaround in the overt nutritional health problems experienced earlier in the century (Chart 1). At the turn of the century, and again today, deaths from pellagra (a major vitamin deficiency disease) were almost unknown in this country. Yet, in the late 1920's and 1930's, there was a very high death rate, particularly in the Southern States. Large numbers also died from scurvy due to a deficiency of vitamin C. Doctors then could readily find cases of beriberi due to thiamine deficiency, cases of xerophthalmia from a deficiency of riboflavin, or cases of rickets due to a vitamin D deficiency. Today these major vitamin deficiency diseases have been eradicated so successfully in the United States that many doctors never see them and would not recognize them.

Poor nutrition is now more frequently seen in the many health problems where nutrition has a more subtle involvement but is at least implicated in playing a role. Diet, and especially the lipid components, is one of the identified factors in serum lipid levels that are listed as a major risk factor in heart disease. Diet, and particularly the caloric intake, is clearly implicated in the major health problem of obesity in our population. A number of diet interrelationships seem to have some role in the problem of osteoporosis encountered in the elderly. The current thrust of this conference suggests that nutrition may indeed play a role in the incidence of some cancers in man.

Marginal Nutritional Status

During the period from 1947 to 1958 a sizeable number of regional nutritional status studies were sponsored by the USDA[1] and summarized in a publication (12). The biochemical, clinical, and dietary studies indicated that the average nutritional health for various population groups was good. Less than recommended dietary intakes were most frequently found for both children and adults for vitamin A, ascorbic acid, and iron. Rural, low-income families had diets containing the lowest nutritive value. Adolescent girls and especially older people tended to be overweight, and Spanish American and Indian children

---

Presented at the Conference on Nutrition in the Causation of Cancer, May 19 to 22, 1975, Key Biscayne, Fla.

From the United States Department of Agriculture, Agricultural Research Service, National Program Staff, Beltsville, Maryland 20705.

[1] The abbreviations used are: USDA, United States Department of Agriculture; DHEW, Department of Health, Education and Welfare.

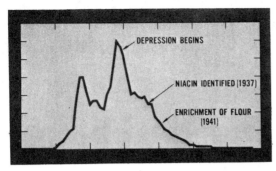

Chart 1. Pellagra death rates in the United States.

frequently had lower heights than average for the population. The hemoglobin content of the blood in nearly all the people examined was fair to excellent (11).

A nationwide survey of the nutritional status of preschool children in the United States was conducted in 1968 to 1970. A summary of this study (14) suggested that those children at nutritional risk were mostly clustered among preschool children of lower socioeconomic status. The major nutritional problem confronting those children appeared to be insufficient food rather than the nutritional quality of the food consumed. The authors noted the fact that a great many preschool children whose diets seemed to be quite adequate were regularly taking vitamin supplements in addition. Other surveys show the same.

At about the same time, the Federal Government conducted a nutritional status survey encompassing all age groups, using a sample drawn from the lowest average income districts in 10 states (5). One major finding in the Ten-State Survey was a high prevalence of low vitamin A values among Mexican Americans. There was a greater prevalence of unsatisfactory nutritional status among adolescents, whereas the elderly showed evidence of general undernutrition. Obesity was very frequently observed, and in some age groups more than 50% of adult women were found to be obese. Iron deficiency anemia was identified as a widespread problem. Such nutrients as vitamin C, thiamine, and iodine did not seem to pose a major problem among any of the groups studied.

In 1971 to 1972, a nationwide survey, Health and Nutrition Examination Survey (HANES) of the nutritional status of the United States population, ages 1 through 74 years, was undertaken (1). The early, still preliminary data that have been reported gave evidence of iron deficiency at all age levels. A few population groups, especially children, showed some biochemical evidence of inadequate vitamin A. For the most part, however, all age groups (and for both race and income levels) had apparently adequate intakes of protein, calcium, vitamin A, and vitamin C.

Because of the close geographical location and a similarity of eating habits and life-styles of Canadians and of population groups in the United States, it is interesting to note the recent Nutrition Canada national survey (13). Some similarities and some differences are seen as compared with similar surveys in the United States. The

problem of overweight was evident in a large proportion of adults. Moderate iron deficiency was also widespread and was observed as a problem for men as well as for infants and women. Some biochemical evidence of a protein deficit was seen in pregnant women. Apparently, many girls and pregnant women had diets with inadequate calcium and vitamin D, but the severity was not such as to lead to rickets. Moderate deficits of calcium, vitamin A, and vitamin C were particularly noted in the Eskimo and Indian populations. By contrast, 1 of 5 Eskimo adult men was receiving approximately 4 times the protein intake considered to be adequate.

Nutrients in the Daily Food Supply

The major sources of data on diets of various United States population groups have been the studies conducted by the USDA and the DHEW. The DHEW data represent dietary intake information taken during the 3 major nutritional status surveys previously mentioned: the survey of preschool children, the Ten-State Survey, and the HANES survey. For the most part, the limited dietary intake information obtained in the DHEW nutritional status surveys tended to confirm more detailed and extensive data in the USDA statistical compilations and nationwide surveys on food consumption.

Two different approaches have been followed by USDA. Using a food balance sheet, the Economic Research Service regularly makes national per capita estimates of food disappearing into United States consumption. From these statistics, estimates are then made of the amount of the various foods available for use by the civilian population (6, 7). Scientists in the Agricultural Research Service can then obtain the nutritive value of the per capita food supply and thus be able to study trends over many years (10). Annual food disappearance and nutrient estimates are available starting in 1909. The figures, of course, do not show which population groups were most affected by observed shifts in consumption.

The other source of data is the periodic nationwide food consumption surveys conducted by the USDA's Agricultural Research Service. The 1st such nationwide survey based on a statistical sampling of households was made in 1936 to 1937. Since then 4 large-scale studies were made in 1942, 1948, 1955, and 1965 to 1966 (4). Currently, plans are being made for the next survey, possibly in 1976 to 1977. All of these surveys have included assessing food used by households, and the most recent survey also developed information on the food intake of individuals in the household (2). Data were thus provided on the total nutritive value of the diets and on the contribution of major food groups to the total of both households and individuals. The sampling allowed a breakdown into subgroups of different incomes, different regions of the United States, and rural and urban people.

What have been the trends during this century in the nutrients in the United States daily food supply? The trends in food uses of protein, fat, and carbohydrate during the past 60 years are shown in Table 1 and Chart 2. The

Table 1
Nutrients contributing food energy available for consumption/day, 1909–1974[a]

Year	Food energy (calories)	Carbo-hydrate (g)	Protein Total (g)	Protein Animal (g)	Protein Vegetable (g)	Fat (g)
1909	3530	497	104	54	50	127
1910	3490	495	102	52	50	124
1911	3470	488	101	52	48	126
1912	3470	490	102	53	49	124
1913	3460	489	100	52	48	125
1914	3440	483	98	51	47	127
1915	3430	481	97	50	47	126
1916	3380	470	96	50	46	126
1917	3330	469	96	50	46	122
1918	3380	464	97	52	45	129
1919	3440	478	97	52	45	130
1920	3290	457	93	51	43	123
1921	3200	441	91	50	41	122
1922	3430	480	94	51	42	129
1923	3440	466	96	53	43	135
1924	3460	474	96	53	43	135
1925	3450	474	95	52	43	134
1926	3460	478	94	52	43	133
1927	3470	477	95	52	43	134
1928	3490	482	94	51	43	135
1929	3460	471	94	51	43	137
1930	3440	474	93	51	42	134
1931	3390	460	92	50	42	135
1932	3320	448	91	50	41	133
1933	3280	436	90	51	39	133
1934	3260	429	91	52	39	134
1935	3200	436	88	48	39	127
1936	3290	438	91	51	40	133
1937	3260	433	90	51	39	133
1938	3260	433	90	51	40	133
1939	3340	439	92	53	39	139
1940	3350	429	93	54	39	143
1941	3410	443	94	55	39	144
1942	3320	425	97	56	41	140
1943	3360	428	100	59	41	142
1944	3350	426	99	60	39	142
1945	3300	418	102	62	40	138
1946	3320	412	102	63	39	143
1947	3290	412	97	62	35	143
1948	3200	397	94	60	34	140
1949	3200	399	94	60	34	140
1950	3260	402	94	60	34	145
1951	3160	391	93	59	34	139
1952	3190	389	94	61	33	143
1953	3170	386	95	62	32	142
1954	3150	380	94	63	32	142
1955	3180	378	95	64	32	146
1956	3180	378	96	65	31	146
1957	3110	372	95	64	31	141
1958	3120	375	94	63	31	142
1959	3170	376	95	64	31	147
1960	3140	375	95	64	31	143
1961	3120	374	95	64	31	142
1962	3120	373	94	64	31	142
1963	3140	371	96	65	31	145
1964	3180	374	97	66	31	147
1965	3140	371	96	65	30	145
1966	3170	371	97	67	30	147
1967	3210	373	98	68	31	150
1968	3260	378	99	69	31	154
1969	3280	381	100	69	31	154
1970	3300	380	100	70	30	157
1971	3320	380	101	71	30	158
1972	3320	381	101	71	30	158
1973	3300	385		68	31	155
1974[b]	3350	388		70	31	158

[a] Quantities of nutrients computed by USDA, Agricultural Research Service, Consumer and Food Economics Institute, on the basis of estimates of per capita food consumption (retail weight), including estimates of produce of home gardens, prepared by the Economic Research Service. No deduction made in nutrient estimates for loss or waste of food in the home, use for pet food, or for destruction or loss of nutrients during the preparation of food. Civilian per capita only, 1941 to date (6, 7, 10).

[b] Preliminary.

available supply of calories shows minimal change, and the proportion of this derived from protein also has not changed much. What is clear is that we have steadily been consuming more fat and less carbohydrates in the United States.

The declining intake of carbohydrate was also accompanied by a shift in the nature of the carbohydrate (Chart 3). Starch has dropped off at a much more rapid rate than the total carbohydrate during these 6 decades. The rather marked rise in sugars and in refined sugar that occurred during the 1920's has (after a decline during World War 2) been maintained in the years subsequent to this.

Similarly, we find that the increased amount of fat in our food balance sheets has been accompanied by a shift in the type of fat consumed (Table 2). There has been only a small change in saturated fatty acids in the food supply during the past several decades. A rather modest increase in polyunsaturated fatty acids (linoleic acid) is seen prior to 1940, and a noticeable increase in the polyunsaturated fatty acids during the last 20 years relates to the increase in our consumption of edible oils, margarine, and shortening.

There now are data showing who is taking this fat into the day's diet (Chart 4). Dietary fat is peaking in the age 12 to 14 group for women and falls fairly steadily thereafter throughout life. By contrast, men do not reach their maximum fat intake until near the end of adolescence, the amount dropping off only after age 20.

Cholesterol appears to have risen to a current level only 10% above that in United States diets at the turn of the century (Table 2). During the past 25 years there has been a declining use of eggs, lard, butter, and various dairy

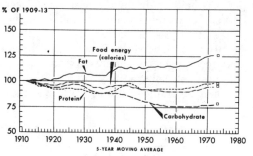

Chart 2. Changes in per capita civilian consumption (disappearance) of food energy, protein, fat, and carbohydrate, 1909 to 1973. □, preliminary.

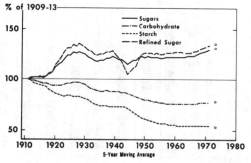

Chart 3. Changes in per capita civilian consumption (disappearance) of sugars, starch, and carbohydrate, 1909 to 1973. □, preliminary.

Table 2

Crude fiber and food lipids available per capita per day in the United States food supply

Years	Total nutrient fat[a] (g)	Fatty acids[a]			Choles- terol[c] (mg)	Crude[b] fiber[c] (g)
		Saturated (g)	Oleic acid (g)	Linoleic acid (g)		
1909–1913	125	50.3	51.5	10.7	509	6.1
1925–1929	135	53.3	55.2	12.5	524	5.8
1935–1939	133	52.9	54.5	12.7	493	5.5
1947–1949	141	54.4	58.0	14.8	577	4.9
1957–1959	143	54.7	58.2	16.6	578	4.4
1965	145	53.9	58.8	19.1	540	4.2
1970[c]	157	55.9	63.1	23.3	556	4.2
1974[c, d]	158	56.0	62.9	24.2		4.3

[a] Ref. 9.
[b] Refs. 6 and 7, Table 40; Ref. 8.
[c] B. Friend, unpublished data.
[d] Preliminary.

products but an increased intake of various meat and poultry products; thus the cholesterol level has remained fairly steady during this period.

Our vitamin and mineral consumption has held up well during this century (Table 3). Calcium, vitamin C, and vitamin A are at higher levels in our food supply than they were 65 years ago (Chart 5). We also can see the very marked improvement that enrichment of cereals has made in B-vitamins and iron going into our food supply (Chart 6). In 1941, these 4 nutrients (iron, riboflavin, niacin, and thiamin) were added to enriched flour, resulting in a quite marked increase in the per capita availability of these nutrients that has held up during the past quarter century.

The USDA survey on nutrient intake of individuals shows who is getting some of these minerals (Chart 7). It is quite evident that, prior to menopause, females take in substantially less than recommended amounts of iron. On the other hand, males take in substantially larger amounts and approximate their recommended nutrient levels from teen-age and on.

There is a different story for calcium in diets of men, women, and children (Chart 8). For females, all age groups from age 9 and on are substantially below recommended daily intakes. Young adult males appear to have adequate calcium, but many other age groups show less than recommended intakes.

Foods Used as Nutrient Sources

The calculations for nutrients in the daily food supply are based on composition of the various foods used (15). Over the years, these foods have changed considerably (Chart 9). Previously mentioned data (Chart 2) indicated that per capita consumption of protein today is similar to that in 1910. Early in this century, about one-half of the protein came from animal products (Table 1), whereas today 70% of protein showing up in the food balance sheets comes from meat, poultry, fish, dairy products, and eggs. The major shift in the diet is in the marked decrease in consumption of flour and cereal products.

Previously mentioned data also showed a continual rise in the daily use of fat in our diet (Chart 2). Again, as can be seen in Chart 10, there have been marked shifts in the sources of fat (3). During the period 1940 to 1965, there was a steady drop in the consumption of pork and milk fat. On the other hand, there was a steady and marked rise in the use of margarine and other shortenings, of various salads and cooking oils (notably soybean oil), and in the fat associated with a marked increase in consumption of beef.

One can look at long-term trends in consumption of major commodities (Chart 11). There has been a fairly steady decline in consumption of cereal products. The very marked decline in consumption of potatoes began to reverse itself some years ago as a result of innovations in processing and marketing and the introduction of dehydrated and frozen products. Note the rather marked shift over the years in the per capita consumption of eggs.

These trends in the major commodities can hide shifts in food consumption of the individual food items in the major groups (Chart 12). During the past 15 years, a marked increase in the consumption of meat products is largely associated with an increased intake of beef and a very marked increase in poultry. The processing and marketing innovations in the broiler industry have led to a rather dramatic increase in consumption of poultry products.

The USDA survey of food intake of individuals in the United States (Ref. 2, Report 11) gives us a picture of who is consuming these various food products. Consumption of milk and milk products (Chart 13) falls off after age 8 for females but stays quite high through age 19 for males. Consumption of animal products (Chart 14) does not change greatly for females throughout the teen-age years and most of the adult life. However, it continues to rise very markedly through age 34 for men.

Grains, fruits, and vegetables may be of special interest to cancer epidemiologists because of the hypothesis that dietary fiber may play a role in cancer in man. Again, beginning at teen-age, females start consuming less grain products/day (Chart 15). Males reach their peak consump-

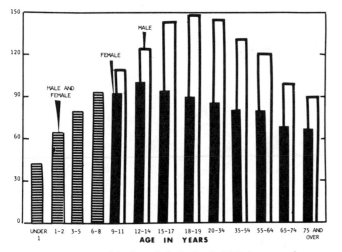

Chart 4. Grams of fat from 1 day's diet in 1965, by age and sex.

Table 3
Mineral and vitamin nutrients available for consumption/day 1909–1974[a]

Year	Calcium (g)	Phos-phorus (g)	Iron (mg)	Mag-nesium (mg)	Vitamin A value[b] (IU)	Thiamin (mg)	Riboflavin (mg)	Niacin (mg)	Ascorbic acid[c] (mg)	Vitamin B$_6$ (mg)	Vitamin B$_{12}$ (mg)
1909	0.83	1.58	15.5		7,800	1.68	1.88	9.5	105		
1910	0.80	1.55	15.3		7,600	1.63	1.82	19.3	107		
1911	0.78	1.52	15.2		7,500	1.63	1.80	18.7	99		
1912	0.85	1.57	15.2		7,600	1.65	1.88	19.0	104		
1913	0.83	1.54	14.8		7,400	1.63	1.84	18.6	103		
1914	0.80	1.49	14.5		7,300	1.58	1.78	18.1	100		
1915	0.80	1.50	14.6		7,600	1.60	1.79	18.3	105		
1916	0.79	1.47	14.3		7,500	1.57	1.77	17.9	96		
1917	0.81	1.50	14.7		7,800	1.54	1.79	18.2	98		
1918	0.86	1.54	15.3		7,700	1.60	1.87	18.3	102		
1919	0.84	1.51	15.1		8,000	1.55	1.83	18.5	100		
1920	0.84	1.47	14.6		7,900	1.52	1.82	17.5	104		
1921	0.83	1.44	14.0		7,800	1.50	1.79	17.1	104		
1922	0.84	1.48	14.5		8,300	1.53	1.83	17.5	104		
1923	0.84	1.51	14.8		8,100	1.62	1.85	18.5	109		
1924	0.85	1.51	14.7		7,800	1.60	1.86	18.2	108		
1925	0.85	1.48	14.3		7,700	1.54	1.84	17.9	106		
1926	0.85	1.48	14.4		8,000	1.51	1.84	17.6	104		
1927	0.86	1.50	14.4		8,200	1.55	1.84	17.8	105		
1928	0.86	1.49	14.4		7,900	1.57	1.84	17.7	105		
1929	0.88	1.51	14.3		8,300	1.57	1.86	17.9	111		
1930	0.87	1.48	14.2		8,000	1.54	1.84	17.3	103		
1931	0.86	1.47	14.1		8,200	1.55	1.84	17.6	109		
1932	0.86	1.45	13.7		8,400	1.53	1.82	17.2	107		
1933	0.86	1.43	13.6		8,100	1.50	1.80	17.1	105		
1934	0.86	1.44	14.0		8,300	1.48	1.81	17.3	108		
1935	0.87	1.42	13.5		8,300	1.39	1.78	16.7	112		
1936	0.89	1.46	13.9		8,000	1.42	1.81	17.3	109		
1937	0.89	1.45	13.6		8,400	1.42	1.83	16.9	110		
1938	0.90	1.46	13.7		8,400	1.44	1.83	17.0	114		
1939	0.91	1.48	14.0		8,600	1.50	1.87	17.3	116		
1940	0.92	1.50	14.2		8,500	1.55	1.90	17.8	115		
1941	0.93	1.51	14.4		8,700	1.64	1.92	18.3	115		
1942	0.98	1.56	15.4		9,100	1.83	2.00	18.7	117		
1943	0.99	1.60	16.1		9,500	2.05	2.15	20.0	115		
1944	1.00	1.60	17.5		9,700	2.09	2.37	22.5	125		
1945	1.06	1.66	17.9		10,000	2.06	2.46	22.7	125		
1946	1.08	1.69	18.2		9,600	2.15	2.48	23.1	123		
1947	1.02	1.57	17.2		9,100	1.94	2.33	21.5	119		
1948	0.99	1.53	16.4		8,700	1.89	2.26	20.8	112		
1949	0.98	1.52	16.4		8,500	1.89	2.25	20.8	109		
1950	0.99	1.53	16.5		8,400	1.90	2.29	20.2	105		
1951	0.98	1.51	16.1		8,000	1.90	2.27	19.9	107		
1952	1.00	1.53	16.2		8,000	1.90	2.31	20.1	105		
1953	0.98	1.52	16.3		8,100	1.85	2.30	20.5	106		
1954	0.98	1.51	16.0		8,000	1.81	2.28	20.1	105		
1955	1.00	1.53	16.2		8,200	1.87	2.31	20.3	106		
1956	0.99	1.54	16.4		8,200	1.87	2.32	20.7	105		
1957	0.98	1.52	16.1		8,100	1.83	2.29	20.5	107		
1958	0.97	1.50	16.1		8,000	1.82	2.27	20.5	102		
1959	0.98	1.52	16.2		8,100	1.88	2.29	20.8	106		
1960	0.97	1.51	16.3		8,000	1.85	2.28	20.8	108		
1961	0.96	1.50	16.4		7,800	1.84	2.26	20.9	107		
1962	0.96	1.49	16.5		7,800	1.86	2.27	21.1	107		
1963	0.96	1.50	16.6		7,800	1.87	2.28	21.5	101		
1964	0.96	1.51	16.8		7,700	1.87	2.29	21.7	100		
1965	0.95	1.50	16.6		7,700	1.81	2.27	21.5	101		
1966	0.95	1.50	16.5		7,800	1.80	2.29	21.6	102		
1967	0.94	1.52	17.2	343	7,900	1.91	2.33	22.4	108	2.18	9.5
1968	0.95	1.53	17.4		8,100	1.91	2.35	22.7	109		
1969	0.94	1.53	17.6		8,100	1.93	2.35	22.8	111		
1970	0.93	1.52	17.8		8,200	1.93	2.35	23.1	114		
1971	0.94	1.53	17.9		8,200	1.97	2.37	23.3	115		
1972	0.94	1.54	18.0	346	8,100	1.94	2.35	23.4	115	2.29	9.8
1973	0.95	1.52	17.9	346	8,100	1.90	2.32	22.9	118	2.24	9.5
1974[d]	0.95	1.54	18.3	348	8,200	1.94	2.33	23.4	119	2.28	9.7

[a] Quantities of nutrients computed by USDA, Agricultural Research Service, Consumer and Food Economics Institute, on the basis of estimates of per capita food consumption (retail weight), including estimates of produce of home gardens, prepared by the Economic Research Service. No deduction has been made in nutrient estimates for loss or waste of food in the home, use for pet food, or for destruction or loss of nutrients during the preparation of food. Civilian per capita only, 1941 to date. Data for iron, thiamine, riboflavin, and niacin include estimates of the quantities of these nutrients added to flour and cereal products (6, 7, 10).
[b] Includes estimates of quantities added to margarine and to milk of all types.
[c] Includes estimates of quantities added to fruit juices and drinks.
[d] Preliminary.

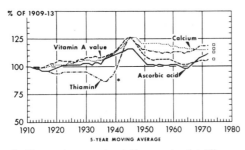

Chart 5. Changes in per capita civilian consumption (disappearance) of calcium, vitamin A, thiamin, and ascorbic acid, 1909 to 1973. *, enrichment initiated; □, preliminary.

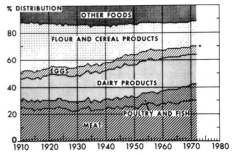

Chart 9. Diet sources of protein, 1910 to 1972. Per capita civilian food supply, 1972, preliminary. *, total animal sources.

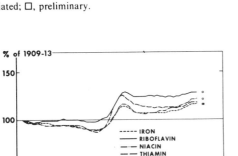

Chart 6. Changes in per capita civilian consumption (disappearance) of vitamin B and iron, 1909 to 1973. □, preliminary.

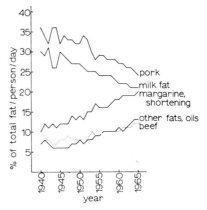

Chart 10. Diet sources of fat, 1940 to 1965. Data from Ref. 3.

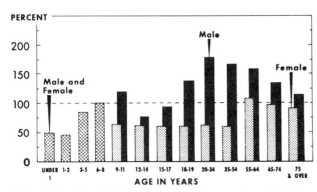

Chart 7. Iron from 1 day's diet in 1965, by age and sex of the National Academy of Science-National Research Council (1968).

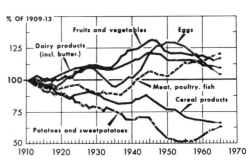

Chart 11. Trends in United States eating habits. Changes in per capita civilian consumption (disappearance) of major food commodities, 1909 to 1965.

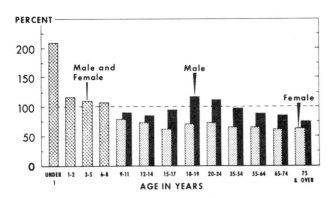

Chart 8. Calcium from 1 day's diet in 1965, by age and sex of National Academy of Sciences-National Research Council (1968).

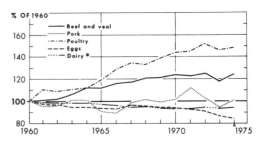

Chart 12. Changes in per capita consumption (disappearance) of selected livestock products, 1960 to 1974. *, includes butter; Δ, preliminary.

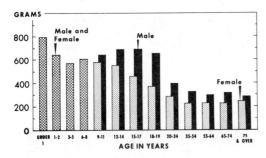

Chart 13. Milk and milk products (calcium equivalent) in 1 day's diet in 1965, by age and sex.

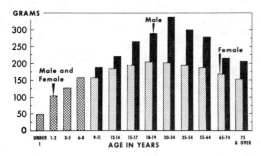

Chart 14. Meat and poultry and fish in 1 day's diet in 1965, by age and sex.

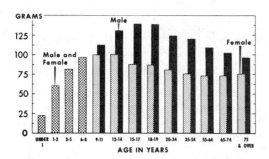

Chart 15. Grain products (flour equivalent) in 1 day's diet in 1965, by age and sex.

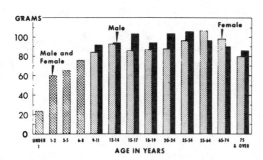

Chart 16. Tomatoes and citrus fruit in 1 day's diet in 1965, by age and sex.

tion of grain products much later, at about age 19.

A very different consumption pattern is seen for various fruits and vegetable products. For tomatoes and citrus fruit (Chart 16), males and females consume comparable quantities/person each day, and there is no tendency for this to change for any of the age groups after late childhood. On the other hand, while the same statement would also apply to the green and yellow vegetables (Chart 17), one may note from the quantity/person that these commodities contribute to the daily diet that they constitute a small fraction of the amount that grain products or tomatoes and citrus fruit contribute.

Potato consumption shows a real difference associated with age and sex (Chart 18). For females, it remains at about 50 g daily from early childhood on. For males, the consumption rises to twice this amount by age 34 and diminishes thereafter.

Unfortunately, neither the food balance sheets (disappearance data) nor the dietary surveys of households or individuals in the United States have been used to come up with solid information on the dietary fiber consumption. B. Friend[2] has estimated that the level of crude fiber in the food supply dropped from about 6 g per capita per day around 1910 to a little over 4 g in 1974 (Table 2). The decline may relate to a decreased consumption of potatoes and grain products. Although the crude fiber composition has not been tabulated for a great many foods, Watt and

---

[2] B. Friend. Changes in the U. S. Diet Caused by Alterations in Food Intake Patterns. Paper for the Food and Drug Administration Conference on the Changing Food Supply in America, Arlington, Virginia, May 22, 1974.

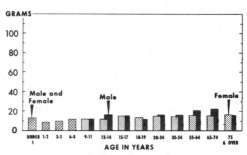

Chart 17. Dark green and yellow vegetables in 1 day's diet in 1965, by age and sex.

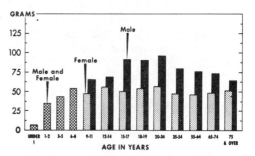

Chart 18. White potatoes in 1 day's diet in 1965, by age and sex.

Merrill (15) include a column listing fiber for a considerable number of foods. There one can see that the fiber content of cereal products runs somewhat lower than that of many fruits and that vegetables as a class have substantially more fiber than do either cereals or fruits. Since much of the cereal consumption in the United States is of white wheat flour with perhaps only 0.3% fiber, it is obvious that an appreciable part of the dietary fiber of the United States may come from noncereal products. Potatoes may be an important source of fiber but the green and yellow vegetables may not be, as their relatively low daily consumption offsets the higher fiber content in vegetables. None of this material dealing with "crude fiber" relates to individual fiber components such as pectins, pentosans, cellulose, or lignin, some of which may be far more important in cancer epidemiology.

Discussion

There is very little basis to relate the current nutritional status of United States population groups to changes over an appreciable period of time.

The food disappearance data do give useful information on changes in nutrients in our food supply during this century and on changes in the foods that provide nutrients to the population. Finally, the study of the dietary intake of individuals helps to define which age and sex groups are taking in the different foods. The data thus also tell how effective these dietary patterns are in meeting the recommended nutrient intakes of the different population groups.

In all of the studies I have referred to, we are talking only of averages. Usually, we do not know or are not told what the range is, what the degree of clustering may be, what the extremes encompass, and how many individuals may be near those extremes in foods or nutrients consumed or in clinical or biochemical or anthropometric tests of "nutritional risk." A person with his head in the oven and his feet in the freezer may be comfortable "on the average;" many of the data defining "Nutrition USA" are similarly comforting to the health scientist, on the average.

An encouraging exception is the series of reports issued in the Canadian survey (Nutrition Canada, 1975; Ref. 13). Their tables show the percentage distribution of dietary intake of various nutrients and also the level for the lowest and for the highest 5% and 25% of the population. The same is presented for many biochemical values relating to nutritional status. Thus, one can see that, while the lowest 5% of the Canadian teen-age males had dietary protein of only four-fifths of the recommended "adequate" intake, the upper 5% of this population group were consuming more than 4 times the amount of protein needed for good nutrition.

Hopefully, the data described in this paper can at least lead the epidemiologist to sources of information dealing with food and nutrition that can be examined relative to the changes in various diseases, including the various forms of cancer.

References

1. Abraham, S., Lowenstein, F. W., and Johnson, C. L. Preliminary Findings of the First Health and Nutrition Examination Survey, United States 1971-72: Dietary Intake and Biochemical Findings. Publication No. (HRA) 74-1219-1. Washington, D.C.: Department of Health, Education and Welfare, 1974.
2. Agricultural Research Service. Household Food Consumption Survey 1965-66, Report Nos. 1 to 18. Washington, D.C.: United States Department of Agriculture, 1968-1974.
3. Call, D. L., and Sanchez, A. M., Trends in Fat Disappearance in the United States, 1909-65. J. Nutr., *93* (suppl.): 1-28, 1967.
4. Clark, F. Recent Food Consumption Surveys and Their Uses. Federation Proc., *33:* 2270-2274, 1974.
5. Department of Health, Education and Welfare. Ten-State Nutrition Survey, 1968-1970. Publication Nos. (HSM) 72-8130, 72-8131, 72-8132, 72-8133, 72-8134. Washington, D.C.: Department of Health, Education and Welfare, 1972.
6. Economic Research Service. Food Consumption, Prices, and Expenditures. Agricultural Economic Report 138. Washington, D.C.: United States Department of Agriculture, 1968.
7. Economic Research Service. Food Consumption, Prices, and Expenditures. Agricultural Economic Report 138. Supplement. Washington, D.C.: United States Department of Agriculture, 1974.
8. Feeley, R. M., Criner, P. E., and Watt, B. K. Cholesterol Content of Foods. J. Am. Dietet. Assoc., *61:* 134-149, 1972.
9. Friend, B. Nutrients in the United States Food Supply. A Review of Trends, 1909-1913 to 1965. Am. J. Clin. Nutr., *20:* 907-914, 1967.
10. Friend, B., and Marston, R. Nutritional Review. National Food Situation (USDA). *150:* 26-32, 1974.
11. Kelsay, J. L. A Compendium of Nutritional Status Studies and Dietary Evaluation Studies Conducted in the United States (1957-1967). J. Nutr., *99:* 119-166, 1969.
12. Morgan, A. F. Nutritional Status U.S.A. Calif. Agr. Exptl. Station Bull. 769, 1959.
13. Nutrition Canada. Nutrition: A National Priority. Report by Nutrition Canada to the Department of National Health and Welfare, Ottawa, Canada: Information Canada, 1973. (In 1975 this material is detailed in 12 survey reports covering Alberta, British Columbia, Eskimos, Indians, Manitoba, New Brunswick, Newfoundland, Nova Scotia, Ontario, Prince Edward Island, Quebec, and Saskatchewan survery areas).
14. Owen, G. M., Kram, K. M., Garry, P. J., Lowe, J. W., and Lubin, A. H. A Study of Nutritional Status of Preschool Children in the United States, 1968-1970. Pediatrics, *53:* 597-646, 1974.
15. Watt, B. K., and Merrill, A. L. Composition of Foods-Raw, Processed, Prepared. Agriculture Handbook No. 8. Washington, D.C.: United States Department of Agriculture, 1963.

Environmental Factors and Cancer Incidence and Mortality in Different Countries, with Special Reference to Dietary Practices

by Bruce Armstrong and Richard Doll

Incidence rates for 27 cancers in 23 countries and mortality rates for 14 cancers in 32 countries have been correlated with a wide range of dietary and other variables. Dietary variables were strongly correlated with several types of cancer, particularly meat consumption with cancer of the colon and fat consumption with cancers of the breast and corpus uteri. The data suggest a possible role for dietary factors in modifying the development of cancer at a number of other sites. The usefulness and limitations of the method are discussed.

The correlation of incidence and mortality rates with the prevalence of environmental agents in various geographical areas has provided useful pointers for the study of environmental factors in the aetiology of cancer. Such studies may be conducted either within defined regions of a single country or across several countries. The former approach has the advantage of more uniform data sources, but is limited in that subdivision to allow sufficient observations for analysis may so reduce the size of the population in each region that the rates become unstable; moreover, differences within a country are likely to be less than those between countries. The correlation of cancer rates with the prevalence of environmental agents in different countries may therefore be a worthwhile exercise in spite of the fact that the apparent distribution of both the cancer and the agent may be significantly affected by differences in the quality of the data available.

Correlation studies of cancer incidence or mortality with various environmental agents have been reported previously over a wide range of countries. Most were conducted before incidence figures became readily available (UICC, 1966, 1970) and before the usefulness was recognized of truncated age-standardized rates as descriptors of international variations (Doll and Cook, 1967). Most of the studies were restricted to a few selected cancers and environmental agents and the analyses limited to calculation of simple correlation coefficients. Only male rates have usually been used except where cancers of the female breast or genital organs have been studied, and often rates have been included for countries for which the mortality data were unreliable.

With the increasing interest in possible environmental causes of human cancer and the availability of incidence data and a wider range of

From the Department of the Regius Professor of Medicine, Radcliffe Infirmary, Oxford OX2 6HE, England.

mortality data, it seemed that a further international correlation analysis would be justified. In this study we have used cancer incidence data from 23 countries and mortality data from 32 countries and have correlated most discrete cancer sites in men and women with a wide range of dietary and other variables. The usefulness of partial correlation analysis has been explored as a means of identifying the relationships most likely to be worthy of further study.

DATA AND METHODS

Cancer incidence data were taken from UICC, 1966 and 1970. The truncated age-standardized incidence rates for ages 35-64 years were used with the "world population" as a standard. The advantages of this age-range are that at these ages cancer is common enough to produce stable rates even in quite small populations; that the relationship between incidence and age is similar through this age range in nearly all countries; and that it reduces the inaccuracies introduced by using data from older age groups in which cancer registration may be very incomplete. The countries from which data were used and the years covered by these data are shown in Table I. All countries were included from which the data available might reasonably have been considered to be representative of the country as a whole. For countries in which data were available from two or more cancer registries, a mean incidence rate was calculated, weighted

for the population in the age-group 35-64 years in each registration area. The person/years of experience for the periods studied ranged from 0.17 to 16.2 million years for men and from 0.21 to 16.9 million years for women.

Cancer mortality data were taken from Segi *et al.* (1969) and WHO (1967-1969, 1970). Truncated age-standardized mortality rates for ages 35-64 years were calculated, using as a standard the same world population as was used for the incidence rates. The countries from which data were used, and the years covered by these data, are shown in Table I. Countries were included in the analysis only if less than 15% of the deaths in 1965 were attributed to senility or ill-defined causes. The person/years of experience for the periods studied ranged from 0.71 to 61.3 million years for men and from 0.71 to 65.0 million years for women.

The 27 types of cancer studied are shown in Table II. Data for each cancer were not available in all countries. Incidence data were available for cancer of the liver and cancer of the gall-bladder and biliary tract in only 21 out of the 23 countries. Mortality data were available for cancer of the pancreas in 23 out of the 32 countries and for cancers of the ovary, kidney and bladder in 21 countries.

International *per caput* commodity consumption and other data were derived from various sources (Food and Agriculture Organization, 1959, 1960, 1971; Statistical Office of the United

TABLE I

YEARS FOR WHICH CANCER INCIDENCE AND MORTALITY DATA WERE USED
IN THE COUNTRIES STUDIED

Country	Incidence data	Mortality data	Country	Incidence data	Mortality data
Nigeria [1]	1960-65 [2]		German Fed. Repub. [1]	1963-66	1964-65
Canada [1]	1963-66	1964-65	German Dem. Repub.	1964-66	
Chile	1959-61	1964-65	Greece		1964-65
Colombia [1]	1962-66	1964-65	Hungary [1]	1962-66	1964-65
Jamaica [1]	1964-66		Iceland	1955-63	
Puerto Rico	1964-66		Ireland		1964-65
USA [1]	1959-66	1964-65	Italy		1964-65
Taiwan		1965-66	Netherlands [1]	1960-62	1964-65
Hong Kong		1965-66	Norway	1964-66	1964-65
Israel	1960-66	1964-65	Poland [1]	1965-66	1964-65
Japan [1]	1962-64, 66	1964-65	Portugal		1964-65
Philippines		1965-66	Rumania [1]	1967	1965-66
Austria		1964-65	Sweden	1962-65	1964-65
Belgium		1964-65	Switzerland		1964-65
Bulgaria		1965-66	United Kingdom [1]	1963-66	1964-65
Czechoslovakia		1964-65	Yugoslavia [1]	1961-65	1964-65
Denmark	1958-62	1964-65	Australia		1964-65
Finland	1962-65	1964-65	New Zealand	1962-66	1964-65
France		1964-65			

[1] Incidence data available for only part of the country.
[2] 1960-65 etc. means all years in the inclusive range 1960 to 1965.

Nations Organization, 1960, 1970; Beese, 1972; Cartographic Department of the Clarendon Press, 1972). The variables studied are listed in Table IV. Except where specified otherwise, the figures used were measurements *per caput* in 1963-65. These data were available for all the countries studied except for tea consumption in Colombia, Puerto Rico and Iceland, coffee consumption in Nigeria and Taiwan and cigarette consumption in 1953-55 in Puerto Rico.

Product-moment simple and first-order partial correlation coefficients between the cancer rates and the environmental variables were calculated using SPSS package programmes (Nie *et al.*, 1970) on the Oxford University ICL 1906A computer. Countries with missing data were excluded separately from the calculation of all correlation coefficients involving the missing variable. The product-moment correlation method was used in preference to a rank correlation method as it provides the most satisfactory partial correlation coefficients. Even when the variables being correlated are both normally distributed, the product-moment correlation coefficient is a useful measure of the association between them which, in contrast to ranking methods, makes use of all the information in the data.

Preliminary analyses

As an aid to interpreting the correlations between the cancer rates and the environmental variables, some preliminary analyses were performed. These are shown in Tables II-IV.

Table II shows the correlation between male and female incidence and mortality rates for the cancer sites common to both sexes. A low correlation between male and female rates may suggest either that different aetiological factors are responsible for the cancer in the two sexes, or that the ratio of male to female exposure or sensitivity to a common aetiological factor differs significantly from country to country; or that random factors are significantly affecting the rates. It is probable, therfore, that the most useful inferences can be drawn from data for cancers in which the male and female rates are highly correlated.

Table III shows the correlations between cancer incidence and mortality rates in the 18 countries for which both rates were available. Clearly, many factors may account for a low correlation between incidence and mortality rates, particularly when the case fatality rate for the cancer site in question is low. From an aetiological point of view, correlations between incidence rates and environmental variables ought to be the more revealing, provided that the incidence data are reliable.

Table IV shows the intercorrelations between all the environmental variables which were highly

TABLE II

SIMPLE CORRELATION COEFFICIENTS BETWEEN MALE AND FEMALE RATES FOR CANCER INCIDENCE AND MORTALITY AT VARIOUS SITES

Cancer site [1]	Incidence rates	Mortality rates
Oesophagus (150)	0.93	0.41
Stomach (151)	0.97	0.95
Small intestine (152)	0.66	—
Colon (Inc. 153; Mort. 152-3)	0.98	0.94
Rectum (154)	0.90	0.93
Liver (155.0)	0.96	—
Gall bladder etc. (155.1)	0.76	—
Pancreas (157)	0.46	0.69
Nose (160)	0.84	—
Larynx (161)	0.10	0.12
Lung (162-3)	0.54	0.28
Kidney (180)	0.81	0.88
Bladder (181)	0.70	0.75
Nervous system (193)	0.94	—
Thyroid (194)	0.73	—
Bone (196)	0.75	—
Connective tissue (197)	0.42	—
Lympho- and reticulosarcoma (200)	0.85	—
Hodgkin's disease (201)	0.62	—
Myeloma (203)	0.93	—
Leukaemia (204)	0.49	0.90

[1] ICD 7th Revision rubrics in parentheses. Where no coefficient is given, mortality data for that cancer were not available in the sources used. Incidence and mortality rates for cancer of the breast (170), cervix uteri (171), and ovary (175) were studied in women and for cancer of the prostate (177) in men. Incidence rates only were studied for cancer of the corpus uteri (172) and other genitalia (176) in women and for cancer of the testis (178) and other genitalia (179) in men.

TABLE III

SIMPLE CORRELATION COEFFICIENTS BETWEEN INCIDENCE AND MORTALITY RATES OF CANCER AT VARIOUS SITES IN 18 COUNTRIES

Cancer site	Men	Women
Oesophagus	0.89	0.96
Stomach	0.88	0.89
Colon	0.92	0.95
Rectum	0.77	0.62
Pancreas [1]	0.70	0.64
Larynx	0.82	0.36
Lung	0.91	0.68
Breast	—	0.90
Cervix	—	0.53
Ovary [2]	—	0.84
Prostate	0.57	—
Kidney [2]	0.78	0.50
Bladder [2]	0.56	0.59
Leukaemia	0.58	0.66

[1] 15 countries.
[2] 14 countries.

correlated with at least one of the rates over the 32 countries with mortality data. This Table is of the familiar triangular form produced when a set of variables are correlated with one another, except that the " tail " of the triangle has been

TABLE IV

CORRELATION COEFFICIENTS BETWEEN ENVIRONMENTAL VARIABLES

Environmental variables [1]	GNP	Physician density	Cereals	Potatoes etc.	Sugar	Pulses etc.	Vegetables	Fruits	Meat	Eggs	Fish	
Liquid energy 1955-57	0.83	0.20	-0.62	-0.06	0.58	-0.20	0.00	0.26	0.61	0.59	0.04	
Solid energy 1955-57	0.42	0.33	-0.35	0.44	0.45	-0.42	0.01	-0.06	0.54	0.40	-0.23	
Population density 1965 [2]	-0.18	-0.32	0.05	-0.34	-0.23	0.18	-0.04	-0.13	-0.12	-0.02	0.33	
Tea 1955-57	0.14	-0.10	-0.29	0.06	0.48	-0.17	-0.09	-0.16	0.52	0.42	-0.10	
Coffee 1955-57	0.69	-0.03	-0.64	0.32	0.46	-0.36	-0.31	0.11	0.19	0.23	0.25	
Cigarettes 1963-65	0.24	0.08	0.02	-0.40	0.12	0.10	0.11	0.02	0.36	0.28	-0.21	
Total fat	0.82	0.39	-0.72	0.34	0.76	-0.55	-0.03	0.35	0.81	0.74	-0.16	
Total protein	0.53	0.56	-0.11	0.08	0.34	-0.24	0.36	0.32	0.65	0.56	-0.34	
Animal protein	0.85	0.33	-0.76	0.28	0.78	-0.55	0.00	0.30	0.87	0.77	-0.08	
Calories	0.57	0.50	-0.24	0.27	0.56	-0.45	0.14	0.22	0.72	0.58	-0.42	
Fats and oils	0.64	0.44	-0.59	0.39	0.55	-0.46	0.08	0.41	0.52	0.62	-0.06	
Fish	-0.01	-0.31	-0.14	-0.06	-0.24	0.27	-0.02	-0.12	-0.35	-0.11		
Eggs	0.69	0.60	-0.61	0.08	0.63	-0.24	0.21	0.46	0.72		0.70	Calories
Meat	0.75	0.38	-0.59	0.10	0.71	-0.48	0.08	0.26		0.74	0.72	Animal protein
Fruits	0.38	0.61	-0.29	-0.25	0.16	0.15	0.40		0.69	0.91	0.61	Total protein
Vegetables	0.03	0.42	0.24	-0.30	-0.28	0.52		0.70	0.93	0.82	0.89	Total fat
Pulses etc. [3]	-0.34	-0.10	0.51	-0.56	-0.67		-0.18	0.53	0.09	0.49	0.16	Cigarettes
Sugar	0.66	0.22	-0.80	0.43		-0.30	0.53	0.09	0.49	0.16	0.55	Coffee
Potatoes etc. [4]	0.09	-0.10	-0.41		-0.30	0.40	0.35	0.25	0.42	0.40	0.06	Tea
Cereals	-0.71	-0.07		0.08	-0.16	0.38	-0.17	-0.28	-0.16	-0.31	-0.11	Population density
Physician density 1965	0.36		-0.13	0.25	0.10	0.20	0.50	0.33	0.43	0.46	0.46	Solid energy
GNP 1965 [5]		0.20	-0.13	0.15	0.57	0.28	0.58	0.32	0.65	0.34	0.38	Liquid energy
	Liquid energy	Solid energy	Population density	Tea	Coffee	Cigarettes	Total fat	Total protein	Animal protein	Calories	Fats and oils	

[1] Also total energy (1955-57), cigarettes (1953-55) and milk.
[2] Per square kilometre of land.
[3] Pulses, nuts and seeds.
[4] Potatoes, starchy and other staple foods.
[5] GNP = Gross national product.

inverted and placed beneath the diagonal line to save space; the columns beneath the diagonal should be read with the column labels at the bottom of the Table and the row labels to the right. From this Table, environmental variables may be identified which are highly correlated with one another. Thus other variables may be identified which could explain an association between one variable and a cancer rate.

RESULTS AND DISCUSSION

The number of correlation coefficients produced in these analyses is very large and we are therefore reporting in detail only those data that relate to cancers which show a pattern of correlation coefficients unlikely to have occurred by chance and which are common in, or limited to, only one sex or whose incidence and mortality rates are closely correlated in both sexes (coefficient >0.80, Table II). The simple correlation coefficients for these cancers which are numerically greater than 0.50 are shown in Tables V to X with only the highest coefficients for cancers of the nose, cervix uteri and other genitalia in Table XI.

The assignment of statistical significance to individual correlation coefficients in this study is complicated by the large number of coefficients which has been calculated, making it likely that some extreme associations will have occurred by chance. We have, therefore, calculated an F ratio ($F_{4, \infty}$; see Appendix) for each set of simple correlation coefficients from which an estimate has been made of the probability that the pattern of coefficients observed might have occurred by chance on the null hypothesis that no real associations exist. The F ratios and probabilities referred to in Tables V-XI therefore relate not to individual coefficients but to the complete set of coefficients for the incidence or mortality of a particular cancer in one or other sex. We have, however, selected the numerically highest coefficients for detailed attention in the subsequent discussion because they are the coefficients most likely to provide useful information.

TABLE V

SIMPLE CORRELATION COEFFICIENTS BETWEEN INCIDENCE AND MORTALITY RATES OF CANCER OF THE STOMACH AND ENVIRONMENTAL VARIABLES

Environmental variable	Incidence		Mortality	
	Men	Women	Men	Women
GNP	-0.38	-0.42	-0.44	-0.54
Meat	-0.43	-0.51	-0.47	-0.58
Animal protein	-0.18	-0.28	-0.43	-0.57
Total fat	-0.48	-0.56	-0.48	-0.63
F ratio	2.1	3.0 [1]	3.6 [2]	6.1 [3]

[1] $p<0.05$.
[2] $p<0.01$.
[3] $p<0.001$.

TABLE VI

SIMPLE CORRELATION COEFFICIENTS BETWEEN INCIDENCE AND MORTALITY RATES
OF CANCERS OF THE COLON AND RECTUM AND ENVIRONMENTAL VARIABLES

Environmental variable	Colon				Rectum			
	Incidence		Mortality		Incidence		Mortality	
	Men	Women	Men	Women	Men	Women	Men	Women
GNP	0.81	0.82	0.77	0.69	0.74	0.64	0.58	0.44
Cereals	−0.52	−0.51	−0.70	−0.67	−0.32	−0.28	−0.49	−0.37
Sugar	0.55	0.56	0.63	0.65	0.48	0.34	0.53	0.41
Meat	0.85	0.89	0.85	0.84	0.83	0.68	0.67	0.57
Eggs	0.69	0.71	0.69	0.70	0.71	0.70	0.59	0.52
Milk	0.58	0.62	0.62	0.62	0.57	0.38	0.53	0.45
Fats and oils	0.49	0.53	0.67	0.60	0.54	0.41	0.68	0.62
Calories	0.60	0.66	0.63	0.62	0.75	0.56	0.64	0.59
Animal protein	0.74	0.80	0.86	0.84	0.71	0.53	0.68	0.59
Total protein	0.54	0.62	0.53	0.53	0.64	0.44	0.51	0.48
Total fat	0.74	0.78	0.85	0.81	0.76	0.60	0.74	0.64
Cigarettes 1963-65	0.53	0.54	0.26	0.20	0.63	0.49	0.12	0.04
Tea	0.50	0.55	0.48	0.59	0.50	0.40	0.34	0.30
Cigarettes 1953-55	0.40	0.41	0.22	0.24	0.51	0.35	0.03	−0.02
Total energy	0.68	0.67	0.69	0.62	0.65	0.53	0.57	0.49
Solid energy	0.34	0.30	0.49	0.37	0.48	0.41	0.63	0.59
Liquid energy	0.59	0.63	0.63	0.66	0.43	0.32	0.30	0.20
F ratio	12.0 [1]	15.0 [1]	21.5 [1]	18.5 [1]	12.0 [1]	6.1 [1]	11.2 [1]	7.4 [1]

[1] $p < 0.001$.

TABLE VII

SIMPLE CORRELATION COEFFICIENTS BETWEEN INCIDENCE AND MORTALITY RATES
OF CANCERS OF THE FEMALE BREAST, CORPUS UTERI AND OVARY AND ENVIRONMENTAL VARIABLES

Environmental variables	Breast		Corpus uteri	Ovary	
	Incidence	Mortality	Incidence	Incidence	Mortality
GNP	0.83	0.72	0.82	0.44	0.64
Cereals	−0.64	−0.70	−0.58	−0.43	−0.78
Sugar	0.70	0.74	0.62	0.43	0.78
Pulses etc.	−0.43	−0.46	−0.62	−0.41	−0.53
Fruits	0.64	0.44	0.54	0.16	0.31
Meat	0.78	0.74	0.78	0.40	0.53
Eggs	0.71	0.80	0.68	0.28	0.51
Milk	0.66	0.73	0.64	0.47	0.66
Fats and oils	0.63	0.80	0.76	0.40	0.66
Calories	0.57	0.71	0.65	0.36	0.51
Animal protein	0.77	0.83	0.74	0.45	0.71
Total protein	0.49	0.57	0.50	0.32	0.33
Total fat	0.79	0.89	0.85	0.53	0.79
Coffee	0.42	0.37	0.43	0.50	0.50
Total energy	0.70	0.60	0.77	0.31	0.45
Solid energy	0.30	0.40	0.55	0.06	0.23
Liquid energy	0.70	0.62	0.55	0.43	0.53
F ratio	14.0 [2]	24.0 [2]	14.9 [2]	3.2 [1]	9.0 [2]

[1] $p < 0.05$.
[2] $p < 0.001$.

Although the incidence rates for lympho- and reticulo-sarcoma and for myeloma are highly correlated in both sexes, they show a pattern of coefficients which might have occurred by chance and these cancers are therefore not considered further. For those types of cancer which are not highly correlated between the sexes but show a pattern of coefficients for at least one of the rates which is unlikely to have occurred by chance, we give only the highest simple correlation coefficients in Table XI.

Some of the relationships between cancer rates and environmental variables are plotted in Figures 1-5. Examination of the graphed data is important, as it allows assessment of the contri-

TABLE VIII

SIMPLE CORRELATION COEFFICIENTS BETWEEN
INCIDENCE AND MORTALITY RATES OF CANCERS
OF THE PROSTATE AND TESTIS AND
ENVIRONMENTAL VARIABLES

Environmental variables	Prostate		Testis
	Incidence	Mortality	Incidence
GNP	0.43	0.69	0.54
Cereals	−0.50	−0.60	−0.50
Sugar	0.33	0.63	0.60
Pulses etc.	−0.15	−0.59	−0.61
Meat	0.37	0.60	0.50
Milk	0.25	0.66	0.57
Fats and oils	−0.04	0.70	0.76
Calories	−0.05	0.61	0.54
Animal protein	0.25	0.67	0.59
Total protein	−0.11	0.50	0.34
Total fat	0.20	0.74	0.76
Coffee	0.43	0.57	0.45
Population density	−0.54	−0.29	−0.08
Total energy	0.30	0.60	0.43
Liquid energy	0.44	0.54	0.37
F ratio	2.0	12.9 [1]	6.9 [1]

[1] $p < 0.001$.

TABLE IX

SIMPLE CORRELATION COEFFICIENTS BETWEEN
INCIDENCE AND MORTALITY RATES OF CANCER
OF THE KIDNEY AND ENVIRONMENTAL
VARIABLES

Environmental variables	Incidence		Mortality	
	Men	Women	Men	Women
GNP	0.73	0.67	0.62	0.49
Cereals	−0.57	−0.41	−0.71	−0.62
Sugar	0.60	0.45	0.65	0.51
Pulses etc.	−0.72	−0.62	−0.56	−0.55
Vegetables	−0.16	−0.02	−0.43	−0.51
Meat	0.70	0.73	0.44	0.21
Milk	0.74	0.73	0.56	0.53
Fats and oils	0.68	0.57	0.64	0.56
Calories	0.55	0.64	0.37	0.18
Animal protein	0.81	0.83	0.59	0.44
Total protein	0.55	0.70	0.21	0.04
Total fat	0.77	0.74	0.69	0.53
Coffee	0.62	0.40	0.56	0.68
Total energy	0.62	0.43	0.44	0.19
Liquid energy	0.62	0.52	0.48	0.37
F ratio	11.9 [2]	10.3 [2]	6.2 [2]	4.1 [1]

[1] $p < 0.01$.
[2] $p < 0.001$.

bution of extreme values to the size of the calculated coefficient.

Cancer of the stomach

A negative correlation with total fat consumption is the strongest association with gastric cancer (Table V). Controlling for total fat

TABLE X

SIMPLE CORRELATION COEFFICIENTS BETWEEN
INCIDENCE RATES OF CANCERS OF THE LIVER
AND NERVOUS SYSTEM AND ENVIRONMENTAL
VARIABLES

Environmental variables	Liver		Nervous system	
	Men	Women	Men	Women
GNP	−0.42	−0.53	0.59	0.54
Physician density	−0.53	−0.55	0.65	0.62
Potatoes etc.	0.71	0.69	−0.44	−0.37
Sugar	−0.68	−0.66	0.62	0.50
Pulses etc.	0.50	0.49	−0.56	−0.42
Fruits	−0.38	−0.46	0.52	0.52
Meat	−0.40	−0.47	0.50	0.37
Eggs	−0.49	−0.57	0.60	0.58
Milk	−0.51	−0.57	0.69	0.58
Fats and oils	−0.47	−0.57	0.65	0.56
Calories	−0.53	−0.60	0.56	0.41
Animal protein	−0.59	−0.67	0.69	0.59
Total protein	−0.46	−0.54	0.54	0.45
Total fat	−0.49	−0.59	0.71	0.58
Cigarettes	−0.52	−0.51	0.16	0.08
Coffee	−0.17	−0.23	0.52	0.51
Liquid energy	−0.25	−0.31	0.50	0.51
F ratio	6.1 [1]	7.7 [1]	8.5 [1]	5.8 [1]

[1] $p < 0.001$.

consumption reduces the partial correlation coefficients with meat consumption and GNP (gross national product) to negligible levels, but strengthens a positive association between incidence rates and fish consumption (r_0, 0.43 and 0.37; r_1, 0.60 and 0.58). r_0 refers to the simple (zero order) coefficient, and r_1 to a first-order partial correlation coefficient. Controlling for meat consumption reduces the partial correlation with total fat consumption to low levels in the same way (r_1 varies from −0.25 to −0.32). An examination of Figure 1 shows that extreme values weaken rather than strengthen the negative association with total fat consumption, whereas a similar plot for fish consumption (not shown) shows that the positive relationship is entirely dependent on the extreme values for Japan and Iceland; fish consumption is therefore unlikely to contribute significantly to international variation in gastric cancer rates.

Case-control studies have not produced a strong association between gastric cancer and any dietary variable. The most convincing finding has been a protective effect of raw vegetable consumption (Graham *et al.*, 1972; Haenszel *et al.*, 1972) but this is not seen in the correlation data (r_0 for vegetables from 0.12 to 0.20). What data there are on fat and meat consumption suggest a weakly positive rather than a negative relationship (Higginson, 1966).

Other geographical correlation studies have shown a positive association with cereal consump-

TABLE XI

SIMPLE CORRELATION COEFFICIENTS BETWEEN OTHER CANCER INCIDENCE AND MORTALITY RATES
IN EACH SEX AND THEIR MOST HIGHLY CORRELATED ENVIRONMENTAL VARIABLE

Cancer	Sex/Rate [1]	Environmental variable	Coefficient	F ratio
Small intestine	MI	Sugar	0.45	1.2
	FI	Liquid energy	0.73	5.9 [4]
Pancreas	MI	Eggs	0.61	4.3 [3]
	MM	Animal protein	0.80	9.1 [4]
	FI	Eggs	0.56	2.0
	FM	Sugar	0.64	4.5 [3]
Nose	MI	Pulses etc.	0.60	3.3 [3]
	FI	Pulses etc.	0.61	2.7 [2]
Larynx	MI	Fish	−0.54	1.1
	MM	Vegetables	0.52	1.4
	FI	Potatoes etc.	0.58	2.6 [2]
	FM	GNP	−0.40	1.6
Lung	MI	Solid energy	0.69	4.3 [3]
	MM	Solid energy	0.67	8.3 [4]
	FI	Tea	0.60	3.3 [3]
	FM	Population density	0.75	3.5 [3]
Cervix uteri	FI	Total protein	−0.66	3.8 [3]
	FM	Fruit	−0.42	1.3
Other genitalia	MI	Total protein	−0.60	2.8 [2]
	FI	Eggs	−0.59	3.2 [2]
Bladder	MI	GNP	0.59	3.8 [3]
	MM	Fats and oils	0.66	2.2
	FI	Cereals	−0.54	1.6
	FM	Fats and oils	0.67	3.6 [3]
Leukaemia	MI	Population density	−0.44	1.1
	MM	Calories	0.75	13.7 [4]
	FI	Sugar	−0.36	0.5
	FM	Fats and oils	0.72	11.3 [4]

[1] MI = male incidence; MM = male mortality; FI = female incidence; FM = female mortality.
[2] $p < 0.05$.
[3] $p < 0.01$.
[4] $p < 0.001$.

tion (Hakama and Saxén, 1967) and a negative association with animal protein consumption (Gregor *et al.*, 1969). In our data, the former association is weak (r_0 from 0.37 to 0.48) and can be accounted for by the negative association with total fat consumption (r_1 from 0.05 to 0.12).

Cancers of the colon and rectum

The environmental variables most highly correlated with colon cancer rates are meat and animal protein consumption (Table VI). Controlling for one or other of these in the calculation of first-order partial correlation coefficients substantially reduces the correlation with all the other variables (*e.g.* r_1 for total fat varies from 0.11 to 0.24), whereas no other variable can reduce the correlation between meat consumption and incidence rates to less than 0.70. The pattern for rectal cancer is not quite as clear; total fat consumption is more highly correlated with the mortality rates (Table VI) but this correlation is

substantially reduced by controlling for animal protein consumption (r_1 0.41 and 0.33). Total fat, meat and animal protein consumption are, of course, highly correlated with one another (Table IV). Figure 2 shows that the association between meat consumption and colon cancer is quite plausible.

Previous studies of colon cancer have emphasized the correlation with total fat consumption, although animal protein consumption has also been mentioned (Gregor *et al.*, 1969; Drasar and Irving, 1973). As a result of these studies, the possible role of dietary fat in the production of potential faecal carcinogens has been extensively investigated (Drasar and Hill, 1972).

Until recently, case-control studies have not shown any association between meat or fat consumption and cancer of the colon and rectum (Higginson, 1966; Wynder and Shigematsu, 1967; Wynder *et al.*, 1969). Haenszel *et al.* (1973),

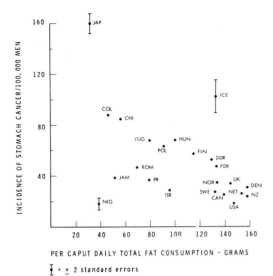

$\mathbf{I}$ = ± 2 standard errors

FIGURE 1

Correlation between incidence of cancer of the stomach in men and *per caput* total fat consumption in 23 countries. NIG = Nigeria; CAN = Canada; CHI = Chile; COL = Colombia; JAM = Jamaica; PR = Puerto Rico; USA = United States of America; ISR = Israel; JAP = Japan; DEN = Denmark; FIN = Finland; DDR = German Democratic Republic; FDR = Federal German Republic; HUN = Hungary; IRE = Ireland; NET = Netherlands; NOR = Norway; POL = Poland; ROM = Rumania; SWE = Sweden; UK = United Kingdom; YUG = Yugoslavia; NZ = New Zealand.

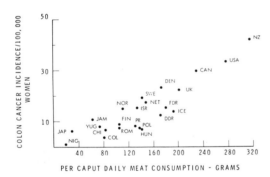

FIGURE 2

Correlation between incidence of colon cancer in women and *per caput* daily meat consumption in 23 countries.

however, have reported a positive association between meat consumption and large-bowel cancer in Hawaiian Japanese. A positive result may have been obtained in this study whilst the others were negative because of the considerable dietary heterogeneity in the Hawaiian Japanese population.

One of the most publicized associations with colon cancer is the negative relationship with

fibre consumption, cereal fibre generally being considered to be the most important (Burkitt, 1971). In our data, the negative correlation with cereal consumption is readily accounted for by the positive association with meat (r_1 for cereals, controlling for meat or animal protein varies from −0.10 to −0.20).

Cancers of the breast, corpus uteri and ovary

The correlation between breast cancer and total fat consumption is the best documented of any such association (Lea, 1966; Carroll, 1968; Drasar and Irving, 1973). This correlation is seen here in the mortality data ($r_0 = 0.89$, Table VII) but not as strongly in the incidence data ($r_0 = 0.79$) in which GNP is more highly correlated and can explain the correlation with total fat consumption (r_1 for total fat controlling for GNP is 0.35). In this situation, GNP may reflect some other variable correlated with economic development (such as animal protein or total fat consumption with which it is highly correlated, $r_0 = 0.85$ and 0.82). Alternatively, it may suggest that the quality of the cancer incidence data is significantly affected by economic factors, particularly as controlling for any of the food consumption variables can reduce the correlation with GNP only to 0.52 (controlling for animal protein).

Total fat consumption is also the variable most highly correlated with cancers of the corpus uteri and ovary (Table VII). The association between total fat consumption and cancer of the corpus uteri is shown in Figure 3.

There is evidence from case-control and prospective studies that both cancer of the breast and cancer of the corpus uteri are associated with obesity (Marks, 1960; Mackay and Khoo, 1969; Lin *et al.*, 1971; de Waard and Baanders van Halewijn, 1974). By implication, therefore, both may be associated with overnutrition. Recent experimental data have demonstrated an enhancing effect of a high-fat diet on 7,12 dimethylbenzanthracene induction of mammary cancer in rats (Chan and Cohen, 1974). This effect appeared to be mediated through alterations in circulating levels of prolactin.

Cancers of the prostate and testis

Mortality from cancer of the prostate is highly correlated with total fat consumption, whereas the incidence is not (Table VIII). In this case, the mortality rates are probably more reliable as the correlation between incidence and mortality rates is fairly low (0.57, Table III) and ascertainment of the true incidence of prostatic cancer is likely to be deficient, varying from country to country according to diagnostic practices. In this respect, it may be relevant that the incidence of

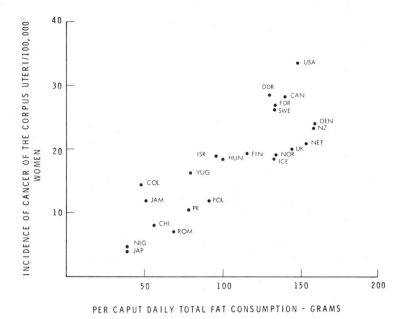

FIGURE 3

 Correlation between incidence of cancer of the corpus uteri and *per caput* daily total fat consumption in 23 countries.

latent cancer of the prostate in Japan and in Japanese in Hawaii may be quite similar whereas the mortality is very much lower in Japan (Akazaki and Stemmerman, 1973). Environmental factors may therefore affect the rate of progression of the latent cancer.

A previous report has been made of the correlation between mortality from prostatic cancer and coffee consumption (Takahashi, 1964; see also Table VIII). This association may, however, be accounted for by the positive correlation with total fat consumption (r_1 coffee, total fat controlled, 0.32 and 0.31).

Cancer of the testis is also positively correlated with total fat consumption (Table VIII). It may be that cancers of the testis and prostate are influenced by hormonal factors which, as with breast cancer, may be affected by the level of dietary fat.

Cancer of the kidney

The positive correlation between renal cancer mortality and coffee consumption (Table IX) has been reported previously (Shennan, 1973). A similar correlation is seen with the incidence rates (r_0 0.40 and 0.62) but the variable correlated most highly with these rates is animal protein consumption (r_0 0.81 and 0.83). The correlation with animal protein consumption can explain the correlations with coffee consumption and with total fat consumption, which has the second highest correlations with the incidence rates

(r_1 coffee 0.31 and −0.18, r_1 total fat 0.00 and 0.18) and can itself be partly explained by the correlation with total fat consumption (r_1 0.42 and 0.55).

Apart from a weak association with cigarette smoking (Bennington and Laubscher, 1968), little is known of the aetiology of renal adenocarcinoma (the major component of renal cancer rates). From Figure 4, it appears that the association with animal protein consumption is plausible and warrants investigation by other methods.

Cancer of the liver

The common view that primary hepatoma is associated with nutritional deficiency (Wynder and Mabuchi, 1972) is supported by the significant negative correlation with consumption of calories, animal protein, total protein and total fat (Table X). The most strongly positive association is with potatoes, starchy and other staple foods (r_0 0.69 and 0.71). These and the other correlations must be interpreted with great care, however, as they are largely (and in the case of potatoes etc., entirely) dependent upon the extreme values for Nigeria, where the incidence of liver cancer in men is three times greater than the next highest rate (Figure 5).

Cancers of the nervous system

Cancers of the nervous system are a heterogeneous group which has seldom been studied

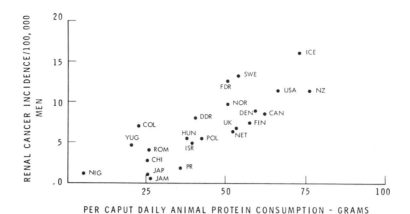

FIGURE 4

Correlation between incidence of renal cancer and *per caput* daily animal protein consumption in 23 countries.

epidemiologically. The highest correlations in this study (Table X) are with the major dietary variables (*e.g.* r_0 0.71 and 0.58 for total fat consumption). An interesting point is raised by the positive correlation with the number of physicians per unit of population (r_0 0.65 and 0.62). This is in part due to the extreme position occupied by Israel on both axes (physician density, 24.5/10,000; incidence of cancers of the nervous system in men aged 35-64 years, 18.3/100,000), but it may be also that the positive correlation reflects the importance of adequate medical services in detecting these diseases.

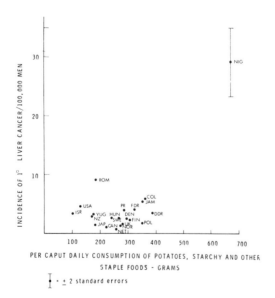

FIGURE 5

Correlation between incidence of primary liver cancer and *per caput* daily consumption of potatoes, starchy and other staple foods in 21 countries.

Other cancers

Cigarette consumption is not, as might have been expected, the variable most highly correlated with male lung-cancer incidence rates (Table XI) and the coefficient is higher with the 1963-65 consumption figures ($r_0 = 0.44$) than with the 1953-55 figures ($r_0 = 0.38$). The correlation is substantially higher ($r_0 = 0.71$), however, when the incidence rates are correlated with cigarette consumption in 1925-29 in the 11 countries for which these data were available. This suggests that the rapid changes in cigarette consumption which occurred between 1925 and 1955 could have substantially altered the relative positions of the countries in relation to *per caput* cigarette consumption so as to obscure an association with lung-cancer rates. Prolonged smoking is needed to produce a high incidence (Doll, 1971) and in these circumstances it may be that a closer association would be found with consumption figures for the more distant past than for the more recent. Other reasons for the low correlation of lung cancer rates with the recent cigarette consumption figures may be the inadequacy of total *per caput* cigarette consumption as a measure of separate male or female smoking habits, or the presence of substantial differences between countries in the methods of smoking (Doll, 1968). The failure of this study to show a strong correlation between cigarette smoking and lung cancer emphasizes the point that a weak or absent correlation between two variables in populations does not necessarily mean that they are not associated in individuals.

Stocks (1970) has previously reported the correlation between solid energy consumption (Table XI) and lung cancer mortality and has suggested that the association is through air pollution from burning solid fuels. He has also produced evidence of a direct association between air pollution and mortality from lung cancer (Stocks, 1960).

It is generally though, however, that the contribution of air pollution to lung cancer is quite small (Waller, 1972).

Bladder-cancer rates are not highly correlated with either of the variables in our study which have been associated with bladder cancer by Cole and others (Cole, 1971; Cole *et al.*, 1971) in case-control studies (cigarette consumption, r_0 from -0.08 to 0.44; coffee consumption, r_0 from 0.17 to 0.39). The highest correlation in our data is between bladder-cancer mortality rates and consumption of fats and oils (Table XI). This is not seen with the incidence rates (r_0, 0.25 and -0.12) and in view of the low correlation between incidence and mortality rates (0.56), no meaning can be readily attached to it.

Some of the other cancers listed in Table XI also show quite strong associations with environmental variables (*e.g.* leukaemia mortality rates). In most cases, however, the lack of consistency in the associations shown by incidence and mortality rates and the low correlation between male and female rates for these cancers makes them difficult to interpret in the absence of more specific hypotheses.

CONCLUSIONS

There are clearly ways in which these analyses might be improved; for example, the inclusion of environmental data recorded at various intervals before the period to which the cancer rates refer. Most of these data, however, are not readily available; moreover, there are seldom objective criteria for deciding the length of latent period to allow. If such analyses were performed, they might reveal other strong correlations which would nonetheless require confirmation by other means, as is the case with our analyses.

It is doubtful whether additional statistical analysis would clarify the associations further than is done by calculating simple and first-order partial correlation coefficients. We have calculated several higher orders of partial correlation coefficients and performed multiple regression analyses, but are not convinced of their value. In any case, with the limited number of observations available, it is possible that calculation of even one order of partial correlation coefficients is not statistically valid, much less the calculation of higher orders or the performance of multivariate regression (Finney, 1974).

The strongest points to emerge from these analyses are the suggestions of associations between cancers of the colon, rectum and breast and dietary variables—particularly meat (or animal protein) and total fat consumption.

Examination of a large number of environmental variables and the calculation of partial coefficients increases the probability that these associations are not just secondary to an association with some other variable. In the case of colon cancer, this suggests that meat consumption may be more strongly associated than total fat consumption, which has received the greatest attention so far.

Given the many weaknesses of this method in terms of the quality of the data, allowances for latent periods and the uncertainty as to whether the most relevant environmental variables have even been included in the correlation matrices, it is clear that these and other correlations should be taken only as suggestions for further research and not as evidence of causation or as bases for preventive action. Nonetheless, we are impressed by the large number of strongly positive and negative relationships between cancer rates and dietary variables. While it is possible that all these relationships might be explained by secondary associations with other environmental agents or by economic effects on the quality of the data, this seems unlikely, particularly as the economic variables are rarely as highly correlated as the dietary ones. It is possible, therefore, that diet may have an effect upon many cancers, perhaps by affecting the metabolism of various carcinogens, as has been suggested by McLean (1973), or by altering the body's capacity to deal with malignant cells. Animal data have been available for many years which demonstrate a general effect of diet upon tumour production (Tannenbaum and Silverstone, 1957). The subject warrants more attention in humans.

ACKNOWLEDGEMENTS

We gratefully acknowledge the advice of Mr. Richard Peto in all aspects of the study. Bruce Armstrong was supported by an F. A. Hadley Scholarship of the University of Western Australia and a National Health and Medical Research Council of Australia Clinical Sciences Fellowship in Epidemiology.

APPENDIX

Overall test of association (by Richard Peto)

Suppose we have a given $n \times m$ matrix z_{ij} (dietary data) and a random $m \times 1$ vector y_j (cancer rates) where the elements of y are mutually independent with variance v and fourth central moment $v^2 (3+k)$. Define $\bar{z}_i = \Sigma_{j=1}^m z_{ij}/m$, $ss_i = \Sigma_{j=1}^m (z_{ij}-\bar{z}_i)^2$ and p_{ck} (c, $k = 1, \ldots, m$) as $\Sigma_{i=1}^n (z_{ic}-\bar{z}_i)(z_{ik}-\bar{z}_i)/n.ss_i$. The regression coefficient b_i of y_j on z_{ij} is $\Sigma_{j=1}^m y_j (z_{ij}-\bar{z}_i)/ss_i$ and the variance, v_i, of b_i equals v/ss_i. The b_i will not in general be statistically independent of each other, and as a test of whether the set of b_is differ significantly from zero, the statistic $B^2 = \frac{1}{n} \Sigma^n_{i=1} b_i^2/v_i$ may be examined. It has exactly unit expectation, and its distribution may reasonably be approximated by the Γ-distribution with the same mean and variance. This is the F-test with $v_2 = \infty$, $v_1 = 2/\text{var}(B^2)$. $\text{var}(B^2)$ can be shown to equal $2\Sigma\Sigma p_{ck}^2 + k\Sigma p_{cc}^2$, which for our data is approximately $0.5+0.05k$, both for "all countries" and for the subset of countries with incidence data. We have therefore approximated the distribution of B^2 in our data by the distribution of $F_{4, \infty}$, and tests of significance based on this approximation are cited in Tables V-XI.

FACTEURS ÉCOLOGIQUES ET TAUX D'INCIDENCE ET DE MORTALITÉ DE CERTAINS CANCERS DANS DIVERS PAYS, PARTICULIÈREMENT DU POINT DE VUE DES HABITUDES ALIMENTAIRES

Les taux d'incidence de 27 types de cancer dans 23 pays et les taux de mortalité concernant 14 types de cancer dans 32 pays ont été mis en corrélation avec une large gamme de variables alimentaires et autres. On a constaté une corrélation très nette entre les variables alimentaires et plusieurs types de cancer, notamment entre la consommation de viande et le cancer du côlon et entre la consommation de graisses et les cancers du sein et du corps utérin. Les statistiques conduisent à penser que les facteurs alimentaires jouent peut-être un rôle dans le développement d'un certain nombre d'autres types de cancers. Les auteurs analysent l'utilité et les limites de la méthode.

REFERENCES

AKAZAKI, K., and STEMMERMAN, G. N., Comparative study of latent carcinoma of the prostate among Japanese in Japan and Hawaii. *J. nat. Cancer Inst.*, **50**, 1137-1144 (1973).

BEESE, D. H., (ed.), *Tobacco consumption in various countries*, Tobacco Research Council, Tobacco Research Paper 6, 3rd ed., Research Council, London (1972).

BENNINGTON, J. L., and LAUBSCHER, F. A., Epidemiologic studies on carcinoma of the kidney. I. Association of renal adenocarcinoma with smoking. *Cancer*, **21**, 1069-1071 (1968).

BURKITT, D. P., Epidemiology of cancer of the colon and rectum. *Cancer*, **28**, 3-13 (1971).

CARROLL, K. K., GAMMAL, E. B., and PLUNKETT, E. R., Dietary fat and mammary cancer. *Canad. med. Ass. J.*, **98**, 590-594 (1968).

CARTOGRAPHIC DEPARTMENT OF THE CLARENDON PRESS, *Oxford economic atlas of the world*, 4th ed., Oxford University Press, Oxford (1972).

CHAN, PO-C., and COHEN, L. A., Effect of dietary fat, antioestrogen and antiprolactin on the development of mammary tumours in rats. *J. nat. Cancer Inst.*, **52**, 25-30 (1974).

COLE, P., Coffee-drinking and cancer of the lower urinary tract. *Lancet*, **1**, 1335-1337 (1971).

COLE, P., MONSON, R. R., HANING, H., and FRIEDELL, G. H., Smoking and cancer of the lower urinary tract. *New Engl. J. Med.*, **284**, 129-134 (1971).

DE WAARD, F., and BAANDERS-VAN HALEWIJN, E. A., A prospective study in general practice of breast cancer risk in postmenopausal women. *Int. J. Cancer*, **14**, 153-160 (1974).

DOLL, R., The geographical distribution of cancer. *T. norske Laegoren*, **88**, 1160-1165 (1968).

DOLL, R., The age distribution of cancer: implications for models of carcinogenesis. *J. roy. stat. Soc.*, Series A, **134**, 133-155 (1971).

DOLL, R., and COOK, P., Summarizing indices for comparison of cancer incidence data. *Int. J. Cancer*, **2**, 269-279 (1967).

DRASAR, B. S., and HILL, M. J., Intestinal bacteria and cancer. *Amer. J. clin. Nutr.*, **25**, 1399-1404 (1972).

DRASAR, B. S., and IRVING, D., Environmental factors and cancer of the colon and breast. *Brit. J. Cancer*, **27**, 167-172 (1973).

FINNEY, D. J., Problems, data and inference. *J. roy. stat. Soc.*, Series B, **137**, 1-19 (1974).

FOOD AND AGRICULTURE ORGANIZATION OF THE UNITED NATIONS, *The world coffee economy*, F.A.O., Rome (1959).

FOOD AND AGRICULTURE ORGANIZATION OF THE UNITED NATIONS, *Tea trends and prospects. Commodity Bulletin Series*, F.A.O., Rome (1960).

FOOD AND AGRICULTURE ORGANIZATION OF THE UNITED NATIONS, *Production yearbook*, Vol. **24**, F.A.O., Rome (1971).

GRAHAM, S., SCHOTZ, W., and MARTINO, P., Alimentary factors in the epidemiology of gastric cancer. *Cancer*, **30**, 927-938 (1972).

GREGOR, O., TOMAN, R., and PRUSOVA, F., Gastrointestinal cancer and nutrition. *Gut*, **10**, 1031-1034 (1969).

HAENSZEL, W., BERG, J. W., SEGI, M., KURIHARA, M., and LOCKE, F. B., Large-bowel cancer in Haiwaiian Japanese. *J. nat. Cancer Inst.*, **51**, 1765-1779 (1973).

HAENSZEL, W., KURIHARA, M., SEGI, M., and LEE, R. K. C., Stomach cancer among Japanese in Hawaii. *J. nat. Cancer Inst.*, **49**, 969-988 (1972).

HAKAMA, M., and SAXÉN, E. A., Cereal consumption and gastric cancer. *Int. J. Cancer*, **2**, 265-268 (1967).

HIGGINSON, J., Aetiological factors in gastrointestinal cancer in man. *J. nat. Cancer Inst.*, **37**, 527-545 (1966).

LEA, A. J., Dietary factors associated with death-rates from certain neoplasms in man. *Lancet*, **2**, 332-333 (1966).

LIN, T. M., CHEN, K. B., and MACMAHON, B., Epidemiologic characteristics of cancer of the breast in Taiwan. *Cancer*, **27**, 1497-1504 (1971).

MACKAY, E. V., and KHOO, S. K., Altered carbohydrate metabolism and other constitutional stigmata and adenocarcinoma of the uterine body. *Med. J. Aust.*, **1**, 724-728 (1969).

MCLEAN, A. E. M., Diet and the chemical environment as modifiers of carcinogenesis. *In:* R. Doll and J. Vodopija (ed.), *Host environment interactions in the etiology of cancer in man*, p. 223-230, I.A.R.C., Lyons (1973).

MARKS, H. H., Influence of obesity on morbidity and mortality. *Bull. N.Y. Acad. Med.*, **36**, 296-312 (1960).

NIE, N. H., BENT, D. H., and HULL, C. H., *Statistical package for the social sciences*, McGraw Hill, New York (1970).

SEGI, M., and KURIHARA, M., *Cancer mortality for selected sites in 24 countries*, No. 5, Department of Public Health, Tohoku University School of Medicine, Sendai, Japan (1969).

SHENNAN, D. H., Renal carcinoma and coffee consumption in 16 countries. *Brit. J. Cancer*, **28**, 473-474 (1973).

STATISTICAL OFFICE OF THE UNITED NATIONS, *World energy supplies 1955-58*, Statistical papers series J, No. 3, United Nations Organization, New York (1960).

STATISTICAL OFFICE OF THE UNITED NATIONS, *Statistical yearbook 1969*, United Nations Organization, New York (1970).

STOCKS, P., On the relations between atmospheric pollution in urban and rural localities and mortality from cancer, bronchitis and pneumonia, with particular reference to 3:4 benzopyrene, beryllium, molybdenum, vanadium and arsenic. *Brit. J. Cancer*, **14**, 397-418 (1960).

STOCKS, P., Cancer mortality in relation to national consumption of cigarettes, solid fuel, tea and coffee. *Brit. J. Cancer*, **24**, 215-225 (1970).

TAKAHASHI, E., Coffee consumption and mortality for prostate cancer. *Tohoku J. exp. Med.*, **82**, 218-223 (1964).

TANNENBAUM, A., and SILVERSTONE, H., Nutrition and the genesis of tumours. *In:* R. W. Raven (ed.), *Cancer*, Vol. 1, p. 306-334, Butterworth & Co., London (1957).

UICC, *Cancer incidence in five continents*, Springer-Verlag, Berlin (1966).

UICC, *Cancer incidence in five continents*, Vol. II, Springer-Verlag, Berlin (1970).

WALLER, R. E., The combined effects of smoking and occupational or urban factors in relation to lung cancer. *Ann. occup. Hyg.*, **15**, 67-72 (1972).

WORLD HEALTH ORGANIZATION, *World Health Statistics Annual*, Vol. **1**, 1964, 1965 and 1966, WHO, Geneva (1967-1969).

WORLD HEALTH ORGANIZATION, *Mortality from malignant neoplasms 1955-65*, WHO, Geneva (1970).

WYNDER, E. L., KAJITANI, T., ISHIKAWA, S., DODO, H., and TAKANO, A., Environmental factors of cancer of the colon and rectum, II. Japanese epidemiological data. *Cancer*, **23**, 1210-1220 (1969).

WYNDER, E. L., and MABUCHI, K., Etiological and preventive aspects of human cancer. *Prev. Med.*, **1**, 300-334 (1972).

WYNDER, E. L., and SHIGEMATSU, T., Environmental factors of cancer of the colon and rectum. *Cancer*, **20**, 1520-1561 (1967).

The Role of Migrant Population in Studies of Selected Cancer Sites: A Review

by Janez Kmet, M.D.

International Agency for Research on Cancer
Lyon, France

INTRODUCTION

THIS paper does not pretend to be complete. The appraisal of study opportunities in cancer epidemiology connected with inter-country and intergroup variations in risk for selected cancer sites would be an enormous task requiring an entire volume. In addition to a brief review of findings from migrant population studies based mainly on Haenszel's papers, I propose to discuss and illustrate with a few examples some pertinent problems in the future strategy of cancer epidemiology.

A basic fact of cancer epidemiology is that all cancer sites show marked geographical variations presumably caused by differences in environmental characteristics. Observations on migrant populations are at best an indication, though not very precise, of existing environmental differences, which may be used in formulating working hypotheses on the etiology of specific cancer sites.

In his review of cancer mortality among the foreign-born in the United States, Haenszel stated, "It is surprising how little analysis of mortality by country of birth of the decedent has been attempted in the United States, the destination of one of the greatest population movements of modern times." [1]. It is not less surprising that so many years after Haenszel said this, how little interest has been shown in utilizing the interesting opportunities provided by the findings of migrant studies—to deepen the research into the detailed environmental characteristics of the countries of origin. I would like to stress this because a weak point in most migrant studies is the fact that migrants only were studied and the populations in the countries of origin excluded. It is obvious that migrants have taken with them to the new country only their genetic background and social characteristics, such as dietary and other habits and customs, leaving behind the environment in the broadest sense of the word, which we would probably all agree, has determined the cancer patterns in specific areas. Other weak points often mentioned include the selective factors of economic, political and other nature, that determine the composition of migrants and make them less representative of the original population in the old country. It would not be surprising, therefore, if the working hypotheses raised under such circumstances prove to be neither numerous nor very productive.

Migrants in their new environment are often referred to as Nature's unplanned experiment, but there is a basic difference to be taken into account. In an experiment we should know the precise conditions over the entire time period, but in migrant studies the first part of the experiment, the stay in the old country, was practically out of our reach and the second part of the experiment, the period of stay in the new country, usually involved conditions in a highly civilized environment that are so complex as to defy complete understanding. Migrants who move for economic reasons go as a rule from under-developed to highly-developed areas.

To illustrate the onesidedness of recent efforts in this field one may refer to the tragic and heroic history of the Jewish people. Ailon Shiloh [2] describing the happenings after the Diaspora concluded: "Two millenia later, when an independent Israel was able to welcome these Jews home, it was realized that they possessed striking differences in physical make-up, language, dress, diet, health and ill-health behaviour, and numerous other cultural manifestations acquired and developed during the centuries of the Diaspora." In epidemiological language this means that Jewish immigrants from different parts of the world brought with them a reflection, but unfortunately no more than a reflection, of the environmental conditions in the countries where they spent so many centuries. To exaggerate only slightly, in studies of Jews from Morocco in Israel every effort should be made to study simultaneously the environment of the Berber population in the Atlas mountains. The fear of great expense involved in such studies should not inhibit in advance efforts along these lines. Nobody has yet placed on the scale the costs and returns for the different disciplines in cancer research. The studies proposed should be judged on their merits by the same criteria applied to other areas of cancer research.

SELECTED CANCER SITES

Oral cavity

Findings on oral cavity, unlike those on stomach, esophagus and large intestine, have not been very provocative. Haenszel [1] in his analysis of cancer mortality among foreign-born in the United States, considered high oral cancer rates in Irish migrants and low rates in persons from USSR to be consistent with the association between this site and excess consumption of alcohol, the evidence for which includes the higher risks for persons engaged in the alcoholic beverage trade. In this connection he quotes Davis [3] who was impressed by the extremely high mortality from alcoholism among Irish in Boston. The low risk among migrants from USSR reflected the very large Jewish component among the Russian-born in the United States and the finding agreed with MacMahon's data [4] on the low risk of oral cancer among Jews.

Haenszel [1] further comments on the low male and high female risk for oral and pharyngeal cancer in Swedish migrants and points to the parallel situation in Sweden where an apparent association of buccal and pharyngeal cancer in women with Plummer–Vinson disease has been observed [5, 6].

Esophagus

One of the most prominent epidemiologic features of esophageal cancer has been the extreme variability in sex ratio apparent in both incidence and mortality data [7]. Haenszel [1] found this characteristic to be present in the U.S. migrant populations. All the foreign-born males in Haenszel's material had substantially greater rates for esophageal cancer than native whites, with the highest values noted for males from Poland, Czechoslovakia and Ireland. The pattern in females was quite different, with women from USSR having much the highest rates. In addition, migrants from Czechoslovakia and Ireland displayed high rates in both sexes. The Irish experience agreed with the Boston findings for buccal cavity and esophagus described earlier by

Lombard and Doering [8]. Both sources reported high rates for Russian women. Haenszel further comments on the low male–female ratio observed in Finland [9, 10] and discusses the possibility that similar relationships may exist in other East European countries. The depressed sex ratio for esophagus death rates in Israel [11] he considers to be consistent with the U.S. observations on Jews, who were also heavily represented among migrants from USSR.

Staszewski and Haenszel [12] in their study of cancer among Polish-born in the United States found no remarkable difference in age-specific mortality for cancer of the esophagus between U.S. native whites and native Poles for either sex, but did observe a strikingly higher mortality at all ages for male migrants, whose rates were more than double those of the sedentes of the two countries. Haenszel and Kurihara [13] in their U.S.–Japanese migrant study, also found that Issei males over 65, experienced higher mortality from cancer of the esophagus than either home or host populations of comparable age, a pattern not reproduced in the data for females; the Japanese results thus appear to be consistent with observations on migrants from Poland and other European countries reported by earlier studies [14, 15]. The high Issei risks have not carried over to Nisei males under 65, whose experience resembled that of white males. One may expect therefore, that Nisei males will continue to experience risks below those established for Japan and Issei males.

Wynder *et al* [16] have suggested that alcohol has a role in cancer of the esophagus; Haenszel considers that the findings in migrants point in the same direction and notes in this connection that the site distribution of excess risk among the Irish in cancer of the buccal cavity, esophagus, intestine and rectum, but not stomach to the same degree, precisely parallels that found in persons employed in alcoholic beverage trade [17].

In South Africa, Dean [18] observed cancer of the esophagus to be more common among native white males than among white immigrants or in England and Wales, the country of origin for the most of the immigrants. Kallner [19] from material based on the Cancer Registry in Israel found her figures on esophageal cancer to be very low, and the results therefore "erratic", but the rates for Yemenites were extraordinarily high, and there was an indication of high rates for persons migrating from Iran. Similar findings have been reported by Steinitz [20].

Stomach

Haenszel in his classic migrant study [1] has shown the stomach cancer rates in all ethnic groups studied in the U.S. to be well above those for native whites. A close sex correspondence in rankings by country of origin indicated that the relatively stable sex ratio for this site known to hold in a wide variety of populations [21] irrespective of the absolute magnitude of the incidence and mortality rates, prevailed here as well. The highest risks were recorded for migrants from Poland, Czechoslovakia, Norway and USSR. While the Irish had above-average risks, they did not stand out in this respect as for other sites within the digestive tract. The rates for Italians for both sexes were comparatively low. Comparing his results with data available from the countries of origin, Haenszel found the migrant experience to resemble that of the parent population. It may be noted that the results for Jews in the United States did not reflect the low rates in the Israeli population. Haenszel did not comment on this point, but the underlying reason for the relatively low stomach cancer rates in Israel is probably the high proportion of its population that has come from low stomach cancer risk areas.

The ranking by ethnic groups as estimated by Haenszel, would support the impression of greater risk in countries in the more northern latitudes. Commenting on the lowest risk found for the southernmost country, Italy, Haenszel did not mention the likelihood that the bulk of migrants from Italy were Sicilians and others from the extreme South, where stomach cancer rates are relatively low [22].

Haenszel further found that regional variation in urban–rural ratios for this disease within the United States can be resolved by control for nativity; when this is done a picture of minimal urban–rural differences in risk emerges. Changes in the nativity composition of the population, with continued diminution of the foreign-born at ages over 40 when stomach cancer becomes a more frequent disease, has also contributed to the rapid decline of stomach cancer mortality in the United States during the past three decades.

Staszewski and Haenszel [14] confirmed anew the fact that stomach cancer mortality among Polish migrants of both sexes tends to approximate the rates in the home country. The risks among Polish migrants exceeded by a substantial margin those for U.S. whites and the authors are sure that for stomach cancer, rates for migrants are closely connected with mortality prevailing in Poland. They feel the collective evidence suggests that persons leaving areas of high stomach cancer risk continue to display high rates for this site, little modified by the changes introduced in the new country and that the persistence of characteristic dietary customs and habits among migrants in the United States might be one of the factors responsible for this situation.

Haenszel and Kurihara [16] in their U.S.–Japanese migrant study found that the Issei experience coincided with other U.S. migrant groups in indicating that stomach cancer mortality relates better to country of origin than to country of destination. Nisei rates while lower than those prevailing in Japan, still exceeded those of the U.S. whites. Since the projections of mortality in early adult life are usually a reliable guide to the subsequent stomach cancer experience of a cohort, Haenszel and Kurihara believe that extrapolation of the Nisei curves suggests that the Nisei males will maintain lower rates than the Issei, an observation in agreement with Buell and Dunn's findings in California [23].

Prudente and Mirra in their study of Japanese migrants in the State of Sao Paulo, where most of the Japanese migrants to Brazil are concentrated, found support for their belief that stomach cancer rates for Japanese in Brazil closely resemble those in Japan. Only Japanese born in Japan were considered by them and observations on Japanese born in Brazil remain to be undertaken [24].

Smith [25–27] has published several papers on cancer mortality among minor racial groups within the United States and Hawaii. Stomach cancer was not uniformly high among Orientals and the mortality was considerably greater among Japanese and Hawaiians than among Chinese and Filipinos. Quisenberry in his studies of ethnic differences in cancer in Hawaii [28, 29] also reported cancer of the stomach to occur more frequently in Japanese than in any other ethnic group. Quisenberry feels that rates for Hawaiian males may be substantially increased in recent years, while those for Japanese remained stable and for Caucasians decreased somewhat. Among females there appears to be relatively little change, though the Caucasian rates have dropped a little. As to the possible role of diet in stomach cancer etiology, Quisenberry remarked that many Orientals in Hawaii, especially older people, eat diets peculiar to their own ethnic groups, a practice probably more pronounced among Japanese who consume large amounts of rice. Since it has been shown that people who eat a high carbohydrate diet need a vitamin B intake higher than average [30], Quisenberry believes that this may be a relevant factor. Other items of interest include hot tea, hot sake and several pickled vegetables. The food contains little animal protein other than fish and is unusually low in dairy products. Shoyu sauce and miso soup, which are made from soy beans fermented with the aid of a fungus, *Aspergillus oryzae*, are often eaten. Quisenberry further noted that a high percentage of Hawaiian food is composed of carbohydrates and is relatively low in protein. A principal source of carbohydrates is poi made from the root of the taro plant.

Tulchinsky and Modan in their study of gastric cancer in Israel [31] observed considerable differences among migrants from a number of European countries as well as between European and African countries. Incidence among persons coming from Poland and Russia was only intermediate whereas the North African State of Morocco was in third place after Rumania and Germany. On the other hand, the incidence was low in immigrants from all Asian countries, particularly Iraq and Yemen, as well as among Israeli-born residents. The authors stress the limitations of their observations due to the small numbers of patients involved. Calculating the mean annual incidence rates according to time of immigration to Israel, they found in all categories—each continent of origin and each age group—that the incidence was higher among the "new" immigrants (arriving after 1952). Tulchinsky and Modan considered their major analytical difficulties to be the lack of comparative incidence data from Eastern Europe, North Africa and the Near East, which are either scarce or missing. The frequent changes in geopolitical maps of Europe during the present century was another problem. Tulchinsky and Modan stress particularly the high stomach cancer incidence observed in Jews from Morocco "a country that constitutes a sizeable proportion of the so-called Oriental population." The authors did not mention that part of the Moroccan Jews originated in the Berber country of the Atlas Mountains.

In Kallner's material from Israel [19], Morocco appears at the bottom of the list, next to Iraq, the country with the lowest rate. The contradictory data represent one of those difficult instances in migrant studies that remain to be resolved.

Dean [15] found higher rates for stomach cancer in South African-born white men than in England and Wales. British male immigrants have shown only about 60 per cent of the rates typical for South African-born white males. For female immigrants the corresponding figure was 59.

Large intestine and rectum

Haenszel and Dawson [32] in their study of the mortality from cancer of the rectum and colon in the United States drew attention to a new point. By cross-classifying current residence with place of birth the colon and rectum cancer experienced for persons migrating within the U.S. could be demonstrated to conform more closely to the risk characteristic of the most recent residence than of place of birth. The probability that risk for cancer of the colon and rectum might be conditioned more by events associated with current residence than by earlier experience had already been suggested by earlier studies of migrants to the United States [1]. In 12 ethnic groups studied, mortality for these sites generally approached that recorded for U.S. native whites and migrants from 4 countries—Italy, Norway, Poland and USSR—had rates more characteristic of the United States than of their original countries.

Staszewski and Haenszel [14] also noted that mortality from colon and rectum among Polish migrants deviated sharply from the experience in Poland and the risks were more closer aligned to those prevailing in the U.S. Given the pattern of regional variation in the United States [33], part of the excess rate for Polish migrants may be attributed to their concentration in the high-risk North East and North Central States. These findings differ from the pattern for stomach cancer, where nearly all foreign-born groups experienced higher risks than U.S. native whites, and which tended to approximate those in country of origin. The findings differ also from the typical pattern for esophageal cancer in which migrants displayed risks higher than for either home or host country.

Haenszel and Dawson found no relationship between level of risk and site localization similar to that for countries of high incidence of cancer of the large bowel, where lesions appear predominantly in the left side of the colon and in the rectum [34]. On the contrary, their data indicated the differences in risk to be reflected throughout the intestinal tract and not concentrated at certain anatomical sites. The authors feel that further inquiry into intergroup differences according to localization within the colon and rectum are indicated for the foreign-born and other groups within the United States. They also stressed the importance of studying populations known to have high gastric cancer risk and low risks for large intestine and rectum, like the American Indians, Japanese, Norwegians, Poles, etc. Discussing the theoretical implications, the authors feel that the migrant findings argue against host factors as an important determinant in risks for colon and rectum. The strong effects linked with current residence seem not to be in accord with prevailing concepts on the role of prolonged exposure in tumor induction and a long latent period between carcinogenic stimulus and response. Such concepts would fit more closely the picture for stomach cancer.

Haenszel and Kuruhara in their U.S.–Japanese study [16] reported that the curves depicting mortality by age for cancer of the intestine among Issei and Nisei males have risen to approach that for white males and that a similar, although smaller, translation has also occurred in females. The Japanese experience for colon was deemed consistent with observations on other migrant populations, although quantitatively the Issei had not made as complete a transition within one generation a migrants from Norway and Poland. The Nisei experience, while inconclusive, suggests that the displacement to higher risk continues in the second-generation Japanese. The authors comment on Stemmermann's discovery of clinically unsuspected cancer of large intestine in about 3½ per cent of Japanese patients over 70 autopsied in a Honolulu hospital [35]. Stemmermann believes that "careful autopsy study of the large intestine in all Japanese dying after 70 might double the yield of new tumors in this age group". The migrant effect for this site may then have been partially expressed late in life as small, asymptomatic tumors.

According to Haenszel and Kurihara [16], the U.S.–Japan differential has never been marked for cancer of the rectum. They had therefore not expected any changes among the Japanese migrants and their material confirmed this point. They comment further on the distribution within the intestinal tract in Japan where the colon cancer death rate is about 70 per cent of that for rectum cancer, a feature quite different from other countries where a colon–rectum ratio of less than unity has not been observed. Although the Japanese findings might represent a reporting and classification artifact, the authors believe that their migrant materials favor a true difference in distribution within the intestinal tract between whites and Japanese, since the colon–rectum ratios for Issei and Nisei combined remained well below the norm for whites. In this respect the Japanese and Polish migrants differ; the Poles show a substantial rise for both colon and rectum over the low rates recorded in Poland in contrast to the selective effects within the intestinal tract for the Japanese. Haenszel and Kurihara stress the need for detailed classification of rectum and colon cancer in morbidity and mortality reports and its significance for epidemiological research.

Dunn [36] recently presented age-standardized mortality rates from cancer of the large bowel and stomach cancer among Japanese living in California, that update previous findings by Buell and Dunn [23]. A marked decline in stomach cancer and a sharp increase in colon cancer for the U.S.-born Japanese was evident.

Kallner [19] in Israel found an excessive Occidental (country of origin) preponderance for cancer of the colon and even more so for cancer of the rectum, the difference however being reduced between 1950–1954 and 1958–1961.

Pancreas

Haenszel [1] found mortality from cancer of the pancreas to be slightly greater among foreign-born whites than among U.S. native-born, but considered the quality of data to be inadequate for definite statements, since cancer of the pancreas presents great diagnostic difficulties. He singled out USSR migrants as possibly having above-average rates, which corresponds with MacMahon's finding [4] of higher rates of pancreas cancer in Jews of both sexes in New York City.

The fact that the mortality in the United States for whites and nonwhites was among the highest recorded anywhere [11] may mean only that pancreatic cancer is diagnosed more frequently in the United States than elsewhere.

Bladder

Haenszel [1] found the results for bladder cancer in the foreign-born in the United States "most provocative". Males displayed minimum ethnic group variability, a not unexpected result since no substantial differences among the countries concerned in exposures to known carcinogens were suspected. Among women the results were quite different with substantially lower rates found in several migrant ethnic groups. No explanation was attempted by Haenszel.

Prostate

Haenszel found no striking departure from the native white experience in ethnic group distribution of prostatic cancer in the United States [1] and the variations were regarded as only suggestive. The use of mortality, rather than incidence data, may have some advantage for this site, since the former presumably represent clinically active cases and not merely lesions uncovered by histologic examination of operative specimens. The low risk for migrants from USSR may warrant investigation, since New York City data [4] pinpointed a low Jewish risk for this site, and the low risk for Italian migrants may be placed in the same category. Internationally, Italy and Israel have the lowest rates [11].

Staszewski and Haenszel [14] later reported prostatic cancer mortality to be exceptionally low in Poland, Japan being the only country with a lower rate. This site, a disease of older men on whom statistical information is not very reliable, was reported with less than average frequency among older Polish migrants in the United States, an observation in agreement with the data from Poland. Haenszel and Kurihara [16] found the upward displacement in risk for prostatic carcinoma among Japanese migrants to be in line with the experience of Polish migrants, the only other group studied for whom the rate observed in the country of origin deviated greatly from that in the United States. The U.S.–Japanese mortality ratios are effectively determined by the experience at ages 65–74 and 75 and over, but review of the age-specific rates showed that the rise in mortality among Issei males is evident before age 75. Any rise in prostatic cancer among Japanese migrants not attributable to diagnostic artifacts might be the male counterpart of changes noted for corpus uteri and ovary.

Discussing these findings Haenszel says that the variation in risk for prostate within the U.S. was not overly impressive and was more reminiscent of that noted for breast, ovary, intestines, and rectum than for esophagus, stomach and lung. Since evidence for environmental effects is lacking, no occupational exposure has been incriminated [37] and the urban–rural and geographic variations are relatively modest [11, 38], Haenszel was not inclined to consider that exogenous factors played an important role in this site. He did raise the possibility that the pronounced variations in risk among whites, Negroes and Orientals might "reflect in a more dilute form effects of endogenous factors governing the racial distribution of prostatic cancer".

Ovary

Haenszel [1] was unable to demonstrate striking departures from the native white experience in ovarian cancer risk for the migrant groups in the United States. The only statistically significant difference was the higher mortality for women from Italy, but Italy has rates much lower than those typical for other West European countries [11].

Haenszel and Kurihara observed that mortality from ovarian tumors has risen among Japanese migrants and their descendants [13]. They noted that in all populations studied the risks for ovary, corpus and breast cancer tend to be closely correlated and to exhibit similar types of change among migrant populations. The Japanese migrants followed the usual pattern for ovary and corpus. This conformity, they feel, underscores still more the deviant behavior of breast cancer, which had *not* risen among the Japanese migrants.

Dean [15] found cancer of the ovary to be less common in South Africa than in England and Wales or in immigrants from the United Kingdom. However, he believes that factors responsible could be obscured by differences in diagnostic practices. Steinitz [20] described a large difference among the morbidity rates in Israel, where Jewesses from Middle and Eastern Europe have rather high morbidity. She too, considered the findings not very reliable in view of the uncertainties in diagnostic criteria. Kallner [19] remained impressed by the extreme Occidental preponderance in ovarian cancer in Israel, since it ranked first in this respect among all sites in her mortality and morbidity material.

Breast

In Haenszel's study [1] the native white breast cancer mortality was in line with the highest foreign-born rates. The differences among native whites and migrants from Canada, the British Isles and several West European countries were trivial. Substantially reduced risks were found among women from Italy and Poland and confirmed previous findings in Boston [8]. The mortality for Italian migrants was thought to agree with the situation in Italy [11]. Haenszel feels that the low rates for Mexican women were consistent with Steiner's Los Angeles autopsy series [39], and with observations on the American Indians [41].

In discussing his materials, Haenszel commented on Clemmesen's findings of a drop in breast cancer incidence between ages 45–49 and 50–54 with resumption of an upward trend at older ages [42], a finding later confirmed by similar data from England, Norway and the United States [42–44]. He noted Dorn and Cutler's inability to confirm completely Clemmesen's findings; when Haenszel re-examined their data from the U.S. in light of the nativity contrasts, he found that the menopausal break in incidence rates was pronounced in populations with a substantial foreign-born component and virtually absent in Iowa where the number of foreign-born was negligible. The question remains why the menopausal break should be more pronounced in the migrants and some ethnic groups in Europe than in U.S. native whites.

Staszewski and Haenszel [14] found a sharp contrast in breast cancer experience between U.S. native whites and females in Poland, and among migrants from Poland mortality from this site at ages over 35 substantially exceeded that for urban or rural Poland. So far as contrasts with U.S. native whites were concerned, the differential was negligible between ages 35 and 65, but thereafter the risks rose more sharply among native whites. A similar concordance up to age 55 between migrants from Italy and native whites has been found. The open question posed by Haenszel is: does the age curve for Polish migrants represent a cohort effect linked with time of migration, differences in composition of the migrant population at older ages, changes in breast-feeding practices or other ethnic group characteristics.

Quisenberry [27] estimated the rates of breast cancer for Japanese women over 55 in Hawaii to be lower than for younger women, which he thinks might be linked with the former breast-feeding practices of older Japanese women. When comparing rates for 1960–1962 with 1947–1954, he found some increase in all racial groups, but greatest among Japanese and least among Caucasians. However, the rank order did not change and the increases were much less marked than for such sites as lung and bronchus.

Haenszel and Kurihara [16] have stressed the failure of breast cancer rates in Japanese migrants to approach those of the host population at any point in the lifespan, although minor differences between Issei and Nisei women were indicated by review of age-specific rates. They found the slope of the curves for U.S. Japanese after the age of 50 less steep than for white women. The slower rate of increase after menopause was very pronounced in Japan and this feature has been retained in the migrant experience. The authors suggest that risks among Nisei females have stabilized and that further drift to the host population level is not assured. Although comparable data on descendants of migrants from Europe are not available, Haenszel and Kurihara feel that the Nisei experience will probably not be reproduced in the other ethnic groups available for study. The persistent low breast cancer rates among the second generation Nisei would suggest a role of genetic factors, and the rarity of male breast cancer in Japan is noteworthy in this connection. It is of utmost interest that the Japanese migrant findings for other cancer sites agree qualitatively in their site-specific nature with those for other groups migrating to the United States.

Kallner [19] found for both mortality and morbidity from breast cancer in Israel, a definite and typical excess risk for newcomers.

Dean [15] found no striking differences in breast cancer experience between South Africa, England and Wales, and immigrants from the United Kingdom and elsewhere to South Africa, although breast cancer was less common as a cause of death in South Africa than in England and Wales. This disease was relatively uncommon in the Colored, Asian and Bantu populations.

Uterus

A basic, often-mentioned difficulty in migrant studies on uterine cancer experience is the imprecise statement on localization within the uterus; cervix and corpus cancer must therefore be discussed together.

Haenszel [1] found the low USSR and high Mexican rates for cervical cancer to be prominent features of the U.S. foreign-born experience and also pointed out the possible below average cervical cancer risk among Italian migrants. The low Russian values reflect the known low incidence of cervical cancer in Jews, while the high Mexican rates appear consistent with the high risks among American Indians [41]. The apparent low risk for cervix in Italian migrants is an anomaly that does not correspond well with the Italian vital statistics [11].

Staszewski and Haenszel [14] comment on the variable ratio of cervix to corpus cancer, which in case report material ranges from 5–8:1 in Poland [45] to about 2:1 for U.S. white females [43]. They believe that part, but not all, of this difference can be ascribed to the younger age composition of the population in Poland, since cervical cancer is seen frequently in women under age 50. Death certificates in Poland did not distinguish as a rule between cervix and corpus cancer but based on indirect evidence from case reports, the authors are convinced that deaths ascribed to uterine cancer are predominantly cervical cancer. They felt that corpus cancer rates were probably higher among migrants than in Poland, although the degree of displacement was uncertain, and for this inference relied on the substantially higher overall uterine cancer mortality among female migrants compared to that reported in Poland. There was an apparent parallel upturn in risk for breast and endometrial cancer among Polish migrants, but the inverse relationship between cancer of the breast and of the cervix, which apparently holds true within Poland and has been observed to prevail in other populations, seems not to have persisted among women migrating to the United States.

Haenszel and Kurihara [16] described a downward displacement in cervical cancer mortality among U.S. Japanese females. For most ages their risks remained well below Japan; only at ages over 75 did the experience of migrants and the population of origin correspond closely. The authors emphasize that high mortality from uterine cancer recorded in Japan is due to cervix, localizations elsewhere in the uterus are uncommon.

Steinitz [20] found low rates for cervical cancer in Israel. Corpus cancer was reported to be more common in groups with low cervical cancer risk. Yemenites were at the bottom of the list for both sites. Kallner [19] believes in Israel that the diagnosis of cervical cancer has often been influenced by "the absence of more intimate knowledge of the case or—possibly—owing to a preconceived idea that Jewish women do not usually have cervical cancer. Therefore, the figures obtained for cervix must actually be accepted as minimum figures . . ."

Dean [15] found cancer of the uterus to be more common in the South African-born women than in immigrants from England and Wales, but had difficulty in distinguishing between cervix and corpus cancer in the statistical material. Oettle [46] reported African white women to follow the pattern of westernized nations with, however, a slightly higher death rate from cancer of the cervix and the body of the uterus. The "Colored" and Bantus have a very high mortality from cancer of the cervix, as high as Negroes in the United States, although they have a low death rate for corpus cancer.

Lung and bronchus

Haenszel [1] found the migrants from countries that experience higher or lower lung cancer rates than the U.S. to exhibit a typical displacement in risk toward a position intermediate between home and host countries. This would suggest a role for environmental exposures early in life as an important determinant for the subsequent lung cancer experience. The U.S. data on lung cancer for migrants from England agrees with reports from New Zealand [47] and South Africa [48]. Haenszel had no specific information on age of entry or duration of residence in the United States and unable to expand on Eastcott's finding of a smaller deviation from the experience in England among persons migrating after the age of 30. Haenszel feels that the ethnic group data might be regarded as consistent with the universally observed urban–rural differences in the sense that both suggest still unidentified environmental factors other than cigarette smoking.

Staszewski and Haenszel [14] in their paper on cancer in Polish-born in the United States indicated the experience of Polish migrants to be an exception to the usual pattern of displacement to an intermediate position. The very high lung cancer risks in the U.S. corresponded much more closely to the pattern presented by esophagus and larynx in which the high rates for male migrants overshadowed those in both home and host countries.

Haenszel and Kurihara [16] found high lung cancer rates among Issei males and females over the age of 65 in the United States. They feel that since the fine-cut tobacco required for Japanese pipes was not obtainable in the United States, the adoption of cigarette smoking by male migrants was probably accelerated by migration. Haenszel and Kurihara were inclined to believe after examination of the age-specific mortality curves that future Nisei cohorts will not experience higher risks than Issei. The higher Issei rates could be the result of more intensive exposure to cigarettes, and to other risks which persons moving from farm to city may be subject; similar elevated risks of lung cancer among persons moving from farm to city have been reported within the United States. Polish migrants to the United States include many from rural areas and they have also experienced much higher risks than their counterparts in the home country [14].

Quisenberry [27] found that Japanese men and women in Hawaii had a considerably lower incidence of lung cancer than Caucasians and Hawaiians as of 1947–1954. The overall rates observed in 1960–1963 were more than double and the increase was greatest among Hawaiians and least for Caucasians. The steeper increase in Hawaiians and Japanese was probably due to more recent changes in cigarette smoking habits.

Steinitz [20] and Kallner [19] both comment on the relatively high lung cancer rates in some Jewish groups in Israel, and also on the extremely low rates for Yemenites, but Steinitz does not believe that a satisfactory explanation can be advanced without a thorough study of smoking habits.

Leukemia

A firmly-established feature in Haenszel's U.S. foreign-born study [1] was an excess risk for leukemia in male and female migrants from USSR, which was in agreement with the earlier findings of high mortality from this disease among Jews in New York City [4]. In another study in the same city MacMahon and Koller noted that the excess among Jews was manifest in each of three common varieties: acute myeloid, chronic myeloid, and chronic lymphatic. The high USSR risk in the United States seems consistent with the elevated leukemia mortality recorded in Israel, particularly for females.

Haenszel thought that the above-average mortality for leukemia among USSR migrants might tie in with reports of greater exposure of Jews to diagnostic and therapeutic radiation which is considered to be luekemogenic [49, 50]. Exception for the USSR group and the low-risk Mexicans, the range of ethnic group variation in his material was small and did not suggest the operation of other environmental factors that would discriminate among ethnic groups.

Jim [51] found in his series of 134 cases of leukemia in Hawaii a predominance of chronic myeloid leukemia in Filipinos. In general, leukemia occurred with about the same frequency in the Japanese, Filipinos and Caucasians, and with somewhat higher frequency in Chinese.

Haenszel and Kurihara [16] feel that their summary ratios indicating higher leukemia mortality among the U.S. Japanese than in Japan reflected the experience of older age groups. The low mortality from leukemia among older persons in Japan ascribed to the infrequent appearance of chronic lymphatic leukemia could be an artifact due to underdiagnosis of leukemia in older persons and they suspect that the observed increment in Issei risk might represent better diagnosis of the disease in the United States. The recently observed risk of leukemia in Japan for persons over 55 would support this view.

Lymphomas

In Haenszel's foreign-born study [1], three migrant groups from USSR, Poland and Austria, have shown above-average lymphoma risks. MacMahon's findings in Brooklyn [52] have revealed a Jewish excess in all lymphoma categories (Hodgkin's disease, lymphosarcoma, reticulum cell sarcoma, multiple myeloma; since excess risks for USSR migrants and Jews persisted within all the major subtypes of leukemia, it is perhaps not surprising that the same phenomenon for USSR migrants carried over to the several lymphoma categories as well.

Haenszel and Kurihara [16] found that unlike leukemia, the differences between Japan and U.S. whites in mortality from lymphomas and related diseases persisted at all ages—the rates being low for Japanese.

DISCUSSION

Attention has been drawn to one important aspect of epidemiological research on migrant populations, broad environmental research in the countries of origin, which has not been properly exploited. The lack of such information represents a serious handicap in the conduct of future migrant studies, and to epidemiological research in general.

Little is known of the mechanisms through which environment determines particular cancer-site patterns in different parts of the world. Epidemiology has provided the key to identification and elimination of many industrial carcinogens, and has been successful in resolving the smoking-lung cancer issue, in large measure because cigarette smoking represented a dominant single factor. The latter situation represents the exception, rather than the rule, in cancer epidemiology. However, neither industrial carcinogens nor cigarette smoking are the full answer to questions of cancer etiology. Industrial carcinogens represent just a part of the etiological complex for the sites affected and smoking does not completely determine the lung cancer pattern. Additional factors in our environment obviously contribute to the final outcome of the complex process called by some "cancerization of the tissue."

Migrant populations take with them a reflection of the environment of their countries of origin. Moving mostly from less- to more highly-developed areas, they have entered very complex environments where it is difficult, if not impossible, to investigate the relationship between specific factors and a specific disease. The observational situation remains more favorable in areas where the conditions of life have not yet lost their "natural" character and where one may have a better opportunity to identify mechanisms for relationships between 'the soil' in the broadest sense of this work, and the human organism. Understanding of the extrinsic factors and their interactions with intrinsic population characteristics, that produce in a group of people precancerous conditions, which in individuals either disappear or change into full-blown cancer, may open new avenues. Migrant studies are particularly valuable in indicating areas and populations of special importance for individual cancer sites.

It has been repeatedly stressed that migrant groups are as a rule not completely representative of populations in the countries of origin. Furthermore, countries of origin are sometimes hard to establish because of political changes and it is often difficult to pinpoint areas where migrant groups have spent part of their lives en route to their final destination, e.g. movement of Jewish groups inside Europe prior to arrival in Israel. But the much more serious problem is the identification of detailed places in the old country where the migrants originated. Peculiarities in detailed geographical distribution of individual cancer sites require analysis of materials by geographical sub-regions. National rates are often meaningless and do not convey any information on the sometimes substantial differences in distribution of risks for individual cancer sites within a country. To take an extreme example, interpretation of cancer data for Yugoslav migrants requires that we know that persons migrating to Canada and the United States came mostly from the former Austrian provinces, particularly westernmost Slovenia and the Adriatic coast and islands, whereas migrants to Turkey were exclusively members of the Turkish minority from the former Turkish provinces in Macedonia. Those migrating to West Germany were Germans forced to leave the country after World War II and the group moving recently to Australia was a mixture of political refugees from all parts of the country.

To place migrant studies in the context of other ongoing work, I will draw on examples from cancer of the oral cavity, esophagus and stomach, which are familiar to me from my recent field studies.

In oral cancer we are not dependent on migrant studies for the discovery of new working hypotheses. From existing knowledge we can plan rather precise field studies in strategic localities. First, chewing habits are known to be closely related with disease incidence; a site and dose relationship between several ingredients in the quid and the subsequent oral lesions has also been demonstrated. Second, in Central and Southeast Asia high incidence areas have been defined, where local site-specific patterns correspond well with local chewing habits. In addition, areas of low incidence have been identified, where wide-spread chewing habits do not cause much apparent harm to the population (Afghanistan) in contrast to other areas with identical habits (Bihar, India). Third, oral inspection with subsequent cytological and histological examination represents a precise diagnostic tool easily applied to study populations. We are thus faced with a peculiar situation in oral cancer, that may have implications for future migrant studies. If different risks despite similar chewing habits are confirmed by current detailed studies in India and Afghanistan, the presence of important environmental factors other than chewing will be further corroborated. The situation is not unique to oral cancer and is reminiscent of lung cancer, for which evidence from migrant studies has suggested that differences in risk among populations cannot be ascribed solely to differences in smoking habits. Under the less sophisticated conditions of Northern India and Afghanistan, it may be easier to identify those additional environmental factors that are determining the different outcomes of interaction between oral mucosa and the tobacco and lime contained in the Khaini and nasswar mixtures.

In esophageal cancer, on the other hand, no profitable working hypotheses have been advanced which would enable us to understand better its etiology. Alcohol and tobacco are only part of the etiological complex and can not account for some very high incidence areas, as in parts of Iran. Fortunately, in esophageal cancer a feature has been identified, more promising than could have been anticipated from the current migrant study results—sharp borderlines between high- and low-incidence areas in such countries as Iran, Soviet Central Asia, Kenya and South Africa. These sharp borderlines seem to be typical for esophageal cancer, together with extremely large differences in incidence rates among several countries. This situation has stimulated broad environmental studies of the physical, biotic and cultural characteristics in several areas simultaneously to seek differences of potential etiological significance.

As to the possible relationship between 'soil' and esophageal cancer, speculations have been raised to the effect that zinc deficiency might affect esophageal physiology in humans as it does in experimental animals. In Iran zinc deficiency has been shown to be one of the causes of dwarfism, hypogonadism, hepatosplenomegaly and iron deficiency anemia, and patients have dramatically improved following administration of therapeutic doses of zinc. If additional findings support such theories, new and promising lines of research will be opened, departing somewhat from the conventional concepts on the role of extrinsic carcinogenic substances. The different trends observed for cancers of the stomach and the large intestine in migrant populations may point in the same direction, cancer of the large intestine presumably having more direct and immediate links with environmental factors than stomach cancer.

The study of detailed geographical features might be of great help in stomach cancer; this site has pronounced geographical characteristics, being generally more common in the countries distant from the Equator as well as in the mountainous areas of the world. Haenszel has shown very low stomach cancer rates for Italians in the United States. Such data are not in agreement with the vital statistics information that indicate stomach cancer mortality to vary substantially within Italy, being high in the North and low in the South. The findings would therefore suggest, and this is consistent with other evidence, that the bulk of Italian immigrants came from Southern Italy including Sicily. Priority for investigations in Southern Italy is the logical consequence of such findings, and it might well turn out that differences in diet will not emerge as the most profitable working hypothesis and that deeper environmental studies will be the obvious choice, A probable first step would be detailed studies of differences in gastric physiology in precisely identified areas of high and low incidence in Italy. It is there we should seek knowledge about those ecological laws which are determining the peculiar local pattern of stomach cancer.

One of the conference participants, Dr. John Berg has proposed that the role of pathologist in cancer research should be that of morphologist in the full sense of the work and not merely that of a microscopist. May I extend that thought to suggest that cancer epidemiologist should regard himself as a cancer ecologist in addition to being a cancer statistician.

REFERENCES

1. Haenszel W: Cancer mortality among the foreign-born in the United States. **J Nat Cancer Inst** 26: 37–132, 1961
2. Shiloh A: The ethnic groups of Israel. **Cancer Mortality and Morbidity in Israel.** Edited by Gertrude Kallner, WHO/CAN/66–68, Part II, Geneva 1968

3. Davis WH: The relation of the foreign population to the mortality rates of Boston. **Bull Am Acad Med** 14: 19–54, 1913

4. MacMahon B: The ethnic distribution of cancer mortality in New York City, 1955. **Acta UICC** 16: 1716–1724, 1960

5. Ahlbom HE: Simple achlorhydric anaemia, Plummer–Vinson syndrome and carcinoma of the mouth, pharynx and oesophagus in women; observations at Radium-hemmet. **Brit Med J** 2: 331–333, 1936

6. Wynder EL, Bross IJ, Feldman RM: A study of the aetiological factors in cancer of the mouth. **Cancer** 10: 1300–1323, 1957

7. Tuyns A: The state of the present knowledge in the epidemiology of oesophageal cancer, I.A.R.C. **Expert Group Meeting on Oesophagus**, Working paper, Lyon, July 1968

8. Lombard HL and Doering CR: Cancer studies in Massachusetts. Cancer mortality in nativity groups. **J Prev Med** 3: 343–361, 1929

9. Kiviranta UK: Carcinoma of the esophagus, its incidence, age and sex distribution, and prognosis in Finland. **Acta Oto-Laryngol** 42: 73–88, 1952

10. Saxén E and Korplea A: Cancer incidence in Finland, 1954. **Ann Chir Gynaec Fenn** 47: 1–32 (Suppl. 79), 1958

11. Segi M: **Age Adjusted Death rates for Malignant Neoplasms, for Selected Sites by Sex in 24 Countries, in 1952–53, 1954–55 and 1956–57,** Department of Public Health, Tohoku University School of Medicine, Sendai, Japan, 1959

12. Staszewski J, Haenszel W: Cancer mortality among Polish-born in the United States. **J Nat Cancer Inst** 35: 291–297, 1965

13. Haenszel W, Kurihara M: Studies of Japanese migrants. I. Mortality from cancer and other diseases among Japanese in the United States. **J Nat Cancer Inst** 40: 43–68, 1968

14. Mancuso TF, Cutler EJ: Cancer mortality among native white, foreign-born white, and non-white male residents of Ohio: Cancer of the lung, larynx, bladder and central nervous system. **J Nat Cancer Inst** 20: 79–105, 1958

15. MacMahon B, Koller EK: Ethnic differences in the incidence of leukemia. **Blood** 12: 1–10, 1957

16. Wynder EL, Bross IL: Study of aetiological factors in cancer of oesophagus. **Cancer (Philad)** 14: 389–413, 1961

17. Registrar-General of England and Wales: **The Registrar-General's Decennial Supp., England and Wales, 1951. Occupational Mortality,** 1957

18. Dean G: The causes of death among the South African-born and immigrants to South Africa. **S Afr Med J** 39: (Suppl): 1–20, 1965

19. Kallner G: **Cancer Mortality and Morbidity in Israel 1950–1961.** WHO/CAN/66–68, Part I. Geneva 1968

20. Steinitz R: **The Israel Cancer Registry. New Cases of Malignant Neoplasms in 1960 and 1961.** Ministry of Health, 1963

21. Haenszel W: Variation in incidence of and mortality from stomach cancer with particular reference to the United States. **J Nat Cancer Inst** 21: 213–262, 1958

22. Sepilli A, Candeli A: Indagini statistiche sulla mortalità per tumori maligni in Italia. II. Rafronto della mortalità per alcune classi di tumori, tra il 1931 e il 1951 **Ann Sanita Pubblica** 19: 703–717, 1958

23. Buell P, Dunn JE Jr: Cancer mortality among Japanese Issei and Nisei of California. **Cancer (Philad)** 18: 656–664, 1965

24. Prudente A, Mirra AO: Gastric cancer in Japanese people living in Brazil. **Acta UICC** 17: 851–857, 1961

25. Smith RL: Recorded and expected mortality among the Japanese of the United States and Hawaii, with special reference to cancer. **J Nat Cancer Inst** 17: 459–473, 1956

26. Smith RL: Recorded and expected mortality among the Chinese of Hawaii and the United States with special reference to cancer. **J Nat Cancer Inst** 17: 667–676, 1956

27. Smith RL: Mortality attributed to cancer among Hawaiians and Filipinos of Hawaii and other racial groups of the United States and Hawaii. **J Nat Cancer Inst** 18: 397–405, 1957

28. Quisenberry WB, Bruyere PT, Rogers MG: Ethnic differences in cancer in Hawaii. **Milit Med** 131: 222–233, 1966

29. Quisenberry W: Gastro-intestinal cancer in Hawaii. **Acta UICC** 17: 324–329, 1961

30. McLester JS, Darby WJ: **Nutrition and Diet in Health and Disease,** Ed 6. Philadelphia. Saunders, 1952

31. Tulchinsky D, Modan B: Epidemiological aspects of cancer of the stomach in Israel. **Cancer** 20: 1311–1317, 1967

32. Haenszel W and Dawson EA: A note on mortality from cancer of the colon and rectum in the United States. **Cancer (Philad)** 18: 265–272, 1965

33. Gordon T, Crittenden M and Haenszel W: Cancer mortality trends in the United States, 1930–1955. **Nat Cancer Inst Monogr** 6: 131–350, 1961

34. Report of the International Working Party of the World Organization of Gastro-enterology: The epidemiology of gastro-intestinal cancer with special reference to causation. **Gut** 5: 3–7, 1964

35. Stemmerman GN: Cancer of the colon and rectum discovered at autopsy in Hawaiian Japanese. **Cancer (Philad)** 19: 1567–1572, 1966

36. Dunn JE Jr: Gastro–intestinal cancer among various ethnic groups in California. **Proceedings of the Third World Congress of Gastroenterology**, Tokyo, September 1966
37. Hueper WC: **Occupational Tumors and Allied Diseases.** Springfield, Illinois, Charles C. Thomas, 1942
38. Levin ML, Haenszel W, Carroll BE, *et al*: Cancer incidence in urban and rural areas of New York State. **J Nat Cancer Inst** 24: 1243–1257, 1960
39. Steiner PE: **Cancer: Race and Geography.** Williams & Wilkins, Baltimore, 1954
40. Smith RL: Recorded and expected mortality among the Indians of the United States with special reference to cancer. **J Nat Cancer Inst** 18: 385–396, 1957
41. Clemmesen J: Carcinoma of the breast. I. Results from statistical research. **Brit J Radiol** 21: 583–590, 1948
42. Pedersen E, Magnus K: **Cancer Registration. Incidence of Cancer in Norway, 1953–1954.** The Cancer Registry of Norway, Monogr No 1, 1959
43. Dorn HF, Cutler SJ: **Morbidity from Cancer in the United States.** Pub Health Monogr No 56, Pub Health Ser Publ No 590, Washington, 1959
44. McKenzie A: Cancer of the female breast, mortality and the menopause. **Lancet** 2: 1129–1130, 1955
45. Staszewski J: Cancer in Poland in 1959. **Brit J Cancer** 18: 1–13, 1964
46. Oettlé G: Malignant neoplasms of the uterus in the white, coloured, Indian and Bantu races of the Union of South Africa. **Acta UICC** 17: 915–933, 1961
47. Eastcott DF: **Report of the B.E.C.C. (N.Z.) Branch, Cancer Registration Scheme.** Department of Health, Wellington, New Zealand, 1954
48. Dean G: Lung cancer among white South Africans. **Brit Med J** 2: 852–857, 1959
49. Hueper WC: Environmental factors in the production of human cancer. **Cancer** (Raven RW, ed.) London, Butterworths, 1957
50. Court-Brown WM, Doll R: **Leukemia and Aplastic Anaemia in the Patients Irradiated for Anklosing Spondilitis.** London, Her Majesty's Stationery Office, 1957
51. Jim RTS: Incidence of acute leukemia in Hawaii. **Lancet** 1: 115–116, 1957 (Letters to the Editor)
52. MacMahon B: Epidemiological evidence on the nature of Hodgkin's disease. **Cancer (Philad)** 10: 1045–1054, 1957

APPENDIX

SUMMARY OF CANCER RISK IN MIGRANTS

Cancer site	Outstanding references	From	To	Outstanding features	Suspected factors
Oral cavity	Haenszel [1] Davis [3] MacMahon [4]	Several European Countries	USA	Higher risk in Irish migrants, lower in Jewish groups* High female risk in Swedish migrants	Alcohol Plummer–Vinson syndrome
Esophagus	Haenszel [1]	Several European Countries	USA	Higher male risk in all migrants, particularly in Polish, Czechoslovakia, and Irish groups* Higher risk in women from USSR*— Higher risk in Swedish women*	Alcohol Plummer–Vinson syndrome
	Staszewski and Haenszel [14]	Poland	USA	Higher risk in male migrants	Alcohol
	Haenszel and Kurihara [16]	Japan	USA	Higher Issei male risk in age group 65 and over*	—
	Kallner [19] Steinitz [20]	European Asian African countries	Israel	Higher risk in migrants from Yemen and Iran	—
Stomach	Haenszel [1]	Several European countries	USA	Higher risk in all migrant groups, highest for Poland, Czechoslovakia, USSR. In Italians relatively low*	Diet

Cancer site	Outstanding references	From	To	Outstanding features	Suspected factors
	Staszewski and Haenszel [14]	Poland	USA	Higher risk in migrants*	Diet
	Haenszel and Kurihara [16]	Japan	USA	No substantial decline in Issei risk, more pronounced decline in Nissei*	Diet
	Quisenberry [27]	Japan	Hawaii	No substantial decline in risk for migrants*	Diet
	Tulchinsky and Modan [30]	European African Asian countries	Israel	Low risk in migrants from Yemen and Iran. Low risk in Israel-born residents, higher in "new" immigrants arriving after 1952	—
	Prudente and Mirra [31]	Japan	Brazil	Persistent high risk in migrants	Diet
	Dean [15]	England and Wales	South Africa	Lower risk in migrants than South African born Whites	—
Large intestine and rectum	Haenszel and Dawson [32]	Internal migration within USA	USA	Migrant risks more closely associated with those prevailing in place of residence than in birthplace. The patterns differ from the experience in gastric cancer where no substantial differences were observed in the risks between the "old" and the "new" countries	—
	Haenszel and Kuirhara [16]	Japan	USA	Rise in risk for migrants (little decline in gastric cancer)	—
	Dunn [35]	Japan	USA (California)	Sharp increase in colonic cancer and a decline in gastric cancer	—
	Staszewski and Haenszel [14]	Poland	USA	Rise in risk among migrants	—
	Kallner [19]	European African Asian countries	Israel	"Occidental" preponderence in for colon and rectum cancer	—
Bladder	Haenszel [1]	Several European countries	USA	Lower female risk in several migrant groups	—
Prostate	Staszewski and Haenszel [14]	Poland	USA	Upward trend in migrants	—
	Haenszel and Kurihara [16]	Japan	USA	Upward trend in Issei	—
Ovary	Haenszel and Kurihara [16]	Japan	USA	Rise in risk in migrants	—
	Kallner [19]	European Asian African countries	Israel	"Occidental preponderance" for ovary cancer	—

Cancer site	Outstanding references	From	To	Outstanding features	Suspected factors
Breast	Haenszel [1]	Several European countries	USA	Lower risk in Italians and Polish migrants than in U.S.-born whites. "Menopausal break" much more pronounced in the migrants from Europe than in the U.S. native whites	Breast-feeding
	Staszewski and Haenszel [14]	Poland	USA	Higher rates in migrants than in the native Polish population	Breast-feeding
	Haenszel and Kurihara [16]	Japan	USA	"Failure" of breast cancer rates in Japanese women to approach those of the host population in contrast to the experience in ovary and corpus cancer. Male breast cancer in Japanese also low	Genetic factors
	Quisenberry [27]	Japan	USA Hawaii	Higher risk in younger Japanese migrants. Lower rates in Hawaiian and Japanese than whites	Breast-feeding
	Kallner [19]	European African Asian countries	Israel	Excess breast cancer risk in "Newcomers"	—
Uterus	Haenszel [1]	European countries, Mexico	USA	Very high cervical cancer rates Mexicans, very low in USSR migrants (Jewish component)	—
	Staszewski and Haenszel [14]	Poland	USA	Higher risk for endometrial (and breast) cancer in migrant than in Poland	—
	Haenszel and Kuirhara [16]	Japan	USA	Downward displacment of cervical cancer risk among migrants	—
	Steinitz [20]	European African Asian	Israel	Corpus cancer more common in groups with low cervical cancer risk	—
Lung and Bronchus	Haenszel [1]	Several European countries	USA	Displacement in rates in either direction to a position intermediate between home and host countries	Role of environmental experience early in life in addition to smoking
	Staszewski and Haenszel [14]	Poland	USA	Higher rates in migrants than in both home and host countries	—
	Dean [15]	England and Wales	South Africa	Lower rates in migrants from UK than for men who remained behind	—
	Quisenberry [27]	Japan	USA Hawaii	Steep increase in risk for Hawaiians and Japanese	Cigarette smoking
	Haenszel and Kurihara [16]	Japan	USA	High risk in Issei male and female over 65	Cigarette smoking
Leukemia	Haenszel [1]	Several European countries	USA	Excess risk in Jews	Radiation

*When compared with the native white population.

Time Trends in Colo-Rectal Cancer Mortality in Relation to Food and Alcohol Consumption: United States, United Kingdom, Australia and New Zealand

by A. J. McMichael, J. D. Potter and B. S. Hetzel

Recent epidemiological and experimental research has implicated dietary factors, including alcoholic drinks, in cancers of the colon and rectum. Analysis of time trends in cancer mortality since 1921, in the United States, England and Wales, Australia, and New Zealand, in relation to changes in per capita consumption of foodstuffs and alcohol reveals some support for the protective effect of fibre, but an inconsistent role for fat and meat in colon cancer. For rectal cancer, and to a lesser extent colon cancer, the most consistent correlate in comparisons across time, and between place, sex, and age-group, is beer consumption. Possible reasons for this correlation within this data set are discussed.

Cancer of the colon is increasingly viewed as diet-related (1). A rise in incidence may result from an increased consumption of fibre-depleted, refined carbohydrates (2), or of high-fat diets (3). Internationally, colon cancer rates correlate most strongly with consumption of saturated fat (1). Experimental and 'metabolic' studies indicate that a high-fat, low-fibre diet may alter bile secretion, bowel flora composition, and the intraluminal binding and degradation of the biliary sterols, thereby producing chemical promoters, if not initiators of colon cancer (1, 3).

Other dietary factors have also been implicated. Vitamin A may render the bowel mucosa less susceptible to neoplastic change (4), accounting for an apparently protective effect of raw vegetables (5). One case-control study implicated beer in colo-rectal cancer (6), whereas 3 others did not (7, 8, 9). Follow-up of 12 000 Norwegian men showed a dose-response relationship between

colo-rectal cancer and alcohol consumption, particularly beer (10).

However, there is epidemiological evidence that cancers of the colon and rectum have different aetiologies. Although dietary factors in rectal cancer have been relatively little studied, an association with beer drinking has been reported in both follow-up and population correlation studies (11, 12). Further, the observed correlation of the male—female ratio for rectal cancer with mean per capita beer consumption accords with the relatively heavier beer consumption by men in high consumption populations (13, 14). Brewery workers, display a pattern of increased risk of rectal, but not colon, cancer, suggesting that differences in brewing practices may be important (15).

The current upturn in colo-rectal cancer mortality in many Western countries may reflect recent dietary changes. This paper examines time trends in colo-rectal cancer death rates in the United States, England and Wales, Australia and New Zealand in relation to changes in eating and drinking habits. Whereas most prior correlation studies of diet and disease have been cross-sectional, drawing

Division of Human Nutrition Commonwealth Scientific and Industrial Research Organization, Kintore Avenue, Adelaide, South Australia, 5000.

on data from many countries but ignoring secular trends and lag periods, this analysis concentrates on time trends in diet and disease in 4 countries. This approach allows comparisons between places, times, sexes, and age-groups, and enables flexibility in the consideration of cancer latency periods.

METHODS

Age-sex-specific death rates were obtained for cancers of the colon and rectum separately. Published rates for England and Wales were available for the whole period 1921 to 1974 (16). For the United States, Australia, and New Zealand, rates since 1950 have been published by WHO (17). Earlier data were obtained from separate sources for each of these 3 countries (18–21). Death rates for US whites and non-whites combined, prior to 1950, were calculated using weights derived from census data (22). Before 1970, the New Zealand rates are for non-Maoris only; but since Maoris account for only 4% of the population aged over 35, the discrepancy between rates before and after 1970 is negligible.

Age-standardised death rates, for ages 35–74, were calculated by the direct standardisation procedure, employing the 'world population' as standard (23).

Per capita food consumption data from the 1930s onwards were obtained from Food Balance Sheets published by the Food and Agricultural Organisation (FAO) since 1949 (24). These were crosschecked against various national governmental and other publications (25–28).

Additional information on trends in consumption of crude fibre (an index of total dietary fibre) in the U.K. and the U.S. was obtained from separate sources (29, 30). Crude fibre accounts for about one-third of total dietary fibre, and variations in its consumption, underestimate the relative magnitude of variations in dietary fibre consumption by about 50% (31).

Data on the per capita consumption of alcohol, overall, and by type of drink, since 1950 were obtained from a comprehensive WHO-supported survey (32), and crosschecked against FAO figures (24). Information on pre-1950 consumption came from separate sources for each country (33–36).

It should be noted that official statistics on consumption of food and alcohol are based predominantly on commercial transactions. Measures of actual household or personal consumption are not systematically available, and the influences of private production, wastage, and storage are therefore not accounted for. Further, per capita figures necessarily ignore intra-population consumption differences.

INTERPRETATION OF MORTALITY RATES

The interpretation of variations in cancer death rates with time, sex, age, and place, must allow for changes in the definition, diagnosis, recording and treatment of cancer. In general, the death certification of cancer within the past 50 years has had good validity, and the concurrence rate between clinicians and pathologists, for cancers of both colon and rectum, has been approximately 70%–85% in recent decades (37).

Successive revisions of the International Statistical Classification of Diseases, Injuries, and Causes of Death (ICD) have altered the rules for assigning the 'underlying' cause of death. Before 1950, almost all death certificates mentioning cancer as a contributory cause led to a cancer assignation. Since the Sixth Revision of the ICD (1950), the certifying doctor's preference has largely determined the assignment. This change resulted in some decreases, mostly above age 75, in the numbers of deaths assigned to colo-rectal cancers (37).

Survival rates for both colon and rectal cancers have improved moderately since 1940, but most of this occurred prior to 1960 (38). Thus, changes in death rates since 1960 are not biased by changes in survival, whereas declines occurring between the 1940s and 1950s must derive at least partly from enhanced survival.

RESULTS

Time trends in age-standardised death rates from colon cancer are shown, for men and women separately, in Figure 1. The overall pattern in the 4 countries comprises a rise during the 1920s, a plateau in the 1930s, a marked decline during the 1940s and 1950s, and a subsequent flattening out, followed, more recently, by an upturn (particularly in males).

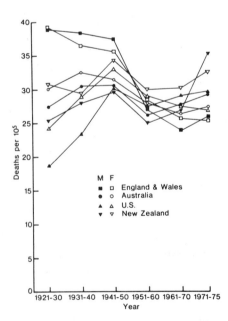

FIGURE 1 *Time trends in age-standardised death rates from colon cancer, ages 35–74, by sex, 1921–75: England and Wales, Australia, U.S. and New Zealand.*

British colon cancer mortality was much higher than in Australia, New Zealand, or the U.S. during the period 1921–50, but has subsequently fallen below those 3 countries.

The longstanding preponderance of female deaths relative to male deaths (i.e. prior to around 1960 — except in the U.K.) has recently been reversed.

Although not shown here, time trends in age-specific colon cancer death rates within any one country have moved in parallel, following this overall age-standardised pattern. In contrast to a staggered sequence of age-specific mortality changes (i.e. a 'cohort effect'), which would suggest that successive generations had experienced different lifetime cancer risks, this observed cross-sectional pattern of change suggests that risk variations were mainly shared simultaneously across the whole community.

Table 1 shows the age-specific changes in colon cancer mortality, by sex, over the decade 1960–64 to 1970–74. For men, the rates have increased at every age, particularly in New Zealand. For women, the rates have generally declined at younger ages, while increasing slightly at older ages.

Time trends in age-standardised rectal cancer mortality (Figure 2) show an overall pattern similar to that of colon cancer. In the most recent decade, the U.S. rates have continued to decline, British rates have been stable, while Australian and New Zealand rates have increased for both sexes. In the first half of the century, the British rates were

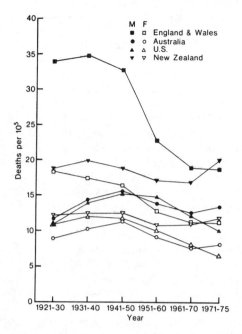

FIGURE 2   *Time trends in age-standardised death rates from rectal cancer, ages 35–74, by sex, 1921–75: England and Wales, Australia, U.S. and New Zealand*

approximately twice those of Australia and the U.S. As with colon cancer, the rates in these 3 countries have subsequently converged, again including a sharp decline in the British rates.

TABLE 1   *Changes in colon cancer mortality, by sex and age, between 1960–64 and 1970–74, by country (deaths per 100,000 p.a.)*

Age, by country	Males			Females		
	1960–64	1970–74	% change	1960–64	1970–74	% change
U.S.						
35–44	3.3	3.4	+ 3%	4.2	3.7	−12%
45–54	12.3	13.1	+ 7%	15.0	13.6	− 9%
55–64	38.2	42.4	+11%	39.0	37.0	− 5%
65–74	89.1	99.7	+12%	80.6	82.1	+ 2%
ENGLAND & WALES						
35–44	3.3	4.1	+24%	4.1	3.8	− 7%
45–54	10.4	11.8	+13%	13.0	12.9	− 1%
55–64	31.2	34.0	+ 9%	33.5	34.0	+ 1%
65–74	78.5	85.5	+ 9%	72.2	71.6	− 1%
AUSTRALIA						
35–44	4.3	5.1	+19%	5.2	5.0	− 4%
45–54	11.5	13.6	+19%	15.6	16.3	+ 4%
55–64	36.0	40.5	+13%	34.0	38.2	+12%
65–74	83.8	91.2	+ 9%	80.8	80.4	N.C.
NEW ZEALAND*						
35–44	5.0	7.1	+42%	8.1	7.9	− 2%
45–54	13.3	19.8	+49%	16.8	20.0	+ 19%
55–64	36.0	43.8	+22%	43.0	46.2	+ 8%
65–74	76.4	103.2	+35%	78.5	87.7	+ 12%

* Because of small population size (3.1m), rates for New Zealand are for 1958–67 and 1968–75.

However, the sex ratio for rectal cancer mortality has differed from that for colon cancer. Male rates have been consistently higher than female rates. Further, as the British rates have declined, the marked male preponderance there has lessened; whereas with increasing rates in Australia (1921–50, 1961–74) and in New Zealand 1921–40, 1961–74), the male preponderance has increased.

Again, the underlying age-specific time trends in rectal cancer mortality exhibit a predominantly cross-sectional pattern of change, consistently similar to those in Figure 2. However, the recent age-specific changes (Table 2) suggest the beginning of a possible cohort effect in Australia and New Zealand, with the proportional increases having been much greater in younger males.

Changes in per capita consumption of major dietary components are shown in Table 3. Both the U.S. and U.K. have almost doubled their meat consumption since the 1930s, whereas in Australia and New Zealand it has changed little. Egg consumption has been consistently highest in the U.S., although declining recently; meanwhile New Zealand consumption of eggs has recently increased. Milk and cheese consumption, initially highest in the U.S., has declined recently in the U.S., the U.K., and Australia, in contrast to the increasing, and high, consumption in New Zealand. Butter consumption has been markedly higher in New Zealand and lower in the U.S. than in the U.K. or Australia.

Consumption of total oils and fats has been consistently lower in Australia than in the U.S., the U.K. and New Zealand. Consumption in the U.K. increased sharply in the Depression, but subsequently declined temporarily during and immediately after World War II. For animal oils and fats, however, New Zealand shows the consistently highest consumption; while the U.S., until the 1960s, was the lowest — a position now occupied by Australia.

Consumption of refined sugar fell temporarily in the 1940s in the U.K. (and, to a lesser extent, in the U.S.); otherwise, sugar consumption has been similar in the 4 countries. Since World War II, consumption of cereals, roots, tubers and pulses has been highest in the U.K. and lowest in the U.S. The reverse has been true for fruit and vegetables. Crude fibre consumption (a rough index of dietary fibre) was initially low in the U.K., and temporarily increased during the 1940s in response to wartime rationing. During those same early decades, fibre consumption declined in the U.S., and, since around 1950, has been similar to that in the U.K. Figures are not available for Australia and New Zealand.

Figure 3 shows changes in consumption of alcohol in beer since 1900. (Alcohol in beer has consistently accounted for 60%–80% of total alcohol consumption in the U.K., Australia and New Zealand, and approximately 50% in the U.S., decreasing to 40% recently.) While beer consumption in the U.K. was 3 times higher than elsewhere early

TABLE 2   *Changes in rectal cancer mortality, by sex and age, between 1960–64 and 1970–74, by country (deaths per 100,000 p.a.)*

Age, by country	Males			Females		
	1960–64	1970–74	% change	1960–64	1970–74	% change
U.S.						
35–44	1.5	1.1	−27%	1.4	0.8	−43%
45–54	5.9	4.4	−25%	4.8	3.1	−35%
55–64	17.9	14.2	−21%	11.2	8.6	−23%
65–74	39.8	31.9	−20%	22.8	17.6	−23%
ENGLAND & WALES						
35–44	2.0	1.9	− 5%	1.9	1.6	−16%
45–54	7.6	8.1	+ 7%	6.5	6.0	− 8%
55–64	26.0	25.0	− 4%	15.4	15.2	− 1%
65–74	71.5	62.5	−13%	33.7	32.1	− 5%
AUSTRALIA						
35–44	1.6	1.9	+18%	1.5	1.5	N.C.
45–54	5.8	6.6	+14%	4.2	5.3	+26%
55–64	17.5	18.2	+ 4%	9.3	10.2	+10%
65–74	39.5	40.8	+ 3%	21.5	22.0	+ 2%
NEW ZEALAND*						
35–44	2.1	2.9	+38%	2.3	2.7	+15%
45–54	7.8	10.9	+40%	6.5	6.2	− 4%
55–64	21.5	25.8	+19%	17.0	16.5	− 3%
65–74	49.0	57.2	+17%	23.0	30.9	+34%

* Because of small population size (3.1m), rates for New Zealand are for 1958–67 and 1968–75.

TABLE 3   Changes, by decade, in estimated consumption of major dietary ingredients, by country (Kg per head p.a.)

	1920's	1930's*	1940's*	1950's	1960's	1970's
Meat						
U.S.	75	70	80	90	98	126
U.K.	—**	55	45	62	80	94
Aust.	—	119	103	112	99	113
N.Z.	—	109	95	105	112	110
Eggs						
U.S.	20	18	22	24	21	17
U.K.	—	13	11	14	15	14
Aust.	—	12	13	10	13	12
N.Z.	—	13	13	14	17	17
Milk and cheese						
U.S.	160	177	213	254	170	165
U.K.	—	110	147	157	166	164
Aust.	—	117	152	142	145	132
N.Z.	—	136	196	223	206	214
Butter						
U.S.	8	6	5	4	3	2
U.K.	—	11	5	7	9	8
Aust.	—	14	11	13	10	8
N.Z.	—	19	13	20	19	17
Total oils, fats						
U.S.	18	19	20	22	23	25
U.K.	15	21	16	22	23	24
Aust.	—	17	14	19	17	16
N.Z.	—	21	18	23	23	24
Oils and fats — animal						
U.S.	—	13	11	12	16	15
U.K.	—	15	11	14	17	15
Aust.	—	15	13	15	12	10
N.Z.	—	21	15	22	22	21
Refined Sugar						
U.S.	55	51	45	48	51	57
U.K.	—	52	33	55	52	53
Aust.	—	51	57	53	52	55
N.Z.	—	50	47	46	45	42
Cereals, roots and tubers, pulses						
U.S.	170	161	145	123	120	116
U.K.	—	176	220	192	181	170
Aust.	—	152	162	157	148	131
N.Z.	—	140	142	143	155	139
Fruit and vegetables						
U.S.	175	184	202	175	160	200
U.K.	—	113	100	104	107	115
Aust.	—	140	154	115	135	140
N.Z.	—	132	119	128	152	138
Crude fibre***						
U.S.	2.2	2.0	1.8	1.7	1.6	1.6
U.K.	1.3	1.4	1.7	1.6	1.5	1.5
Aust.	—	—	—	—	—	—
N.Z.	—	—	—	—	—	—

*   Estimates for latter half of decade
**   Estimates not available
*** See comment, and data source, in Methods

in the century, consumption since 1950 has been highest in Australia and New Zealand. Since the 1930s, beer consumption in the U.S. has been much lower than elsewhere.

Table 4 shows that, although per capita consumption of total alcohol has increased by approximately one-third in each country since 1950—52, the proportional increase in beer consumption has varied

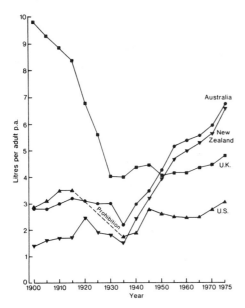

FIGURE 3   Time trends in adult per capita consumption of alcohol in beer, 1900–75: Australia, New Zealand, U.K. and U.S.

during the period 1950–52 to 1970–72 and the proportional changes in colo-rectal cancer mortality, at ages 35–54. Since young adults (ages 15–34) are presumed to have participated centrally in the post-World War II upturn in beer consumption, that generation, aged 35–54 in the 1970s, is most likely to exhibit any beer-related increase in cancer risk. A positive relationship between increases in beer consumption and bowel cancer is evident, particularly for rectal cancer. No such obvious relationship is apparent between these recent trends in colo-rectal cancer mortality and the trends in consumption of major food groups listed in Table 3.

DISCUSSION

To seek single dietary factors responsible for these observed changes in colo-rectal cancer mortality would be misguided. The daily diet affords to the bowel mucosa a multiplicity of mixed exposures, and the resultant nutritional and intraluminal physico-chemical changes may affect tissue susceptibility to carcinogenesis, or either the initiation or promotion of cancer.

The several relationships observed within these data apply at the population level, but do not necessarily apply at the individual level. Further, in this type of comparative time trend analysis, the apparent influence of a particular dietary item upon cancer mortality may well be due to co-existent effects of other dietary and non-dietary items that

considerably. Both absolute and relative consumption of beer has increased most in New Zealand and least in the U.S.

Table 5 shows the relationship, by sex, between the proportional increase in beer consumption

TABLE 4   Absolute and proportional (%) changes per capita consumption of alcohol (beer and total) between 1950–52 1970–72, by country

Country	Litres of beer				Litres of total alcohol			
	1950–52	1960–62	1970–72	% increase	1950–52	1960–62	1970–72	% increase
U.S.	63.5	57.0	71.3	12.3%	4.9	4.8	6.5	32.7%
U.K.	84.7	85.6	104.2	23.0%	4.9	5.3	6.6	34.7%
Australia	91.9	101.5	125.1	36.1%	6.3	6.5	8.3	31.7%
New Zealand	86.1	110.2	119.8	39.1%	5.7	6.8	7.8	36.8%

TABLE 5   Percentage change in per capita beer consumption, 1950–52 to 1960–62, and in death rates from colon and rectal cancer at ages 35–54, 1960–64 to 1970–74: New Zealand, Australia, England and Wales, and U.S.A.

Country	% Change in beer alcohol per capita 1950–52 to 1960–62	% Change in cancer mortality at ages 35–54: 1960–64 to 1970–74			
		Colon		Rectum	
		M	F	M	F
New Zealand*	+28%	+47%	+12%	+40%	+ 2%
Australia	+19%	+19%	+ 3%	+15%	+19%
England and Wales	+ 1%**	+16%	− 3%	+ 4%	−10%
U.S.	−10%	+ 6%	−10%	−26%	−37%

*   Because of small population size (3.1m), mortality data for New Zealand are for 1958–67 and 1968–75.

**   Refers to consumption in total U.K.

are also varying by place and time.

The high colon cancer mortality in the U.K. before 1950, together with the low mortality in the U.S., accord with the higher crude fibre intake in the U.S. during the 1920s and 1930s. Further, during the 1930s and 1940s, consumption of animal fats was higher in the U.K. However, the fact that New Zealand, with the consistently highest animal fat consumption, had a colon cancer death rate until 1950 that was similar to that of the U.S., with the lowest consumption of animal fat, casts some doubt upon the suggested aetiological importance of animal fats.

The consistently low consumption of meat in the U.K., particularly before 1950, does not accord with the proposition that meat per se increases colon cancer risk. However, it is possible that relatively greater dietary differences between British socio-economic classes early this century, compared with elsewhere, resulted in a sufficient concentration of above-threshold dietary 'affluence' to produce relatively more cases of colon cancer. That is, discrepancies in the association of national indices of consumption of fat and meat, for example, with national colon cancer rates could reflect internal distributional differences between countries.

Since 1950, the high rates of colon cancer in New Zealand match the continued high consumption of animal fats. However, animal fat consumption has noticeably declined, since 1950, in Australia, but not in the U.S., yet colon cancer has increased more in Australia than in the U.S.

The greater decline in colon cancer mortality in England and Wales than elsewhere between the 1940s and 1950s may reflect beneficial effects of the British wartime low-fat, low-sugar, high-fibre diet. However, this decline also followed, albeit by 20–30 years, the very sharp reduction in British beer (and total alcohol) consumption. Further, prior to 1950, England and Wales alone had had a colon cancer sex ratio greater than unity (see Figure 1). Elsewhere, women had been at noticeably greater risk than men. This greater risk in British men accords with an aetiological role for beer, given a greater relative consumption of beer by men than women in high-consumption populations.

Other similarities between the graphs in Figures 1 and 3 can be seen. The approximately 70% increase in beer consumption between 1935 and 1945, in the U.S., Australia and New Zealand, was followed by an increase in male colon cancer mortality after 1950. Beer consumption stabilised in the U.S. after 1945, and so did U.S. male colon cancer mortality after the 1960s. However, in Australia and New Zealand, where beer consumption continued to climb after 1945, so too has the male colon cancer mortality. Indeed, in both these countries, the rises have been proportionally greatest in males aged 35–54 – the generation of 'affluent-living' young adults from the 1950s, referred to in

Table 5. In the U.K., however, beer consumption rose by only about 10% between 1935 and 1945, and then declined again, and, unlike elsewhere, no rise in male colon cancer mortality occurred in the 1950s.

Beer consumption could increase the risk of colon cancer by several biological mechanisms. The alcohol component is unlikely to have a direct effect on the colonic mucosa, since most of it is absorbed in the upper gastrointestinal tract. However, other ingredients in beer may be carcinogenic (15, 39). Alternatively, ethanol has been shown, in human volunteer subjects, to increase the hepatic production of bile acids (40) – now widely thought to be involved in colon carcinogenesis.

Rectal cancer appears, from Figures 1 and 2, likely to share some aetiological factors with colon cancer. Since the majority of colon cancers are in the distal (particularly the sigmoid) colon (1), this is not surprising. However, unlike colon cancer, the sex ratio for rectal cancer has been consistently greater than unity. From 1921 to 1940, the sex ratio was highest in England and Wales (approximately 2.0) and lowest in Australia and the U.S. (approximately 1.3), thereby demonstrating a direct correlation between sex ratio and per capita beer consumption. Enstrom noted that the sex ratio for rectal cancer approached unity in areas of low beer consumption in the U.S., but approached 2.0 in high consumption areas (14).

From 1921 to 1940, rectal cancer death rates in England and Wales, compared with the other 3 countries, were approximately double in men, and 50% higher in women. Similarly, there had been a two- to three-fold higher consumption of beer in the U.K. early in the century. Although U.K. consumption of beer and total alcohol fell below that of Australia and New Zealand after 1950, rectal cancer mortality in the U.K. is still higher than in Australia and is approximately equal to that of New Zealand. This could reflect differences in beer composition, or if, as suggested by the colon cancer mortality data, there is a 20–30 year lag period between trends in beer consumption and cancer mortality, then Australian rates would be expected to overtake British rates within the next decade.

The recent sharp increase in rectal cancer mortality in New Zealand may reflect their greater increase in beer consumption. The fact that the rise in New Zealand has been similarly sharp for both colon and rectal cancers, that it has been essentially confined to males, and that, in males, it clearly exceeds the rises in the other 3 countries, holds obvious promise for further clues in understanding the dietary aetiology of colo-rectal cancers.

While the number of countries included in this analysis is small, it is of interest that an approach that emphasises time trends between countries provides less support for dietary fat and meat in colon carcinogenesis than have the more usual multi-country cross-sectional analyses. Cancer time trends may be more sensitive to changes in population exposure to cancer 'initiating' agents than in exposure to cancer 'promoting' agents (e.g. bile acid derivatives). If so, this could indicate that certain components of beer may act as an initiating agent.

However, it must be noted also that the major characteristics of the modern 'affluent' diet were established in these 4 western countries by early in this century, as were relatively high rates of large bowel cancer. In cross-sectional comparisons between western and other countries, these dietary characteristics have therefore been associated with the high rates of colon cancer in western countries. Perhaps the residual differences in large bowel cancer between 4 such western countries, since 1921, reflect major changes in consumption of factors, such as alcohol, that are superimposed on their otherwise qualitatively similar diets.

Finally, the correlation over time between beer consumption and colo-rectal cancer is of a similar form to that demonstrated previously for alcohol consumption and oesophageal and laryngeal cancers in Australia and England and Wales (41, 42). The aetiological role of alcohol in these 2 cancers is now widely recognised.

REFERENCES

(1) Correa P and Haenszel W. The Epidemiology of Large Bowel Cancer. In: Klein G and Weinhouse S (eds.) Advances in Cancer Research, vol 26, pp 1–141 Academic Press, San Francisco, 1978.

(2) Burkitt D P. Large bowel carcinogenesis: An epidemiologic jigsaw puzzle. *Journal of the National Cancer Institute* 54: 3–6, 1975.

(3) Hill M J. Metabolic epidemiology of dietary factors in large bowel cancer. *Cancer Research* 35: 3398–3402, 1975.

(4) Newberne P M and Suphakarn V. Preventive role of Vitamin A in colon carcinogenesis in rats. *Cancer* 40: 2553–2557, 1977.

(5) Graham S and Mettlin C. Diet and colon cancer. *American Journal of Epidemiology* 109: 1–20, 1979.

(6) Wynder E L and Shigematsu T. Environmental factors of cancer of the colon and rectum. *Cancer* 20: 1520–1561, 1967.

(7) Bjelke E. Case-control study of cancer of the stomach, colon and rectum. In Oncology 1970: Proceedings of the Tenth International Cancer Congress, vol 5, pp 320–334. Yearbook Medical Publications, Chicago, 1971.

(8) Higginson J. Etiological factors in gastrointestinal cancer in man. *Journal of the National Cancer Institute* 37: 527–545, 1966.

(9) Pernu J. An epidemiological study on cancer of the digestive organs and respiratory system. *Annales Medicine Internae Fenniae* 49, Suppl. 33: 1–117, 1960.

(10) Bjelke E. Epidemiologic studies of cancer of the stomach, colon and rectum, with special emphasis on the role of diet. Ph.D. dissertation, vols I–IV. University of Michigan, University microfilms, Minnesota, 1973.

(11) Sundby P. Alcoholism and Mortality. p 107. Rutgers Center on Alcohol Studies, New Brunswick, New Jersey. 1967.

(12) Breslow N E and Enstrom J E. Geographic correlations between cancer mortality rates and alcohol-tobacco consumption in the United States. *Journal of the National Cancer Institute* 53: 631–639, 1974.

(13) McMichael A J. Alimentary tract cancer in Australia in relation to diet and alcohol. *Nutrition and Cancer* 1: 82–89, 1979.

(14) Enstrom J E. Colorectal cancer and beer drinking. *British Journal of Cancer* 35: 674–683, 1977.

(15) MacLennan R. Colon cancer epidemiology and possible causation. *Nutrition and Cancer* 1: 64–66, 1979.

(16) Registrar General's Annual Statistical Review, 1921–74, Her Majesty's Stationery Office, London.

(17) World Health Organization. Epidemiological and Vital Statistics Report, and World Health Statistics Annuals, WHO, Geneva, 1950–74.

(18) Gordon T, Crittenden M and Haenszel W. Cancer mortality trends in the United States, 1930–1955. In End Results and Mortality Trends in Cancer. National Cancer Institute (DHEW) Monograph No. 6, pp 131–150, Washington DC. 1961.

(19) Gover M. Cancer Mortality in the United States. 1. Trend of Recorded Cancer Mortality in the Death Registration States of 1900 from 1900 to 1935. Public Health Bulletin No. 248, U.S. Government Printing Office, Washington, DC. 1939.

(20) Australian Bureau of Statistics. Annual Publications on demography and mortality, since 1921.

(21) Donovan J W. Cancer mortality in New Zealand: 2. Digestive System. *New Zealand Medical Journal* 72: 104–108, 1970.

(22) Department of Commerce (U.S.). Statistical Abstract of the United States, 1952. U.S. Government Printing Office, Washington, DC. 1952.

(23) Waterhouse J, Muir C, Correa P and Powell J. Cancer Incidence in Five Continents, vol. 3, IARC, Lyon, 1976.

(24) Food and Agricultural Organization of the United Nations. Food Balance Sheets: 1949, 1955, 1958, 1971, 1977 (provisional), FAO. Rome.

(25) Gortner W A. Nutrition in the United States, 1900 to 1974. *Cancer Research* 35: 3246–3253, 1975.

(26) Friend B. Nutrients in United States food supply. A review of trends, 1909–1913 to 1965. *American Journal of Clinical Nutrition* 20: 907–914, 1967.

(27) Australian Bureau of Statistics. Apparent Consumption of Foodstuffs and Nutrients: Australia 1974–75. ABS Publication, Series 10.10, Canberra, 1977.

(28) Ministry of Agriculture, Fisheries and Food. Domestic Food Consumption and Expenditure: 1957. Annual Report of the National Food Survey and Committee, Her Majesty's Stationery Office, London, 1963.

(29) Robertson J. Changes in the fibre content of the British diet. *Nature (London)* 238: 290–292, 1972.

(30) Heller S N and Hackler L R. Changes in the crude fiber content of the American diet. *American Journal of Clinical Nutrition* 31: 1510–1514, 1978.

(31) Scala J. Fiber: The forgotten nutrient. *Food Technology* 28: 34–36, 1974.

(32) The Finnish Foundation for Alcohol Studies. International Statistics on Alcoholic Beverages: Production, Trade and Consumption, 1950–72. Vol 27, Forssa, Finland, 1977.

(33) Spring J A and Buss D H. Three centuries of alcohol in the British diet. *Nature (London)* 270: 567–572, 1977.

(34) Rorabaugh W J. Estimated U.S. Alcoholic Beverage Consumption, 1790–1860. *Journal of Studies on Alcohol* 37: 357–364, 1976.

(35) Drew L H R. A proposal concerning a national policy on alcohol. In: Proceedings of National Alcohol and Drug Dependence Multidisciplinary Institute, Australian Foundation, Alcohol and Drug Dependence, Canberra, p 6, 1975.

(36) Salmond G C. (Department of Health, New Zealand). Personal communication.

(37) Donovan J W. Cancer mortality in New Zealand: 1. General. *New Zealand Medical Journal* **72**: 9–14, 1970.

(38) Cutler S J, Myers M H and Green S B. Trends in survival rates of patients with cancer. *New England Journal of Medicine* **293**: 122–124, 1975.

(39) McGlashan N D, Walters C L and McLean A E M. Nitrosamines in African alcoholic spirits and oesophageal cancer. *Lancet* **ii**: 1017, 1968.

(40) Nestel P J, Simons L A and Homma Y. Effects of ethanol on bile acid and cholesterol metabolism. *American Journal of Clinical Nutrition* **29**: 1007–1015, 1976.

(41) McMichael A J and Hetzel B S. Time trends in upper alimentary tract cancer mortality and alcohol consumption in Australia. *Community Health Studies* **1**: 43–47, 1978.

(42) McMichael A J. Increases in laryngeal cancer in Britain and Australia in relation to alcohol and tobacco consumption trends. *Lancet* **i**: 1244–1247, 1978.

The Epidemiology of Cancer in China

by Bruce Armstrong

China has made impressive progress in unravelling the causes of certain cancers. It is expected that this knowledge will contribute greatly to the understanding of cancer etiology in other parts of the world.

Data on the incidence of cancer in China have been derived from a number of sources, mainly:

(1) a retrospective survey of mortality from all causes in the whole of mainland China in the period 1973–75;

(2) comprehensive cancer registries established in some of the main cities;

(3) registries devoted to single cancers in areas with particularly high rates of the cancer concerned;

(4) special surveys of cancer incidence or mortality in particular areas.

Dr Armstrong is with the NH & MRC Research Unit in Epidemiology and Preventive Medicine, Department of Medicine, University of Western Australia, The Queen Elizabeth II Medical Centre, Nedlands, Western Australia. The article is from *International journal of epidemiology*, Vol. 9 (1980). © Oxford University Press 1980. By permission of Oxford University Press.
The original paper was based on data presented at an international course on cancer epidemiology in Beijing, 1979, by Drs Li Ping, Li Jun-Yao, Zhou Yu-Shang, Tu Qi-Tao, Hsui Hai-Hsio, Gu Xing-Yuan, Gao Yu-Tang, Hu Men-Xie, Zeng Yi, and Calum Muir. Additional data were obtained from Drs Gao Ru-Nie (Shanghai) and Zhao Eu-Sheng (Hangzhou).

This review is based largely on the retrospective survey of cancer mortality with additional data where available on the main cancer sites. Two other reviews have been published in English recently (*1, 2*).

Cancer Mortality in China

The retrospective survey of all deaths in mainland China in 1973–75 was organized by the Chinese National Office of Cancer Control with local organizing groups in each province and most cities and counties. The local groups enlisted the aid of medical workers (particularly the barefoot doctors) who determined the name, age, sex, and date of death of each deceased person in the survey period, together with any information on cause of death which was recorded. A meeting was than held in each production brigade attended by the organizing group, local officials, the barefoot doctors, members of the deceased's families, and older women from the brigade. The cause of death of each of the deceased was assigned following discussion at this meeting. For cancer deaths, the place of final diagnosis or treatment and basis for the diagnosis were also recorded. The number of deaths surveyed was checked against the number registered with the county, and brigades providing returns which attributed greater than 10% of deaths to unknown causes were subject to further investigation.

A total of 18 439 072 deaths were surveyed and 1 868 310 (10.1%—11.3% in males and 8.8% in females) were attributed to cancer. The highest level of diagnosis and treatment and the best available criterion for the diagnosis of cancer are summarized in Table 1.

Nearly 80% of those dying from cancer were diagnosed or treated at the county hospital level or above. In just over 70% of cases, the diagnosis was based on some form of special investigation, although cytologic or histologic confirmation was available in only 17%.

For all sites of cancer together the estimated mortality rates in China are modest at 119.6 per 100 000 in males and 80.7 in females, adjusted to the age distribution of the "world" population (3). Although likely to be underestimated, these rates compare favourably with those of developed countries (e.g., Britain, 192.4 and 128.3 per 100 000 in males and females respectively and the United States, 162.7 and 108.4 per 100 000). Within these relatively low overall rates, however, there are some very high rates at particular sites and substantial geographic variation within the country. For some sites, the highest rates in particular counties are probably the highest in the world.

Mortality rates for the sites of cancer classified separately in the survey are shown in Table 2. Cancer of the stomach was commonest in both sexes, followed by cancer of the oesophagus in males and cancer of the cervix in females. Cancer of the liver (presumed primary) also ranks high in both sexes. This pattern is similar to that seen in other developing countries (2).

The survey results have now been mapped and published in an Atlas of Cancer Mortality in the People's Republic of China, prepared and edited by the National Cancer Control Office of the Ministry of Health and the Nanjing Institute of Geography of the Chinese Academy of Sciences (5). This Atlas is discussed in an article by Li Jun-Yao et al. (6).

Cancer of the Oesophagus

Cancer of the oesophagus has a long history in China having been referred to as "Ye ge" (difficulty with swallowing) for more than 2000 years. A number of historical documents attributed the disease to excessive consumption of alcohol or very hot foods. According to Yen Yung Ho's pharmacopoeia (Ge Sung Fone) written in the Sung Dynasty (960–1279 AD), "eat, and drink alcohol, in moderation (not in excess, not at a rapid rate, not foods which are too hot and not overly hard foods), maintain an even temperament, eat a good diet and Ye ge will not develop".

Among countries reporting mortality by site of cancer, China has the highest mortality from oesophageal cancer with annual rates, standardized to the age distribution of the "world" population, of 31.7 per 100 000 in males and 15.9 per 100 000 in females. The next highest rates are in males in Singapore (14.4 per

Table 2. Rates of mortality from cancer at various body sites in China in 1973-75

Sites	Annual mortality per 100 000	
	Males	Females
Stomach	20.9	10.2
Oesophagus	19.7	9.8
Liver	14.5	5.6
Cervix	—	10.0
Lung	6.8	3.2
Intestines	4.1	3.0
Leukaemia	2.8	2.2
Nasopharynx	2.5	1.3
Breast	0.1	2.6
Brain	1.4	1.1
Lymphoma	1.4	1.0
Bladder	0.8	0.3
Penis	0.4	—
Chorionepithelioma	—	0.2
Other sites	4.8	3.8
All sites	80.2	54.3

Adjusted to the age distribution of the Chinese population in 1964.

Table 1. Percentage distribution of cancer deaths in China in 1973–75 by highest level of diagnosis and treatment and best available criterion for the diagnosis

Diagnosis/treatment level	%	Main diagnostic criterion	%
No treatment	2.8	Supposition after death	6.0
Clinic	18.1	Clinical signs or symptoms	23.5
Hospital	79.2	Special investigations	70,5

100 000) and females in Puerto Rico (5.2 per 100 000).

Within China, oesophageal cancer mortality varies very widely (more than 600-fold in both sexes) with high rates concentrated on the Tai-hang mountains at the border of Henan, Hebei, and Shanxi provinces in North China; northern Sichuan; the Da-bie mountains on the border of Anhui and Hubei provinces; southern Fujian and regions of north-eastern Guangdong; northern Jiangsu; and northern Xinjiang.

From these centres mortality decreases in irregular concentric belts. The high rate areas tend to be dry, infertile and poor, providing a limited food supply, particularly in respect of vegetables and fruit. Lin Xian county in Henan province, has the highest rates in both sexes (161.3 per 100 000 in males and 102.9 per 100 000 in females) which, at least in males are equal to or higher than those in the Gonbad region of Iran and the adjacent parts of the USSR and may, therefore, be the highest rates in the world.

Among the larger minority nationalities in China, oesophageal cancer rates are highest in the Kazaks of northern Xinjiang and lowest in the Miao who live in the more fertile areas of the south. Even within Xinjiang the rates in the Kazaks are three times higher than in the Uygurs and Mongols who live in close proximity to them.

Work on the epidemiology of cancer of the oesophagus in China has concentrated on the high-rate area, Lin Xian county in Henan province. A number of interesting observations have been made.

(1) High mortality rates from oesophageal cancer are associated with a high prevalence of oesophageal dysplasia which is believed to be a premalignant lesion. Observation of some cases suggests that the progression from severe dysplasia to cancer takes about four years.

(2) Cancers of the pharynx and gullet are more common in chickens in areas of high incidence of oesophageal cancer than in areas of low incidence. In Lin Xian county the chickens are kept only for their eggs and remain as household pets after they stop laying. They may, therefore, live for over 10 years.

(3) Oesophageal cancer mortality has not fallen in a group of 100 000 residents of a high-rate area in Henan province who were moved to a low-rate area in Hebei province when their land was flooded by a new reservoir about 10 years ago.

Theories about the etiology of oesophageal cancer in China relate mainly to diet—either nutrient insufficiency or ingestion of carcinogens or carcinogen precursors. With respect to nutrient insufficiency, poor diet is a common feature of high-risk groups in China. The Kazaks of Xinjiang have a much more limited diet than their near-neighbour Uygurs, and studies of the migrant and native populations in Hebei province have shown that the former have retained their pre-migration dietary habits.

With respect to dietary carcinogens, interest has focused on the consumption of pickled vegetables which are heavily contaminated with various moulds (including *Aspergillus flavus*). Extracts of these vegetables have been found to be mutagenic and have produced oesophageal dysplasia and liver tumours in a small number of rats. Mouldy foods are also commonly eaten by other high-risk groups.

In many respects the areas of high oesophageal cancer mortality in China are similar to those of the Caspian littoral in Iran (7). They are arid and their populations are poorly nourished relative to those of low-incidence areas. There are also rapid changes in mortality over relatively short distances.

Cancer of the Stomach

Cancer of the stomach is the most common form of cancer leading to death in China. The mortality rates, standardized to the age distribution of the "world" population, are 32.4 and 15.9 per 100 000 in males and females respectively. These rates are high by world standards but substantially lower than those in Japan (54.5 per 100 000 in males and 27.5 per 100 000 in females).

The areas of highest mortality from gastric cancer are similar in distribution but not identical to those of oesophageal cancer. The counties with highest rates are in the eastern area. The high rate areas are generally in arid and semi-arid regions. The Kazaks of Xinjiang have the highest rates of this cancer, as they do for oesophageal cancer. It is not surprising, therefore, that their mortality from cancer at all sites is the highest of any minority group.

The rates of gastric cancer in Kazaks are more than double those of the Mongols and Uygurs living in close proximity to them. It is thought that these differences and also the differences in rates of cancer of the oesophagus may be explained by differences in diet between the groups. The Uygurs work mainly in agriculture and eat more vegetables than the Kazaks. The Mongols, however, are similar to the Kazaks in living mainly from animal husbandry. In general, low consumption of fresh fruit and vegetables, meat, and eggs and high consumption of salted and pickled vegetables and sweet potato are characteristic of regions in China in which gastric cancer is common.

Cancer of the Liver

Liver cancer (presumed primary) is the third most important cancer as a cause of death in China (third in males at 14.5 per 100 000 and fourth in females at 5.6 per 100 000) and accounts for 15% of all cancer deaths. It may be of more social significance than gastric and oesophageal cancer because in high-incidence areas the age at which the incidence is highest is in the fifth or sixth decade of life compared with the eighth decade for other sites.

The geographic distribution of areas of high incidence of liver cancer is different to that of gastric and oesophageal cancers. It is mainly concentrated in the south-east, in the warm, humid areas along the coast. The highest rates are seen in the Chang Jiang (Yangtse) river delta with rates of, for example, 76.3 and 21.6 per 100 000 in males and females respectively in Qidong county. The incidence rates are not believed to have changed greatly in recent years although analysis of death rates in Shanghai suggests a graded increase in mortality from 11.2 per 100 000 to 25.0 per 100 000 between 1963 and 1977.

Populations migrating from high- to low-mortality areas have shown a fall in incidence and vice versa. Observations on the migrant populations were based on some 75 000 and 60 000 person years respectively.

Migrants from both high- and low-rate areas to an area of intermediate rate showed changes in mortality toward the intermediate level.

The epidemiology of liver cancer in domestic animals has also been studied in high-incidence areas. Ducks were found to have a high prevalence of cholangiocellular carcinoma, which rose to 56% in those aged 5 years and over. There was a correlation between the prevalence of this cancer in ducks and mortality from liver cancer in humans. The predominant form of human liver cancer in these areas, however, is hepatocellular carcinoma, not cholangiocarcinoma.

In analytic studies, liver cancer has been related to occupation, family history, consumption of food contaminated with aflatoxin B_1, infection with hepatitis B virus, nature of the water supply, parasitic infection, environmental contamination with pesticides, and presence of nitrosamines in food.

On present evidence it appears most likely that the high incidence of liver cancer in the south-east of China is due to an interaction between hepatitis B virus and an environmental carcinogen, probably aflatoxin B_1. This is the currently favoured hypothesis for high liver cancer rates elsewhere in the world (*8*).

Cancer of the Cervix

Cancer of the cervix is the fourth most common cause of death from cancer in China. In women, it is second only to cancer of the stomach, with a mortality of 10.1 per 100 000 per year. The mortality rates are generally higher in rural than in urban areas. The provinces with highest rates are Inner Mongolia (Nei Monggol), Shanxi, Shaanxi, Hubei, Hunan, and Jiangxi. The highest rate of 66.0 per 100 000 is in a county in Hubei. The minority nationalities with the highest rates are the Uygurs and Mongols (17.3 and 15.7 per 100 000 respectively).

In Shanghai, mortality rates from cancer of the cervix have been reported for each year from 1964 to 1977. There was a graded decline in mortality from 19.9 per 100 000 in 1964 to 9.5 per 100 000 in 1977. Most other cancer sites showed stable or increasing rates over the same period and none showed a fall of this magnitude. It is therefore likely that this decline in mortality is real. The greatest decline was in women aged 35 to 64 years (45.1 per 100 000 to 12.3 per 100 000). This point may be of special interest because Shanghai has been particularly active in providing mass-screening with cervical cytology. This programme began in 1958 among textile workers and has been expanded gradually to other employed groups. The greatest decline in mortality would be expected in women of working age, as has been seen.

Cancer of the Lung

In the 1973–75 mortality survey, lung cancer ranked fourth in males and fifth in females among cancers as a cause of death. Its geographic distribution within China is unremarkable.

Interest in lung cancer in Chinese populations outside China has focused on the unusually high rates in Chinese women (Table 3).

The incidence rate recorded by the Shanghai cancer registry for women in 1975 was 17.8 per 100 000 and the mortality from lung cancer in Hong Kong women in 1970–72 was 19.7 per 100 000. These rates are similar to those in Table 3.

An unusual feature of the high rate of lung cancer in Chinese women (particularly Cantonese women) is the relatively high propor-

Table 3. The ten highest ranking populations for lung cancer in women

Population	Lung cancer incidence per 100 000 women
New Zealand, Maoris	35.4
USA, San Francisco Bay, Chinese	22.2
Hawaii, Hawaiians	20.6
USA, San Francisco Bay, Whites	19.1
USA, Hawaii, Filipinos	19.1
USA, Hawaii, Caucasians	18.9
USA, Alameda County, Blacks	18.9
USA, San Francisco Bay, Blacks	18.5
Singapore, Chinese	17.3
USA, Hawaii, Chinese	17.0

tion of the tumours which are adenocarcinomas. This is as high as 46% in Cantonese women in Singapore (9).

Lung cancer rates in Chinese men although high (for example, 60.0 per 100 000, 56.9 per 100 000, and 50.2 per 100 000 in San Francisco Bay, Singapore, and Shanghai respectively), do not rank among the top 10 in the world. They are, however, higher than in many North American and European populations and Japanese men.

Reasons for the relatively high rates of lung cancer in Chinese women have been sought in both Singapore and Hong Kong (10, 11). Smoking is a risk factor in both groups but may explain only 40–50% of the disease. The use of kerosene stoves for cooking may also be a risk factor. Both, however, appear to influence the risk of cancers other than adenocarcinomas. In Chinese men in both Singapore and Hong Kong, cigarette smoking is sufficient to explain some 80% of lung cancers.

The epidemiologists to whom I spoke felt that smoking was very likely to be a cause of lung cancer in China although unlikely to explain the high rates in women, who are said to smoke little. The Ministry of Health has recently begun an extensive anti-smoking campaign.

Cancer of the Large Bowel

Cancer of the large bowel is the sixth most common cause of cancer death in China (fifth in males, sixth in females) with mortality rates of 4.1 and 3.0 per 100 000 in males and females respectively. The county with highest rates (23.6 per 100 000 in males and 22.7 per 100 000 in females) is an area of endemic schistosomiasis in Zhajiang province. Elsewhere the rates in Zhajiang are comparatively low (4 to 5 per 100 000). This variation appears to

correlate with prevalence of infestation with *Schistosoma japonicum,* as it does also in rural Shanghai. Overall in China, rates of large-bowel cancer are higher in rural than in urban areas and, in the high-incidence areas where schistosomiasis is endemic, the peak of incidence with age is some 5–10 years earlier than it is in Western countries. In the cities this cancer tends to be more common among the better educated classes.

Tumours associated with *S. japonicum* tended to be well differentiated and had a lower prevalence of metastases at diagnosis and a better overall prognosis than tumours without this association.

Nasopharyngeal Cancer

Nasopharyngeal cancer is eighth among cancers as a cause of death in China, seventh in males and ninth in females (3.1% and 2.3% of cancer deaths in them respectively). The age adjusted annual death rates from nasopharyngeal cancer for the whole of China are 2.5 per 100 000 in males 1.3 per 100 000 in females. In most other parts of the world, annual incidence and mortality rates are both less than 1 per 100 000.

The geographic distribution of nasopharyngeal cancer within China is quite remarkable, with a very high incidence area centred on Guangdong province in the south. From Guangdong, the incidence decreases in concentric bands in all directions. Expatriate Chinese populations also have high rates, the highest being among those resident in Hong Kong, Singapore, and San Francisco. High rates have also been observed in populations closely associated with the Chinese (e.g., the Malays of Singapore and Selangor and the Polynesian Hawaiians).

Following Chinese migration to Singapore, the rates of nasopharyngeal cancer have not fallen. In contrast, in the USA there is evidence of decline in its incidence in second- and third-generation Chinese. It is said, however, that an increase in the proportion of northern (low risk) Chinese in the population may explain this change.

Current theories of the etiology of nasopharyngeal cancer invoke three possibilities.

(1) A genetic predisposition of southern Chinese to the disease.

(2) Exposure to environmental chemical carcinogens, although no carcinogen has been identified in the environment of the southern Chinese which could explain their very much increased risk of nasopharyngeal cancer.

(3) Infection with Epstein-Barr virus. High titres of antibodies to viral capsid antigen are consistently found in a high proportion of patients with nasopharyngeal cancer and are otherwise rare in the populations concerned. The etiological significance of these findings is unclear.

Internal migration within China shows retention of the nasopharyngeal cancer rate of the home area rather than deviation toward that of the host area. Occupational studies have not shown any association with exposure to dust or fumes, and the other environmental associations have not been established with any certainty.

Other Cancer Sites

Apart from the basic descriptive data of the retrospective survey of cancer mortality, no detailed information about other types of cancer was obtained. This should not be taken to imply however that they have not been studied in China.

Conclusions

Prevention is accorded a high priority in modern Chinese medicine and it is not surprising therefore that efforts are being made to unravel the causes of China's main cancer problems. Progress is limited because China is a developing country and resources, particularly of trained and experienced personnel, are meagre in comparison with the size of the task. Considering these limitations, what has been achieved is very impressive.

Opportunities for study, however, are abundant with well-defined geographic gradients in cancer risk; populations that have migrated along these gradients; and, above all, a large and accessible population. The organization of Chinese society and its health services facilitate epidemiological studies. It may be expected therefore, that study of the epidemiology of cancer in China will contribute substantially to knowledge in the future, particularly in relation to cancers of the oesophagus, liver, and nasopharynx. Much of this will be applicable to other populations in which these cancers are a problem.

REFERENCES

1. MILLER, R. W. Epidemiology. In: Kaplan, H. S. & Tsuchitani, P. J., ed. *Cancer in China,* New York, Liss, 1978, p. 39.

2. HENDERSON, B. *National Cancer Institute monograph,* **53**: 59 (1979).

3. DOLL, R. Comparisons between registries, age-standardized rates. In: Waterhouse, J. et al., ed. *Cancer incidence in five continents.* Lyons, International Agency for Research on Cancer, 1976, vol. 3, p. 453.

4. DOLL, R. & ARMSTRONG, B. Cancer. In: Trowell, H. C. & Burkitt, D. P., ed. *Western diseases: their emergence and prevention.* London, Arnold 1981, p 93.

5. THE NATIONAL CANCER CONTROL OFFICE OF THE MINISTRY OF HEALTH. *Investigation of cancer mortality in China.* Beijing, People's Health Publishing House, 1980.

6. LI JUN-YAO ET AL. *International journal of epidemiology,* **10** : 127 (1981).

7. COOK-MOZAFFARI, P. J. ET AL. *British journal of cancer,* **39**: 293 (1979).

8. LINCELL, C. A. & PEERS, F. G. Field studies on liver cancer. In: Watson, J. D. et al., ed. *Origins of human cancer,* New York, Cold Spring Harbor Laboratory, 1977, p. 549.

9. LAW, C. H. ET AL. *International journal of cancer,* **17**: 304 (1976).

10. MACLENNAN, R. ET AL. *International journal of cancer,* **20**: 854 (1977).

11. LEUNG, J. S. M. *British journal of the diseases of the chest,* **21**: 273 (1977).

Seneca County, New York: An Area with Low Cancer Mortality Rates

by Birger Jansson, Ph.D.

The combined mortality rates for all high-rate neoplasms and for all malignant neoplasms combined are considerably lower in Seneca County, New York, than in its surrounding counties. The possibility that these lower rates are attributable to the geochemical uniqueness of the two lakes that enclose the county, availability and concentration of selenium, high salinity of the lakes, and high concentration of potassium cations is discussed.
Cancer 48:2542–2546, 1981.

SENECA COUNTY, NEW YORK, is a small rural county located in the Finger Lakes region, where it lies between Seneca and Cayuga Lakes. The population, which was about 35,000 in 1970 (including 1.5% nonwhites), is expected to drop to 32,000 in 1980. The portion of the 1970 population over 65 years of age was 12.6%, compared with 10.8% in New York state and 9.9% in the United States as a whole. Furthermore, during the 1960s, there was a net emigration from Seneca County of persons over 70 years of age who wanted better housing. Without this departure, and combined

From the National Large Bowel Cancer Project and the Department of Biomathematics, The University of Texas System Cancer Center, M.D. Anderson Hospital & Tumor Institute, Texas Medical Center, Houston, Texas.

Supported by NCI Grants no. CA-14140 and CA-11430.

Address for reprints: Birger Jansson, PhD, National Large Bowel Cancer Project, The University of Texas System Cancer Center, M.D. Anderson Hospital & Tumor Institute, 6723 Bertner Drive, Texas Medical Center, Houston, TX 77030

The author gratefully acknowledges the assistance in collecting information on Seneca County given by Mr. David L. Rotz, President of the Church of Latter Day Saints, Fayette Branch, New York, and his wife, Barbara; by Dr. Peter Greenwald, New York State Department of Health, Albany, New York, and his co-workers; and by the staff of CORE Laboratories, Inc., Houston, Texas, who provided information on subsurface saline water in Texas.

with a net immigration of persons under 70 years, the percentage of elderly residents would have been still higher. The income level of the county is low to medium, with the median family income being $9600 in 1970.[1]

Seneca County stirred our interest while we were conducting an epidemiologic study of the geographic distributions of colon and rectum cancers. Using the cancer mortality rates by U. S. counties published in 1974 by Mason and McKay,[2] we mapped the distributions of these cancers and found that the northeast part of the United States had an especially high mortality for colorectal cancer, with a coastal strip from the Canadian border to New Jersey having the highest rates.[3] Besides this "hot spot" region, the investigation also revealed that Seneca County was a "cold spot" (low mortality) for cancers of the colon and rectum. When the U. S. counties were ranked from highest (Rank 1) to lowest (Rank 3056), we found rank differences of about 1000 places between Seneca County and its six neighboring counties.[4,5]

Suspecting that this could be an improbable random event, we compared the mortality rates for cancer at sites other than the colon and rectum. The results are shown in Table 1 for all such site–sex combinations for

TABLE 1. Mortality Rates/100,000/year 1950–1969 in New York State and Seneca County

Site	ICD*	Mortality Rate, White				Rank of Seneca County among the 58 counties in New York State	
		N.Y. State		Seneca County			
		Males	Females	Males	Females	Males	Females
Mouth, Tongue	141–145, 148	5.29	1.13	1.9	0.6	57	50
Esophagus	150	5.44	1.39	3.0	0.5	45	53
Stomach	151	18.52	9.78	11.2	6.5	53	57
Colon	153	21.66	19.55	13.0	15.8	57	58
Rectum	154	11.48	6.75	5.6	2.8	58	56
Liver	155	5.51	5.60	3.4	2.2	42	58
Pancreas	157	10.58	6.70	5.7	3.3	55	57
Larynx	161	3.41	—	3.5	—	10	—
Lung	162, 163	43.77	7.20	23.4	5.1	58	37
Breast	170	—	31.53	—	21.7	—	58
Cervix	171	—	6.64	—	7.4	—	41
Uterus	172–174	—	6.09	—	5.9	—	42
Ovary	175	—	10.00	—	6.4	—	58
Prostate	177	16.80	—	14.6	—	57	—
Kidney	180	4.31	2.20	2.2	1.1	57	56
Bladder	181	8.64	2.73	8.2	2.4	24	41
Melanoma	190	1.52	1.01	0.3	2.2	58	1
Skin	191	1.13	—	0.5	—	56	—
Brain	193	4.59	2.98	4.0	2.6	22	19
Bone	196	1.35	—	0.8	—	54	—
Hodgkin	201	2.59	1.59	1.8	1.3	46	37
Lymphoma	200, 202, 205	5.46	3.66	3.3	3.7	54	21
Myeloma	203	1.84	1.34	1.0	1.2	54	31
Leukemia	204	8.90	5.98	5.1	5.9	56	15
White, all malignant neoplasms	140–205	199.24	148.01	125.2	108.0	58	58
Nonwhite, all malignant neoplasms	140–205	95.50	96.48	67.8	19.2	51	55

* ICD—International Classification of Diseases.[6]

which the state rates are more than 1/100,000/year. The rates in Seneca were shown to be unexpectedly low, not only for colon and rectum cancers but for almost all other cancers, especially those cancers for which the rates in New York state are high. The eight highest rates among the 58 counties in New York are 43.77, 31.53, 21.66, 19.55, 18.52, 16.80, 11.48, and 10.00; the corresponding ranks for Seneca County are, respectively, 58, 58, 57, 58, 53, 58, and 58. Thus, in New York, Seneca has among the very lowest mortality rates for all high-rate cancer sites. The same is true for most low-rate cancer sites.

Interestingly, Seneca females have the highest and Seneca males the lowest mortality rates for melanoma in New York. This is most likely a random event made possible by the low melanoma rates. For other skin cancers, the rank for males is 56 and for females 51.

When mortality rates for all malignant neoplasms are taken together, Seneca has the lowest rates for white males and white females. The corresponding rates are also low for nonwhites, with ranks of 51 and 55 for males and females. Because the nonwhite population is only about 500, these figures are less reliable.

The rates for all counties in New York for colon, rectum, and breast cancers and for all malignant neoplasms taken together are displayed in Figure 1. Here the outstandingly low rates in Seneca County are obvious.

The low rates for almost all cancer sites in Seneca County males and females seem to rule out randomness and favor some systematic and rational explanation. Hypotheses based on weaknesses in the reporting system, such as deaths being mistakenly reported in the county of death and not in the county of residence, do not seem to be valid. Some cancers, especially of the larynx, bladder, and brain, rank in the upper half of the scale, which most likely would not happen if systematic misreporting had occurred.

Cancer Mortality Rates For The Counties In New York State
→○ Seneca County

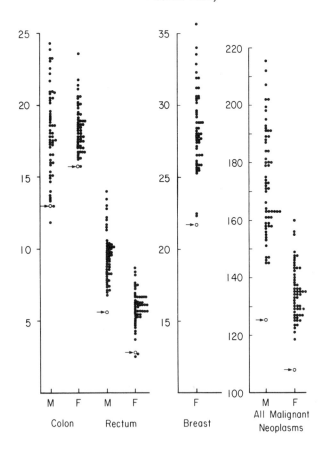

FIG. 1. Cancer mortality rates for counties in New York State. ○ Seneca County, ● other counties, M = Males, F = Females.

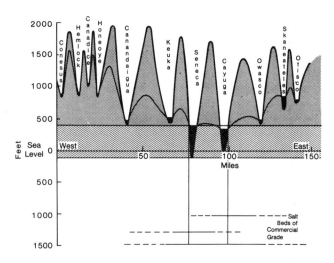

FIG.2. Profile of the lakes in the Finger Lakes region and of the land between the lakes. The thin line represents the land profile at the north end of the lakes and the thick line that at the south end (Modified from Berg[7]).

An explanation for the low rates of cancer in Seneca County may be the unique geographic and geochemical nature of the area. It is located between the two deepest lakes in the Finger Lakes region, Seneca and Cayuga Lakes. Moreover, these two lakes are the lowest in elevation. For a profile of the lakes and the area between them, see Figure 2, modified from Berg.[7] The low, thinner profile in the figure indicates the heights of the land in the north ends of the lakes, while the high, thicker profile indicates the heights in the south ends. Northern Seneca County is largely a low region not reaching much above the levels of Cayuga and Seneca Lakes. Horizontal salt strata formed during the Paleozoic era underlie the Finger Lakes region. These strata contain high-quality salt that has been commercially mined from the lakes' shores. Due to their low elevation and depth, Seneca and Cayuga Lakes penetrate strata not reached by the other lakes. Berg mentions the possibility that salt beds not satisfying the commercial standards of purity for extraction may be intersected by the two lakes, thereby making them geochemically unique, and

he concludes that "the great depths of Cayuga and Seneca Lakes may expose them to influences from which the shallower lakes of the region are effectively isolated."

Figure 3, based on a table by Berg, presents the "conductivity" and concentrations of the ions of sodium plus potassium, chloride, calcium, and sulfate in eight of the lakes. (Berg did not, in his table, separate the concentrations of sodium and potassium.)

It can be seen that the concentrations of sodium plus potassium, and chloride are extremely high in Seneca and Cayuga Lakes when compared with the other Finger Lakes and with almost all New York lakes listed by Berg. (The one exception is the small Onondaga Lake in the New York limestone belt, which has still higher concentrations of these ions. According to Berg, this is caused partly by domestic and industrial pollution.) The chloride concentration, listed by Berg as 125 ppm, has increased since his report and is now approaching 200 ppm.[8]

Besides high concentrations of sodium, potassium, and chloride ions, the concentration of sulfate ions is also higher in Seneca and Cayuga Lakes than in the other Finger Lakes and most New York lakes. This may be important because of a high sulfur concentration may also be indicative of a high selenium concentration.

When the sizes of populations served by different water sources are used as weights in the determination of these concentrations, we find that the concentration of the trace element selenium in the waters in Seneca is about 1.6 times the mean concentration in New York. Moreover, the soil in Seneca is alkaline, while the soil in the northeast United States is generally acid (personal communication, Department of Health, State of New York). The alkalinity of the soil increases the availability of selenium for plants and animals, which,

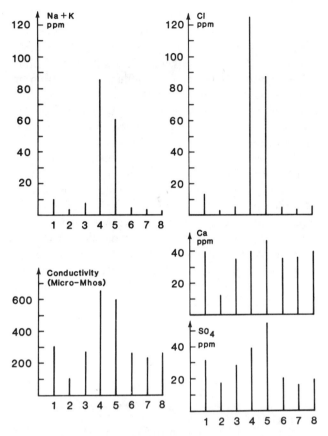

FIG. 3. The conductivity and the concentrations of some chemical ions from west to east in (1) Conesus, (2) Canadice, (3) Canandaigua, (4) Seneca, (5) Cayuga, (6) Owasco, (7) Skaneateles, and (8) Otisco Lakes.

in combination with the rather high concentration, may be a protective factor against carcinogenicity. That selenium acts as an anticarcinogen has been demonstrated in a number of animal experiments; that it also acts as an antimutagen has been shown by bacterial tests. Furthermore, in epidemiologic studies, an association between selenium-deficient areas and high-cancer-rate areas has been observed.[9]

That potassium cations play a vital role in the salification of the hydrogen bonds in all living structures has been postulated by Pantellini.[10] According to his theory, this salification is especially important for the bases of DNA and RNA, in which its lack leads to opening of the valences and distortion of the genetic information, and ultimately to the formation of neoplasms. Pantellini declares that this chemical–physical mechanism is the same for all tumors, with differences due only to different protein syntheses.

If Pantellini's hypothesis proves true, one might expect lower incidence rates of tumors in areas where the environment contains sufficient amounts of potassium. This might then be part of the explanation for the low cancer rates in Seneca County.

A superficial reading of limnologic and "salt" literature reveals a number of saline (i.e. chloride-rich) lakes and salt playas. It is of interest to compare the cancer mortality rates in counties with such formations to the rates in other counties within the same state (Table 2). We find that in the salt-rich counties, the cancer mortality rate is among the lowest and often the very lowest in the state.

Combining information on subsurface saline water[19] by county in Texas with the United States rank for the same counties of colon plus rectum plus breast cancers

TABLE 2. Rank Within State for All Malignant Neoplasms, White, Males + Females among All Counties in the State for Counties with Salt Lakes or Salt Playas

Lake	County	Comments	References	County rank in state among all counties in the state
Seneca Cayuga	Seneca, NY		7, 11	58/58
Devil's Lake	Ramsey, ND	Salinity increased since last century	12	76/83
Devil's Lake	Benson, ND	Salinity increased since last century	12	82/83
Soap Lake	Okanogan, WA	High concentration of K^+	13	31/39
Soap Lake	Grant, WA	High concentration of K^+	13	39/39
—	Esmeralda, NV	Salt playas	14, 15	17/17
Zuni Salt Lake	Catron, NM	Salt has for centuries been gathered in this lake	14, 15	32/32
Mono Lake	Mono, CA	High concentration of K^+	16	58/58*
Goose Lake	Modoc, CA	Large saline lake	17	57/58
—	Culberson, TX	Salt lake	18	245/255
—	Hudspeth, TX	Salt flats	18	240/255

* Mono Lake has much lower rate for all malignant neoplasms combined for white males than all other California counties. White females in this county, however, have the highest cancer mortality rates in the United States for a number of rare sites combined into one group (ICD 147, 152, 158, 159, 164, 165, 176, 178, 179, 198, 199). This high rate is most likely an error, if not it indicates an interesting clustering of rare cancers in a small region. If these rare cancer sites are omitted, the male plus female cancer rate in Mono County is the lowest in California.

further supports a relation between salinity and cancer rates. The results are presented in Table 3, in which the counties are dichotomized regarding water salinity and cancer rank. A cancer rank above the cut-off point 2700 corresponds approximately to a rate among the 10% lowest in the country. We note that 48% of the saline counties fall in the low rate group compared to only 18% among the nonsaline counties and that this difference is highly significant.

Finally, an observation from Evans County, Georgia, indicates the role of potassium as an anticarcinogen. Grim *et al.*[20] estimated the dietary intake of sodium and potassium for whites and blacks living in this county in order to test the hypothesis that the greater prevalence of hypertensives among the blacks depended on a greater intake of sodium. Contrary to the hypothesis, they found that whites had a greater sodium intake and above all a much greater potassium intake than did the blacks. The potassium dietary intake was shown to be 2.3 times higher for white males than for black males, while the corresponding figure for females was 1.6. The cancer mortality rate for all malignant neoplasms in Evans County for black men is 243.3/100,000/year and for white men, 156.1. The corresponding state rates in Georgia are 152 and 154, respectively. For females, the rates in Evans County agree well with the rates in Georgia, with black women having somewhat higher cancer mortality rates than white women. Is the low potassium intake among black men related to their high cancer rate?

A more thorough study of regions in which the biota comes into contact with potassium-rich brines or superficial layers of potash may confirm or refute the hypothetical relation between potassium and cancer rates.

The geochemical uniqueness of Seneca County should be further studied to clarify its role in the low cancer rates. Unfortunately, Berg[7] did not separate sodium and potassium ions in his table of ion concentrations in Seneca and Cayuga Lakes. Later determinations compiled by Oglesby[11] show that, in Cayuga Lake, sodium ions are about 30 times as abundant as potassium ions.

In contrast, the proportion of sodium to potassium is about 20 to 1 in the saline lakes in the western United States. The absolute concentration of sodium plus potassium, that is, 100–200 ppm in Seneca and Cayuga Lakes, is 10 to 100-fold higher in the western saline lakes, such as Mono Lake in California. In nonsaline lakes in the Finger Lakes region, as well as in other parts of the country, it is generally lower than 10 ppm.

The relative freedom from industrial pollution in Seneca County, enhanced by the fact that the north-south water divider passes through it, reducing the inflow of polluted water, may also contribute to the low cancer rate.

Our observation of the very low cancer rates in Seneca County when compared to the surrounding counties led us to some hypothetical explanations. Prevalence and availability of selenium, high salinity of the water and especially high concentrations of potassium cations may belong to the anticarcinogenic factors contributing to the low rates. These and other factors are leads that should be further investigated and that may provide us with information leading to an increased understanding of the etiology of cancer.

TABLE 3. Rank of Colon + Rectum + Breast Cancer, White Males + Females, among U. S. Counties in Relation to Subsurface Water Salinity in Texas Counties

	Rank		
	>2700	<2700	TOTAL
Saline counties*	27	29	56
Nonsaline counties+	35	164	199
TOTAL	62	193	255

* Depth to saline water <300 feet and concentration of Cl^- >300 ppm.
+ All others.
$\chi^2 = 21$ with $P = 0.00001$.

REFERENCES

1. Stevens KB. Seneca County Housing Plan. 1976; Seneca-NYP 1100-5.3.
2. Mason TJ, MacKay FS. U. S. Cancer Mortality by County 1950–1969. 1974, DHEW Publication No. (NIH) 74-615.
3. Jansson B, Malahy MA, Seibert GD. Geographical distribution of gastrointestinal cancer and breast cancer and its relation to selenium deficiency. Proceedings of the Third International Symposium on Detection and Prevention of Cancer. New York: Marcel Dekker, 1976:1161–1177.
4. Jansson B. The geographical distribution of colorectal cancer in the United States. *Med Biolog Environ* 1976; 4:119–123.
5. Jansson B, Jacobs MM. Selenium—a possible inhibitor of colon and rectum cancer. Proceedings of the Symposium on Selenium-Tellurium in the Environment. Pittsburgh: Industrial Health Foundation, Inc., 1976:326–340.
6. Manual of the International Statistical Classification of Diseases, Injuries, and Causes of Death. Sixth Revision of the International List of Diseases and Causes of Death, Adopted 1948, vol. 1, Geneva, Switzerland: World Health Organization, 1948:79–89.
7. Berg CO. Middle Atlantic States. In: Frey DG, ed. Limnology in North America. Madison: The University of Wisconsin Press, 1963:191–237.
8. Ahrnsbrak WF. Saline infusion into Seneca Lake, New York. *Limn Ocean* 1975; 20:275–278.
9. Jansson B. The role of selenium as a cancer-protecting trace element. In: Sigel H, ed. Carcinogenicity and Metal Ions, vol. 10 in the series Metal Ions in Biological Systems. New York: Marcel Dekker, 1980:281–311.
10. Pantellini VG. Hydrogen (H) bonds and their salification by potassium (K) in the structuring of living matter. *Med Biolog Environ* 1976; 4:467–472.
11. Oglesby RT. The limnology of Cayuga Lake. In: Bloomfield JA, ed. Lakes of New York State, vol. 1. New York: Academic Press: 1978:1–20.
12. Eddy S. Minnesota and the Dakotas. In: Frey DG, ed. Limnology in North America. Madison: The University of Wisconsin Press, 1963:301–315.

13. Edmondson WT. Pacific Coast and Great Basin. In: Frey DG, ed. Limnology in North America. Madison: The University of Wisconsin Press, 1963:371–392.

14. Landes KK. Salt deposits of the United States. In: Kaufmann DW, ed. Sodium Chloride. New York: Reinhold Publishing, 1960:70–95.

15. Lefond SJ. Handbook of World Salt Resources. New York: Plenum Press, 1969.

16. Altman PL, Dittmer DS. Environmental Biology. Bethesda, Maryland: Federation of American Societies for Experimental Biology, 1966.

17. Geraghty JJ, Miller DW, van der Leeden F, Troise FL. Water Atlas of the United States. Port Washington, New York: Water Information Center, Inc., 1973.

18. Texas Almanac and State Industrial Guide 1974–1975. Dallas, Texas: A.H. Belo Corporation, 1973.

19. CORE Laboratories, Inc., Dallas, Texas. Chemical analysis of saline water. In: A Survey of the Subsurface Saline Water in Texas, vol. 2. Austin, Texas: Texas Water Development Board, Report 157, September 1972.

20. Grim CE, Luft FC, Miller JZ, Meneely GR, Battarbee HD, Hames CG, Dahl LK. Racial differences in blood pressure in Evans County, Georgia: relationship to sodium and potassium intake and plasma renin activity. *J Chron Dis* 1980; 33:87–94.

Statistics and Trends by Cancer Site with
Population Correlatives

Diet in the Etiology of Oral and Pharyngeal Cancer among Women from the Southern United States

by Deborah M. Winn,[1] Regina G. Ziegler, Linda W. Pickle, Gloria Gridley, WIlliam J. Blot, and Robert N. Hoover

ABSTRACT

A case-control interview study involving 227 women in North Carolina with oral cavity or pharyngeal cancer and 405 matched controls showed a protective effect of a usual adult diet high in fruits and vegetables. The relative risks of 0.65 for moderate and 0.52 for high (relative to 1.0 for infrequent) consumption of fruits and vegetables were statistically significant and remained after controlling for demographic characteristics, tobacco and alcohol use, relative weight, and intake of other food groups. Risks were lower with higher bread and cereal intake but higher for those women with the lightest weights, adjusted for height. The inverse associations between oral and pharyngeal cancer and intake of fruits and vegetables and intake of breads and cereals could not be attributed to an association with general nutritional status, since meat and fish consumption was related to an increased risk of oral and pharynx cancer. Moreover, dairy and egg consumption was generally unrelated to cancer risk. The reduction in risk with greater fruit and vegetable consumption is consistent with the hypothesis that vitamin C and/or β-carotene intake is associated with a reduced risk of oral and pharyngeal cancer.

INTRODUCTION

Mortality rates from oral cavity and pharyngeal cancer among white women are higher in the Southeast than elsewhere in the United States (24). We conducted a case-control study among women in North Carolina to identify life-style, occupational, and medical characteristics contributing to the high female mortality rate for oral cavity and pharyngeal cancer in the region. Snuff dipping, cigarette smoking, and alcohol consumption were strongly related to oral and pharyngeal cancer in the study population; findings concerning these risk factors as well as dental, mouthwash, and occupational associations have been described elsewhere (4, 37–39). In this report, using the interview data on food consumption from the case-control study, the role of diet in the etiology of oral and pharyngeal cancer among women in North Carolina is evaluated.

Recent findings (21) suggest that indices of vitamins A and C intake may be inversely associated with epithelial cancers in the oral cavity. We were interested not only in exploring the relationship between these cancers and intake of food groups which are typically high in selected vitamins but also in examining some food preparation methods and overall dietary patterns. As a consequence of the persuasive findings for snuff and cigarettes, we were interested also in interactions between diet and these 2 tobacco habits, which appear to act on/at the site of physical contact.

MATERIALS AND METHODS

Female oral cavity and pharyngeal cancer cases were identified through review of hospital discharges at 5 North Carolina hospitals, supplemented with tumor registry listings in 3 of the hospitals, occurring over a 3-year period ending in August 1978. Included were 156 incident and prevalent cases with cancers of the tongue, gums, buccal mucosa, floor of mouth, palate, tonsils, or pharynx and hypopharynx [International Classification of Diseases, Eighth Revision (27) Codes 141, 143 to 146, 148, 149]. Two controls per case were sought from the same hospital as the case, matched on age (± 5 years), race, and county of residence.

From the Environmental Epidemiology Branch, National Cancer Institute, Bethesda, Maryland 20205.

[1] *To whom requests for reprints should be addressed, at the Environmental Epidemiology Branch, Landow Building 3C09, Bethesda, MD 20205.*

Controls with a major oral or pharyngeal disease, cancer of the esophagus or larynx, or a mental disorder were ineligible. An additional 99 female residents who died in North Carolina of oral or pharyngeal cancer over a 2.5-year concomitant period were obtained from Vital Statistics listings and were each matched with 2 controls from the same source using the same age, race, residence, and diagnostic criteria as for hospitalized subjects. Hospital controls were obtained by review of hospital admissions subsequent to the case; death certificate controls were ascertained from lists of deaths occurring subsequent to the case's death.

Of the 405 controls, 98 (24%) had diseases of the heart as the first listed discharge diagnosis or underlying case of death; 70 (17%) had a malignant neoplasm (12, digestive system; 16, respiratory system; 25, genitourinary system; and 17, other sites); 41 (10%) had cerebrovascular disease; 31 (8%) had diseases of the digestive system; 25 (6%) had musculoskeletal system conditions; 20 (5%) had nervous system or sense organ diseases; 19 (5%) were victims of accidents, poisonings, or violence; and 101 (25%) had other conditions.

A questionnaire was administered to the study subject or her next of kin by a trained interviewer in the home of the respondent. Interviews were conducted with the closest possible next of kin when the study subject was deceased or unable to provide an interview. Information recorded on each subject included demographic characteristics, tobacco habits, occupation, medical history, and dental status.

The dietary section of the questionnaire asked about the subject's usual adult diet. At the start of the diet history section, the interviewer stated, "This section will ask for information about your diet history from the time you were 20 years old until 1975. We are mainly concerned with your most usual diet as an adult." Frequency of consumption was determined for 21 food items. Also included were questions concerning usual adult height and weight, special diets, meal patterns (*e.g.*, the number of meals per day), and methods of preparation of meat and fish (*e.g.*, smoking). Three ordinal levels of frequency of consumption, high, moderate, and low, for each of the food items were created by dividing the total (cases plus controls) distribution into approximate thirds. Food groups based on traditional food groupings (*e.g.*, fruits and vegetables) or food preparation methods (*e.g.*, smoked meats and fish, nitrite-containing meats) were created by summing the usual weekly consumption of appropriate individual food items. The food group distributions were stratified into the lowest 25%, middle 50%, and highest 25%.

RRs,[2] estimated by odds ratios (20), were calculated for high and for moderate consumption relative to low consumption. Confidence intervals were calculated using the method of Gart (11). Mantel's (19) extension test was used to test (one-tailed) the progressive dependence (trend) of the odds ratio on the amount of consumption of food items or groups. Adjusted summary odds ratios (RRs) were computed from a stratified analysis according to the method of Gart (11). In addition to the stratified analysis, the logistic model (7, 31) was used to examine further the interrelationships among food groups and case-control status and to adjust for potential risk factors simultaneously. In developing the final logistic model, the statistical significance of potential correlates of exposure were evaluated by examination of the *t* statistics, as well as likelihood differences when parameters were deleted.

Relative weight was obtained by dividing the subject's reported usual adult weight by height raised to the 1.5 power ($W/H^{1.5}$). The power of 1.5 for the body mass index for women had been derived empirically in a survey of a sample of the United States population (1). Subjects were divided into 4 groups: those much heavier than "typical"; those centered around the typical value; those centered at an "ideal" value; and those much lighter than the ideal. Typical weight was based on the race- and age group-specific median weights for United States women obtained from the Health and Nutrition Examination Survey I (28). The "ideal" relative weight for adult women, 0.23 lb/inch$^{1.5}$ (= 26.5 kg/m$^{1.5}$), was

[2] The abbreviation used is: RR, relative risk.

obtained from the Recommended Dietary Allowances (10).

Included in the analysis were 227 cases and 405 controls; 59% of the interviews were conducted with next of kin (husbands, 28%; children, 49%; siblings, 11%; other, 12%). More case (69.6%) than control (53.1%) interviews were with next of kin due to the fatal or disabling nature of oral and pharyngeal cancer; thus, respondent status was a key adjustment factor. The next of kin of 5 cases and 5 controls failed to respond to at least 25% of the questions in the diet section of the questionnaire; these study subjects have been excluded from the analysis. In the remaining informative questionnaires, the median intake for monthly consumers of that food item replaced the unknown value when persons were known to eat an item but with an unknown frequency per month. Substituted values accounted for not more than 2.5% of the responses to any given food item.

RESULTS

Table 1 describes general charcteristics and established risk factors for oral and pharyngeal cancer in this study population.

Food Groups

Fruits and Vegetables. Table 2 shows that the estimate of the relative risk for fruits and vegetables was 0.7 for moderate and 0.5 for high consumption, a highly statistically significant trend ($p = 0.002$). In addition, for each of the 3 food items included in the fruits and vegetables grouping, lower risks were seen among both moderate and heavy consumers. The lower risks associated with fruit and vegetable consumption were

Table 1

Odds ratios for selected oral cavity and pharynx risk factors

Factor	Cases (n = 227)	Controls (n = 405)	RR	95% confidence interval
Age				
<65	96	163	(Matching factor)	
65	131	242		
Race				
White	193	344	(Matching factor)	
Black	34	68		
Education				
Grade 6	63	103	1.0	
Grades 7–11	80	139	0.9	0.6–1.5
Grade 12	71	145	0.8	0.5–1.3
Missing	13	18	1.2	0.5–2.8
Tobacco and alcohol use				
No tobacco and alcohol habits	37	136	1.0	
Snuff dipper only	81	78	3.8	2.3–6.3
Snuff and cigarettes only	6	6	3.7	1.0–13.9
Snuff and alcohol only	10	26	1.4	0.6–3.4
All 3 habits	10	13	2.8	1.0–7.6
Cigarettes only	19	48	1.5	0.7–2.9
Alcohol only	4	30	0.5	0.1–1.6
Cigarettes and alcohol	60	68	3.2	1.9–5.5
Wearing of dentures (as indicator of oral problems)				
No	85	172	1.0	
Yes	142	232	1.2	0.9–1.8
Mouthwash[a]				
No	109	201	1.0	
Yes	92	149	1.1	0.8–1.6

[a] Variable available on only a subset of study subjects.

consistently observed within almost every demographic subgroup examined (*e.g.*, racial, educational, regional, urban-rural).

No differences (of more than 0.15 odds ratio units) between the adjusted and unadjusted estimates of effect for the fruit and vegetables grouping were observed for any of the potential confounders examined individually. The confounders which were evaluated included: race; education; cigarette smoking-snuff dipping; ethyl alcohol consumption; the relationship of the respondent to the study subject (self or next of kin); relative weight; presence or absence of dentures; whether 10 or more teeth were missing; reported gum-tooth quality; regular or not regular use of mouthwash; whether 3 or more meals were eaten per day; residence inland or on the coast; usual residence in a farming, rural, or urban area; and the other major food groups. The final logistic model for each food group, which adjusted for the potential confounders simultaneously, yielded adjusted RRs not different from the crude RRs.

This absence of confounding also generally held for the other major food groups examined in detail (breads and cereals, dairy products and eggs, pork products, and fish and shellfish); differences which did occur will be noted explicitly.

Snuff dipping and cigarette smoking were 2 strong independent risk factors for oral and pharyngeal cancer in this study (39). The relationship between these 2 habits and oral and pharyngeal cancer risk was evident among low, moderate, and high consumers of each food group. As shown in Table 3, high but not moderate intake of fruits and vegetables was associated with a reduced RR in those with no tobacco habits; decreasing RRs with increasing intake of fruits and vegetables were evident in those who used cigarettes only or cigarettes and snuff.

Breads and Cereals. The complex carbohydrate food group included whole-grain breads and cereals, white bread, and corn-meal or grits products. As shown in Table 4, the inverse trend of risk with bread and cereal intake was statistically significant. Lower odds ratios with increasing bread and cereal consumption were evident in nonusers of tobacco as well as in snuff dippers and cigarette smokers. Intake of white bread and cornbread-grits appeared to be unrelated to oral and pharyngeal cancer risk, while consumption of whole-grain breads and cereals (moderate RR, 0.8; high RR, 0.7) was associated with lower risk. However, the odds ratio for high whole-grain breads and cereals intake was closer to 1.0 after adjustment for smoking and snuff dipping (moderate RR, 0.8; high RR, 0.9). Unlike the fruit and vegetable items, which were all positively correlated with one another, whole-grain bread consumption was negatively correlated with white bread intake, and both items were unrelated to the consumption of cornbread.

Meat and Fish. Table 5 shows that for several (not mutually exclusive) combinations of the meat and fish items there is an

Table 2

Odds ratios for consumption of fruits and vegetables

	Times consumed/wk	Median weekly intake	Odds ratio	95% confidence interval	*p* for χ^2 trend test
Fruits and vegetables	Low (0–10.9)	8	1.0		0.002
	Moderate (11.0–20.9)	15	0.7	0.4–1.0	
	High (≥21.0)	21	0.5	0.3–0.8	
Fresh fruit	Low (0–1.0)	0.2	1.0		0.001
	Moderate (1.1–6.9)	3	0.7	0.5–1.2	
	High (≥7.0)	7	0.6	0.4–0.8	
Green leafy vegetables	Low (0–2.0)	1	1.0		0.06
	Moderate (2.1–6.9)	3	0.7	0.5–1.1	
	High (≥7.0)	7	0.7	0.5–1.1	
Other vegetables	Low (0–6.9)	2	1.0		0.08
	Moderate (7.0)	7	0.7	0.5–1.1	
	High (≥7.1)	14	0.7	0.4–1.3	

Table 3

Odds ratios for tobacco habits and fruit and vegetable intake

Fruit and vegetable intake	None No.	None RR	None 95% CI[a]	Snuff only No.	Snuff only RR	Snuff only 95% CI	Cigarettes only No.	Cigarettes only RR	Cigarettes only 95% CI	Both No.	Both RR	Both 95% CI
Low												
Cases	9	1.0[b]		24	3.8	1.4–10.7	28	4.4	1.6–12.3	10	9.4	2.0–47.8
Controls	34			24			24			4		
Medium												
Cases	18	1.1	0.4–2.9	39	2.8	1.1–7.2	35	2.5	1.0–6.4	3	1.4	0.2–7.9
Controls	64			52			53			8		
High												
Cases	14	0.8	0.3–2.2	28	3.8	1.4–10.3	16	1.6	0.6–4.4	3	1.6	0.3–9.3
Controls	68			28			39			7		

[a] CI, confidence interval.
[b] Referent.

Table 4

Odds ratios for consumption of breads and cereals

	Times consumed/wk	Median weekly intake	Odds ratio	95% confidence interval	p for trend test
All breads and cereals	Low (0–8.5)	7	1.0		0.02
	Moderate (8.6–17.0)	14	0.9	0.6–1.3	
	High (>17.0)	22	0.6	0.4–1.0	
White bread	Low (0–6.9)	0.2	1.0		0.34
	Moderate (7.0–9.9)	7	1.1	0.7–1.7	
	High (≥10.0)	14	0.9	0.6–1.5	
Whole-grain breads and cereals	Low (0)	0	1.0		0.06
	Moderate (0.1–6.9)	1	0.8	0.5–1.2	
	High (≥7.0)	7	0.7	0.5–1.1	
Cornbread and grits	Low (0–1.9)	1	1.0		
	Moderate (2.0–3.9)	2	1.0	0.7–1.5	0.33
	High (≥4.0)	7	1.1	0.7–1.7	

Table 5

Odds ratios for consumption of meat and fish subgroups by consumption level

	Times consumed/wk	Median weekly intake	Odds ratio	95% confidence interval	p for trend test
All meat and fish	Low (0–7.5)	5	1.0		0.09
	Moderate (7.6–15.0)	11	1.2	0.8–1.9	
	High (>15.0)	19	1.4	0.9–2.2	
Pork products (ham or pork dried meats, bacon, sausage, brains, lunch meat, frankfurters, canned meats)	Low (0–4.9)	3	1.0		0.05
	Moderate (5.0–11.5)	8	1.3	0.8–2.0	
	High (>11.5)	16	1.5	0.9–2.4	
Fish and shellfish	Low (0–0.3)	0.2	1.0		0.04
	Moderate (0.4–1.0)	0.8	1.4	0.9–2.2	
	High (>1.0)	2	1.6	1.0–2.5	
Expensive meat (other beef or veal, pork or ham)	Low (0–1.9)	1	1.0		0.44
	Moderate (2.0–4.0)	3	1.4	0.9–2.1	
	High (>4.0)	6	1.0	0.6–1.7	
Convenience meat (lunch meat, canned meats, frankfurters)	Low (0–0.2)	0	1.0		0.10
	Moderate (0.3–2.0)	1	1.5	1.0–2.3	
	High (>2.0)	4	1.3	0.8–2.1	
Breakfast meat (bacon, sausage)	Low (0–2.0)	1	1.0		0.35
	Moderate (2.1–7.0)	5	1.2	0.8–1.9	
	High (>7.0)	9	1.1	0.7–1.8	
Nitrite-containing meats (corned beef, lunch meat, frankfurters, canned meat, bacon)	Low (0–2.0)	1	1.0		0.31
	Moderate (2.1–7.5)	4	1.0	0.6–1.5	
	High (>7.5)	9	1.1	0.7–1.9	

increasing oral and pharyngeal cancer risk with increasing consumption. The pork products and fish-shellfish categories, as well as the total meat and fish group, show dose-response gradients. Individual food items in the meat-fish category for which more frequent consumption was associated with a higher, although not statistically significant, risk of mouth and throat cancer included frankfurters, luncheon meats, corned beef-pastrami, sausage, brains-chitterlings, ham or pork, fish, and shellfish.

Associations for pork products, which were sometimes obtained from the subjects' own farms, and for the total meat and fish group were modified by other variables, particularly socioeconomic status. The increasing risk with increasing pork prod-

ucts consumption was limited to women with less than a seventh grade education (moderate RR, 1.9; high RR, 3.4); in contrast, the RRs for those with a high school education were in the opposite direction (moderate RR, 0.9; high RR, 0.4), making adjustment by education inappropriate. The RRs were reduced from 1.5 to 1.3 for high consumption when adjustment was made for the relationship of the respondent to the study subject. The estimated risks for fish and shellfish consumption were similar in magnitude and direction to the risks for pork products. High fish and shellfish consumers had 1.6 times the risk of low consumers; only adjustment for overall tooth and gum condition, 1 of 3 dental variables, had an impact on the magnitude of the RR leading to a change from 1.6 to 1.8. No elevated odds ratios were observed for moderate intake of either fish or shellfish, the 2 contributors to the category; however, for both items the RR for high intake was 1.4.

Only 10% of women were reported to consume pickled meats and fish; smoked meat and fish (49%) and charcoal-grilled meat and fish (37%) were more commonly consumed. There was little or no evidence for any overall association with charcoal-grilled or with pickled meats or fish. Elevated risks were seen for smoked beef (RR, 1.8; $p = 0.13$), which was eaten by 26 women; smoked poultry (RR, 3.7; $p = 0.03$); and smoked fish (RR, 3.3; $p = 0.03$), although fewer than 20 respondents reported consumption of the latter 2 foods. However, the smoking of meats and fish was not consistently related to risk, since the RR for the 302 persons who ate smoked pork was only 1.1.

Dairy Products and Eggs. High or moderate consumption of dairy products and eggs was not related to oral and pharyngeal cancer risk. The food items contributing to this food group also showed no consistent patterns of risk with consumption. Adjustment by cigarette smoking and snuff changed the odds ratios for dairy and egg consumption slightly from 0.9 for moderate and 1.0 for high intake to 1.0 and 0.8, respectively.

General Nutritional and Medical Status

The white women in the study were lighter in relative weight than other United States women of comparable age. Sixty-seven % of the total white cases and 66% of white controls had usual adult relative weights less than the median for United States women of the same race and comparable to the case's age at hospitalization or death. More black controls were lighter than the United States median relative weight for blacks (72% were below the median), but only 47% of all black cases were below the median. Overweight women had the same oral and pharyngeal cancer risk as did those close to the United States median weight, while those with ideal or very low weights had race-adjusted relative risks (compared to those of typical weight) of 1.8 and 1.3, respectively, a statistically significant trend ($p = 0.03$). Women who usually ate 3 or more meals per day experienced a nonsignificant decreased risk relative to those who ate less often (RR, 0.8; $p = 0.24$). Although relative weight and meals per day were positively correlated, the RRs for each factor did not change with adjustment for the other factor. Relative weight was positively correlated with intake of each of the food groups, but adjustment by each of the food groups did not diminish the elevated odds ratio for underweight women. In addition, the RRs were not altered when we adjusted for tobacco use, denture wearing, or education.

Information had been obtained by questionnaire regarding diseases previously linked with oral cancer occurrence in the literature. However, only one case and one control were reported to have had syphilis, and none of the women were said by the respondent to have Plummer-Vinson syndrome. A diet predisposing to pellagra and consisting primarily of fatback, cornmeal, and molasses was first identified in the southeastern United States in the early 1900's (12). After elevated risks for pork products were observed, a "pellagra-prone" index based on bacon, sausage, ham-pork, and cornbread intake was created. The RR of 1.3 for high consumption was less than the comparable RR for the pork products groups, and no trend with increasing intake was observed.

Eating Style and Spices and Condiments

Whether fluids were consumed with meals was unrelated to oral and pharyngeal cancer risk (RR, 1.0). Eating faster than other people (RR, 0.4; $p = 0.05$) and drinking beverages that are very hot (RR, 0.7; $p = 0.24$) were inversely related to risk.

Moderate (RR, 1.0) or heavy (RR, 0.9) use of condiments (mustard, ketchup, steak sauce) and spices (pepper, hot peppers, curry powder, chili sauce, hot sauce) was not significantly related to cancer risk, nor was the use of any individual condiment or spice. Only 38% of the study population used "hot" spices, a category which included hot peppers, chili sauce, or hot sauce, with an associated risk of 0.9 ($p = 0.5$).

Case and Control Subpopulations

Minimal changes in the estimated RRs were evident when the case and the control series were restricted to subsets of the study population likely to have different relationships with dietary factors (see Table 6). Relative risks for fruits and vegetables, breads and cereals, and dairy products and eggs were virtually unchanged when the 100 cases identified through death certificates and the 10 prevalent cases (those hospital cases initially diagnosed prior to the 1975–1978 study period) were excluded from the analysis. When the 117 hospitalized incident cases were compared with only the 361 controls with conditions unrelated to diet ("acute" conditions[3]), the patterns originally present in the total population also remained evident for the most restrictive case and control definitions. Slightly stronger associations for fish-shellfish were observed when the case and control definitions were more restricted.

When oral cavity cancer cases and their matched controls were examined separately from pharyngeal cancer cases and controls, the direction of the odds ratios remained consistently above 1 for pork products and below 1 for fruits and vegetables and for cereals and breads; for the latter 2 food groups, the RRs were even lower for the pharyngeal cancer cases than for the oral cavity cancer cases. Elevated RRs for the oral cavity but not for the pharynx were observed with intake of fish and shellfish.

DISCUSSION

This study of diet and oral and pharyngeal cancer revealed clear differences in adult food consumption between women with cancer and controls, suggesting that nutritional factors may play an important role in the origins of these neoplasms.

The most compelling findings concerned the dose-dependent reduction in risk associated with fruit and vegetable consumption, with the high consumers (21 or more portions per week) at approximately one-half the risk of low consumers (less than 11 portions per week). The reduced risks with increasing consumption of the fruit and vegetable food group were consistently observed for the individual food items composing the food group and within subgroups reflecting a wide variety of demographic and life-style characteristics (e.g., education, race), although the

---

[3] Excluded were women with chronic conditions which might significantly influence or are influenced by dietary patterns (neoplasms of the digestive system, ulcers, diabetes, diseases of the intestine, cholelithiasis, dental and facial anomalies, esophageal inflammatory disease, and nutritional deficiencies).

Table 6
Odds ratios[a] with case and control series restrictions

| | Consumption level | All cases (N = 227) vs. all controls (N = 405) | Hospital incident cases[b] (N = 117) vs. all controls (N = 405) | Hospital incident cases (N = 117) vs. acute controls[c] (N = 361) | Anatomic site | |
					Oral cavity cases (N = 157) vs. matched controls (N = 294)	Pharynx cases (N = 69) vs. matched controls (N = 110)
Fruits and vegetables	Moderate	0.7	0.5	0.6	0.9	0.3
	High	0.5	0.5	0.5	0.6	0.4
Bread and cereals	Moderate	0.9	0.8	0.8	0.9	0.8
	High	0.6	0.6	0.6	0.6	0.5
Pork products	Moderate	1.3	1.5	1.5	1.3	1.2
	High	1.5	1.5	1.5	1.6	1.3
Fish and shellfish	Moderate	1.4	1.8	2.0	1.6	1.0
	High	1.6	1.9	1.9	1.9	0.9
Dairy products and eggs	Moderate	0.9	0.9	0.9	0.8	1.4
	High	1.0	1.0	1.0	0.9	1.1

[a] Relative to low consumption.
[b] Cases ascertained from participating hospitals and initially diagnosed during 3-year study period.
[c] Controls with diagnoses unrelated to or unaffected by diet.

reduction was most prominent among smokers. None of the many factors that we examined separately (in the stratified analysis) or together (in the logistic analysis) introduced any substantial confounding of the RR estimates.

The apparent protective effect noted for high consumption of total fruits and vegetables is consistent with several biological mechanisms. Fruits and vegetables are the primary source of β-carotene, which is metabolized to retinol (vitamin A) in humans. Numerous animal and cell culture studies have shown cancer inhibition by retinoids (34), and evidence is mounting from epidemiological studies of several epithelial cancers that high intake of vitamin A-containing foods may be protective (2, 14, 15, 25). There is also evidence that mean serum retinol levels are lower in those who ultimately develop cancer (17, 36).

β-Carotene itself, the level of which in serum is far more closely related to dietary intake than is retinol, has been postulated to have an effect independent of that for retinol (30). One small follow-up survey implicated dietary β-carotene, rather than retinol, in the reduced risk of lung cancer (33). We did not obtain information on all major retinol- and carotene-containing foods and could not develop indices of consumption to evaluate adequately the relative contributions of these 2 micronutrients. However, retinol is present in substantial amounts in milk, cheese, and eggs, whereas β-carotene is present in fruits and vegetables. Our finding of a very weak and inconsistent association between oral and pharyngeal cancer and dairy products and eggs suggests that retinol may not be a protective factor.

Vitamin C also has been suggested as an anticancer agent primarily because it inhibits the formation of nitrosamines from amines (or amides) and nitrite (26). Vitamin C is found almost exclusively in fruits and vegetables. Since we asked only about the consumption of fresh fruit, green leafy vegetables, and other vegetables, we were unable to examine separately the contributions of total fruits and vegetables, vitamin C, and β-carotene.

The inverse association between intake of the breads and

cereals food group and cancer risk was close in magnitude to that for fruits and vegetables and appeared independent of the effect of the other food groups including fruits and vegetables. This absence of confounding implies that the distribution of other food groups cannot account for this association. However, the effect seemed to be limited to whole-grain breads and cereals. One hypothesis that could account for an apparent protective effect of both fruits and vegetables and bread and cereals is that the bulk and fiber of these foods may cleanse the mouth and throat of ingested carcinogens.

In contrast to the apparent reduction in risk with high fruit and vegetable and high bread and cereal consumption, increasing consumption of pork products and of fish and shellfish were related to increasing oral and pharyngeal cancer risk. The association with pork consumption was inconsistent, the positive association coming entirely from a strong relationship among the lowest social class while those in the highest social class who consumed a large amount of pork were actually at a decreased risk. This inconsistency casts doubt on the association. Alternatively, the form of pork consumed or a pork preparation or storage method used by the least educated might account for the increased risk, since many study subjects ate pigs which had been killed and prepared on their own farms. Thus, while the pork products and fish-shellfish associations persisted after controlling for fruit and vegetable intake, the biological meaningfulness of these associations is unclear.

There are several studies of nutrition and oral cancer with which to compare our findings. No differences were found between oral cancer cases and controls in the percentage of patients with an "adequate diet" (9), in the intake of a number of specific food items in a New York study (13), or in a population based study of oral cavity, pharyngeal, and esophageal cancer in Puerto Rico (23). In a case-control study of oral cavity cancers in New York (40), no consistent patterns of risk in both men and women were observed for specific food items and food groups.

However, Marshall *et al.* (21) did find in their questionnaire survey lower dietary intake of vitamins A and C in cases compared to non-cancer controls. Studies in India have shown that serum vitamin A and carotene levels are lower in oral and oropharyngeal cancer cases than in controls (5, 35); however, changes in serum vitamin A levels as a consequence of the cancer cannot be ruled out.

A common criticism of case-control studies of diet and cancer is that differences between cases and controls may be a consequence of the disease process in the cases. Cancer in general and oral and pharyngeal cancer in particular may interfere with the patient's ability to eat and may lead to dietary disturbances. To avoid this form of bias, the questionnaire was oriented to usual adult dietary patterns and not to recent habits. In addition, we analyzed subsets of the cases and controls in several ways because of our concerns that the cases' or controls' dietary patterns may have changed due to the symptoms of disease. The associations observed with the entire case group were observed in those whose onset of disease was most recent (the incident cases). In addition, the associations were specific for certain food groups, while one might expect more of an across-the-board effect resulting from disease symptomatology.

When a hospital control group is used, there is a possibility that the conditions of the patients in the control group may have influenced their diet, or conversely dietary factors may have contributed to disease occurrence in some members of the control group. However, we found no substantial differences in the relative risks even when we further restricted the study population by including in the control series only those with "acute" conditions presumably unrelated to dietary factors.

Two other concerns in the interpretation of case control investigations of nutrition and cancer are the validity of the diet history method of data collection and the value of interviews conducted with next of kin rather than with the subject herself. In a review of dietary assessment methods, Block (3) suggests that diet history methods, like the one used here, usually are in reasonable agreement with results obtained from other dietary methods (*e.g.*, 24-hr recall) and with certain clinical measurements (*e.g.*, serum vitamin C). Moderately high correlations for dietary items are observed with reinterview of study subjects, especially when the interval between interviews is relatively short (*e.g.*, 6 months) (8, 16, 29), indicating that diet history methods can provide acceptable test-retest reliability. Surveys of comparability of responses between subjects and surrogates also have generally shown adequate agreement on dietary or height and weight questions when the surrogates are close relatives (18, 22, 32). Most surrogate respondents in our research were close relatives of the study subjects who would be expected to be familiar with the subjects' dietary habits. In addition, our estimates of risk adjusted for respondent type were virtually the same as the initial estimates. Because next of kin were respondents for some of the cases (and also because the dietary component of the questionnaire was designed to generate rather than test hypotheses), portion size information was not collected. However, since the study population of women was relatively homogeneous in age and region of the country, it was assumed that food frequencies would vary more than portion size.

Finally, any misclassification of dietary habits due to deficiencies in the method or recall of the subjects is likely to be random (*i.e.*, similar for cases and controls), since the study population was unaware of the specific suspicions about links between diet and oral cancer. Such random misclassification could not produce a spurious association but could tend to obscure a real one (6). Thus, while such difficulties could have caused us to miss an important finding, they are unlikely to be responsible for the observed associations.

In summary, the reduction in risk associated with fruit and vegetable consumption is dose dependent and unconfounded by other aspects of life-style. Risks are of modest magnitude, which may be expected in a population which is relatively homogeneous with respect to diet. However, the association has biological plausibility and is consistent with findings for epithelial cancer in other studies. Although this study does not provide definitive answers, it does add to the enthusiasm for additional work to confirm and refine our understanding of the role of diet and micronutrients in cancer etiology.

ACKNOWLEDGMENTS

We thank Westat, Inc., Rockville, MD, for data collection activities; ORI, Inc., Bethesda, MD, for computer programming support; the Environmental Epidemiology Section of the National Cancer Institute's Environmental Epidemiology Branch for their insightful comments; and Theresa Pino and Michele Rasa for valuable secretarial support.

REFERENCES

1. Abraham, S., Carroll, M., Najjar, M., and Fulwood, R. Obese and overweight adults in the U.S. (Vital and Health Statistics; Ser. 11, Data from the National Health Surveys No. 230). DHHS Publication No. (PHS) 83-1680. Hyattsville, MD: National Center for Health Statistics, 1983.
2. Bjelke, E. Dietary vitamin A and human lung cancer. Int. J. Cancer, *15:* 561–565, 1975.
3. Block, G. A review of validations of dietary assessment methods. Am. J. Epidemiol., *115:* 492–505, 1982.
4. Blot, W. J., Winn, D. M., and Fraumeni, J. F., Jr. Mouthwash and oral cancer. J. Natl. Cancer. Inst., *70:* 251–253, 1983.
5. Chaudhy, N. A., Jafarey, N. A., and Ibrahim, K. Plasma vitamin A and carotene levels in relation to the clinical stages of carcinoma of the oral cavity and oropharynx. JPMA, *30:* 221–223, 1980.
6. Copeland, K. T., Checkoway, H., McMichael, A. J., and Holbrook, R. H. Bias due to misclassification in the estimation of relative risk. Am. J. Epidemiol., *105:* 488–495, 1977.
7. Cox, D. R. The Analysis of Binary Data. London: Methuen, 1970.
8. Dawber, T. R., Pearson, G., Anderson, P., Mann, G. V., Kannel, W. B., Shurtleff, P., and McNamara, P. Dietary assessment in the epidemiologic study of coronary heart disease: the Framingham study. II. The reliability of measurement. Am. J. Clin. Nutr., *11:* 226–234, 1962.
9. Feldman, J. G., and Hazan, M. A case-control investigation of alcohol, tobacco, and diet in head and neck cancer. Prev. Med., *4:* 444–463, 1975.
10. Food and Nutrition Board. Recommended Dietary Allowances, Revised Ed. 9. Washington, D.C.: National Academy of Sciences, 1980.
11. Gart, J. J. The comparison of proportions: review of significance tests, confidence intervals, and adjustments for stratification. Rev. Int. Statist. Inst., *39:* 148–169, 1971.
12. Goldberger, J. The cause and prevention of pellagra. *In:* M. Terris (ed.), Goldberger on Pellagra, pp. 23–26. Baton Rouge, LA: Lousiana State University Press, 1964.
13. Graham, S., Dayal, H., Rohrer, T., Swanson, M., Sultz, H., Shedd, D., and Fischman, S. Dentition, diet, tobacco, and alcohol in the epidemiology of oral cancer. J. Natl. Cancer Inst., *59:* 1611–1618, 1977.
14. Graham, S., Mettlin, C., Marshall, J., Priore, R., Rzepka, T., and Shedd, D. Dietary factors in the epidemiology of cancer of the larynx. Am. J. Epidemiol., *113:* 675–680, 1981.
15. Hirayama, T. Diet and cancer. Nutr. Cancer, *1:* 67–81, 1979.
16. Jain, M., Howe, G. R., Johnson, K. C., and Miller, A. B. Evaluation of diet history questionnaire. Am. J. Epidemiol., *111:* 212–219, 1980.
17. Kark, J. D., Smith, A. H., Switzer, B. R., and Hames, C. G. Serum vitamin A (retinol) and cancer incidence in Evans County, Georgia. J. Natl. Cancer Inst., *66:* 7–16, 1981.
18. Kolonel, L. N., Hirohata, T., and Nomura, A. Adequacy of survey data collected from substitute respondents. Am. J. Epidemiol., *106:* 476–484, 1977.

19. Mantel, N. Chi-square tests with one degree of freedom, extensions of Mantel-Haenszel procedure. J. Am. Statist. Assoc., *58:* 690–700, 1963.

20. Mantel N, and Haenszel W. Statistical aspects of the analysis of data from retrospective studies of disease. J. Natl. Cancer Inst., *22:* 719–748, 1959.

21. Marshall, J., Graham, S., Mettlin, C., Shedd, D., and Swanson, M. Diet in the epidemiology of oral cancer. Nutr. Cancer, *3:* 145–149, 1982.

22. Marshall, J., Priore, R., Haughey, B., Rzepka, T., and Graham, S. Spouse-subject interviews and the reliability of diet studies. Am. J. Epidemiol., *112:* 675–683, 1980.

23. Martinez, I. Factors associated with cancer of the esophagus, mouth, and pharynx in Puerto Rico. J. Natl. Cancer Inst., *42:* 1069–1094, 1969.

24. Mason, T. J., McKay, F. W., Hoover, R., Blot, W. J., and Fraumeni, J. F., Jr. Atlas of Cancer Mortality for U. S. Counties, 1950–1969. DHEW Publication No. (NIH) 75-780. Washington, DC: Government Printing Office, 1975.

25. Mettlin, C., and Graham, S. Dietary risk factors in human bladder cancer. Am. J. Epidemiol., *110:* 255–263, 1979.

26. Mirvish, S. S., Wallcave, L., Eagen, M., and Shubik, P. Ascorbate-nitrite reaction: possible means of blocking the formation of *N*-nitroso compounds. Science (Wash. DC), *177:* 65–68, 1972.

27. National Center for Health Statistics. Eighth Revision International Classification of Diseases (Adapted for Use in the United States), Vol 1. DHEW Publication No. (PHS) 1693. Washington, DC: Government Printing Office, 1968.

28. National Center for Health Statistics. Overweight Adults in the United States. Advance data, No. 51. Hyattsville, MD: National Center for Health Statistics, 1979.

29. Nomura, A., Hankin, J. H., and Rhoads, G. G. The reproducibility of dietary intake data in a prospective study of gastrointestinal cancer. Am. J. Clin. Nutr., *29:* 1432–1436, 1976.

30. Peto, R., Doll, R., Buckley, J. D., and Sporn, M. B. Can dietary beta-carotene materially reduce human cancer rates. Nature (Lond.), *290:* 201–208, 1981.

31. Prentice, R. Use of the logistic model in retrospective studies. Biometrics, *32:* 599–606, 1976.

32. Rogot, E., and Reid, D. D. The validity of data from next-of-kin in studies of mortality among migrants. Int. J. Epidemiol., *4:* 51–54, 1975.

33. Shekelle, R. B., Liu, S., Raynor, W. J., Lepper, M., Maliza, C., Rossof, A. H., Paul, O., Shryock, A. M., and Stamler, J. Dietary vitamin A and the risk of cancer in the Western Electric study. Lancet, *2:* 1185–1189, 1981.

34. Sporn, M. B., Dunlop, N. M., Newton, D. L., and Smith, J. M. Prevention of chemical carcinogenesis by vitamin A and its synthetic analogs (retinoids). Fed. Proc., *35:* 1332–1338, 1976.

35. Wahi, P. N., Kehar, U., and Lahiri, B. Factors influencing oral and oropharyngeal cancers in India. Br. J. Cancer, *19:* 642–660, 1965.

36. Wald, N., Idle, M., Boreham, J., and Bailey, A. Low serum-vitamin-A and subsequent risk of cancer. Lancet, *2:* 813–815, 1980.

37. Winn, D. M., Blot, W. J., and Fraumeni, J. F., Jr. Snuff dipping and oral cancer. N. Engl. J. Med., *305:* 230–231, 1981.

38. Winn, D. M., Blot, W. J., Shy, C. M., and Fraumeni, J. F., Jr. Occupation and oral cancer among women in the South. Am. J. Indust. Med., *3:* 161–167, 1982.

39. Winn, D. M., Blot, W. J., Shy, C. M., Pickle, L. W., Toledo, A., and Fraumeni, J. F., Jr. Snuff dipping and oral cancer among women in the southern United States. N. Engl. J. Med., *305:* 745–749, 1981.

40. Wynder, E. L., Bross, I. J., and Feldman, R. M. A study of the etiologic factors in cancer of the mouth. Cancer (Phila.), *10:* 1300–1323, 1957.

Nasopharyngeal Carcinoma in Chinese—Salted Fish or Inhaled Smoke?

by Mimi C. Yu, John H. C. Ho, Ronald K. Ross, and Brian E. Henderson

The role of two proposed risk factors for nasopharyngeal carcinoma (NPC) in Chinese was examined by comparing incidence rates (1974–1975) of NPC among Chinese in Hong Kong with those in Los Angeles County (1972–1976) by age, sex, birthplace, and occupation. In Hong Kong, incidence rates for NPC were highest for persons born outside of the Chiu Chau region in Kwangtung Province. In Los Angeles County, the highest rates were observed for immigrant Chinese followed by indigenous Chinese. The high rates in Hong Kong-born Chinese and in Hong Kong boat people and the much higher rates in men compared with women do not support an inhaled carcinogen as the major risk factor for NPC in southern Chinese. The incidence data coupled with available experimental evidence are most consistent with consumption of Cantonese salted fish as the major etiologic factor.

INTRODUCTION

The exceptionally high incidence of nasopharyngeal cancer (NPC) among southern Chinese both in China and abroad and the intermediate rates among populations admixed with southern Chinese have been well documented (3, 4, 17, 26, 29–32). The epidemiological evidence suggests that the development of NPC in these high risk people is largely due to environmental factors. Two basic hypotheses for the etiology of NPC have been proposed and debated (13). One hypothesis is that NPC is caused by carcinogens in inhaled smoke. Alternatively, Ho suggested that ingestion of Cantonese salted fish is a major risk factor for NPC in southern Chinese. The present study further examines the role of these two proposed risk factors in southern Chinese by comparing incidence rates (1974–1975) of NPC among Chinese in Hong Kong with those in Los Angeles County (1972–1976) by such factors as age, sex, birthplace, and occupation.

Mimi C. Yu, Ronald K. Ross, and Brian E. Henderson are with the Department of Community and Family Medicine, University of Southern California School of Medicine, 2025 Zonal Avenue, Los Angeles, California 90033.

John H. C. Ho is with the Medical and Health Department Institute of Radiology and Oncology, Queen Elizabeth Hospital, Kowloon, Hong Kong.

Requests for reprints should be addressed to Mimi C. Yu.

This work was supported by grants (CA 14089 and CA 17054) from the National Cancer Institute of the National Institutes of Health.

MATERIALS AND METHODS

Hong Kong data. During the period 1974–1975, 2,041 new cases of NPC in Chinese residents of Hong Kong were diagnosed. Patients who came from outside Hong Kong for medical consultation or treatment were excluded. Ninety-one percent of these diagnoses were made at government-operated or university-affiliated institutions: 228 (11%) at the radiotherapy department, and 52 (3%) from discharge records of Queen Mary Hospital; 1,058 (52%) at the radiotherapy department, 373 (18%) from discharge records, and 54 (3%) from the Pathology Institute of Queen Elizabeth Hospital; 42 (2%) at the Sai Ying Pun Pathology Institute; and 45 (2%) at the Hong Kong University Pathology Institute. The remaining 189 (9%) cases were voluntary cancer notifications submitted by private hospitals and physicians. The registration rate was believed to be nearly complete (19). Most of the cases diagnosed in Queen Mary and Queen Elizabeth Hospitals were reviewed by one of us (J.H.C.H.). Information on birthplace and occupation were routinely recorded only for those cases who attended the radiotherapy departments of Queen Mary Hospital and Queen Elizabeth Hospital.

We were unable to ascertain the sex of one patient, so the case was dropped from the analysis. Information on age at diagnosis was missing on 30 men and 21 women; these cases were also dropped. Of the remaining 1,404 male patients, 499 (36%) had unknown birthplace, as did 239 of the 585 (41%) female patients. The seven places of birth used by the Hong Kong 1971 Census (33) were defined as follows (see Fig. 1): (1) Hong Kong (Xianggang), including the Tanka boat people from the waters of Hong Kong, (2) Canton (Guangzhou)—Canton, Macao, and adjacent areas, (3) Sze Yap (Siyi), (4) Chiu Chau (Chaozhou), (5) Kwangtung (Guangdong)—other, (6) China—other, and (7) Outside China.

Age and sex distribution of the cases with unknown birthplace were found to be similar to those with known birthplace. It is, therefore, unlikely that the missing values were associated with particular birthplaces. Thus, within each age group, the cases with unknown birthplace were allocated according to the known birthplace distribution.

Population figures used in the computation of incidence rates were based on an estimated total Hong Kong population on January 1, 1975. Using the Hong Kong 1971 Census (33) and 1976 By-Census data (courtesy of the Commissioner for Census and Statistics, Hong Kong), the total population in 1975 by age by birthplace was estimated by linear interpolation. A small percentage of the population in Hong Kong is non-Chinese (1.7% in the 1971 Census); thus the population at

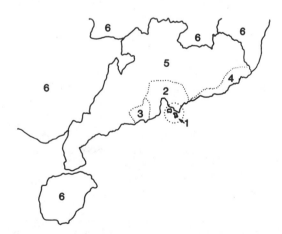

Fig. 1. Places of birth used by the Hong Kong 1971 Census: 1—Hong Kong; 2—Canton, Macao, and adjacent areas; 3—Sze Yap; 4—Chiu Chau; 5—elsewhere in Kwangtung; 6—elsewhere in China.

risk would be slightly overestimated. Census data showed that there had been very little change in the China-born population between 1971–1976. Since the 1976 By-Census did not distinguish birthplace within China, we further assumed that for each age group, the 1975 estimated population had the same distribution by birthplace inside China as the 1971 Census population.

Occupational information was available from 845 men and 350 women; 102 other women listed their occupation as housewife. In the calculation of standardized incidence ratios by occupational groups according to their last occupation, we defined expected number of cases for an occupational group as the total number of cases times the proportion of the working population in that occupational group based on the Hong Kong 1971 Census. This was necessary due to lack of information on occupation by age in the population.

Los Angeles County data. Incidence data in Los Angeles County were available from the population-based Los Angeles County Cancer Surveillance Program (14). Between 1972 and 1976, 138 male and 67 female cases of NPC were first diagnosed. Population figures used in the computation of incidence rates were based on the 1970 Census adjusted for undercounting and postcensal change (28).

RESULTS

Hong Kong Data

Age-sex-specific incidence rates per 100,000 person-years by place of birth are shown in Table 1. Age-standardized (based on a standard World population) (35) rates were also computed by sex for each place of birth.

For both sexes, the overall incidence rates began to rise after age 24, reached a plateau around age 55, and then declined. The overall standardized rate for males

TABLE 1
AGE-SEX-SPECIFIC INCIDENCE RATES BY PLACE OF BIRTH FOR NASOPHARYNGEAL
CANCER IN HONG KONG (1974–1975)[a]

Age	Place of Birth							
	M	F	M	F	M	F	M	F
	Hong Kong		Canton		Sze Yap		Chiu Chau	
0–14	0.4(5)	0.2(2)	0.0	0.0	0.0	0.0	0.0	0.0
15–24	2.9	2.4	1.9(1)	5.1(4)	32.6(7)	11.2(2)	21.1(3)	0.0
25–34	24.9	9.4	16.0	16.9	20.9(9)	14.1(4)	22.2(9)	24.0(6)
35–44	83.4	44.7	71.7	27.8	92.7	35.0	48.7	10.4(3)
45–54	111.0	40.9	110.4	44.5	130.8	52.9	55.2	26.0(8)
55–64	118.7	52.9	94.6	30.4	98.7	45.7	59.5	15.3(3)
65–74	22.5(3)	53.3	80.6	45.9	49.6(9)	5.4(1)	51.2(4)	14.5(1)
75+	0.0	0.0	48.9(8)	31.3	102.1(8)	0.0	0.0	30.5(1)
Total[b]	36.9	18.5	35.9	16.8	46.4	17.8	25.9	10.0
	Kwangtung—Other		China—Other		Outside China		Total	
0–14	0.0	0.0	0.0	0.0	0.0	0.0	0.4(5)	0.2(2)
15–24	0.0	0.0	0.0	0.0	0.0	0.0	3.7	2.7
25–34	57.4	13.0(1)	24.5(6)	12.3(3)	23.0(6)	0.0	22.5	12.4
35–44	96.0	36.4(6)	26.3(7)	9.8(3)	67.8	28.2(4)	74.0	30.6
45–54	161.5	45.5(8)	21.3(8)	0.0	75.6(9)	18.6(1)	103.2	38.8
55–64	142.7	32.6(4)	20.5(6)	19.7(4)	52.7(3)	28.7(1)	90.3	33.8
65–74	91.8(7)	42.2(3)	66.7(7)	34.8(3)	0.0	0.0	65.5	35.6
75+	0.0	37.4(1)	0.0	0.0	0.0	0.0	46.2	19.3
Total	53.3	16.7	13.9	6.2	23.9	7.7(6)	35.5	15.1

[a] If the rate is based on fewer than 10 cases, the actual number of cases is shown in parentheses.
[b] Standardized to the World population.

was 35.5, and 15.1 for females. The overall sex ratio was 2.4:1, with the sex ratio of age-standardized rates by birthplace ranging from 2.0 in Hong Kong to 3.2 in Kwangtung—other. The sex ratio by age group ranged from 1.4 for those under 25 years to 2.7 for those between the ages 45 and 64.

Persons born inside China but outside of Kwangtung Province had the lowest age-standardized incidence rates. Within Kwangtung, those born in the Chiu Chau region had rates of NPC 40% lower than those born in the rest of the province. Hong Kong, which is geographically part of Canton region, had rates very similar to Canton. For men only, those born in "Kwangtung-other" had an incidence rate 50% higher than the ones born in Canton. The rate for the Sze-Yap-born was intermediate between those born in Canton and "Kwangtung-other."

For the outside-China-born, the rates were intermediate between those from the Kwangtung Province and elsewhere in China. Of the 23 men born outside of China, 21 were born in Southeast Asia. Three of the twenty-three men claimed that their families were originally from Fukien (Fujien) province, while 18 claimed Kwangtung as their place of origin. For the five women born outside of China, three were born in Southeast Asia, three claimed Kwangtung, and one claimed Fukien as her place of origin.

Table 2 shows standardized incidence ratios (SIR) of high-risk (SIR greater than or equal to 1.3) occupational groups. For men, occupational groups at increased risk were farmhands (SIR = 2.7), fishermen (SIR = 3.5), unskilled laborers (SIR = 2.9), food and beverage workers (SIR = 1.8), carpenters (SIR = 1.5), and painters (SIR = 1.3). For women, they were farm hands (SIR = 4.5), fishermen (SIR = 1.9), and food and beverage workers (SIR = 4.4). Of the 19 men who were food and beverage workers, 7 worked with the preparation of traditional Chinese foods, 5 were bakers, 4 were meat roasters, and the remaining 3 were a butcher, a candy maker, and a flour maker. The 5 female food and beverage workers worked with the preparation of traditional Chinese foods. Within each of these high-risk occupational groups, the percentage of people born in high-risk areas (Hong Kong, Canton, Sze Yap, Kwangtung-other) was not different from the rest of the occupational groups. No excess risk was observed for any one of the following occupational categories: skilled service workers, unskilled service workers, transport and communication workers, clerical and sales workers, administrative and managerial workers, artists, and professional staff and qualified technologists.

Los Angeles County Data

Table 3 shows the age-standardized (35) incidence rates of NPC per 100,000 person-years in Los Angeles County by race and sex. For Chinese, the foreign

TABLE 2
STANDARDIZED INCIDENCE RATIO BY OCCUPATION, BY SEX FOR
NASOPHARYNGEAL CANCER IN HONG KONG (1974–1975)

	Male			Female		
Occupation	Mean age	No. of cases	SIR[a]	Mean age	No. of cases	SIR[a]
Farm hands, gardeners (public parks)	50	26	2.7	58	20	4.5
Fishermen, fish hatchers	50	43	3.5	51	12	1.9
Carpenters, wood workers	50	30	1.5	—	0	0.0
Painters	39	10	1.3	—	0	0.0
Food and beverage workers	52	19	1.8	51	5	4.4
Unskilled laborers	49	83	2.9	56	10	0.8

[a] Expected number of cases = proportion of working population in that occupational category times total number of cases with known occupation.

TABLE 3
Age-Standardized Incidence Rates for Nasopharyngeal Cancer in
Los Angeles County (1972–1976) by Racial Groups[a]

	Male		Female	
Race	No. of cases	Age-standardized rate	No. of cases	Age-standardized rate
Non-Spanish surnamed white	90	0.6	44	0.3
Spanish surnamed white	11	0.6	4	0.2
Black	10	0.5	8	0.4
Japanese	2	0.9	1	0.3
Chinese—immigrant	16	13.9	3	3.3
Chinese—indigenous	1	3.5	2	4.4
Other nonwhite	8	3.6	5	2.3

[a] Standardized to the world population using the age groups 0–14, 15–24, 25–34 . . . 75+.

born are listed separately from the local born.

The foreign-born Chinese were clearly at high risk compared with the other racial groups. Of the nine foreign-born Chinese patients of known birthplace, there were six from Kwangtung, two from Taiwan, and one from Kwangsi.

There were one male and two female cases of NPC in the U.S.-born Chinese population. All three patients were interviewed. The 77-year-old man was born in Hawaii, but lived in Chungshan, Kwangtung, from age 2 to 25 before returning to Hawaii. The two women were a 26-year-old born in Utah and a 25-year-old born in California. The parents of the 26-year-old woman were immigrants from Sze Yap, Kwangtung, and she grew up on a traditional southern Chinese diet. The 25-year-old woman was a third generation Chinese-American whose grandparents were all from Sze Yap, Kwangtung. Both the 77-year-old man and the 26-year-old woman claimed to eat salted fish quite regularly.

The "Other Non-Whites" had rates intermediate between the high rates in foreign-born Chinese and the low rates in whites. The eight men in this category were all Filipino. Of the five women, three were Filipino and two were Korean.

DISCUSSION

The age-standardized incidence rates for Hong Kong (35.5 for men, 15.1 for women) are 45% higher than the rates previously reported for the period 1965–1969 (17). We cannot distinguish whether this represents a true secular increase or simply more comprehensive cancer registry coverage.

In Hong Kong, Chinese born in the province of Kwangtung have almost three times the rate of NPC as those born elsewhere in China. This is in general agreement with Liang's (26) findings. Kaplan and Tsuchitani (25) reported an age-standardized incidence rate of 3.3 for men in Shanghai for the year 1975, which is 1/10th the rate of Kwangtung-born men in Hong Kong.

Within Kwangtung, previous reports (1, 15, 17, 30–32) which analyzed incidence rates by place of origin for Chinese in Malaysia, Hong Kong, and Singapore have shown that the Chiu Chau (called Teochew in Singapore and Malaysia) people have lower rates of NPC than those from the rest of the province. Present analysis by place of birth and by place of origin (data not shown) shows a similar pattern. In fact, incidence rates for the Chiu Chau people resemble closely the rate for the Fukienese (called Hokkien in Singapore and Malaysia) in the neighboring province (30, 31). It is interesting to note that the Chiu Chau people are culturally closer to the Fukienese than those from the rest of Kwangtung.

On the other hand, the Hakkas who migrated from northeast China to south China about 700 years ago, have an incidence rate of NPC comparable with the rates for the other dialect groups of south China, even though they can be considered genetically distinct since intermarriages with other dialect groups have been rare (1).

For the Chinese immigrants living in Los Angeles County, the risk for NPC is less than half that experienced by the Hong Kong Chinese. This lower rate could be partly due to an increase in the proportion of central and northern Chinese immigrants to the U.S. following 1945. Prior to this period, immigration was largely confined to high-risk southern Chinese. However, the slight decrease in proportion of southern Chinese within the immigrant population cannot possibly account for all the reduction in NPC incidence rates within this group. Among the U.S. born Chinese, two of the three cases of NPC grew up in a traditional southern Chinese environment. Had the indigenous Chinese experienced the same risk for NPC as the Hong Kong Chinese, we would expect to find about 16 male cases and 5 female cases between 1972 and 1976. In fact, there were only one male and two female cases during this 4-year period. These results are consistent with Buell's observations that Chinese migrants to California show a decreasing rate of NPC in succeeding generations (3, 4). Much of the above evidence suggests that the risk of NPC in Chinese is related to some environmental factors inherent in the traditional culture of south China.

Inhalation of carcinogen-containing smoke has been proposed as a possible cause of nasopharyngeal cancer. Dobson (7) was the first to notice the heavy exposure to smoke from wood and charcoal fires used for indoor cooking in the chimneyless houses of south China. In Kenya, inhalation of wood fire smoke has also been suggested as a possible factor (5). A number of case-control studies have reported elevated risk ratios in persons exposed to fumes, dust, or smoke. Henderson *et al.* (12) reported a significant positive association between occupational exposure to smoke and fumes and risk for NPC in both Chinese and non-Chinese; the relative risk was 7.5 for more than 10 years of smoke exposure. Hu and Huang (22) found that working as a chef for any time was a significant risk factor (RR = 2.7) for NPC. They suggested that this was due to exposure to cooking fires and fumes. Djojopranoto and Soesilowati (6) found a significantly greater use of wood fires for cooking by nasopharyngeal cancer patients. Lin *et al.* (27) found a strong association (RR = 2.6) between NPC and working in poorly ventilated places.

However, the incidence data in Hong Kong do not support the hypothesis that the primary cause of NPC is carcinogens contained in inhaled smoke. If exposure to smoke in the chimneyless houses of south China was an important risk factor in southern Chinese, we would expect a lower NPC rate in the Hong Kong born Chinese whose houses are quite well ventilated. On the contrary, the incidence rates for this group are as high as for those born in the neighboring rural regions of Kwangtung province. Also, Ho (17) has found that women who are more heavily exposed to cooking fires have less than half the risk for NPC than men. Finally, the fishermen who live on boats in Hong Kong and cook their food in the open air have high rates of NPC (15, 20).

Our occupational data, however, do suggest that inhaled carcinogens may play a role in the etiology of nasopharyngeal cancer. In Hong Kong, carpenters, painters, bakers, and meat roasters were found to have excess risk of NPC. These high-risk occupational groups belonged to the same social class, and did not contain a disproportionate number of persons from the high-risk areas. We have no reason to think that diet or life-style in general, were different between the groups. Among the Los Angeles NPC patients, there were two bakers and three cooks. Bakers, cooks, and meat roasters would be exposed to fumes and cooking fires; carpenters would be exposed to wood dust; and painters to fumes. But the number of excess NPC cases in these occupational groups is small. Therefore, even though inhaled carcinogens may be the cause of elevated risk in these occupations, it is not a major risk factor for NPC in south China.

Alternatively, consumption of Cantonese salted fish has been suggested by Ho (16, 18, 20) as a risk factor in southern Chinese. As noted above, the fishermen who live on boats in Hong Kong have high rates of NPC; our occupation data confirm excess risk among fishermen. Accordingly to Ho, these boat people eat a large quantity of salted fish, preferring to sell their fresh-caught fish. Ho reported that for both sexes the age-specific incidence curve shows a steep rise after the age of 20–24 suggesting that the critical period of exposure might be in early childhood. Salted fish added to soft rice, a mushy form of rice, is a common food fed to southern Chinese in the weaning and post-weaning period (34). In a case-control study in Hong Kong, Geser *et al.* (11) found a positive association between exposure to salted fish during the weaning period and risk for NPC (RR = 2.6). Henderson and Louie (13) observed a significant positive association between frequency of current consumption of Cantonese salted fish and risk for NPC (RR = 3.1). Interestingly, salted fish is also a traditional food item among Filipinos in the Philippines. Our data show that Filipinos residing in Los Angeles County have an incidence rate for NPC six times as high as that for whites in the county. The rate in these immigrants is intermediate between the high rate in the Philippines (2) and the low rate in whites in Los Angeles.

There is also experimental evidence in support of Ho's hypothesis that consumption of salted fish in early life may be a cofactor in the genesis of NPC in southern Chinese. Volatile nitrosamines known to be powerful carcinogens in animal models have been found in Cantonese salted fish (8, 9, 23). However, the observed levels were no higher than those encountered in cured meats consumed in Europe where the incidence of NPC is very low. A number of animal studies have produced some very interesting findings. WA rats fed with salted fish were found to pass mutagenic urine (10, 21). Huang *et al.* (24) reported that 4 of 20 rats fed with Cantonese salted fish developed carcinomas in the nasal and paranasal regions; in addition, in the same series of experiments 14 rats were administered oral *N*-nitrosodiethylamine (NDEA) and three developed carcinoma in the nasal cavity. NDEA was later detected in low levels (less than 1 μg/kg) in some salted fish samples (Huang, unpublished data). Whether NDEA is the sole etiologic agent, whether some interaction between nitrosamine precursors takes place on ingestion, or whether some other carcinogen present in salted fish is responsible requires further study.

In Hong Kong, there is a definite upward trend in male NPC incidence rates proceeding from low rates associated with birthplace in Canton, to intermediate rates for birthplace in Sze Yap, to high rates for "Kwangtung-other." Canton is the richest region in Kwangtung, whereas "Kwangtung-other" consists mainly of mountainous areas not well suited to agriculture. Traditionally, salted fish has been among the least expensive foods (besides rice) available to the southern Chinese, so it is conceivable that consumption of salted fish would be higher in the poorer regions. In fact, salted fish is the only source of marine fish for the inland people of "Kwangtung-other." Geser *et al.* (11) found that in Hong Kong, those in the four lowest occupational classes had a significant excess risk of NPC (RR = 3.2). This is consistent with our findings of increased risk among unskilled laborers and farmers. For those poor people, salted fish is likely to be a frequent dish. Males play a dominant role in traditional Chinese families. It is conceivable that female babies may get less salted fish when a limited quantity is available.

In summary, inhaled carcinogens is not a major risk factor for NPC in southern Chinese, although it may account for some excess risk among selected occupational groups. Ingestion of Cantonese salted fish as a causative factor for NPC in southern Chinese has gained considerable support from recent experimental studies, and it is the hypothesis most consistent with our incidence data from Hong Kong.

ACKNOWLEDGMENTS

We wish to thank Mrs. E. Louie for coding and checking the Hong Kong data.

REFERENCES

1. Armstrong, R. W., Kutty, M. K., and Dharmalingam, S. K. Incidence of nasopharyngeal carcinoma in Malaysia, with special reference to the State of Selangor. *Brit. J. Cancer* 30, 86–94 (1974).
2. Basa, G. F., Hirayama, T., and Cruz-Basa, A. G. Cancer epidemiology in the Philippines, *in* "Epidemiology and Cancer Registries in the Pacific Basin," National Cancer Institute Monograph 47, pp. 45–56. National Cancer Institute, Bethesda, Md., 1975.
3. Buell, P. Nasopharynx cancer in Chinese of California. *Brit. J. Cancer* 19, 459–470 (1965).
4. Buell, P. The effect of migration on the risk of nasopharyngeal cancer among Chinese. *Cancer Res.* 34, 1189-1191 (1974).
5. Clifford, P. Carcinogens in the nose and throat: Nasopharyngeal carcinoma in Kenya. *Proc. Roy. Soc. Med.* 65, 682–686 (1972).
6. Djojopranoto, M., and Soesilowati. Nasopharyngeal cancer in East Java (Indonesia), *in* "Cancer of the Nasopharynx" (C. S. Muir and K. S. Shanmugaratnam, Eds.), UICC Monograph Series 1, pp. 43–46. UICC, Copenhagen, 1967.
7. Dobson, W. H. Cervical lympho-sarcoma. *Chinese Med. J.* 38, 786–787 (1924).
8. Fong, Y. Y., and Walsh, E. O. Carcinogenic nitrosamines in Cantonese salt-dried fish. *Lancet* 2, 1032 (1971).
9. Fong, Y. Y., and Chan, W. C. Dimethylnitrosamine in Chinese marine salt fish. *Food Cosmet. Toxicol.* 11, 841–845 (1973).
10. Fong, L. Y. Y., Ho, J. H. C., and Huang, D. P. Preserved foods as possible cancer hazards: WA rats fed salted fish have mutagenic urine. *Int. J. Cancer* 23, 542–546 (1979).
11. Geser, A., Charney, N. D., Day, N. E., Ho, H. C., and De-The, G. Environmental factors in the etiology of nasopharyngeal carcinoma: Report on a case-control study in Hong Kong, *in* "Nasopharyngeal Carcinoma: Etiology and Control" (G. De-The and Y. Ito, Eds.), IARC Scientific Publication No. 20, pp. 213–230. IARC, Lyon, 1978.
12. Henderson, B. E., Louie, E., Jing, J. S., Buell, P., and Gardner, M. B. Risk factors associated with nasopharyngeal carcinoma. *New Engl. J. Med.* 295, 1101–1106 (1976).
13. Henderson, B. E., and Louie, E. Discussion of risk factors for nasopharyngeal carcinoma, *in* "Nasopharyngeal Carcinoma: Etiology and Control" (G. De-The, and Y. Ito, Eds.), IARC Scientific Publication No. 20, pp. 251–260. IARC, Lyon, 1978.
14. Hisserich, J. C., Martin, S. P., and Henderson, B. E. An areawide cancer reporting network. *Publ. Health Rep.* 90, 15–17 (1975).
15. Ho, J. H. C. Nasopharyngeal carcinoma in Hong Kong, *in* "Cancer of the Nasopharynx" (C. S. Muir and K. Shanmugaratnam, Eds.), UICC Monograph Series 1, pp. 58–63. UICC, Copenhagen, 1967.
16. Ho, J. H. C. Genetic and environmental factors in nasopharyngeal carcinoma (NPC), *in* "Recent Advances in Tumor Virology and Immunology" (W. Nakahara, N. Nishioka, T. Hirayama, and Y. Ito, Eds.), Proc. 1st Int. Cancer Symp. Princess Takamatsu Cancer Research Fund, pp. 275–295. University Park Press, Baltimore, Md., 1971.
17. Ho, J. H. C. Nasopharyngeal carcinoma (NPC). *Advan. Cancer Res.* 15, 57–92 (1972).
18. Ho, J. H. C. Epidemiology of nasopharyngeal carcinoma. *J. Royal Coll. Surg. Edin.* 20, 223–235 (1975).
19. Ho, J. H. C. Current status of the cancer registry and population-based studies in Hong Kong, *in* "Epidemiology and Cancer Registries in the Pacific Basin," National Cancer Institute Monograph 47, pp. 57–60. National Cancer Institute, Bethesda, Md., 1977.
20. Ho, J. H. C. An epidemiologic and clinical study of nasopharyngeal carcinoma. *Int. J. Radiat. Oncol. Biol. Phys.* 4, 181–198 (1978).
21. Ho, J. H. C., Huang, D. P., and Fong, Y. Y. Salted fish and nasopharyngeal carcinoma in southern Chinese. *Lancet* 2, 626 (1978).
22. Hu, M. S., and Huang, H. L. Retrospective study on the etiological factors of nasopharyngeal carcinoma. *New Med.* (*Canton*) 12, 10 (1972). (in Chinese).
23. Huang, D. P., Ho, H. C., Gough, T. A., and Webb, K. S. Volatile nitrosamines in some traditional southern Chinese food products. *J. Food Safety* 1, 1–5 (1977).

24. Huang, D. P., Ho, J. H. C., Saw, D., and Teoh, T. B. Carcinoma of the nasal and paranasal regions in rats fed Cantonese salted marine fish, *in* "Nasopharyngeal Carcinoma: Etiology and Control" (G. De-The, and Y. Ito, Eds.), IARC Scientific Publication No. 20, pp. 315–328. IARC, Lyon, 1978.

25. Kaplan, H. S., and Tsuchitani, P. J. (Eds.) "Cancer in China," p. 47. Liss, New York, 1978.

26. Liang, P. C. Studies on nasopharyngeal carcinoma in the Chinese: Statistical and laboratory investigations. *Chinese Med. J.* **83**, 373–390 (1964).

27. Lin, T. M., Chen, K. P., Lin, C. C., Hsu, M. M., Tu, S. M., Chiang, T. C., Jung, P. F., and Hirayama, T. Retrospective study on nasopharyngeal carcinoma. *J. Nat. Cancer Inst.* **51**, 1403–1408 (1973).

28. Siegel, J. S. "Estimates of Coverage of the Population by Sex, Race and Age in the 1970 Census." Annual Meeting Population Assoc. America, New Orleans, 1973.

29. Shanmugaratnam, K., and Tye, C. Y. A study of nasopharyngeal cancer among Singapore Chinese with special reference to migrant status and specific community (dialect group). *J. Chron. Dis.* **23**, 433–441 (1970).

30. Shanmugaratnam, K. Cancer in Singapore — Ethnic and dialect group variations in cancer incidence. *Singapore Med. J.* **14**, 69–81 (1973).

31. Shanmugaratnam, K., and Wee, A. "Dialect group" variations in cancer incidence among Chinese in Singapore, *in* "Host-Environmental Interactions in the Etiology of Cancer in Man" (R. Doll and I. Vodopija, Eds.), IARC scientific Publication No. 7, pp. 67–82. IARC, Lyon, 1973.

32. Shanmugaratnam, K. Variations in nasopharyngeal cancer incidence among specific Chinese communities (dialect groups) in Singapore, *in* "Nasopharyngeal Carcinoma: Etiology and Control" (G. De-The and Y. Ito, Eds.), IARC Scientific Publication No. 20, pp. 191–198. IARC, Lyon, 1978.

33. Topley, K. W. J. "Hong Kong Population and Housing Census, 1971: Main Report." Census and Statistics Department of Hong Kong Government, 1971.

34. Topley, M. Cultural and social factors related to Chinese infant feeding and weaning, *in* "Growing Up in Hong Kong" (C. E. Field and F. M. Barbaer, Eds.), pp. 56–65. Hong Kong Univ. Press, Hong Kong, 1972.

35. Waterhouse, J., Muir, C., Correa, P., and Powell, J. "Cancer Incidence in Five Continents," Vol. III. IARC Scientific Publication No. 15, IARC, Lyon, 1976.

Stomach Cancer Among Japanese in Hawaii[1,2]

by William Haenszel, Minoru Kurihara,[3] Mitsuo Segi,[4] and Richard K. C. Lee[5,6]

SUMMARY—Study of 220 Japanese stomach cancer patients and 440 hospital controls in Hawaii revealed that migrants (Issei) from prefectures with the highest stomach cancer risks in Japan continued to display an excess risk in Hawaii, but this effect did not persist among their Nisei offspring. Lower risks were suggested for Nisei, but not Issei adhering to Western-style diets. These nativity distinctions are consistent with other studies suggesting that early exposures are critical. Associations of stomach cancer with consumption of specific foods were noted. Elevated risks were described for Issei and Nisei users of pickled vegetables and dried/salted fish, the most frequent consumers having the highest risks. Since similar associations did not appear for raw fish and unprocessed vegetables, suspicion is directed to methods of preparation. Low risks were suggested for several Western vegetables, many of which are eaten raw. The associations for uncooked vegetables appeared independent of those found for pickled vegetables; both persisted after control for other facets of vegetable consumption. Associations for tobacco, liquor, coffee, and milk were observed only in the Issei population. Points of consistency between the Hawaii findings and those assembled in Japan are cited. Experimental evidence bearing on the epidemiologic data for processed fish and vegetables is mentioned.—J Natl Cancer Inst 49: 969–988, 1972.

[1]*From the Biometry Branch, National Cancer Institute, Bethesda, Maryland 20014.*

[2]*Conduct of field work was supported in part by a National Cancer Institute research contract PH43-63-558 with the University of Hawaii.*

[3]*Department of Public Health, Tohoku University School of Medicine, Seiryomachi, Sendai, 980, Japan.*

[4]*Now emeritus professor, Tohoku University.* Present address: *Aichi Cancer Center, Research Institute, Chikusaku, Nagoya, 464, Japan.*

[5]*School of Public Health, University of Hawaii, Honolulu, Hawaii 96817.*

[6]*We acknowledge the many contributions of the late Dr. Ishiko Mori and Mr. Ernest Fuginaga to development and refinement of the questionnaire and interviewing procedures.*

[7]*National Institutes of Health, Public Health Service, U.S. Department of Health, Education, and Welfare.*

EPIDEMIOLOGIC observations have supplied a few leads on the etiology of stomach cancer. The significance of host factors is suggested by the association of pernicious anemia and stomach cancer (*1*), risks for relatives of stomach cancer patients 2–3 times those for relatives of index controls (*2–5*), and the 15–25% higher risks among persons of blood group A than of group O (*6–10*). Other features of stomach cancer—the marked intercountry differences in risk, the rapid decline in incidence and mortality during the past quarter-century in many countries, the omnipresent social-class gradient (*11, 12*)—tend to implicate environmental factors.

While many investigators have entertained the possibility of etiologies linked to diet and nutrition, such studies have been unrewarding. In retrospect this outcome is not surprising. Diet inquiries present formidable problems of informant recall and are complicated by the inability to quantitate food intake precisely, particularly when interest is directed to earlier practices. Attempts to reduce the diet to the constituent proteins, fats, and carbohydrates do not improve matters, since other characteristics of the foods and their preparation may be responsible for any carcinogenic properties. Finally, as emphasized by Wynder et al. (*13*), studies of homogeneous populations in a single locale cannot be expected to incriminate an agent to which all members have been exposed.

The Japanese migrant offers attractive opportunities to reexamine dietary hypotheses. There are distinct differences between Japanese and Western foods; many Japanese migrating to Hawaii and the continental United States have adopted Western-style diets, and it is an advantage that the timing and degree of transition have varied within this group. The sharp demarcation between Japanese and Western foods eases the collection of information on discontinuance of some foods and introduction of others. As emphasized by Steiner, and others, the choice of a migrant population facilitates assessments of the relative contributions of host characteristics and environmental exposures as determinants of stomach cancer risk (*14*). International comparisons place Japan with such other high-risk countries as Chile, Finland, and Iceland (*15, 16*), so that the migration of Japanese to Hawaii, beginning in the latter part of the 19th century, provides information on the history of this disease in a high-risk group settling in a low-risk area.

From necropsy studies, Steiner was impressed by the high relative frequency of stomach cancer among U.S. Japanese compared to other ethnic groups (*14*). While Steiner's data could not directly position the U.S. Japanese experience against Japan and U.S. whites, Smith reported the stomach cancer mortality of U.S. Japanese in 1949–52 to be about 80% of that in Japan and over 3 times that for the host U.S. white population (*17*). The 1959–62 mortality data, which distinguished between migrants (Issei) and their offspring (Nisei) born in the United States, and more recent incidence data assembled by the Hawaii Tumor Registry have confirmed and elaborated the earlier observations (*16, 18, 19*). The Issei experience conformed to the characteristic displacement pattern for stomach cancer noted for European populations coming to the United States, risks lower than in the country of origin but still more closely aligned to home than to host population (*20, 21*). The 1959–62 data indicated Nisei rates were lower than those for Issei at comparable ages in the lifespan, though the Nisei rates remained above the prevailing U.S. white level (*18*).

The evidence pinpoints an effect, a decline in stomach cancer among Japanese migrants more marked for Nisei than Issei, for which a cause should be sought. Case-control studies and household surveys were initiated in Hawaii, California, and Japan to identify contributing factors. The present paper reports on the study of patients of Japanese ancestry in Hawaii. Subsequent publications will review and collate the findings obtained in Hawaii and Japan.

MATERIAL AND METHODS

Field work in Hawaii was directed by Dr. Lee. Begun in mid-1963, interviews of 220 patients and 440 hospital controls were completed in the ensuing 6 years. Interviewing was effectively limited to residents of the island of Oahu (Honolulu). The original plan contemplated interviewing on both Oahu and Hawaii, but the yield from Hawaii was incommensurate with costs, and work was discontinued after a trial period. Kuakini Hospital, Honolulu, was the source of 71% of the patients in the study series, a figure reflecting the prevailing pattern of hospital utilization by the Japanese community.

Two controls were designated for each patient, the selection rule being the next older and next younger Japanese of the same sex in the same hospital service at the time of interview. Persons hospitalized with diagnoses of gastric ulcers, other diseases of the stomach, or other cancers of the digestive system were excluded from the control series. Japanese comprised only a fraction of the patients in some hospitals, so that controls were sometimes drawn from other hospital services, but always in a way that identified controls without ambiguity. Patients and controls were not matched on nativity; Issei patients could have Nisei controls and vice versa.

The content of the questionnaires was the same in Hawaii, California, and Japan. Bilingual schedules were used in Hawaii and interviews were conducted in both English and Japanese. Shades of meaning are difficult to convey in translation, and this practice contributed to interarea comparability of data. A major portion of the interview was devoted to diet history, but residence and migration history, tobacco use, occupation, living customs, reproductive history, previous illnesses, and dental health were also covered. "Frequency of use"—the number of times the item was taken on the average over a specified time interval—was the basic device for quantitating food intake. The questions on foods were designed to elicit the subject's practices over a sustained period and to ignore departures from normal occasioned by parties, restaurant dining, etc.

Most stomach cancer diagnoses were confirmed by microscopic examination of tissue. Histologic types other than carcinoma were excluded from the study series and only 9 patients (4%) had no histologic diagnosis. The anatomical localizations of the tumors were distributed as follows: cardiac orifice, 14; fundus, 17; prepyloris, 23; antrum, 72; lesser curvature, 44; greater curvature, 12; other, 12; unknown, 26.

A diagnostic record covering the standard range of clinical information, supplemented by a special pathology protocol for the available surgical and necropsy specimens (developed by K. Akazaki, formerly of Tohoku University School of Medicine; K. Herrold, National Cancer Institute; G. Stemmermann, Kuakini Hospital, Honolulu) was completed for each stomach cancer patient. Typing of stomach cancers as intestinal or diffuse, following Lauren's criteria as modified by Correa and Muñoz (22), was done by Stemmermann. Other investigators will report the pathology protocol findings for tumors and adjacent gastric mucosa.

The associations between stomach cancer and food history and selected demographic variables were described in the form of relative risks and tested for statistical significance by standard statistical techniques (23).

Confounding variables.—Upper limits to food intake presumably exist and high consumption of some foods may imply reduced use of others, so that case-control differences for some foods may reflect indirect associations with other etiologically more relevant factors. Cross-classification was introduced to control for some potentially confounding variables. However, extensive application of procedures to estimate separate, independent effects for individual foods would not have been rewarding. Using the initial 171 cases and matched controls, Hankey (24) developed a discriminant function to calculate regression slopes (a measure closely allied to relative risk) for individual foods, with and without statistical control for other food variables, and found generally close correspondence between the crude slope estimates (without adjustment for other foods) and the adjusted slope estimates. Hankey's results suggest that intercorrelations among foods differentiating between case and control experience are weak and/or not easily detectable in the data available. The latter possibility is related to a general problem of biologic data, in which addition of independent variables past the first 3 or 4 in a regression equation rarely improves the correspondence between observation and prediction. In examining this question, Cochran concluded that inability to incorporate profitably more variables in regression equations was due to poor precision in their measurement (25), precisely the situation presented by the interview data.

Given these circumstances, we relied primarily on case-control comparisons for individual items without adjustments for other food variables, with emphasis on the detection of important differences supplemented by a search for gradients in risks with frequency of use.

RESULTS

Table 1 supplies background information on patient and control characteristics. Use of sex and age as criteria for the designation of controls forced close agreement on these attributes. Drawing of controls from the same hospital service also contributed to similar case-control distributions for other variables not strongly associated with stomach cancer. Since sex and age are matching variables, they can serve only as control variables in the analysis.

Nativity

The sharp demarcation in the age distributions of Issei and Nisei means that control on age and

TABLE 1.—*Selected characteristics of gastric cancer patients and matched hospital controls*

	Cases		Controls	
	Number	Percent	Number	Percent
A. Sex and age				
Males, total	*135*	*61. 4*	*270*	*61. 4*
<50 yr	27	12. 3	61	13. 9
50–59 yr	34	15. 5	68	15. 5
60–69 yr	35	15. 9	66	15. 0
70+ yr	39	17. 7	75	17. 0
Females, total	*85*	*38. 6*	*170*	*38. 6*
<50 yr	26	11. 8	53	12. 0
50–59 yr	11	5. 0	29	6. 6
60–69 yr	28	12. 7	54	12. 3
70+ yr	20	9. 1	34	7. 7
B. Nativity and age				
Issei (born in Japan), total	*120*	*54. 5*	*229*	*52. 0*
<60 yr	15	6. 8	31	7. 0
60+ yr	105	47. 7	198	45. 0
Nisei and Sansei (born in U.S.), total	*100*	*45. 5*	*211*	*48. 0*
<60 yr	83	37. 7	180	40. 9
60+ yr	17	7. 7	31	7. 0
C. Year left Japan (Issei), total	*120*	*100. 0*	*229*	*100. 0*
Before 1898	1	0. 8	3	1. 3
1898–1907	45	37. 5	84	36. 7
1908–17	47	39. 2	97	42. 4
1918–27	23	19. 2	34	14. 8
1928 or later	4	3. 3	11	4. 8
D. Residence on arrival in Hawaii (Issei), total	*120*	*100. 0*	*229*	*100. 0*
Oahu	56	46. 7	115	50. 2
Hawaii	29	24. 2	48	21. 0
Maui	17	14. 2	37	16. 2
Kauai	18	15. 0	29	12. 7
E. Marital status, total	*220*	*100. 0*	*440*	*100. 0*
Never married	12	5. 5	12	2. 7
Married	165	75. 0	339	77. 0
Widowed, divorced, other	43	19. 5	89	20. 2
F. Education				
In Japan, total	*111*	*50. 5*	*213*	*48. 4*
None, not reported	20	9. 1	42	9. 5
Elementary	82	37. 3	154	35. 0
Middle school	8	3. 6	16	3. 6
College	1	0. 5	1	0. 2
In United States, total	*109*	*49. 5*	*227*	*51. 6*
Elementary	52	23. 6	116	26. 4
High school	47	21. 4	89	20. 2
College	10	4. 5	22	5. 0
G. Religion, total	*220*	*100. 0*	*440*	*100. 0*
Buddhist	174	79. 1	346	78. 6
Christian	27	12. 3	55	12. 5
Other	19	8. 6	39	8. 9

nativity is roughly equivalent. As a quasimatched factor the nativity data cannot be used to estimate Issei-Nisei differences in stomach cancer risk; this represents no loss, since mortality and incidence data provide direct information on this point.

Year of Migration

Migration of Japanese to Hawaii reached a peak before 1920 and most Issei interviewed had resided in the State over 40 years. The case and control distributions for year of departure from Japan were remarkably similar and, given the correspondence in current ages, one may safely infer virtually identical distributions for age at departure from Japan. Under these circumstances, indirect associations with time and/or age of migration can be ruled out as an explanation for any findings described here.

Residence on Arrival

Many Japanese were recruited as farm laborers for large plantations and roughly half the Issei patients and controls first resided on Hawaii, Maui, and Kauai. Since nearly all Issei lived on Oahu at the time of interview, the case-control experience accurately reflects the substantial population movement to Honolulu from the other islands.

Marital Status

A small preponderance of never-married in the case series was in the direction expected. Mating selection generally operates to leave a residuum of single persons with higher mortality for many diseases, of which stomach cancer is only one (*26*).

Education

The close correspondence between cases and controls for amount of education in Japan and in the United States means that indices based on attained education would reveal no social-class gradient for stomach cancer among Japanese migrants. This outcome is not surprising, since the predominantly middle-class Hawaii Japanese have few highly educated professionals and managers. The education received by the remainder did not appear important in determining subsequent occupation—shop owner, skilled tradesman versus laborer, service worker. Data on occupation have been used to investigate the social-class gradient in risk.

Illnesses and Symptoms

Cases and controls supplied a history of illnesses and symptoms. Table 2 compares the affirmative patient replies with the numbers expected based on control experience for selected conditions. Pernicious anemia, a disease associated with subsequent development of stomach cancer (*1*), was reported by 3 patients versus .5 expected. Diabetes and gallbladder disease were less frequent among patients. Stomach cancer patients reported an excess of conditions linked with previous illnesses of the stomach and duodenum. Little or no difference between patients and controls was noted for previous surgery or abdominal X-rays.

We turn now to information assembled on birthplace, occupation, tobacco use, and food habits in search of items that discriminate between patients and controls. Table 3 specifies the nature of the contrast, the group considered (all Japanese, Issei,

Nisei), the variables controlled, and the observations from which the relative risk estimate was derived.

Prefecture of Origin

Issei patients and controls were distributed by prefecture of birth, and we extended this classification to Nisei by considering the parents' birthplace. The latter presented no difficult problems in classification, since the parents almost invariably came from the same or a neighboring prefecture; if one parent was born in Hawaii, the assignment was to the birthplace of the Issei parent. The heavy representation of Hiroshima, Yamaguchi, and Kumamoto prefectures in the control series was compatible with other sources describing the predominant stream of migration to Hawaii to have originated in southern Honshu and Kyushu.

The top 50% of the prefectures in the Segi et al. ranking of gastric cancer mortality in Japan for 1950–59 (*27*) was designated as "high-risk" and the remainder as "low-risk." A significantly elevated relative risk (1.8) was observed for Issei coming from prefectures with above-average gastric cancer mortality, but place of origin did not discriminate for the second-generation Nisei. An alternative approach, based on the concentration of high-risk prefectures in northern Honshu, contrasted northern Honshu against the rest of Japan, with the same outcome. Parenthetically, the experience of migrants from Okinawa resembled that of persons from southern Honshu and Kyushu.

The failure of the "place of origin" effect for Issei to persist among Nisei seems consistent with other evidence; we have remarked that migrants from Japan and European countries with high stomach cancer mortality have continued to display risks characteristic of the country of origin, and their descendents born in the United States have stomach cancer mortality resembling that of other native-born. This nativity gap in stomach cancer risk, less completely expressed among the Japanese than for other migrants (*18*), suggests early exposures as critical in the etiology of gastric cancer. Apart from the substantive issues of interpretation, the findings underline the importance of routine inspection of the separate Issei and Nisei data.

Socioeconomic Class

The major lifetime occupations of the respondents were coded according to a standard classification of the U.S. Bureau of the Census and then reduced to socioeconomic classes: professional, administrative,

TABLE 2.—*Number of gastric cancer patients reporting history of selected illnesses, symptoms, and procedures compared with expected numbers based on control experience*

Illness	Observed	Expected
Ulcer—stomach	41	10. 5
Ulcer—duodenal	9	3
Diabetes	12	21
Gallbladder disease	5	8
Pernicious anemia	3	0. 5
Cirrhosis of liver	3	0
Gastritis	16	5
Colitis	0	0. 5
"Weak stomach"	24	12
Previous surgery	95	111
Abdominal X-ray	76	74. 5

TABLE 3.—*Relative risks of gastric cancer for selected contrasts of place of origin, occupation, smoking history, and food habits*

Contrast	Relative risk [1]		
	Hawaiian Japanese	Issei	Nisei
A. Place of origin			
Birthplace (Issei)			
High [2] vs. low-risk prefecture		1.8*(33, 63; *40, 139*)	
Birthplace of parents (Nisei)			
High vs. low-risk prefecture			0.84(11, 66; *27, 136*)
B. Occupation			
"Low" [3] vs. "high" socio-economic class			
Both sexes	1.51*(114, 106; *183, 257*)	1.44(68, 52; *109, 120*)	1.6 (46, 54; *74, 137*)
Males	1.8* (66, 69; *93, 177*)	1.7 (42, 34; *62, 83*)	2.1*(24, 35; *31, 94*)
Females	1.15 (48, 37; *90, 80*)	1.14(26, 18; *47, 37*)	1.16(22, 19; *43, 43*)
C. Smoking history			
Any tobacco vs. no tobacco use			
Both sexes	1.45*(95, 125; *157, 283*)	1.9*(50, 70; *67, 162*)	1.11(45, 55; *90, 121*)
Males	1.36 (76, 59; *132, 138*)	1.9*(44, 32; *60, 85*)	0.87(32, 27; *72, 53*)
Females	1.7 (19, 66; *25, 145*)	1.7 (6, 38; *7, 77*)	1.8 (13, 28; *18, 68*)
Cigarette smokers only—males			
20+ vs. <20 cigarettes daily	0.87 (48, 25; *88, 37*)		
D. Food habits			
+Japanese style meals daily vs. none [4]			
At time of interview	1.11 (148, 72; *284, 156*)	0.76(94, 26; *189, 40*)	1.5 (54, 46; *95, 116*)
As of 1940	1.24 (177, 39; *339, 94*)	0.69(106, 13; *209, 18*)	1.6 (71, 26; *130, 76*)

[1] In terms of unit risk for last-named group in each contrast; *denotes risks significantly different from unity at the 5% level. Relative risks for total Hawaiian Japanese are adjusted for sex and nativity; those for Issei and Nisei are adjusted for sex. Figures in parentheses report the basic data for each relative risk estimate; the first pair gives the numbers of cases in the two categories contrasted and the second pair, in italics, the corresponding information on controls.

[2] The upper 50% in ranking of prefectures in Japan by gastric cancer mortality by Segi et al. (*27*).

[3] Includes semiskilled factory workers, laborers, and domestic and service workers.

[4] Relative risks are also adjusted for age.

etc. The limited material forced a simple contrast of "high" versus "low" socioeconomic class. Semi-skilled factory workers, laborers (including farm and plantation laborers), and domestic and service workers were assigned to the latter group. Higher relative risks were observed for both Issei and Nisei in the lower socioeconomic stratum. The difference was concentrated among males; however, women were assigned to their reported occupations rather than to those of their husbands (housewives with no history of gainful employment were arbitrarily assigned to "high" socioeconomic class) and the possibility that husband's occupation may be a more efficient discriminator is not excluded. An inverse social-class gradient has always been a prominent feature of stomach cancer and its presence among Hawaiian Japanese is consistent with other findings from the United States and Japan (*28, 29*). We know of no counter examples of populations in developed countries that do not display this feature.

Smoking History

Issei males accounted for the significant excess risk among smokers, no difference on this score being evident for Nisei males. The meaning of this result is further clouded by the absence of a regular gradient in risk by amount of tobacco used, the secondary contrast of males smoking 20+ and ≤20 cigarettes daily being essentially negative. Curiously, these findings parallel those obtained from prospective studies conducted in the U.S. white population which have described risks about 40% higher for smokers, not accompanied by a gradient in risk with amount used (*30, 31*). Two of the three studies conducted in Japan also suggested that male cigarette smokers have higher stomach cancer risks (*9, 32*). Cigarette smoking, as it bears on the etiology of stomach cancer, is not a primary concern here and we note merely the compatibility of these data with other studies.

Nutritional Status

Information on dental health and age at menarche (not shown) was reviewed on the premise that these items provide indirect measures of nutritional status and thus are of possible relevance for the study of stomach cancer. Nothing of note was uncovered.

Diet

The opening question on food habits, "Generally speaking, which of your meals are prepared in Japanese-style and which in Western-style?" identified respondents who regularly ate only Western-style meals at time of interview (before present illness) and as of 1940. Contrasts of current and past status pointed to lower risks among Nisei eating Western-style meals only, but not for Issei. Although the individual results were not statistically significant, the different behavior of the Issei and Nisei data is provocative. If one accepts the critical nature of exposures in early life, the failure to detect a higher risk for Issei persisting in the custom of Japanese-style meals might have been predicated *a priori*, due to dilution of the Issei contrasts by the more homogeneous background of food practices in Japan.

The potential ability of a crude, summary classification of diet to discriminate between patients and controls raises the possibility that larger contrasts linked with individual items may be present. As a first step in locating more specific effects, relative risks based on dichotomies of above- and below-average frequency of use were computed for the individual foods and beverages included in the questionnaire. The candidates surviving the initial screen, those displaying relative risks deviating from unity by a specified amount—≥ 1.35 and ≤ .75 for Hawaiian Japanese; ≥ 1.50 and ≤ .65 for Issei and Nisei—are arranged in table 4 by descending order of relative risk for Japanese and Western foods. (The limits stated are approximately symmetrical for percentage deviations from unit risk.) Subsequent presentation and discussion will focus primarily on this candidate list of foods and beverages.

Before detailed review, the pattern in table 4 merits comment. A diet-related decline in stomach cancer risk among Hawaiian Japanese might arise in two ways: reduced exposure to Japanese foods that promotes development of the disease or increased use of Western foods that protects against it. One may first ask if two table quadrants, high-risk Japanese and low-risk Western foods,

display a more distinctive pattern than their opposites. The configuration of the presumptive high-risk Japanese foods would support this conjecture, the most striking aspect being the prominent presence of foods with a high salt content: dried/salted fish, Japanese radish pickled in salt brine, shoyu; neither raw fish nor unprocessed vegetables appear in this category. No simple label can be applied to the few low-risk Japanese foods, and their scarcity may have significance. Fresh vegetables predominate among the low-risk Western foods, and this list appears more homogeneous than the high-risk Western foods which present no obvious theme.

Dried and Salted Fish

Table 5 elaborates the results for dried and salted fish by inclusion of more details on frequency of use. The risk for dried and salted fish relative to non-users reached a peak in the highest use category, 4+ times/month, and rising gradients in risk, analogous to a dose-response relationship, were suggested. Elevated risks for the more frequent users prevailed among both Issei and Nisei, with slightly more pronounced effects in the former group. When the information on frequency of use for both forms was pooled, the results followed the pattern for dried and salted fish, but with no apparent enhancement in risk. Earlier patient-control studies conducted in Japan did not distinguish between the consumption of raw and preserved fish, so that no comparable findings for the latter commodity can be cited. Sato et al. (*33*) surveyed selected districts in Japan with high and low stomach cancer mortality and found consumption of salted fish and vegetables more prevalent in the high-risk districts. The excess intake of

TABLE 4.—*List of Japanese and Western foods with suggestive high or low relative risks: Hawaiian Japanese (1.35⁺, ≤.75), Issei and/or Nisei (1.50⁺, ≤.65)*

High risk						Low risk					
Hawaiian Japanese		Issei		Nisei		Hawaiian Japanese		Issei		Nisei	
Japanese											
Dried fish	1.8	Dried fish	2.0	Pickled J radish.	1.7	Chinese peas	0.72	Chinese peas	0.59	Persimmon	0.50
Salted fish	1.6	Shoyu	1.7	Dried fish	1.7	Bean curd	.69				
Shoyu	1.5	Salted fish	1.6	Salted fish	1.5						
Sake	1.42	Salted fish guts	1.6								
Pickled J radish.	1.41	Rice	1.6								
Salted fish guts	1.40										
Western or both											
Candies	2.1	Coffee	2.0	Candies	2.2	Corn	0.73	Corn	0.63	String beans	0.64
U.S. pear	1.7	Candies	2.0	Cherries	2.0	Eggplant	.72	Cucumber	.63	Green onions	.61
Butter	1.49	Butter	1.9	U.S. pear	2.0	Milk	.72	Tomatoes	.54	Lettuce	.61
		Beer	1.9	Cake, pie	1.8	Cucumber	.69	Milk	.44	Sweet potatoes	.60
				Peaches	1.7	Green onions	.65			Tomatoes	.48
				Watermelon	1.5	Celery	.64			Celery	.45
						Tomatoes	.51				

TABLE 5.—*Relative risks for selected contrasts of dried and salted fish*

Contrast		Relative risk [1]		
		Hawaiian Japanese	Issei	Nisei
Dried fish				
Use		1.8*(174, 46; *298, 142*)	2.0*(96, 24; *154,* 75)	1.6 (78, 22; *144, 67*)
1 time/month		1.48(79, 46; *166, 142*)	1.5 (38, 24; *79,* 75)	1.46(44, 22; *87, 67*)
2–3 times/month	vs. non-use	1.6 (32, 46; *63, 142*)	1.8 (20, 24; *35,* 75)	1.31(12, 22; *28, 67*)
4+ times/month		2.8*(63, 46; *69, 142*)	3.0*(38, 24; *40,* 75)	2.6*(25, 22; *29, 67*)
Salted fish				
Use		1.6*(147, 73; *249, 191*)	1.6 (73, 47; *112, 117*)	1.5 (74, 26; *137, 74*)
1 time/month		1.36(84, 73; *165, 191*)	1.34(38, 47; *70, 117*)	1.38(46, 26; *95, 74*)
2–3 times/month	vs. non-use	2.0*(31, 73; *42, 191*)	2.0 (18, 47; *22, 117*)	2.0 (13, 26; *20, 74*)
4+ times/month		2.0*(32, 73; *42, 191*)	2.1 (17, 47; *20, 117*)	1.9 (15, 26; *22, 74*)
Combined use				
Use both		2.0*(132, 31; *205,* 98)	2.3*(66, 17; *92,* 55)	1.8 (66, 14; *113, 43*)
Total 2 times/month		1.5 (44, 31; *97,* 98)	1.6 (19, 17; *35,* 55)	1.38(25, 14; *62, 43*)
Total 3–5 times/month	vs. non-use	2.5*(48, 31; *60,* 98)	2.4*(23, 17; *31,* 55)	2.6*(25, 14; *29, 43*)
Total 6+ times/month		2.6*(40, 31; *48,* 98)	3.0*(24, 17; *26,* 55)	2.2 (16, 14; *22, 43*)

[1] *See* table 3 footnote 1.

TABLE 6.—*Relative risks for selected contrasts of pickled vegetables*

Contrast		Relative risk [1]		
		Hawaiian Japanese	Issei	Nisei
Individual vegetables				
Pickled Japanese radish				
Use		1.41 (185, 35; *349,* 91)	1.28(95, 25; *171,* 58)	1.7 (90, 10; *178, 33*)
1–10 times/month		1.04 (99, 35; *249,* 91)	0.91(46, 25; *117,* 58)	1.32(53, 10; *132, 33*)
11–20 times/month	vs. non-use	2.1 (36, 35; *46,* 91)	1.8 (20, 25; *25,* 58)	2.6 (16, 10; *21, 33*)
21+ times/month		2.7* (50, 35; *54,* 91)	2.7*(29, 25; *29,* 58)	2.7 (21, 10; *25, 33*)
Pickled hakusai				
Use		1.10 (181, 39; *356,* 84)	1.18(97, 23; *179,* 50)	1.01(84, 16; *177, 34*)
1–10 times/month		0.91 (109, 39; *259,* 84)	1.01(54, 23; *115,* 50)	0.80(55, 16; *144, 34*)
11–20 times/month	vs. non-use	1.33 (33, 39; *54,* 84)	1.38(21, 23; *33,* 50)	1.25(12, 16; *21, 34*)
21+ times/month		2.2* (39, 39; *43,* 84)	3.4*(22, 23; *31,* 50)	1.7 (17, 16; *12, 34*)
Pickled plum				
Use		1.26 (164, 56; *307, 133*)	1.30(91, 29; *162,* 67)	1.23(73, 27; *145,* 66)
1–5 times/month	vs. non-use	1.14 (112, 56; *233, 133*)	1.16(59, 29; *118,* 67)	1.12(53, 27; *115,* 66)
6+ times/month		1.7 (52, 56; *74, 133*)	1.7 (32, 29; *44,* 67)	1.6 (20, 27; *30,* 66)
Pickled cucumber				
Use		1.10 (145, 75; *281, 159*)	0.98(75, 45; *144,* 85)	1.26(70, 30; *137,* 74)
1–5 times/month	vs. non-use	1.00 (98, 75; *212, 159*)	0.95(50, 45; *99,* 85)	1.05(48, 30; *113,* 74)
6+ times		1.45 (47, 75; *69, 159*)	1.06(25, 45; *45,* 85)	2.2*(22, 30; *24,* 74)
Pickled eggplant				
Use		0.87 (135, 85; *285, 155*)	0.85(68, 52; *139,* 90)	0.90(67, 33; *146,* 65)
1–5 times/month	vs. non-use	0.86 (100, 85; *216, 155*)	0.89(50, 52; *97,* 90)	0.83(50, 33; *119,* 65)
6+ times/month		0.92 (35, 85; *69, 155*)	0.74(18, 52; *42,* 90)	1.23(17, 33; *27,* 65)
Combined use				
Number of pickled vegetables used				
Use 3+ vs. <2		1.09 (171, 49; *336, 104*)	1.11(90, 30; *167,* 62)	1.06(81, 19; *169,* 42)
Number of pickled vegetables used				
21+ times/month				
1+		1.47*(72, 148; *109, 331*)	1.34(41, 79; *64, 165*)	1.7 (31, 69; *45, 166*)
1 only		1.02 (35, 148; *76, 331*)	1.02(20, 79; *41, 165*)	1.01(15, 69; *35, 166*)
2+	vs. non-use	2.7* (37, 148; *33, 331*)	2.3*(21, 79; *23, 165*)	3.9*(16, 69; *10, 166*)
2+(adj.)[2]		2.6* (37, 148; *33, 331*)	1.9 (21, 79; *23, 165*)	4.9*(16, 69; *10, 166*)

[1] *See* table 3 footnote 1.
[2] Relative risks are adjusted, in addition, for frequency of use of the following fresh vegetables: tomatoes, celery, green onion, cucumber, eggplant.

salted foods in the high-risk districts appeared real, since the authors could account for it on the basis of such local conditions as inadequate rail transport facilities, low income, and climatic influences on the type and annual number of crops.

Pickled Vegetables

Table 6 pursues the lead suggested by the case-control difference for Japanese radish pickled in salt brine. The absence of effects for unproc-essed Japanese vegetables directs suspicion to the pickling process, so the analysis was extended to cover all pickled vegetables (radish, hakusai, plum, cucumber, eggplant).

When the detailed frequency data were reviewed, a definite gradient in risk with amount of use emerged for pickled radish and hakusai, and a lesser one for pickled plum. The effects for hakusai and radish were concentrated in the highest frequency range, 21+ times/month, where significant, over 2-fold risks were estimated relative to non-users. The results for pickled cucumber may be discounted in view of the unimpressive gradient in risk and they may reflect indirect associations with pickled radish and hakusai, which are consumed in much greater amounts.

Since the pickling process may be more critical than the identity of the vegetables, the indicated next step was to consolidate the information on all pickled vegetables. Contrasts based solely on the number used were negative, and discrimination in risk was not achieved until data on the amount of use were introduced. Both Issei and Nisei, using at least 2 pickled vegetables (radish and hakusai were the most common combination) each at a rate of 21+ times/month, displayed significant and substantially elevated relative risks. The absence of an effect when only 1 vegetable was consumed at this level suggests a multiple-use effect underlies the individual findings for radish and hakusai. The requirement of frequent consumption of 2 or more pickled foods to produce an effect strengthens the impression of an underlying dose-response relationship. The results for pickled vegetables, including the Issei and Nisei effects, closely parallel those described for salted and dried fish.

The indicated lower risks among users of fresh vegetables (table 4) raise the possibility that the high risk for pickled vegetables might be attributable to low consumption of fresh vegetables. The data yielded no evidence of negative correlations between these two classes of foods; if anything, they tended to be positively correlated, so that control for Western vegetables left the relative risk estimates for pickled vegetables virtually unchanged.

These findings on pickled vegetables among Hawaiian Japanese have counterparts in the literature from Japan. For example, Hirayama in his case-control study was impressed by the strong association between stomach cancer and an excess intake of highly salted pickles (*34*). The geographic comparisons of Sato et al. (*33*), mentioned in connection with dried and salted fish, also tend to support the associations of stomach cancer and salted pickles.

Shoyu

Like pickled vegetables and dried/salted fish, shoyu has a high salt content. A risk of 1.6, not statistically significant, was estimated for persons currently taking shoyu with their meals, relative to those not following this custom. The relative risk was the same for Issei and Nisei and the absence of a nativity differential follows the pattern presented by the high-salt preserved fish and pickled vegetables. The question did not lend itself to quantitation and it could not be ascertained if a larger, significant effect prevailed among persons with high intake. The latter line of inquiry might have been unproductive, since the study of Segi et al. in Japan did not detect an excess number of heavy users of shoyu among stomach cancer patients. (*9*).

"Western" Vegetables

Table 4 lists 9 Western vegetables, including some known in Japan, for which relative risks substantially below unity for above-average users were described for Issei and/or Nisei. The inverse associations with stomach cancer are reinforced by the collective tendency of items in this category to exhibit low relative risks. When the 9 items surviving the initial screen were scrutinized in detail, 3 (tomato, celery, corn) exhibited definite gradients, with the lowest risks appearing among frequent users; 2 others (lettuce, onion) were marginally suggestive in this respect. The findings are given in table 7. No strong Issei-Nisei differences appeared in this collection, as can be demonstrated by the simple average of the 5 summary relative risks: Hawaii Japanese, .67; Issei, .75; Nisei, .63.

Information on the 5 vegetables was combined to see if the case-control differences would be reinforced in subgroups with highest overall exposure. Two approaches, one based on a straightforward summation of frequencies of use and the other on characterizing a relative profile of use for each item (high, moderate, same, low) yielded similar results (table 7). Neither approach strongly enhanced the low risks noted for individual vegetables.

Adjustment for consumption of pickled vegetables left the combined relative risk estimate unchanged, which argues against viewing the Western vegetable effect as a mirror image of the pickled-vegetable effect and favors instead the alternative of two distinct, independent components.

The meaning of these observations is hard to assess in the absence of comparable findings from other U.S. or Japanese populations. In studies of diet and stomach cancer at Roswell Park Memorial Institute, Graham et al. did not cover the vegetables mentioned here, except to note a reduced risk for frequent users of lettuce (*35*); they did consider several vegetables that are normally cooked and found no noteworthy case-control differences, and these results parallel those for cooked vegetables

TABLE 7.—*Relative risks for selected contrasts of Western vegetables*

Contrast	Relative risk [1]		
	Hawaiian Japanese	Issei	Nisei
Individual vegetables			
Tomatoes			
Use 4+	0.51*(162, 58; *372, 68*)	0.54*(92, 28; *197, 32*)	0.48*(70, 30; *175, 36*)
4-10 } vs. <4 times/month	0.61*(111, 58; *214, 68*)	0.77 (67, 28; *102, 32*)	0.47*(44, 30; *112, 36*)
11+	0.39*(51, 58; *158, 68*)	0.31*(25, 28; *95, 32*)	0.49 (26, 30; *63, 36*)
Celery			
Use 4+	0.64*(133, 87; *311, 129*)	0.83 (72, 48; *147, 82*)	0.45*(61, 39; *164, 47*)
4-10 } vs. <4 times/month	0.77 (94, 87; *181, 129*)	1.03 (54, 48; *88, 82*)	0.52*(40, 39; *93, 47*)
11+	0.44*(39, 87; *130, 129*)	0.54 (18, 48; *59, 82*)	0.36*(21, 39; *71, 47*)
Corn			
Use	0.73 (181, 39; *381, 59*)	0.63 (90, 30; *189, 40*)	1.00 (91, 9; *192, 19*)
1-7 times/month } vs. non-use	0.79 (163, 39; *319, 59*)	0.69 (83, 30; *161, 40*)	1.07 (80, 9; *158, 19*)
8+ times/month	0.45*(18, 39; *62, 59*)	0.32*(7, 30; *28, 40*)	0.68 (11, 9; *34, 19*)
Lettuce			
Use 11+	0.83 (173, 47; *359, 81*)	1.09 (97, 23; *182, 47*)	0.61*(76, 24; *177, 34*)
11-20 } vs. <11 times/month	0.93 (76, 47; *142, 81*)	1.30 (42, 23; *66, 47*)	0.63 (34, 24; *76, 34*)
21+	0.77 (97, 47; *217, 81*)	0.97 (55, 23; *116, 47*)	0.59 (42, 24; *101, 34*)
Onions, including green onions			
Use 8+	0.72 (182, 38; *383, 57*)	0.84 (100, 20; *196, 33*)	0.59 (82, 18; *187, 24*)
8-20 } vs. <8 times/month	0.79 (153, 38; *290, 57*)	0.91 (82, 20; *148, 33*)	0.67 (71, 18; *142, 24*)
21+	0.48*(29, 38; *93, 57*)	0.67 (18, 20; *48, 33*)	0.31*(11, 18; *45, 24*)
Combined use			
Use 60+ vs. <40 times/month [2]	0.39*(58, 71; *194, 103*)	0.38*(30, 36; *106, 57*)	0.40*(28, 35; *88, 46*)
"High" vs. "low" use of each vegetable	0.51*	0.55*	0.46*

[1] *See* table 3 footnote 1.
[2] Adjusted, in addition, for frequency of use of pickled vegetables.

eaten by Hawaiian Japanese. We note parenthetically that, of the 5 vegetables pinpointed here as displaying the most prominent effects, all except corn are often eaten raw.

Fruits

Efforts to uncover effects for fruits paralleling those described for Western vegetables were negative; no case-control differences worthy of comment were found.

Rice

No report on stomach cancer in the Japanese is complete without mention of rice. The relative risk estimate in table 4 was derived from the contrast of persons currently eating rice at least 2 times daily

against all others. To elaborate on this result, quantitative data on number of bowls consumed daily (currently and as of 1940) were reviewed, with the outcome shown in table 8. The impression of a higher risk confined to Issei persisted in the second set of data, but introduction of amount consumed did not enhance the case-control difference. Nor was the association sharpened by reference to status as of 1940. The composite results reinforce the effect concentrated among Issei. Hirayama referred to an earlier study of Hawaii Japanese that found only a small excess frequency in rice intake among patients, but these data did not report on Issei and Nisei separately (*36*). The present Issei results agree with those from the counterpart case-control study undertaken in Miyagi Prefecture (*37*). The Miyagi findings remained substantially unchanged with control for social class and urban-

TABLE 8.—*Relative risks for selected contrasts of rice and butter*

Contrast	Relative risk [1]		
	Hawaiian Japanese	Issei	Nisei
A. Rice			
Frequency of use			
At time of interview			
2+ vs. <2 meals daily	1.25 (144, 76; *264, 175*)	1.6 (89, 31; *148, 80*)	1.00 (55, 45; *116, 95*)
As of 1940			
3+ vs. <3 meals daily	1.03 (38, 179; *73, 363*)	1.04 (28, 91; *52, 176*)	1.01 (10, 88; *21, 186*)
Amount used			
At time of interview			
2+ vs. <2 bowls daily	1.48*(151, 69; *263, 177*)	1.8*(86, 34; *134, 95*)	1.19 (65, 35; *129, 82*)
As of 1940			
4+ vs. <4 bowls daily	1.22 (131, 86; *241, 194*)	1.42 (83, 36; *141, 87*)	1.03 (48, 50; *100, 107*)
B. Butter on bread			
Use vs. non-use	1.49*(155, 65; *269, 167*)	1.9*(87, 33; *133, 94*)	1.14 (68, 32; *136, 73*)

[1] *See* table 3 footnote 1.

rural residence. On the other hand, Hirayama's prospective study in Japan to date has identified no noteworthy excess of stomach cancer deaths among cohort members with the highest rice intake (*38*).

The 1953–55 study by Segi described a substantially higher proportion of patients than controls reporting rice to be their sole staple food (*4*). The thrust of Segi's inquiry was directed, not to amount of rice, but rather to dietary deficiencies. Segi's results might be construed as consistent with the views of Gregor et al. who have associated stomach cancer with deficient intake of animal proteins (*39*). The present Hawaii series was reviewed for evidence on the latter point, with negative results, the level of total meat and fish consumption being about equal for patients and controls.

The Hawaii Japanese findings on rice deviate from those for dried/salted fish and pickled vegetables, which indicated an association in both nativity groups. Two differently phrased explanations, both having a similar content, might account for the nativity difference: *a*) greater susceptibility of the Issei gastric mucosa due to a background of nutritional deficiencies or other environmental insults, or *b*) stronger indirect Issei associations of rice consumption with the responsible etiologic factor(s). Either could operate if Issei consuming the most rice represented adherents to other traditional Japanese practices.

Merliss speculated that asbestos contamination of rice treated with talc may be responsible for the high stomach cancer risks among Japanese (*40*). As noted by Merliss, rice grown in California for the U.S. Japanese market continues to have talc addi-

tives, but this method was generally replaced in Japan during the immediate post-war interval by mechanical milling processes. The sustained, modest reduction in stomach cancer risk among U.S. Japanese relative to Japan (*18*) during the continued exposure of U.S. Japanese to talc-treated rice detracts from Merliss' hypothesis. The absence of a case-control difference in rice consumption of Nisei, who share with Issei a common exposure to talc-treated rice, casts further doubt on the conjecture that asbestos residues in rice are responsible for the high Japanese stomach cancer risks.

Butter

An elevated relative risk for Issei using butter as a spread for bread followed the general rule that, when the experience of the two nativity groups differed, case-control discrimination was concentrated among the Issei. The question on butter did not lend itself to further refinement by frequency or amount of use, and this result may represent nothing more than sampling variation.

Alcoholic Beverages

Sake and beer were the 2 alcoholic beverages that discriminated most between patients and controls. Except for sake, Japanese women consumed little alcohol and the detailed comparisons in table 9 were restricted to males. The contrast of current users of any liquor versus non-users yielded a significantly higher relative risk for Issei males only. Other variants intended to pinpoint groups

TABLE 9.—*Relative risks for selected contrasts of alcoholic and other beverages*

Contrast	Relative risk [1]		
	Hawaiian Japanese	Issei	Nisei
A. Alcoholic beverages			
Any alcoholic beverage			
Use vs. non-use	**1.39**(102, 118; *174, 266*)	**2.1***(63, 57; *84, 145*)	**0.84**(39, 61; *90, 121*)
Use vs. non-use, males	**1.26**(83, 52; *151, 119*)	**2.3***(52, 24; *70, 75*)	**0.60**(31, 28; *81, 44*)
Beer			
Use vs. non-use	**1.17**(75, 145; *137, 302*)	**1.9***(47, 73; *63, 165*)	**0.67**(28, 72; *74, 137*)
Use ⎱ vs. non-use, males	**1.19**(69, 66; *126, 143*)	**2.1***(44, 32; *57, 87*)	**0.60**(25, 34; *69, 56*)
1–5 times/month ⎰	**1.16**(31, 66; *58, 143*)	**2.1***(23, 32; *30, 87*)	**0.47**(8, 34; *28, 56*)
6+ times/months	**1.19**(38, 66; *68, 143*)	**2.1** (21, 32; *27, 87*)	**0.68**(17, 34; *41, 56*)
Sake			
Use vs. non-use	**1.42**(47, 173; *71, 369*)	**1.48**(37, 83; *54, 175*)	**1.29**(10, 90; *17, 194*)
Use ⎱	**1.47**(40, 95; *60, 210*)	**1.6** (31, 45; *44, 101*)	**1.23**(9, 50; *16, 109*)
Less than daily ⎰ vs. non-use, males	**1.02**(17, 95; *37, 210*)	**0.98**(10, 45; *23, 101*)	**1.09**(7, 50; *14, 109*)
At least daily	**2.2***(23, 95; *23, 210*)	**2.2***(21, 45; *21, 101*)	**2.2** (2, 50; *2, 109*)
B. Other beverages			
Coffee			
2+ vs. <2 cups daily	**1.21**(102, 118; *186, 253*)	**2.0***(53, 67; *67, 161*)	**0.74**(49, 51; *119, 92*)
Milk			
Use ⎱	**0.73**(111, 109; *257, 183*)	**0.44***(52, 68; *145, 84*)	**1.27**(59, 41; *112, 99*)
Less than daily ⎰ vs. non-use	**0.67**(24, 109; *65, 183*)	**0.31***(7, 68; *27, 84*)	**1.12**(17, 41; *38, 90*)
At least daily	**0.76**(87, 109; *192, 183*)	**0.47***(45, 68; *118, 84*)	**1.37**(42, 41; *74, 90*)

[1] *See* table 3 footnote 1.

with above-average exposure (use of 2 or more alcoholic beverages, daily use of at least 1, etc.) did not materially sharpen the distinction between cases and controls. The information on beer drinking was mainly responsible for the 2 features just noted—an effect limited to Issei and the absence of a clear relationship between risk and frequency of use.

For sake drinkers, the Issei-Nisei disparity in relative risk estimates was at best suggestive and neither risk was statistically significant. The weak Issei result for sake is not grossly at variance with information from Japan. While Segi et al. did find a substantial excess proportion of heavy sake drinkers, more specifically for those who habitually drank sake before the evening meal, among patients compared to hospital controls (9), the later case-control and prospective studies of Hirayama have not adequately confirmed the Segi et al. report (34, 38). Wynder et al. also found no noteworthy case-control differences in type or quantity of alcohol consumption in their investigations in Japan and 3 other countries (13).

Beverages

A low relative risk for Issei milk drinkers, not reproduced among Nisei, is another example of divergent nativity findings. The Issei results, however, revealed no gradient in risk by amount consumed. A failure to demonstrate a "dose-response" relationship is one reason Hirayama's report of lower stomach cancer mortality among milk drinkers in Japan (36) has not commanded wide acceptance (the other being the well-known fact that milk is an important staple food in some high-risk countries). Nevertheless, the replication among Issei of Hirayama's findings in Japan may warrant pursuit of this lead, with emphasis on reasons for the expression of a "protective" effect limited to Issei.

Coffee also behaved differently for Issei and Nisei, with only the former presenting an elevated risk. The restricted range of amounts consumed by Hawaiian Japanese precluded further assessment of this association.

Type

Muñoz, using a modified Laurens classification to type in stomach cancers, described high-risk populations as presenting more intestinal-type carcinomas (22) and concluded that the intestinal type accounts for the major share of interpopulation

variability in total stomach cancer incidence. Intestinal metaplasia has been proposed as a precursor lesion of the intestinal type (41). This configuration of evidence raises the possibility of an environmental etiology for intestinal-type tumors.

If a relationship between intestinal type and environmental factors exists, one might expect case-control discrimination (relative risk) for diet and other environmentally determined factors to be enhanced for these lesions. The present material, providing type information for 162 of the 220 cases studied, can be examined from this point of view. The intestinal/diffuse ratio rises with age and the present series displays this feature: under 60 years $19/54 = 0.35$; 60 years and over $55/35 = 1.57$. However, the overall I/D ratio (.83) seems atypically low when compared with other high-risk populations. This may be a general Japanese characteristic and not a peculiarity of the present data, since Yamamoto and Kato reported similar results for a Hiroshima necropsy series (42).

For the 10 case-control contrasts yielding relative risks significant at the 5% level, table 10 gives the risk estimates for the corresponding subsets of intestinal and diffuse tumors. With one major exception, dried fish, the results conformed to the *a priori* prediction of stronger positive or negative associations for intestinal-type lesions and in this sense support the notion of environmental etiologies for the intestinal type. The sparse data in hand convey little conviction and this must remain a subject for further inquiry.

DISCUSSION

While the favorable setting of the Hawaii Japanese simplified the collection of diet histories, the complications introduced by changes in food habits over time remain. Observations of current conditions can discriminate for our purposes only insofar as they convey information on past status. Also, data on individual foods may conceal important differences in composition or preparation. Given the background noise arising from the inability to collect very precise and specific data, one would not anticipate strong effects of a magnitude so as to be self-interpreting. A more probable outcome was that differences in risk related to specific foods might survive in diluted form.

Although the magnitude and coherence of the risks estimated for dried/salted fish and pickled vegetables perhaps exceeded expectations, the assessment of these and other findings must invoke

TABLE 10.—*Relative risks for selected contrasts involving subsets of intestinal (I) and diffuse (D) type lesions*

Contrasts		Type	Relative risk [1]
A. Prefecture of origin:			
high risk vs. low risk	Issei	I	2.5*
		D	1.41
B. Occupation:			
"low" vs. "high" socioeconomic class	All males	I	2.0*
		D	1.7
C. Smoking history:			
any tobacco vs. no tobacco use	Issei males	I	1.9
		D	1.6
D. Dried fish:			
4+ times/month vs. non-use	Total group	I	2.6*
		D	3.2*
E. Pickled vegetables:			
(combined use) 2+ used 21+ times/month vs. none	Total group	I	2.7
		D	2.0
F. Western vegetables (total frequency use):			
60+ times/month vs. <40 times/month	Total group	I	0.46*
		D	0.44*
G. Rice:			
2+ vs. <2 bowls daily	Issei	I	1.7
		D	1.7
H. Beer:			
use vs. non-use	Issei males	I	2.6*
		D	1.9
I. Sake:			
use daily vs. non-use	Issei males	I	2.7
		D	1.4
J. Coffee:			
2+ cups daily vs. <2 cups daily	Issei	I	2.0
		D	2.0
K. Milk:			
use vs. non-use	Issei	I	0.34*
		D	0.55*

[1] *See* table 3 footnote 1.

collateral evidence represented by internally consistent patterns. We believe patterns have emerged which offer leads and which may narrow the field of search.

The major finding, the elevated relative risks among Issei and Nisei for pickled vegetables and dried/salted fish, is enhanced by its specificity, the absence of similar effects for fresh vegetables and raw fish, and by the rough equivalent of a "dose-response" phenomenon. Points of consistency with data from Japan have been noted. Consumption of these items is substantially lower in Hawaii than in Japan, and the ability to detect an effect in the lower range of usage in Hawaii may be significant.

Review of more detailed tabulations gave no reason to believe that dried/salted fish could account for the pickled vegetable result or vice-versa. The inability to incriminate fresh vegetables and raw fish directs attention to a common property, their high salt content.

Experimental support for the epidemiologic findings can be cited. Sato fed salted codfish and yukari (salted leaves of a plant used to color salted plums) to mice and found both to provoke bleeding

in the glandular stomach within 7 days (*43*). MacDonald took 3 men adhering to Western diets, with normal control biopsies of the gastric antrum, and added selected Japanese foods to their diet. One test item, salted vegetables in soy sauce (fukujin-zuke) was assessed by biopsies of the antrum on the 4th day and all subjects showed abnormalities of the surface epithelium and a markedly increased mytotic count (*44*). Neither experiment demonstrates carcinogenicity, but they do indicate that abnormal responses in the gastric mucosa can be elicited quickly. A rapid cell turnover in the gastric mucosa has been advanced as one reason for doubting local action of a carcinogen in this site, and the rapid cellular response may lessen the force of this argument.

Sato suggested that bleeding in stomachs of his mice was mediated through high osmotic pressure from salt concentrates. Since Sato and MacDonald tested foods, pure NaCl is not necessarily incriminated and other food-related properties might be considered. Bacterial toxins in foods pickled in brine seem unlikely candidates, since bacterial growth is inhibited by 3.5% brine concentrations and 5% concentrations are lethal.

Nitrosamines might be considered. The distribution of secondary amines, a known precursor of nitrosamines, in foods corresponds well to the epidemiologic picture; raw fish, beef, pork, and chicken for which the case-control results were negative, are low in secondary amines (*45*). Dried fish have high concentrations of secondary amines (*45*, *46*). Kawamura also described boiled cuttlefish canned in shoyu to be exceptionally rich in secondary amines. Nitrosamines may also be present, since Fong and Walsh have identified nitrosamines in Cantonese salt-dried fish (*47*). Other evidence hinting indirectly at nitrosamine activity might be assembled. For example, Drasar et al., in commenting on Stalsberg's finding of a high number of gastric cancer patients with a history of an operation for gastric or duodenal ulcers more than 25 years before death, noted that the colonized stomach would provide a suitable site for in vivo synthesis of nitrosamines (*48*).

Pickled vegetables do not appear to have been studied intensively for nitrites and secondary amines, and we have found no reported data on this point. The chemistry of pickled vegetables warrants more attention.

The argument for a protective effect conferred by consumption of selected vegetables is more speculative in the absence of evidence that the present data replicate other work. Nor do we have any ideas on a mechanism of action. Given the diversity in environmental background, including diet, for populations at high risk to stomach cancer, we can believe that multiple etiologies are involved. For example, even if nitrosamines should prove the major factor in gastric cancer among Japanese, this would not mean that the long-term decline of stomach cancer mortality among U.S. whites can be accounted for by a parallel decline in exposure to foods rich in secondary amines. The unanticipated finding for vegetables may later dovetail more closely with the epidemiologic pattern for U.S. whites.

Certain case-control differences limited to the Issei population—tobacco, liquor (beer), coffee, milk—and reinforced on some points by the correspondence of the Issei findings with Japan, raise the possibility that observational associations are not reproducible in all populations. Issei stomachs, sensitized by more prolonged exposure to salted foods and other agents, may respond to insults or protective factors without effect on more normal Nisei or White gastric mucosa.

The list given above has at least one common thread: Their use is thought to influence adversely, beneficially for milk, the clinical course of gastric and duodenal ulcers. This point comes to mind, when we recall that some, but not all, Japanese pathologists, impressed by appearance of gastric cancers in ulcer margins, believe that the two diseases are associated (*49–51*), while American pathologists have not thought the two diseases to be associated in U.S. populations (*52, 53*). Stout, for example, states ". . . the association is so uncommon that benign peptic ulcer of the stomach can not be regarded as a precancerous lesion." The divergence in views between two groups of observers may mean that gastric cancer is presented differently in the two populations. The speculation that Issei may share with people in Japan an ulcer-related pathway for the malignant transformation of cells in the gastric mucosa emphasizes the need for more attention to the epidemiology and pathology of precursor lesions along lines initiated by Correa (*41*).

The case-control findings call for expansion of studies of the chemistry of suspect Japanese foods and intensified efforts to refine and modify feeding experiments and to develop new animal models.

Meanwhile, the study potential of the Japanese migrants for stomach cancer has not been exhausted. Priority was accorded to the data for Hawaii Japanese in the hope that a population in transition might yield the more provocative contrasts. We plan to return to the case-control data assembled in Japan to consider how the consolidated Hawaii-Japan findings tie in with the changed food and cultural practices of the migrants and their descendents. New case-control and prospective studies to probe more specific exposures and effects, such as those linked with dried/salted fish and pickled vegetables, are also under way.

REFERENCES

(*1*) State D, Varco RL, Wangensteen OH: Attempt to identify likely precursors of gastric cancer. J Natl Cancer Inst 7:379–384, 1947

(*2*) Graham S, Lilienfeld AM: Genetic studies of gastric cancer in humans: An appraisal. Cancer 11:945–958, 1958

(*3*) Macklin MT: Role of heredity in gastric and intestinal cancer. Gastroenterology 29:507–511, 1955

(*4*) Videbaek A, Mosbech J: Aetiology of gastric carcinoma elucidated by study of 302 pedigrees. Acta Med Scand 149:137–159, 1954

(*5*) Woolf CM: Further study on familial aspects of carcinoma of stomach. Am J Human Genet 8:102–109, 1956

(*6*) Aird I, Bentall HH, Roberts JAF: A relationship between cancer of stomach and the ABO blood groups. Br Med J 1:799–801, 1953

(7) BILLINGTON BP: Gastric cancer-relationships between ABO bloodgroups, site, and epidemiology. Lancet 2:859–862, 1956

(8) BUCKWALTER JA, WOHLWEND CB, COLTER DC, et al. The association of the ABO blood groups to gastric carcinoma. Surg Gynecol Obstet 104: 176–179, 1957

(9) SEGI M, FUKUSHIMA I, FUJISAKU S, et al: An epidemiological study on cancer in Japan. Gann (Suppl) 48: 1957

(10) WHITE C, EISENBERG H: ABO blood groups and cancers of the stomach. Yale J Biol Med 32:58–61, 1959

(11) DOLL R: Environmental factors in the aetiology of cancer of the stomach. Gastroenterologia 86:320–328, 1956

(12) HAENSZEL WM: Variation in incidence of and mortality from stomach cancer, with particular reference to the United States. J Natl Cancer Inst 21:213–262, 1958

(13) WYNDER EL, KMET J, DUNGAL N, et al: An epidemiological investigation of gastric cancer. Cancer 16:1461–1496, 1963

(14) STEINER PE: Cancer: Race and Geography. Baltimore, Williams & Wilkins Co., 1954, 363 pp

(15) SEGI M, KURIHARA M: Cancer Mortality for Selected Sites in 24 Countries, No. 4 (1962–1963). Sendai, Japan, Dept. of Public Health, Tohoku Univ School Med, 1966, 358 pp

(16) DOLL R, MUIR C, WATERHOUSE J (eds.): Cancer Incidence in Five Continents, Vol II. Geneva, UICC, 1970, 388 pp

(17) SMITH RL: Recorded and expected mortality among Japanese of the United States and Hawaii, with special reference to cancer. J Natl Cancer Inst 17:459–473, 1956

(18) HAENSZEL WM, KURIHARA M: Studies of Japanese Migrants. I. Mortality from cancer and other diseases among Japanese in the United States. J Natl Cancer Inst 40:43–68, 1968

(19) Hawaii Tumor Registry: Cancer in Hawaii, Morbidity and Treatment: Five Years—1960–1964. Hawaii Med J 27:409–456, 1968

(20) HAENSZEL WM: Cancer mortality incidence among the foreign-born in the United States. J Natl Cancer Inst 26:37–132, 1961

(21) STASZEWSKI J, HAENSZEL W: Cancer mortality among the Polish-born in the United States. J Natl Cancer Inst 35:291–297, 1965

(22) MUÑOZ N, ASVALL J: Time trends of intestinal and diffuse types of gastric cancer in Norway. Int J Cancer 8:144–157, 1971

(23) MANTEL N, HAENSZEL WM: Statistical aspects of the analysis of data from retrospective studies of disease. J Natl Cancer Inst 22:719–748, 1959

(24) HANKEY BF: Application of multivariate risk function in considering the association between food consumption and risk of stomach cancer. PhD dissertation. Univ Pittsburgh, Pittsburgh, Pa., 1970

(25) COCHRAN WG: Some effects of errors of measurement on multiple correlation. J Am Statis Assoc 65:22–34, 1970

(26) US Dept Health, Education, and Welfare, National Office Vital Stat: Mortality from selected causes by marital status. United States, 1949–1951. Vital Statistics Special Report 39, 303–429, 1956

(27) SEGI M, KURIHARA M, MATSUYAMA T: Cancer Mortality in Japan (1899–1962). Sendai, Japan, Dept. of Public Health Tohoku Univ School Med, 1965

(28) DORN HF, CUTLER SJ: Morbidity from cancer in the United States. Publ Health Monogr 56: 1–207, 1959

(29) HIRAYAMA T, YUSA Y: The occupational-social class risks of cancer in Japan. Jap J Cancer Clin 9:66–74, 1963

(30) KAHN HA: The Dorn study of smoking and mortality among U.S. veterans: Report on eight and one-half years of observation. Natl Cancer Inst Monogr 19: 1–125, 1966

(31) HAMMOND EC: Smoking in relation to the death rates of one million men and women. Natl Cancer Inst Monogr 19:127–204, 1966

(32) HIRAYAMA T: Smoking in relation to the death rates of 265,118 men and women in Japan. A report on five years of follow-up. Report presented to American Cancer Society (Miami), Mar 1972

(33) SATO T, FUKUYAMA T, SUZUKI T, et al: Studies of the causation of gastric cancer. 2. The relation between gastric cancer mortality rate and salted food intake in several places in Japan. Bull Inst Publ Health 8:187–198, 1959

(34) HIRAYAMA T: The epidemiology of cancer of the stomach. Itocho 3:787–795, 1968

(35) GRAHAM S, LILIENFELD AM, TIDINGS JE: Dietary and purgation factors in the epidemiology of gastric cancer. Cancer 20:2224–2234, 1967

(36) HIRAYAMA T: A study of the epidemiology of stomach cancer, with special reference to the effect of the diet factor. Bull Inst Publ Health 12:85–96, 1963

(37) HAENSZEL W, SEGI M: Stomach cancer among the Japanese. UICC Monogr Ser 10 (Harris RJ, ed.). Ninth International Cancer Congress, 1967

(38) HIRAYAMA T: Epidemiology of stomach cancer. Gann Monogr 11:3–19, 1971

(39) GREGOR O, TOMAN R, PRŮŠOVÁ F: Relation of gastrointestinal cancer mortality to cancer mortality in general. Scand J Gastroenterol 9:79–85, 1971

(40) MERLISS RR: Talc-treated rice and Japanese stomach cancer. Science 173:1141–1142, 1971

(41) CORREA P, CUELLO C, DUQUE E: Carcinoma and intestinal metaplasia of the stomach in Colombian migrants. J Natl Cancer Inst 44:297–306, 1970

(42) YAMAMOTO T, KATO H: Two major histological types of gastric carcinoma among the fixed population of Hiroshima and Nagasaki. Gann 62:381–387, 1971

(43) SATO T, FUKUYAMA T, URATA G, et al: Studies of the causation of gastric cancer. 1. Bleeding in the glandular stomach of mice by feeding with highly salted foods, and a comment on salted foods in Japan. Bull Inst Public Health 8:10–13, 1959

(44) MACDONALD WC, ANDERSON FH, HASHIMOTO S: Histological effect of certain pickles on the human gastric mucosa: A preliminary report. Canad Med Assoc J 96:1521–1525, 1967

(45) KAWAMURA T, SAKAI K, MIYAZAWA F, et al: Studies on nitrosamines in foods (IV). Distribution of secondary amines in foods. J Food Hyg Soc Japan 12: 192–197, 1971

(46) ISHIDATE M: Secondary amine and nitrate contents of Japanese foods. Paper presented at Second International Symposium of the Princess Takamatsu

Cancer Research Fund (Tokyo), Nov. 1971

(47) FONG YY, WALSH EO'F: Carcinogenic nitrosamines in Cantonese salt-dried fish. Lancet Nov 6:1032, 1971

(48) DRASAR BS, HILL MJ, HAWKSWORTH G: Stomach cancer after gastric operations for benign conditions. Lancet Dec 11:1317, 1971

(49) OOTA K: On the nature of the ulcerative changes in early carcinoma of the stomach. Proc Int Conf Gastric Cancer. Gann Mongr 3:141–151, 1968

(50) MURAKAMI T: Significance of ulcers. Proc Int Conf Gastric Cancer. Gann Mongr 3:153–155, 1968

(51) SANO R: Significance of ulcers. Proc Int Conf Gastric Cancer. Gann Mongr 3:155–156, 1968

(52) STOUT AP: Tumors of the stomach. *In* Atlas of Tumor Pathology, sect VI, fasc 19. Washington, D.C., Armed Forces Inst Pathol, 1953

(53) EWING J: Neoplastic Diseases, a Treatise on Tumors, 4th ed. Philadelphia, W.B. Saunders Co., 1941, 1160 pp

Developments in the Epidemiology of Stomach Cancer over the Past Decade

by William Haenszel and Pelayo Correa

Biometry Branch, National Cancer Institute, NIH, Bethesda, Maryland 20014 [W. H.], and Department of Pathology, Louisiana State University Medical School, New Orleans, Louisiana 70112 [P. C.]

Summary

The history of stomach cancer epidemiology is reviewed. The introduction of migrant population studies in the 1960 decade that described the critical role of exposures to this disease in early life was a key event. Companion pathology studies have indicated different epidemiological patterns for 2 histological entities, intestinal and diffuse type carcinomas, and confirmed an excess of intestinal metaplasia in populations at high risk to stomach cancer. Recent results suggest that epidemiology of stomach cancer can be transformed into the epidemiology of precursor lesions, and introduction of the fiberoptic gastroscope makes technically feasible detailed studies of the relationship of precursor lesions to suspect factors, including diet, in selected geographic areas. Nitroso compounds have been identified as candidate carcinogens and the epidemiological, pathological, and chemical data display signs of internal consistency. Feeding experiments with N-methyl-N'-nitro-N-nitrosoguanidine have led to animal models that permit a coordinated epidemiological-experimental approach to stomach cancer.

The epidemiology of stomach cancer has been the subject of several reviews. Barrett's (2) comprehensive review, published in 1946, summarized the information available up to that time. Later reviews by Doll (8) in 1956 and by Haenszel (15) in 1958 utilized the more extensive and

Presented at the Conference on Nutrition in the Causation of Cancer, May 19 to 22, 1975, Key Biscayne, Florida, by William Haenszel.

reliable data on cancer mortality and incidence accumulated in the years following World War II. A survey of the literature appearing after Barrett's publication was included in the 1963 report by Wynder *et al.* (40) on case-control studies of stomach cancer in Japan, Iceland, Slovenia, and the United States. The most recent compilation and appraisal of the relevant epidemiological data on gastrointestinal cancers was carried out by Bjelke (3).

This paper will attempt to place in perspective developments of the past decade, and for this purpose the summary by a panel of experts assembled under the auspices of the World Organization of Gastroenterology in 1964 provides a useful benchmark and point of departure (4). The characteristics of stomach cancer epidemiology established beyond dispute at that time were as follows.

1. There was marked intercountry variation in stomach cancer mortality, the rates in high-risk countries being approximately 5 times those in low-risk areas. Japan, Chile, Costa Rica, Iceland, and Finland had been identified as high-risk populations, while United States whites and Commonwealth countries, particularly Australia and New Zealand, were at the opposite end of the risk spectrum. However, the geographical comparisons of mortality did not suggest racial immunity to stomach cancer, and for all races subpopulations at high or low risk could be identified. The inferences drawn from the mortality data appeared consistent with the incidence data available from cancer registries in selected localities.

2. The marked intercountry variation in risk was accompanied by variation within countries, the general rule being that northern and/or colder regions had the higher risks,

one well-known example being the higher stomach cancer rates in the mountainous region of Slovenia (Yugoslavia) as contrasted with the lower risks in the Adriatic coastal zone.

3. A rather stable male:female ratio of risks had been observed to prevail within all populations, the overall female rate being roughly one-half to two-thirds of the corresponding male rate.

4. A marked inverse socioeconomic gradient in risk was a prominent characteristic of this disease, the risks for the lower classes being roughly 2.5 times those for the highest socioeconomic class.

5. No consistent gradient in risk between urban and rural populations was demonstrable, and this did not appear to be an important epidemiological characteristic.

6. Within the United States the foreign-born displayed higher mortality than the native-born, the excess being most pronounced among migrants from Japan and certain European countries.

7. A steady downward trend in stomach cancer mortality had been underway for many years, a feature noticed first in the United States and later in several European countries.

8. Observations on the high risk of stomach cancer patients with pernicious anemia had firmly established the premalignant role of pernicious anemia.

These undisputed facts were accompanied by other pieces of evidence of more uncertain pedigree, the interpretation of which was subject to discussion and caveats. The latter included the following.

1. A role for genetic factors was suggested by the familial clustering of disease and by the excess number of patients in Blood Group A. Since familial aggregation is a necessary, but not sufficient, condition for a genetic factor, familial aggregation could also reflect exposure to a common environment. The excess stomach cancer risk of patients in Blood Group A was small (a risk of 1.2 relative to Blood Group O was suggested by the composite evidence). What seemed clear was the inability of a genetic factor to account for a substantial portion of the interpopulation variation in stomach cancer risk.

2. While several authorities were of the opinion that chronic atrophic gastritis and intestinal metaplasia were precancerous conditions, the information in hand seemed inconclusive and more epidemiological studies were needed to clarify the issue.

3. The social class gradient in risk was not accompanied by consistent patterns of excess risks in specific occupations. Miners, fishermen, and agricultural workers were implicated by several studies, but the evidence was anecdotal in character.

4. The belief that occupations involving close contact with the soil carried higher risks was widely held. Some studies had associated soil composition with gastric cancer risk, although the nature of the relationship varied from place to place. Most of the findings were based on a search for coincidences in maps of geological formation and soil contents and maps of stomach cancer risks. Soils with a high content of peat and other organic matter were incriminated in Great Britain, peat and clay soils in the Netherlands, and ill-drained alluvial and acidic soils in Japan. These geochemical studies also attempted to correlate the distribution of trace elements with stomach cancer risks. In Wales an excess of chromium and deficiency of

nickel, vanadium, and lead were linked to high stomach cancer mortality. By contrast, in Devonshire nearly all trace elements had high mean values in the high-risk areas with significant excesses noted for cobalt, nickel, and iron. Some results of case-control studies were available. In Wales the largest differences were found in concentrations of chromium, cobalt, and zinc when soils in gardens of families of persons with gastric cancer were compared with gardens of controls (35). It was well known, although never the subject of a systematic investigation, that active volcanos and soils of volcanic origin were present in several countries with high stomach cancer risks (Japan, Chile, Costa Rica, Iceland).

5. The observations on diet and gastric cancer assembled prior to 1964 were varied in nature. Some represented observations of unusual customs in high-risk populations, others were based on contrasts in food practices between high- and low-risk populations, and a few were derived from case-control studies. Rice was suspected in Japan, fried foods in Wales, potatoes in Slovenia, grain products in Finland, spices in Java, and smoked fish in Iceland. Some epidemiologists viewed starchy foods as a potential common denominator. Time trends represented another axis for comparisons of stomach cancer and food consumption. In the United States the decline in stomach cancer mortality, for example, coincided with decreased consumption of cabbage and increased consumption of lettuce and citrus fruits. Haenszel's (14) review commented on weaknesses in the available data due in part to inadequacies in study design and also to the fact that the operative dietary factors might have occurred many years earlier, thus magnifying the problems of accurate recall by individuals under study.

Even so, the configuration of evidence had led most epidemiologists to believe that the environmental factors in the etiology of stomach cancer were probably related to diet. The underlying chain of reasoning was never clearly specified, but the controlling elements probably were: (a) the very large intercountry differences in risk accompanied by striking differences in food intake; and (b) a plausible pathway, since the stomach is a digestive organ in immediate contact with ingested food, and the absence of simple alternatives that could account for the enormous interpopulation variation in risk. While the search for leads had to continue, irrespective of the hypotheses they might support, 3 general classes of diet effects had been enumerated: (a) presence of a carcinogen in food; (b) introduction of carcinogens during food preparation; and (c) the absence of protective factors in some foods (14). None of the 3 alternatives had been elaborated into well-structured etiological hypotheses as of 1964, and their development was probably inhibited by the lack of suitable animal models to test hunches or impressions. The glandular mucosa of the stomachs of experimental animals was resistant to methylcholanthrene and the other potent carcinogens then available for feeding experiments.

Recent History

We now turn to recent developments. New data on cancer incidence and mortality from many areas throughout the world have elaborated and refined earlier reports (9) on intercountry and regional variation in stomach cancer risks.

The high risks in the altiplano of Costa Rica have been confirmed (36). Certain cities in the tropical zone of Latin America, Bogota, Cali, Guatemala, and Lima, were described to have elevated risks for stomach cancer (30). The pattern that emerged indicated populations in the central Andean region to be at high risk while residents of the tropical coastal zones in Latin America tended to be at low risk. The latter feature was suggested by observations on migrants to Cali, Colombia, which has received an influx of population from both low-lying and mountainous areas of Colombia (6).

The decline in stomach cancer risks has continued unabated in the United States and western Europe. A recent downturn in stomach cancer mortality has been suggested by the vital statistics from Japan (32), and examination of the age-specific rates indicates this feature to be most pronounced in the age group under 65 years.

The male:female ratio for stomach cancer has been investigated in depth by Griffith (13) and has been shown to be age dependent. The ratio is close to unity at ages under 35, reaches a peak of about 2:1 around age 55, and thereafter declines to about 1.3 to 1.5:1 at the oldest ages. It was suggested that this specific pattern might be linked to sex differences in food and caloric intake. However, as noted later, the findings may be better reconciled with histological-type differences in age- and sex-specific rates. The behavior of the sex ratios provides support for the thesis that gastric carcinoma is not a homogeneous entity but is composed of at least 2 distinctive etiological components.

Migrant Studies

The major advances in stomach cancer epidemiology over the past 10 to 15 years have come from utilization of the natural experiment of human migration. The migrant population approach dates from the observation (15) that the United States foreign-born coming from countries with high risks for stomach cancer continued to experience the risks characteristic of the population of origin. The presentation of risks characteristic of the host population of United States whites was delayed to the succeeding generation of United States-born offspring. This phenomenon was general and not peculiar to any single migrant group, nor was it a feature common to all cancer sites. For example, the risks for large bowel cancer among these same migrants rose during their lifetime to approximate the risk characteristic of the United States white host population. The observations on stomach cancer are not confined to the United States and similar findings have been reported from Australia (33). Nor does the stream of migration need to cross national boundaries. The cancer registry in Cali, Colombia, has described a marked excess of stomach cancer cases among migrants born in the department of Nariño, a mountainous region bordering Ecuador (6).

The strong correlation of stomach cancer with birthplace found in the migrant studies offers a possible explanation for the absence of striking urban-rural differentials in risk. Large-scale farm to city migration means that urban populations represent a mixture of individuals with different birthplaces and exposures; when the decisive events occur elsewhere, the urban rates will represent a weighted average of risks for its constituent migrant and native-born groups.

Histology

Investigations of migrant populations benefited from close coordination in the collection of epidemiological and pathological observations. The need for companion pathology studies had been suggested by the work of Järvi (22), Lauren (25), and Muñoz et al. (29) who had applied the Järvi-Lauren type criteria to stomach cancers in Latin American populations at high and low risk to the disease. They reported the intestinal type to constitute the greater proportion of cases in high-risk areas from which they inferred the intestinal type to be an "epidemic" component of stomach cancer responsible for much of the difference between high- and low-risk areas. Typing of stomach cancers in Cali indicated that the intestinal-type tumors accounted for most of the excess incidence in the subpopulations of migrants at highest risk (6), and the Cali results appeared consistent with the earlier, broadly based geographic comparisons within Latin America.

The typing of cases in Miyagi prefecture and Hawaii by 3 collaborating pathologists has elaborated previous findings (7). Tumor registries provided incidence data for Japanese populations in both localities, and the substantial number of cases typed permitted estimation of type- and age-specific incidence rates. The incidence for diffuse carcinomas differed little between the 2 areas and the disparity in overall incidence was concentrated in the intestinal, mixed, and other types, thus providing additional documentation for the conjecture of Muñoz et al. The age detail in the Miyagi-Hawaii comparisons represents the most substantial body of evidence now available on type-specific differences in incidence among populations at varying levels of risk. The data suggest the age curves of log incidence to have distinctive slopes for the diffuse and intestinal types, the risk for the diffuse type rising more slowly with age in both Japan and Hawaii. A steeper gradient in log incidence for the intestinal type appeared in both areas, the difference between Miyagi and Hawaii being expressed as a lateral displacement of the curve to the right (to older ages) in Hawaii. For both areas the rise in the female curves for intestinal type occurred at older ages than for males, and this feature could account for the characteristic peak in the male:female ratio of stomach cancer risk around age 55 noted by Griffith.

The constant slope values for the intestinal type suggest that the forces contributing to the rise in incidence with age are of the same magnitude once a critical age has been attained in each population. The displacement of the Hawaii curves could reflect either a later exposure to carcinogens or a longer latent period. Given the evidence for the close link between intestinal metaplasia and intestinal-type tumors, the latter appears more plausible.

The differences in type distribution have been more clearly expressed for the more extreme contrasts in stomach cancer risks represented by intercountry comparisons. While Kubo (24) has reported data that cast doubt on the hypothesis that the intestinal type is the variable component in contrasts of high- and low-risk populations, his classification criteria are not identical with those of Correa et al.;

further checks and standardization of criteria for use in interpopulation comparisons are needed. For the smaller risk differentials encountered in intracountry comparisons, the use of typing in studies of time trends and case-control analyses has been less informative and the findings more equivocal (16, 27, 28) [1]

Precursor Lesions

Epidemiology-pathology studies in migrant populations have strengthened the case for intestinal metaplasia as a precursor lesion. In Cali, Colombia, autopsy studies have demonstrated a greater prevalence of intestinal metaplasia among migrants from Nariño (6). Also, among the several migrant groups in Cali, the prevalence of intestinal metaplasia appeared more closely correlated with the incidence of intestinal-type stomach cancer than with incidence of the diffuse type. Review of autopsy materials collected in several localities have confirmed an excess of intestinal metaplasia in populations at high risk to stomach cancer (5). Other observations (coincidence in sites of maximal intestinalization and gastric cancer, description of transitional states between metaplasia and cancer, etc.) provide corroborative detail implicating intestinal metaplasia as a precursor lesion (34).

Introduction of the fiber-optic gastrocamera has added another dimension to the study of intestinal metaplasia. The cancer registry and autopsy observations on the Nariño-born in Cali indicated the need for field work in the place of origin. Although the risks in Nariño are exceptionally high, equal to or exceeding those in Japan and the altiplano of Costa Rica, preliminary inquiries suggested clustering of cases in certain localities. Review of hospital admissions and discharges confirmed the clinical impressions of local physicians on clustering (C. Cuello, personal communication) and this information was taken into account in the survey design. Samples of apparently well individuals were gastroscoped to identify individuals with IM [2] and CAG and to determine the prevalence of these lesions. All persons examined were asked to report on residence history, food history, and soures of water supply. When the population was classified by birthplace, the distribution of IM and/or CAG coincided closely with the distribution previously delineated for stomach cancer cases (C. Cuello, P. Correa, W. Haenszel, *et al.*, unpublished data). The prevalence of IM and/or CAG for stomach cancer was under 25% in low-risk communities and close to 50% in high-risk communities. The excess prevalence of intestinal metaplasia persisted among individuals born in high-risk (by Nariño standards) communities who had later moved to low-risk areas, a feature that reinforced the pervasive epidemiological theme on the important role for exposures in early life for stomach cancer. The comparison of findings on Nariño residents and Nariño migrants to Cali raises the possibility that the prevalence of CAG may be diminished, and hence reversible, by removal to a different environment, but this possibility does not extend to the later stage of intestinal metaplasia. The consistency between the survey findings and earlier autopsy studies enhances the case for IM and CAG as precursor lesions.

It would be difficult to overemphasize the importance of the fiber-optic gastroscope for epidemiologically oriented studies of the gastric mucosa. More indirect measures of intestinalization of the gastric mucosa, gastrin, parietal cell antibodies, and pepsinogen I and II, have been made in studies of the Hawaiian Japanese, but the sensitivity and specificity of the latter tests do not permit an adequate classification of individuals by presence and degree of intestinal metaplasia (G. N. Stemmermann, personal communication). Direct visual and histological surveillance of the gastric mucosa via endoscopy seems required.

Geochemistry

The major new impetus in geochemical studies has come from the discovery of the mutagenic and carcinogenic properties of nitroso compounds. Hill *et al.* (20) have reported an association between high nitrate ingestion and high gastric cancer in Worksop, England. This clue is being pursued in Colombia (Nariño) where samples of well water have been collected and analyzed for nitrate and nitrite content (18). The local surface water supplies have negligible nitrate and nitrite content. Wells with nitrate-rich water are a distinctive feature of several of the high-risk communities in Nariño. However, the finding that nonusers and users of nitrate-rich wells in these same communities have the same prevalence of precursor lesions raises questions about the meaning of this observation (C. Cuello, personal communication). A modified hypothesis that well water is an index of local soil content, implying that locally grown foods are the source of nitrates, may still be viable, since elevated urinary nitrate levels (an index of nitrate intake) have been reported for residents of high-risk areas who do not use well water (C. Cuello, personal communication). While elevated nitrate intake may prove to be correlated with precursor lesions and stomach ulcer in Nariño, additional studies must be carried out before accepting this conclusion.

A case-control study in Japan describing an elevated risk of stomach cancer for well water users, particularly among farmers in Miyagi prefecture, provides another indication that associations with nitrates are worth pursuing. [3] Studies of nitrates are attractive since they offer plausible pathways for production of carcinogenic effects. Weisburger (39) has pointed out that bacterial conversion of nitrates in foods stored at room temperatures to nitrites opens the way to the synthesis of nitroso compounds but that either ascorbic acid or refrigeration blocks nitrosamine formation in stored foods. MNNG has been shown to induce cancer of the glandular stomach in rats (38), and Sugimura has stated that administration of low dosages of MNNG produces intestinal metaplasia.

Foods

The findings on diet from case-control studies of stomach cancer have been reviewed by Bjelke (3), and Table 1 draws on this source for the summary of results for nonmigrant populations published since 1964. Japanese and Norwegian

---

[1] W. Haenszel, M. Kurihara, F. B. Locke, K. Shimuzu, and M. Segi, unpublished manuscript.

[2] The abbreviations used are: IM, intestinal metaplasia; CAG, chronic atrophic gastritis; MNNG, *N*-methyl-*N'*-nitro-*N*-nitrosoguanidine.

Table 1
Summary of findings on food intake of stomach cancer patients and controls

Author, yr of publication	Study locale	Findings
Wynder *et al.*, 1963 (40)	Iceland, Japan, Slovenia, United States	No noteworthy case-control differences
Meinsma, 1964 (26)	Holland	Higher consumption of bacon by cases; lower intake of citrus fruits (and ascorbic acid) by cases
Acheson and Doll, 1964 (1)	England	No significant case-control differences
Higginson, 1966 (19)	Kansas City (United States)	More frequent use of fried foods by cases (bacon drippings and animal fats used for cooking)
Graham *et al.*, 1967 (11) Reanalyzed, 1972 (12)	Buffalo (United States)	Smaller proportion of cases using raw vegetables (lettuce, tomatoes, cole slaw)
Hirayama, 1967 (21)	Japan (Kanagawa prefecture)	Daily milk drinking less frequent and daily use of salted foods more frequent among cases

migrants to the United States have been the most intensively studied and a brief recapitulation of the findings follows.

The Hawaiian Japanese study revealed that migrants from the Japanese prefectures with highest stomach cancer risks continued to exhibit higher risks in Hawaii, a relationship that did not persist for their Nisei offspring (16). Lower risks were also suggested for the Nisei but not for the original migrants (Issei), who had adopted Western-style diets. These nativity distinctions were consistent with other evidence on the critical nature of exposures in early life.

The favorable observational situation presented by the Hawaiian Japanese, distinctive Japanese and Western foods, heterogeneity in food habits arising from variation in timing, and degree of transition from Japanese to Western-style customs, facilitated detection of case-control differences for some food items. Elevated stomach cancer risks were described for users of pickled vegetables and dried, salted fish, and a rise in risks with increased frequency of use was suggested. In the absence of similar associations for raw fish and unprocessed vegetables, suspicion is directed to methods of preparation. Low risks were described for several Western-type vegetables (lettuce, celery, corn, etc.), and the latter effects appeared to be independent of the associations with pickled Japanese foods, suggesting possible protective effects. The companion case-control studies conducted in Japan (Hiroshima and Miyagi prefectures) did not reproduce the associations with pickled vegetables and salted, dried fish reported for the Hawaiian Japanese.[3] A homogeneous background of food habits in early life prior to World War II may have operated against their detection. The greater use of lettuce and celery reported by controls in Japan reinforced the Hawaiian Japanese results on possible protective effects.

The Norwegian migrant studies included collection of diet data by mail questionnaires from representative samples of Norwegian-born men in the United States and Norway. Case-control studies of stomach cancer using a common protocol were also conducted in Norway and in Minnesota (for persons mostly of Scandinavian descent). Bjelke's findings (3) are quoted below.

Norway. (*a*) Recent use of cooked cereals, fruit, soup, and salted fish was somewhat higher among stomach cancer patients than among controls. The data for salted fish suggest greater case-control difference for former use, an observation consistent with the greater use of this item among siblings of index patients with stomach cancer compared to control siblings. (*b*) More pronounced case-control differences were shown by a number of vegetables and fruits, which were used less frequently by the stomach cancer patients. The greatest deviations from the controls were shown for the indices for total vegetables and vitamin C intakes, for which the relative deviations were greatest among young patients and women. (*c*) The negative associations with vegetables and, more clearly, with vitamin C were more pronounced for diffuse than for intestinal-type carcinoma. (*d*) The negative association with vitamin C was seen most strongly in the subsets of individuals whose risks otherwise were relatively low due to absence of previous gastric surgery, Blood Group O (women), or infrequent use of salted fish. Salted fish and vitamin C appeared to interact also with respect to the histological expression of the carcinomas. (*e*) As reported earlier, the 3 variables, ABO blood group, history with respect to gastric surgery, and intakes of fruits and vegetables as summed up in the vitamin C index, were all independently associated with case-control status and constituted the most powerful discriminators between cases and controls.

United States. (*a*) Recent use of cooked cereals, smoked fish, and canned fruits was higher and intakes of lettuce and tomatoes were lower among stomach cancer patients than among controls. (*b*) While total intakes of cereal products and fish were only slightly higher than among the controls, the index for total vegetables was considerably lower and the vitamin C index was moderately lower among the stomach cancer patients. (*c*) As in Norway, the lower vegetable and vitamin C intakes among stomach cancer patients had persisted over a long period, were more pronounced among women, and, in both sexes, were mainly a feature of the diffuse carcinomas.

The long interval between exposure and onset of disease complicates the collection of reliable and relevant histories of food practices. Two remedies are possible. One is to collect diet histories prospectively and to observe the subsequent disease experience of the cohort members. This approach has, in fact, been taken in ongoing studies of Hawaiian Japanese males, male residents of Norway, and insurance policyholders of Scandinavian descent in the United States. Another alternative is to reduce the interval between exposure and onset of disease by substituting a precursor lesion as an observational end point. The transformation of stomach cancer epidemiology into the epidemiology of intestinal metaplasia was 1 objective of the Hawaiian Japanese male cohort study. This objective has not been completely satisfied because, as has been noted, the indices available on degree of intestinalization do not permit an adequate classification of the status of individual members.

The transformation to epidemiology of intestinal metaplasia is off to a more promising start in Nariño, where population screening with gastroscopy has opened the door to a contrast of diet histories between individuals with chronic atrophic gastritis and/or intestinal metaplasia. The results will be reported elsewhere (W. Haenszel *et al.*, unpublished data) and we comment here on the findings for 2 foods, lettuce and corn. A negative association with lettuce described by the low prevalence of IM and/or CAG among regular users is the latest in a series of similar observations from many populations (1, 4, 16, 28) and the repeated detection of a "protective" effect warrants more attention to the chemical and nutritional properties of lettuce. Corn is of interest because it has been the most important staple food in high-risk communities. More than 80% of persons born in high-risk areas eat corn as a staple diet item *versus* 50% of natives of low-risk areas. While above- and below-average use of corn as a discriminant for prevalence of IM and/or CAG was weakened when birthplace was controlled in the analysis, the omission of information on methods of preparation may be responsible, since much of the corn in Nariño is prepared by the Indian technique of alkali cooking (with wood ashes) (23). This point will be investigated in later work.

The collective information from diet studies lends itself to some tentative generalizations. Given the diverse foodstuffs consumed in populations with a high risk of stomach cancer, no single food or class of foods displays a 1:1 correspondence with the geographic distribution of stomach cancer. A relationship, if it exists, seems more likely to be linked with the treatment of foods (salting or smoking of fishes, meats, and vegetables for preservation and storage; alkali cooking of corn to enhance the biological availability of certain amino acids).

Discussion

Reviews of stomach cancer epidemiology prior to 1964 leave the reader with the impression that work in populations sharing homogeneous backgrounds of exposures had come to a dead end. Migrant population studies emphasizing a combined epidemiology-pathology approach have infused new life into this subject. Their great virtue has been the ability to correlate observations over a wide spectrum of exposures in home and host populations, which has emphasized the critical role of exposures in early life and the search for etiological factors in places of origin. The results were achieved by straightforward epidemiological methods demanding no novel analytical techniques. The new elements were selection of observational settings that might be expected to yield fruitful leads. In turn, the stage has been set for transformation of the epidemiology of stomach cancer into the epidemiology of intestinal metaplasia and allied precursor lesions. While the latter will depend on direct observation of the gastric mucosa, it will make technically feasible studies of variability within small geographic areas and detailed consideration of suspect factors, including diet, in local environments.

Recent experimental advances make possible a coordinated epidemiological-experimental approach to stomach cancer. Sugimura's (37) feeding experiment with MNNG has led to animal models that may yield information on how the chain of events culminating in stomach cancer may be interrupted.

To close this review we summarize our reading of the facts in hand bearing on the etiology of stomach cancer and propose a model that may fit the facts.

1. Environmental factors play an overriding role in gastric cancer etiology. The declining incidence and mortality rates observed in recent decades is the most eloquent evidence of this assertion.

2. The initiating event in the carcinogenic process occurs early in life. This is best indicated by the prevailing high incidence in migrants from high-risk countries to low-risk environments. Our studies in Colombia indicate that the experience of the 1st decade of life determines the magnitude of the risk at later years.

3. A long latent period, 30 to 50 years, corresponds to the natural evolution of precursor lesions in the gastric mucosa: chronic atrophic gastritis and its frequent companion, intestinal metaplasia. The process begins as an inflammatory change leading to atrophy of the normal gastric mucosal epithelium and its gradual replacement by cells that are foreign to the stomach but occur normally in the intestine: goblet cells, absorptive cells, Paneth cells, and argentaffin cells. These metaplastic cells show, with time, different degrees of atypia which gradually progress until they become autonomous.

4. The series of mutations or cell transformations from gastric to intestinal to atypical to invasive epithelial cell may be accomplished by a ubiquitous low-dose mutagen-carcinogen. The agent may be a nitrosamine synthesized somewhere between the oral and the gastric cavities from the nitrite normally found in the saliva and the amines present in food. *In vivo* formation of nitrosamines from nitrites and secondary amines has been well documented, and their intragastric synthesis and potential carcinogenic role have been suggested (17, 31). Endo and Takahashi (10) have shown that methylguanidine, a compound present in several foods, is converted into a potent mutagen after exposure to sodium nitrite in both simulated and real human gastric juice environment.

5. Synthesis of the agent is dependent on food intake. Correlations between some foods and gastric cancer risk have been reported, but no food can be identified that is common to all high-risk populations. More consistent results have been obtained for foods associated with a decrease risk, such as lettuce. A complex interaction of food items in the microenvironment of the stomach may be involved. The forces favoring induction may include abra-

sive or irritant items such as vegetables with hard cortex or fiber or items with a high salt concentration. On the protective side, we may have fresh vegetables and fruits rich, among other things, in vitamin C. Such foods may condition the effectiveness of a carcinogen.

6. Intercountry comparisons of autopsy series have described 2 major types of stomach cancer, intestinal and diffuse. The risk of the diffuse type appears less variable among countries and it is the predominant type at younger ages. However, the intestinal-diffuse distinction apparent in interpopulation contrasts has not been well demonstrated in studies of time trends or by case-control studies of suspect factors conducted within a single population. We speculate that the different behavior of type distinctions in inter- and intrapopulation contrasts might arise in the following manner. Synthesis of suspect nitroso compound(s) may be promoted by a low-pH gastric environment, so that vulnerable individuals not developing the intestinalization response continue to have a low-pH-favoring synthesis and tend to present diffuse-type carcinoma at young ages, the experimental counterpart being early induction of carcinoma of the glandular stomach by high dosages of MNNG. Individuals manifesting intestinalization followed by an elevated pH may be exposed to lower doses over the longer term and tend to present intestinal-type carcinomas at older ages, the experimental counterpart being slower induction of intestinal metaplasia by low dosages of MNNG.

In this situation the intracountry findings would not discriminate well between intestinal and diffuse types because the same environmental factors underlie both types and the diffuse response at an early age would reflect primarily host characteristics. The intercountry differences in presentation of intestinal-type tumors would, on the contrary, be sensitive to interpopulation differences in dietary and nutritional factors that enhanced or retarded the formation and activity of a mutagen-carcinogen within the stomach. Variations in environmentally modulated effective exposures would be a major determinant of latent period (and age of expression) of extensive intestinalization and intestinal-type tumors.

The general subject of the rate of formation and stability of various nitroso compounds in different pH environments and the conditions that affect their biological activity within the stomach need investigation in suitable animal models.

References

1. Acheson, E. D., and Doll, R. Dietary Factors in Carcinoma of the Stomach: A Study of 100 Cases and 200 Controls. Gut, *5:* 126–131, 1964.
2. Barrett, M. K. Avenues of Approach to Gastric-Cancer Problem. J. Natl. Cancer Inst., *7:* 127–157, 1946.
3. Bjelke, E. Epidemiologic Studies of Cancer of the Stomach, Colon, and Rectum; with Special Emphasis on the Role of Diet. Scand. J. Gastroenterol., *9* (Suppl. 31): 1–253, 1974.
4. Boyd, J., Langman, M., and Doll, R. The Epidemiology of Gastrointestinal Cancer with Special Reference to Causation. Gut, *5:* 196–200, 1964.
5. Correa, P. I.A.P. Maude Abbott Lecture. Geographic Pathology of Cancer in Colombia. Intern. Pathol., *11:* 16–22, 1970.
6. Correa, P., Cuello, C., and Duque, E. Carcinoma and Intestinal Metaplasia of the Stomach in Colombian Migrants. J. Natl. Cancer Inst., *44:* 297–306, 1970.
7. Correa, P., Sasano, N., Stemmermann, G. N., and Haenszel, W. Pathology of Gastric Carcinoma in Japanese Populations: Comparisons between Miyagi Prefecture, Japan, and Hawaii. J. Natl. Cancer Inst., *51:* 1449–1459, 1973.
8. Doll, R. Environmental Factors in the Aetiology of Cancer of the Stomach. Gastroenterologia, *86:* 320–328, 1956.
9. Doll, R., Payne, P., and Waterhouse, J. Cancer Incidence in Five Continents. A Technical Report. Unio Intern. Contre Cancrum Monograph Ser., 78–83, 1966.
10. Endo, H., and Takahashi, K. Methylguanidine, a Naturally Occurring Compound Showing Mutagenicity after Nitrosation in Gastric Juice. Nature, *245:* 325–326, 1973.
11. Graham, S., Lilienfeld, A. M., and Tidings, J. E. Dietary and Purgation Factors in the Epidemiology of Gastric Cancer. Cancer, *20:* 2224–2234, 1967.
12. Graham, S., Schotz, W., and Martino, P. Alimentary Factors in the Epidemiology of Gastric Cancer. Cancer, *30:* 927–938, 1972.
13. Griffith, G. W. The Sex Ratio in Gastric Cancer and Hypothetical Considerations Relative to Aetiology. Brit. J. Cancer, *22:* 163–172, 1968.
14. Haenszel, W. Variation in Incidence of and Mortality from Stomach Cancer, with Particular Reference to the United States. J. Natl. Cancer Inst., *21:* 213–262, 1958.
15. Haenszel, W. Cancer Mortality among the Foreign-born in the United States. J. Natl. Cancer Inst., *26:* 37–132, 1961.
16. Haenszel, W., Kurihara, M., Segi, M., and Lee, R. K. C. Stomach Cancer among Japanese in Hawaii. J. Natl. Cancer Inst., *49:* 969–988, 1972.
17. Hawksworth, G. M., and Hill, M. J. Bacteria and the *N*-Nitrosation of Secondary Amines. Brit. J. Cancer, *25:* 520–526, 1971.
18. Hawksworth, G., Hill, M. J., Gordillo, G., and Cuello, C. Possible Relationship between Nitrates, Nitrosamines and Gastric Cancer in Southwest Colombia. *In*: P. Bogovski and E. A. Walker (eds.), *N*-Nitroso Compounds in the Environment. Proceedings of the Third International Meeting on the Analysis and Formation of *N*-Nitroso Compounds. IARC Sci. Publ. No. 9, pp. 229–234. Intern. Agency for Res. on Cancer, Lyon, France: 1975.
19. Higginson, J. Etiological Factors in Gastro-intestinal Cancer in Man. J. Natl. Cancer Inst., *37:* 527–545, 1966.
20. Hill, M. J., Hawksworth, G., and Tattersall, G. Bacteria, Nitrosamines and Cancer of the Stomach. Brit. J. Cancer, *28:* 562–567, 1973.
21. Hirayama, T. The Epidemiology of Cancer of the Stomach in Japan with Special Reference to the Role of Diet. Unio Intern. Contre Cancrum Monograph Ser., *10:* 37–48, 1967.
22. Järvi, O. A Review of the Part Played by Gastrointestinal Heterotopias in Neoplasmogenesis, Proc. Finnish Acad. Sci., pp. 151–187, 1962.
23. Katz, S. H., Hediger, M. L., and Valleroy, L. A. Traditional Maize Processing Techniques in the New World. Science, *184:* 765–773, 1974.
24. Kubo, T. Geographical Pathology of Gastric Carcinoma. Acta Pathol. Japon., *24:* 465–479, 1974.
25. Lauren, P. The Two Histological Main Types of Gastric Carcinoma: Diffuse and So-called Intestinal-type Carcinoma. An Attempt at a Histo-clinical Classification. Acta Pathol. Microbiol. Scand., *64:* 31–49, 1965.
26. Meinsma, L. Voeding en Kanker. Voeding, *25:* 357–365, 1964.
27. Muñoz, N., and Asvall, J. Time Trends of Intestinal and Diffuse Types of Gastric Cancer in Norway. Intern. J. Cancer, *8:* 144–157, 1971.
28. Muñoz, N., and Connelly, R. Time Trends of Intestinal and Diffuse Types of Gastric Cancer in the United States. Intern. J. Cancer *8:* 158–164, 1971.
29. Muñoz, N., Correa, P., Cuello, C., and Duque, E. Histologic Types of Gastric Carcinoma in High- and Low-risk Areas. Intern. J. Cancer, *3:* 809–818, 1968.
30. Puffer, R. R., and Griffith, G. W. Patterns of Urban Mortality. Pan Am. Health Organ. Sci. Publ. *151:* 1–353.

31. Sander, J. Kann Nitrit in der menschlichen Nahrung Ursache einer Krebsentstehung durch Nitrosaminbindung sein? Arch. Hyg. Bakteriol., *151:* 22–28, 1967.

32. Segi, M., and Kurihara, M. Cancer Mortality for Selected Sites in 24 Countries. No. 6 (1966–1967), pp. 1–137. Tokyo: Japan Cancer Soc., 1972.

33. Staszewski, J., McCall, M. G., and Stenhouse, N. S. Cancer Mortality in 1962–66 Among Polish Migrants to Australia. Brit. J. Cancer, *25:* 599–610, 1971.

34. Stemmerman, G. N. The Epidemiologic Pathology of Gastric Carcinoma. Excerpta Med., in press.

35. Stocks, P., and Davies, R. I. Epidemiological Evidence from Chemical and Spectrographical Analysis That Soil is Concerned in the Causation of Cancer. Brit. J. Cancer, *14:* 8–22, 1960.

36. Strong, J. P., Baldizon, C., Salas, J., McMahan, C. A., and Mekbel, S. Mortality from Cancer of the Stomach in Costa Rica. Cancer, *20:* 1173–1180, 1967.

37. Sugimura, T., Fujimura, S., and Baha, T. Tumor Production in the Glandular Stomach and Alimentary Tract of the Rat by *N*-Methyl-*N'*-nitro-*N*-nitrosoguanidine. Cancer Res., *30:* 455–465, 1970.

38. Weisburger, J. H. Chemical Carcinogenesis in the Gastrointestinal Tract. Can. Cancer Conf. *7:* 465–473, 1973.

39. Weisburger, J., and Raineri, R. Assessment of Human Exposure and Response to *N*-Nitroso Compounds. A New View on the Etiology of Digestive Tract Cancers. Toxicol. Appl. Pharmacol., *31:* 369–374, 1975.

40. Wynder, E. L., Kmet, J., Dungal, N., and Segi, M. An Epidemiological Investigation of Gastric Cancer. Cancer, *16:* 1461–1496, 1963.

Nutritional Factors and Etiologic Mechanisms in the Causation of Gastrointestinal Cancers

by John H. Weisburger, Ph.D., M.D.(hc), Ernst L. Wynder, M.D., with Clara L. Horn, B.A., M.T.

The etiologic factors and mechanisms related to each kind of gastrointestinal cancer are complex. An analysis of these elements and an understanding of the relevant mechanisms leads to suggested interventions of a nutritional nature that should be effective both in primary and in secondary prevention. Agents involved in the carcinogenic process can be classified into genotoxic carcinogens and epigenetic agents. Their mode of action is distinct, especially with regard to dose–response effects and reversibility. Analysis of the etiologic cause of each kind of gastrointestinal cancer in terms of the types of agents associated with cancer causation and development provides a basis for risk reduction, and hence, prevention. Cancer of the esophagus in the Western world involves excessive smoking and alcohol consumption. Current research investigates whether nutritional factors, particularly relative deficiencies in specific vitamins, may exacerbate the cocarcinogenic action of alcohol with genotoxic carcinogens in tobacco smoke. The intake of highly salted, pickled food or smoked food, particularly fish or beans, is a risk factor for glandular gastric cancer, caused by an as yet unknown genotoxic carcinogen, which can be prevented by foods containing vitamin C. Cancer of the pancreas has multiple etiologic factors involving typically a Western high-fat diet, cigarette smoking; and coffee drinking, which remains to be validated. While the exact mechanisms are not yet known, several animal models have shown that dietary fat augments the risk for pancreas cancer. Cancer of the colon and rectum have different etiologic causes, the former being associated with nutritional elements such as high fat, high cholesterol intake, and relative lack of dietary fiber, possibly modulated by low intake of nutrients such as selenium salts. Reducing the concentration of bile acids by lowering dietary fat and cholesterol, or by increasing dietary fiber, effectively lowers the risk for disease as a primary prevention tool, and importantly, should lower the risk of recurrence in individuals who have had colon cancer. Current research explores whether the dark parts of fried or broiled foods, particularly meats, contains the genotoxic carcinogens for colon cancer.

Cancer 50:2541–2549, 1982.

V ARIOUS EVIDENCE and multidisciplinary approaches suggest environmental causes for the majority of human cancers.[1-4] The environment is certainly complex. In relation to the cancer question, it is often construed to mean ubiquitous chemicals, and, more specifically, those due to modern technology and industrial development. It is true that a number of food additives, pesticides, insecticides, and industrial chemicals introduced commercially in the last 40 years have exhibited carcinogenic properties in animal models.[5] Historically, it is also true that chemical exposure due to occupation or to drugs has caused human cancers.[1-4,6-8] Thus, it is important to identify the actual causes of cancer as a rational, effective basis for prevention. Insight into the complex causes of cancer requires a detailed analysis of the factors inherent in the occur-

Presented at the American Cancer Society National Conference on Gastrointestinal Cancer, December 8–10, 1981, Miami Beach, Florida.

From The American Health Foundation, Valhalla, New York.

Supported by National Cancer Institute Grants CA-12376 and CA-29602, U.S. Department of Health and Human Services, and USPHS grants CA-15400, CA-16382, and CA-24217 through the National Large Bowel Cancer Project of the National Cancer Institute.

Address for reprints: John Weisburger, PhD, MD, American Health Foundation, Valhalla, NY 10595–1599.

rence of each specific type of cancer.

In this report, we develop the theme that most of the main human cancers in the world do not stem from intentional or even inadvertent chemical contaminants in the environment. From worldwide statistics on time trends and the incidence of diverse cancers, as well as the altered risk for migrants from areas of high to low incidence over several generations, and the corresponding analysis of data obtained under controlled conditions in animal models, a picture emerges permitting delineation of the multiple causative factors involved in each of the main human cancers. It will be noted that lifestyle, especially tobacco use, and broad nutritional factors are important, as described by Dr. Miller in this conference.[9] Prior to a consideration of the relevant mechanisms, it will be useful to consider current concepts of the mechanisms of carcinogenesis, and then see how those can be applied to an evaluation of the role of nutritional factors in the causation of cancers in the gastrointestinal tract.

Mechanisms of Carcinogenesis

Considerable advances have been achieved in studies on the mechanisms of carcinogenesis. Cancer causation and development involves a series of steps. It is likely that neoplasia stems from a somatic mutation involving an alteration of the genetic material.[10-14] This has been a controversial topic for over 100 years. Multidisciplinary approaches and various lines of evidence have provided a sound scientific basis for this concept, as a first event in the overall carcinogenic process.

Genotoxic Events

A change in the genetic material can arise through a number of mechanisms: (1) The genetic material can be changed through a direct attack by radiation, chemicals, or viruses. Radiation or chemicals can damage the genetic material at a number of loci along the DNA chain that are converted to permanent alterations by mispairing of bases during replication of the damaged regions. With viruses, a more specific insertion of DNA segments or, through reverse transcriptase, of RNA sequences takes place through the operation of specific polymerases, and hence, yields an abnormal DNA containing new information.[15] (2) Faulty operation of DNA polymerase during DNA synthesis, resulting in an inaccurate transcription of the parent DNA segment, can produce abnormal DNA. Certain carcinogenic metal ions may have this effect.[16,17] (3) Abnormal DNA can also ensue, especially during postreplicative DNA synthesis, through the errors introduced by specific DNA polymerases concerned with DNA repair.[18-20] The infidelity of DNA polymerases may lead to further ab-

normalities in the DNA produced during the replication of early tumor cells, and thus, may represent the means whereby tumor cells progress to less differentiated, more malignant cancer types during their growth and development.

Nongenotoxic or Epigenetic Events

Abnormal DNA obtained by any of the above mechanisms is only the first step in a long sequence of events terminating in a malignant invasive neoplasm. An important element is the ability of an abnormal cell population to achieve a selective growth advantage in the presence of surrounding normal cells. The cell duplication process is highly dependent on a number of endogenous and exogenous controlling elements operating by epigenetic mechanisms. Two such elements are promoters or inhibitors of growth which either enhance or retard the process.

As numerous experiments documenting this phenomenon indicate, promoters do not lead to the production of an invasive cancer in the absence of an antecedent cell change.[14,21-23] Thus, in exploring the causes of any specific human cancer, consideration must be given both to the agents leading to an abnormal genome and to any other agents possibly involved in the growth and development of the resulting abnormal neoplastic cells and their further progression to malignancy.

Classification of Carcinogens

Chemical carcinogens have been classified into eight classes that, in turn, belong to two main groups: genotoxic carcinogens and agents, including promoters, operating by nongenotoxic or epigenetic pathways (Table 1).[24] In relation to an understanding of the relevant mechanisms, this classification is important in dissecting the complex causes of diverse kinds of cancer and arriving at a delineation of the role of each agent—genotoxic carcinogen, cocarcinogen, or promoter—in the overall carcinogenic process for each kind of cancer. This aspect will now be discussed in relation to important, nutritionally linked cancers.

Genotoxic Carcinogens in Upper Gastrointestinal Tract Cancer

Nitrosamines as possible human carcinogens: There are certain tobacco-specific nitrosamines, such as nitrosonornicotine, which form a substantial part of the genotoxic carcinogens in tobacco smoke and in tobacco chews.[25] Specific association of these kinds of carcinogens with cancer at sites related to the use of tobacco, such as cancer of the lung, pancreas, kidney, urinary bladder, and also, the oral cavity and esophagus in the presence of heavy alcohol intake, remains to be fully

TABLE 1. Classes of Carcinogenic Chemicals[14]

Type	Mode of action	Example
Genotoxic		
1. Direct-acting or primary carcinogen	Electrophile, organic compound, genotoxic, interacts with DNA.	Ethylene imine bis(chloromethyl)ether
2. Procarcinogen or secondary carcinogen	Requires conversion through metabolic activation by host or *in vitro* to type 1.	Vinyl chloride, benzo(a)pyrene, 2-naphthylamine, dimethylnitrosamine
3. Inorganic carcinogen	Not directly genotoxic, leads to changes in DNA by selective alteration in fidelity of DNA replication.	Nickel, chromium
Epigenetic		
4. Solid-state carcinogen	Exact mechanism unknown; usually affects only mesenchymal cells and tissues; physical form vital.	Polymer or metal foils, asbestos.
5. Hormone	Usually not genotoxic; mainly alters endocrine system balance and differentiation; often acts as promoter	Estradiol, diethylstilbestrol
6. Immunosuppressor	Usually not genotoxic; mainly stimulates "virally induced," transplanted, or metastatic neoplasms.	Azathioprine, antilymophocytic serum
7. Cocarcinogen	Not genotoxic or carcinogenic, but enhances effect of type 1 or type 2 agent when given at the same time. May modify conversion of type 2 to type 1	Phorbol esters, pyrene, catechol, ethanol, n-dodecane, SO_2
8. Promoter	Not genotoxic or carcinogenic, but enhances effect of type 1 or type 2 agent when given subsequently.	Phorbol esters, phenol, anthralin, bile acids, tryptophan metabolites, saccharin.

documented.[26,27] It is reasonable to assume, however, that these carcinogens play a role in cancer in these target organs that accounts for a substantial part of the cancers in various countries.

In addition, in certain parts of the world, such as Eastern Iran, Southern Soviet Union, and Central China, cancer of the esophagus is seen in people who do not appear to smoke and drink heavily. Despite extensive cooperative efforts between investigators in Iran and the International Agency for Research on Cancer, the etiology of esophageal cancer in Iran remains obscure. Nitrosamines have been suspected as etiologic factors but as yet have not been found. Nonetheless, the nutritional intake is poor in terms of green and yellow vegetables, fruits, and other vitamin C and E containing antidotes to nitrite, and thus, through this association, the endogenous formation of nitrosamines cannot be ruled out. This is especially true inasmuch as recent data from China,[28-30] the easternmost extension of the belt of esophageal cancer incidence, suggests that nitrosamines are present in that environment. The next few years may well provide conclusive evidence on this point.

Nitrosamides as possible human carcinogens: While attempting to examine the question whether some powerful bacterial mutagens, in this instance N-methyl-N′-nitro-N-nitrosoguanidine (MNNG), were carcinogenic, Sugimura and Kawachi[31] administered this mutagen, a water-soluble, rather polar substance, to rats in drinking water. The important discovery was made that this mutagen was not only a powerful carcinogen but reliably induced cancer in the glandular stomach, mimicking accurately the disease seen in humans. A detailed study of the pathogenesis of this then new animal model revealed that this chemical, taken orally, not only induced the invasive neoplasm but also induced all the antecedent and accompanying lesions such as gastritis and intestinalization of the gastric epithelium, as seen in humans.[31-33]

We,[34] and also Mirvish,[35] have linked the gastric cancer model of Sugimura and Kawachi to the examination of the occurrence of human gastric cancer and to consideration of the underlying mechanisms. Between 1900 and 1950, gastric cancer was one of the major types of cancer in the United States. Its incidence and mortality have decreased sharply since 1950,[36] and the concepts presented in this report account for this decline. In other parts of the world, including Japan, the mountainous interior regions of central and western Latin America, and in northern and eastern Europe, as well as in Iceland, gastric cancer remains one of the major cancers, but even there, there is a beginning indicator of a decrease. There is a north–south gradient, or south–north in the southern hemisphere, with a greater incidence in more frigid or mountainous zones.

High risk foods include dried, salted, pickled, or smoked fish, or other pickled foods.[2,33,37] Also, there usually is a variable intake of fresh fruits and vegetables, namely, a seasonal low consumption of such foods during winter and spring. The geochemistry often involves elevated soil nitrate and, thus, foods and water rich in nitrate.[38,39]

We have suggested that an alkylnitrosoureido type of compound, such as the one developed by Sugimura and Kawachi,[31] which induces glandular gastric cancer in animal models, may be involved in human gastric carcinogenesis,[34] and Mirvish[35] has proposed a similar scheme. We used an experimental model, the fish *Sanma hiraki*, which is eaten in a region of Japan at high risk for gastric cancer. Treatment of homogenates of this fish with nitrite at pH 3 led to the development of a direct-acting mutagen for *Salmonella typhimurium* TA 100. The formation of mutagens could be completely blocked by vitamin C. Mirvish[35] discovered that the formation of nitroso compounds could be inhibited by vitamin C and Mergens and Newmark[40] noted that vitamin E also has such properties. In view of the similarity of the behavior of the mutagens in nitrite-treated fish, it would seem logical that they are compounds with a nitrosamide type of functional group. *Sanma, Aji,* and *Iwashi* yielded more mutagenic activity than other types of fish, but it is important that several types of meat failed to produce such direct-acting mutagens. We also found that similar pickling of beans, as eaten in high-risk Latin America, or of borscht, as consumed in eastern Europe, led to mutagenic activity.[34] Yano[41] noted alkylating activity towards 4-(p-nitrobenzyl)pyridine in nitrite treated or smoked fish.

We demonstrated that the mutagenic activity from the reaction of nitrite and *Sanma* was not only carcinogenic but specifically induced glandular stomach cancer in rats.[34] Since the formation of the mutagen can be blocked by vitamin C, it would seem that the formation of glandular stomach cancer can also be so inhibited. Thus, treatment of fish of a type eaten in Japan, a high-risk region for gastric cancer, with nitrite at pH 3 yielded not only an extract with mutagenic activity, but one which induced cancer in the glandular stomach. Glandular stomach cancer is rare in rats; the control group had no neoplastic lesions in the stomach. Also, a high incidence of epithelial hyperplasia or intestinalization of glandular stomach cancer was observed only in the experimental group. Thus, the neoplastic lesions in the

glandular stomach were no doubt due to the treatment administered. As is true for rats given MNNG,[31] we also noted tumors in the small intestine and in the pancreas.

The nature of the mutagen responsible for carcinogenesis is not yet known and is being investigated. It is clear from the inhibition of its formation by vitamin C and from the fact that like alkylnitrosoureido compounds, it produced cancer in the glandular stomach, that we are dealing with this kind of compound. However, in contrast to compounds such as methylnitrosourea, we noted that the mutagenic activity was rather stable at pH 3 and even at higher pH values. Nonetheless, Mirvish *et al.*[42] have evidence that *Bonito* fish contains some nitrosatable alkylureas. Perhaps nitroso derivatives of Maillard-type products in fish and other foods deserve consideration.

Comment: Upper gastrointestinal tract carcinogens: Migrants maintain their risk for gastric cancer when changing residence from high-risk to low-risk regions.[2,37,43] Thus it may be that the nature of the carcinogens operating in man is similar to what we have identified through mutagen and carcinogen bioassays. With such compounds, exposure throughout life is not required to yield eventual stomach cancer. It follows that for effective gastric cancer prevention, exposure to agents causing this disease must be minimized or avoided from the earliest age. This means, in turn, that foods providing the necessary vitamin C, such as fresh fruits, vegetables, and salad, or supplementary vitamin C, ought to be consumed with every meal.

It is known that some vegetables and salads are also good sources of nitrate, but they are eaten fresh and are usually refrigerated, so that their content in bacterially-produced nitrite is minimal. The nitrite, possibly stemming from reduction of nitrates in vegetables in the oral cavity,[39] is not important in this case, since those foods contain substantial amounts of the antidotes, vitamins C and E, and also phenolic inhibitors.[44,45]

Salt has a promoting effect in gastric carcinogenesis,[46] although in some areas of the world it may also lead to mucosal damage, gastritis, rise in stomach pH, bacterial overgrowth, and thence to another source of nitrite through bacterial reduction of nitrate in the stomach.[32] However, in the MNNG model, the antecedent precancerous lesions occur with or without salt,[47,48] and thus we believe that salt use augments the risk through promotion rather than causes gastric cancer. Nonetheless, a lowered salt intake would not only reduce the risk of gastric cancer, but also lower the occurrence of hypertension and stroke associated with salt in genetically sensitive individuals.[34,49,50]

If the concepts and facts presented are correct, a major kind of human cancer in many regions of the world, cancer of the stomach, is due to a type of nitroso compound, a nitrosoureido derivative. Similarly, esophageal

TABLE 2. Current Concepts on Colon Cancer Causation and Development[54]

Risk factors: Diets high in fat, cholesterol, fried foods, and low in fiber

Established mechanisms
    High fat ⟶ High cholesterol biosynthesis ⟶ High gut bile acid levels
                 High dietary cholesterol ⟶
    Low fiber ⟶ High concentration of gut bile acids (low dilution through lack of bulk)
    High bile acid concentration ⟶ Promoting effect in colon carcinogenesis

Mechanisms under study
    Fried food ⟶ Mutagens ⟶ Colon carcinogens?
    Role of micronutrients (vitamins and minerals) and different types of fiber in production and metabolism of carcinogens, bile acids, promoters?

Mechanisms of promotion?

cancer may be due to a nitrosamine. It is quite certain that the formation of such compounds can be blocked by vitamins C and E, as well as by some other nitrite-trapping agents such as gallates. Thus, the primary prevention of cancers of the upper GI tract caused by nitroso compounds can be achieved through an adequate intake of such harmless inhibitors with every meal from infancy onwards, and through the avoidance of highly salted, pickled foods.

Genotoxic Carcinogens for Cancer of the Colon

Until recently there were no data as to the genotoxic carcinogens responsible for nonoccupational human cancer in the general public in western countries, except for those found in tobacco smoke.[2,25,51] This is especially so for nutritionally linked cancers such as colon, breast, prostate, or perhaps pancreatic cancer.

A key event in the search for the nature of such carcinogens was the discovery that charcoal broiling of meat or fish yielded mutagenic activity for *Salmonella typhimurium* TA-98.[52,53] Since mutagenic activity is often an indicator of carcinogenic activity, the development of mutagenic activity as a function of mode and temperature of cooking was studied under typical realistic cooking conditions.[54] Frying meat mixed with soy protein flour or a small amount of the antioxidant BHA yielded less mutagenic activity.[55]

The principal mutagenic components from fried beef were resolved into two major fractions. Those from fried fish could be separated into more fractions and included small amounts of compounds such as the amino acid pyrolysates TRP-1 and TRP-2.[53] One of the main components in fried sardines is identical to one of the mutagens in beef. Its structure, 2-amino-3-methyl-imidazo-[4,5-d]quinoline is similar sterically and structurally to known homocyclic carcinogenic arylamines, such as 3,2'-dimethyl-4-aminobiphenyl, which are colon, mammary gland, and prostate carcinogens in rodents.[56]

The main mutagens in fried meat or fish most likely do not derive only from the pyrolysis of amino acids or peptides but from the formation of heterocyclic compounds from carbohydrate components and amino acids, as formed in a model system for browning reactions involving the reaction of sugars with ammonium ions.[57,58]

Nongenotoxic or Epigenetic Agents in Nutritionally-Linked Cancers

Delineating the epigenetic promoting effects relevant to cancers in the GI tract and in the endocrine-controlled organs is important. For cancers in the colon, breast, and prostate, promoting effects appear to be decisive, because whether or not overt invasive disease is seen depends a great deal on epigenetic promoting factors. For example, in the case of prostate cancer, *in situ* lesions have been found in diverse populations in the world,[59–61] but the clinical invasive disease affects only populations consuming higher levels of dietary fat.[62,63] The following discussion will emphasize the rationale for epigenetic actions. Colon cancer should be considered distinct from rectal cancer on the basis of several lines of evidence, including international and intranational incidence patterns, sex ratio, and age distribution. For example, for left-sided colon cancer, the ratio of incidence rates between a Western high-risk country such as the US and a low-risk country such as Japan is about 6:1, but for rectal cancer the ratio is only 2.8:1. The male/female ratio for colon cancer is 1:1, for rectal cancer 1.4:1.[64] Time trends in the US show a slightly increasing incidence for colon cancer and a decreasing one for rectal cancer.[64] Not much is known about risk factors for rectal cancer, but ale or stout is one element incriminated.[65]

For colon cancer, the specific relevant dietary elements are the amounts of dietary fat and fiber as shown by studies in man and in animal models[66,67] (Table 3). One of the best arguments for these concepts is the changing incidence of colon cancer in Japan in recent years as the Japanese nutritional intake became pro-

TABLE 3. Comparison of High and Low Risk Dietary Factors for Cancer in Specific Organs

Organ	Population lower risk	Dietary factors lower risk	Population higher risk	Dietary factors higher risk
Esophagus	US: Utah; Rural Norway	Low alcohol and smoking habits	France: Calvados, Normandy	Extensive alcohol and smoking
Esophagus	Idem	Idem	US: lower socioeconomic groups	Alcohol and smoking
Esophagus	Idem	Idem	Eastern Iran, Southern Soviet Union	Low micronutrient vitamin C intake
Esophagus	Idem	Idem	Central China	Dietary carcinogen? low vitamin C intake
Stomach	US	Fresh fruit, salad, vitamins C and E	Japan, Chile, Colombia	Salted, pickled foods, geochemical & water nitrate, low vitamin C, E
Pancreas	Bombay, India	Low risk diet, low smoking habits	US, California black	Early start smoking habit, Western style high fat-cholesterol diet, coffee drinking?
Colon	Japan	Low fat diet	US, Western Europe, New Zealand, Australia, Scandinavia	High fat & cholesterol, low fiber diets; fried food
Colon	Mormons 7th Day Adventists	Higher fiber Low or no fried food, higher fiber	US in general US in general	Idem Idem
Colon	Finland	Higher fiber, lower fried food	US in general, Denmark	Idem

gressively westernized.[68] In addition, in many areas of the world, an association exists between colon cancer and coronary heart disease, where the amount of dietary fat and cholesterol have been shown to relate to risk for heart disease. An interesting exception to this rule is Finland where the risk for heart disease is high and that for colon cancer low, and we, as well as the IARC, have obtained some evidence that the lower risk of Finnish people for colon cancer, despite a high fat intake, is due to their consumption of foods high in fiber, especially cereal bran fiber.[69-71]

Laboratory research by a number of groups, particularly by Reddy et al.[70] and by Nigro,[72] yields insight into the mechanism whereby fat and cholesterol promote colon cancer risk and fiber inhibits colon carcinogenesis. The main effect of dietary fat appears to reside in a direct association between endogenous cholesterol biosynthesis, which when combined with exogenous cholesterol intake, in turn, leads to increased bile acid biosynthesis. Bile acids have been shown to be effective promoters for colon cancer and their role would seem to be to act as epigenetic agents in the overall carcinogenic process.[70] The effect of some dietary fibers, such as cereal brans, is to increase intestinal and stool bulk, which reduces the *concentration* of promoters, thereby

effectively lowering the risk for development of colon cancer. The lower colon cancer incidence in populations such as the Mormons and the Finns, who consume fried meat and other sources of genotoxic carcinogens and promoters but who also eat sizable amounts of cereal grains, may be thus explained (Table 3).

Recently, during reexamination of the prospective study of diet and coronary heart disease in Framingham, Massachusetts, Williams et al.[73] noted that a small number of men (28 men in a total of 5209 subjects) had a relatively low serum cholesterol, and therefore, a presumably low risk for arteriosclerosis and heart disease, but they had developed colon cancer. Interestingly, such a finding was not made in respect to other nutritionally linked cancers such as breast cancer, nor was there a significant excess of colon cancer in women. Thus, it could be that the small number of males with a low serum cholesterol and colon cancer are exceptional cases that may relate to an above average conversion of cholesterol to bile acids by the liver of these individuals. As we discussed, the higher bile acid levels would tend to promote colon cancer and account for the higher risk and disease incidence. There are no data on fecal bile acid levels in individuals on a Western diet who show a low serum cholesterol, a gap that needs to be filled.

In any case, increasing intake of cereal fiber, with a consequent rise in stool bulk, would tend to lower colon cancer risk, even in such individuals.

Epilogue and Prospects

Based on developments over the last ten years obtained through multidisciplinary approaches, the concepts outlined in this paper indicate lifestyle, especially nutrition and specific nutritional components as well as dietary habits in various parts of the world, plays a crucial role as risk factor for a number of important cancer types. Thus, nutrition may relate directly to the occurrence of 30–40% of cancers in men and 50–60% of cancers in women in the US and other Western countries.[71] Because of the rapid westernization of nutritional customs in Japan, there have been parallel alterations in the incidence of specific cancers due to this change.[68] We have dissected the overall carcinogenic process into a number of sequential steps, all of which are required for the occurrence of a clinical, invasive cancer. This sequence has been demonstrated in numerous studies in animal models, and there is no reason to assume that this sequence would not also hold for the initiation, development, and progression of human cancers.

We have outlined the essence of the concept that early lesions are the result of neoplastic changes caused by genotoxic carcinogens for cancers of the colon, breast, prostate, and perhaps even the pancreas. The pancreas may be subject also to carcinogens from tobacco smoke[74] and possibly from coffee.[75,76] We have noted that mutagens which may be carcinogenic are seen at the surface of fried, broiled, or roasted foods such as meat, fish, or even coffee. It is clear that this concept needs further validation through research being performed in a number of laboratories in Japan and in the United States. On the other hand, gastric cancer appears to have a totally distinct risk factor, namely pickled and salted fish or beans and also residence in areas with geochemical or agriculture sources of nitrate intake, not balanced by the presence of vitamin C, vitamin E, or certain phenolic antioxidants and nitrite traps such as pyrogallol or tannins. The possible genotoxic carcinogen is postulated to be of an alkylnitrosamide type. Cancer of the esophagus in countries such as China, southern Soviet Union, and eastern Iran may stem from an alkylnitrosamine stemming from similar processes, but with a different substrate subject to nitrosation. The formation of such compounds is inhibited by vitamin C, vitamin E, and certain antioxidants. This fact can be used to deliberately decrease the risk for gastric or esophageal cancer, as has been discussed.

Epigenetic agents play a major role in the development of cancer of the colon, and incidentally also of the breast, and prostate. These stem from the intake of appreciable amounts of dietary fat which are responsible for the endogenous production of specific nongenotoxic, epigenetic agents associated with increased risk. Modulators of promotion, such as stool bulk due to adequate fiber intake, reduce the risk of colon cancer. More research is also needed on modulators and inhibitors such as micronutrients, vitamins, and minerals that would eventually find application in lowering human disease risk.

These facts are excellent evidence for the rationale presented in this paper, namely that the mode of cooking and the level of dietary fat and fiber are associated with the occurrence of cancers of the colon, breast, and perhaps of the prostate and pancreas. This evidence can be the basis for suggesting relatively minor alterations in dietary habits, involving mainly a lower fat intake and a higher fiber consumption.

Since these elements operate through epigenetic mechanisms, their action is, by definition, dose- and time-dependent. Thus, a reduction in effective dose, by whatever means, would be expected to lead to rather rapid lowering of risk, and hence of incidence. This applies even to patients with such diseases, where dietary intervention promises to be an effective adjuvant therapy. When the postmenopausal use of estrogen drugs such as premarin was discontinued, there was a rapid decline in endometrial cancer, witness that epigenetic phenomena are reversible.

If current research does document further that the mode of cooking, especially frying and broiling, yields carcinogens for these kinds of cancers, means of preventing formation of such carcinogens may be found, and hopefully, would eventually yield a lower risk. Research on optimal levels of vitamins, minerals, antioxidants, and other micronutrients in the current diet would provide a broad basis for chemoprevention. Over the last several years, research has provided new perspectives on the causes and modifiers of the main premature killing diseases. Data in this report specifically record experimentation designed to yield understanding of underlying mechanisms as a sound reliable basis for prevention of many important kinds of human cancer and for the long-term goals of disease prevention generally.

REFERENCES

1. Doll R, Peto R. The causes of cancer: Quantitative estimates of avoidable risks of cancer in the United States today. *J Natl Cancer Inst* 1981; 66:1191–1308.
2. Hiatt HH, Watson JD, Winsten JA, eds. Origins of Human Cancer. Cold Spring Harbor, NY: Cold Spring Harbor Laboratory, 1977.
3. Higginson J. Proportion of cancers due to occupation. *Prev Med* 1980; 9:180–188.
4. Wynder EL, Gori GB. Contribution of the environment to cancer incidence: An epidemiologic exercise. *J Natl Cancer Inst* 1977; 58:825–832.
5. IARC Monographs series. On the evaluation of the carcinogenic

risk of chemicals to humans. Lyon: International Agency for Research on Cancer 1971–1980.

6. Saffiotti U, Wagoner JK. Occupational carcinogenesis. *Ann NY Acad Sci* 1976; 271:1–516.

7. Shimkin M. Industrial and lifestyle carcinogens. In: Burchenal JH, Oettgen, HF, eds. Cancer: Achievements, Challenges, and Prospects for the 1980s, vol. 1. New York: Grune & Stratton, 1981; 255–268.

8. Vaino H, Sorsa M, Hemminki K, eds. Occupational cancer and carcinogenesis. *J Toxicol Environ Health* 1980; 6(5–6):921–1335.

9. Miller AB. Risk factors from geographic epidemiology for gastric cancer. *Cancer* 1982; 50:2533–2540.

10. Burchenal JH, Oettgen HF, eds. Cancer: Achievements, Challenges and Prospects for the 1980s. New York: Grune & Stratton, 1981.

11. Emmelot P, Kriek E, eds. Environmental Carcinogenesis: Occurrence, Risk Evaluation and Mechanisms. Amsterdam: Elsevier/North Holland, 1979.

12. Griffin AC, Shaw CR, eds. Carcinogens: Identification and Mechanisms of Action. New York: Raven Press, 1979.

13. Straus DS. Somatic mutation, cellular differentiation, and cancer causation. *J Natl Cancer Inst* 1981; 67:233–241.

14. Weisburger JH, Williams GM. Chemical carcinogenesis. In: Doull J, Klaassen C, Amdur M, eds. Toxicology: The Basic Science of Poisons, ed. 2. New York: Macmillan, 1980; 84–138.

15. Berg P. Dissection and reconstruction of genes and chromosomes. *Science* 1981; 209:296–303.

16. Costa M. Metal Carcinogenesis Testing. Clifton: The Humana Press, 1980.

17. Tkeshelashvii LK, Shearman CW, Zakour RA, Koplit, M, Loeb LA. Effects of arsenic, selenium, and chromium on the fidelity of DNA synthesis. *Cancer Res* 1980; 40:2455–2460.

18. Cleaver JE. DNA damage, repair systems and human hypersensitive diseases. *J Environ Pathol Toxicol* 1980; 3:53.

19. Roberts JJ. Carcinogen-induced DNA damage and its repair. *Br Med Bull* 1980; 36:25–27.

20. Setlow RB. Different basic mechanisms in DNA repair. *Arch Toxicol* 1980; (Suppl) 3:217–225.

21. Pitot H, Sirica A. The stages of initiation and promotion in hepatocarcinogenesis. *Biochem Biophys Acta* 1980; 605:191.

22. Slaga TJ, Sivak A, Boutwell RK, eds. Mechanisms of Tumor Promotion and Cocarcinogens. New York: Raven Press, 1978.

23. Weinstein IB, Lee LS, Fisher PB, Mufson A, Yamasaki H. The mechanism of action of tumor promoters and a molecular model of two stage carcinogenesis. In: Emmelot P, Kriek E, eds. Environmental Carcinogenesis: Occurrence, Risk Evaluation and Mechanisms. Amsterdam: Elsevier/No. Holland, 1979; 265–286.

24. Weisburger JH, Williams GM. Carcinogen testing: Current problems and new approaches. *Science* 1981; 214:401–407.

25. Hoffmann D, Adams JD. Carcinogenic tobacco specific N-nitrosamines in snuff and in the saliva of snuff dippers. *Cancer Res* 1981; 41:4305–4308.

26. Alcohol and cancer workshop. *Cancer Res* 1979; 39:2853–2908.

27. McCoy GD, Hecht SS, Wynder EL. The roles of tobacco, alcohol, and diet in the etiology of upper alimentary and respiratory tract cancers. *Prev Med* 1980; 9:622–629.

28. Cheng S-J, Sala M, Li MH, Wang M-Y, Pot-Deprun J, Chouroulinkov I. Mutagenic, transforming and promoting effects of pickled vegetables from Linxian county, China. *Carcinogenesis* 1980; 1:685–692.

29. Huang DP, Ho JHC, Webb KS, Wood BJ, Gough TA. Volatile nitrosamines in salt-preserved fish before and after cooking. *Food Cosmet Toxicol* 1981; 19:167–171.

30. Lu SH, Camus A-M, Wang YL, Wang MY, Bartsch H. Mutagenicity in *Salmonella typhimurium* of N-3-methyl-butyl-N-1-methylacetonyl-nitrosamine and N-methyl-N benzylnitrosamine, N-nitrosation products isolated from corn-bread contaminated with commonly occuring moulds in Linshien county, a high incidence area for oesophageal cancer in Northern China. *Carcinogenesis* 1980; 1:867–870.

31. Sugimura T, Kawachi T. Experimental stomach carcinogenesis. In: Lipkin M, Good R, eds. Gastro-intestinal Tract Cancer Carcinogenesis. New York: Plenum, 1978; 327–341.

32. Cuello C, Lopez J, Correa P, Murray J, Zarama G, Gordillo G. Histopathology of gastric dysplasias: Correlations with gastric juice chemistry. *Am J Surg Pathol* 1979; 3:491–500.

33. Piper DW. Stomach cancer. UICC Tech. Rept. 34. Geneva: Union Internationale contre le Cancer, 1978; 1–138.

34. Weisburger JH, Marquardt H, Mower HF, Hirota N, Mori H, Williams G. Inhibition of carcinogenesis: Vitamin C and the prevention of gastric cancer. *Prev Med* 1980; 9:352–361.

35. Mirvish SS. Inhibition of the formation of carcinogenic N-nitroso compounds by ascorbic acid and other compounds. In: Burchenal JH, Oettgen HF, eds. Cancer: Achievements, Challenges, and Prospects for the 1980s, vol. 1. New York: Grune & Stratton, 1981; 557–588.

36. Devesa SS, Silverman DT. 1981: Trends in incidence and mortality in the United States. *J Environ Pathol Toxicol* 1981; 3:127–156.

37. Fraumeni JF Jr, ed. Persons at High Risk of Cancer. New York: Academic Press, 1975.

38. Armijo R. Epidemiology of cancer in Chile. *Natl Cancer Inst Monogr* 1979; 53:115–118.

39. Tannenbaum SR, Moran D, Rand W, Cuello C, Correa P. Gastric cancer in Colombia. IV: Nitrate and other ions in gastric contents of residents from a high-risk region. *J Natl Cancer Inst* 1979; 62:9–12.

40. Mergens WJ, Newmark HL. Blocking nitrosation reactions in vivo. In: Scanlan RA, Tannenbaum SR, eds. *N-Nitroso Compounds*. ACS Symposium Series 174. Washington, DC: American Chemical Society, 1981; 193–206.

41. Yano K. Alkylating activity of processed fish products treated with sodium nitrite in simulated gastric juice. *Gan* 1981; 72:451–454.

42. Mirvish SS, Karlowski K, Cairnes DA, Sams JP, Abraham R, Nielsen J. Identification of alkylurea after nitrosation–denitrosation of a bonito fish product, crab, lobster, and bacon. *J Agric Food Chem* 1980; 28:1175–1182.

43. McMichael AJ, McCall MG, Hartsthorne JM *et al*. Patterns of gastro-intestinal cancer in European migrants to Australia: The role of dietary change. *Int J Cancer* 1980; 25:431–437.

44. Kurechi T, Kikugawa K, Fukuda S. Nitrite reacting substances in Japanese radish juice and their inhibition of nitrosamine formation. *J Agric Food Chem* 1980; 28:1265–1269.

45. Walker EA, Griciute L, Castegnaro M, Börzsönyi M, Davis W, eds. N-Nitroso Compounds: Analysis, Formation and Occurrence, vol. 31. Lyon: International Agency for Research on Cancer, 1980.

46. Tatematsu M, Takahashi M, Fukushima S, Hanaouchi M, Shirai T. Effects in rats of sodium chloride on experimental gastric cancers induced by N-methyl-N'-nitro-N-nitrosoguanidine or 4-nitroquinoline-1-oxide. *J Natl Cancer Inst* 1975; 55:101–104.

47. Matsukura N, Itabashi M, Kawachi T, Hirota T, Sugimura T. Sequential studies on the histopathogenesis of gastric carcinoma in rats by a weak gastric carcinogen, N-propyl-N'-nitro-N-nitrosoguanidine. *J Cancer Res Clin Oncol* 1980; 98:153–163.

48. Quimby GF, Eastwood GL. Effect of N-methyl-N'nitro-N-nitrosoguanidine on gastroduodenal epithelial proliferation in Wistar/Lewis rats. *J Natl Cancer Inst* 1981; 66:331–337.

49. Joossens JV, Kesteloot H, Amery A. Salt intake and mortality from stroke. *N Engl J Med* 1979; 300:1396.

50. Meneely GR, Battarbee HD. High sodium–low potassium environment and hypertension. *Am J Cardiol* 1976; 38:768–781.

51. Wynder EL, Hoffmann D. Tobacco and health: A societal challenge. *N Engl J Med* 1979; 300:894–903.

52. Shelby MD, Matsushima T. Mutagens and carcinogens in the diet and digestive tract. *Mutat Res* 1981; 85:177.

53. Sugimura T, Kawachi T, Nagao M, Yahagi T. Mutagens in food as causes of cancer. In: Newell GR, Ellison NM, eds. Nutrition and Cancer: Etiology and Treatment. New York: Raven Press, 1981; 59–71.

54. Weisburger JH, Reddy BS, Spingarn NE, Wynder EL. Current views on the mechanisms involved in the etiology of colorectal cancer. In: Winawer S, Schottenfeld D, Sherlock P, eds. Colorectal Cancer: Prevention, Epidemiology, and Screening. New York: Raven Press, 1980; 19–41.

55. Weisburger JH, Horn C. Nutrition and cancer: Mechanisms of genotoxic and epigenetic carcinogens in nutritional carcinogenesis.

Bull NY Acad Med 1982; 58:296–312.

56. Weisburger JH, Spingarn NE, Wang YY, Vuolo LL. An assessment of the role of mutagens and endogenous factors in large bowel cancer. *Cancer Bull* 1981; 33:124–129.

57. Shibamoto T, Nishimura O, Mihara S. Mutagenicity of products obtained from a maltol-ammonia browning model system. *J Agric Food Chem* 1981; 29:641–646.

58. Spingarn NE, Garvie CT. Formation of mutagens in sugar-ammonia model systems. *J Agric Food Chem* 1979; 27:1319–1321.

59. Akazaki K, Stemmermann GN. Comparative study of latent carcinoma of the prostate among Japanese in Japan and Hawaii. *J Natl Cancer Inst* 1973; 50:1137–1141.

60. Guileyardo JM, Johnson WD, Welsh RA, Akazaki K, Correa P. Prevalence of latent prostate carcinoma in two U. S. populations. *J Natl Cancer Inst* 1980; 65:311–315.

61. Hirayama T. Epidemiology of prostate cancer with special reference to the role of diet. *Natl Cancer Inst Monogr* 1979; 53:149–155.

62. Hill P, Garbaczewski L, Helman P, Walker ARP, Garnes H, Wynder EL. Environmental factors and breast and prostatic cancer. *Cancer Res* 1981; 41:3817–3818.

63. Hill P, Wynder EL, Garnes H, Walker ARP. Environmental factors, hormone status, and prostatic cancer. *Prev Med* 1980; 9:657–666.

64. Schottenfeld D. Cancer Epidemiology and Prevention. Springfield: Charles C Thomas, 1975.

65. Editorial: Beer and bowel cancer. *Lancet* 1980; 1:1396–1397.

66. Modan B, Barell V, Lubin F, Modan M, Greenberg RA, Graham S. Low-fiber intake as an etiologic factor in cancer of the colon. *J Natl Cancer Inst* 1975; 55:15–18.

67. Reddy BS. Dietary fat and its relationship to large bowel cancer. *Cancer Res* 1981; 41:3700–3705.

68. Hirayama T. Diet and cancer. *Nutr Cancer* 1979; 1:67–78.

69. Jensen OM, McLennan R. Dietary factors and colorectal cancer in Scandinavia. *Isr J Med Sci* 1979; 15:329–336.

70. Reddy BS, Cohen LA, McCoy GD, Hill P, Weisburger JH, Wynder EL. Nutrition and its relationship to cancer. *Adv Cancer Res* 1980; 32:237–345.

71. Wynder EL, McCoy GD, Reddy BS *et al.* Nutrition and metabolic epidemiology of cancers of cancers of the oral cavity, esophagus, colon, breast, prostate, and stomach. In: Newell GR, Ellison NM, eds. Nutrition and Cancer. New York: Raven Press, 1981; 11–48.

72. Nigro ND. Animal studies implicating fat and fecal steroids in intestinal cancer. *Cancer Res* 1981; 41:3769–3770.

73. Williams RR, Sorlie PD, Feinleib M, McNamara PM, Kannel WB, Dawber TR. Cancer incidence by levels of cholesterol. *JAMA* 1981; 245:247–252.

74. Wynder EL. An epidemiological evaluation of the causes of cancer of the pancreas. *Cancer Res* 1975; 35:2228–2235.

75. MacMahon B, Yen S, Trichopoulos D, Warren JL, Nardi G. Coffee and cancer of pancreas. *N Engl J Med* 1981; 304:630–634.

76. Nagao M, Takahashi U, Yamanaka H *et al.* Mutagens in coffee and tea. *Mutat Res* 1979; 68:101–106.

Epidemiology of Cancer of the Colon and Rectum

by Denis P. Burkitt

The close relationship between bowel cancer and other non-infective diseases of the bowel, such as benign tumor, diverticular disease, and appendicitis, indicates that these conditions may have a common or related etiology. Their close association with the refined diet characteristic of economic development suggests that the removal of dietary fiber may be a causative factor. These diseases are all rare in every community examined which exists on a high residue diet, and common in every country where a low residue diet has been adopted. Dietary fiber has been shown to regulate the speed of transit, bulk, and consistency of stools, and together with other dietary factors is probably also responsible for the changes which have been demonstrated in the bacterial flora of feces. It seems likely that carcinogens produced by the action of an abnormal bacterial flora when held for a prolonged period in a concentrated form in contact with the bowel mucosa may account for the high incidence of these diseases in economically developed countries.

IN MOST OF THE WESTERN WORLD TODAY, THE large bowel is, after the bronchi, the next most common site for cancer in men.

The evidence discussed here would suggest that this high incidence of cancer of the bowel may, like that of lung cancer, be a relatively recent development, for both these tumors are still rare in developing countries.

As Higginson[26] has pointed out, the incidence of bowel cancer is related to economic development, and no other form of cancer is so closely linked to the alterations in dietary habits with which this is usually associated.

The rates for cancer of the colon and rectum in men per 100,000 standardized for 35–64 years of age[19] arranged in order of

incidence clearly indicate this relationship to economic development (Fig 1). Kampala (Uganda), serving a largely rural African community, is at the bottom of the list.

For most of Africa, incidence rates are not available, but the general rarity of bowel cancer can be judged from its proportion of total cases of cancer recorded.

Table 1 summarizes the frequency of cancer of the colon and rectum in published reports from different countries in Africa together with figures obtained from doctors in up-country hospitals with whom a liaison has been established and from whom regular reports have been received. Four other small series, from Uganda,[7] Tanzania,[22] Acornhoek, South Africa,[64] and Lambarene,[16] each with a total of less than 300 cases, reported a frequency of large bowel cancer varying from 0.2% to 4.4% of the total. Bremner and Ackerman[6] have re-

Presented at the National Conference on Cancer of the Colon and Rectum, San Diego, Calif., January 7–9, 1971.

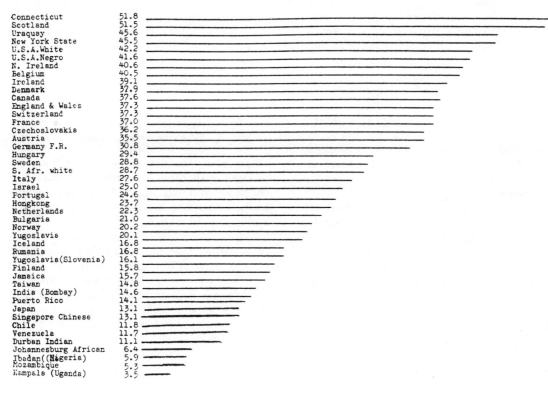

Fig. 1. Age-standardized incidence rates for cancer of the colon and rectum in men 35-64 years of age arranged in order of incidence (modified from Doll[10]).

TABLE 1. Proportion of Cancer of the Colon and Rectum to Total Cancer in Different Parts of Africa

Place	Period	Total Series	Percent of total cancer of colon and rectum	Reference
	Reported Series			
Johannesburg (S. Africa)	1952–54	1076	2.6	54
do. do.	1962–64	2407	2.4	54
Durban (S. Africa)	1964–66	1040	2.1	55
Lourenço Marques (Mozambique)	1956–60	603	1.3	49
Sudan	1954–61	2234	2.8	38
Accra (Ghana)	1942–55	1192	1.8	21
Kampala (Uganda)	1954–60	615	2.8	15
Nairobi (Kenya)	1957–63	4206	2.5	37
Dakar (Senegal)	1955–64	1838	2.5	13
Salisbury (Rhodesia)	1963–65	1415	1.6	58
Ilesha (Nigeria)	1954–67	465	5.8	42
Stanleyville (Congo Kinshasa)	1939–55	2536	1.1	65
M. R. C. Survey of Up-Country Hospitals				
	Hospitals			
Kenya	5	934	1.5	
Uganda	7	613	2.1	
Tanzania	23	1743	2.3	
Malawi	22	827	1.7	

cently reported the rarity of large bowel cancer and the extreme rarity of intestinal polyps in Johannesburg Bantu. The most remarkable feature is the low and uniform figure of around 2% obtained from each series, with the single exception of Ilesha (Nigeria).[42] This percentage corresponds to the lowest in the world list (Fig. 1) and would appear to represent the basic minimum incidence of this form of cancer. In contrast to certain other diseases associated with Western civilisation, there is as yet no obvious increase in urban relative to rural communities.

Replies to questionnaires received from 34 up-country government and mission hospitals in rural Africa further indicate the great rarity of cancer of the colon and rectum in developing countries. Twenty-one of these hospitals saw an estimated one case, or no case, of large bowel cancer annually. Six stated it was rare or very rare and in only one hospital were as many as 4 cases seen annually.

The age-adjusted incidence rates (Fig. 1) suggest that in industrialized Western countries, bowel cancer is more than ten times more common than it is in the African countries listed and, since the frequency in these centres corresponds to that in all other areas investigated in Africa, it can be assumed that a difference of this magnitude exists between Africa as a whole and the industrialized West.

It has been considered advisable to study tumors of the colon and rectum together since many of the variations in relative incidence can be accounted for by tumors near the pelvirectal junction which might be classified in either group. Moreover, as will be discussed below, there are probably common etiological factors.

INCIDENCE CHANGES RESULTANT ON EMIGRATION

The factor which best emphasizes the environmental, rather than the genetic, dependence of bowel cancer is the contrast between the situation in American Negroes, who now have an incidence comparable to that of Caucasians, and that of Africans. Environmental influences are also apparent, although to a lesser extent, in the raised incidence of bowel cancer in the Japanese who have emigrated to America compared with that observed in Japan. Second generation immigrants to California[71] and Hawaii[61] have nearly reached the incidence of their Caucasian compatriots. These migrants have for the most part accepted the dietary customs of their country of adoption, whereas rice has continued to be the basic diet of indigenous Japanese, particularly in rural areas. The rapidly changing dietary pattern in Japan, particularly in urban areas, is being reflected by an increase in large bowel disease.[61]

ASSOCIATION WITH OTHER NON-INFECTIVE DISEASES OF THE BOWEL

Cancer of the colon and rectum is closely associated with other non-infectious disease of the bowel and with hemorrhoids, in geographical distribution, historical rise in incidence, and in individual patients.[8–10]

Similar geographical distribution: Diverticular disease, adenomatous polyps, appendicitis, ulcerative colitis, and hemorrhoids are all rare in those populations in which cancer of the bowel is rare and have their highest incidence in those areas in which bowel cancer is most prevalent.[8,44] Large bowel cancer [20] and colon diverticula[33] are, for instance, both three times as common in industrialized Sweden as in more rural Finland. Adenomatous polyps of the bowel are even more rare in Africa than are malignant tumors. Bremner and Ackerman[6] found only 6 in a review of surgical specimens received over 13 years in a 2,000-bed hospital. No polyps were found in a series of 1,000 autopsies in which the bowel had been routinely opened and inspected. Parker and Skinner[6] found no case in over 13,000 autopsies in Rhodesia. Hutt and Templeton[31] reported only 2 in over 40,000 surgical specimens in Uganda, and none in 2,000 autopsies in which the bowel was routinely opened.

Historical appearances: Chronologically, an increase in the incidence of diverticular disease apparently followed the increase in the incidence of bowel cancer. It may be assumed that initially both diverticula and cancer of the large bowel were rare in American Negroes, as they still are in Africans today. Some 30 years ago, much of the gap between the incidence of both these conditions in the Caucasian and Negro population was already partly bridged. Kocour[32] reported that diverticula were only two thirds as common in Negroes as in Caucasians. In 1936, Lawrence[36] reported that both cancer and polyps of the colon were much more common in the Caucasian than in the Negro population. In 1946, Quinland and Cuff,[51] reporting on 300 cases of primary cancer in the Negro, recorded only 10 tumors of the large bowel—8 in the rectum and 2 in the colon. In 1947, cancer of the colon was nearly twice as common in American Caucasians as in Negroes, and rectal cancer was 40% more common.[50] Steiner,[60] surveying a series between 1918 and 1947, also concluded that cancer of the large intestine was considerably less common in the Negro than in the Caucasian.

These racial differences have now almost disappeared in America. In India, the incidence of bowel cancer is significantly higher than in Africa but very much lower than in the Western world. Diverticular disease is still very rare. A possible explanation will be suggested here in relating cancer to changes in both bacterial flora and cellulose deficiency and attributing diverticular disease to gross cellulose deficiency alone. In Puerto Rico, the age-adjusted incidence rates for cancer of the bronchus rose by 117% and for the colon by 95%, between 1950 and 1968. The overall increase for all forms of cancer was 40%.[40] The rise in bronchial carcinoma accompanied an increase in cigarette smoking, and likewise the rise in colon carcinoma accompanied a progressive adaptation to North American type of diet.

Appendicitis appears at least a generation earlier than the other non-infective bowel diseases associated with Western civilization, just as its age distribution reaches its peak nearly 50 years earlier than that of the other conditions.

Association in individuals—cancer and adenomatous polyps: Strongly positive correlations have been shown between bowel cancer and both adenomatous polyps and villous papillomas. Morson and Bussey[41] consider these benign tumors to be fundamentally part of the same disease, and state that approximately one third of all specimens of bowel removed for cancer have also benign tumors. If the whole of the large bowel could have been examined in each case, the proportion would have almost certainly been considerably higher. Rider et al.[52,53] and Bockus et al.[5] produce abundant evidence of a strongly positive association between benign and malignant tumors of the bowel. Moreover, bowel cancer occurs in nearly half of all patients with familial polyposis.

Cancer and ulcerative colitis: There is a well-recognized association between bowel cancer and ulcerative colitis.

Bowel cancer and hemorrhoids: An association between these conditions has been accepted.

Cancer and appendicitis: Since appendicitis occurs in a much younger age group and is of short duration, an association in the same individuals between this condition and diseases of later adult life would be unlikely even if caused by related factors. Nevertheless, McVay[39] has shown a weak association between bowel cancer and previous appendicectomy.

INVESTIGATING THE COMMON RATHER THAN THE RARE

The geographical association between different non-infective bowel diseases, both in their historical appearance and in individual patients, strongly suggests common or related causative factors. It may, of course, be that it is only one or some of many co-factors responsible for these diseases that are related or common. However, this does imply that a successful search for the cause of one of these diseases may provide clues as to the cause of the others, and the more common diseases—appendicitis, adenomatous polyps, and diverticula—provide greater opportunities for investigation than do the rarer partners of the group—cancer and ulcerative colitis.

ASSOCIATION WITH DISEASES NOT AFFECTING BOWEL

Not only are there possible leads from the observed association between cancer and other non-malignant diseases of the colon, but clues might also be found from an observed association with other conditions.[9] Communities little influenced by Western customs not only have a very low incidence of non-infective disease of the bowel but also have a low incidence of diabetes, a condition which rises steeply on adoption of Western food and of atherosclerosis which may be attributed to similar dietary habits. These two conditions are closely associated both in geographical distribution and in their tendency to be found concurrently in individual patients. Diabetes and atherosclerosis, like the non-infective diseases of the bowel, have a comparable incidence in American Negroes and Caucasians in contrast to their rarity in rural Africa. Moreover, both these conditions, like the non-infective diseases of the bowel, are relatively rare in Japan, but have increased in incidence in Japanese who have emigrated to the U.S.A.[61] Bowel cancer has also been related to obesity which is closely associated with both diabetes and atherosclerosis.[61,72] Diverticular disease, which has a similar geographical distribution to that of bowel cancer, has been shown to have a strongly positive association with both diabetes and atherosclerosis in individual patients.[56]

RELATIONSHIP TO DIET

It would seem reasonable to assume that the conditions prevailing within the lumen of the bowel are the factors most responsible for the environment of bowel mucosa. However, this does not preclude the possibility of other factors playing a part, such as substances reaching the bowel through the bloodstream.

As has been emphasized, there is a close relationship between bowel cancer and economic development, and the operative factors are probably alterations in dietary patterns. The bridging of the gap between the incidence of non-infective disease in American Negroes and Caucasians during the last 40 years relates to the lessening of dietary differences. Similarly, the low frequency of about 1% of all malignant tumors given for bowel cancer in Egypt, in 1924,[18] was considered to be related to the then prevailing diet. In contrast, Nasr,[43] nearly half a century later, reported from Cairo a frequency of 6%, a figure three times greater than that pertaining in sub-Saharal Africa. Wynder et al.[72] have, moreover, pointed out that bowel cancer in Japan is more common among those on a more Westernized diet.

EFFECT OF DIET ON INTESTINAL TRANSIT TIME, STOOL BULK, AND CONTENT

One of the most notable differences between the diet of the Western world where bowel cancer is most prevalent, and that of less-developed communities where it has its lowest incidence, are the proportions of unabsorbable fiber and refined carbohydrate in the food ingested.[14] Reduction in fiber and, therefore,

in bulk inevitably results in an increased consumption of refined carbohydrate. Changes in cellulose content of food alter colonic activity, intestinal transit time, and stool bulk and consistency,[66-69] and excess carbohydrate has been shown to alter the bacterial content of the feces.[29]

It is noticeable that the stools of those eating high residue diets are almost invariably bulky, soft, and non-odorous in contrast to the formed and often faceted motions so common in communities eating highly processed food.[14] The relative absence of fetid smell in the stools of people in developing communities and in the stools of wild animals[14] is also significant and is believed to indicate a lower rate of bacterial decomposition compared to that occurring in Western countries.

Following the example of Walker[66,68] in South Africa, I have enlisted the cooperation of workers in many countries in Africa and elsewhere to measure intestinal transit times using the method advocated by Hinton et al.[28] This entails swallowing radiopaque plastic pellets which can be detected in the stools either by x-ray or by washing a stool through a wire mesh.[69] The time the pellets are swallowed and the time each stool is passed are recorded. There is a clear correlation between intestinal transit time and stool bulk, and the fiber content of food. The intestinal transit time and stool weights measured for African villagers, boys in an African boarding school on semi-European type diet, and boys in an English boarding school are shown in Figs. 2 and 3.[11] The effect of diet cellulose on intestinal transit time has also been estimated by Holmgren and Mynors,[30] who gave capsules of carmine to 3 groups of Africans living on un-

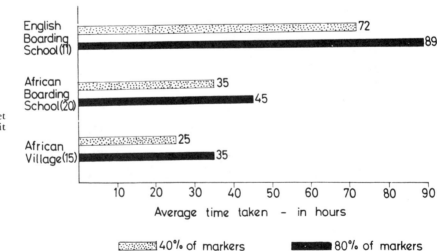

FIG. 2. Effect of diet on intestinal transit time.

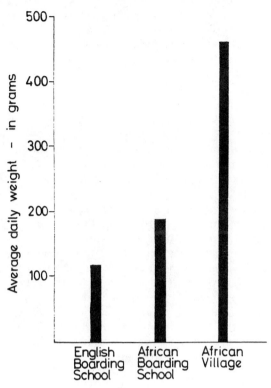

FIG. 3. Effect of diet on stool weight.

refined, mixed, and refined diets. The average time that lapsed before the appearance of the dye in the stools in the miners on traditional diet was 14.5 hours. For the African trainee-teachers on a mixed diet, it was 20.6 hours, and for the medical students on a refined diet 28.4 hours.

Measurement of the bacterial flora is much more difficult. Comparisons between English and African stools were made by Aries et al.[3] who compared a group of Londoners with some Uganda adults and found the main differences in the increase in bacteroides and bifidobacteria and decrease in streptococci and lactobacilli in the English compared to the Ugandan stools. Hoffman[29] reported a higher bacteria content in volunteers on a high carbohydrate diet than in those on high fat or protein diet.

The rarity of pyelitis in rural Africans, together with the observation that toxemia from gangrenous bowel and the mortality from bowel surgery are both much less in Africans than in Caucasians, certainly suggest differences in intestinal flora between the two groups.

It can be concluded that diet affects intestinal transit time, and the bulk, consistency, and bacterial flora of the feces. It seems al-most certain that it also determines intralumen pressures.

Experimentally, it is easy to demonstrate the effect of increased roughage on bowel activity by adding bran to one's diet; not only is this an effective preventative of constipation[63,70] but it has been found therapeutically effective for relieving the symptoms of piles[17] and diverticular disease, which is now believed to result from the high pressures associated with low residue diet.[46,47]

BOWEL CANCER RELATED TO FECAL CONTENT

Anatomical distribution: The fact that most non-infective diseases of the large bowel have their greatest incidence in the segment of bowel in which both fecal arrest and bacterial proliferation are maximum suggests a relationship between these diseases and bowel content.

Absence of tumors in short-circuited bowel loop: The former concept that the pelvic colon was a reservoir for feces, while the rectum remained empty, has been challenged by Halls[25] who has shown that the rectum is not normally empty. The close epidemiologic association between cancer of the colon and rectum increases the suspicion that retained feces may be etiologically related to these tumors.

The evidence that a loop of bowel short-circuited from the stream of feces remains free of tumors induced experimentally in other parts of the intestine supports this concept.[59]

Rarity of tumors in other body canals: Of all the epithelial-lined channels of the body, only the bowel and the bronchi are highly prone to malignant change. These are also the only ones in which the content can be readily controlled. The large bowel is unique in its high bacterial content. Tumors of the ureter, urethra, common bile ducts, or salivary gland ducts are exceedingly rare, and there is no evidence that the incidence varies in different communities.

Rarity in primitive communities and animals: A further factor which suggests that alterations in diet may be responsible for increase in bowel cancer is its rarity, not only in all communities living on relatively unprocessed food, but also in all animals.

RELATED CAUSATIVE FACTORS IN CANCER AND OTHER NON-INFECTIVE DISEASES OF THE LARGE BOWEL

Malignant and benign tumors: The following evidence indicates that both bowel cancer and adenomatous polyps must have a closely related or common cause.

1. They are closely associated both epidemiologically[8-10] and in individals.[5,41,53]

2. They have a similar anatomical distribution in the large bowel.

3. They have a similar age distribution except that there is approximately a 5-year shift to the left for benign, compared with malignant tumors.

4. They can both be produced experimentally by the same procedures.[41,71,72]

5. The sex distribution with a 3:2 female preponderance is the same for each condition.[4]

6. The fact that at least 3.5% of patients who have had colon or rectal cancer removed surgically will develop a second primary growth, and the observation that the chance of a further primary tumor developing is doubled if polyps are associated with the cancer at the first operation[41] suggests a factor acting generally on the bowel mucosa to produce either benign or malignant tumors.

7. The very high risk of colon cancer developing in patients with familial polyposis suggests that some hereditary factor may render affected individuals particularly susceptible to a common factor responsible for both diseases. The observation that both the benign and malignant tumors in these patients tend to occur at an earlier age than usual with these lesions, supports this contention. Morson and Bussey[41] state "the experimental evidence to date suggests only that there is a common factor in the aetiology of adenomas and carcinoma not that carcinomas are usually or always preceded by a benign lesion."

Cancer and ulcerative colitis: These conditions are closely associated in their geographical distribution.

They are closely associated in individuals, patients with ulcerative colitis having a greatly increased risk of developing bowel cancer. It seems more reasonable to postulate associated factors than a cause and effect relationship, as it is very rare for an inflammatory process to give rise to malignant change. For example, there is no evidence that chronic bowel ulcers caused by schistosomiasis or amoebiasis predispose to bowel cancer. It may be that some factor responsible for both conditions is operating with undue intensity or on a particularly susceptible patient.

Cancer and diverticula: The close epidemiologic association is the strongest argument for a related causative factor.

Cancer and hemorrhoids: It is much more likely that both conditions are the result of common or related causative factors than that hemorrhoids are the result of cancer. Although the former have a positive association with the latter, the vast majority of patients with hemorrhoids never develop bowel cancer.

BACTERIAL CHANGES IN FECES IN INDUCING TUMORS OF LARGE BOWEL

Small bowel exemption: Epithelial tumors are very rare in the small intestine which has a much lower bacterial content than the colon.

Cancer suppressed in germ-free rats: Cole[72] showed that a carcinogen capable of inducing bowel cancer in normal rats produced no tumore in germ-free animals. Stewart[62] confirms this evidence, reporting that cycasin given by mouth produces tumors, chiefly in the colon, in experimental animals, but does not have this effect if fed to germ-free rats. He interprets the observation that nearly all the ingested cycasin can be recovered from the urine and feces in germ-free rats and only 15–35% of it from normal rats as an indication that it is broken down in the bowel by bacteria with production of carcinogens.

Bile salts in stools: It has been postulated that altered bacterial flora may lead to degradation of bile salts with resultant formation of carcinogens.[71]

Hill et al.[27] believe that there are less bile salts in stools from Africa compared with England but have shown that stools from Western communities, where bowel cancer is common, contained more bacteria capable of causing degradation of bile salts than did stools from Indians and Africans. They have also shown that there are more products of bile degradation in Western stools than in stools from regions where bowel cancer is rare. They blame increased consumption of fat rather than of refined carbohydrates. In this connection, it is of interest that the total per capita increase in consumption of fats in the U.S.A. between 1909 and 1961 rose only 12%, and the increase in saturated fatty acids was only 7%. The increase in the consumption of sugars and syrups over the same period was 218%.[1] Moreover, bowel cancer tends to be more common in urban than in rural communities, although the latter usually have a higher fat consumption.

It seems likely that bacterial changes will be accepted as probable causative factors in bowel cancer, though the reason for the bacterial changes may be disputed.

A number of bile acids have, in fact, been

shown to be carcinogenic. Lacassagne et al.[34] showed that apocholic acid, a product of mild dehydration of cholic acid, one of the two main bile acids, could definitely be carcinogenic. Later,[35] they reported the sarcomagenic activity of a product of the artificial oxidative degradation of bile acids.

Haddow[24] has stated that "the recognition . . . of the nature of the steroid skeleton . . . at once suggested the possibility . . . of the formation of small amounts of potent carcinogens within the body from such naturally occurring molecules as the bile acids." He had previously reported[23] that the bile acid deoxycholic acid could be chemically converted into a potent carcinogen, 3-methylcholanthrene.

Antonis and Bersohn[2] provided further evidence suggesting that this may in fact occur. They showed that the quantity of bile acids in the stools is greater in Africans on a high residue diet than in Europeans on diets with reduced fiber content, which suggests that in the latter group a proportion of the bile acids had been destroyed in the gut. This evidence might suggest that in the case of patients on low residue diet a proportion of the bile acids had been altered, possibly by abnormal or excessive bacterial flora, to products with carcinogenic activity. In keeping with this are the observations referred to above, that the amount of ingested cycasin which can be recovered from the feces is greater in germ-free rats without bowel tumors than in normal rats with tumors. The disappearance of part of the cycasin in one case and of the bile salts in the other, in the presence of bacteria, suggests that the latter play a part in the production of carcinogens.

These observations parallel the production of carcinogens formed from cycads which are also believed to depend on bacterial activity as mentioned previously.

Differences in bowel flora: In at least some Africans, bowel flora is different from that of Europeans.[1]

Most chemical compounds which are carcinogens in the gastrointestinal tract produce tumors in the proximal rather than in the distal bowel where bacterial action is maximal.

FACTS IN FORMULATING AN HYPOTHESIS OF CAUSE OF BOWEL CANCER

1. The close association both epidemiologically and in individual patients with other non-infective diseases of the bowel.

2. The geographical association between non-infective disease of the bowel and some other conditions, such as diabetes, atherosclerosis, and obesity.

3. The association between diet and bowel behavior and content.

4. The epidemiologic association between non-infective diseases of the bowel and low residue diet.

5. The rarity of epithelial tumors in the small intestine and all other epithelial-lined canals except the bronchi.

6. The role played by bacteria in producing bowel cancer in experimental models.

SUGGESTED HYPOTHESIS

It is a bold move to suggest an explanation for the frequency of large bowel tumors in Western countries, particularly in view of the fact that most cancer is probably multifactoral in origin. It may seem even more daring to suggest a similar cause for such common diseases as appendicitis and diverticular disease, but I am convinced that these diseases must be considered together. The adoption of a refined carbohydrate diet appears the most important, though probably not the only, responsible factor, and this hypothesis is consistent with the clinical, epidemiologic, and experimental evidence.

Diverticular disease: This is easy to explain on the basis of a cellulose-depleted diet.[47,48] Diverticula can be produced in experimental animals fed for prolonged periods on a low-residue diet. A high-residue diet alleviates the disease.

The prevalence of diverticular disease in a community does not appear to rise until sometime after a rise in cancer incidence. Dietary cellulose is usually not significantly depleted until some time after refined carbohydrates, which affect bowel bacterial flora, have been added to the diet.

Appendicitis: There is abundant epidemiologic evidence relating appendicitis to both the removal of fiber from diet[57] and the addition of sugar.[12,14] The former results in raised intralumen pressures in the colon, in general, but particularly in the appendix when blocked with fecoliths which are peculiar to constipated bowels. This may cause devitalization of the mucosa while the excess sugar alters the bacterial flora in the feces which is probably chiefly responsible for the inflammatory process.

Diseases associated with refined carbohydrate: The association between conditions believed to be partly or largely due to low residue diet on the one hand and those believed by many to be due to excess consumption of refined carbohydrates, such as diabetes, atherosclerosis, and obesity on the other, can be readily explained by the fact that removing unabsorbable fiber from carbohydrate foods results in increased consumption of the refined product to satisfy appetite.[10,14] Cleave et al.[14] argue persuasively that these and other diseases are due primarily to refining carbohydrate, and they recommend the inclusive term "Saccharine Disease"* for all the conditions.

Tumors: With regard to benign and malignant tumors, there are at least two ways in which a refined carbohydrate diet could be responsible (Fig. 4).

Any carcinogen ingested or formed in the gut would, in refined carbohydrate eaters, not only be present in a more concentrated form in small stools, but would be held in contact with the mucosa for a prolonged period in a constipated colon.[45,71] An additional factor responsible for retention of stools in the distal colon and rectum in economically developed communities is the social custom which precludes bowel evacuation unless facilities are readily available. Walker et al.[69] have commented on the ability of the African to empty his bowel at will.

The most likely cause of bowel tumors

* Saccharine, meaning related to sugar, is to be pronounced to rhyme with the river Rhine, to distinguish it from the chemical sweetener.

seems to be carcinogens produced by bacterial action on bile salts or other normal bowel constituents. The degradation of bile salts by bacteria could explain the reduced quantity of those salts in people prone to bowel cancer on a Western diet compared to that found in South African Bantu, whose bowel cancer incidence is very low. A hypothesis incriminating both bacterial activity and colonic stasis could account for the anatomical distribution of benign and malignant tumors which are found maximally in the area where fecal retention is most prolonged and bacterial action most pronounced.

Conclusions

All experimental studies in cancer are eventually aimed at limiting or curing the disease. When relationships have been established between environmental factors and the incidence of a particular disease, whether benign or malignant, evasive action can be taken before the actual causative agents or mode of action is understood. Cholera was evaded by the avoidance of sewage-contaminated water a century before the v. cholera was identified as the cause of the disease. Lung cancer can largely be avoided by abstinence from smoking cigarettes, although the carcinogenic mechanism whereby tobacco smoke causes cancer is not yet understood. A relationship can be demon-

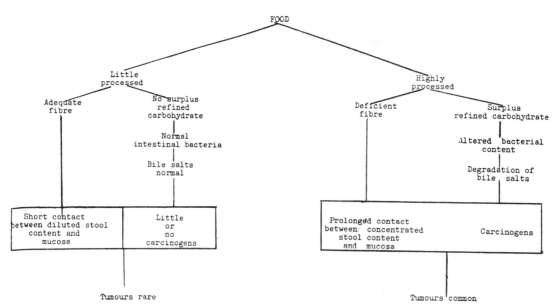

FIG. 4. Diagrammatic representation of possible relationship between diet and cancer of the bowel.

strated between certain bowel diseases and diet, and although this has not yet been shown to be causative in the case of cancer, the relationship between an over-refined diet and diverticular disease can now be considered established. In view of the evidence, it seems justifiable to issue a warning against the removal of so much of the unabsorbable fiber from our food, and the associated over-ingestion of refined carbohydrates.

REFERENCES

1. Antar, M. A., Ohlson, M. A., and Hodges, R. E.: Perspectives in nutrition. Changes in retail market food supplies in the United States in the last seventy years in relation to the incidence of coronary heart disease with special reference to dietary carbohydrates and essential fatty acids. *Amer. J. Clin. Nutr.* 14:169–178, 1964.

2. Antonis, A., and Bersohn, I.: The influence of diet on faecal lipids in South African white and Bantu prisoners. *J. Clin. Nutr.* 11:142–155, 1962.

3. Aries, V., Crowther, J. S., Drasar, B. S., Hill, M. J., and Williams, R. E. O.: Bacteria and the aetiology of the large bowel. *GUT* 10:334, 1969.

4. Bacon, H. E.: Cancer of the Colon, Rectum and Anal Canal. Philadelphia, J. B. Lippincott & Co., 1964.

5. Bockus, H. L., Tschdjian, V., Ferguson, L. K., Mouhran, Y., and Chamberlain, C.: Adenomatous polyp of colon and rectum; its relation to carcinoma. *Gastroenterology* 41:225–232, 1961.

6. Bremner, C. G., and Ackerman, L. V.: Polyps and carcinoma of the large bowel in the S. African Bantu. *Cancer* 26:991–999, 1970

7. Buckley, R. M.: Patterns of cancer at Ishaka Hospital in Uganda. *E. Afr. Med. J.* 44:465–468, 1967.

8. Burkitt, D. P.: Related disease—related cause? *Lancet* 2:1229–1231, 1969.

9. ———: Relationship as a guide to etiology of disease. *Int. Path.* 11:3–5, 31–32, 1970.

10. ———: Relationship as a clue to causation. *Lancet* 2:1237–1240, 1970.

11. ———: Some leads to the aetiology of cancer of the large bowel. *Proc. Roy. Soc. Med.* (In press).

12. ———: The aetiology of appendicitis. *Brit. J. Surg.* (In press).

13. Camain, R., and Lambert, D.: Les hematosarcomes en Afrique Noire Occidentale et Centrale francophone. *In* The Lymphoreticular Tumours in Africa. (A symposium organized by UICC. Basel, S. Karger, 1964, pp. 42–53.

14. Cleave, T. L., Campbell, G. D., and Painter, N. S.: Diabetes, Coronary Thrombosis and the Saccharine Disease. Bristol, John Wright & Sons Ltd., 1969.

15. Davies, J. N. P., Knowelden, J., and Wilson, B. A.: Incidence rates of cancer in Kyandondo County, Uganda, 1954–60. *J. Nat. Cancer Inst.* 35:789–821, 1965.

16. Denues, A. R. T., and Munz, W.: Malignancies at the hospital of Dr. Albert Schweitzer, Lambarene, Gabon, 1950–65. *Int. J. Cancer* 2:406–411, 1967.

17. Dimock, E. M.: The prevention of constipation. *Brit. Med. J.* 2:906–909, 1937.

18. Dolbey, R. V., and Mooro, A. W.: The incidence of cancer in Egypt. *Lancet* 1:587–590, 1924.

19. Doll, R.: The geographical distribution of cancer. *Brit. J. Cancer* 23:1–8, 1969.

20. Doll, R., Payne, P., and Waterhouse, J., Eds.: Cancer Incidence in Five Continents. UICC Report. Heidelberg, Springer-Verlag, 1966.

21. Edington, G. M.: Malignant disease in the Gold Coast. *Brit. J. Cancer* 10:595–608, 1956.

22. Eshleman, J. L.: A study of the relative incidence of malignant tumours seen at Shirati Hospital in Tanzania. *E. Afr. Med. J.* 43:273–283, 1966.

23. Haddow, A.: Chemical carcinogens and their modes of action. *Brit. Med. Bull.* 14:79–92, 1958.

24. ———: The possible causes of cancer—our present knowledge. Abbottempo, Bk. 4, Abbott Universal Ltd., 1970, pp. 8–11.

25. Halls, J.: Bowel content shift during normal defaecation. *Proc. Roy. Soc. Med.* 58:859–860, 1965.

26. Higginson, J.: Etiology of gastrointestinal cancer in man. *In* Tumors of the Alimentary Tract in Africans. Nat. Cancer Inst. Monograph 25. (A symposium organized by UICC). Bethesda, Nat. Cancer Inst., 1967, pp. 191–198.

27. Hill, M. J., and Crowther, J. S., Drasar, B. S., Hawksworth, G., Aries, V., and Williams, R. E. O.: Bacteria and aetiology of cancer of large bowel. *Lancet* 1:95–99, 1970.

28. Hinton, J. M., Lennard-Jones, J. E., and Young, A. C.: A new method for studying gut transit times using radio-opaque markers. *Gut* 10:842–847, 1969.

29. Hoffman, K.: Untersuchungen uber die Zusammensetzung der Stuhlflora Wahrend eines langdauernden Erhahrungsversuches mit kohlenhydratreicher, mit fettreicher und mit eiweissreicher Kost. *Zbl. Bkt. l Abt. Orig.* 192:500–508, 1964.

30. Holmgren, G. O. R., and Mynors, J. M.: Personal communication, 1970.

31. Hutt, M. S. R. and Templeton, A. C.: Personal communication, 1970.

32. Kocour, E. J.: Diverticulosis of the colon. *Amer. J. Surg.* 37:430–436, 1937.

33. Kohler, R.: The incidence of colonic diverticulosis in Finland and Sweden. *Acta. Chir. Scand.* 126:148–155, 1963.

34. Lacassagne, A., Buu-Hoï, N. P., and Zajdela, F.: Carcinogenic activity of apocholic acid. *Nature* 190:1007–1008, 1961.

35. ———, ———, and ———: Carcinogenic activity in situ of further steroid compounds. *Nature* 209:1026–1027, 1966.

36. Lawrence, J. C.: Gastrointestinal polyps. Statistical study of malignancy incidence. *Amer. J. Surg.* 31:499–505, 1936.

37. Linsell, C. A.: Cancer incidence in Kenya 1957–64. *Brit. J. Cancer* 21:465–473, 1967.

38. Lynch, J. B., Hassan, A. M., and Omar, A.: Cancer in the Sudan. *Sudan Med. J.* 2:29–37, 1963.

39. McVay, J. R., Jr.: Association of Appendectomy and Neoplastic Disease. Summary of Scientific Exhibit Presented at Tenth International Cancer Congress, Houston, May 1970.

40. Martinez, I.: Cancer in Puerto Rico. Report from the Central Cancer Registry, Department of Health, Puerto Rico, 1968; Personal communication, 1970.

41. Morson, B. C., and Bussey, H. J. R.: Predisposing causes of intestinal cancer. Current problems in surgery—a series of monthly clinical monographs. Chi-

cago, Year Book Medical Publishers Inc., February 1970.

42. Mulligan, T. O.: The pattern of malignant disease in Ilesha, Western Nigeria. *Brit. J. Cancer* 24:1–10, 1969.

43. Nasr, A. L. Aboul: Epidemiology of cancer of the gastrointestinal tract in Egyptians. *In* Tumors of the Alimentary Tract in Africans. Nat. Cancer Inst. Monograph 25 (A symposium organized by UICC). Bethesda, Nat. Cancer Inst., 1967, pp. 1–6.

44. Oettle, A. G.: Cancer in Africa, especially in regions south of the Sahara. *J. Nat. Cancer Inst.* 33: 383–439, 1964.

45. ———: Primary neoplasms of the alimentary canal in Whites and Bantu of the Transvaal, 1949–1953. A histopathological series. *In* Tumors of the Alimentary Tract in Africans. Nat. Cancer Inst. Monograph 25 (A symposium organized by UICC). Bethesda, Nat. Cancer Inst., 1967; pp. 97–110.

46. Painter, N. S.: Diverticular disease of the colon. A disease of this century. *Lancet* 2:586–588, 1969.

47. ———: Diverticular Disease of the Colon—A Disease of Western Civilization. Disease-a-Month Series. Chicago, Year Book Medical Publishers Inc., 1970.

48. Painter, N. S., and Burkitt, D. P.: Diverticular disease—a deficiency disease of civilization. Brit. Med. J. (In press).

49. Prates, M. D., and Torres, F. O.: A cancer survey in Lourenço Marques, Portuguese East Africa. *J. Nat. Cancer Inst.* 35:729–757, 1965.

50. Public Health Monograph: Morbidity from cancer in the United States, 1956.

51. Quinland, W. S., and Cuff, J. R.: Primary cancer in the negro. Anatomic distribution of 300 cases. *Arch. Path.* 30:393–402, 1940.

52. Rider, J. A., Kirsner, J. B. Moeller, H. C., and Palmer, W. L.: Polyps of the colon and rectum. *Amer. J. Med.* 16:555–564, 1954.

53. ———, ———, ———, and ———: Polyps of the colon and rectum. *J. Amer. Med. Ass.* 170:633–638, 1959.

54. Robertson, M. A.: Clinical observations on cancer patterns at the non-white hospital, Baragwanath, Johannesburg, 1948–1964. *S. Afr. Med. J.* 43:915–931. 1969.

55. Schonland, M., and Bradshaw, E.: Cancer in the Natal African and Indian 1964–66. *Int. J. Cancer* 3:304–316, 1968.

56. Schowengerdt, C. G., Hedges, G. R., Yaw, P. B., and Altemeier, W. A.: Diverticulosis, diverticulitis and diabetes. A review of 740 cases. *Arch. Surg.* 98:500–504. 1969.

57. Short, A. R.: The causation of appendicitis. *Brit. J. Surg.* 8:171–186, 1920.

58. Skinner, M. E. G.: Malignant disease of the gastrointestinal tract in the Rhodesian African, with special reference to the urban population of Bulawayo. A Preliminary Report. *In* Tumors of the Alimentary Tract in Africans. Nat. Cancer Inst. Monograph 25 (A symposium organized by UICC). Bethesda: Nat. Cancer Inst. 1967, pp. 57–71.

59. Spjut, H. J., and Spratt, J. S., Jr.: Endemic and morphological similarities existing between spontaneous neoplasms in man and 3:2'-dimethyl-4-aminodiphenyl induced colonic neoplasms in rats. *Ann. Surg.* 161:309–324, 1965.

60. Steiner, P. E.: Cancer: Race and Geography. Baltimore, The Williams & Wilkins Co., 1954.

61. Stemmermann, G. N.: Patterns of disease among Japanese living in Hawaii. *Arch. Environ. Health* 20:266–273, 1970.

62. Stewart, H. L.: Experimental alimentary tract cancer. *In* Tumors of the Alimentary Tract in Africans. Nat. Cancer Inst. Monograph 25. (A symposium organized by UICC). Bethesda, Nat. Cancer Inst. 1967, pp. 199–217.

63. Streicher, M. K., and Quirk, R. M.: Constipation: clinical and roentgenologic evaluation of the use of bran. *Amer. J. Dig. Dis.* 10:179–181, 1943.

64. Sutherland, J. C.: Cancer in a mission hospital in South Africa. *Cancer* 22:372–378, 1968.

65. Thijs, A.: Considérations sur les tumeurs malignes des indigenes du Congo belge et du Ruanda-Urundi. A propos de 2,536 cas. *Ann. Soc. Belg. Med. Trop.* 37:483–514, 1957.

66. Walker, A. R. P.: The effect of recent changes of food habits on bowel motility. *S. Afr. Med. J.* 21:590–596, 1947.

67. Walker, A. R. P.: Crude fibre, bowel motility and pattern of diet. *S. Afr. Med. J.* 35:114–115, 1961.

68. Walker, A. R. P., Walker, B. F., and Richardson, B. D.: Bowel transit times in Bantu population. *Brit. Med. J.* 3:238, 1969.

69. Walker, A. R. P., Walker, B. F., and Richardson, B. D.: Bowel transit times in Bantu population. *Brit. Med. J.* 3:48–49, 1970.

70. Wozasek, O., and Steigmann, F.: Studies on colon irritation. III. Bulk of faeces. *Amer. J. Dig. Dis.* 9:423–425, 1942.

71. Wynder, E. L., and Shigamatsu, T.: Environmental factors of cancer of the colon and rectum. *Cancer* 20:1520–1561, 1967.

72. Wynder, E. L., Kajitani, T., Ishikawa, S., Dodo, H., and Takano, A.: Environmental factors of cancer of the colon and rectum. II. Japanese epidemiological data. *Cancer* 23:1210–1220, 1969.

Epidemiologic and Dietary Evidence for a Specific Nutritional Predisposition to Esophageal Cancer

by Schalk J. Van Rensburg

ABSTRACT—A total of 21 different regions were found to have a very low relative frequency and/or low incidence rates of esophageal cancer (the male mean being 0.6 and the range being 0.1-1.0/100,000 per annum). In all these areas the dietary staples were either sorghum, millet, cassava, yams, or peanuts or a combination of these items. In another 17 areas that had a high risk for esophageal cancer (the male mean being 41.3 and the range being 16.5-86.0/100,000 per annum), the dietary staple was invariably corn or wheat. It is calculated that dietary staples associated with a high risk for esophageal cancer will be marginal or deficient particularly in riboflavin, nicotinic acid, magnesium, and zinc, whereas dietary staples associated with a low risk for esophageal cancer will be rich in these substances. The evidence presented supports the concept that these high rates of esophageal cancer in diverse peoples are associated with long-standing deficiencies of a few micronutrients and explains epidemiologic features such as geographic variation, recent emergence of the disease in Africa, and the role of alcohol abuse.—JNCI 1981; 67:243-251.

The remarkable geographic and regional variations in the incidence of esophageal cancer have been documented in many parts of the world (*1, 2*) and remain largely unexplained. In general, the male age-standardized incidence rates for esophageal cancer reported for affluent Western populations are less than 5/100,000 p.a., and the major risk factors for the development of esophageal cancer are alcohol abuse and smoking (*3*).

At the other extreme are a few localities such as those in Kazakhstan (U.S.S.R.), northeastern Iran, Henan Province of China, and southern Transkei where the male rates of esophageal cancer exceed 100/100,000 p.a. and as such equate with the male rates for heart disease in the West, the major single cause of adult deaths. No evidence for a role of alcohol abuse has emerged from these areas; however, exceedingly mutagenic pyrolysis products of opium and tobacco are ingested in Iran and Transkei, respectively (*4*). Smoking of home-grown tobacco and marijuana, both of which produce pyrolysates that are more mutagenic than is any commercially available tobacco (*5*), is traditional in Transkei and can hardly account for the increased incidence of esophageal cancer in recent years. Some evidence of a suboptimal geochemical environment has emerged from Transkei (*6*), Iran (*7*), China (*8*), and even the United States (*9*). Mineral element deficiencies may account for increased fungal invasion and mycotoxin contamination of corn, which have been reported in areas of Transkei with populations at high risk for esophageal cancer (*10*). Currently, we are exploring other possible interactions with the environment that may account for increased exposure to carcinogens (*11*).

Large populations, particularly in Africa and Asia, have esophageal cancer rates intermediate between the low rates of affluent Western countries and the extremely high rates in some rural localities mentioned

ABBREVIATIONS USED: kcal=kilocalories; p.a.=per annum; R.D.A.= recommended dietary allowance(s).

Schalk J. van Rensburg is with the National Research Institute for Nutritional Diseases of the South African Medical Research Council, P. O. Box 70, Tygerberg 7505, South Africa.

Reprinted with permission from *Journal of the National Cancer Institute,* Vol. 67, No. 2, August 1981, pp. 243-251.

above. Intermediate rates can be found in diverse groups, some of whom are urbanized, such as black males living in Soweto who now have an esophageal cancer rate of 24/100,000 black males (*12*). Interspersed among areas in Africa with populations at high risk for esophageal cancer are communities with a very low incidence of esophageal cancer. We became familiar with two such regions (northern Namibia and central Mozambique) where alcohol abuse, smoking, and malnutrition did not seem less than elsewhere, yet considerably fewer esophageal cancers than would be expected among affluent whites were diagnosed. The possibility that a deficiency in a few critical protective micronutrients is the unifying factor in the etiology of the disease among diverse people in different geographic regions was therefore further examined.

Vitamin A has often been suggested as being deficient in populations at high risk for esophageal cancer, but this has never been convincingly demonstrated. Furthermore, our unpublished epidemiologic and experimental data, as well as the data of others (*3*), are not consistent with a prophylactic effect of vitamin A on esophageal carcinogenesis. Vitamin C may well be important where exposure to carcinogens or their precursors is unusual, but there are populations with a very low risk of developing esophageal cancer in whom scurvy is not rare (*13*).

Riboflavin deficiency has long been known to promote hepatic and skin carcinogenesis in certain animal models and to cause extensive lesions in the esophageal epithelium of humans and animals (*14*). Zinc levels may be lower in esophageal cancer patients than in healthy controls (*15*), and the zinc levels in the hair of Iranians at high risk for esophageal cancer are very low (*16*). Experimentally, severe zinc deficiency increased the incidence of methylbenzylnitrosamine-induced esophageal cancers in rats (*17*). When rats were rendered subclinically zinc-deficient by being fed low levels of dietary phytate, the sizes of the methylbenzylnitrosamine-induced esophageal tumors were increased (*18*).

In this study some basic differences in dietary practices of populations all over the world at high and low risks of developing esophageal cancer are explored, and the likelihood of intermittent deficient intakes of riboflavin, nicotinic acid (niacin), zinc, and magnesium is calculated. Agreement of the principal results with relevant distinctive epidemiologic features is also examined.

MATERIALS AND METHODS

Esophageal cancer occurrence data.—We preferred to use incidence rates from recognized cancer registries when available, but we supplemented these data with data from a few sporadic studies that are referenced in table 1. A second method used was the use of the relative frequency, defined as the percentage of total tumors diagnosed that represented esophageal carcinomas. The two decades extending from 1950 to 1970

generally represent a good period as far as medical services are concerned (particularly in Africa); therefore, only published series embracing parts of this period were accepted. Obviously, the relative frequency is liable to many more pitfalls than are actual incidence rates, but it does provide useful corroborative data (table 2) in view of the limited availability of statistics on incidence.

Dietary staples.—Dietary items for a particular area were accepted only if the weight of evidence indicated that the staple had been a major item in the diet for at least three decades prior to assessment of esophageal cancer frequency. A number of reviews (*1, 19–22*) provided data on the cultivation and use of dietary staples in Africa. These reviews were supplemented by our considerable experience in southern Africa, which included projects involving food surveys in northern Namibia (*23*), central Mozambique (*24*), and recently in Transkei. Some information on China was obtained from the reports given in (*25, 26*). Further information on China and some on Curaçao appeared in a study of plant usage and esophageal cancer zones (*27*). Historical dietary practices in Kazakhstan were described by Dr. L. Gricute and extensive dietary studies in Iran have been reported (*28*). It was also verified that rice is a prominent dietary item in the following groups at high risk of developing esophageal cancer: Japanese (*29, 30*), Puerto Ricans (*31*), and Singapore Chinese (*32*).

Composition of foods.—Nutrient composition was ascertained from standard tables (*33, 34*). As far as possible, the zinc content was read from provisional standard tables (*35*), but in a few instances of African items (sorghum, millet, and cassava) the mean of at least five samples analyzed by atomic absorption spectrophotometry for zinc in our laboratory was used. For more common items such as locally produced corn or wheat, our zinc and magnesium analyses yielded results similar to published U.S. values. Dietary staples from areas with populations at exceptionally high risk of developing esophageal cancer have, however, not been analyzed and since a suboptimal geochemical environment is evident in some such areas, the use of standard tables may overestimate their nutrient intakes.

R.D.A. were those approved by the National Academy of Sciences in 1980. In general, calculations were for young men, and we assumed a daily energy requirement for these subjects of 3,000 kcal.

RESULTS

Occurrence of Esophageal Cancer and Use of Dietary Staples

Similar patterns emerged when cancer occurrence was assessed by the use of actual esophageal cancer rates (table 1) or when the relative frequency of esophageal cancer to total tumors diagnosed (table 2) was used. Esophageal cancer seemed to be rare in a total of 21 different localities, and the main dietary staple in all of these areas was either sorghum, millet,

TABLE 1.—*Major dietary staples and incidence rates (per 100,000 p.a.) of esophageal cancer*

Locality	Date	Source	Male rate	Male & female rate	Female rate	Major dietary staples
Nigeria, Ibadan	1960–62	(*36*)	0.4		0.1	Sorghum, millet, yams
	1960–70	(*37*)	0.3		0.3	Sorghum, millet, yams
Uganda, Kyadondo	1954–60	(*36*)	1.0		0.5	Millet, sorghum
Namibia, Owambo	1968–72	(*13*)	0.1		0	Millet, sorghum
Mozambique:						
Inhambane	1968–72	*a*	<1.0		0	Cassava, sorghum, peanuts
Maputo	1956–60	(*36*)	2.6		0	Cassava, peanuts, corn
China, Shantung	1959–60	(*38*)		0.32		Sorghum, millet
Japan	1968–71	(*37*)	7.9		3.4	Rice
Singapore (Chinese)	1968–72	(*37*)	11.1		4.4	Rice
India, Bombay	1968–72	(*37*)	6.6		5.1	Rice
United States, Puerto Rico	1968–72	(*37*)	12.9		4.8	Rice
Iran:						
Gilan	1960–61	(*7*)	16.0		5.5	Rice
West Mazandaran	1960–61	(*7*)	25.4		18.0	Wheat, rice
East Mazandaran	1960–61	(*7*)	86.0		87.1	Wheat
U.S.S.R., Kazakhstan	1959	(*39*)		75.6		Wheat
	1965	(*39*)	43.5		49.7	Wheat
China, Linxian	1959–70	(*8*)		108.6		Corn, wheat
Zimbabwe, Bulawayo	1968–72	(*37*)	16.5		0.8	Corn
South Africa:						
Soweto	1966–75	(*12*)	23.7		4.2	Corn, wheat
Durban	1964–66	(*40*)	24.9		7.3	Corn
Transkei:						
Whole	1955–59	(*41*)	37.2		21.1	Corn
Whole	1965–69	(*41*)	34.9		19.3	Corn
Butterworth	1965–69	(*41*)	79.4		36.5	Corn
Bizana	1965–69	(*41*)	11.5		5.2	Corn, sorghum
Curaçao	1960–65	(*42*)		20.9		Corn

a Simpson RL: Personal communication.

cassava, or yams or a combination of these staples. The association may not be limited to western and central Africa, since in one study in China the lowest esophageal cancer rate was found in Shantung (*38*), a province that has been mentioned as a chief producer of sorghum (*27*). A further dietary item that may be associated with a low risk for esophageal cancer is peanuts, known to be used in most areas of Africa with populations at low risk of developing esophageal cancer and not to any significant extent in any of the regions with populations at high risk for esophageal cancer.

Esophageal cancer rates that shall be referred to as moderate (8–16/100,000 p.a. for males) were invariably found for rice-eating populations. This association seems to apply to the Middle East, Asia, and possibly even Puerto Rico.

If a high risk for males is arbitrarily defined as an esophageal cancer rate of 17 or higher, then the data in table 1 show that in all 10 localities where corn and/or wheat are the main dietary staples, the populations may be classed as having a high risk for esophageal cancer. The high relative risk for esophageal cancer (table 2) of corn- and wheat-consuming populations also did not overlap with the risk of the groups at moderate or low risk for esophageal cancer. The two

sets of data encompass 17 high-risk regions where the male esophageal cancer rate seems remarkably constant, probably most being in the region of 20–25, except for four regions. Extraordinarily high rates seem to be limited to Kazakhstan, Mazandaran, Linxian, and Transkei.

The relative contribution of nutrition and carcinogen exposure to such high esophageal cancer rates is of interest. To explore the relationship, we plotted the data on bread consumption and esophageal cancer from Iran (*28*) (text-fig. 1). There appears to be a linear increase of cancer rate with increasing bread consumption up to a moderate truncated rate of approximately 120, but higher cancer rates are apparently dependent on other factors. Exactly the inverse type of relationship may be demonstrated if one plots the rice consumption data against the same cancer incidence data. Of considerable interest in text-figure 1 is the absence of very high cancer rates in persons consuming less than approximately 400 g bread/day and consequently using relatively more rice. Some of these populations likely were also exposed to a hypothesized extraordinary source of carcinogens; therefore, a potent protective effect of diet may be operative. However, the extent to which a poor diet can promote carcinogenesis is probably limited in the presence of average carcinogen

TABLE 2.—*Major dietary staples and the relative frequency (% of total tumors diagnosed) of esophageal cancer*

Locality	Date	Source	No. of esophageal tumors/ total No. of tumors	Relative frequency	Major dietary staples
Senegal	1950–53	(22)[a]	0/1,183	0	Sorghum, millet
Ghana	1942–55	(22)	0/243	0	Yams, millet
	1923–55	(22)	1/149	0.7	Yams, millet
Nigeria:					
Ibadan	1962–64	(22)	3/318	0.9	Sorghum, millet, yams
Ilesha	1954–67	(22)	0/239	0	Sorghum, millet, yams
Cameroon	1946–52	(22)	0/132	0	Cassava, sorghum, yams
Gabon, Lambarene	1950–65	(22)	0/97	0	Cassava, yams
Congo	1965–66	(22)	0/243	0	Cassava, yams
Zaire	1939–55	(22)	0/1,161	0	Cassava, yams
	1953–60	(22)	0/207	0	Cassava, yams
Angola	1966–72	(13)	0/35	0	Millet, sorghum
Namibia (Southwest Africa)	1966–72	(13)	1/305	0.3	Millet, sorghum
Sudan	1935–54	(22)	1/1,337	0.1	Millet, sorghum
Uganda:					
Northwest	1966–69	(43)	3/153	2.0	Sorghum, millet
Northeast	1964–67	(22)	0/99	0	Millet, cassava
Southwest	1964–67	(22)	1/172	0.6	Millet, sorghum
Tanzania:					
Mvumi	1966–69	(43)	0/100	0	Millet, sorghum
Mtwara	1964–67	(22)	1/112	0.9	Sorghum
Shiriti	1966–69	(43)	1/95	1.1	Millet
Rwanda and Burundi	1968–69	(43)	0/64	0	Millet, cassava
Mozambique, Maputo	1956–60	(22)	7/405	1.7	Cassava, sorghum, corn
India, south		(44)		5.6	Rice
Japan, Tokyo		(45)		5.3	Rice
Kenya:					
Kisumu	1965–68	(22)	116/394	29.4	Corn
Maseno	1950–64	(22)	30/134	22.4	Corn
Central	1964–69	(22)	114/475	24.0	Corn
Tanzania, Tanga	1966–69	(43)	10/101	9.9	Corn
Malawi:					
North	1967–69	(43)	9/119	7.6	Corn, millet
South	1967–69	(43)	74/371	19.9	Corn
Zimbabwe, Bulawayo	1963–67	(22)	73/450	16.2	Corn
South Africa:					
Johannesburg	1953–55	(22)	55/491	11.2	Corn
Johannesburg	1962–64	(22)	371/1,350	27.5	Corn, wheat
Durban	1964–66	(40)	136/687	19.8	Corn
Ciskei	1960–63	(22)	25/139	18.0	Corn
Transkei	1958–65	(22)	136/259	52.5	Corn
Transkei, west	1964–71	(46)	167/361	46.3	Corn
Transkei, central	1965–69	(41)	496/1,038	47.8	Corn
U.S.S.R., Kazakhstan	1959–65	(39)	1,426/4,737	30.1	Wheat

[a] Cited in review.

exposure. The same interaction of diet could account for the rarity of esophageal cancer in pre-1940 Transkei where a particularly mutagenic tobacco (5) had been used extensively but together with a sorghum-based diet for at least a century.

The principal results of the diet association study are summarized in table 3. An outstanding feature is the difference in esophageal cancer risk between populations subsisting on sorghum, millet, cassava, yams, or peanuts and those living on corn and/or wheat. On the basis of incidence rates for both sexes, the difference in the risk is 92 times, whereas the relative frequency shows a difference in the risk of 81 times. Most significantly, all the evidence indicates a considerably reduced risk for esophageal cancer among African populations living in a traditional manner and not using wheat or corn, as compared to the risk of affluent Western populations

The preponderance of male cases over female cases generally seems most evident in Western populations. Elsewhere, as shown in table 3, the sex ratio decreases with increasing risk. It has long been known that in all of the highest incidence areas of the world, the sex ratio tends to approach unity.

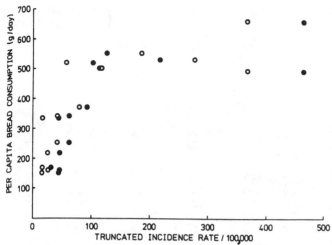

TEXT-FIGURE 1.—Relationship between bread consumption and the incidence rate of esophageal cancer. ●, males; ○, females. As bread consumption decreases, rice consumption increases. *Note* the absence of very high incidence rates when <400 g of bread/day is eaten. The similar susceptibility of males and females is possibly due to the absence of any significant role of conventional smoking and alcohol use. Data from the Caspian littoral of Iran (*28*).

Chemical Composition of Foods

Nutrient concentrations of dietary staples are readily available from published tables (*33–35*), and the available data for those staples under discussion and for some other items of interest have for selected nutrients been compiled in table 4. Those familiar with Africa know that many communities will subsist for considerable periods on virtually a single dietary staple. Such a situation has been documented in Transkei (*47*) and in a region of Iran with a population at high risk for esophageal cancer (*28*) where at times total energy requirements may be derived almost exclusively from corn and wheat products, respectively. The incidental intake of micronutrients would then depend on their concentration in relation to the calorific value of the staple food.

Simple calculations made on the data in table 4 show that if total energy is derived from refined wheat or corn products, then the individual would be in a positive total protein balance. Protein intake would be inadequate only in the cases of bananas, cassava, and yams, and indeed in regions of West Africa with a low esophageal cancer risk cases of clinical protein deficiency are not rare. Such an assessment of the role of protein naturally does not consider the quality that could conceivably be important in improving the resistance to esophageal cancer.

Similarly, although wheat, white corn, sorghum, and cassava contain virtually no vitamin A, yellow corn, which is commonly used in regions of Transkei with a high esophageal cancer risk, contains more than adequate amounts of carotene. In addition, the cancer incidence is not associated with the ascorbic acid content of staple foods. Scurvy has been reported by early Portuguese writers to be common among the sorghum- and millet-eating populations of southern Angola and quite recently in populations immediately to the south in northern Namibia (*13*) where the esophageal cancer risk is exceedingly low.

The composition of whole or processed wheat and corn differs greatly as far as the remaining nutrients listed in table 4 are concerned. The vitamins and minerals are largely associated with the husks; therefore, even slight refinement from, for example, wholemeal to brown bread meal will drastically reduce the content of these nutrients. In text-figure 2 the differences in the amount of riboflavin, nicotinic acid, zinc, and magnesium contributed by the equivalent of 3,000 kcal of each staple are illustrated.

The riboflavin content of staples associated with low, moderate, or high risks of esophageal cancer is not a good indicator of esophageal cancer risk. The extensive studies in Iran also did not demonstrate clear

TABLE 3.—*Summary of main results from the study on diet and its association with esophageal cancer occurrence*

Parameters	Low risk	Moderate risk	High risk	Utah, 1966–70[a]	Detroit (black), 1969–71[a]
Mean cancer rate:[b]					
No.[c]	5	5	9		
Male	0.56	10.90	41.27	1.7	12.7
Female	0.18	4.64	27.02	0.4	3.3
Male:female	3.11	2.37	1.53	4.2	3.8
Relative frequency	0.33 (20)[d]	5.50 (2)[d]	26.78 (14)[d]		
Dietary staples	Sorghum Millet Cassava Yams Peanuts	Rice	Corn Wheat	Mixed Western	Mixed Western with alcohol

[a] Utah and Detroit data are extremes for U.S. cancer registries (*37*).
[b] Per 100,000 p.a., all ages.
[c] No. of localities for which means were calculated.
[d] *No. in parentheses* indicate No. of localities for which means were calculated.

TABLE 4.—*Chemical composition (per 100 g) of foods used by populations at high and low risks of developing esophageal cancer*[a]

Food	Moisture %	Kcal	Vitamin A, IU	Ascorbic acid, mg	Riboflavin, mg	Nicotinic acid, mg	Zinc, mg	Magnesium, mg	Calcium, mg	Phosphorus, mg	Protein, g
Wheat:											
Whole	12	333	0	0	0.12	4.3	2.4	113	41	372	13.3
Flour	12	363	0	0	0.05	0.9	0.8	25	16	87	10.5
Corn:											
White whole	12	351	0	0	0.14	1.45	2.1	94	4.1	219	9.4
Flour	12	368	0	0	0.08	0.7	0.4	16	2.2	148	7.5
Rice:											
Brown	12	360	0	0	0.05	4.7	1.8	119	32	221	7.5
Polished	12	362	0	0	0.03	1.6	1.3	28	24	94	6.7
Sorghum	11.7	349	0	0	0.19	3.9	2.1	161	29	324	12.1
Millet (dehusked)	12.4	356	220	0	0.16	3.2	3.2	125	42	269	11.6
Cassava flour	14.2	320	0	14	0.07	1.6	3.0		148	104	1.7
Yams (mean, three types)	73.0	101	502	0.3	0.18	0.9		34	43	43	1.7
Potatoes	79.8	76	35	20	0.04	1.2	0.3	27	14	53	2.1
Peanuts	1.8	582	360	0	0.13	17.1	3.0	181	74	407	26.2
Beans	11.6	338	0	2	0.22	2.1	2.8	132	106	429	21.3
Milk	88.5	64	140	1	0.15	0.07	0.4	13	133	88	3.2
Meat (lean rib)	66.8	193	20	0	0.18	5.0	4.2	24	12	208	20.7
Spinach	90.7	26	8,100	51	0.20	0.6	0.8	62	106	51	3.2
Pumpkins	95.0	15	1,600	9	0.11	0.6	0.09	12	21	44	0.8
Bananas	75.7	85	190	10	0.06	0.6	0.2	31	8	26	1.1

[a] Data taken from standard international tables (*33, 35*) as far as possible and supplemented by a local source (*34*) for sorghum, millet, cassava, and yams. In areas of poor agricultural potential, the use of these tables may overestimate some intakes.

differences in the incidence of angular stomatitis between bread- and rice-eating populations (*48*), but there is some evidence that esophageal cancer patients from both populations had a lower intake of riboflavin than did controls (*49*). Since the vitamin is uniformly low in staples associated with high and moderate risks of esophageal cancer, it may well play some role.

Deficient intakes of nicotinic acid, zinc, and magnesium from either a corn- or wheaten bread-based diet would largely depend on the extraction rate of the flour. In southern Africa most of these products are consumed after processing at least to the level of the flour or meal (text-fig. 2). The values for whole wheat will be considerably reduced also in Iran even if a flour having a high extraction rate is used. Binding elements such as fiber and phytate will naturally reduce further the availability of zinc and magnesium.

The composition of brown rice would indicate that it is likely to be a staple associated with a low risk of esophageal cancer, whereas the process of polishing reduces the magnesium, zinc, and nicotinic acid to levels similar to those of staples associated with a high risk. Final assessment of risk associated with rice clearly awaits more detailed studies on specified types of rice.

If one considers the above evidence, there seems to be a good inverse relationship between the esophageal cancer risk and the amount of magnesium, zinc, and nicotinic acid in the diet. The only likely exception is the nicotinic acid content of a brown bread diet where the intake may be marginally adequate; the availability of magnesium in an unrefined diet is questionable (*50, 51*), and we have confirmed the low magnesium levels in various cornmeals used by the Soweto population.

Numerous dietary studies conducted on populations at high risk for esophageal cancer have invariably revealed low intakes of green leafy vegetables and animal products. In Africa, however, there are virtually vegetarian societies who supplement their diet with peanuts and have a very low risk of esophageal cancer. The question arises: Will a modest portion of green vegetable (e.g., spinach) and either meat or peanuts rectify the deficient intake of those nutrients considered important? The data in table 5 show that clinical signs of deficiencies will probably develop with a diet of corn or wheaten flours and that addition to the diet of a portion of green leafy vegetable and a modest portion of meat or peanuts will prevent both clinical and biochemical signs of deficiencies in the case of riboflavin, nicotinic acid, zinc, and magnesium.

DISCUSSION

The two approaches used to assess esophageal cancer risk have pitfalls, and the published data are not always strictly comparable. Yet the methods were independent of each other, and both demonstrated marked differences associated with the nature of the staple diet. Of particular interest was the exceedingly low risk of esophageal cancer, lower than that for affluent Western societies, for some African communities living in a traditional manner where malnutrition

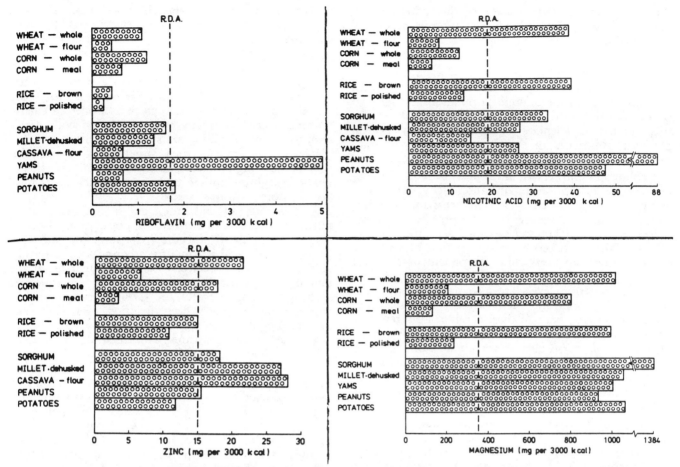

Text-figure 2.—The amount of riboflavin, nicotinic acid, zinc, and magnesium that would be ingested if total energy were derived from each dietary staple. Wheat and corn are considered staples associated with high risk of esophageal cancer, rice is associated with an intermediate risk, and sorghum, millet, cassava, yams, and peanuts are associated with a low risk. *Note* that much of the zinc and magnesium in whole wheat and corn are known to be unavailable.

Table 5.—*Nutrient content of cereal diets associated with a high risk of esophageal cancer when supplemented with spinach, meat, or peanuts*

Source of kcal[a]	Riboflavin, mg[b]	Nicotinic acid, mg[c]	Zinc, mg[d]	Magnesium, mg[e]
Wheaten flour, 100%	0.41	7.4	6.6	206
Cornmeal, 100%	0.65	5.7	3.3	130
Cornmeal, 87.5%; meat, 10%; spinach, 2.5%	1.43	14.4	19.4	330
Wheaten flour, 87.5%; meat, 10%; spinach, 2.5%	1.22	15.9	22.3	418
Wheaten flour, 87.5%; peanuts, 10%; spinach, 2.5%	1.01	17.0	17.35	452
Cornmeal, 87.5%; peanuts, 10%; spinach, 2.5%	1.22	15.5	14.5	386

[a] A total of 3,000 kcal/day: 10% meat = 155 g lean beef, 10% peanuts = 52 g roasted, and 2.5% spinach = 288 g (91% moisture).
[b] R.D.A. = 1.7 mg.
[c] R.D.A. = 19 mg.
[d] R.D.A. = 21 mg.
[e] R.D.A. = 350 mg.

is not rare. The sex ratios of patients with esophageal cancer from both the Western communities and the African communities at low risk for esophageal cancer were high, which suggests that factors such as alcohol abuse and smoking, which impinge largely on the male, are particularly responsible for the few cases that do occur.

Without a single exception, all of the many communities found to be living mostly on wheat or corn had a considerable esophageal cancer risk. Thus either there is, on an universal basis, a unique carcinogen peculiar to wheat and corn, or commonly occurring carcinogens (e.g., polycyclic aromatic hydrocarbons, nitrosamines in food and drink, and tobacco smoke carcinogens) are, at the levels to which most people are exposed, collectively adequate to induce transformation in the nutritionally predisposed esophageal epithelial tissue, resulting in moderately high cancer rates.

If a good diet has such a potent protective effect, then in practice the nutritional status of a population will be the main determinant of esophageal cancer rates and should explain some of the more unusual epidemiologic phenomena, such as the role of alcohol and also the emergence of esophageal cancer in Africa during the last few decades.

Increased esophageal cancer risk with alcohol consumption and smoking can be readily demonstrated only in lower socioeconomic populations, which can be explained by the hypothesis that alcohol acts by precipitating deficiencies of one or a few critical protective nutrients that are usually taken in marginally adequate amounts by the population.

Alcohol abuse lowers vitamin status by reducing vitamin intakes, absorption, and metabolic activation as well as by increasing the tissue requirements for vitamins. There is ample evidence for the prevalence of deficiencies of riboflavin and nicotinic acid in alcoholics (52, 53). Many workers have shown that plasma zinc concentrations are very low in patients with liver cirrhosis of alcoholic origin (54). Low serum levels and increased excretion levels are also seen in some non-cirrhotic alcoholics and in individuals suffering from acute alcoholism; both of these levels readily revert to normal after abstinence from alcohol (55). Hypomagnesemia is, of course, also present in alcoholic patients. Ethanol promotes urinary excretion of magnesium in both normal and alcoholic subjects, but also important are excessive fecal losses superimposed on a dietary deficiency of magnesium (56).

Apart from increasing the requirements for all four nutrients under discussion, acute and chronic consumption of alcohol can have extensive metabolic consequences (57, 58). Some attractive hypotheses on alcohol-related biochemical changes at the intracellular level have been proposed (59, 60) that would go far to explain some characteristics of alcohol-related cancers such as site specificity. Nutritional deficiency involvement, however, remains an integral component.

In central and southern Africa, within four decades esophageal cancer emerged from a virtually unknown disease to attain almost epidemic proportions, an increase that has been well documented in at least a dozen regions (1, 22, 61). Rural as well as urban groups were involved; concurrently the esophageal cancer rates of U.S. blacks increased substantially (62). Again, the only logical explanation for the same phenomenon in diverse groups seems to lie in changing circumstances that have resulted in modulation of nutritional status.

Animal protein sources have relatively declined since the turn of the century. From that time there has been no increase in southern African domestic animal populations and there has been a dramatic decline in indigenous fauna, concurrent with a several-fold increase in the human populations. Those people continuing to subsist on sorghum, millet, peanuts, yams, and cassava seemed to have retained considerable resistance to esophageal cancer, but in all high esophageal cancer regions the traditional African crops have given way to the exotic high-yielding and easily cultivated corn and, to a much lesser extent, to wheat. Esophageal

cancer patients today are usually 50–70 years old; in a review of traditional crops (19), evidence is discussed showing that corn cultivation was unknown or of recent origin 50–70 years ago in areas where the cancer rate is now high. The time sequence fits best if it is assumed that prolonged exposure to a predominantly corn diet dating from childhood is necessary to ensure a high esophageal cancer rate in middle-aged or elderly persons. Currently, many communities in both Africa and, for example, China are still in transition as far as dietary staples are concerned, largely due to the promotion of new high-yielding corn and wheat varieties to replace sorghum, millet, and cassava; such areas have been ignored in this study.

A deficiency of nicotinic acid is the outstanding nutritional feature of corn-eating populations. Corn is also deficient in the precursor, tryptophan, and what little nicotinic acid it contains is bound in an unavailable form, unless treated with alkali such as in the making of tortillas in South America. In countries such as the United States and Great Britain, corn and wheat products have been fortified ever since the availability of the vitamin, which was referred to as niacin to avoid confusion with nicotine of tobacco origin. Pellagra emerged as a common disease in Transkei around 1930, some 25 years before esophageal cancer emerged as a frequent cancer (1). Clinically, pellagrins usually have an esophageal mucosa intensely hyperemic and sometimes edematous; some pellagrins develop secondary ulcerations, constrictions, and dysphagia (1). Signs of esophagitis were also found in 80% of individuals among the population of Iran at high risk for esophageal cancer (63).

The magnesium content of African and Asian dietary staples seemed to correlate best with esophageal cancer risk, and in the West the most common cause of hypomagnesemia is alcoholism. In common with the availability of zinc, the availability of magnesium in unrefined diets is poor (50, 64) and when cereals are processed into flours, most of the magnesium is lost. Several epidemiologic and animal studies have suggested an anticarcinogenic effect of magnesium (65). There are many possibilities regarding the biologic plausibility of such an action. These range from the stabilization of DNA replication to the reported ability of magnesium to metabolize the prevalent carcinogen benzo[a]pyrene into a nonharmful form (65).

The immense diversity of cultural and ethnic groups afflicted by high rates of esophageal carcinoma points to a multifactorial etiology as far as carcinogen exposure is concerned. The dominant and unifying factor in the etiology seems to be the nutritional status. Most evidence suggests that a chronic low status of zinc, magnesium, riboflavin, and nicotinic acid, together with an adequate energy and protein intake, will increase the predisposition of the esophageal epithelium to neoplastic transformation and promote tumor growth. Such a mechanism would apply equally to alcoholics in New York (66, 67) as it does to Iranians, Chinese, or Africans at high risk for esophageal cancer.

REFERENCES

(1) WARWICK GP, HARINGTON JS. Some aspects of the epidemiology and etiology of esophageal cancer with particular emphasis on the Transkei, South Africa. Adv Cancer Res 1973; 17:82-215.

(2) DOLL R. Geographical variation in cancer incidence: A clue to causation. World J Surg 1978; 2:595-602.

(3) TUYNS AJ, PÉQUIGNOT G, HENSEN DM. Role of diet, alcohol and tobacco in oesophageal cancer, as illustrated by two contrasting high-incidence areas in the north of Iran and west of France. Front Gastrointest Res 1979; 4:101-110.

(4) HEWER T, ROSE E, GHADIRIAN P, et al. Ingested mutagens from opium and tobacco pyrolysis products and cancer of the oesophagus. Lancet 1978; 2:494-496.

(5) WEHNER FC, VAN RENSBURG SJ, THIEL PG. Mutagenicity of marijuana and Transkei tobacco smoke condensates in the Salmonella/microsome assay. Mutat Res 1980; 77:135-142.

(6) BURRELL RJ, ROACH WA, SHADWELL A. Esophageal cancer in the Bantu of the Transkei associated with mineral deficiency in garden plants. J Natl Cancer Inst 1966; 36:201-214.

(7) KMET J, MAHBOUBI E. Esophageal cancer in the Caspian littoral of Iran: Initial studies. Science 1972; 175:846-853.

(8) The Coordinating Group for Research on Etiology of Esophageal Cancer in North China. The epidemiology and etiology of esophageal cancer in north China: A preliminary report. Chin Med J [Engl] 1975; 1:167-183.

(9) BERG JW. Diet. In: Fraumeni JF Jr, ed. Persons at high risk of cancer. New York: Academic Press, 1975:201-219.

(10) MARASAS WF, VAN RENSBURG SJ, MIROCHA CJ. Incidence of *Fusarium* species and the mycotoxins, deoxynivalenol and zearalenone, in corn produced in esophageal cancer areas in Transkei. J Agric Food Chem 1979; 27:1108-1112.

(11) LAKER MC, HENSLEY M, DE L BEYERS CP, VAN RENSBURG SJ. Environmental associations with oesophageal cancer: An integrated model. S Afr Cancer Bull 1980; 24:69-70.

(12) ISAACSON CI, SELZER G, KAYE V, et al. Cancer in the urban blacks of South Africa. S Afr Cancer Bull 1978; 22:49-84.

(13) GILDENHUYS J. Die siekteprofiel van die Owambo en ń oorsig van die belangrikste voorkomingsmaatreëls. Thesis. Pretoria: Univ Pretoria, 1974.

(14) FOY H, MBAYA V. Riboflavin. Prog Food Nutr Sci 1977; 2:357-394.

(15) LIN HJ, CHAN WC, FONG YY, NEWBERNE PM. Zinc levels in serum, hair and tumors from patients with esophageal cancer. Nutr Rep Int 1977; 15:635-643.

(16) MOBARHAN S, DOWLATSHAHI K, DIBA YY. Hair zinc levels from a normal population of north east Iran with a high incidence of esophageal carcinoma. Am J Clin Nutr 1980; 33:940.

(17) FONG LY, SIVAK A, NEWBERNE PM. Zinc deficiency and methyl-benzylnitrosamine-induced esophageal cancer in rats. JNCI 1978; 61:145-150.

(18) VAN RENSBURG SJ, DU BRUYN DB, VAN SCHALKWYK DJ. Promotion of methylbenzylnitrosamine-induced esophageal cancer in rats by subclinical zinc deficiency. Nutr Rep Int 1980; 22:891-899.

(19) QUIN PJ. Foods and feeding habits of the Pedi with special reference to identification, preparation and nutritive value of the respective foods. Johannesburg: Witwatersrand Univ Press, 1959.

(20) MURDOCH GP. Africa: Its peoples and their culture history. New York: McGraw-Hill, 1959.

(21) ———. Staple subsistence crops of Africa. Geogr Rev 1960; 50:523-540.

(22) COOK P. Cancer of the oesophagus in Africa: A summary and evaluation of the evidence for the frequency of occurrence, and a preliminary indication of the possible association with the consumption of alcoholic drinks made from maize. Br J Cancer 1971; 25:853-880.

(23) RABIE CJ, VAN RENSBURG SJ, VAN DER WATT JJ, LÜBBEN A. Onyalai—the possible involvement of a mycotoxin produced by *Phoma sorghina* in the aetiology. S Afr Med J 1975; 49:1647-1650.

(24) VAN RENSBURG SJ, KIRSIPUU A, PEREIRA COUNTINHQ L, VAN DER WATT JJ. Circumstances associated with the contamination of food by aflatoxin in a high primary liver cancer area. S Afr Med J 1975; 49:877-883.

(25) KAPLAN HS, TSUCHITANI PJ. Cancer in China. New York: Alan R. Liss, 1978.

(26) American Plant Studies Delegation. Plant studies in the Peoples Republic of China. Washington, D.C.: National Academy of Sciences, 1975:67-73.

(27) MORTON JF. Tentative correlations of plant usage and esophageal cancer zones. Econ Bot 1970; 24:217-226.

(28) Joint Iran-International Agency for Research on Cancer Study Group. Esophageal cancer studies in the Caspian littoral of Iran: Results of population studies—a prodrome. J Natl Cancer Inst 1977; 59:1127-1138.

(29) TAKANO K, OSOGOSHI K, KAMIMURA N, et al. Epidemiology of cancer of the esophagus. Jpn J Clin Med 1968; 26:1823-1828.

(30) MARUCHI N, AOKI S, TSUDA K, TANAKA Y, TOYOKAWA H. Relation of food consumption to cancer mortality in Japan, with special reference to international figures. Gan 1977; 68:1-13.

(31) MARTÍNEZ I. Factors associated with cancer of the esophagus, mouth, and pharynx in Puerto Rico. J Natl Cancer Inst 1969; 42:1069-1094.

(32) DE JONG UW, BRESLOW N, HONG JG, SRIDHARAN M, SHANMUGARATNAM K. Aetiological factors in oesophageal cancer in Singapore Chinese. Int J Cancer 1974; 13:291-303.

(33) DIEM K, LENTNER C. Scientific tables. Basel: Ciba-Geigy 1970: 499-515.

(34) FOX FW. Studies on the chemical composition of foods commonly used in southern Africa. Johannesburg: S Afr Institute for Medical Research, 1966.

(35) MURPHY EW, WILLIS BW, WATT MK. Provisional tables on the zinc content of foods. J Am Diet Assoc 1975; 66:345-355.

(36) DOLL R, PAYNE P, WATERHOUSE J, eds. Cancer incidence in five continents. Vol I. Berlin, Heidelberg, and New York: Springer-Verlag, 1966.

(37) WATERHOUSE J, MUIR CS, CORREA P, POWELL J, eds. Cancer incidence in five continents. Vol III. IARC Sci Publ No. 15, 1976.

(38) LI KH, KAO JC, WU YK. A survey of the prevalence of cancer of the esophagus in North China. Chin Med J [Engl] 1962; 81:489-494.

(39) BASHIROV MS, NUGMANOV SN, KOLYCHEVA NI. Epidemiology of esophageal cancer in the Aktrubinsk of Kazakh SSR. Vopr Onkol 1968; 14:3-6.

(40) SCHONLAND M, BRADSHAW E. Cancer in the Natal African and Indian, 1964-66. Int J Cancer 1968; 3:304-316.

(41) ROSE EF. Esophageal cancer in the Transkei: 1955-69. J Natl Cancer Inst 1973; 51:7-16.

(42) EIBERGEN R. Kanker op Curaçao. Thesis. Groningen: J. B. Walters, 1961.

(43) COOK PG, BURKITT DP. Cancer in Africa. Br Med Bull 1971; 27:14-20.

(44) SHANTA V, KRISHNAMURTHI S. Further study in aetiology of carcinomas of the upper alimentary tract. Br J Cancer 1963; 17:8-23.

(45) STEINER PE. Cancer, race and geography; some etiological, environmental, ethnological, epidemiological and statistical aspects in Caucasoids, Mongoloids, Negroids and Mexicans. Baltimore: Williams & Wilkins, 1954.

(46) VON ZEYNEK ER. Survey of cancer of the oesophagus in relation to other malignant neoplasms. S Afr Med J 1973; 47:325-331.

(47) ROSE EF. Some observations on the diet and farming practices of the people of the Transkei. S Afr Med J 1972; 46:1353-1358.

(48) SIASSI F, McLAREN DS, VAGHEFI S, GHADIRIAN P, KEIGHOBADI K, AGHELI N. Nutritional status of vulnerable groups in the Caspian littoral of Iran: Clinical and anthropometric evaluation. In: Proceedings of the third international symposium on oncology. Tehran: Pahlavi Medical School, 1978:81.

(49) SIASSI F. Riboflavin and oesophageal cancer. Fed Proc 1980; 3 (part 1):654.

(50) KELSAY JL, BEHALL KM, PRATHER S. Effect of fiber from fruits and vegetables on metabolic responses of human subjects. II. Calcium, magnesium, iron and silicon balances. Am J Clin Nutr 1979; 32:1876-1880.

(51) SLAVIN JL, MARLETT JA. Influence of refined cellulose on human bowel function and calcium and magnesium balance. Am J Clin Nutr 1980; 33:1932-1939.

(52) LEEVY CM, THOMPSON A, BAKER H. Vitamins and liver injury. Am J Clin Nutr 1970; 23:493-498.

(53) DASTUR DK, SANTHADEVI N, QUADROS EV, et al. The B-vitamins in malnutrition with alcoholism. Br J Nutr 1976; 36:143-159.

(54) REINHOLD JG. Trace elements—a selective survey. Clin Chem 1975; 21:476-500.

(55) BURCH RE, HAHN HK, SULLIVAN JF. Newer aspects of the roles of zinc, manganese and copper in human nutrition. Clin Chem 1975; 21:501-520.

(56) FANKUSHEN D, RASKIN D, DIMICH A, WALLACH S. The significance of hypomagnesemia in alcoholic patients. Am J Med 1964; 37:802-812.

(57) LIEBER CS, TESCHKE R, HASUMURA Y, DECARLI LM. Differences in hepatic and metabolic changes after acute and chronic alcohol consumption. Fed Proc 1975; 34:2060-2074.

(58) VON WARTBURG JP. Metabolic consequences of alcohol consumption. Nutr Metab 1977; 21:153-162.

(59) McCoy GD. A biochemical approach to the etiology of alcohol related cancers of the head and neck. Laryngoscope 1978; 88(1 Pt 2 Suppl 8):59-62.

(60) McCoy GD, WYNDER EL. Etiological and preventive implications in alcohol carcinogenesis. Cancer Res 1979; 39:2844-2850.

(61) KEEN P. The epidemiology of oesophageal cancer in S.A. In: Silber W, ed. Carcinoma of the oesophagus. Cape Town: A. A. Balkema, 1978:4-9.

(62) SCHNEIDERMAN MA. Epidemiology, carcinogenicity and virology: Time trends: United States 1953-1973. Laryngoscope 1978; 88(1 Pt 2 Suppl 8):44-49.

(63) CRESPI M, MUNOZ N, GRASSI A, et al. Oesophageal lesions in northern Iran: A premalignant condition? Lancet 1979; 2:217-221.

(64) SLAVIN JL, MARLETT MS, MARLETT JA. Influence of refined cellulose on human bowel function and calcium and magnesium balance. Am J Clin Nutr 1980; 33:1932-1939.

(65) BLONDELL JM. The anticarcinogenic effect of magnesium. Med Hypotheses 1980; 6:863-871.

(66) WYNDER EL, BROSS IJ. A study of etiological factors in cancer of the esophagus. Cancer 1961; 14:389-413.

(67) LEEVY CM, BAKER H, TEN HOVE W, FRANK O, CHERRICK GR. B-complex vitamins in liver disease of the alcoholic. Am J Clin Nutr 1965; 16:339-346.

Esophageal Cancer Among Black Men in Washington, D.C. I. Alcohol, Tobacco, and Other Risk Factors

by Linda M. Pottern, M.P.H., Linda E. Morris, M.P.H., William J. Blot, Ph.D., Regina G. Ziegler, Ph.D., and Joseph F. Fraumeni, Jr., M.D.

ABSTRACT—A case-control study involving interviews with the next of kin or close friends of 120 black males who recently died of esophageal cancer and 250 similarly aged black males who died of other causes was undertaken to discover reasons for the exceptionally high mortality from this cancer in Washington, D.C. The age-adjusted annual death rate in Washington, D.C., for nonwhite males, 1970–75, was 28.6/100,000, far higher than the national rate of 12.4/100,000 and the rates in other metropolitan areas of the country. The major factor responsible for the excess was alcoholic beverage consumption, with an estimated 81% of the esophageal cancers attributed to its use; high use of alcoholic beverages was also found among the controls. The relative risk (RR) of esophageal cancer associated with use of alcoholic beverages was 6.4 (95% confidence interval = 2.5, 16.4). The RR increased with amount of ethanol consumed and was highest among drinkers of hard liquor, although the risk was also elevated among consumers of wine and/or beer only. The RR associated with cigarette smoking was 1.9 (1.0, 3.5) when controls with smoking-related causes of death were excluded but declined to 1.5 (0.7, 3.0) when adjusted for ethanol consumption. Significant differences of approximately twofold were found between low and high levels of a) consumption of fresh or frozen meat and fish, fruits and vegetables, and dairy products and eggs and b) relative weight (wt/ht²). The inverse trends with these general measures of nutritional status were not explained by alcoholic beverage consumption or socioeconomic status as measured by educational level.—JNCI 1981; 67:777–783.

ABBREVIATIONS USED: fl oz = fluid ounce(s); RR = relative risk(s).

Environmental Epidemiology Branch, Division of Cancer Cause and Prevention, National Cancer Institute (NCI), National Institutes of Health, Public Health Service, U.S. Department of Health and Human Services, Bethesda, Md. 20205.

We thank Dr. Jack White, Director of Cancer Research, Howard University Hospital, for his aid in initiating this study; the D.C. Department of Human Resources for supplying death certification information; Ms. Violette Kasica of NCI for data review; Dr. Linda W. Pickle and Dr. B. J. Stone (NCI) for technical assistance; Westat, Inc., for data collection and preparation; and Mrs. Theresa McKinney for manuscript preparation.

Mortality rates for esophageal cancer among black male residents of Washington, D.C., are among the highest in the United States (1). To identify the risk factors that may be responsible, we conducted a case-control interview study with the next of kin of black males who had died of esophageal cancer.

MATERIALS AND METHODS

To update esophageal cancer mortality statistics reported for 1950–69 (1), we computed mortality rates for 1970–75 by sex, race (white, nonwhite), and age for D.C., other metropolitan areas, and the entire United States, with the use of data from the National Center for Health Statistics and the Bureau of the Census. Deaths for 1972 were not recorded at the national level and are not included in the calculations. Methods of calculation for age-adjusted rates are described in (1).

Reprinted with permission from *Journal of the National Cancer Institute*, Vol. 67, No. 4, October 1981, pp. 777-783.

Subjects for the case-control study were identified from a computerized mortality tape from the D.C. Department of Human Resources. All deaths among black male residents attributed to primary esophageal cancer [code No. 150 (2)] during the years 1975–77 were selected as cases. Controls were randomly selected from among other causes of death (excluding oral, pharyngeal, and laryngeal cancers). The controls were black males of similar age and year of death and were twice the number of cases. Identifying information from death certificates was used to locate the next of kin or close friend of the subjects with esophageal cancer and of the controls for interview. For the purposes of this paper the respondent will be referred to as the next of kin.

Personal interviews of the next of kin were conducted in 1979 by local interviewers under the supervision of a professional survey organization. The interviewers were unaware of the case–control status of the study subjects. The questionnaire used sought information on usual lifetime tobacco consumption (cigarettes, cigars, pipes, chewing tobacco, and snuff); usual lifetime alcohol consumption (beer, wine, and hard liquor) prior to 1974 (i.e., prior to onset of disease); other beverage consumption (carbonated beverages, coffee, and tea); usual dietary patterns during adult life prior to 1974 (frequency of consumption of certain hot spices and sauces, 31 food items, unusual substances eaten, number of meals per day, and methods of cooking); usual adult weight prior to 1974; medical and dental history; lifetime occupational history; highest level of school completed; and residential history (state of birth, childhood state of residence, and length of time living in D.C.).

Quantitative indices of consumption were calculated for several variables. We estimated average daily ethanol intake, assuming 1 fl oz of beer, wine, and hard liquor yields, respectively, 1.1, 2.9, and 9.4 g ethanol (3). We then calculated total ethanol consumption by summing the amounts from all three types of alcoholic beverages. The summation was then converted into hard liquor equivalents for ease of interpretation.

All dietary responses were converted to the number of times the food item was eaten per week. Certain food items were combined to form food groups, such as fresh or frozen meat and fish (beef, chicken, lamb, fish, and shellfish) and precooked or cured meat and fish (bacon, sausage, frankfurters, lunch meat, canned meat, and canned fish). We quantitatively measured the intake of selected micronutrients (e.g., vitamin A and riboflavin) by summing the micronutrient content of each of the food items consumed. Three consumption categories—light, moderate, and heavy—were created for each food item, food group, and micronutrient by the division of the frequency distribution of the variable approximately into thirds.

For the identification of risk factors for esophageal cancer in this population, the interview responses for cases and controls were compared. The measure of strength of association used was the RR, approximated by the odds ratio (4). Associations were further examined by calculation of the odds ratios stratified by various factors, particularly ethanol consumption, with summary RR estimated and tested for significance by the Mantel-Haenszel method (5) and with confidence intervals calculated as described by Rothman and Boice (6). A prospective logistic model was used to adjust for confounding and to test for interaction among risk factors (7).

The Mantel extension test (8) was used to test risk factors for trend. For alcohol consumption, known to be causally related to esophageal cancer (9), attributable risk estimates and associated approximate confidence limits were also calculated (10, 11). Student's t-tests were used to compare mean weight and height between cases and controls (12).

RESULTS

Mortality from esophageal cancer among nonwhite males during 1970–75, 1972 excluded, was higher in D.C. than in other large metropolitan areas of the United States and exceeded that for most urban centers by 50% or more (table 1). The age-adjusted rate of 28.6 deaths/year/10^5 was more than double the U.S. rate of 12.4 for nonwhite males and seven times the national rate of 4.1 for white males. The elevation in mortality was apparent at all ages (text-fig. 1). Esophageal cancer in this period accounted for more deaths (279) among D.C. nonwhite males than all cancers except those of the lung (812 deaths) and prostate gland (320 deaths). Among nonwhite males in the suburban counties surrounding D.C., mortality from esophageal cancer was also high. The age-adjusted rates for Montgomery and Prince Georges Counties in Maryland and Arlington and Fairfax Counties in Virginia were, respectively, 19.6, 23.5, 25.9, and 34.8.

During 1975–77, 190 deaths among black male resi-

TABLE 1.—*Age-adjusted esophageal cancer mortality rates, 1970–75,[a] among nonwhite males in the 10 U.S. locations with the largest nonwhite populations*

Location[b]	No. of deaths	Mortality rate, death/yr/10^5
Washington, D.C.	279	28.6
Baltimore City, Md.	153	20.0
Essex County, N.J. (Newark)	78	19.0
New York City, N.Y.	499	17.1
Cook County, Ill. (Chicago)	334	16.4
Philadelphia, Pa.	202	15.7
Cuyahoga County, Ohio (Cleveland)	93	14.7
Wayne County, Mich. (Detroit)	198	13.7
Harris County, Tex. (Houston)	70	11.3
Los Angeles, Calif.	176	10.3

[a] Deaths (and populations) for the yr 1972 were excluded because all deaths in this yr were not recorded by the National Center for Health Statistics.
[b] Major city *in parentheses.*

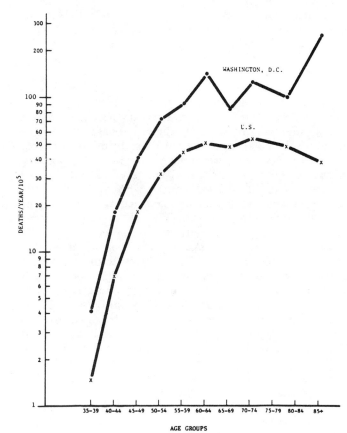

TEXT-FIGURE 1.—Age (yr)-specific esophageal cancer mortality rates in 1970-75 for nonwhite males in Washington, D.C., and the United States.

dents of D.C. were attributed to primary esophageal cancer. These individuals comprised the eligible case group for the interview study. The controls numbered 380 and represented deaths from the following causes: other cancer (28%), heart and circulatory diseases (42%), cirrhosis (8%), respiratory diseases (4%), accidental or violent deaths (6%), and other causes (12%).

Interviews were completed for 67% of the cases and 71% of the controls. The primary reasons for no interview were the inability to locate the next of kin (19%) and respondent refusal to be interviewed (7%). Information was considered to be incomplete for 4.5% of the interviews. These were excluded from the analysis, as well as the 2.5% of the study subjects who had lived in Washington, D.C., less than 4 years. The final study population on which the analyses were based, therefore, consisted of 120 cases and 250 controls. The next of kin interviewed for cases and controls, respectively, were wives (45%, 45%), relatives (siblings, children, parents, and other relatives) (48%, 48%), and friends (6%, 7%). Most of the study subjects were longtime residents of the D.C. area (median, 39 yr). The median ages for the cases and controls were 59 and 60 years, respectively.

The major risk factor for esophageal cancer was alcoholic beverage consumption. Ninety-six percent of the subjects with esophageal cancer drank some type of alcoholic beverage compared to 78% of the controls (RR, 6.4; $P<0.001$), yielding an attributable risk of 81% ($\approx$95% confidence interval, 52-91%) from alcohol consumption.

The RR tended to increase with amount of ethanol consumed (table 2). The RR were 4.0 for those who drank less than 6 fl oz in hard liquor equivalents/day, 5.5 for those who drank 6-15 fl oz/day, and 7.6 for those who drank more than 15 fl oz/day, a significant ($P<0.001$) trend. The RR was highest for those who drank hard liquor; however, the RR were also elevated for those who drank wine only, wine and/or beer only, and beer only (table 3). The higher RR asociated with hard liquor use was not solely related to higher ethanol content. As shown in table 4, the RR for hard liquor drinkers of less than 6 fl oz/day was higher than that for wine and/or beer drinkers who drank the ethanol equivalent of 6 or more fl oz of hard liquor/day. The subjects with esophageal cancer drank hard liquor in straight rather than mixed form more often than did

TABLE 2.—*RR of esophageal cancer by daily amount of ethanol consumed in hard liquor equivalents*

Hard liquor equivalents, fl oz/day	No. of cases[a]	No. of controls[a]	RR[b] (95% confidence interval)
None[c]	5	55	1.0 —
1.0–5.9	16	44	4.0 (1.4–12.0)
6.0–14.9	25	50	5.5 (2.0–15.0)
15.0–29.9	25	36	7.6 (2.7–22.0)
30.0–80.6	19	28	7.5 (2.5–22.0)

[a] Excludes 4 cases and 5 controls with unknown drinking status and 26 cases and 32 controls reported to have drunk alcoholic beverages but in unknown amounts.
[b] All risks relative to risks for nondrinkers.
[c] Never drank more than 5 shots or glasses of alcoholic beverages/wk for a period >1 mo.

TABLE 3.—*RR of esophageal cancer by type of alcoholic beverage consumed*

Type of beverage	No. of cases[a]	No. of controls[a]	RR[b] (95% confidence interval)
None[c]	5	55	1.0 —
Any type[d]	111	190	6.4 (2.5–16.4)
Hard liquor only	32	48	7.3 (2.6–20.3)
Hard liquor plus wine or beer	67	106	7.0 (2.7–18.5)
Wine only	2	5	4.4 (0.7–28.8)
Wine and/or beer only[e]	8	29	3.0 (0.9–10.0)
Beer only	3	19	1.7 (0.4–7.8)

[a] Excludes 4 cases and 5 controls with unknown drinking status.
[b] All risks relative to risks for nondrinkers.
[c] Never drank more than 5 shots or glasses of alcoholic beverages/wk for a period of >1 mo.
[d] Includes 4 cases and 7 controls reported to have drunk alcoholic beverage, but information incomplete.
[e] Includes persons who drank wine only, beer only, or both wine and beer.

TABLE 4.—*RR of esophageal cancer according to type and amount of alcoholic beverages consumed*

Hard liquor equivalents, fl oz/day	Alcoholic beverage	No. of cases[a]	No. of controls[a]	RR[b] (95% confidence interval)
0.1–5.9	Wine and/or beer only[c]	4	17	2.6 (0.6–10.8)
	Hard liquor only	6	11	6.0 (1.6–23.2)
	Hard liquor plus wine or beer	6	16	4.1 (1.1–15.2)
≥6.0	Wine and/or beer only[c]	4	12	3.7 (0.9–15.9)
	Hard liquor only	17	28	6.7 (2.2–20.0)
	Hard liquor plus wine or beer	48	74	7.1 (2.6–19.0)

[a] Excludes 30 cases and 37 controls with unknown amount of alcoholic beverages consumed.
[b] All risks relative to risks for nondrinkers.
[c] Includes persons who drank wine only, beer only, or both wine and beer.

the controls (68 vs. 57%). Whiskey (including bourbon) was drunk by a greater percentage of the subjects with esophageal cancer (67%) than by the controls (56%).

The RR for cigarette smoking according to amount smoked are presented in table 5. Eighty-three percent of the subjects with esophageal cancer and 79% of the controls were reported to have smoked cigarettes during their lifetime. Smokers were at increased risk [RR = 1.3 (0.7, 2.3); $P = 0.65$], with the greatest risk [RR = 1.6 (0.8, 3.3)] for those usually smoking two or more packs per day. These risks faded after adjustment for ethanol consumption [overall RR = 1.0 (0.5, 1.8)] (table 5). However, the ethanol-associated risk remained high after we controlled for cigarette smoking. For the nonsmokers (20 cases, 53 controls), the RR associated with consumption of alcoholic beverages was 19.9 (2.4, 166.4). The RR for cigarette smoking were also calculated with the use of only the controls whose causes of death were not known to be related to smoking. Thus lung, pancreas, and bladder cancers, heart disease, and chronic lung diseases were

TABLE 5.—*RR of esophageal cancer by cigarette smoking categories*[a]

Amount smoked/day	No. of cases	No. of controls	RR[b]	RR adjusted for ethanol consumption
Nonsmoker[c]	20	53 (30)	1.0 (1.0)	1.0 (1.0)
Smoker[d]	99	195 (78)	1.3 (1.9)	1.0 (1.5)
<½ pack	12	25 (13)	1.3 (1.4)	1.1 (1.0)
½–1½ packs	56	117 (51)	1.3 (1.7)	0.8 (1.2)
≥2 packs	22	37 (10)	1.6 (3.3)	0.9 (2.1)

[a] *Numbers in parentheses* refer to numbers of controls with non-smoking-related causes of death and corresponding RR.
[b] All risks relative to risks for nonsmokers.
[c] Never smoked 100 or more cigarettes during their lifetime.
[d] Includes 9 cases and 16 controls known to have smoked but in unknown amounts. Excludes 1 case and 2 controls with unknown smoking status.

excluded. Their deletion raised the overall RR for smoking to 1.9 (1.0, 3.5) (table 5). However, the overall RR was reduced to 1.5 (0.7, 3.0) when adjusted for ethanol consumption, and the trend with increasing amounts smoked was marginally significant ($P = 0.06$).

A comparison of other forms of tobacco revealed no increases in risk. Only a small percentage of the subjects with esophageal cancer had smoked cigars (14%), smoked pipes (13%), chewed tobacco (3.3%), or used snuff (1.7%). For each of these forms of tobacco, except the last, the percentage of ever users was slightly higher among the controls. However, 13 of the 20 subjects with esophageal cancer who did not smoke cigarettes smoked pipers or cigars compared to 22 of the 53 nonsmoking controls. The RR for pipe or cigar smoking among noncigarette smokers was 2.6 (0.9, 7.6).

Differences in food consumption were observed between cases and controls. The subjects with esophageal cancer ate more bacon, sausage, frankfurters, lunch meat, canned meat, canned fish, liver, and potatoes but less beef, chicken, lamb, fish, eggs, milk, vegetables, and fruit. As can be seen in table 6, a greater proportion of the subjects with esophageal cancer than the controls ate fewer than three meals a day [RR = 1.8 (1.1, 3.0)] but slightly more precooked or cured meat and fish. The RR associated with low compared to high consumption of 1) fresh or frozen meat and fish, 2) dairy products and eggs, and 3) fruits and vegetables were about twofold and were not substantially altered when adjusted for ethanol consumption or level of education. While the RR for consumption of vitamin A, vitamin C, riboflavin, and thiamine increased with decreased intake, the trends for the 3 food groups were more impressive. No clear association with nitrite-containing foods was observed. A trend of increasing RR was seen with a decrease in relative weight, although very few of the subjects with esophageal cancer were especially light in weight. The average adult weight for the cases (162.8 lb) was significantly less than that of the controls (171.0 lb) ($P = 0.009$), but their average heights were similar, 68.4 and 68.1 inches, respectively.

Analyses with the use of linear logistic models that simultaneously considered the factors of age, alcohol, smoking, and diet tended to show independent effects associated with the nutritional indices. For example, we found the RR for consumption of moderate and low levels of fresh or frozen meat and fish to be 1.6 (0.85, 3.0) and 2.3 (1.1, 4.4), respectively, after adjusting for these other factors. This same analysis yielded RR for the five ethanol categories (table 2) of 1.0, 4.2 (1.4, 13.0), 6.5 (2.2, 19.5), 8.1 (2.7, 24.2), and 9.2 (2.9, 29.1).

The RR for consumption of hot spices and sauces, such as chili peppers, red peppers, and hot sauce, revealed no significant trends for the four levels of consumption—never, rarely, occasionally, and often. No significant differences were observed between cases and controls in the consumption of carbonated beverages, coffee (any and "burning hot"), and tea (any,

TABLE 6.—*RR of esophageal cancer by selected nutritional indices*

Nutrition index	RR: Consumption level			RR adjusted for ethanol, consumption level			RR adjusted for education,[a] consumption level		
	High	Moderate	Low	High	Moderate	Low	High	Moderate	Low
Food groups									
Fresh or frozen meat and fish	1.0	1.5	2.1[b]	1.0	1.6	2.2[b]	1.0	1.6	2.1[b]
Dairy products and eggs	1.0	1.6	2.0[b]	1.0	1.7	1.9[b]	1.0	2.0	2.1[b]
Fruits and vegetables	1.0	2.1	2.4[c]	1.0	1.7	2.0[b]	1.0	2.0	2.8[c]
Precooked or cured meat and fish	1.0	0.9	0.8	1.0	0.9	0.9	1.0	0.8	0.6
Nitrite-containing foods	1.0	1.1	0.8	1.0	1.1	1.0	1.0	1.0	0.7
Micronutrients									
Vitamin A	1.0	1.4	1.5	1.0	1.5	1.5	1.0	1.4	1.4
Vitamin C	1.0	1.3	2.1[c]	1.0	1.2	1.8[b]	1.0	1.2	2.1[c]
Riboflavin	1.0	1.1	1.6	1.0	1.0	1.7[b]	1.0	1.2	1.7
Thiamine	1.0	1.2	1.1	1.0	1.2	1.2	1.0	1.2	1.1
Other									
Relative wt	1.0	1.6	2.4[c]	1.0	1.5	2.1[c]	1.0	1.7	2.6[c]
Meals per day	1.0	—	1.8	1.0	—	1.6	1.0	—	1.9

[a] Excludes persons with unknown educational status.
[b] Significant (*P*<0.05) trend.
[c] Significant (*P*<0.01) trend.

burning hot, and herbal). No significant case–control differences were observed for the following dental health indices: the condition of teeth and gums, the number of teeth lost due to decay, the wearing of false teeth, and the number of times permanent teeth were brushed per week. Also, there were no clear case-control differences for ever having had anemia, arthritis, or thyroid disease. Review of the occupational histories revealed no significant differences when jobs were grouped by major industry (e.g., construction, transportation, and military and other government services) and by level of skill (e.g., unskilled, skilled, or professional).

The esophageal cancer subjects tended to have less formal education than did the controls. There was a trend of increasing risk with decreasing level of education (RR = 1.0, 1.3, and 1.5, respectively, for ≥12, 8–11, and <8 yr of school completed). These risks were not affected by the adjustment for ethanol consumption.

Approximately half of our study population was born in the D.C. area, including parts of Maryland and Virginia. A higher percentage of the subjects with esophageal cancer than the controls was born in either Georgia [RR = 1.3 (0.8, 2.8)] or North Carolina [RR = 1.5 (0.5, 3.3)], but there was no excess risk associated with either being born or spending one's childhood in South Carolina, where a cluster of high rates for esophageal cancer has been identified (*13*).

DISCUSSION

Esophageal cancer varies more worldwide than any other neoplasm, with annual rates exceeding 100 per 100,000 population for both males and females in parts of northern China, Iran, and the Soviet Union (*14*).

Reasons for the exceptional risk in these areas are obscure. In western countries, the major risk factors are alcohol consumption and cigarette smoking, which probably account for the higher rates in cities and in males (*15, 16*). In the United States, the rates are much higher in blacks than in whites, particularly in the urban areas (*16*). The present study was conducted among black men in Washington, D.C., where the death rate for esophageal cancer (28.6/10^5) is especially high, exceeding the national level for nonwhite males by over twofold and for white males by sevenfold.

The major risk factor was found to be ethanol consumption (RR = 6.4), which was estimated to be causally associated with about 80% of the neoplasms among the esophageal cancer subjects.[1] Nearly all the esophageal cancer subjects drank alcoholic beverages, usually in very high quantities.

The controls drank more than expected when compared to males of the populations surveyed in other studies. Forty-six percent consumed six or more alcoholic drinks per day, whereas only 4.4% of the 5,000 black males enrolled in the Kaiser-Permanente health plan in the Oakland–San Francisco area drank this amount (*18*). In addition, a national survey conducted in 1972–74 showed that less than 15% of males 40 years of age or over drank 1 or more oz of ethanol/day (*19*). These data suggest that blacks in D.C. drink more than

---

[1] It is likely that the consumption of alcoholic beverages among our mortality series of controls is greater than that of the living Washington, D.C., black male population inasmuch as drinking contributes to many causes of death. If this is the case, then the relative and attributable risks of esophageal cancer due to ethanol consumption would actually be higher in a population of living subjects than calculated for our study group.

blacks in other areas of the United States. Although our study differed from other studies in the phrasing of the questions asked, in second-party versus direct reporting, and in obtaining information about deceased rather than about living individuals, such study differences seem unlikely to account for the substantially higher consumption reported in D.C. Other evidence exists of high alcoholic beverage consumption in D.C. The per-capita "apparent consumption" of alcoholic beverages on the basis of tax revenues for D.C. surpasses the national level by nearly fourfold for hard liquor and about threefold for wine (19), although part of the excess is related to purchases by nonresidents. In addition, the computation of age-adjusted mortality rates from cirrhosis of the liver for the years 1965-71 revealed that nonwhite males in D.C. had rates about 2.5 times higher than those of U.S. nonwhite males.

Although an increased risk of esophageal cancer in this study was associated with all forms of alcoholic beverages, the excess was greatest for hard liquor, particularly whiskey or bourbon. A gradient in risk according to ethanol concentration was evident with straight liquor having the highest relative risk, mixed liquor and wine having an intermediate risk, and beer having the lowest risk. This finding, together with the gradient in risk observed with increasing amounts of ethanol consumed, is consistent with a causal effect of alcohol consumption.

Cigarette smoking is regarded as a major risk factor for esophageal cancer, and some studies have shown a synergism between tobacco and ethanol consumption (14). In contrast, the overall data from our case-control study revealed no significant risk associated with cigarette smoking and also no consistent enhancement of risk following exposure to both alcoholic beverages and cigarette smoking. The discrepancy in part relates to different comparison groups. Controls in our study included persons who died from lung cancer and heart disease, conditions known to be induced by cigarette smoking, whereas some other studies (15) excluded as controls persons who died from smoking-related conditions. When we restricted our comparisons by using only those controls who died of illnesses not known to be linked to smoking, a 90% increased risk of esophageal cancer and a dose-response relationship were observed for smokers. However, this smoking-associated risk was considerably reduced when we controlled for ethanol intake. Possibly, the consumption of such large amounts of alcoholic beverages by our study population overwhelmed the risk that would have been due to cigarette smoking in a population consuming lesser amounts.

Whereas esophageal cancer has been related to pipe smoking, cigar smoking, tobacco chewing, and other smokeless tobacco products in various populations (14), the percentage of D.C. residents using a tobacco product other than cigarettes was small. Only among noncigarette smokers was an association found with pipe and cigar smoking.

Review of the dietary information revealed an increased risk of esophageal cancer associated with poor nutritional status. The esophageal cancer subjects were approximately the same height as controls but their usual adult weight before onset of cancer was less, although very few were seriously underweight. They were reported to eat fewer meals per day and less dairy products and eggs, fruits and vegetables, and fresh or frozen meat and fish. Although food intake can be limited by alcoholic beverage consumption, twofold differences between high and low consumption of the food variables were seen after adjustment for ethanol and social staus. Specific indices of vitamin A, vitamin C, riboflavin, and thiamine showed patterns similar to the general nutritional measures, although of a lower order of magnitude. These findings, consistent with those of other studies (14), suggest that poor nutrition, possibly involving complex dietary deficiencies, is involved in the development of esophageal cancer.

These results may be influenced by a case recall bias. Despite an attempt to assess dietary patterns predating the disease (i.e., prior to 1974), it is possible that the next of kin recalled a decrease in food consumption caused by the esophageal cancer instead of by the study subjects' usual lifetime dietary patterns. This possibility seems unlikely, however, since a history of low food intake among the esophageal cancer subjects did not apply to all food items (e.g., the esophageal cancer subjects did eat more of the precooked and cured varieties of meat and fish), and these esophageal cancer subjects were not found to be underweight when compared to black males 55-64 years of age who participated in the 1971-74 U.S. Health and Nutrition Examination Survey (Abraham S: Personal communication). Furthermore, although knowledge of the diets of cases and controls by next of kin may have been incomplete, when the RR for each of the major food groups were calculated separately by respondent type, the RR determined from the wife's responses (considered to be most accurate) showed good agreement with the RR determined from the responses of other relatives.

Information was obtained on several potential risk factors (including consumption of coffee, tea, and burning hot liquids; history of certain medical conditions; and occupation), but no significant case-control differences were observed. While the present study showed no association between poor oral hygiene and increased risk of esophageal cancer, next-of-kin responses may not have been adequate to assess the dental health of the study subjects. One hypothesis under test concerned migration from other areas, especially coastal South Carolina where mortality from esophageal cancer has been extremely high among blacks at least since the early 1950's (17). A higher proportion of esophageal cancer subjects than controls was born in the Deep South, but there was no excess of migrants from South Carolina.

In this case-control study, with information obtained

from next of kin of deceased patients, we had an overall response rate of 70%. Nonresponse was primarily related to difficulty in locating the next of kin of the decedents. Although information is limited on the characteristics of the nonrespondents, we suspect that they may have represented study subjects who were poor and without close friends or family ties. This type of response bias might affect the comparisons made but would not materially reduce the RR presented. We made the decision to interview relatives because esophageal cancer is a highly fatal disease [the median survival for blacks nationwide is 4 mo (20)] and because establishing a rapid reporting system for interviewing a high percentage of newly diagnosed patients proved not to be feasible. Lack of knowledge or difficulty in recall by the next of kin may have influenced the responses but probably not differentially between cases and controls because the questions were asked in a similar manner by interviewers "blind" to the disease status of the study subjects. Comparison of self versus next-of-kin interviews in other studies has revealed generally good concordance for broadly defined variables, including smoking (21–23), alcohol intake and dietary history (21), and usual occupation (22).

Despite the limitations of a case–control study involving next-of-kin respondents in a difficult-to-locate population, the data gathered appeared adequate to identify alcoholic beverage consumption as the major factor responsible for the elevated risk of esophageal cancer among black males in D.C. and also to contribute some intriguing hypotheses regarding the role of poor nutrition in the origins of this cancer.

REFERENCES

(1) MASON TJ, MCKAY FW. U.S. cancer mortality by county 1950–69. Washington, D.C.: U.S. Govt Print Off, 1973 [DHEW publication No. (NIH)74-615].

(2) National Center for Health Statistics. International Classification of Diseases. Eighth revision. Washington, D.C.: U.S. Govt Print Off, 1967 (PHS publication No. 1693).

(3) ADAMS CF. Nutritive value of American foods in common units. Washington, D.C.: U.S. Govt Print Off, 1975 (USDA agriculture handbook No. 456).

(4) FLEISS JL. Statistical methods for rates and proportions. New York: Wiley, 1973.

(5) MANTEL N, HAENSZEL W. Statistical aspects of the analysis of data from retrospective studies of disease. J Natl Cancer Inst 1959; 22:719–748.

(6) ROTHMAN KJ, BOICE JD. Epidemiologic analysis with a programmable calculator. Washington, D.C.: U.S. Govt Print Off, 1979:5–6. [U.S. DHEW publication No. (NIH)79-1649].

(7) PRENTICE RG, PYKE R. Logistic incidence disease models and case-control studies. Biometrika 1969; 66:408–412.

(8) MANTEL N. Chi-square tests with one degree of freedom; extensions of the Mantel-Haenszel procedure. J Am Stat Assoc 1963; 58:690–700.

(9) ROTHMAN KJ. Alcohol. In: Fraumeni JF Jr, ed. Persons at high risk of cancer: An approach to cancer etiology and control. New York: Academic Press, 1975:139–148.

(10) MACMAHON B, PUGH TF. Epidemiology principles and methods. Boston: Little, Brown & Co., 1970:273–275.

(11) WALTER SD. The estimates and interpretation of attributable risk in health research. Biometrics 1976; 32:829–849.

(12) SNEDECOR GW, COCHRAN WG. Statistical methods. Ames, Iowa: Iowa State Univ Press, 1967:59–60.

(13) BATES DC, CASTON JC, O'BRIEN P, SANDIFER SH. Carcinoma of the esophagus in South Carolina. J SC Med Assoc 1971; 67:453–456.

(14) DAY NE, MUNOZ N. Cancer of the esophagus. In: Schottenfeld D, Fraumeni JF Jr, eds. Cancer epidemiology and prevention. Philadelphia: Saunders In press.

(15) WYNDER EL, BROSS IJ. A study of etiological factors in cancer of the esophagus. Cancer 1961; 14:389–413.

(16) SCHOENBERG BS, BAILAR JC III, FRAUMENI JF JR. Certain mortality patterns of esophageal cancer in the United States, 1930-67. J Natl Cancer Inst 1971; 46:63–73.

(17) FRAUMENI JF JR, BLOT WJ. Geographic variation in esophageal cancer mortality in the United States. J Chronic Dis 1977; 30:759–767.

(18) KLATSKY AL, FRIEDMAN GD, SIEGELAUB AB, GERALD MJ. Alcohol consumption among white, black or oriental men and women; Kaiser Permanente multiphasic health examination data. Am J Epidemiol 1977; 105:311–322.

(19) KELLER M, ed. Second special report to the U.S. Congress on alcohol and health. Washington, D.C.: U.S. Govt Print Off, 1975 [DHEW publication No. (ADM)75-212].

(20) AXTELL LM, ASIRE AJ, MYERS MH, eds. Cancer patient survival. Washington, D.C.: U.S. Govt Print Off, 1976 [Report No. 5. DHEW publication No. (NIH)77-992].

(21) KOLONEL LM, HIROHATA T, NOMURA AM. Adequacy of survey data collected from substitute respondents. Am J Epidemiol 1977; 106:476–483.

(22) ROGOT E, REID DD. The validity of data from next-of-kin in studies of mortality among migrants. Int J Epidemiol 1975; 4:51–54.

(23) BLOT WJ, HARRINGTON JM, TOLEDO A, HOOVER R, HEATH CW JR, FRAUMENI JF JR. Lung cancer after employment in shipyards during World War II. N Engl J Med 1978; 299:620–624.

Esophageal Cancer Among Black Men in Washington, D.C. II. Role of Nutrition

by Regina G. Ziegler, Ph.D., Linda E. Morris, M.P.H., William J. Blot, Ph.D., Linda M. Pottern, M.P.H., Robert Hoover, M.D., and Joseph F. Fraumeni, Jr., M.D.

ABSTRACT—A case-control study of esophageal cancer was conducted among the black male residents of Washington, D.C., to find reasons for the exceptionally high risk in this population. The next of kin of 120 esophageal cancer cases who died during 1975-77 and of 250 D.C. black males who died of other causes were interviewed. Five indicators of general nutritional status—fresh or frozen meat and fish consumption, dairy product and egg consumption, fruit and vegetable consumption, relative weight (wt/ht²), and number of meals eaten per day—were each significantly and inversely correlated with the relative risk of esophageal cancer. Associations with other food groups were not apparent. The least nourished third of the study population, defined by any of these five measures, was at twice the risk of the most nourished third. None of these associations was markedly reduced by controlling for ethanol consumption, the other major risk factor in this population; smoking; socioeconomic status; or the other nutrition measures. When the three food group consumption measures were combined into a single overall index of general nutritional status, the relative risk of esophageal cancer between extremes was 14. Estimates of the intake of vitamin A, carotene, vitamin C, thiamin, and riboflavin were inversely associated with relative risk; but each micronutrient index was less strongly associated with risk than were the broad food groups that provide most of the micronutrient. Thus no specific micronutrient deficency was identified. Instead, generally poor nutrition was the major dietary predictor of risk and may partially explain the susceptibility of urban black men to esophageal cancer.—JNCI 1981; 67:1199-1206.

ABBREVIATIONS USED: fl oz = fluid ounce(s); kcal = kilocalorie(s); RR = relative risk(s).

Environmental Epidemiology Branch, Division of Cancer Cause and Prevention, National Cancer Institute, National Institutes of Health, Public Health Service, U.S. Department of Health and Human Services, Bethesda, Md. 20205.

We are grateful to Ms. Patricia Strasser and Dr. Linda Pickle for their advice on epidemiologic methods and to Ms. Nancy Guerin, Ms. Theresa McKinney, and Mr. Todd Ostrow for their assistance in manuscript preparation.

A case-control study of esophageal cancer was initiated among black male residents of Washington, D.C., the U.S. metropolitan area with the highest esophageal cancer mortality rate for nonwhite males for 1970-75 (*1*). In an earlier paper, alcoholic beverage consumption was identified as the dominant risk factor; but poor nutrition was also implicated (*1*). In the present paper the role of nutritional status in esophageal cancer is further assessed.

MATERIALS AND METHODS

The 120 cases in the study were all black male residents of Washington, D.C., who died during 1975-77 of primary esophageal cancer [code No. 150 (*2*)]. The 250 controls were randomly selected from among D.C. black males of the same age who died of other causes during the same time period, after oral, pharyngeal, and laryngeal cancer were excluded. Next of kin were identified from the death certificates and interviewed in 1979 about the dietary patterns, cooking practices, alcohol consumption, and tobacco use of the study subjects. Interviews were completed for 67% of the cases and 71% of the controls. The next of kin interviewed were wives (45%, 45%), other relatives (48%, 48%), and friends (6%, 7%) for the cases and controls (respectively). Further details are given elsewhere (*1*). An earlier attempt to interview esophageal cancer patients directly had floundered because of the small number of incident cases that could be prospectively identified and the advanced disease in these patients once located.

The dietary section of the interview asked about the usual adult frequency of consumption, prior to 1974, of 31 food items. Answers were converted to the number of times a food item was eaten per week. To explore the basic dietary patterns associated with esophageal cancer, measures of consumption of food groups were created by summing responses for individual food items. Traditional food groups, such as green vegetables, fruit, and meat-fish, were formed, as well as less traditional groups, such as nitrite-containing foods (bacon, frankfurters, lunch meat, corned beef-pastrami, and canned meat). Beef, chicken, lamb, fresh or frozen fish, and shellfish were combined into a food group of relatively "affluent" foods called "fresh or frozen meat and fish"; and frankfurters, lunch meat, canned meat, canned fish, bacon, and sausage were combined into a food group of generally cheaper foods called "precooked or processed meat and fish."[1]

Indices of micronutrient intake for vitamin A, carotene, vitamin C, thiamin, and riboflavin were created by weighting and summing responses for the appropriate individual food items. Each weight was the quantity of the micronutrient in a typical serving of the food item and was derived from U.S. Department of Agriculture food composition data (3, 4). To form the vitamin A index, carotene- and retinol-containing foods were weighted according to the number of retinol equivalents that they contain (5).

Five cases (4%) and 25 controls (10%) were excluded from all the dietary analyses because few of the food frequency questions could be answered by their next of kin. The remaining next of kin of the cases and of the controls could both answer quantitatively an average of 96% of the food frequency questions. To form the food group and micronutrient variables, any response in which it was not known whether an individual food item was eaten was coded as "0"; and any response in which a food item was known to be eaten but with unknown frequency was replaced with the study sample median, which was calculated after nonconsumers had been eliminated from the distribution. Three consumption categories—low, moderate, and high—were created for each food item, food group, and micronutrient index by dividing the frequency distribution of the variable into approximate thirds.

A simple measure of relative weight was formed by dividing usual adult weight (prior to 1974), in pounds, by the square of adult height, in feet. The study sample was divided into four strata on the basis of ideal and typical relative weights for this population:

those lighter than ideal (wt/hr$^2 \le 4.32$), those centered around the ideal relative weight ($4.32 < wt/ht^2 \le 4.84$), those centered around the typical relative weight ($4.84 < wt/ht^2 \le 5.72$), and those heavier than typical (wt/ht$^2 > 5.72$). An ideal relative weight of 4.52 was derived from the National Academy of Sciences Food and Nutrition Board's recommendation for adult men (5). A median or typical relative weight of 5.04 was calculated from data obtained for black males, 55–64 years of age, in the 1971–74 U.S. Health and Nutrition Examination Survey (6).

Usual alcoholic beverage consumption was measured in terms of grams of ethanol and calories. Total ethanol intake was calculated by summing the intake of beer (1.1 g ethanol/fl oz), wine (2.9 g ethanol/fl oz), and hard liquor (9.4 g ethanol/fl oz) (3). Total calorie intake was also calculated by summing the intake of beer (13 kcal/fl oz), wine (25 kcal/fl oz), and hard liquor (65 kcal/fl oz) (3).

RR were estimated by the odds ratio (7), and associations were further examined by calculating odds ratios stratified by various factors, with summary RR estimated by the Mantel-Haenszel method (8). Adjustment for ethanol consumption was routinely done over six strata, identified in table 2 of (1), and over nine strata for the five primary nutrition indices. Unless otherwise noted, ethanol-adjusted RR presented in this paper are those calculated over six strata. Confidence intervals were calculated as described by Rothman and Boice (9). Tests for significance of trend used the Mantel extension test (10). Pairwise correlations were calculated for the primary nutrition indices (11).

In general, controls with nutrition-related causes of death were not excluded from the dietary analyses. Nearly all major causes of death are believed to be associated with one dietary pattern or another, and selective exclusion might well compromise the broad representativeness of the control series. Relative weight, however, was analyzed with and without exclusion of obesity-related deaths from the control series.

RESULTS

The RR of esophageal cancer by consumption of the 31 individual food items are shown in table 1. RR tended to increase with decreasing consumption of beef, chicken, lamb, fresh or frozen fish, eggs, butter or margarine, fruit (excluding citrus fruit), bananas, leafy green vegetables, other green vegetables, and yellow vegetables (excluding corn). The RR tended to decrease with decreasing consumption of bacon, sausage, frankfurters, lunch meat, canned meat, liver, canned fish, and potatoes. Adjusting the RR for the individual food items for ethanol consumption did not markedly alter them.

The RR of esophageal cancer by consumption of various food groups and micronutrients are shown in table 2. The ethanol-adjusted RR increased with decreasing consumption of dairy products and eggs,

---

[1] Four meats did not clearly belong in one or the other of these 2 subgroups and were excluded from both: liver, pastrami-corned beef, brains-chitterlings, and ham-pork. The interview question about ham-pork was considered ambiguous since chops and pigs' feet had been given as examples. The "precooked or processed meat and fish" group was referred to as the "precooked or cured meat and fish" group in the earlier paper (1).

TABLE 1.—*RR of esophageal cancer by consumption of specific foods*

Food item	RR by consumption level[a]		
	High	Moderate	Low
1. Beef or veal	1.0	1.3	1.5
2. Chicken	1.0	1.0	1.3†
3. Lamb	1.0	3.0	3.0†
4. Ham or pork	1.0	1.5	1.0
5. Bacon	1.0	0.6	0.7*
6. Sausage	1.0	0.8	0.4†
7. Frankfurters	1.0	0.9	0.9
8. Lunch meat, e.g., salami, bologna	1.0	0.7	0.8
9. Corned beef or pastrami	1.0	1.0	1.0
10. Canned meat, e.g., Spam, Treet	1.0	0.7	0.6*
11. Liver	1.0	0.7	0.8
12. Brains or chitterlings (intestines)	1.0	1.3	1.0
13. Shellfish	1.0	1.5	0.8
14. Canned fish, e.g., tuna, sardines	1.0	0.9	0.4‡
15. Fresh or frozen fish, e.g., flounder, catfish	1.0	1.5	1.7
16. Eggs	1.0	1.3	1.5*
17. Cheese	1.0	1.3	0.9
18. Milk	1.0	1.7	1.4
19. Butter or margarine	1.0	1.0	1.2
20. Leafy green vegetables, e.g., spinach, kale	1.0	1.3	1.6*
21. Other green vegetables	1.0	1.2	1.3
22. Corn	1.0	1.0	0.9
23. Other yellow vegetables, e.g., carrots, squash	1.0	1.3	1.9†
24. Citrus fruits or juices	1.0	1.6	1.2
25. Bananas	1.0	1.8	1.7†
26. Other fruits, e.g., peaches, pears	1.0	1.4	2.5‡
27. Whole grain breads or cereals	1.0	1.2	1.1
28. Cornbread, corn mush, corn grits, etc.	1.0	1.1	0.9
29. Potatoes	1.0	1.1	0.7
30. Potato chips, fried potatoes, or fried onions	1.0	1.4	1.0
31. Peanuts or peanut butter	1.0	1.4	0.9

[a] Statistical significance of trend: *, $P<0.10$; †, $P<0.05$; ‡, $P<0.01$.

fruits and vegetables, vegetables alone, and fruits alone but were not markedly associated with carbohydrate or bread consumption. Nor was there a clear trend with total meat and fish consumption. However, the ethanol-adjusted RR increased with decreasing consumption of fresh or frozen meat and fish and tended to decrease slightly with decreasing consumption of precooked or processed meat and fish. The fresh or frozen meat and fish group, relative to the precooked or processed meat and fish group, contains foods that tend to be more expensive, more typical of an affluent diet, less processed, and less easily prepared. Although precooked or processed meat and fish consumption was slightly associated with esophageal cancer, consumption of nitrite-containing meats was not associated. Adjusting each of the food group and micronutrient RR for ethanol consumption produced no striking changes, as shown in table 2, nor did adjustment for cigarette smoking.

For fresh or frozen meat and fish, dairy products and eggs, and fruits and vegetables, the RR associated with low consumption was about twice that for high consumption. The approximate third of the study subjects who were categorized as low consumers of fresh or frozen meat and fish had 1-3 servings a week; the third categorized as high consumers had 6-18 servings a week. Low dairy product and egg consumption was 0-7 servings a week; high was 14-28 servings a week. Low fruit and vegetable consumption was 1-12 servings a week, and high was 20-43 servings a week. The ethanol-adjusted trends in RR for the three food groups were statistically significant and of similar magnitude. However, when consumption was divided into six levels rather than three, fresh or frozen meat and fish showed the clearest dose-response relationship, with the ethanol-adjusted RR of those with the lowest intake being 3.3, relative to those with the highest intake.

Risk was elevated among individuals with a low intake of vitamin A but there was no clear gradient; and the risk was less than that for low consumption of dairy products and eggs or fruits and vegetables, which are the major sources of vitamin A. Similarly, risk was elevated among those with a low intake of vitamin C or carotene; but the risk was somewhat less than that for low consumption of fruits and vegetables, the food group that provides vitamin C and carotene. Risk was elevated among those with a low intake of riboflavin, but not as markedly as among those with low consumption of dairy products and eggs, the major sources of riboflavin.

Esophageal cancer was also associated with two indirect measures of diet. Relative weight (wt/ht^2) was inversely related to risk, with the RR of the lightest third of the study sample being 2.4 that of the heaviest third ($P<0.01$, for trend). The ethanol-adjusted RR was 2.1. The number of meals usually eaten per day was also inversely related to risk, with those eating two meals a day (51 cases, 78 controls) having 1.8 times the risk of those eating three or more meals a day (55, 147, respectively) and those eating one meal a day (8, 9, respectively) having a risk of 2.4 relative to the same group ($P<0.01$, for trend). The ethanol-adjusted RR were 1.6 and 1.7, respectively. Adjustment for cigarette smoking did not markedly change these RR.

The RR for fresh or frozen meat and fish consumption, fruit and vegetable consumption, dairy product and egg consumption, usual number of meals eaten per day, and relative weight were controlled for socioeconomic status, as measured by education, and were not markedly changed. These results are shown in (*1*). The RR associated with less than 8 years of school, relative to 12 or more years, was 1.5, less than the risk associated with poor nutrition measured by any of the five nutrition indices. Occupation, another possible measure of socioeconomic status, was not related to esophageal cancer in this study (*1*).

The inverse association of esophageal cancer with relative weight was further examined by grouping the

TABLE 2.—*RR of esophageal cancer by consumption of food groups and micronutrients*

Nutrition index[a]	RR by consumption level[c]			RR adjusted for ethanol, by consumption level[c]		
	High	Moderate	Low	High	Moderate	Low
Food groups[b]						
Meat, fish, eggs, and cheese (1–17)	1.0	1.7	1.1	1.0	1.7	1.3
Meat and fish (1–15)	1.0	1.3	0.9	1.0	1.3	1.2
Dairy products and eggs (16–18)	1.0	1.6	2.0†	1.0	1.7	1.9†
Fruits and vegetables (20–26)	1.0	2.1	2.4‡	1.0	1.7	2.0†
Vegetables (20–23)	1.0	1.7	1.8†	1.0	1.5	1.6*
Green vegetables (20, 21)	1.0	1.2	1.5*	1.0	1.0	1.3
Yellow vegetables (22, 23)	1.0	1.0	1.2	1.0	1.0	1.7
Fruits (24–26)	1.0	2.8	2.4‡	1.0	2.4	2.0†
Carbohydrates (22, 27–30)	1.0	1.1	1.2	1.0	1.1	1.2
Bread (27, 28)	1.0	1.1	1.2	1.0	1.1	1.1
Fresh or frozen meat and fish (1–3, 13, 15)	1.0	1.5	2.1†	1.0	1.6	2.2†
Precooked or processed meat and fish (5–8, 10, 14)	1.0	0.9	0.8	1.0	0.9	0.9
Nitrite-containing foods (5, 7–10)	1.0	1.1	0.8	1.0	1.1	1.0
Micronutrients						
Vitamin A	1.0	1.4	1.5	1.0	1.5	1.5
Carotene	1.0	1.4	1.6*	1.0	1.3	1.3
Vitamin C	1.0	1.3	2.1‡	1.0	1.2	1.8†
Thiamin	1.0	1.2	1.1	1.0	1.2	1.2
Riboflavin	1.0	1.1	1.6*	1.0	1.0	1.7†

[a] Includes all food groups and micronutrients analyzed.
[b] Specific food items combined to form each food group are indicated by the *numbers in parentheses*, which refer to table 1.
[c] Statistical significance of trend: *, $P<0.10$; †, $P<0.05$; ‡, $P<0.01$.

study subjects into four categories: those lighter than ideal, those close to the ideal relative weight, those close to the typical or median relative weight, and those heavier than typical. Table 3 shows that a slightly higher percentage of cases than controls were in each of the two lighter categories, but only 11% of the cases were actually in the lightest category. In comparison, 15% of U.S. blacks, 55–64 years of age, had relative weights in this range in the 1971–74 U.S. Health and Nutrition Examination Survey (Abraham S: Personal communication). There was only a small RR, about 1.2, for those especially light in weight relative to those of typical weight; but the RR for those who were especially heavy was 0.4. This reduced RR remained after exclusion of the 95 controls who died of

TABLE 3.—*RR of esophageal cancer by relative weight*

Relative weight	No. of cases (% of all cases)	No. of controls (% of all controls)	RR[a] (95% confidence interval)	RR, excluding obesity-related deaths from controls[a] (95% confidence interval)
Light	13 (11)	19 (8)	1.2 (0.5–2.6)	0.9 (0.4–2.1)
Ideal	32 (28)	52 (22)	1.1 (0.6–1.9)	1.1 (0.6–2.1)
Typical	55 (48)	99 (42)	1.0	1.0
Heavy	15 (13)	64 (27)	0.4 (0.2–0.8)	0.6 (0.3–1.2)

[a] All risks relative to those of typical relative weight.

obesity-related diseases (myocardial infarction, hypertensive heart disease, and diabetes). Adjustment for ethanol consumption did not change the pattern.

Table 4 shows the interrelationships among the five primary measures of nutritional status and ethanol consumption. The nutrition indices were positively, but weakly, correlated with each other. Thus there was sufficient variety of diet within the study population to allow each nutrition index to be adjusted for the others. When the ethanol-adjusted RR for fresh or frozen meat and fish consumption, fruit and vegetable consumption, and dairy product and egg consumption were adjusted for each other, separate effects for all three were evident. The ethanol-adjusted RR for fresh or frozen meat and fish consumption were the only RR for consumption of a food group to remain unchanged after controlling for consumption of another food group, with the RR of the low consumers, relative to high consumers, remaining about 2.2. Controlling the ethanol-adjusted RR for fruit and vegetable consumption or dairy product and egg consumption for another food group reduced the gradients, with the risk of the low consumers, relative to high consumers, falling from about 2.0 to about 1.6.

Fresh or frozen meat and fish consumption, fruit and vegetable consumption, and dairy product and egg consumption seemed to be relatively independent measures of dietary patterns, all similarly related to the risk

TABLE 4.—*Correlation matrix for the five primary nutrition indices and ethanol consumption*

Nutrition index	Fresh or frozen meat and fish	Fruits and vegetables	Dairy products and eggs	Relative weight	Meals/ day	Ethanol, g
Fresh or frozen meat and fish	1.0	0.26	0.18	0.02	0.06	0.06
Fruits and vegetables		1.0	0.40	0.10	0.24	−0.13
Dairy products and eggs			1.0	0.04	0.21	0.00
Relative weight				1.0	0.13	−0.09
Meals/day					1.0	−0.26
Ethanol, g						1.0

of esophageal cancer. The ethanol-adjusted RR of individuals with low intake of two of the food groups was generally four times the risk of those with high intake of the same two food groups: the RR were 4.2, 3.9, or 2.8, depending on the pair of food groups being considered. The three food group consumption measures were then combined into a single measure of overall nutritional status. The RR for combinations of high, moderate, and low consumption of the three food groups are shown in table 5. The risk of esophageal cancer decreased steadily with improving patterns of food consumption. Relative to those who consumed high quantities of all three food groups (HHH), those who consumed low quantities of all three (LLL) had 14 times the risk. Adjustment for ethanol, across only two strata because of sparse numbers in the extreme nutrition categories, did not reveal any confounding, as shown in table 5.

With this overall measure of food consumption

TABLE 5.—*RR of esophageal cancer by an overall measure of food consumption patterns*

Food consumption pattern[a]	No. of cases	No. of controls	RR[b] (95% confidence interval)	RR, adjusted for ethanol[b,c]
HHH	2	20	1.0	1.0
HHM HMM	24	65	3.7 (0.8–17.0)	3.8
HHL MMM HML HLL	32	68	4.7 (1.0–21.4)	4.5
MML MLL	36	46	7.8 (1.7–35.7)	6.7
LLL	11	8	13.8 (2.5–76.4)	15.0

[a] Concurrent level of consumption of fresh or frozen meat and fish, fruits and vegetables, and dairy products and eggs, each rated as high (H), moderate (M), or low (L). For example, HML indicates high consumption of 1 of the 3 food groups, moderate consumption of a 2d, and low consumption of a 3d.
[b] All risks relative to those consuming high quantities of all 3 food groups (HHH).
[c] The categories of ethanol consumption were 0–5.9 and 6.0–80.0 fl oz of hard liquor equivalents/day.

patterns as the nutrition index, the interaction of nutritional status and ethanol intake was examined. As shown in table 6, the risks for poor nutrition and ethanol intake remained distinct and seemed to be multiplicative. With different divisions of the nutrition and ethanol variables or different nutrition indices, other patterns emerged, with combined effects often being less than multiplicative. Nonetheless, the elevated risk associated with poor nutrition could be detected across each level of ethanol consumption considered. It was not possible to determine whether poor nutrition was a risk factor among those unexposed to ethanol, since only 5 cases did not drink.

Beer, wine, and hard liquor provide almost none of the daily requirements for micronutrients and protein and therefore can be considered empty calories. Alcoholic beverage intake for the study subjects was converted to empty calorie intake and related to the risk of esophageal cancer, as shown in table 7. The RR rose steadily from 1.0 to 4.1 to 6.4 as the percent of the estimated caloric need of the average adult male, 51–75 years of age, that was being supplied by alcoholic beverages rose from less than 0.03% to 0.03–20% to 21–80%. When each study subject's intake of empty calories was divided by his usual adult weight, the gradient in RR became somewhat smoother. Dividing intake of empty calories by height produced similar results.

Information was collected on whether the usual method of cooking meat and fish was frying, baking, broiling, or a combination. Most of the study population (51%) fried their meat, and most (83%) fried their fish. The RR dropped to 0.6 (95% confidence interval = 0.3–1.1) when meat was usually baked rather than fried and to 0.3 (0.2–0.7) when meat was usually broiled. Those who usually baked or broiled fish rather than fried it showed similarly reduced RR of 0.8 (0.3–2.3) and 0.2 (0.1–0.6), respectively, although the numbers were sparse. These associations of esophageal cancer with the cooking method were not markedly reduced when adjusted for ethanol consumption, fresh or frozen meat and fish consumption, or education.

DISCUSSION

Poor nutrition is suspected to be a cause of esophageal cancer for several reasons. 1) In Iran (*12*), the

TABLE 6.—*RR of esophageal cancer by nutritional status and ethanol consumption*

Ethanol consumption, in hard liquor equivalents	Nutritional status[a]		
	High	Moderate	Low
0–5.9 fl oz/day	1.0[b] (6, 43)[c]	1.7 (6, 25)	3.0 (8, 19)
6.0–80.0 fl oz/day	2.7 (13, 34)	4.1 (21, 37)	8.0 (29, 26)

[a] Concurrent level of consumption of fresh or frozen meat and fish, fruits and vegetables, and dairy products and eggs. High, moderate, and low nutritional status were defined as food consumption patterns HHH, HHM, and HMM; patterns HHL, MMM, HML, and HLL; and patterns MML, MLL, and LLL, respectively.
[b] All risks relative to those who drank <6 fl oz/day and were of high nutritional status.
[c] *Numbers in parentheses* are numbers of cases and controls. Excluded from analysis were those of unknown nutritional status or with unknown ethanol intake.

Soviet Union (*13*), and China (*14*) esophageal cancer is endemic in regions with limited diets and impoverished agriculture. 2) Case–control studies in the United States (*15, 16*) and Iran (*17*) and a prospective cohort study in Japan (*18*) have demonstrated an association between reduced consumption of certain basic food groups, notably vegetables and fruits, and esophageal cancer. These studies, as well as case–control studies in Puerto Rico (*19*) and Singapore (*20*), have also shown an association between low socioeconomic status and esophageal cancer. 3) Within the United States mortality rates for esophageal cancer are inversely related to county socioeconomic indices and are higher among blacks than whites (*21*). 4) Until recently, esophageal cancer was unusually common in women from the rural, northern areas of Sweden, many of whom also had the Plummer-Vinson (or Paterson-Kelly) syndrome, which is associated with iron and other micronutrient deficiencies (*22, 23*). 5) Esophageal cancer has been reported as a sequel of celiac disease, a malabsorption

disorder of the small intestine (*24, 25*).

Several micronutrients can be postulated to play a role in the etiology of esophageal cancer. In experimental animals very large doses of analogs of vitamin A have been shown to protect against the development of cancer, whereas vitamin A deficiency often increases the risk (*26*). Either dietary vitamin A or dietary carotene could be the protective agent. Vitamin C is known to block the formation of N-nitroso compounds (*27*), carcinogens that can be formed in food or in the digestive tract once nitrite is present. Riboflavin, niacin, and vitamin B_6 are all essential for the health and integrity of the epithelium, particularly along the upper digestive tract (*28*). Thiamin deficiency is common among chronic alcoholics, and iron deficiency appears to be partly responsible for the Plummer-Vinson syndrome (*22*).

In this case-control study of an urban black male population with strikingly high mortality from esophageal cancer, poor nutrition was identified as a primary risk factor. Consumption levels of fresh or frozen meat and fish (beef, chicken, lamb, fish, shellfish), fruits and vegetables, and dairy products and eggs were inversely associated with esophageal cancer. For each of these measures of food group consumption, there were statistically significant trends in RR, with the least nourished third of the study population having twice the risk of the most nourished third. Individuals who consumed low levels of any two of these three specific food groups had about four times the risk of those who consumed high levels of the same two food groups. When the three food group consumption measures were combined into a single comprehensive nutrition index, the RR between extremes was 14, with a 95% confidence interval of 2.5–76. In addition, there were statistically significant inverse trends in RR, with gradients around twofold, for two indirect measures of nutritional status: relative weight (wt/ht^2) and number of meals eaten per day. All of these nutrition-related RR are adjusted for ethanol consumption.

The association of esophageal cancer with poor nutrition appeared to be independent of any associa-

TABLE 7.—*RR of esophageal cancer by consumption of the empty calories in alcoholic beverages*

kcal of beer, wine, and hard liquor consumed weekly	Percent of caloric needs filled by alcoholic beverages[a]	No. of cases	No. of controls	RR by empty calories[b] (95% confidence interval)	RR by empty calories/weight[b,c] (95% confidence interval)
<500	<0.03	5	55	1.0	1.0
500–3,360	0.03–20	16	43	4.1 (1.4, 12.1)	4.5 (1.5, 13.2)
3,361–6,720	21–40	18	31	6.4 (2.1, 18.8)	5.6 (1.9, 16.2)
6,721–13,440	41–80	28	49	6.3 (2.3, 17.6)	6.4 (2.3, 18.2)
>13,440	>80	23	35	7.2 (2.5, 20.8)	7.1 (2.5, 20.4)

[a] Daily caloric need of each individual was assumed to be 2,400 kcal, on the basis of the National Academy of Sciences' recommendation for U.S. males, 51–75 yr of age (*5*).
[b] All risks relative to those who drank <500 kcal of beer, wine, or hard liquor/wk.
[c] Empty calories/weight was cut into strata that were almost identical in size to those chosen for empty calories.

tions with alcohol consumption (the other major risk factor in these urban black men), with smoking, or with socioeconomic status. Adjustment for these potential confounders did not markedly change the relationships between the various nutrition measures and esophageal cancer risk; and the associations were consistently seen across the various levels of ethanol consumption, smoking, and socioeconomic status. Because the association of esophageal cancer with poor nutrition was independent of socioeconomic status, it seems unlikely that unidentified aspects of life-style, correlated with dietary patterns, are primarily responsible.

Before interpreting these associations between diet and esophageal cancer, it is necessary to assess their validity. Esophageal cancer might restrict food consumption through dysphagia or anorexia and thus influence the dietary history of the cases. Therefore, in this study next of kin were deliberately asked about the subjects' usual adult diet several years prior to death. The specificity of the associations that emerged suggests that the disease process itself did not create the differences in dietary patterns between cases and controls nor did it bias the recall of diet by the next of kin. Although consumption of 11 food items decreased with increasing risk, consumption of 8 other food items increased with increasing risk; and no association was seen for consumption of the other 12 food items. As for the food groups, cases were reported to eat significantly less fresh or frozen meat and fish, fewer fruits and vegetables, and fewer dairy products and eggs than the controls but similar amounts of carbohydrates and precooked or processed meat and fish. Thus consumption of a few food groups, typically associated with a sensible diet, was selectively reduced. In addition, the usual adult weight, several years prior to death, recalled by the next of kin, indicated a smaller percentage of very light individuals among the cases than that reported for blacks ot similar age in the 1971–74 U.S. Health and Nutrition Examination Survey. Thus there is no suggestion of a general decrease in total food consumption among the cases, which might have resulted from preclinical cancer.

Information on dietary patterns is occasionally criticized as imprecise and of limited value, especially if obtained from next of kin. However, in this study relatively strong associations with clear gradients were repeatedly noted; and the relationship that emerged was internally consistent. First of all, poor nutrition, whether measured by consumption of certain specific food groups, anthropometry, or frequency of eating, was repeatedly associated with increased risk of esophageal cancer. Second, similar food items, such as the various individual fruits and vegetables, were similarly associated with risk. Random misclassification of exposure might obscure a true association, but it does not generate a false association.

To help evaluate the validity and reliability of the

next of kin responses, the RR for several of the nutrition measures were calculated separately for interviews of wives and of other next of kin. They were generally comparable. For example, for the general measure of nutritional status defined in table 6, the RR rose, as nutrition declined, from 1.0 to 1.4 and 3.0 among the subjects whose wives were interviewed and from 1.0 to 1.7 and 2.8 among the other subjects.

The relationships identified in this study suggest that general malnutrition, probably of a mild form, increases the susceptibility of urban black men to esophageal cancer. No direct evidence for a specific nutritional deficiency was found. Estimates of the intake of vitamin A, carotene, vitamin C, thiamin, and riboflavin were each less strongly associated with esophageal cancer than was consumption of the basic food groups that provide most of each micronutrient. In addition, the micronutrient indices were not as strongly associated as such general measures of nutritional status as relative weight and meals eaten per day. However, the micronutrient estimates were constrained by the food frequencies actually asked in the interview. For example, no information on tomato consumption could be incorporated into the vitamin C estimates; and no information on fortified bread and cereal consumption could be incorporated into the thiamin and riboflavin estimates. A niacin index was not formed because of the difficulty of estimating the contribution of tryptophan intake (5), and an iron index was not formed because of uncertainty about the degree of absorption of iron in different foods and at different meals (29).

Consumption of bacon, frankfurters, lunch meats, and canned meats was more frequent among the cases than the controls and suggested exposure to nitrites and possible formation of endogenous N-nitroso compounds. However, canned fish, which contains no nitrite, and breakfast sausage, which usually contains no nitrite either, were also consumed more frequently by the cases. Thus esophageal cancer seemed more closely associated with precooked or processed meat and fish consumption than with nitrite intake.

The inverse association with relative weight resulted primarily from a reduced risk among heavy individuals. The RR for heavy subjects was approximately half that for those of typical weight. Risk was not markedly elevated among light subjects. It is plausible that in this study population, with its high intake of alcoholic beverages and the resultant empty calories, only those who regularly consumed more than their daily caloric needs and thus maintained excess weight were able to approach reasonable intakes of a variety of nutritious food groups.

The mechanism by which alcohol increases the risk of esophageal cancer is not known, and attempts to produce cancer in well-nourished laboratory animals by prolonged ingestion of ethanol have failed (30). Since poor nutrition is a risk factor for esophageal cancer, it is conceivable that alcohol increases risk, in part, by reducing nutrient intake. Beer, wine, and hard liquor provide a share of the daily caloric needs and consequently reduce appetite but provide almost none of the daily requirements for micronutrients and protein. In this study the risk of esophageal cancer increased sharply with heavy consumption of alcoholic beverages, whether measured as intake of empty calories or grams of ethanol.

Among these urban black men the risk of esophageal cancer associated with alcoholic beverage consumption seemed relatively independent of the association with poor nutrition. Alcohol consumption was only weakly correlated with the primary nutrition indices. Nonetheless, it is possible that alcohol consumption functions by a nutritional mechanism. Alcohol intake could be a partial measure of the underlying dietary determinants of esophageal cancer in much the same way as fresh or frozen meat and fish consumption and fruit and vegetable consumption are only partially correlated with each other, and yet each partially measures overall nutritional status and the related risk of esophageal cancer.

The usual method of cooking was also related to risk of esophageal cancer. Those who usually baked or broiled meat or fish were at less risk than those who usually fried meat and fish. Cooking practices are often influenced by the type of foods purchased. In this study population, however, the usual method of cooking was not consistently correlated with consumption of either the fresh or frozen or the precooked or processed meat and fish groups. The implications of the risk associated with frying foods are not clear and suggest further study.

This study was unable to identify a specific nutritional deficiency associated with the high risk of esophageal cancer among urban black men. However, a provocative pattern of generally poor nutrition was clearly associated with risk; a complex nutritional deficiency, involving several micronutrients or food groups, may be involved. A precedent exists for this hypothesis since many of the nutritional deficiencies observed in humans, such as protein–calorie malnutrition, encompass multiple inadequacies (31).

The nutrition-related associations identified in this study were relatively strong, graded with respect to exposure level, internally consistent, and specific, all of which was reassuring in view of the difficulties inherent in the study design. Information on usual diet several years earlier was obtained from next of kin, and occasionally close friends, for persons who often had limited education, histories of heavy drinking, and thus presumably erratic life-styles. Future studies involving a large number of study subjects and more detailed and varied questions about diet might narrow the associations indicated by this study and further clarify the role of nutrition in the development of esophageal cancer.

REFERENCES

(1) POTTERN LM, MORRIS LE, BLOT WJ, ZIEGLER RG, FRAUMENI JF JR. Esophageal cancer among black men in Washington, D.C. I. Alcohol, tobacco, and other risk factors. JNCI 1981; 67:777-783.

(2) National Center for Health Statistics. International classification of diseases. Eighth revision. Washington, D.C.: U.S. Govt Print Off, 1967 (PHS publication No. 1693).

(3) U.S. Department of Agriculture. Nutritive value of American foods, in common units. Agriculture handbook No. 456. Washington, D.C.: U.S. Govt Print Off, 1975.

(4) U.S. Department of Agriculture. Composition of foods: Raw, processed, prepared. Agriculture handbook No. 8. Washington, D.C.: U.S. Govt Print Off, 1963.

(5) Food and Nutrition Board. Recommended dietary allowances. Ninth revision. Washington, D.C.: National Academy of Sciences, 1980.

(6) National Center for Health Statistics. Weight by height and age for adults 18-74 years: U.S., 1971-74. Hyattsville, Md.: DHEW, 1979 (Vital and Health Statistics 11-208).

(7) FLEISS JL. Statistical methods for rates and proportions. New York: Wiley, 1973.

(8) MANTEL N, HAENSZEL W. Statistical aspects of the analysis of data from retrospective studies of disease. J Natl Cancer Inst 1959; 22:719-748.

(9) ROTHMAN KJ, BOICE JD. Epidemiologic analysis with a programmable calculator. Washington, D.C.: U.S. Govt Print Off, 1979 [DHEW publication No. (NIH) 79-1649].

(10) MANTEL N. Chi-square tests with one degree of freedom: Extensions of the Mantel-Haenszel procedure. J Am Stat Assoc 1963; 58:690-700.

(11) SNEDECOR GW, COCHRAN WG. Statistical methods. Ames: Iowa State Univ Press, 1967.

(12) Joint Iran–International Agency for Research on Cancer Study Group. Esophageal cancer studies in the Caspian Littoral of Iran: Results of population studies—A prodrome. J Natl Cancer Inst 1977; 59:1127-1138.

(13) KOLYCHEVA NI. Epidemiology of esophageal cancer in the USSR. In: Levin DL, ed. Cancer epidemiology in the USA and the USSR. Washington, D.C.: DHHS, 1980 (DHHS publication No. 80-2044).

(14) WEINSTEIN IB. Chemical and viral carcinogenesis. In: Kaplan HS, Tsuchitani PJ, eds. Cancer in China. New York: Alan R. Liss, 1978:58-67.

(15) WYNDER EL, BROSS IJ. A study of etiological factors in cancer of the esophagus. Cancer 1961; 14:389-413.

(16) METTLIN C, GRAHAM S, PRIORE R, SWANSON M. Diet and cancer of the esophagus. Am J Epidemiol 1980; 112:422-423.

(17) COOK-MOZAFFARI PJ, AZORDEGAN F, DAY NE, RESSICAUD A, SABAI C, ARAMESH B. Oesophageal cancer studies in the Caspian Littoral of Iran: Results of a case–control study. Br J Cancer 1979; 39:293-309.

(18) HIRAYAMA T. Diet and cancer. Nutr Cancer 1979; 1:67-81.

(19) MARTÌNEZ I. Factors associated with cancer of the esophagus, mouth, and pharynx in Puerto Rico. J Natl Cancer Inst 1969; 42:1069-1094.

(20) DE JONG UW, BRESLOW N, HONG JG, SRIDHARAN M, SHANMUGARATNAM K. Aetiological factors in oesophageal cancer in Singapore Chinese. Int J Cancer 1974; 13:291-303.

(21) FRAUMENI JF JR, BLOT WJ. Geographic variation in esophageal cancer mortality in the United States. J Chronic Dis 1977; 30: 759-767.

(22) LARSSON LG, SANDSTRÖM A, WESTLING P. Relationship of Plummer-Vinson disease to cancer of the upper alimentary tract in Sweden. Cancer Res 1975; 35:3308-3316.

(23) DAY NE, MUÑOZ N. Esophagus. In: Schottenfeld D, Fraumeni JF Jr, eds. Cancer epidemiology and prevention. Philadelphia: Saunders, 1982:596-623.

(24) HARRIS OD, COOKE WT, THOMPSON H, WATERHOUSE JA. Malignancy in adult coeliac disease and idiopathic steatorrhoea.

Am J Med 1967; 42:899–912.

(25) HOLMES GK, STOKES PL, SORAHAN TM, PRIOR P, WATERHOUSE JA, COOKE WT. Coeliac disease, gluten-free diet, and malignancy. Gut 1976; 17:612–619.

(26) SPORN MB, DUNLOP NM, NEWTON DL, SMITH JM. Prevention of chemical carcinogenesis by vitamin A and its synthetic analogs (retinoids). Fed Proc 1976; 35:1332–1338.

(27) MIRVISH SS, WALLCAVE L, EAGEN M, SHUBIK P. Ascorbate–nitrite reaction: Possible means of blocking the formation of carcinogenic N-nitroso compounds. Science 1972; 177:65–67.

(28) BOGERT LJ, BRIGGS GM, CALLOWAY DH. Nutrition and physical fitness. 9th ed. Philadelphia: Saunders, 1973.

(29) MONSEN ER, HALLBERG L, LAYRISSE M, et al. Estimation of available dietary iron. Am J Clin Nutr 1978; 31:134–141.

(30) SCHOTTENFELD D. Alcohol as a co-factor in the etiology of cancer. Cancer 1979; 43:1962–1966.

(31) Joint Food and Agriculture Organization and World Health Organization Expert Committee on Nutrition. Protein-calorie malnutrition, eighth report. Geneva: WHO, 1971 (WHO technical report series No. 477).

Dietary Aflatoxins and Human Liver Cancer. A Study in Swaziland

by F. G. Peers[1,3]*, G. A. Gilman*[1,4]*, and C. A. Linsell*[2]

F. G. Peers [1, 3], G. A. Gilman [1, 4] and C. A. Linsell [2]
[1] *Tropical Products Institute, 56-62, Grays Inn Road, London, England; and* [2] *Nairobi Research Centre, International Agency for Research on Cancer, P.O. Box 46831, Nairobi, Kenya*

Summary. *A study in Swaziland to assess the possible relationship of aflatoxin contamination and the incidence of primary liver cancer is reported. Aflatoxin ingestion levels have been determined in "food from the plate" samples collected over a 1-year period. A significant correlation between the calculated ingested daily dose and the adult male incidence of primary liver cancer in different parts of Swaziland has been established. Samples of food-stuffs other than the plate samples also reflected the correlation of aflatoxin contamination and liver cancer. This study extends and amplifies the findings of an earlier study in the Murang'a district of Kenya and supports the hypothesis that aflatoxin ingestion is a factor in the genesis of primary liver cancer in Africa.*

An evaluation of the contamination of diets by aflatoxin and the primary liver cancer incidence in the African population of the Murang'a district of Kenya established a statistically significant correlation (Peers and Linsell, 1973). The distribution of medical facilities in the Murang'a study and the low number of cancer cases recorded in some of the altitude areas of the district might have contributed a bias to the correlation. A further study in Africa was therefore carried out to test the strength and consistency of the association.

In Swaziland it had already been reported (Keen and Martin, 1971a) that the risk of developing liver cancer varied with altitude as in Kenya. Stored groundnuts, a popular food in Swaziland, were often contaminated with aflatoxin and the occurrence of such contamination was associated with an increased liver cancer frequency (Keen and Martin, 1971a, b). It was not possible, however, to infer dietary exposure levels of aflatoxin from these data.

The main medical facilities in Swaziland are located in the areas of lower liver cancer frequency where it was assumed that cancer case catchment would be more effective: the reverse of the potential bias present in the Kenya study. Primary liver cancer was also more frequent, 4.9/100,000 crude rate for all ages in Swaziland, 1964-1968, compared with 3.3/100,000 crude rate for all ages, in Murang'a, 1967-1970. The African population of Swaziland was approximately the same as in the Kenya study area (Murang'a 344,858 and Swaziland 362,367) although the area of the latter is 10 times greater.

Additional advantages of Swaziland as the site of the second study were that the country is naturally divided into four well-defined altitude areas which, it was suspected, would reflect varying levels of

---

[3] On detached duty with Nairobi Research Centre of the International Agency for Research on Cancer.

[4] On detached duty in Swaziland.

aflatoxin contamination of food staples and the distribution of liver cancer cases as reported in the independent study by Keen and Martin (1971a) between these areas was significantly different from that expected on a population basis.

Topography

Swaziland is a landlocked, independent kingdom of 17,422 km² in southern Africa bounded on the north, south and west by the Transwaal province of the Republic of South Africa and on the east by Mozambique and Natal province of South Africa.

The country is divided naturally into four well-defined altitude regions which extend north and south in roughly parallel belts. The highveld, in the west, the middleveld and the lowveld are more or less of equal breadth, while the Lebombo, in altitude similar to the middleveld, is a markedly narrower strip along the eastern border.

The location of the medical facilities available in 1964, shown in Figure 1, were obtained from the Swaziland Ministry of Health.

The highveld averages 1,000-1,350 m in altitude and occupies some 4,900 km². It is mountainous and split by numerous river valleys and gorges. There are good pastures for summer grazing and considerable areas are covered by pine and eucalyptus forests. Arable production is generally confined to the gentler slopes and valleys.

The middleveld averages 650-750 m in altitude and is undulating to hilly, occupying an area of about 4,700 km². Although the soil fertility is often not particularly good, the physical aspects of the land render it suitable for arable production. There is also much natural grassland and the grazing is good in summer.

The gently undulating lowveld averages 150-300 m in altitude and covers more than 6,500 km². It is seldom a true plain as isolated knolls and ridges rise above the general level. It has a distinctive " bush " vegetation which ranges from dense, thorny thicket, to more open parkland savannah with large trees. The underlying grass has a high food value which makes it excellent for cattle ranching. Apart from some irrigated areas, arable production is often sparse, especially in the low-rainfall areas.

The Lebombo range in the extreme east of the country has an impressive western escarpment. This region approximates to the middleveld in altitude although it resembles the lowveld in many places with respect to vegetation. There is good, mixed farming country but the chief type of individual holding is the cattle ranch.

Climate

The highveld in general has a near-temperate climate with warm summers while the lowveld is sub-tropical and semi-humid. Rainfall decreases from an average of 1,270 mm in the highveld to some 660 mm in the lowveld, higher in the north than the south, and most of this falls in the summer between early October and the end of March. The lowveld has a mean maximum temperature of 29° C, which is some 6° C higher than that for the highveld. Frosts are common in the winter in the highveld and occur, to a lesser extent, in the lowveld.

Population

The Report on the 1966 census enumerated a total resident population of 374,571 of which 93.9% were Swazis living predominantly in rural areas. In the northern lowveld and Lebombo there are some Shangaans from the eastern Transvaal who work mainly on estates. The middleveld is the most densely populated area with 41.6% of the population or an average of 338 persons per km².

Crops, storage methods and fungal deterioration

Maize is the staple diet but sorghum, groundnuts, jugo beans *(Voandzeia subterranea)* and various

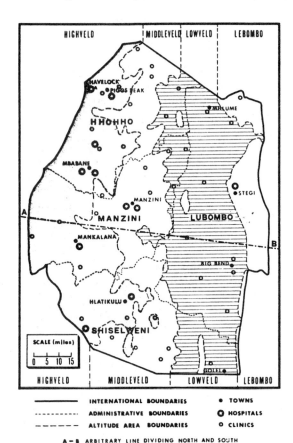

FIGURE 1

Swaziland—medical facilities, 1964.

pulses including the cowpea *(Vigna sinensis)*, the kidney bean *(Phaseolus vulgaris)* and the mung bean *(Phaseolus aureus)* are other durable food crops grown for home consumption. The areas under these crops vary with altitude. A recent agricultural Sample Census (1971/2) has shown that the area under maize is over 62,000 hectares, of which a little less than half is in the middleveld. Areas under other durable food crops of lesser importance are groundnuts (5,000 hectares), sorghum (2,500 hectares), jugo beans (2,800 hectares) and beans (2,000 hectares).

In the lower areas especially, maize and sorghum dry out considerably before harvest which is why cribs or grain stores are seldom seen there. Open storage platforms are observed mainly in the lowveld but crude cribs inside huts with open-structured walls are more common in the high- and middlevelds. No mould damage was observed to occur in these structures, but if rain falls on the mature crop prior to harvest, considerable mould damage occurs in the field, especially to maize. Most of this damage is caused by *Fusarium moniliforme* and other typical " field " fungi. *Aspergillus flavus* and other storage species are not common at this time. After 3-4 months, maize and sorghum are shelled and stored as grain in a variety of traditional or imported containers.

One traditional method that might be expected to encourage mould growth in stored grain is the underground pit. Pits are found mainly in the lowveld and on the Lebombo range, but they were once more widely distributed. They represent, in fact, a method of great antiquity used in one form or another in many parts of Africa. Those in Swaziland are narrow-necked, beehive-shaped, and are usually situated in the cattle kraal. Those examined held between 3 and 30 bags of maize and sorghum.

As the pits are not lined except with a thin layer of cattle dung, water rapidly penetrates and is absorbed by the grain. Some mould damage usually occurs in the neck region, if this is filled with grain, or at the rim of surface layers, if the pit is not completely filled. Small quantities of grain in large pits frequently become caked with fungal mycelium. Mouldy grain from pits is sometimes washed and eaten, a factor which could be of some significance in this survey. In full pits the bulk of the grain is reasonably well preserved although it undergoes a partial ensilagement, while changes in colour, flavour and texture, especially in grain near the walls and floor of the pit, are usual.

Insect damage is generally absent from pit-stored maize but in above-ground stores, especially in the lowveld, this is a serious problem, especially as insect-damaged grain is more easily invaded by storage fungi than undamaged seeds.

Other traditional stores with a more general distribution are clay pots and spherical, woven grass baskets. These are used for all crops and are kept under cover. In certain middle-veld areas of northern Swaziland mud and wattle structures are used to store shelled grain but the method is relatively uncommon.

More recent introductions, gradually replacing the traditional methods, are small tins, 200 l drums, sacks and metal silos. The silos are cylindrical and made from corrugated metal, resembling water tanks. Mould damage was seen occasionally in metal silos exposed to direct sunlight.

The groundnut is an important source of protein in Swaziland. The crop is dried in a variety of ways including windrows, platforms and small stacks. After hand picking, the pods are given a further period of sun drying prior to storage.

A more detailed account of storage and handling methods used in Swaziland and adjoining territories, particularly in respect of deterioration by fungi, has been published elsewhere (Gilman, 1971; Martin *et al.*, 1971).

Cancer registration

During the 5-year period 1964-1968 a total of 500 primary liver cancers in Africans was registered by the Swaziland Cancer Registry. Using the 1966 Census data this means a crude cancer rate of 27.6 per 100,000/year compared with 19.9 per 100,000/year recorded for the Murang'a district of Kenya. Details of cancer data used in this study were derived from Keen and Martin (1971) and further information from Dr. Keen (personal communications, 1974) on the location, sex and age of previously recorded cases.

Experimental design of the study

Apart from the four topographical zones of Swaziland already described, the country is also divided administratively into four Districts. These are Hhohho (A) in the northwest, Manzini (B) in the centre and west of the country, Shiselweni (C) in the south and Lubombo (D) in the east. The latter district includes the Lebombo range and a large proportion of the lowveld. The study was so designed that, if necessary, a comparison of the administrative districts could also be made.

For sampling, Swaziland was divided as follows into eleven main arable areas to include a range of climates, altitudes, crops and storage and handling methods: Highveld—Oshoek (A), Mankanyane (B) and Hlatikulu (C); Middleveld—Lomati Valley (A), Manzini (B) and Hluti (C); Lowveld—Belgane (A), Ngcina (D), Big Bend/Sipofaneni (D); Lebombo range—Lomashasha (D) and Siteki (D).

In the absence of tax lists and identity numbers, which were available in the Murang'a District of Kenya, a random individual or family sampling was not possible. However, lists of Chiefs and

Indunas, (sub-chiefs) living in the above areas were obtained with the assistance of the Ministry of Local Administration and from these lists Indunas were selected at random, two from each area, to form the focal points of 22 sampling clusters.

It was thought that the socio-economic status of the Indunas used as cluster centres might bias the sampling and to test this, seven householders living progressively further away from the Indunas' homes were chosen to complete each cluster. As holdings are generally well scattered this involved distances of up to 2.4 km from the cluster centre to the last sample in a cluster.

The clusters were sampled every 2 months, though not necessarily in the same order, for a period of 1-year. The 2-month periods constitute arbitrary " seasons " to test seasonal variation within the year of study. This provided a total of 1,056 diets, according to the factorial design: 11 (areas) $\times 2$ (clusters) $\times 6$ (" seasons ") $\times 8$ (samples).

In addition to the diets one sample each of beer (Tswala), sour porridge (Incwancwa), sour drink (Amahhewu) and groundnuts were, if possible, collected separately at each visit as these foodstuffs are often not consumed with the main meal.

Collection of samples

The maize crop in Swaziland is harvested in April/May and shelled in July/August while groundnuts are harvested sooner and are therefore usually in store by the beginning of June. The collection of samples was started in October 1972 at the beginning of the rains and was completed in September 1973. When this survey commenced, therefore, maize had only recently been stored as shelled grain whereas groundnuts had been in store for approximately 6 months.

It was established that the main meal of the day was usually consumed in the morning. This consisted of maize porridge with one or more of the following: vegetables, meat, spinach, groundnuts, sourmilk, pumpkin, sweet potatoes and various kinds of beans and other pulses. Groundnuts are frequently consumed as a relish in powder form, often with a " spinach " prepared from the leaves of a variety of wild and cultivated plants. Occasionally sour porridge or sorghum may be substituted for the normal maize porridge.

The collector visited each cluster the night before a collection was due to take place. This was necessary as extra food had to be cooked. Periodic checks were made to ensure that special meals were not being prepared for the collector. During these preliminary visits certain households were asked to prepare sour drinks, sour porridge and powdered groundnuts if they were not already available. Beer was obtained from the brewing point nearest to the cluster concerned.

Collections were made in the early morning,

visiting each household in turn. If any food remained from the meal of the previous evening this was included in the diet sample. The collector was instructed to purchase a " man-sized " portion of each meal.

The dietary components of the meal, sociological and other data were recorded for each household sampled. Safeguards, such as a record of the altitude, were included to ensure that each cluster was actually sampled and that the diets were not obtained from easier sources.

Also on the first visit to the cluster centre an appropriate number of serially numbered tickets were handed to the Indunas and at every subsequent food collection these were matched with the duplicates.

Inability to collect a particular sample due to illness or absence occurred on a average three times in a " season ". In these instances, adjacent households, not normally included in the cluster, were sampled instead.

The diets were placed in plastic bags, the fluids in 1-litre plastic bottles, and the groundnuts in small plastic cartons. All samples were deep frozen as soon as possible after collection, almost invariably on the same day, insulated cold boxes and " scotch-ice " coolant packs being provided to the field team. On return to the laboratory the samples were deep frozen at $-20°$ C until processed.

Sample processing

In order to obtain representative sub-samples for analysis the diets were homogenized. However, the porridge which formed the bulk of the samples in most cases, assumed a spongy consistency on thawing and could not be easily homogenized. It was therefore often necessary to add water. This was always a known amount, either 25% or 50% of the wet weight of the sample. A potato masher was then used to break up the diet prior to homogenizing. With the beers, sour porridges and sour drinks, homogenization was not necessary but they were shaken vigorously before sampling.

The diet samples were freeze-dried in shallow containers at a shelf temperature of 50° C for 24 h. to enable mycological studies to be made on the beers and sour foods and to prevent sugar inversion these were dried at a shelf temperature of 35° C for 36-48 h. The samples were stored in plastic containers and air freighted to Nairobi for aflatoxin analysis.

Aflatoxin analysis

Aflatoxin analyses were carried out on the lyophilized diet samples by methods previously described (Peers and Linsell, 1973) except that no preliminary drying over silica gel was necessary. The dry residues from the lyophilization of the beer, sour drink and sour porridge samples were processed in the same way. The powdered groundnut samples were analysed by the methods described by Jones (1972).

RESULTS

Table I illustrates the exposure to aflatoxin of the study population of Swaziland using the mean contamination levels of plate samples, including all negative samples, and the frequency of aflatoxin positivity by cluster and individual diet samples. The data have been divided into four altitude areas and six " seasons " of collection.

Table II shows the frequency and mean level of contamination of samples other than whole diet plate samples which were also collected as part of the survey. These dietary items are freely available to the Swazis but it was not possible to assess accurately individual or group consumption. A total of 126 sour drink samples were also collected but all proved negative for aflatoxins at a detection level of 1 μg/litre.

Although the dietary data with a large number

of negative results can be fitted to a Gamma function curve (Berry and Day, 1973) it was decided to express the statistics of the results by more simple methods. In Table III the various frequencies of positivity have been compared by the χ^2 tests and in Table IV the mean contamination levels of the diets have been evaluated for significance using Student's t tests.

Overall, the principal significant factor is that of altitude and this is true for both frequency and mean contamination levels. Since the administrative areas of Swaziland correspond to a large degree to the altitude areas, as opposed to the situation in Murang'a, a significant effect is observed when the frequency distribution of aflatoxin positivity is evaluated by this parameter.

The data have also been evaluated on a north-south division in order to test the conclusion of Keen and Martin (1971a) that liver cancer frequency differed significantly between these two regions of Swaziland. The north-south division was defined by an arbitrary line, based on the 1966

TABLE I

FREQUENCY OF CONTAMINATION OF CLUSTERS AND INDIVIDUAL DIET SAMPLES AND MEAN AFLATOXIN CONTAMINATION LEVELS OF THE DIETS

Season	Highveld			Middleveld			Lowveld			Lebombo		
	Cluster frequency [1]	Sample frequency [2]	Aflatoxin level [3]	Cluster frequency	Sample frequency	Aflatoxin level	Cluster frequency	Sample frequency	Aflatoxin level	Cluster frequency	Sample frequency	Aflatoxin level
A Oct. and Nov. 1972	0/6	0/48	0.000	2/6	2/48	0.188	3/6	3/48	2.750	2/4	2/32	1.375
B Dec. 1972 and Jan. 1973	0/6	0/48	0.000	1/6	1/48	0.208	2/6	4/48	1.135	3/4	4/32	0.641
C Feb. and March 1973	4/6	5/48	0.375	3/6	3/48	0.375	3/6	5/48	1.260	1/4	1/32	0.266
D April and May 1973	2/6	3/48	0.114	3/6	4/48	0.302	6/6	7/48	0.802	2/4	2/32	0.391
E June and July 1973	2/6	2/48	0.406	3/6	3/48	0.542	2/6	6/48	2.063	1/4	1/32	0.391
F Aug. and Sept. 1973	1/6	1/48	0.177	2/6	2/48	0.250	4/6	9/48	1.052	1/4	1/32	0.172
Total	9/36	11/288	0.179	14/36	15/288	0.311	20/36	34/288	1.510	10/24	11/192	0.539

[1] Frequency of positive clusters expressed as the ratio of clusters with one or more positive samples of the total of clusters examined. — [2] Frequency of positive diets expressed as the ratio of positive diets ($\geqq$ 1 μg/kg)/total number of diets analysed. — [3] Mean aflatoxin contamination expressed as μg/kg wet diet including all negative samples.

TABLE II

FREQUENCIES AND MEAN LEVELS OF AFLATOXIN CONTAMINATION
OF SAMPLES COLLECTED OTHER THAN DIETS

Season	Sour drinks		Sour porridges		Beers		Groundnuts	
	n [1]	$\bar{x}$ [2]	n	$\bar{x}$	n	$\bar{x}$	n	$\bar{x}$
A	0/18	0.00	1/8	0.56	4/18	0.67	2/19	18.00
B	0/21	0.00	3/19	0.61	1/20	0.08	2/22	20.09
C	0/22	0.00	1/20	0.05	0/22	0.00	1/2	0.75
D	0/21	0.00	2/23	0.50	1/22	0.07	2/14	3.43
E	0/22	0.00	0/22	0.00	2/20	0.33	2/14	5.54
F	0/22	0.00	1/22	0.61	1/20	0.23	2/22	3.41
Totals	0/126	0.00	8/114	0.37	9/122	0.21	11/93	10.60

[1] n = frequency expressed as number of positives/total analysed. — [2] $\bar{x}$ = mean aflatoxin in μg/kg of material as collected (including negatives).

TABLE III

STATISTICS OF FREQUENCIES OF POSITIVE CLUSTERS, INDIVIDUAL DIET SAMPLES
AND SAMPLES OTHER THAN DIETS

Statistic	Degrees of freedom	χ^2—clusters	χ^2—diets	χ^2—other samples
Altitude areas	3	7.04	17.09 *** [1]	13.63 **
Administration areas	3	10.53 *	14.49 **	7.13 *
Seasons	5	6.61	4.97	2.83 for 2 d.f. [2]
Between samples within clusters [3]	7	—	3.50	—
Within clusters from binomial [4]	2	—	0.74	—
North *vs* South	1	8.23 **	4.51 *	3.88 *
A *vs* B cluster	1	0.50	0.06	0.10

[1] * $0.05 > p > 0.01$; ** $0.01 > p > 0.001$; *** $p < 0.001$. — [2] The low cell expectation for individual seasons was < 5 and hence the seasons have been combined in pairs (*i.e.* A + B, C + D and E + F) to evaluate this statistic. — [3] Starting with the cluster centre (Induna) the set of eight samples was collected progressively further away and sequentially marked stroke 1 to stroke 8. This statistic shows no bias for contamination of the first or any other sample within a cluster. — [4] Using an overall positivity of 6.7% (71/1056) the expectations of multiple contaminated samples within a cluster have been calculated from the binomial expansion.

TABLE IV

STATISTICS OF THE MEAN LEVELS
OF DIETARY AFLATOXINS

Mean values compared [1]	t value	Probability
Season A *vs* season D (widest difference between two seasons)	1.23	$0.3 > p > 0.2$
Highveld *vs* Middleveld	1.17	$0.3 > p > 0.2$
Highveld *vs* Lowveld	3.33	$p < 0.001$
Highveld *vs* Lebombo	1.68	$0.1 > p > 0.05$
Middleveld *vs* Lowveld	2.96	$0.01 > p > 0.001$
Middleveld *vs* Lebombo	0.99	$0.4 > 0 > 0.3$
Lowveld *vs* Lebombo	1.86	$0.1 > p > 0.05$
North *vs* South	1.31	$0.2 > p > 0.1$

[1] Means include all negative results.

census, which avoided passing through any collection area or site of a cancer case. The frequency of aflatoxin positivity from this present study does indeed show significant differences between the north and the south. However, the mean contamination levels of the diet samples including all positives do not show a significant difference. This would imply that the more frequent exposure in the north is at a lower dose level.

The principal results obtained in this study are summarized in Table V and in Figure 2 the calculated exposure data for males (four areas) and females (three areas) have been plotted against the adult liver cancer rates recorded by Keen (personal communications, 1974). The sex ratio (M/F) of the cancer incidence in Swaziland is approximately 5:1 as compared with 2:1 in Kenya and with the small population in the Lebombo area no female cases of liver cancer were recorded in the 5 years of registration, whereas 4 adult male cases were recorded. Hence the two sexes have been treated separately with respect to correlation exercises. The male aflatoxin ingestion data have been obtained assuming 2 kg wet food and 2 litres of beer per day and a mean body weight of 70 kg and this has been evaluated for the four altitude sub-areas. The regression line, $y = 23.84 \log_{10} x - 13.66$, has been drawn in Figure 2 together with the 95% confidence limits: the correlation coefficient for this line is 0.988 for two degrees of freedom ($0.02 > p > 0.01$).

For females the Middleveld and Lebombo data have been combined as one area and the aflatoxin ingestion levels have been calculated assuming a 2 kg wet food intake per day and a 70 kg mean body weight.

TABLE V
SUMMARY OF THE PRINCIPAL RESULTS

	Altitude area									
	Highveld		Middleveld		Lowveld		Lebombo		Swaziland	
	M	F	M	F	M	F	M	F	M	F
Total population (1966 census)	48,628	52,091	69,136	82,294	45,814	45,657	8,713	10,034	172,291	190,076
Population ⩾15 years old (1966 census)	25,658	28,203	32,464	45,225	26,266	24,907	4,279	5,464	88,667	103,799
Primary liver cancer cases ⩾15 years old, 1964-68	9	2	24	5	35	7	4	0	72	14
Adult incidence rates per 100,000 per year	7.02	1.42	14.79	2.21	26.65	5.62	18.65	0.00	16.24	2.70
Frequency of contaminated diets	11/288		15/288		34/288		11/192		71/1,056	
Mean level (μg/kg)	0.179		0.311		1.510		0.539		0.643	
Frequency of contaminated beers	1/31		2/31		5/35		1/25		9/122	
Mean level (μg/l)	0.11		0.19		0.36		0.16		0.21	
Frequency of contaminated groundnuts	0/19		3/26		6/27		2/21		11/93	
Mean level (μg/kg)	0.00		6.94		29.09		0.95		10.60	
Frequency of contaminated porridges	0/31		5/30		3/29		0/24		8/114	
Mean level (μg/kg)	0.00		0.92		0.50		0.00		0.37	
Mean aflatoxin ingested [1]	5.11		8.89		43.14		15.40		24.37	
ng/kg body-weight/day [2]	8.34		14.43		53.34		19.89		18.37	

[1] Calculated assuming 2 kg wet diet intake per day and 70 kg body/weight. — [2] Calculated assuming intake of 2 kg diet and 2 l beer per day and 70 kg body/weight.

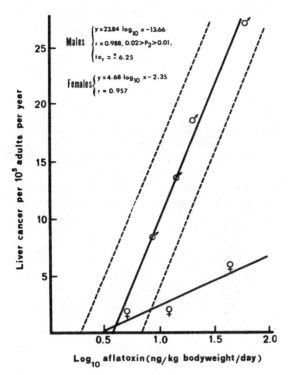

FIGURE 2

Correlation of liver cancer with aflatoxin ingestion.

The correlation line $y = 4.68 \log_{10} X - 2.35$ has been calculated but the correlation coefficient ($r = 0.957$) is not significant for only 1 degree of freedom.

DISCUSSION

This study was undertaken to ascertain whether the relationship between dietary aflatoxin levels and primary liver cancer incidence established in the Murang'a district of Kenya was valid for another area of Africa, specifically where the range of liver cancer incidence was higher than that recorded in Murang'a and where groundnuts were known to be incorporated into the diet.

The foodstuffs referred to in Table III all form part of the Swaziland diet but they were collected separately from the diet plate samples, and it was not possible to assess ingestion levels due to the widely varying quantities and frequencies of consumption. The contamination data from Table III therefore have not been included in the calculation of ingestion levels. Any aflatoxin exposure levels quoted are thus almost certainly minimal ingestion levels. Our experience and that of others (Shank *et al.*, 1972; van Rensburg *et al.*, 1974) would suggest that it is the chronic ingestion levels that more closely parallel liver cancer incidence rather than occasional high exposures.

As in other studies the anomaly of relating current exposure to a suspect carcinogen with retrospective rather than prospective data has been ignored. It has been assumed that the dietary habits and customs of the Swazi people have changed little over the last few decades.

As aflatoxin contamination is mainly related to poor storage the lack of a seasonal effect on the aflatoxin content of the diets was surprising. The data for the groundnut samples in Table III suggest that November to January is the period when high levels of aflatoxins may be encountered in this dietary component but the relative constancy of the exposure from the diet samples suggests that a discriminatory sorting is effected by the housewife as detected in Murang'a (Peers and Linsell, 1973) and Mozambique (van Rensburg *et al.*, 1975).

A comparison of the components of the positive diets with those of the negative diets indicated that groundnuts, beans and cultivated vegetables are included more frequently in the positive diets. Since 98.4% of the plate samples collected contained maize it was not possible to incriminate specifically this diet component. The incrimination of groundnuts was suspected from the work of Keen and Martin (1971a) and is confirmed by the data in Tables II/III.

In Swaziland, tribal custom does not inhibit women from drinking home-brewed beers (tswala) in contrast to the Kikuyu women of Murang'a. These Swazi beers are very popular with the men and the more mature women, but younger women frequently abstain. For the purposes of evaluating minimal aflatoxin ingestion data, however, we have assumed a male preponderance in beer consumption.

Although the trend to increasing incidence of liver cancer with decreasing altitude is reflected in the female data (Table V) the significance of these differing incidences rates cannot be tested statistically as with the male cases because of the small number of cases (Table VII). Experimental work in rats has also shown a sex differential in the toxic and carcinogenic effects of the aflatoxins (Butler, 1964, 1971; Wogan and Newberne, 1967). It is postulated that a sex-linked protection of some kind, among the other factors which play a part in the aetiology of liver cancer, may be present. Whether there is an individual variation, perhaps sex-linked, in the ability of microsomal enzymes of the liver to hydroxylate or otherwise metabolize the aflatoxin B_1 molecule to the proximal carcinogen remains to be proved.

An evaluation of the incidence, by administrative areas or altitude areas, of cancers other than liver cancer was not possible from the Swaziland Cancer Registry as exact home addresses had only been determined for liver, skin and bladder cancers which were of particular interest to the Registry in 1966. Records of tuberculosis patients for 1965 and 1966 were made available by the WHO Epidemiology

Centre in Nairobi and these were examined to assess the availability of medical care for patients suffering from a chronic disease. The data were recorded by centre of first diagnosis rather than home address. In Table VI tuberculosis patients are shown by administrative and altitude areas together with the expected values on a population basis.

The large deviations from probability are due to the siting of the national TB centre in the Middleveld area of Manzini and because the main hospitals obviously drain tuberculosis patients from further afield than the altitude or administrative areas in which they are sited.

In Table VII we have evaluated the significance of the distribution of the liver cancer cases as allocated to the altitude areas.

The major contributions to these χ^2 values derive from the low numbers of cases recorded in the highveld area with more developed medical facilities and the large number of cases recorded in the lowveld area with less comprehensive medical facilities. This can be assessed from Figure 1 and by the details of 1964 medical facilities given in Table VIII.

With such a distribution of medical facilities case catchment is indeed likely to be more efficient in the area of lower cancer incidence where it is important for the present study that no cancer case be overlooked.

Keen and Martin (1971a) suggested that the adult male Shangaans living in Swaziland were at approxi-

mately twice the risk of liver cancer than the indigenous Swazis living in a similar environment. A study of tribal customs showed that they associated this increased risk with the consumption of groundnuts. The age structure of the small Shangaan population living in Swaziland differs from that of the resident Swazis in that a large proportion of this immigrant population consists of adult males recruited for work on the sugar estates around Mhlume and other estates in northern Hhohho. We consider that as actively employed workers they were more likely to reach medical care than resident Swazis. Based on 1966 Census data and further information from Keen, Table IX shows that although the frequency of cases in the Shangaans cannot be evaluated for significance, a χ^2 test of the Swazis *versus* combined Shangaans and other Africans is not significant ($\chi^2 = 2.52$, $0.2 > p_1 > 0.1$). In view of the possible biases mentioned and the low numbers involved, an increased risk for liver cancer in the Shangaans cannot be accepted from these data.

Keen and Martin (1971) noted a lower liver cancer frequency in the south as compared with the north of Swaziland and that this was particularly marked for the High- and Middleveld areas. The aflatoxin ingestion levels north and south of the arbitrary line shown on Figure 1 have been evaluated and whilst a significantly increased frequency of contamination of the diets in the north is recorded, the mean level of contamination is not significant. Using information provided by Keen (personal communication), the 72 adult male liver

TABLE VI

1965 AND 1966 TUBERCULOSIS RECORDS FOR SWAZILAND

| Administrative area | Altitude area | | | | | | | | | |
| | Highveld | | Middleveld | | Lowveld | | Lebombo | | Totals | |
	Obs.	Exp.	Obs.	Exp.	Obs.	Exp.	Obs.	Exp.	Obs.	Exp.
Hhohho	62	111.1	8	103.6	5	41.8	—	—	75	256.5
Manzini	119	87.5	530	170.5	12	13.0	—	—	661	271.0
Shiselweni	198	82.7	36	140.3	0	40.1	—	—	234	263.1
Lubombo	—	—	0	8.5	32	160.5	10	52.4	42	221.4
Totals	379	281.3	574	422.9	49	255.4	10	52.4	1,012	—

TABLE VII

SIGNIFICANCE OF THE DISTRIBUTION OF LIVER CANCER CASES, BY ALTITUDE AREA

	Highveld	Middleveld [1]	Lowveld	Totals	χ^2
Total cases	11	34	44	89	—
Expected from total populations	24.8	41.8	22.5	—	29.7 *** [2]
Adult male cases	9	28	35	72	—
Expected from adult male population	20.9	29.8	21.3	—	15.7 ***

[1] The Lebombo and Middleveld have been combined in this Table due to the low expectation from the small population in the Lebombo. —
[2] *** p<0.001.

cancer cases have been allocated to the two areas as defined by this arbitrary line and the distribution tested statistically in Table X.

TABLE VIII

CLINICS AND HOSPITALS IN SWAZILAND

	Highveld	Middleveld	Lowveld	Lebombo
Clinics	12	13	13	2
Hospitals	8	2	0	1

TABLE IX

TRIBAL DISTRIBUTION OF THE ADULT MALE LIVER CANCER CASES

	Swazis	Shangaans	Other Africans
Adult male population ⩾15	80,369	3,872	4,426
Percentage actively employed	44.9	83.6	67.9
Liver cases 1964-1968	64	7	4
Expected from population	68.0	3.3	3.7
Crude adult male rate per 100,000 per year	15.9	36.2	18.1

TABLE X

SWAZILAND LIVER CANCER INCIDENCE ON A NORTH-SOUTH BASIS

	North	South	χ^2
1964-68 adult male cases	48	24	—
Adult male population	52,834	35,833	—
Expected No. of cases	42.9	29.1	1.5
1964-68 adult female cases	7	7	—
Adult female population	59,230	44,569	—
Expected No. of cases	8.0	6.0	0.29

Hence, although there may be an increased frequency of the disease in the northern as compared with the southern areas of the High- and Middleveld areas, this is not true of the country taken as a whole.

It has been demonstrated in this study that, at least in males, a log relationship exists (Fig. 2) between the liver cancer incidence and the ingestion of aflatoxin (Fig. 2). The range of the observations in Africa of dietary aflatoxin levels and primary liver cancer incidence has been extended to adult male liver cancer rates of 26 per 100,000 per year. The data are consistent with the hypothesis that chronic aflatoxin exposure is related to the incidence of liver cancer within an African population.

ACKNOWLEDGEMENTS

The considerable assistance and co-operation of many members of the Swaziland Ministries of Health, Agriculture and Local Administration are acknowledged.

We are deeply indebted to Dr. Paul Keen of the Cancer Research Unit of the South African Institute for Medical Research for access to unpublished data without which we would not have been able to prepare this manuscript.

We are particularly grateful to Mr. Paul Dlamini, our sample collector, and Mr. R. W. Bell and Mr. P. Jones for laboratory space at the Malkerns Agricultural Research Station. We would also like to thank Mr. Sven Christensen of the WHO Epidemiology Centre, Nairobi, Kenya, for access to the 1965-1966 Swaziland Tuberculosis records, Dr. J. Nabney and Dr. N. R. Jones of the Tropical Products Institute for helpful comments during the preparation of this manuscript, and the Directors of TPL and IARC for permission to publish this paper.

AFLATOXINE DANS L'ALIMENTATION ET CANCER DU FOIE. UNE ÉTUDE EFFECTUÉE AU SWAZILAND

Il est rendu compte d'une étude effectuée au Swaziland pour apprécier l'éventualité d'une relation entre la contamination par l'aflatoxine et l'incidence du cancer primitif du foie. On a déterminé les teneurs en aflatoxine d'échantillons d'aliments " prélevés dans les assiettes " au cours d'une période d'un an. Une corrélation significative a été établie entre la dose journalière ingérée ainsi calculée et l'incidence du cancer primitif du foie chez les hommes adultes au Swaziland. Les échantillons d'aliments autres que ceux prélevés dans les assiettes ont également fait apparaître cette corrélation entre la contamination par l'aflatoxine et le cancer du foie. Cette étude étend et amplifie les conclusions d'une étude menée antérieurement dans le district de Murang'a, au Kenya; elle corrobore l'hypothèse selon laquelle l'ingestion d'aflatoxine est un facteur étiologique du cancer primitif du foie en Afrique.

REFERENCES

AGRICULTURAL SAMPLE CENSUS (Swazi Nation Land), Central statistical office, Mbabane, Swaziland (1971/72).

BERRY, G., and DAY, N. E., The statistical analysis of the results of sampling an environment for a contaminant when most samples contain an undetectable level. *Amer. J. Epidem.*, **97**, 160-166 (1973).

BUTLER, W. H., Acute toxicity of aflatoxin B_1 in rats. *Brit. J. Cancer*, **18**, 756-762 (1964).

BUTLER, W. H., The toxicology of aflatoxin. *In:* I. F. H. Purchase (ed.), *Symposium on mycotoxins in human health*, pp. 141-151, Macmillan Press, London (1971).

GILMAN, G. A., Storage surveys and how they may be used both to detect and estimate fungal contamination in the diet. *In:* I. F. H. Purchase (ed.), *Symposium on mycotoxins in human health*, pp. 133-140, Macmillan Press, London (1971).

JONES, B. D., *Methods of aflatoxin analysis, Report G 70*, 1-57, Tropical Products Institute, London (1972).

KEEN, P., and MARTIN, P., Is aflatoxin carcinogenic in man? The evidence in Swaziland. *Trop. geogr. Med.*, **23**, 44-53 (1971*a*).

KEEN, P., and MARTIN, P., The toxicity and fungal infestation of foodstuffs in Swaziland in relation to harvesting and storage. *Trop. geogr. Med.*, **23**, 35-43 (1971*b*).

MARTIN, P. M. D., GILMAN, G. A., and KEEN, P., The evidence of fungi in foodstuffs and their significance, based on a survey in the Eastern Transvaal and Swaziland. *In:* I. F. H. Purchase (ed.), *Symposium on mycotoxins in human health*, pp. 281-290, Macmillan Press, London (1971).

PEERS, F. G., and LINSELL, C. A., Dietary aflatoxins and liver cancer—A population based study in Kenya. *Brit. J. Cancer*, **27**, 473-484 (1973).

REPORT ON THE 1966 SWAZILAND POPULATION CENSUS, Central statistical office, Mbabane, Swaziland (1968).

SHANK, R. C., GORDON, J. E., WOGAN, G. N., NONDASUTA, A., and SUBHAMANI, B., Dietary aflatoxins and human liver cancer, III. Field survey of rural Thai families for ingested aflatoxins. *Fd. cosmet. Toxicol.*, **10**, 71-84 (1972).

VAN RENSBURG, S. J., KIRSIPUU, A., COUTINHO, L. P., and VAN DER WATT, J. J., Circumstances associated with the contamination of food by aflatoxin in a high primary liver cancer area. *S. Afr. med. J.*, **49**, 877-883 (1975).

VAN RENSBURG, S. J., VAN DER WATT, J. J., PURCHASE, I. F. H., COUTINHO, L. P., and MARKHAM, R., Primary liver cancer rate and aflatoxin intake in a high cancer area. *S. Afr. med. J.*, **48**, 2508a-2508d (1974).

WOGAN, G. N., and NEWBERNE, P. M., Dose-response characteristics of aflatoxin B_1 carcinogenesis in the rat. *Cancer Res.*, **27**, 2370-2376 (1967).

Coffee Drinking and Risk of Bladder Cancer

by Patricia Hartge, Robert Hoover, Dee W. West, and Joseph L. Lyon

ABSTRACT—The relationship between coffee drinking and risk of bladder cancer was assessed with the use of data from a case–control study of bladder cancer. Incident cases (2,982) and general population controls (5,782) were interviewed. Overall, the relative risk (RR) of bladder cancer for subjects who had ever drunk coffee was estimated as 1.4 (95% confidence interval=1.1–1.8). There was no consistent relation between the RR estimate and the current consumption level. Among men who drank coffee, those who drank more than 49 cupfuls of coffee per week had an apparent excess in risk, but women who drank that much had an apparent deficit in risk.—JNCI 1983; 70:1021–1026.

In 1971, a report from a case–control study of bladder cancer (*1*) suggested that coffee might cause human bladder cancer. Several but not all subsequent studies have reported

ABBREVIATIONS USED: CI=confidence interval; RR=relative risk(s).

Patricia Hartge and Robert Hoover are with the Environmental Epidemiology Branch, Division of Cancer Cause and Prevention, National Cancer Institute, Bethesda, Maryland 20205.

Dee W. West and Joseph L. Lyon are with the University of Utah Medical Center, Salt Lake City, Utah 84108.

Address reprint requests to Dr. Hartge, Landow Building, Room C306, National Institutes of Health, Bethesda, Maryland 20205.

We thank Dr. Kenneth Rothman and Dr. Alan Morrison for advice.

Sponsored by the U.S. Food and Drug Administration, National Cancer Institute, and the Environmental Protection Agency.

Research procedures were in accord with the ethical standards of the human subjects' investigation committees of each participating hospital and registry.

an association among men; fewer studies have reported an association among women (*2–12*). The inconsistencies in the data and the apparent lack of a dose response in most studies suggest that coffee drinkers may be at increased risk of bladder cancer but that coffee drinking itself may not cause bladder cancer. Nonetheless, concern about coffee has not been entirely laid to rest, partly because brewed coffee has shown mutagenic activity (*13*) and because caffeine, coffee's principal active constituent, alters susceptibility of various organisms to mutation by other agents (*14–17*). We therefore evaluated the relation between coffee and bladder cancer using interview data from a large case–control study.

METHODS

We interviewed 2,982 cases and 5,782 controls as part of a collaborative population-based case–control study conducted in 10 geographic areas of the United States—Atlanta, Ga.; Connecticut; Detroit, Mich.; Iowa; New Jersey; New Mexico; New Orleans, La.; San Francisco, Calif.; Seattle, Wash.; and Utah (*18*). The case group was composed of all identified residents of the areas who were of ages 21–84 years and who were diagnosed with histologically confirmed bladder cancer in a 1-year period (with the beginning varying among areas from December 1977 to March 1978). Cases were identified from cancer registries, nine of which were part of the Surveillance, Epidemiology, and End Results Program of the National Cancer Institute. The control group was randomly selected from the general population (weighted by the age, sex, and geographic distribution of the cases). Controls aged 21–64 years were selected from 22,633 households chosen by telephone sampling with the use of random-digit dialing (*19*). Controls aged 65–84 years were selected from Health Care Financing Administration rosters.

We identified 4,086 eligible cases and interviewed 2,982 (73%) of them. The remaining 1,104 were not interviewed because of death (282), illness (288), patient refusal (252), physician refusal (128), being identified after the study ended (65), not being found (81), and other reasons (8). A total of 4,057 older controls were eligible, of whom 3,313 (82%) were interviewed. The remaining 744 were not interviewed because of death (94), illness (174), refusal (348), not being found (105), and other reasons (23). From telephone sampling of households, 2,928 people younger than 65 were selected as controls, of whom 2,469 (84%) were interviewed. The remaining 459 were not interviewed because of death (7), illness (23), refusals (335), not being found (87), and other reasons (7). About 75% of the interviewed cases (and controls) were male, and the median age was 67 years.

All subjects were interviewed at home. Interviewers used a questionnaire that included questions about the use of artificial sweeteners, hair dyes, and tobacco products, occupational history, and residential history. In addition, a brief series of questions was asked about each of several other exposures, including exposures to coffee and tea. Respondents were asked whether they had drunk more than 100 cupfuls of coffee in their life ("coffee drinkers") and, if so, how many years they had drunk coffee. For the measurement of recent or "current," prediagnosis coffee consumption, respondents were asked how many cupfuls of various types of coffee (e.g., ground decaffeinated) they typically drank each week in the winter 1 year ago (i.e., before onset of the cases' illness).

The effect of coffee drinking on bladder cancer risk was measured by the maximum likelihood estimate of the RR, controlled for potentially confounding variables by stratification into multiple contingency tables and by entering continuous variables into multiple logistic regression models (*20, 21*).

The estimates are presented separately for males and females. They were adjusted for age (21–44, 45–64, and 65–84 yr), race (white or other), residence (the 10 study areas), and tobacco smoking history (nonsmokers, smokers of pipes or cigars only, ex-smokers of <20 cigarettes/day, ex-smokers of ≥20 cigarettes/day, smokers of <20 cigarettes/day, smokers of 20–39 cigarettes/day, and smokers of ≥40 cigarettes/day). Exceptions are noted in the text. Finer adjustment for amount smoked did not affect the estimates of RR, nor did control for other indices of tobacco exposure. These indices included the usual numbers of filtered cigarettes and unfiltered cigarettes separately, the usual number of cigars or pipes, the lifetime number of packs smoked, the number of years since quitting smoking, the number of years of smoking, and combinations of these variables. The estimates were also not appreciably altered by finer adjustment for age or by adjustment for urinary stones or infections, hair dyeing, fluid intake, artificial sweetener use, urban residence, usual occupation, exposure to suspect chemicals (dye, rubber, leather, ink, or paint), or religion.

RESULTS

Six percent of the subjects in the control group said that they had drunk fewer than 100 cupfuls of coffee in their lives ("nondrinkers"). The coffee drinkers reported consuming 11.8 cupfuls per week of regular (nondecaffeinated) ground coffee, on average. They reported substantially lower consumption of regular instant coffee (5.3 cupfuls/wk), decaffeinated instant coffee (3.2), decaffeinated ground coffee (0.8), coffee with chicory (0.6), and espresso (0.1). All types of coffee were combined to estimate total current consumption, and the four caffeine-containing types were combined to estimate current consumption of caffeinated coffee. Coffee consumption patterns varied with sex, race, age, and tobacco consumption (table 1).

TABLE 1.—*Patterns of coffee consumption within general population control group*

Variables	Percent ever drank coffee	Mean weekly cups of coffee among drinkers
Sex		
Male	94	22
Female	92	20
Age, yr		
21–44	83	24
45–64	94	26
65–84	94	19
Race		
White	94	22
Other	87	15
Area[a]		
Atlanta, Ga.	95	19
Connecticut	95	19
Detroit, Mich.	95	24
Iowa	91	26
New Jersey	95	19
New Mexico	94	23
New Orleans, La.	94	22
San Francisco, Calif.	96	22
Seattle, Wash.	96	27
Utah	72	19
Cigarettes[a]		
Never smoked	88	17
Former smokers, <1 pack/day	95	19
Former smokers, ≥1 pack/day	97	22
Current smokers, <1 pack/day	96	22
Current smokers, ≥1 pack/day	96	28
Job exposure[a]		
Never handled dye, rubber, leather, ink, or paint	94	21
Handled dye, rubber, leather, ink, or paint	93	22
Artificial sweeteners[a]		
Never used	93	22
Used <240 mg/day	95	22
Used ≥240 mg/day	92	25

[a] Standardized to the age, sex, and race distribution of the entire control group.

All Coffees

Table 2 shows the estimated RR of bladder cancer according to history of coffee drinking for men and women separately and for both sexes combined. The overall RR estimate, adjusted only for sex, age, race, and area of residence, was 1.8 for drinkers versus nondrinkers, but this

TABLE 2.—*Estimated RR of bladder cancer according to history of coffee drinking, by sex*

Sex	Coffee	No. of cases	No. of controls	RR[a]	95% CI
Male	Never drank	58	244	1.0	
	Ever drank	2,139	3,942	1.6	1.2–2.2
Female	Never drank	40	121	1.0	
	Ever drank	670	1,347	1.2	0.8–1.7
Both sexes	Never drank	98	365	1.0	
	Ever drank	2,809	5,289	1.4	1.1–1.8

[a] RR estimates are from a logistic regression model including (sex), age, race, geographic area, and tobacco history.

estimate was markedly confounded by the effect of smoking, and the adjusted estimate was 1.4 (95% CI=1.1–1.8). The estimated effect was greater in men than women, but the difference was not statistically significant (*P*=0.39).

Table 3 presents the RR estimated according to duration of coffee drinking. Study subjects who never drank coffee were not included. RR did not vary appreciably according to duration of coffee drinking. As table 4 shows, current drinkers had substantially the same risk as former drinkers.

Table 5 presents RR estimates according to current level of consumption of all types of coffee combined. Because ex-drinkers had the same adjusted RR as current light drinkers, they were combined to form the group of lowest exposure (0–7 current cupfuls/wk) to which all other groups were compared. Among men, RR appeared to be constant for levels up to 49 cupfuls per week, but it was slightly elevated at the highest level (>49 cupfuls/wk). The 87 men who reported more than 84 weekly cupfuls showed an RR of 1.5. Among women, a slight deficit in RR appeared for all levels above 0–7 cupfuls per week, with no evidence of a trend.

We estimated the simultaneous effects of a history of

TABLE 3.—*Estimated RR of bladder cancer among coffee drinkers according to duration of coffee drinking, by sex*

Duration of coffee drinking, yr	Males				Females			
	No. of cases	No. of controls	RR[a]	95% CI	No. of cases	No. of controls	RR[a]	95% CI
<10	32	88	1.0		17	30	1.0	
10–19	55	147	0.9	0.5–1.5	28	65	0.8	0.4–1.7
20–39	462	875	1.1	0.7–1.6	164	322	0.8	0.4–1.6
≥40	1,565	2,781	1.1	0.7–1.6	456	911	0.8	0.4–1.5
(Unknown)	(25)	(51)			(5)	(19)		

[a] RR estimates are from a logistic regression model including age, race, geographic area, and tobacco history.

TABLE 4.—*Estimated RR of bladder cancer among coffee drinkers according to whether drinking recently, by sex*

Recent coffee	Males				Females			
	No. of cases	No. of controls	RR[a]	95% CI	No. of cases	No. of controls	RR[a]	95% CI
Ex-drinker	91	205	1.0		37	73	1.0	
Recent drinker	2,021	3,687	1.1	0.8–1.4	627	1,263	1.0	0.6–1.5
(Unknown)	(27)	(50)			(6)	(11)		

[a] RR estimates are from a logistic regression model including age, race, geographic area, and tobacco history.

TABLE 5.—*Estimated RR of bladder cancer according to recent cupfuls of coffee per week among coffee drinkers, by sex*

Cupfuls of coffee per week	Males				Females			
	No. of cases	No. of controls	RR[a]	95% CI	No. of cases	No. of controls	RR[a]	95% CI
≤7	397	862	1.0		164	331	1.0	
7.1–14	389	842	0.9	0.8–1.1	161	346	0.9	0.7–1.2
14.1–21	381	747	1.0	0.8–1.2	110	237	0.8	0.6–1.1
21.1–35	493	821	1.1	0.9–1.3	133	249	0.9	0.7–1.2
35.1–49	195	329	1.0	0.8–1.3	49	104	0.7	0.5–1.1
49.1–63	109	139	1.2	0.9–1.6	21	31	0.9	0.5–1.7
63.1–155	148	152	1.5	1.1–1.9	26	38	0.8	0.4–1.4
(Unknown)	(27)	(50)			(6)	(11)		

[a] RR estimates are from a logistic regression model including age, race, geographic area, and tobacco history.

coffee drinking (yes/no), duration of coffee drinking (yr), and current consumption (cupfuls/day) using a logistic regression to adjust for age in 5 groups, sex, race, geographic area in 2 groups, and tobacco history in 7 groups. Among men, the RR for ever drinking versus never drinking was estimated as 1.3 (95% CI=0.9–1.9), the estimated multiplication of RR for each year of coffee drinking was 1.00 (95% CI=1.00–1.01), and the estimated multiplication of RR for each cupful per day currently drunk was 1.04 (95% CI=1.01–1.06). Among women, the corresponding estimates were 1.2 (95% CI=0.7–1.9) for ever drinking, 1.00 (95% CI=0.99–1.01) for each year of drinking, and 0.99 (95% CI=0.94–1.03) for each current cupful per day.

Caffeine

When only caffeine-containing coffees were combined, the pattern observed in table 5 among men was virtually unaffected. Among women, those who consumed at the highest level showed a slightly elevated RR, but there was no evidence of a trend. The slight excess RR associated with a history of coffee drinking was not attributable to any particular type of coffee consumed, nor was the slight additional excess RR to men who drank more than 49 cupfuls per week.

Compared to men who never drank any type of coffee, men who were drinking only decaffeinated coffee (ground or instant) had an estimated RR of 1.2 (95% CI=0.8–1.9). The corresponding estimate for women was 1.5 (95% CI=0.9–2.6). Among men who drank only decaffeinated coffee, those who drank more than 49 cupfuls per week showed the highest RR, but there was no consistent relation between the amount of coffee and RR. Among women who drank only decaffeinated coffee, there was also no consistent relation between RR and the amount of coffee, but those who drank most heavily showed the lowest RR. Essentially similar patterns appeared when all of the subjects were included in the analysis and the estimates were adjusted for the effects of consumption of caffeine-containing coffee.

Although 90% of caffeine ingested in the United States comes from coffee (22), some people consume a substantial amount of caffeine from tea and drink little or no coffee. On average, a cupful of tea contains about 60 mg of caffeine, whereas a cupful of coffee contains about 90 mg (22). Among subjects who were currently drinking no more than 7 cupfuls of coffee per week, tea consumption was weakly and inconsistently related to RR of bladder cancer (table 6). In the total study group, tea consumption was weakly related to RR. Women who drank more than 7 cupfuls per week had slightly elevated RR (RR=1.2 for 7.1–14 cupfuls; RR=1.3 for >14 cupfuls). Men who drank more than 14 cupfuls per week had a slightly elevated RR (RR=1.2).

Subgroups

The data in tables 2–5 show three discrete levels of RR for men (nondrinkers, very heavy drinkers, and all others) and two levels for women (nondrinkers and drinkers). To examine how the effects of coffee varied within subgroups,

we considered two contrasts: subjects who ever drank versus those who never drank and subjects who drank very heavily versus all others who ever drank (tables 7, 8). The RR estimates for ever drinking coffee, within the seven tobacco history categories, did not show statistically significant heterogeneity (P=0.81), but the nonsmokers had estimates different from those for the smokers. The estimates for current smokers and for ex-smokers did not depend on the usual amount smoked, so we combined categories and adjusted for the amount smoked. Estimated RR for ever drinking coffee was lower among women and nonsmokers. Excess RR for heavy coffee drinking was absent among women, but it was present among nonsmokers.

Although estimates of RR varied by geographic area, the pattern seen overall was not confined to one area or region. For both sexes combined, the geographic variation was no more than would be expected by chance (P=0.44). The estimated RR for ever drinking also did not vary significantly by race (P=0.43), usual occupation (P=0.65), artificial sweetener use (P=0.18), history of urinary infection (P=0.86), or source of controls (P=0.85).

DISCUSSION

Our data show coffee drinkers to be at apparently greater risk of bladder cancer than nondrinkers, but the data do not show any consistent relationship between the extent of exposure and the degree of risk. We estimated that current and former coffee drinkers had an RR of bladder cancer of 1.4 compared to nondrinkers. Among subjects who never smoked, the estimate was 1.2. We found no consistent pattern of higher RR with higher levels of current coffee consumption. Although men who drank more than 49 cupfuls of coffee per week showed a slightly elevated risk, those who drank 35.1–49 cupfuls of coffee per week showed no elevation. Further, women who drank coffee heavily showed RR below the null value. The number of years that subjects had drunk coffee was apparently unrelated to RR. The patterns of RR within subgroups did not suggest a consistent pattern of interaction with other risk factors for bladder cancer.

Our findings are consistent with findings from earlier epidemiologic studies, many of which have reported slightly and inconsistently elevated risks of bladder cancer among coffee drinkers. Two case–control studies similar in design to the present study have recently been reported. A study by Howe et al. (10) conducted in three Canadian provinces estimated the RR to coffee drinkers as 1.4 (95% CI=0.9–2.0) among males and 1.0 (95% CI=0.5–2.1) among females, with no evidence of a dose response. A study by Morrison et al. (12) conducted in Boston, Mass., Nagoya, Japan, and Manchester, England, estimated the RR as 1.0 (95% CI=0.8–1.2) for both sexes combined, with no evidence of a dose response.

Like the epidemiologic evidence, the laboratory evidence about the possible carcinogenic effects of coffee does not lead to a definite conclusion. It is well established that caffeine can enhance the effects of some mutagens and inhibit the effects of others in a variety of bacterial systems

TABLE 6.—*Estimated RR of bladder cancer according to recent consumption of tea among subjects who drank no more than 7 cupfuls of coffee per week, by sex*

Recent tea—cupfuls per week	Males				Females			
	No. of cases	No. of controls	RR[a]	95% CI	No. of cases	No. of controls	RR[a]	95% CI
0	198	510	1.0		56	163	1.0	
0.1–7	137	322	1.1	0.8–1.4	63	150	1.1	0.7–1.7
7.1–14	59	132	1.1	0.7–1.5	40	57	1.7	1.0–2.9
>14	59	140	1.0	0.7–1.4	44	81	1.2	0.7–2.0
(Unknown)	(2)	(2)			(1)	(1)		

[a] RR estimates are from a logistic regression model including age, race, geographic area, tobacco history, and history of coffee drinking.

TABLE 7.—*Estimated effects of ever drinking coffee and of heavy recent consumption, by sex and tobacco history*

Sex	Tobacco	Ever vs. never[a]			>49 cupfuls/wk vs. less cupfuls[a]		
		No. of subjects who never drank	RR[b]	95% CI	No. of subjects who drank >49 cupfuls/wk	RR[b]	95% CI
Both sexes	All	463	1.4	1.1–1.8	664	1.3	1.1–1.5
Male	All	302	1.6	1.2–2.1	548	1.3	1.1–1.6
Female	All	161	1.2	0.8–1.7	116	1.0	0.7–1.5
Male	Nonsmokers	159	1.5	0.9–2.5	21	4.2	1.7–10.
	Pipes, cigars only	25	2.2	0.6–7.8	17	0.8	0.3–2.7
	Ex-smokers	62	1.4	0.8–2.6	208	1.3	1.0–1.8
	Smokers	56	2.1	1.2–3.9	302	1.2	1.0–1.6
Female	Nonsmokers	121	0.9	0.6–1.5	24	0.4	0.1–1.5
	Ex-smokers	13	3.0	0.8–12.	25	1.7	0.7–4.2
	Smokers	27	1.3	0.6–2.9	67	1.0	0.6–1.7

[a] Subjects who drank >49 cupfuls/wk are compared to all others who ever drank.
[b] RR estimates are from separate logistic regression models with terms for sex, age, race, and amount of tobacco.

TABLE 8.—*Estimated effects of ever drinking coffee and of heavy recent consumption, by sex and geographic area*

Sex	Area	Ever vs. never[a]			>49 cupfuls/wk vs. less cupfuls[a]		
		No. of subjects who never drank	RR[b]	95% CI	No. of subjects who drank >49 cupfuls/wk	RR[b]	95% CI
Male	Atlanta, Ga.	11	—	—	16	1.2	0.4–3.8
	Connecticut	29	3.2	0.9–11.	49	1.6	0.9–2.6
	Detroit, Mich.	27	1.1	0.4–2.6	69	1.1	0.6–1.8
	Iowa	34	2.2	0.8–5.8	95	1.3	0.8–2.1
	New Jersey	74	2.1	1.1–3.9	121	1.3	0.9–2.0
	New Mexico	8	0.7	0.1–4.1	25	3.2	1.1–9.5
	New Orleans, La.	14	0.8	0.2–3.0	14	0.9	0.3–3.0
	San Francisco, Calif.	30	1.4	0.6–3.6	75	1.3	0.8–2.2
	Seattle, Wash.	12	0.3	0.1–1.4	56	1.0	0.5–1.8
	Utah	63	1.5	0.7–3.5	28	2.3	0.9–5.8
Female	Atlanta, Ga.	6	0.7	0.1–8.0	3	[c]	
	Connecticut	18	1.8	0.6–5.6	15	1.5	0.5–4.7
	Detroit, Mich.	17	1.2	0.4–3.6	13	1.2	0.4–4.0
	Iowa	18	2.2	0.5–11.	31	0.8	0.3–2.1
	New Jersey	37	1.0	0.5–2.2	19	0.6	0.2–1.6
	New Mexico	4	[c]		2	[c]	
	New Orleans, La.	3	[c]		2	[c]	
	San Francisco, Calif.	17	0.9	0.3–2.8	17	2.6	0.8–8.5
	Seattle, Wash.	3	[c]		11	0.5	0.1–2.6
	Utah	38	0.5	0.2–1.7	3	[c]	

[a] Subjects who drank >49 cupfuls weekly are compared to all others who ever drank.
[b] RR estimates are from separate logistic regression models including age, race, and tobacco history.
[c] Fewer than 5 subjects exposed or fewer than 5 subjects unexposed.

and cell cultures (*14–17*). The tests of direct effects of caffeine in such systems have been predominantly negative, but positive results have been reported from Ames assays of whole brewed coffee but not of caffeine (*13*). Tests of coffee or caffeine in animals pretreated with known carcinogens showed that the coffee or caffeine either decreased (*23*) or did not alter (*24*) tumor yield. To date, the whole-animal tests of caffeine alone have not shown that caffeine is carcinogenic (*25–27*). A standard National Cancer Institute bioassay of caffeine is under way and will be completed in late 1983. In short, the existing laboratory evidence does not suggest that coffee is likely to be a powerful human carcinogen, but it does suggest two possible mechanisms by which coffee might influence cancer risk, i.e., by the mutagenic action of coffee or by the interaction of caffeine with some other mutagen.

There are several possible interpretations of the current evidence. The patterns observed in this study may be due to a noncausal association between coffee drinking and bladder cancer, to a causal relation, or to chance. Chance is the least likely explanation, in view of the large size of this study and the replication of the finding of a low-level association in many studies.

If the association is causal, one would expect to observe a relation between risk and duration or dose. Our study, like other studies, showed no such relation. It is possible, but not likely, that drinking even modest amounts of coffee for a short period of time raises the risk of bladder cancer, while greater exposure does not further raise the risk, except perhaps at the very extreme. A second possible interpretation is that greater coffee consumption does lead to greater RR but that our dose data were so severely misclassified that the dose-response relation was obscured.

Two possible explanations of a noncausal relation are residual confounding by tobacco and confounding by other correlates of coffee drinking. (Other noncausal interpretations of our findings are also possible, but less likely, in our view. For example, if coffee drinking increased chances of survival from bladder cancer, then the cases available for interview would have had a higher exposure rate than the case group as a whole.)

Confounding by tobacco was present in these data because tobacco is a strong risk factor for bladder cancer and is highly correlated with amount of coffee drunk, in part because caffeine clearance rates are about twice as high in smokers as in nonsmokers (*28*). Adjustment for smoking markedly reduced the estimated RR—from 1.8 to 1.4. Despite our adjustments, residual confounding could have occurred through 1) insufficiently narrow categories of tobacco exposure in the multiple contingency table analysis, 2) misspecification of the analytic models, or 3) random errors (misclassification) in the tobacco data. To reduce the possibility of the first two problems, we examined a wide variety of tobacco exposure indices and analytic models and tried very narrow categories of tobacco exposure. Residual confounding because of misclassification of tobacco was present to the extent that study subjects did not perfectly recall and report tobacco histories. With a sample of respondents, we conducted a brief telephone re-interview. There

was 97% concordance between the history of nonfilter smoking (yes or no) reported in the re-interview and that reported in the original home interview. We do not know whether the more complicated tobacco questions would have shown high accordance, and we do not know if the answers were accurate as well as replicable. Greenland (*29*) discussed the problem of misclassification of covariates leading to residual confounding, and Morrison et al. (*12*) and Morrison (paper presented at the annual meeting of the Society for Epidemiologic Research) discussed the particular implications for coffee, tobacco, and bladder cancer. Whether residual confounding accounts for the entire observed excess RR of 40% cannot be determined.

Confounding by correlates of coffee drinking other than tobacco exposure may also have contributed to the persistent but inconsistent relation between bladder cancer and coffee. As noted, control for a variety of factors did not materially alter the estimates. Overall, people who never drank coffee are a small minority of American adults, and the distinguishing characteristics of this minority are not well understood. They may differ from coffee drinkers on a variety of health-related variables, but it is not clear what other correlates of coffee drinking might be related to bladder cancer.

Further studies of typical U.S. populations are not likely to provide more precise estimates than those from this unusually large study, and they are not likely to avoid the bias created by residual confounding by tobacco. Additional studies of populations with a low prevalence of coffee drinking, e.g., Mormons or Seventh-Day Adventists, may illuminate the comparison of nondrinkers and drinkers. (We are pursuing this possibility by continuing the present study in Utah.) Studies of populations who drink more coffee than the U.S. population, e.g., Scandinavians, may also reveal whether very high doses of coffee affect bladder cancer risk. In addition, the completion of laboratory tests in progress will further our understanding of the effects of coffee. Meanwhile, the available evidence from our study, other epidemiologic studies, and laboratory experiments suggests that coffee plays either a small biologic role in human bladder cancer or no role at all.

REFERENCES

(*1*) COLE P. Coffee-drinking and cancer of the lower urinary tract. Lancet 1971; 1:1335–1337.
(*2*) FRAUMENI JF JR, SCOTTO J, DUNHAM LJ. Coffee drinking and bladder cancer. Lancet 1971; 2:1204.
(*3*) BROSS ID, TIDINGS J. Another look at coffee drinking and cancer of the urinary bladder. Prev Med 1973; 2:445–451.
(*4*) MORGAN RW, JAIN MG. Bladder cancer: Smoking, beverages, and artificial sweeteners. Can Med Assoc J 1974; III:1067–1070.
(*5*) SIMON D, YEN S, COLE P. Coffee drinking and cancer of the lower urinary tract. J Natl Cancer Inst 1975; 54:587–591.
(*6*) WYNDER EL, ONDERDONK J, MANTEL N. An epidemiological investigation of cancer of the bladder. Cancer 1963; 13:1388–1406.
(*7*) MILLER CT, NEUTEL CI, NAIR RC, MARRETT LD, LAST JM, COLLINS WE. Relative importance of risk factors in bladder carcinogenesis. J Chronic Dis 1978; 31:51–56.
(*8*) KESSLER II, CLARK JP. Saccharin, cyclamate, and human bladder cancer. JAMA 1978; 240:349–355.
(*9*) METTLIN C, GRAHAM S. Dietary risk factors in human bladder cancer.

Am J Epidemiol 1979; 110:255–263.

(10) HOWE GR, BURCH JD, MILLER AB, et al. Tobacco use, occupation, coffee, various nutrients, and bladder cancer. JNCI 1980; 64:701–713.

(11) CARTWRIGHT RA, ADIB R, GLASHAN R, GRAY BK. The epidemiology of bladder cancer in West Yorkshire. A preliminary report on non-occupational aetiologies. Carcinogenesis 1981; 2:343–347.

(12) MORRISON AS, BURING JE, VERHOEK WG, et al. Coffee drinking and cancer of the lower urinary tract. JNCI 1982; 68:91–94.

(13) NAGAO M, TAKAHASHI Y, YAMANAKA H, SUGIMURA T. Mutagens in coffee and tea. Mutat Res 1979; 68:101–106.

(14) MAHER VM, OUELLETTE LM, MITTLESTAT M, McCORMICK JJ. Synergistic effect of caffeine on the cytoxicity of ultraviolet irradiation and of hydrocarbon epoxides in strains of Xeroderma pigmentosum. Nature 1975; 258:760–763.

(15) CHANG CC, PHILLIPS C, TROSKO JE, HART RW. Mutagenetic and epigenetic influence of caffeine on the frequencies of UV-induced ouabain-resistant Chinese hamster cells. Mutat Res 1977; 45:125–136.

(16) HAVA P, HEJLOVA A, SOSKOVA L. Antimutagenic effects of caffeine during nitrosoguanidine-induced mutagenesis of *Salmonella typhimurium* cells and phages. Folia Microbiol (Praha) 1978; 23:45–54.

(17) MENNIGMANN HD, PONS FW. Mutation induction by thymidine deprivation in *Escherichia coli* B/r. I. Influence of caffeine. Mutat Res 1979; 60:13–23.

(18) HOOVER RN, STRASSER PH, CHILD MA, et al. Progress report to the Food and Drug Administration from the National Cancer Institute concerning the National Bladder Cancer Study. Bethesda, Md.: National Cancer Institute, 1979.

(19) WAKSBERG J. Sampling methods for random digit dialing. J Am Stat Assoc 1978; 73:40–46.

(20) GART JJ. Point and interval estimation of the common odds ratio in the combination of 2×2 tables with fixed marginals. Biometrika 1970; 57:471–475.

(21) BRESLOW NE, DAY NE. Statistical methods in cancer research. I. The analysis of case-control studies. Lyon, France: IARC, 1980.

(22) GRAHAM DM. Caffeine—its identity, dietary sources, intake and biological effects. Nutr Rev 1978; 36:97–102.

(23) NOMURA T. Diminution of tumourigenesis initiated by 4-nitroquinoline-1-oxide by post treatment with caffeine in mice. Nature 1976; 260:547–549.

(24) HICKS RM, SEVERS N, CHOWANIEC J. Further investigations with a 2-stage model designed to detect low potency bladder carcinogens and cocarcinogens. In: Toxicology research projects directory. Vol 4, issue 10. Springfield, Va.: Natl Technical Information Service, 1979.

(25) JOHANSSON SL. Carcinogenicity of analgesics. Long-term treatment of Sprague-Dawley rats with phenacetin, phenazone, caffeine and paracetomol. Int J Cancer 1981; 27:521–530.

(26) WURZNER HP, LINDSTROM E, VUATAZ L, LAGINBUHL H. A 2-year feeding study of instant coffee in rats. II. Incidence and types of neoplasms. Food Cosmet Toxicol 1977; 15:289–296.

(27) PALM PE, ARNOLD EP, RACHWALL PC, LEYCZEK JC, TEAGUE KW, KENSLER CJ. Evaluation of the teratogenic potential of fresh-brewed coffee and caffeine in the rat. Toxicol Appl Pharmacol 1978; 44:1–16.

(28) PARSONS WD, NEIMS AH. Effect of smoking on caffeine clearance. Clin Pharmacol Ther 1978; 24:40–45.

(29) GREENLAND S. The effect of misclassification in the presence of covariates. Am J Epidemiol 1980; 112:564–569.

Dietary Vitamin A and Risk of Cancer in the Western Electric Study

by Richard B. Shekelle, Shuguey Liu, William J. Raynor, Jr., Mark Lepper, Carol Maliza, Arthur H. Rossof, Oglesby Paul, Anne MacMillan Shryock, and Jeremiah Stamler

Summary Intake of dietary provitamin A (carotene) was inversely related to the 19-year incidence of lung cancer in a prospective epidemiological study of 1954 middle-aged men. The relative risks of lung cancer in the first (lowest) to fourth quartiles of the distribution of carotene intake were respectively, $7 \cdot 0$, $5 \cdot 5$, $3 \cdot 0$, and $1 \cdot 0$ for all men in the study, and $8 \cdot 1$, $5 \cdot 6$, $3 \cdot 9$, and $1 \cdot 0$ for men who had smoked cigarettes for 30 or more years. Intake of preformed vitamin A (retinol) and intake of other nutrients were not significantly related to the risk of lung cancer. Neither carotene nor retinol intake was significantly related to the risk of other carcinomas grouped together, although for men in whom epidermoid carcinomas of the head and neck subsequently developed, carotene intake tended to be below average. These results support the hypothesis that dietary beta-carotene decreases the risk of lung cancer. However, cigarette smoking also increases the risk of serious diseases other than lung cancer, and there is no evidence that dietary carotenoids affect these other risks in any way.

RICHARD B. SHEKELLE   MARK LEPPER
SHUGUEY LIU   CAROL MALIZA
WILLAM J. RAYNOR, JR   ARTHUR H. ROSSOF

Departments of Preventive Medicine and of Medicine, Rush-Presbyterian-St Luke's Medical Center, Chicago, Illinois U.S.A.

OGLESBY PAUL

Department of Medicine, Harvard Medical School, Boston, Massachusetts

ANNE MACMILLAN SHRYOCK

School of Nursing, University of Michigan, Ann Arbor, Michigan

JEREMIAH STAMLER

Department of Community Health and Preventive Medicine, Northwestern University School of Medicine, Chicago, Illinois

Introduction

PROSPECTIVE epidemiological investigations in Norway[1] and Japan[2] and case-control studies in Singapore,[3] the U.S.A.,[4] and the U.K.[5] have shown an inverse association between intake of foods rich in vitamin A and risk of lung cancer. Although some results were presented for selected groups of foods, these studies did not clearly determine whether the risk was associated with intake of preformed vitamin A (described here as retinol), intake of provitamin A (compounds that can be converted to vitamin A in the body, described here as carotene), or intake of both. Retinol occurs naturally only in certain foods of animal origin (chiefly whole milk, cheese, butter, egg yolk, and liver), and the principal sources of carotene are dark-green leafy vegetables, carrots, and certain yellow and red fruits and vegetables. Peto et al.[6] have argued in support of the hypothesis that dietary beta-carotene, but not dietary retinol, reduces the risk of cancers in man. This study was undertaken to investigate the association between intake of carotene and retinol in the diet as assessed in 1959, and the risk of cancer during the following 19 years in a group of men participating in a prospective epidemiological study. Our hypothesis, based on the consistent epidemiological evidence on vitamin A and lung cancer and the arguments of Peto et al.,[6] was that intake of dietary carotene would be inversely related to risk of lung cancer.

Subjects and Methods

In 1957 3102 men were randomly selected for the Western Electric Study from 5397 men aged 40–55 years who had been employed for at least 2 years at the Western Electric Company's Hawthorne Works in the Chicago metropolitan area. 2080 (67·1%) of the selected men agreed to participate. Another 27 men served as a pilot group, bringing to 2107 the total number initially examined from October, 1957, to December, 1958. Approximately 65% were first and second generation Americans, predominantly of German, Polish, or Bohemian ancestry. Most of the other men were descendants of earlier emigrants from the British Isles. The men worked at various occupations associated with the manufacture of telephones and related products. Selection, examination, and follow-up procedures have been described elsewhere.[7]

Two nutritionists obtained information about diet at both the initial examination and the second examination 1 year later. They used a standard 1 h interview and a questionnaire to the homemaker to determine the kinds and quantities of foods and beverages consumed during the previous 28 days. The interview asked about the customary pattern of eating on workdays and weekends, and included a detailed review of 195 specific foods to determine how often each had been eaten and the usual size of portions. Models of common foods and dishes of various sizes were used as aids. Questions about food supplements were asked, but the information was not coded or included in assessments of nutrient intake because they were so rarely used. The data were analysed by a food composition table derived from several sources[8-11] to estimate each participant's usual daily intake of energy and of various nutrients, including total vitamin A—i.e., the sum of retinol and carotene. Re-analysis to estimate carotene intake and retinol intake separately is not now possible because the dietary histories are no longer available. However, at the second examination, in addition to estimation of nutrients, food-profile scores (0–3) were used to indicate consumption of 26 separate foods or food groups formed from the original list of 195 items. The score 0 was always assigned to zero units; other scores were defined by ranges of values. For instance, the food-profile scores for eggs were defined as follows: 0=0, 1=1–11, 2=12–28, and 3=29 or more eggs per 28-day period. Selected food-profile scores were used to estimate the proportional contributions of retinol and carotene to intake of total vitamin A (table I). For this purpose, the range of values that originally defined a food-profile score was replaced by a single characteristic value, shown in parentheses in table I. The amount of vitamin A activity per unit for a group of foods was estimated by averaging the amounts shown in the food composition table for each of the foods in the group. Although some foods in a group were undoubtedly eaten more often than others, data on relative frequency of consumption of foods within a group in this population are not available. Therefore, a simple unweighted mean value was used to avoid the influence of subjective judgment on the results.

The amount of retinol (R) was estimated by multiplying, for each of 8 food groups shown in the upper section of table I, the amount of vitamin A per unit of the food by the number of units consumed, as indicated by the characteristic value of the food-profile score, and summing these products. Carotene (C) was similarly estimated from the 3 food groups shown in the lower section of table I. The proportional contribution of retinol, $R/(R+C)$, was multiplied by the intake of total vitamin A (VITA), estimated by the earlier nutrient analysis of the 28-day diet history taken at the second examination, to calculate the retinol index (RI): $RI = VITA [R/(R+C)]$. The carotene index (CI) was calculated as $CI = VITA - RI$.

Men continuing to participate in this study were re-examined annually until 1969. 9 years later, vital status was determined for all but 3 of the 2107 participants. Death certificates were obtained for all those who had died. We sent all the survivors a questionnaire which included questions on history of diagnosis of cancer; replies were obtained from all but 19 of 1546 survivors. Medical and hospital records were sought, with the permission of the participant or his next-of-kin, for all men with malignant neoplasm indicated on the death certificate or the questionnaire (n=285) and were obtained for 243 of these men (85·3%). This information was reviewed and coded without knowledge of other information about participants.

153 men (7·3% of 2107) were omitted from this analysis for one or more of the following reasons: age at first examination was less than 40 years (1 man); vital status was unknown at the twentieth anniversary (3 men); malignant neoplasm had been diagnosed before the second examination (9); the second examination was not conducted owing to death (14), leaving the company's employment or transfer to another plant (17), or withdrawal from the study (31); and data were missing from the second examination on the food-profile scores (74) or cigarette smoking (6).

Data were analysed by the Statistical Analysis System, Release 79·3A.[12] Proportional hazards (Cox-type) regression analysis was performed by PROC PHGLM.[13,14] Univariate tests for linear trends in incidence and mortality rates were conducted as described by Fleiss.[15]

TABLE I—UNIT OF MEASUREMENT, VITAMIN A PER UNIT, AND NUMBER OF UNITS INDICATED BY EACH FOOD-PROFILE SCORE FOR FOOD GROUPS FORMING RETINOL AND CAROTENE INDICES

Food groups	Unit of measurement	Vitamin A (IU/food unit)	Number of units indicated by food-profile score		
			1	2	3
Forming the retinol index:					
Whole milk	480 ml	780	1–27 (14)	28 (28)	⩾29 (56)
Cream	30 ml	249	1–13 (7)	14–84 (49)	⩾85 (168)
Butter	14 g	460	1–27 (14)	28–84 (56)	⩾85 (140)
Margarine*	14 g	460	1–27 (14)	28–84 (56)	⩾85 (140)
Cheese†	28 g	400	1– 7 (4)	8–16 (12)	⩾17 (32)
Ice cream, custard, pudding	120 ml	330‡	1– 3 (2)	4–12 (8)	⩾13 (24)
Eggs	54 g	550	1–11 (6)	12–28 (20)	⩾29 (56)
Liver§	120 g	52 680	<1 (0·5)	1–2 (1·5)	⩾ 3 (4)
Forming the carotene index:					
Vegetables	100 g	2560¶	1–27 (9)	28–84 (42)	⩾85 (98)
Soup	240 ml	1113‖	1–11 (3)	12–28 (16)	⩾29 (42)
Fruit	100 g	940**	1–27 (9)	28–84 (42)	⩾85 (98)

Food-profile score 0 was used to indicate 0 units. Scores 1–3 were initially defined by ranges of values; to calculate the retinol and carotene indices, these ranges were replaced by characteristic values (in parentheses). *Margarine was fortified with vitamin A, mostly retinyl esters, to the same level as butter. In the late 1950s, 3·3 mg (5500 IU) β-carotene was added as a colouring agent to each pound (453·6 g) in about one-third of margarines. †Value for American cheese used. ‡Mean value for three items comprising this group was assigned. §Value for beef liver used. ¶Nominal value was obtained by averaging value for each of separate items listed in this group: asparagus, green beans, beets, broccoli, cabbage, carrots, cauliflower, corn, eggplant, leafy green vegetables, other green and yellow vegetables, onions, peas, and tomatoes.‖Value for composite soup used. **Nominal value was obtained by averaging value for each of separate items listed in this group: avocado, apple, banana, cantaloupe, citrus fruit, other fresh or canned fruit, and dried fruit.

Results

The mean carotene index was 5543±2769 (1 SD) IU/day. The carotene index was inversely related to the incidence of lung cancer (table II) but apparently was not related to the incidence of other carcinomas grouped together. The relative risks of lung cancer in the first (lowest) to the fourth (highest) quartiles of the carotene index were 7·0, 5·5, 3·0, and 1·0, respectively. Food-profile scores for all 3 food groups used to calculate the carotene index tended to be inversely related to the risk of lung cancer, although only the association with the score for soup was significant at the 5% level. The p values for vegetables, soups, and fruit were 0·225, 0·033, and 0·073, respectively. The small number of men (33) in whom lung cancer developed, and the large proportion of them for whom no information about type was available (see footnote to table II), precluded statistical analysis according to type of lung cancer.

The mean retinol index was 4734±3196 (1 SD) IU/day. The simple coefficient of correlation with the carotene index was 0·285, and the partial correlation coefficient was 0·172 after adjustment for total energy intake. The retinol index was not significantly associated with incidence of lung cancer or of other cancers (table II). 4 of the food groups forming the retinol index (whole milk, cream, butter, and cheese) tended to be inversely related to risk of lung cancer, but no relation was significant; the p values were 0·944, 0·170, 0·798, and 0·824, respectively. The other 4 food groups tended to be positively related to the risk of lung cancer, but only the trend for margarine was significant; the p values for margarine, ice cream/custard/puddings, eggs, and liver were 0·041, 0·190, 0·325, and 0·459, respectively.

The retinol index was not significantly correlated with age, with cigarettes smoked per day, with years of smoking cigarettes, or with serum cholesterol. The carotene index was not significantly correlated with age or with serum cholesterol, but there was a small negative correlation with cigarettes smoked per day ($r = -0·06$) and with years of smoking ($r = -0·06$).

The level of the dietary carotene index and the duration of cigarette smoking were both associated with incidence of lung cancer (fig. 1). Cox-type regression analysis (table III) confirmed that the carotene index had a significant inverse association with incidence of lung cancer after adjustment for duration of cigarette smoking, number of cigarettes smoked per day, the retinol index, and age. Although age and cigarettes smoked per day were significantly and positively associated with risk of lung cancer in univariate analysis (not shown here), these associations were reduced in magnitude and were not significant at the 5% level in multivariate analyses that included duration of smoking.

Men in whom lung cancer developed tended to have had below-average intake of dietary carotene at the beginning of the study; this tendency persisted throughout the 19 years of follow-up (fig. 2). Below-median values of carotene intake had been recorded for 11 of 16 men in whom lung cancer was diagnosed during the first 13 years of follow-up and for 14 of 17 men diagnosed during the 14th−19th years. Overall, 14 men (42% of the 33 with lung cancer) had values of carotene intake below the 25th percentile, and 2 (6%) had values above the 75th percentile.

Fig. 3 shows the mean carotene index, and its 95% confidence interval, for each of 8 categories of carcinomas compared with the mean value for the entire study group of 1954 men. Although the mean carotene index for the men in whom epidermoid carcinomas of the head and neck developed was only slightly higher than that for the men in whom lung cancer developed (4481 *vs* 4342 IU/day), the 95% confidence interval was substantially larger and encompassed the mean value for the total study group owing to a larger standard deviation (2642 *vs* 1886 IU/day) and a smaller number of men. None of the remaining categories of

TABLE II—19-YEAR RISK OF CARCINOMA ACCORDING TO LEVEL OF DIETARY CAROTENE AND RETINOL INDICES IN 1954 MIDDLE-AGED MEN

Mean dietary variable (range)	No. at risk	Mean age (yr)*	19-yr incidence of carcinoma†					
			Lung‡		Other§		Total	
			No.	(%)	No.	(%)	No.	(%)
Quartiles of carotene index (100 IU/day):								
27 (1−37)	488	48·8	14	(2·9)	42	(8·6)	56	(11·5)
45 (38−50)	489	48·9	11	(2·2)	54	(11·0)	65	(13·3)
58 (51−66)	489	48·5	6	(1·2)	38	(7·8)	44	(9·0)
91 (67−320)	488	48·7	2	(0·4)	41	(8·4)	43	(8·8)
Total 55	1954	48·7	33	(1·7)	175	(9·0)	208	(10·6)
Slope			−0·037		−0·011		−0·048	
χ² slope (df=1)			8·688		0·165		2·586	
p			0·003		0·684		0·108	
Quartiles of retinol index (100 IU/day):								
16 (1−22)	488	48·8	5	(1·0)	44	(9·0)	49	(10·0)
32 (23−39)	489	48·5	11	(2·2)	39	(8·0)	50	(10·2)
50 (40−62)	489	48·9	7	(1·4)	48	(9·8)	55	(11·2)
92 (63−255)	488	48·7	10	(2·0)	44	(9·0)	54	(11·1)
Total 47	1954	48·7	33	(1·7)	175	(9·0)	208	(10·6)
Slope			0·009		0·011		0·020	
χ² slope (df=1)			0·781		0·214		0·636	
p			0·377		0·644		0·425	

*Age at the second examination. †Rates have not been age-adjusted because age, within the relatively narrow range studied here, was not correlated with the carotene or retinol indices and, consequently, quartiles did not differ substantially in distribution of age. ‡Lung carcinomas: 4 adenocarcinomas; 2 small-cell; 2 large-cell; 9 epidermoid carcinomas; and 16 bronchogenic carcinomas of unspecified type. §Other carcinomas: 36 non-melanoma skin; 29 colon; 29 prostate; 20 rectum; 19 urinary bladder; 14 epidermoid head and neck; 7 kidney; 5 stomach; 5 pancreas; and 11 patients with generalised carcinomatosis with unknown primary site.

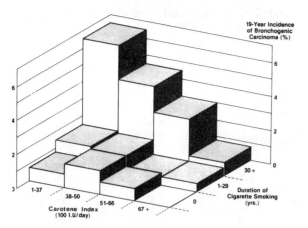

Fig. 1—Bivariate association of carotene index and duration of cigarette smoking with 19-year incidence of lung cancer.

Ratio of cases to number at risk in each quartile of carotene index, low to high, for men who reportedly had never smoked cigarettes was 1/129, 2/139, 1/149, and 0/158; for men smoking 1–29 years, 3/204, 3/218, 1/208, and 1/211; and for men smoking >30 years, 10/155, 6/132, 4/132, and 1/119.

carcinoma had a mean carotene index significantly different from the overall mean value.

The mean intake of dietary carotene was lower in men who subsequently developed lung cancer than in men who did not, but mean intake of retinol, mean energy intake, and mean intake of other nutrients were similar in the two groups (table IV).

The level of the carotene index was significantly inversely related to 19-year mortality from lung cancer but not from other carcinomas, other malignant neoplasms, cardiovascular-renal diseases, or other causes grouped together (table V). In contrast, cigarette-smoking status was strongly associated with risk of death in every category of cause except malignant neoplasms other than carcinomas.

Discussion

Both evidence from animal experimental studies and the epidemiological evidence on vitamin A and risk of cancer have been reviewed in detail.[6,16] The results of our study support the hypothesis of Peto et al. with respect to lung cancer; the dietary variable related to risk of lung cancer is beta-carotene, not retinol. There were no significant differences in mean intake of other nutrients by men in whom lung cancer developed and by those in whom it did not during

19 years of follow-up; this strengthens the view that the risk of lung cancer was specifically related to intake of carotene and not to some other variable associated with eating fruits and vegetables. The long period of follow-up indicates that below-average intake of carotene preceded the carcinoma and was not a consequence of it.

All dietary survey methods have problems with reliability and validity,[17] but the methods for assessing intake of vitamin A in previous epidemiological studies (excepting Gregor's[5]), and of carotene and retinol in our study, were particularly crude. It is not possible, therefore, to estimate whether the values of dietary carotene reported here are higher or lower than the values that would be obtained by chemical analysis of duplicate meals. We believe that the correlation between our estimates of carotene intake and the true values, if they were known, would be moderate at best and that these results should be interpreted with considerable caution.

Other studies[18,19] have shown positive correlations between serum cholesterol concentrations and serum levels of retinol and of beta-carotene. Kark et al.[20] suggested that the inverse relation between serum cholesterol level and risk of cancer found in some populations may be secondary to an inverse relation between serum retinol and risk of cancer coupled with a positive correlation between serum retinol and serum cholesterol levels. Our study showed no association between the level of serum cholesterol and the estimated

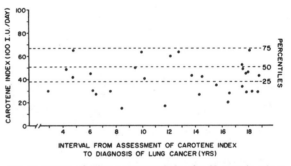

Fig. 2—Values of dietary carotene index for 33 men in whom bronchogenic carcinoma subsequently developed according to time from dietary assessment to diagnosis of cancer.

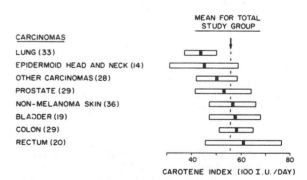

Fig. 3—Mean value of the dietary carotene index and its 95% confidence interval for each of 8 categories of carcinoma which occurred in a group of 1954 men followed for 19 years.

Number of men in each category is shown in parentheses. Group of 28 other carcinomas distributed by site as follows: 7 kidney, 5 stomach, 5 pancreas, and 11 cases of generalised carcinomatosis with primary site unknown. Broken line = mean value for total group of 1954 men; solid bar = mean carotene index; open bar = 95% confidence interval.

TABLE III—PROPORTIONAL HAZARDS (COX-TYPE) REGRESSION OF 19-YEAR INCIDENCE OF LUNG CANCER ON THE CAROTENE AND RETINOL INDICES, THE DURATION AND AMOUNT OF CIGARETTE SMOKING, AND AGE

Regression of 19-year incidence of lung cancer on:	Coefficient	Standard error	χ^2	p
Duration of cigarette smoking (yr)	0·070	0·021	10·94	<0·001
Carotene index (100 IU/day)	−0·024	0·009	7·78	0·005
Retinol index (100 IU/day)	0·009	0·005	3·02	0·082
Age at 2nd examination (yr)	0·079	0·046	2·89	0·089
Number of cigarettes smoked per day most of adult life	−0·012	0·023	0·29	0·590

Results for a total of 1954 men, in 33 of whom lung cancer subsequently developed, were analysed. χ^2 for the overall model with 5 variables was 37·82, which with 5 degrees of freedom is associated with p<0·001.

TABLE IV—DIFFERENCES IN MEAN VALUE OF NUTRITIONAL VARIABLES AT START OF STUDY BETWEEN MEN WHO SUBSEQUENTLY DEVELOPED LUNG CANCER AND THOSE WHO DID NOT DURING 19 YEARS OF FOLLOW-UP

| Dietary variables (units/day)* | Mean value of nutritional variables ±SD | | Difference between means | Student's *t* | p |
	Men with lung cancer (n=33)	All others (n=1921)			
Carotene index (100 IU)	43·4±18·9	55·6±27·8	−12·2	−3·65†	<0·001
Retinol index (100 IU)	52·2±34·5	47·3±31·9	4·9	0·88	0·378
Energy intake (100 kcal)	29·5± 8·7	31·1± 8·4	−1·6	−1·10	0·272
Animal protein (% cal)	11·5± 2·1	11·6± 2·1	−0·1	−0·08	0·933
Vegetable protein (% cal)	3·3± 0·5	3·5± 0·6	−0·2	−1·63	0·102
Animal fat (% cal)	32·9± 5·8	32·7± 5·0	0·2	0·21	0·836
Vegetable fat (% cal)	10·4± 3·9	10·2± 3·7	0·2	0·28	0·781
Carbohydrate (% cal)	36·5± 5·6	38·0± 4·7	−1·5	−1·83	0·067
Calcium (g)	1·02± 0·46	0·92±0·34	0·10	1·63†	0·112
Phosphorus (g)	2·35±0·86	2·18±0·85	0·17	1·13	0·260
Iron (mg)	15·8± 5·4	16·8± 4·4	−1·0	−1·33	0·184
Thiamin (mg)	1·52±0·52	1·63±0·47	−0·11	−1·33	0·185
Riboflavin (mg)	2·26±0·70	2·41±0·78	−0·15	−1·11	0·266
Niacin (mg)	21·0± 6·5	22·8± 6·2	−1·8	−1·63	0·104
Vitamin C (mg)	91·8±31·4	101·0±41·1	−9·2	−1·28	0·200
Vitamin D (IU)	175±117	179±132	−4·0	−0·19	0·848
Cholesterol (mg)	774±472	729±249	45	0·55	0·586

*Carotene and retinol indices were measured only at the second examination. Values of other dietary variables were obtained by averaging measurements made at both the first and second examinations to decrease the effect of intra-individual variation. †For these variables the value of Student's *t* and its degrees of freedom were calculated by the Statistical Analysis System approximation in the case of unequal variances.

TABLE V—19-YEAR MORTALITY RATE PER 100 ACCORDING TO LEVEL OF THE CAROTENE INDEX AND TO CIGARETTE SMOKING STATUS

| | No. at risk | Percentage dead by cause | | | | | |
		Lung cancer	Other cancers	Other malignant neoplasms	Cardio-vascular/renal diseases	Other causes	Total
Quartiles of carotene index (100 IU/day):							
1–37	488	2·7	3·7	1·0	16·0	3·3	26·6
38–50	489	1·8	4·3	1·4	13·9	2·2	23·7
51–66	489	0·6	2·9	1·2	16·4	3·7	24·7
67–320	488	0·2	3·1	0·8	13·7	2·9	20·7
Slope		−0·036	−0·012	−0·004	−0·019	0·000	−0·071
χ^2 slope (df=1)		10·827	0·441	0·176	0·300	0·000	2·993
p		0·001	0·507	0·675	0·584	1·000	0·084
Cigarette smoking:							
Never	575	0·5	2·4	0·9	10·8	1·2	15·8
Former	266	0·0	2·6	1·5	10·5	4·9	19·5
Current, 1–14/day	279	1·1	3·6	2·1	13·6	2·5	22·9
Current, 15–24/day	644	2·3	3·9	0·8	19·6	3·6	30·1
Current, ⩾25/day	190	2·6	6·3	1·0	20·5	4·7	35·3
Total	1954	1·3	3·5	1·1	15·0	3·0	24·0
Slope		0·082	0·118	0·007	0·478	0·103	0·788
χ^2 slope (df=1)		10·519	8·429	0·103	36·675	7·369	69·741
p		0·001	0·004	0·749	<0·001	0·007	<0·001

Total number of deaths in each group were: 26 lung cancers, 68 other cancers, 22 other malignant neoplasms, 293 cardiovascular/renal diseases, and 59 other causes. Mean ages for quartiles of carotene index are shown in table II. For five categories of cigarette smoking (never to ⩾25/day) mean ages were 49·0, 49·3, 49·1, 48·2, and 48·1 years, respectively. Rates have not been age-adjusted because age, within relatively narrow range studied here, was not correlated with carotene index and had only a very small negative correlation with quantity of cigarettes smoked. Consequently, the categories did not differ substantially in distribution of age.

intake of dietary retinol and carotene. However, this finding should also be interpreted cautiously in view of the known difficulties in correlating dietary variables with serum cholesterol concentration.[21,22]

Doll and Peto[23] have shown that the risk of lung cancer depends much more strongly on the number of years that a person has smoked cigarettes than on either chronological age or the number of cigarettes smoked per day. Our results are consistent with their findings.

Many questions remain to be answered, and further studies are required to determine whether increasing the intake of dietary beta-carotene will reduce the risk of lung cancer in man. However, it seems prudent to emphasise that sound nutritional practice, at least for the general populations of countries such as the U.S.A., involves selecting foods from each of several major groups, including the vegetables and fruits that contain substantial amounts of beta-carotene. The consistency of the epidemiological evidence from diverse populations, the graded nature and temporal sequence of the association, its independence from cigarette smoking, and its coherence with the evidence from animals, all suggest that a diet relatively high in beta-carotene may reduce risk of lung cancer even among persons who have smoked cigarettes for many years. It should be emphasised, however, that cigarette smoking increases the risk of other serious diseases, and there is no evidence that dietary carotene affects these other risks in any way.

We thank the officers and employees of the Western Electric Company, in particular, the participants and their families, and all the physicians who were involved in the Western Electric Health Study. We also thank Dr Martha Trulson and Ms Dorothea Turner who helped to prepare the food composition table, Dr Harlley McKean and Mr Daniel Garside who helped to organise the data file, Mr Joseph Costello, Mrs Nancy O'Dell, and Mrs Dolores Vogel who assisted in determining the vital status of participants, and Ms Loralei LeGrady who helped to prepare data tables and manuscript. Dr Charles Hennekens and Mr Richard Peto made helpful suggestions on analysis of data. The Western Electric Study has been supported by the American Heart Association; Mrs Tiffany Blake; Chicago Heart Association; Illini Foundation; Illinois Heart Association; National Heart, Lung and Blood Institute; Research and Education Committee of Presbyterian-St Luke's Hospital; Otho S. Sprague Foundation, and other private donors. This investigation was supported by the Day Fund, the Rush Cancer Center, and the National Cancer Institute (CA 22536).

Correspondence should be addressed to R. B. S., Department of Preventive Medicine, Rush-Presbyterian-St Luke's Medical Center, Chicago, Illinois 60612, U.S.A.

REFERENCES

1. Bjelke E. Dietary vitamin A and human lung cancer. *Int J Cancer* 1975; **15:** 561–65.
2. Hirayama T. Diet and cancer. *Nutr Cancer* 1979; **1:** 67–81.
3. MacLennan R, DaCosta J, Day NE, Low CH, Ng YK, Shanmugaratnam K. Risk factors for lung cancer in Singapore Chinese, a population with high female incidence rates. *Int J Cancer* 1977; **20:** 854–60.
4. Mettlin C, Graham S, Swanson M. Vitamin A and lung cancer. *J Natl Cancer Inst* 1979; **62:** 1435–38.
5. Gregor A, Lee PN, Roe FJC, Wilson MJ, Melton A. Comparison of dietary histories in lung cancer cases and controls with special reference to vitamin A. *Nutr Cancer* 1980; **2:** 93–97.
6. Peto R, Doll R, Buckley JD, Sporn MB. Can dietary beta-carotene materially reduce human cancer rates? *Nature* 1981; **290:** 201–08.
7. Paul O, Lepper MH, Phelan WH, et al. A longitudinal study of coronary heart disease. *Circulation* 1963; **28:** 20–31.
8. Department of Nutrition. Food Composition Table No. 3. Boston: Harvard School of Public Health, 1957.
9. Hayes OB, Rose G. Supplementary Food Composition Table. *J Am Diet Assoc* 1957; **33:** 26–29.
10. Hardinge MG, Crooks H. Fatty acid composition of food fats. *J Am Diet Assoc* 1958; **34:** 1065–71.
11. Bowes A de P, Church CF. Food values of portions commonly used. Philadelphia: JB Lippincott, 1956.
12. Helwig JT, Council KA, eds. SAS User's Guide. Raleigh, North Carolina: SAS Institute, 1979.
13. Kalbfleisch JD, Prentice RL. The statistical analysis of failure time data. New York: John Wiley and Sons, 1980.
14. Harrell F. The PHGLM Procedure. In: Reinhardt PS, ed. The SAS supplemental library user's guide, 1980 edition. Cary, North Carolina: SAS Institute, 1980: 119–31.
15. Fleiss JL. Statistical methods for rates and proportions. 2nd ed. New York: John Wiley & Sons, 1981: 143–46.
16. Sporn MB, Newton DL. Chemoprevention of cancer with retinoids. *Federation Proc* 1979; **38:** 2528–34.
17. Keys A. Dietary survey methods in studies on cardiovascular epidemiology. *Voeding* 1965; **26:** 464–83.
18. Kark JD, Smith AH, Switzer BR, Hames CG. Retinol, carotene, and the cancer/cholesterol association. *Lancet* 1981; i: 1371.
19. Smith AH, Hoggard BM. Retinol, carotene, and the cancer/cholesterol association. *Lancet* 1981; i: 1371–72.
20. Kark JD, Smith AH, Hames CG. The relationship of serum cholesterol to the incidence of cancer in Evans County, Georgia. *J Chron Dis* 1980; **33:** 311–22.
21. Jacobs DR Jr, Anderson JT, Blackburn H. Diet and serum cholesterol: do zero correlations negate the relationship? *Am J Epidemiol* 1979; **110:** 77–87.
22. Liu K, Stamler J, Dyer A, McKeever J, McKeever P. Statistical methods to assess and minimize the role of intra-individual variability in obscuring the relationship between dietary lipids and serum cholesterol. *J Chron Dis* 1978; **31:** 399–418.
23. Doll R, Peto R. Cigarette smoking and bronchial carcinoma: dose and time relationships among regular smokers and lifelong nonsmokers. *J Epidemiol Commun Hlth* 1978; **32:** 303–13.

Trends in Diet and Breast Cancer Mortality in England and Wales 1928-1977

by David M. Ingram

Abstract

Trends in age-adjusted breast cancer mortality and consumption of meat, fat, sugar, cereal, and fruit and vegetables were studied for England and Wales over the 50-year period from 1928 to 1977. At the onset of World War II, there was a marked reduction in both breast cancer mortality and intake of sugar, meat and fat, and an increased consumption of cereals and vegetables. Consumption of these foodstuffs returned to pre-war levels by 1954, but breast cancer mortality did not return to pre-war levels until some 15 years later. The association between the various dietary components and subsequent breast cancer mortality was determined for various lag intervals. Significant correlations were found for cereal, fat, sugar and meat consumption, the correlation being maximal for a diet-breast cancer death lag interval of 12 years.

These findings add weight to the hypothesis that breast cancer development is related to a diet rich in meat, fat and sugar, and that some protection against cancer may be afforded by a reduction in these dietary components and an increase in cereal consumption.

Introduction

It has been suggested that as much as 90% of all cancers may be preventable [1]; that is, there are environmental factors which, if removed, should prevent the occurrence of these cancers. Breast cancer appears to be no exception, as there is now considerable evidence that environmental factors play an important role in its origin [2]. Several epidemiological studies have suggested associations between fat, meat and sugar consumption and breast cancer [3-5].

During World War II, the United Kingdom experienced shortages of dairy products, meat and sugar due to difficulties with supply, and compensated for this lack by increased consumption of cereals and vegetables. We utilized this period of altered diet in a study of breast cancer mortality and diet in England and Wales from World War II to the present.

D.M. Ingram is affiliated with the University Department of Surgery, Queen Elizabeth II Medical Centre, Nedlands, Western Australia 6009.

Copyright © 1981 by The Franklin Institute. All rights reserved. Reprinted with permission from *Nutrition and Cancer,* Vol. 3, No. 2, 1981, pp. 75-80.

Materials and Methods

Female breast cancer mortality in England and Wales was age-standardized against a standard European population [6] and plotted as 2-year averages over the 50-year period from 1928 to 1977 (Figure 1). In a study of cancer epidemiology, it is desirable to use incidence rather than mortality, as death rates are a compound of both incidence rates and fatality rates. Data of breast cancer incidence are not available for the early years of this study, so it has been necessary to use mortality statistics. The need to age-adjust cancer mortality statistics when making comparisons between different populations has been previously emphasized [6]. Data on deaths from breast cancer were obtained from *The Registrar General's Statistical Review of England and Wales* [7].

The civilian consumption of meat, fat, sugar, cereals, and fruit and vegetables per capita per annum was plotted as 2-year averages for as much of the period from 1928 to 1977 as figures were available (Figure 1). These data were not available prior to 1934, and were available only as a 5-year average from 1934 to 1938. Meat consumption included beef, mutton, lamb, pork, ham, bacon and offal; fat consumption included fat from all sources including meat; sugar consumption included granular sugar as well as sugar in jams and other manufactured goods. Data on consumption of foodstuffs were obtained from the *Annual Abstract of Statistics*, Central Statistics Office, London [8].

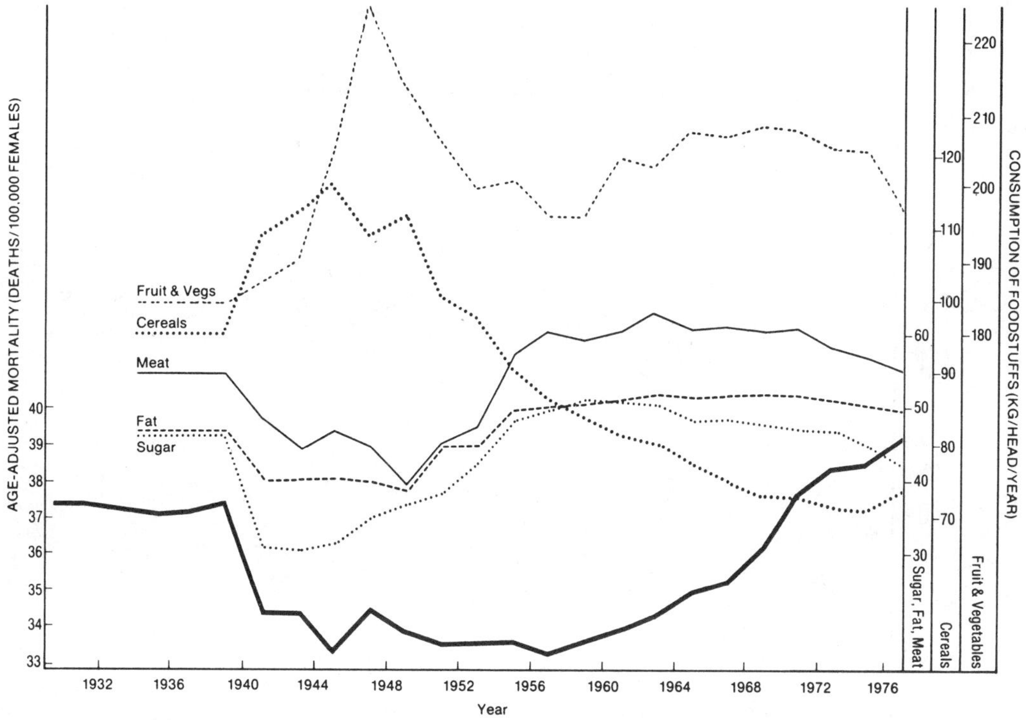

Figure 1. Comparison of 2-year averaged age-adjusted breast cancer mortality (▬▬) and consumption of cereal products (•••••••), fruit and vegetables (-- -- -- --), meat (———), fat (------) and sugar (.......).

Correlation coefficients were computed for breast cancer mortality and the concurrent consumption of each dietary component, as well as for breast cancer mortality and changes in consumption of these foodstuffs in preceding years. These computations were made at 2-year intervals up to a lag interval of 20 years, and plotted so the lag interval of greatest significance could be identified (Figure 2).

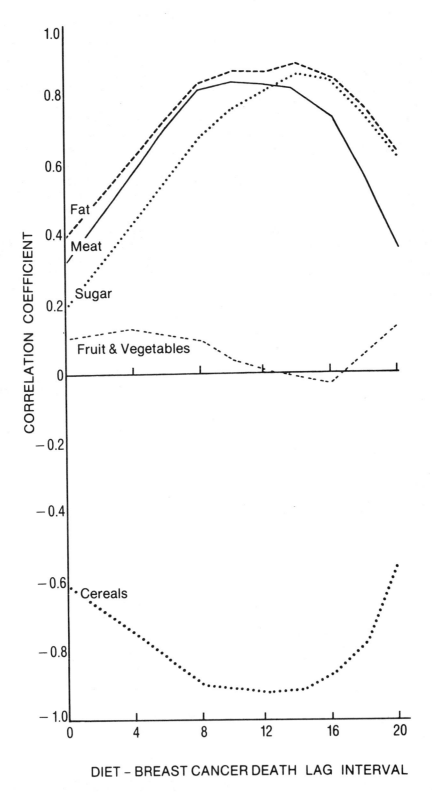

Figure 2. Correlation coefficients computed at various lag intervals between dietary change and subsequent breast cancer deaths for each dietary component. Cereal products (·······), fruit and vegetables (-- -- -- --), meat (———), fat (------) and sugar (········).

Results

Breast cancer mortality fell markedly in England and Wales at the commencement of World War II (average of 39.3 deaths per 100,000 from 1934 to 1938; average of 34.3 deaths per 100,000 from 1940 to 1944), and persisted at this level until 1956. Subsequently, there has been a slow and steady rise reaching pre-war levels in 1970, and continuing to rise up to the present time.

The graphs of meat, fat and sugar consumption followed a similar pattern to that of breast cancer mortality (Figure 1). Coincident with the onset of World War II, there was a marked drop in the consumption of these foodstuffs (maximal decrease from pre-war levels: sugar, 49%; meat, 30%; fat, 18%). This drop was balanced, however, by increased consumption of cereal products (23%) and fruit and vegetables (25%). By 1948 these trends were reversed, and consumption of foodstuffs reached pre-war levels in 1954, remaining relatively stable thereafter.

Highly significant correlation coefficients were found for breast cancer mortality and for each of the foodstuffs studied, with the exception of fruit and vegetable consumption (Table 1). This association was greatest when breast cancer mortality was compared with the dietary changes 10 to 14 years previously (Figure 2). The best correlation was the inverse relationship with cereal consumption at a lag interval of 12 years.

Table 1. The Association of Breast Cancer Mortality and Various Dietary Components

Dietary component	Maximum correlation coefficient	Lag interval (years)	Significance
Cereal	−0.92	12	$P < 0.00001$
Fat	0.87	12	$P < 0.0001$
Sugar	0.86	14	$P < 0.001$
Meat	0.84	10	$P < 0.001$
Fruit and vegetables	0.14	20	N.S.

N.S. = not significant.

Discussion

There is increasing evidence for an association between breast cancer and diet. The evidence includes the following:

1. Major international differences in both nutritional intake and breast cancer incidence have been demonstrated [3-5]. Intakes of fat, meat, dairy products and refined sugar are much higher in the US as compared to Japan, and similarly the US has a much higher incidence of breast cancer as compared to Japan. In addition, migration of Japanese people to the US results in an increase in the incidence of breast cancer among that subpopulation, particularly with an increase in duration of settlement [9].

2. Studies of subgroups within a given population having differing dietary habits have suggested that dietary factors may be important in the development of breast cancer. In Japan, women of high socioeconomic strata who eat meat daily were found to have an 8.5 times higher risk of developing breast cancer than women of low socioeconomic strata who did not eat meat daily [10]. In the US, Seventh-Day Adventist vegetarians have a lower incidence of breast cancer than the rest of the population [11].

3. Subjects with greater than normal weight and height are predisposed to the development of breast cancer [12, 13]. This would suggest that nutrition during growth and development may be important.

4. Studies in rats have found an increased incidence of 7,12-dimethylbenz(α)anthracene-induced breast cancer in animals fed diets high in vegetable fat [14] and sugar [15].

There are several points in the current study that are of particular interest. The marked change in the consumption of foodstuffs at the commencement of the war and an almost simultaneous drop in breast cancer mortality suggests an association. Any postulate of cause and effect cannot, of course, include tumor initiation, as the expected time lag is missing. What is more likely, however, is that dietary alteration has inhibited tumor growth, possibly via a hormonal or immunological mechanism, or simply by a reduction in available nutrition. Dietary studies in humans have demonstrated that consumption of a vegetarian diet results in reduced production of prolactin and estrogen [16, 17], while other studies have found that tumor immunity is increased by reduction in consumption of some amino acids [18]. Animal studies have demonstrated that tumor development and growth are inhibited by undernutrition [19], and that mitotic activity is dependent on carbohydrate and calorie supply [20]. Perhaps attention to diet should be considered more seriously in the treatment of established cancer.

Also demonstrated by this study is the association of breast cancer mortality and consumption of fat, sugar and meat (positive correlation) and cereal products (negative correlation) 10 to 14 years previously. The best correlation was that with cereal consumption. Although the apparently beneficial effect of increased cereal consumption may reflect no more than an increased intake to compensate for reduced consumption of dairy products, meat and sugar, the converse should also be considered, that is, there may be an inherent beneficial effect from the consumption of cereal products themselves.

Conclusion

World War II affected countless facets of everyone's lives in Britain, and there are many possible explanations for the drop in breast cancer mortality during and after World War II. As demonstrated in this study one of these facets was diet, and it is suggested that wartime alteration in the dietary balance of meat, fat and sugar on the one hand, and cereal consumption on the other, played a role in the changes in breast cancer mortality that occurred over the period of this study. While this study provides evidence for a dietary link with breast cancer, further studies are necessary to explore the association.

References

1. "Editorial: Are 90% of Cancers Preventable?" *Lancet* i, 685-687, 1977.
2. Kelsey, JL: "A Review of the Epidemiology of Human Breast Cancer." *Epidemiol Rev* 1, 74-109, 1979.
3. Drasar, BS, and Irving, D: "Environmental Factors and Cancer of the Colon and Breast." *Br J Cancer* 27, 167-179, 1973.
4. Armstrong, BK, and Doll, R: "Environmental Factors and Cancer Incidence and Mortality in Different Countries With Special Reference to Dietary Practices." *Br J Cancer* 15, 617-631, 1975.
5. Hems, G: "The Contribution of Diet and Childbearing to Breast Cancer Rates." *Br J Cancer* 37, 974-982, 1978.
6. Doll, R: "Comparisons Between Registries, Age Standardised Rates." In Waterhouse, J, Muir, CS, Correa, P, and Powell, J (eds): *Cancer Incidence in Five Continents, Vol. 3.* Lyon: International Agency for Research on Cancer, 1976, pp. 453-457.
7. General Registry Office: *The Registrar General's Statistical Review of England and Wales. Part I: Tables, Medical 1927-1977.* London: Her Majesty's Stationery Office.
8. Central Statistics Office: *Annual Abstract of Statistics. 1927-1977. Vols. 84-114.* London: Her Majesty's Stationery Office.
9. Wynder, EL, and Hirayama, T: "Comparative Epidemiology of Cancers of the United States and Japan." *Prev Med* 6, 567-594, 1977.
10. Hirayama, T: "Epidemiology of Breast Cancer With Special Reference to the Role of Diet." *Prev Med* 7, 173-195, 1978.
11. Phillips, RL: "Role of Life-Style and Dietary Habits in Risk of Cancer Among Seventh-Day Adventists." *Cancer Res* 35, 3513-3522, 1975.
12. De Waard, F, and Baanders-Van Halewijn, EA: "A Prospective Study in General Practice on Breast Cancer Risk in Postmenopausal Women." *Int J Cancer* 14, 158-160, 1974.

13. Staszewski, J: "Breast Cancer and Body Build." *Prev Med* **6,** 410-415, 1977.

14. Carroll, KK: "Experimental Evidence of Dietary Factors and Hormone-Dependent Cancers." *Cancer Res* **35,** 3374-3383, 1975.

15. Hoern, SK, and Carroll, KK: "Effects of Dietary Carbohydrate on the Incidence of Mammary Tumours Induced in Rats by 7,12-Dimethylbenz(α)Anthracene." *Nutr Cancer* **1**(3), 27-30, 1979.

16. Armstrong, BK: "Diet and Hormones in the Epidemiology of Breast and Endometrial Cancers." *Nutr Cancer* **1**(3), 90-95, 1979.

17. Hill, P, Chan, P, Cohen, L, Wynder, E, and Kuno, K: "Diet and Endocrine-Related Cancer." *Cancer* **39,** 1820-1826, 1977.

18. Bounous, G, and Kongshavn, PAL: "The Effect of Amino Acids on Immune Reactivity." *Immunology* **35,** 257-266, 1978.

19. Jose, DG: "Dietary Deficiency of Protein, Amino Acids and Total Calories on Development and Growth of Cancer." *Nutr Cancer* **1**(3), 58-63, 1979.

20. Bullough, WS: "Mitotic Activity and Carcinogenesis." *Br J Cancer* **4,** 329-336, 1950.

Epidemiology of Prostate Cancer With Special Reference to the Role of Diet

by Takeshi Hirayama

ABSTRACT—A prospective epidemiologic study of prostate cancer was conducted in Japan. The 10-year follow-up study of 122,261 men aged 40 years and above, who constitute 94.5% of the census population of 29 Health Center Districts, revealed a significantly lower age-standardized death rate for prostate cancer in men who daily ate green and yellow vegetables. This association is consistently observed in each age-group, in each socioeconomic class, and in each prefecture. Selected epidemiologic phenomena, such as the upward trend of the prostate cancer death rate in Japan, intracountry variation of death rate, the significantly lower incidence rate in Japan compared with that of the United States, and elevated risk in Japanese migrants to Hawaii, appear to be explained by the variation in diet and change in amount of green and yellow vegetables ingested. The possible role of vitamin A is considered as a factor in preventing and inhibiting growth of prostate cancer. Most of the other factors studied appear noncontributory, except for marital status; a higher risk was observed in "ever married" men. — Natl Cancer Inst Monogr 53: 149–155, 1979.

Numerous studies have been conducted on the epidemiology of prostate cancer, considering factors such as the relationship to heredity (*1*), blood group (*2*), urban or rural environment (*3*), marital status (*3*), social class (*4*), air pollution (*5*), sexual factors (*6, 7*), effect of migration (*8*), relation to benign prostatic hyperplasia (*9, 10*), physical features (*11*), diet (*12*), smoking, drinking, and other factors (*13*); a review article has also been published (*14*).

Presented at the Second Symposium on Epidemiology and Cancer Registries in the Pacific Basin, Maui, Hawaii, January 16–20, 1978.

Division of Epidemiology, National Cancer Center Research Institute, Tsukiji 5-chome, Chuo-ku, Tokyo 104, Japan.

However, reasons for the striking international differences in incidence and death rates of prostate cancer are still not clear. The present paper proposes a hypothesis derived from preliminary results of a large-scale ongoing study on prostate cancer in Japan with special reference to the risk associated with lower daily intake of green and yellow vegetables.

MATERIALS AND METHODS

Cancer Incidence in Five Continents (*15*), and *Vital Statistics, Causes of Death, Japan, 1950–1975* (*16*), were used for the study of descriptive epidemiology of prostate cancer. Results of the census population-based prospective study initiated in 1965 (*13*) of 122,261 men aged 40 years and over from 29 Health Center Districts in Japan were used to investigate the analytic epidemiology of prostate cancer; these men were followed for 10 years. The age-standardized death rates of the disease were compared by each risk factor under investigation at the time of enrollment.

RESULTS

Incidence Rate

Adjusted incidence rates of prostate cancer in 80 registries in the world (*15*) are shown in text-figure 1. The highest three are for blacks living in the United States and the lowest three are for Japanese in Japan; Japanese in Hawaii rank just between. We explored the reasons for such distinct discrepancies between prostate cancer incidence in United States blacks and Japanese in Japan.

Reprinted with permission from *National Cancer Institute Monograph* No. 53, 1979, 149-155.

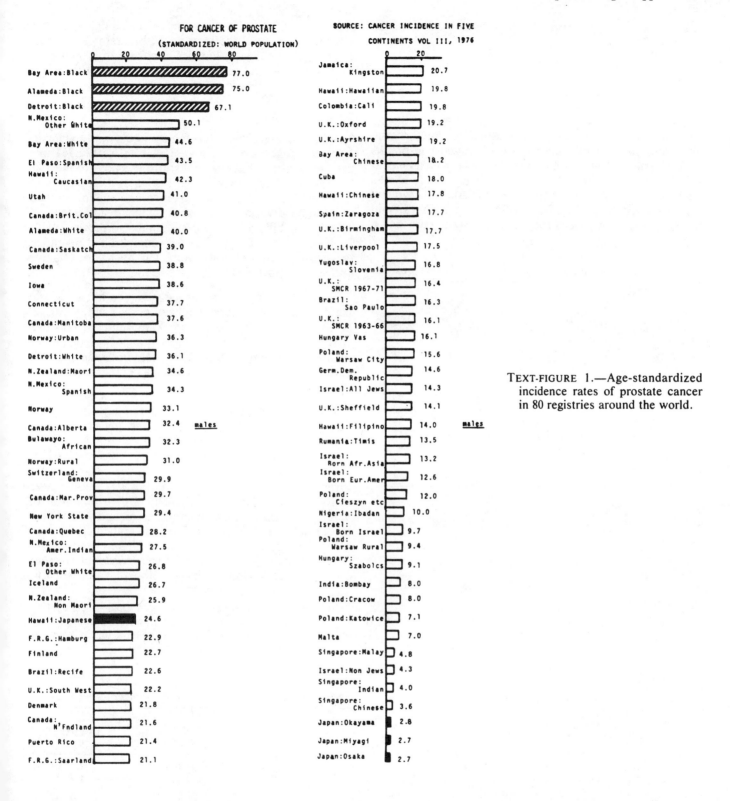

FOR CANCER OF PROSTATE

(STANDARDIZED: WORLD POPULATION)

SOURCE: CANCER INCIDENCE IN FIVE CONTINENTS VOL III, 1976

Registry	Rate
Bay Area:Black	77.0
Alameda:Black	75.0
Detroit:Black	67.1
N.Mexico: Other White	50.1
Bay Area:White	44.6
El Paso:Spanish	43.5
Hawaii: Caucasian	42.3
Utah	41.0
Canada:Brit.Col	40.8
Alameda:White	40.0
Canada:Saskatch	39.0
Sweden	38.8
Iowa	38.6
Connecticut	37.7
Canada:Manitoba	37.6
Norway:Urban	36.3
Detroit:White	36.1
N.Zealand:Maori	34.6
N.Mexico: Spanish	34.3
Norway	33.1
Canada:Alberta	32.4
Bulawayo: African	32.3
Norway:Rural	31.0
Switzerland: Geneva	29.9
Canada:Mar.Prov	29.7
New York State	29.4
Canada:Quebec	28.2
N.Mexico: Amer.Indian	27.5
El Paso: Other White	26.8
Iceland	26.7
N.Zealand: Non Maori	25.9
Hawaii:Japanese	24.6
F.R.G.:Hamburg	22.9
Finland	22.7
Brazil:Recife	22.6
U.K.:South West	22.2
Denmark	21.8
Canada: N'Fndland	21.6
Puerto Rico	21.4
F.R.G.:Saarland	21.1

males

Registry	Rate
Jamaica: Kingston	20.7
Hawaii:Hawaiian	19.8
Colombia:Cali	19.8
U.K.:Oxford	19.2
U.K.:Ayrshire	19.2
Bay Area: Chinese	18.2
Cuba	18.0
Hawaii:Chinese	17.8
Spain:Zaragoza	17.7
U.K.:Birmingham	17.7
U.K.:Liverpool	17.5
Yugoslav: Slovenia	16.8
U.K.: SMCR 1967-71	16.4
Brazil: Sao Paulo	16.3
U.K.: SMCR 1963-66	16.1
Hungary Vas	16.1
Poland: Warsaw City	15.6
Germ.Dem. Republic	14.6
Israel:All Jews	14.3
U.K.:Sheffield	14.1
Hawaii:Filipino	14.0
Rumania:Timis	13.5
Israel: Born Afr.Asia	13.2
Israel: Born Eur.Amer	12.6
Poland: Cieszyn etc	12.0
Nigeria:Ibadan	10.0
Israel: Born Israel	9.7
Poland: Warsaw Rural	9.4
Hungary: Szabolcs	9.1
India:Bombay	8.0
Poland:Cracow	8.0
Poland:Katowice	7.1
Malta	7.0
Singapore:Malay	4.8
Israel:Non Jews	4.3
Singapore: Indian	4.0
Singapore: Chinese	3.6
Japan:Okayama	2.8
Japan:Miyagi	2.7
Japan:Osaka	2.7

males

TEXT-FIGURE 1.—Age-standardized incidence rates of prostate cancer in 80 registries around the world.

Annual Trend

The death rate for prostate cancer is increasing sharply in Japan. The crude death rates in 1950, 1955, 1960, 1965, 1970, and 1975 are 0.2, 0.6, 1.0, 1.4, 1.7, and 2.3, respectively, indicating an increase of 11.50 times during the past 25 years. The age-adjusted death rates are 0.2, 0.5, 0.8, 1.0, 1.1, and 1.3, respectively, a 6.50 times increase. A recent study by the author (*17*) on trends of prostate cancer death rates (1950–74) in each age-group for blacks and Caucasians in the United States and for native Japanese revealed the consistently highest rate to be in blacks and a striking upward trend in Japanese and blacks aged 65–74 years.

Age Distribution

Age-specific incidence rates in Japan are compared with those for Japanese in Hawaii, San Francisco Bay Area whites and blacks, and Chinese, whites, and blacks of Alameda County (table 1; text-fig. 2). Age-specific incidence ratio to the rate in Japan is highest in blacks and is similar in the Bay Area and Alameda, with a peak at age 50–54. The ratio in whites is lower than that in blacks and again is similar in the Bay Area and Alameda whites, with the peak at age 55–59 years. Japanese in Hawaii and Chinese in the Bay Area show a much lower ratio and a

peak at age 60–64. The tendency of the peak is to shift to a younger age with the increase in prostate cancer incidence, which suggests heavier exposure to environmental carcinogens and/or weaker effect or protective factors in communities where prostate cancer is more endemic.

Prospective Study

A large-scale prospective study is currently (January 1978) in progress in Japan (*13*). A total of 122,261 men aged 40 years and above, constituting 94.5% of the 1965 census population in 29 Health Center Districts, were followed for 10 years. From over one million person-years of observation, 63 prostate cancer deaths occurred. The age-specific death rates are similar to those for all of Japan in 1970 (table 2). The age-standardized death rate for prostate cancer was calculated by various factors under study in 1965.

No association was observed with the intake of rice, meat, fish, milk, pickles, soybean paste soup, green tea, or alcohol, or with cigarette smoking (table 3). This table also shows that the rates in married men are much higher than those in single men, which may indicate the influence of marital sexual experience as emphasized in previous reports (*2, 11*).

The most interesting finding was the negative association with the frequency of green and yellow vegetable intake [1] (table 3; text-fig. 3). This association was consistently observed in different age-groups (under 74 yr) and socioeconomic classes, as well as in the various prefectures (text-figs. 4, 5). The association was also observed in the annual trend and geographical distribution of the death rate for prostate cancer and green and yellow vegetable intake (text-figs. 6, 7). The per capita daily intake of green and yellow vegetables in the United States is 20 g (*18*), compared with 52.9 g in Japan (*National Nutrition Survey*, 1965). Therefore, it is possible that at least part of

---

[1] Green and yellow vegetables (more than 1,000 IU/100 g containing carotenoids): carrots, spinach, green pimento, pumpkin, green lettuce, chives, leek (green), turnip leaves, asparagus (green), chicory, parsley, and broccoli.

TABLE 1.—*Age-specific incidence rate for cancer of the prostate*

| Ages, yr | Japan, average of 5 registries, 1972–73 | Bay Area | | | Alameda | |
		Black 1969–73	White 1969–73	Chinese 1969–73	Black 1969–73	White 1969–73
40–44	0.5	2.3	1.5	—	—	1.6
45–49	0.4	10.8	5.4	—	8.7	4.5
50–54	1.0	62.1	14.3	—	73.8	15.3
55–59	3.2	174.2	64.8	9.6	138.6	60.2
60–64	8.3	290.0	153.1	63.4	268.0	144.8
65–69	27.5	418.5	286.4	66.4	409.7	231.4
70–74	51.1	1,007.0	484.9	200.2	1,073.4	458.7
75–79	65.4	1,009.7	721.5	262.0	892.2	684.6
80–84	80.3	1,486.2	909.3	479.5	1,400.0	761.9
85–	110.5	865.4	938.4	843.4	973.5	844.7

TABLE 2.—*Age-specific death rate for cancer of the prostate* [a]

Age-group, yr	Prospective study, 1966–75	All Japan, 1970
45–49	0.6	0.2
50–54	0.5	0.7
55–59	1.0	1.9
60–64	4.2	4.9
65–69	10.7	11.3
70–74	19.3	19.8
75–	44.6	43.9

[a] Total No. of deaths recorded in the 1966–75 study and for all Japan (1970) were 63 and 883, respectively.

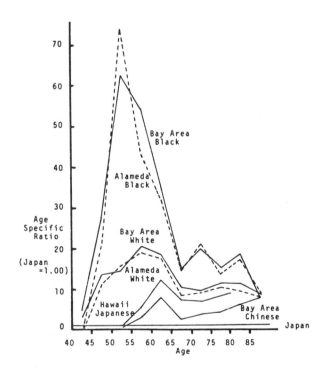

TEXT-FIGURE 2.—Age-specific incidence ratio for cancer of the prostate (Japan = 1.00).

TABLE 3.—*Age-standardized death rate for cancer of the prostate: Prospective study (1966–75)*

Parameter	Daily	Occasionally	Rarely/none	Rare	None	Hot	Average	Married	Divorced/widowed	Single
Rice										
180 cc	5.2									
360 cc	4.6									
540 cc	5.4									
720 cc	6.9									
Twice daily	5.9									
Thrice daily	5.1									
Meat	5.1	5.6	6.3							
Fish	5.7	→ 5.8 ←								
Milk	6.6	3.2	6.7							
Green and yellow vegetables	4.9	7.9	11.8							
Pickles	6.8	3.7	7.6							
Soybean paste soup	5.9	5.0	7.8							
Japanese tea			5.8			4.1	6.1			
Alcohol	6.4	4.9		→ 6.0 ←						
Smoking [a]	5.8	0.0			6.1					
Marital status								6.8	1.1	0.0

[a] Death rate for ex-smokers was 3.7.

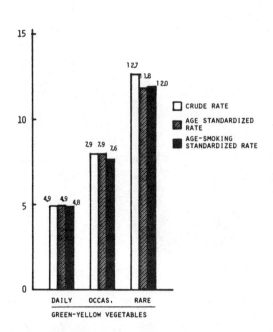

TEXT-FIGURE 3.—Death rate for cancer of the prostate by frequency of green and yellow vegetable intake (prospective study, 1966–75, Japan).

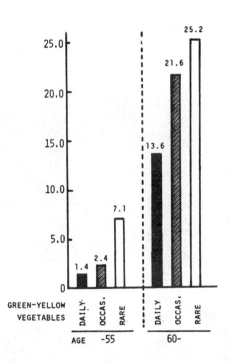

TEXT-FIGURE 4.—Death rate for cancer of the prostate by age-group and frequency of green and yellow vegetable intake (prospective study, 1966–75, Japan).

the difference in prostate cancer incidence rates in Japan and the United States comes from the difference in green and yellow vegetable intake. Since 44% of vitamin A and 23% of ascorbic acid intake came from green and yellow vegetables in 1970 in Japan (table 4), these nutritional ele-

ments provide the most likely explanation for the lower prostate cancer death rate in persons who eat these vegetables daily. Some experimental evidence indicates that vitamin A lowers an individual's risk of developing prostate cancer. The hyperplasia induced in cultured mouse

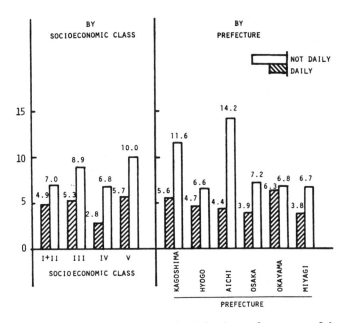

TEXT-FIGURE 5.—Age-standardized death rate for cancer of the prostate by socioeconomic class, prefecture, and frequency of green and yellow vegetable intake (prospective study, 1966–75, Japan).

TEXT-FIGURE 6.—Annual change in intake of green and yellow vegetables and in prostate cancer adjusted death rate, 1949–74, Japan.

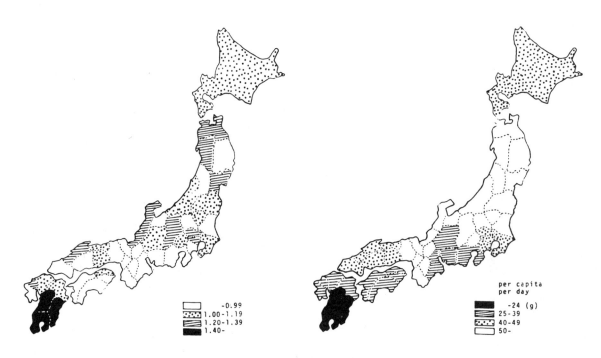

TEXT-FIGURE 7.—Adjusted death ratio for cancer of the prostate (1970–71) and intake of green and yellow vegetables (1967–69) in 46 prefectures in Japan.

prostatic tissue by chemical carcinogens (3-methyl-cholanthrene or *N*-methyl-*N'*-nitro-*N*-nitrosoguanidine) was reported inhibited and reversed by simultaneous treatment with β-retinoic acid (*19*). In this regard, the results of a comparative study of latent carcinoma of the prostate in Japanese in Japan and Hawaii, reported by Akazaki and Stemmermann (*8*), is of particular interest. Although the prevalence of latent cancer did not differ significantly between native and Hawaiian Japanese, the prevalence of the proliferative type of latent carcinoma

TABLE 4.—*Intake of nutrients from green and yellow vegetables in Japan, 1970*

Nutrient	Amount of intake	Percent of total nutrient intake
Energy, kcal	14.9	1
Protein, g	0.9	1
Fat, g	0.1	0
Carbohydrate, g	2.7	1
Calcium, mg	32.2	6
Iron, mg	0.8	6
Vitamin A, IU	640.4	44
" B$_1$, mg	0.03	3
" B$_2$, mg	0.06	7
Ascorbic acid, mg	25.2	23
Total amount of green and yellow vegetable intake, g	48.8	4

was higher in the migrant group. This finding suggested the existence of factors that prevent or slow down the growth of cancer in native Japanese. Vitamin A derived from green and yellow vegetables is the most likely candidate for such a preventive factor, although the role of ascorbic acid cannot be neglected as it could inhibit nitrosamine formation.

DISCUSSION

None of the risk factors of prostate cancer suggested heretofore in the literature appear to explain satisfactorily known epidemiologic characteristics, such as international variation in incidence and death rate, or increasing trend and enhanced risk in Japanese who migrated to the United States.

As shown in numerous studies, including ours, marital sexual experience could be of etiologic importance in prostate cancer. However, the above mentioned demographic pattern is not likely to be fully explained by this alone. Just as with breast and colon cancer, distinctly different dietary patterns in different ethnic groups must seriously be taken into consideration as factors influencing the incidence. The possible influence of meat intake on prostate cancer incidence was suggested by Howell based on an international correlation study (*12*). The results of our ongoing prospective study, however, do not confirm his observation. Rather, a marked lowering of risk by daily intake of green and yellow vegetables was observed. The association was consistent by socioeconomic status and by district. The lower incidence of prostate cancer in vegetarian countries, particularly in younger age-groups, and an upward trend in these populations when a sudden change takes place in dietary pattern appear to be explained by the vitamin A hypothesis. The lower risk of prostate cancer in vegetarians living in the United States, such as the Seventh Day Adventists in California, is also compatible with this hypothesis (*20*).

REFERENCES

(*1*) WOOLF CM: An investigation of the familial aspects of carcinoma of the prostate. Cancer 13:739–744, 1960

(*2*) BOURKE JB, GRIFFIN JP: Blood groups in benign and malignant prostatic hypertrophy. Lancet 2:1279–1280, 1962

(*3*) KING H, DIAMOND E, LILIENFELD AM: Some epidemiological aspects of cancer of the prostate. J Chronic Dis 16:117–153, 1963

(*4*) RICHARDSON IM: Prostatic cancer and social class. Br J Prev Soc Med 19:140–142, 1965

(*5*) WINKELSTEIN W, KANTOR S: Prostatic cancer: Relationship to suspended particulate air pollution. Am J Public Health 59:1134–1138, 1969

(*6*) STEEL R, LESS RE, KRAUS AS, et al: Sexual factors in the epidemiology of cancer of the prostate. J Chronic Dis 24:29–37, 1971

(*7*) WYNDER EL, MABUCHI K, WHITMORE WF: Epidemiology of cancer of the prostate. Cancer 28:344–360, 1971

(*8*) AKAZAKI K, STEMMERMANN GN: Comparative study of latent carcinoma of the prostate among Japanese in Japan and Hawaii. J Natl Cancer Inst 50:1137–1144, 1973

(*9*) ARMENIAN HK, DIAMOND EL, LILIENFELD AM, et al: Relation between benign prostatic hyperplasia and cancer of the prostate: A prospective and retrospective study. Lancet 2:115, 1974

(*10*) GREENWALD P, KIRMSS V, POLAN AK, et al: Cancer of the prostate among men with benign prostatic hyperplasia. J Natl Cancer Inst 53:335–340, 1974

(*11*) GREENWALD P, DAMON A, KIRMSS V, et al: Physical and demographic features of men before developing cancer of the prostate. J Natl Cancer Inst 53:341–346, 1974

(*12*) HOWELL MA: Factor analysis of international cancer mortality data and per capita food consumption. Br J Cancer 29:328–336, 1974

(*13*) HIRAYAMA T: Prospective studies on cancer epidemiology based on census population in Japan. *In* Proceedings of the XIth International Cancer Congress, Florence, Italy, 1974. Amsterdam: Excerpta Medica, 1975, pp 26–35

(*14*) HIGGINS IT: The epidemiology of cancer of the prostate. J Chronic Dis 28:343–348, 1975

(*15*) WATERHOUSE J, MUIR C, CORREA P, et al (eds): Cancer Incidence in Five Continents, vol III. IARC Sci Publ No. 15. Lyon: IARC, 1976

(*16*) Health and Welfare Statistics and Information Department: Vital Statistics, Japan 1950–1975. Tokyo: Minister's Secretariat, Ministry of Health and Welfare, 1976

(*17*) HIRAYAMA T (ed): Comparative Epidemiology of Cancer in the U.S. and Japan Mortality. The USA–Japan Cooperative Cancer Res Program. Tokyo: Japanese Society for the Promotion of Science, January 1977

(*18*) Agricultural Research Service: Household Food Survey 1965–66. ARS Report No. 11. Washington, D.C.: U.S. Govt Print Off, 1968

(*19*) CHOPRA DP, WILKOFF LJ: Inhibition and reversal by β-retinoic acid of hyperplasia induced in cultured mouse prostate tissues by 3-methylcholanthrene or *N*-methyl-*N'*-nitro-*N*-nitrosoguanidine. J Natl Cancer Inst 56:583–589, 1976

(*20*) PHILLIPS RL: Role of life-style and dietary habits in risk of cancer among Seventh Day Adventists. Cancer Res 35:3513–3522, 1975

DISCUSSION

R. Ross: In Los Angeles, blacks have high rates of prostate cancer. Age-adjusted rates in blacks, by the way, are the highest for any site for any single sex or any racial or ethnic group. Most of the rates in populations we discussed are much lower than those of prostate cancer in blacks living in Los Angeles. We see a positive association of prostate cancer rates with social class with blacks and whites and also with occupational class: Managers and professional types have higher rates than expected and laborers and similar workers lower than expected.

A. Smith: I have recently studied the vitamin A levels of residents of Evans County, Georgia. Diet and the serum level of vitamin A are not closely related unless there is a serious depletion of this vitamin in the diet. In the United States, many would consider it unlikely that diets of a population would be depleted enough to affect the serum levels. The dietary intake primarily affects the liver stores of vitamin A. Serum vitamin A levels were higher among the blacks than among the whites, a fact that surprised us, since we were expecting to find the reverse, due to differences in social class. I would be interested to know if you have measured any serum vitamin A levels or if you know of any measurement in Japan of these levels.

D. Austin: We just completed an investigation of socioeconomic status and prostate cancer incidence among blacks and whites in Alameda County, and we noted no straight-line gradient the way there apparently is in Los Angeles. If anything, we observed a U-shaped curve with consistently higher incidence rates in the extremes of low and high socioeconomic classes among both blacks and whites.

Ross: We grouped the upper three social classes together because of low denominators of blacks. It is a fairly clear trend in the lower three social classes in blacks. In whites for the higher four social classes, the gradient shows about a 25% differential between the top social class and social class four.

G. Stemmermann: I would like to go back to the observation that cancer of the prostate is not uncommon in Japan. What is uncommon in Japan is clinical prostate carcinoma or carcinoma of the prostate as a cause of death. When you have a tumor which was present in about 25% of deceased patients who have been autopsied, you are not dealing with a rarity, and this is, in fact, the case in Japan. When one thinks in terms of these small tumors one knows the transformation has already occurred, so the implication of yellow and green vegetables under these circumstances leads one to think they would not have the function of preventing transforma-

tion, since that has already occurred, but rather of having something to do either with promotion or the lack of it. In considering promotion of a tumor of this type, one is forced to think also of steroid metabolism. The steroids that we are dealing with are difficult to measure consistently in large amounts; they are subject to diurnal variation and, moreover, they are subject to intrinsic stimulation, e.g., the male in anticipation of sexual intercourse has a rise in his serum testosterone. We should devise a means of getting a broad-based profile in cases and controls for this tumor.

D. Thomas: Parallel with this kind of investigation, we are now conducting an intensive case–control study with regard to sexual factors and prostate cancer.

A. Nomura: I thought it was interesting that we have a situation here with urinary bladder cancer in which the difference between Hawaii and Japan is about twofold (rate is higher in Japan), and that in this particular cancer, we have a number of leads to work on right now. Then we turn to prostate cancer and we have few leads. If you compare the incidence of prostate cancer between Japanese in Hawaii and in Japan, you would see about a sevenfold to eightfold difference, with more prostate cancer occurring in Hawaii. We are currently conducting a prospective study of the incidence of prostate cancer in Japan and Hawaii. We have approximately 30 incident cases from the population, but we have no specific leads and nothing really to report yet.

P. Correa: The November 1977 issue of *International Journal of Cancer (1)* has an article on the international comparison of prostate carcinoma. The incidence of occult carcinoma, which the author calls nonproliferative, was practically the same all over the world. However, the larger overt carcinomas are the ones that vary in incidence. We recently completed a study in blacks in New Orleans and, again, the results were the same. The important factors that these studies show are that the initiation of cancer in the prostate is similar everywhere, but the promotion is different in various locations. In regard to the theory of the green vegetables, the only thing that strikes me is that the epidemiology of prostate carcinoma is independent of the epidemiology of gastric cancer, in which we have reason to believe that green leafy vegetables play a role.

REFERENCE

(*1*) Breslow N, Chan CW, Dhom G, et al: Latent carcinoma of prostate at autopsy in seven areas. Int J Cancer 20:680–688, 1977

Part 3: Social Marketing and Dietary Cancer Prevention

As illustrated in Parts 1 and 2 of this *Sourcebook,* there is much scientific evidence that cancer is avoidable and that lifestyle factors over which individuals have control contribute greatly to causation and, therefore, to prevention. Recent intervention programs aimed at preventing cardiovascular disease through control of such behavioral factors as diet have demonstrated that it is possible to change health behavior in the name of health promotion and disease prevention.

While it is not yet clear that the same type of intervention can produce a decrease in incidence and mortality rates for cancer, recent trends in health care imply that a similar approach to cancer control may be possible. The articles that follow are intended to review theories, techniques, and issues concerning health behavior change. Social marketing is a relatively new field that has moved extensively into many nontraditional marketing areas. In the field of health, for example, social marketing techniques have been used by individuals in behavioral medicine, health education, and health communication. In the past 30 years, many studies in interrelated disciplines have contributed to our knowledge of health attitudes and what influences health behavior, but the precise connection between the two is still unknown. Experience has shown, in fact, that we still do not know exactly how to elicit sustained health behavior change. Antismoking efforts over the last 20 years have shown that marketing and communication efforts to make consumers aware of the dangers of cigarette smoking have been successful. However, even when consumers know the risks they are taking, many continue to smoke. Campaigns aimed at changing awareness commonly succeed, whereas those aimed at changing behavior often fall short of the desired goals.

Social marketing, the marketing of social causes such as health issues, has emerged in the last 10 years as a possible answer to this problem. Many authorities in public health have come to believe that the field of marketing can play an important role in eliciting important behavior change to promote health and prevent diseases such as cancer. Although the important differences between health marketing and commercial marketing require some adaptation for use in health-related causes, it has been shown that the principles of marketing have much to offer the health professions.

This third part of the *Sourcebook* presents selected information on social marketing as applied to health behavior change. Since dietary guidelines for cancer prevention have been released only recently, few programs have been initiated, and even fewer completed, that focus on changing dietary habits to prevent cancer. Consequently, most of the studies presented concern general cancer prevention or general nutritional change. We have included papers on several programs developed to elicit nutritional and other changes in the name of cardiovascular disease prevention. Since a connection between certain nutritional factors and the cause of cardiovascular disease has long been established, several such studies are currently available; it is hoped that these will serve as examples of how the same marketing techniques can be applied to dietary cancer prevention.

The field of social marketing is not widely known or understood by many in the health professions. The term *social marketing,* in fact, has different meanings for different people. The first section, "Introduction to Social Marketing," presents papers that define social marketing and its role in health behavior change efforts. Here, leading authorities in this burgeoning field review past, present, and future applications of social marketing, its successes and failures. Dietary change is put into context as behavioral change, one of the four general types of social change. This section also illustrates how the "four Ps" of marketing—product, price, place, and promotion—can be applied to efforts to change health behavior.

The second section, "Theories, Techniques, and Issues in Health Behavior Change," is a selection of articles on various facets of social marketing and behavioral medicine that may affect dietary prevention of cancer. While we do not understand the precise relationship between health attitudes and health behavior, it is clear that there is a connection between the two. This section begins with a review of a Health Belief Model that defines consumers' behavior based on three different attitudes toward health. This 20-year-old theory, which is still applicable today, is supplemented by a review of recent developments in health behavior change and a specific example of how these techniques and theories can be applied to health education.
Next, the unique problems of cancer and diet are addressed. If we are to elicit behavior change to prevent cancer, it is important to understand how consumers perceive the threat of this killing disease. It is also crucial here to take into account the unique problems of changing people's food-related habits. How do people select foods and develop food preferences? At issue here are many elusive factors, including cultural factors. Thus, asking people to change food habits may amount to asking them to make a value change as well as a behavioral change. Although it has long been known that nutrition affects overall health, for many reasons physicians often hesitate to give dietary advice in the absence of definite symptoms or conditions that indicate the necessity for dietary change. How this bears on consumers' willingness to change dietary habits is also addressed here.

The second section is concluded with papers discussing the problems social marketers must face, including some brought on by the inherent differences between commercial marketing and health marketing.

The last section, "Dietary Intervention Studies Incorporating Social Marketing Techniques," presents case studies of well-known recent intervention programs. Although only the last paper is related directly to cancer, the case studies chosen for inclusion both involve dietary change and incorporate established social marketing techniques. The MRFIT program is notable as the most extensive—and most expensive—program of its kind ever undertaken in the U.S.; the Stanford Heart Disease Prevention Program is noted as a community program that used many social marketing techniques to its benefit. It is hoped that the same techniques may be applicable to programs aimed at dietary cancer prevention in the future.

William D. Novelli
President
Needham Porter Novelli
Adjuvant Professor
University of Maryland

Introduction to Social Marketing

The Marketing of Social Causes: The First Ten Years

by Karen F. A. Fox and Philip Kotler

URING the past decade the "territory" of marketing has expanded to include the marketing tasks of non-profit organizations and the marketing of worthwhile social causes. Kotler (1979) reviewed the accomplishments in the first area, describing how an increasing number of nonprofit organizations—particularly hospitals, colleges, social service agencies, and cultural organizations—are applying marketing concepts and techniques to improve the marketing of their services. Despite earlier controversy, few marketers dispute the relevance of marketing to the management of nonprofit organizations (Nickels 1974).

The time is now appropriate to evaluate the status of work in the area of social cause marketing—social marketing. Here the applicability of marketing is more hotly contested. Social marketing as a distinct application area for general marketing theory was advanced about a decade ago (Kotler and Zaltman 1971). Since then, various reform groups and government agencies have applied social marketing to such causes as family planning, energy conservation, improved nutrition, antismoking, prevention of alcohol and drug abuse, safer driving, and myriad other causes. Yet no review

of these efforts and of the issues and problems connected with social marketing has been published. In fact, some recent articles—written by academic marketers rather than practitioners—question the appropriateness and ethics of social marketing just as it is being more widely adopted (e.g., Laczniak, Lusch, and Murphy 1979). G. D. Wiebe's (1951–52) question of 30 years ago, "Why can't you sell brotherhood like you sell soap?", persists along with the newer question, "Should you be selling brotherhood?" Furthermore, the whole discussion is plagued by confusion about what social marketing is. As the technology of social marketing will shortly mark its first decade, an assessment of its nature, successes, limitation, and future is now warranted.

As background for such an assessment, we undertook an extensive review of the literature in marketing and in public health (where many of the applications of social marketing have been carried out). We interviewed key people in two leading social marketing firms to learn what problems they have tackled and what successes and frustrations they have encountered, and interviewed people in federal government agencies concerned with health and nutrition about their awareness of and experience with social marketing. Our findings are presented in the form of answers to the following questions.

· What is social marketing?
· What situations call for social marketing?
· What has social marketing accomplished?
· What are the major criticisms of social marketing?
· What are the hurdles in successful social marketing?
· What is the future of social marketing?

Karen F. A. Fox is Assistant Professor of Marketing, The University of Santa Clara. Philip Kotler is the Harold T. Martin Professor of Marketing, Northwestern University. The authors thank those who shared their experiences in social marketing and Phillip White for his helpful comments on a draft.

What is Social Marketing?

Social marketing was originally defined as:

> . . . the design, implementation, and control of programs calculated to influence the acceptability of social ideas and involving considerations of product planning, pricing, communications and marketing research (Kotler and Zaltman 1971, p. 5).

Thus social marketing was conceived to be an application of marketing concepts and techniques to the marketing of various socially beneficial ideas and causes instead of products and services in the commercial sense. Synonymous terms might be "social cause marketing," "social idea marketing," or "public issue marketing."

The term "social marketing" unfortunately has been given different meanings by other writers. For example, Lazer and Kelley (1973) published *Social Marketing: Perspectives and Viewpoints* which includes articles on marketing's social responsibilities and social impacts, as well as the marketing of social ideas, under the term "social marketing." In a recent article entitled "Social Marketing: Its Ethical Dimensions," Laczniak, Lusch, and Murphy (1979) confuse social marketing with nonprofit organization marketing by improperly including the marketing of political candidates and urban police departments as examples of "social marketing." Our position is that social marketing should be distinguished from "societal marketing" on the one hand and "nonprofit organization marketing" on the other.

The Evolution of Social Marketing

One can best understand social marketing by seeing it in relationship to the major broad approaches to producing social change—the legal, technological, economic, and informational approaches. Consider how these approaches apply in inducing people to reduce their cigarette consumption. The *legal* approach is to pass laws that make cigarette smoking either illegal, costly, or difficult (e.g., prohibiting smoking in public places). The *technological* approach is to develop an innovation that will help people reduce their smoking or the harm thereof (e.g., an antismoking pill, a harmless cigarette). The *economic* approach is to raise the price or cost of smoking (e.g., higher cigarette taxes, higher insurance rates for smokers). Finally, the *informational* approach is to direct persuasive information at smokers about the risks of smoking and the advantages of not smoking (e.g., "Warning: The Surgeon General Has Determined That Smoking Is Dangerous to Your Health").

The roots of social marketing lie in the informational approach, in the form known as *social advertising*. Many cause groups, struck by the apparent effectiveness of commercial advertising, began to consider its potential for changing public attitudes and behavior. Family planning organizations in India, Sri Lanka, Mexico, and several other countries have sponsored major advertising campaigns attempting to sell people on the idea of having fewer children. Messages on billboards and over radio tell the public that they can have a higher standard of living with fewer children (India) or be happier (Sri Lanka). Nutrition groups have also used advertising extensively to encourage people to adopt better eating habits. The U.S. Department of Energy has plans for a multimillion-dollar advertising campaign to promote energy conservation to the American people.

Properly designed, these campaigns can influence attitudes and behavior. The problem is that all too often these campaigns are the only step taken to motivate new behavior and, by themselves, are usually inadequate. First, the message may be inadequately researched. For example, media campaigns to encourage people in developing countries to improve their diets miss the point that many people lack knowledge of which foods are more healthful, they may lack the money to buy these goods and, in remote areas, they may not find certain foods available. Second, many people screen out the message through selective perception, distortion, and forgetting. Mass communications have much less direct influence on behavior than has been thought, and much of their influence is mediated through the opinion leadership of other people. Third, many people do not know what to do after their exposure to the message. The message "Stop smoking—it might kill you" does not help the smoker know how to handle the urge to smoke or where to go for help.

As these limitations were recognized social advertising evolved into a broader approach known as *social communication*. Much of current social marketing has moved from a narrow advertising approach to a broad social communication/promotion approach to accomplish its objectives. Social communicators make greater use of personal selling and editorial support in addition to mass advertising. Thus, the family planning campaign in India utilizes a network of agents, including doctors, dentists, and barbers, to "talk up" family planning to people with whom they come in contact. Events such as "Family Planning Day" and family planning fairs, together with buttons, signs, and other media, get across the message.

Only recently has *social marketing* begun to replace social communication as a larger paradigm for effecting social change. Social marketing adds at least four elements that are missing from a pure social communication approach.

One element is sophisticated *marketing research* to learn about the market and the probable effectiveness of alternative marketing approaches. Social advertising amounts to "a shot in the dark" unless it is preceded by careful marketing research. Thus social marketers concerned with smoking would examine the size of the smoking market, the major market segments and the behavioral characteristics of each, and the benefit-cost impact of targeting different segments and designing appropriate campaigns for each.

The second element added by social marketing is *product development*. Faced with the problem of getting people to lower their thermostats in winter, a social advertiser or communicator will see the problem largely as one of exhorting people to lower the thermostat, using patriotic appeals, fuel-cost-saving appeals, or whatever seems appropriate. The social marketer, in addition, will consider existing or potential products that will make it easier for people to adopt the desired behavior, such as devices that automatically lower home heat during the middle of the night or that compute fuel cost savings at various temperature settings. In other words, whenever possible the social marketer does not stick with the existing product and try to sell it—a sales approach—but rather searches for the best product to meet the need—a marketing approach.

The third element added by social marketing is *the use of incentives*. Social communicators concentrate on composing messages dramatizing the benefits or dis-benefits of different kinds of behaviors. Social marketers go further and design specific incentives to increase the level of motivation. For example, social marketers have advised public health officials who are running immunization campaigns in remote villages to offer small gifts to people who show up for vaccinations. Some hospitals in South America run "price specials" on certain days whereby people who come in for health checkups pay less than the normal charge. The sales promotion area is rich with tools that the marketer can use to promote social causes.

The fourth element added by social marketing is *facilitation*. The marketer realizes that people wishing to change their behavior must invest time and effort, and considers ways to make it easier for them to adopt the new behavior. For example, smoking cessation classes must be conveniently located and conducted in a professional manner. Marketers are keenly aware of the need to develop convenient and attractive response channels to complement the communication channels. Thus they are concerned not only with getting people to adopt a new behavior, but also with finding ways to facilitate maintenance of the behavior.

Our discussion of how social marketing goes beyond social advertising and social communication can be summarized by saying that social marketing involves all "four P's," not just one. Social marketing involves coordinating product, price, place, and promotion factors to maximally motivate and facilitate desired forms of behavior. Furthermore, social marketing calls for marketing research and for preparation of a full marketing plan, strategy, and budget to get initial "sales" and to reinforce the new behavior over time.

What Situations Call for Social Marketing?

Social marketing potentially can be applied to a wide variety of social problems. It appears to be particularly appropriate in the following three situations.

When New Information and Practices Need to be Disseminated

In many situations people need to be informed of an opportunity or practice that will improve their lives. In developing nations, social marketers have had to tackle such challenges as:

- Convincing people to boil their water and keep the water supply covered.
- Encouraging people to build and use latrines.
- Explaining to mothers the advantages of continuing to breastfeed their babies instead of switching them to less nourishing gruel at an early age.
- Encouraging people to buy and use iodized salt to prevent goiter.
- Showing parents a simple way to treat infant diarrhea at home—important because infant diarrhea is a major cause of infant mortality in less developed countries.

In industrialized nations the social marketer often must disseminate new information resulting from scientific research, including significant changes in high blood pressure treatment, in childhood immunization, in cancer detection and treatment, and in recommended diet.

Consider the changing concepts of what constitutes a good diet. In the early 1950s American elementary school children were taught about the seven basic food groups and were told to eat foods from each group daily. The 1969 USDA Yearbook entitled *Food For Us All* indicated that the American population was well fed and reported that "sugar or a sweet in some form is a daily necessity" (Mikesh and Nelson 1969, p. 232), Yet in 1979, the Surgeon General's Report on health promotion and disease prevention criticized the typical American diet, linking a diet high in fat, sugar, cholesterol, and salt and low in dietary fiber to heart disease, dental caries, high blood pressure, and colon cancer (U.S. Public Health Service 1979). These shifts in our knowledge of sound health practices suggest that we cannot simply relegate new health information to a slot in the elementary school curriculum, trusting that the next generation will be better informed and thus healthier than their parents. New information must be transmitted much more widely and more rapidly along with facilitation, price, and innovation steps to stimulate and reinforce new behavior.

When Countermarketing is Needed

In various nations of the world, companies are promoting the consumption of products that are undesirable or potentially harmful—for example cigarettes, alcoholic beverages, and highly refined foods which contribute to lung and heart disease, liver damage, overweight, and other problems. The large promotional budgets behind these products tend to crowd out opposing views, because those who disagree are often too fragmented, too few in number, or have inadequate resources to present the counterposition. Social marketing is now viewed by many public interest groups and government agencies as a way to present the other side of the story and stimulate people to adopt more healthful behavior. Sweden, for example, has taken vigorous steps to countermarket alcohol consumption, including running ad campaigns stigmatizing drunk behavior, restricting the availability of alcoholic beverages, raising the prices of alcoholic beverages, establishing stiff penalties for drunken driving, and increasing anti-alcohol school education programs.

Another current example of countermarketing has come in response to the promotion of infant formula in Third World countries. Borden, Nestlé, and other infant formula manufacturers, faced with declining birth rates in developed countries, began aggressive marketing to mothers in Africa, Latin America, and other less developed regions characterized by poverty, illiteracy, lack of pure water, lack of facilities for sterilizing bottles, and lack of refrigeration for storing mixed formula (Post and Baer 1978). Social marketing campaigns have been carried out to counter such powerful slogans as "Give your baby love and Lactogen" and to inform mothers of the advantages of breastfeeding.

When Activation is Needed

Often people know what they should do, but do not act accordingly. For example, nine out of 10 smokers interviewed in a 1975 government survey said they would like to quit, yet 57% expected to be smoking five years later (Fisher 1977). Likewise, many people "know" they should lose weight, get more exercise, floss their teeth, and do other things, but they do not do them. In part their inertia is related to the myriad alternatives they have and the countervailing media messages to enjoy life and maintain current habits ("Have a Coke and a smile" instead!). Furthermore, the benefits may be obtainable only by sustained effort, and the personal "payoff" over a lifetime may be exceedingly difficult to estimate. As one elderly man reportedly said, "If I had known I was going to live this long, I would have

taken better care of my health" (*Forbes* 1979).

In such situations, the task of social marketing is to move people from intention to action. Marketers have studied the many factors that affect the readiness of people to act, and have developed several approaches to motivate and facilitate action. In the future, various national or local emergencies—such as water shortages, oil shortages, and epidemics—may increase the need for public agencies to know how to activate people quickly.

What Has Social Marketing Accomplished?

Although social marketing is an appealing social change approach in theory, to what extent has it been effective in practice? At this time, we can only review the accomplishments of social marketing on an impressionistic basis. The bona fide applications of social marketing—as distinguished from social advertising or social communication—are too few to provide a full data base. Moreover, because social marketing often has been carried out without experimental controls, it is difficult to know whether behavioral changes were due to social marketing efforts or to other factors.

We consider two major areas of application—family planning and motivating healthier life styles—and a sampling of other interventions which reflect elements of a social marketing approach.

Family Planning

Family planning has been a major focus of social marketing efforts, reflected in a growing literature. Roberto (1975) provides an excellent exposition of social marketing theory applied to the problem of family planning. The Population Information Program at The Johns Hopkins University recently published a detailed review of social marketing applications, including information on features of specific programs and their effectiveness (Population Information Program 1980). The report defines the basic goal of such programs as providing contraceptives "efficiently, economically, and conveniently to people who will use them" (p. J-395). The majority of campaigns to market family planning are government-sponsored, motivated by the availability of effective birth control products and by the growing awareness that economic and social gains can be wiped out by rapid population growth. Many of these social marketing campaigns have been successful, as the following cases show.

A successful social marketing campaign in Sri Lanka (formerly Ceylon) was based on principles of marketing research, brand packaging, distribution channel analysis, and marketing management and control. Consumer research prior to the campaign indicated widespread approval of the idea of family planning but little knowledge and use of contraception. The government, in cooperation with several agencies, centered its efforts on achieving widespread usage of condoms as a means of birth control. A brand was developed named "Preethi" (meaning happiness), and was sold in a three-pack for four cents (U.S.), one of the lowest costs in the world. Preethi achieved distribution in more than 3,600 pharmacies, teahouses, grocery and general stores, as well as by direct mail. Literature and order forms for condoms were distributed by agricultural extension workers on their regular visits to farm families. The sale of condoms was supported through a mass media campaign, including newspaper and radio ads, films, and a booklet entitled "How to Have Children by Plan and Not by Chance." Distributors also received large point-of-purchase displays. As a result of this orchestrated marketing approach, Preethi sales grew from 300,000 per month (in mid-1974) to an average of 500,000 per month in 1977. It was estimated that 60,000 unwanted pregnancies were averted by this social marketing project (Population Services International 1977).

Similar campaigns have been successful in parts of India, Thailand, Bangladesh, and other countries. For example, in Bangladesh this type of campaign resulted in the monthly use of more than 1.5 million condoms and about 100,000 cycles of oral contraceptives, providing full contraceptive protection for approximately 400,000 couples at a yearly cost of about $4 per couple. In Thailand, the Community-Based Family Planning Services marketing program for promoting birth control includes some novel features. The agency stages contests with prizes to the person who inflates the biggest "balloon"—a condom—as a way to break down taboos about contraception. Contraceptives are accepted in rural villages, where villagers often ask local Buddhist monks to bless newly arrived shipments of contraceptives. The agency has recruited 5,000 rural distributors, including rice farmers, shopkeepers, village elders, and others who receive a one-day training course on selling condoms and keeping records, for which they receive a modest commission. The cost of all this effort is $3.50 per recipient per year, less than half of the cost of a similar government program in Thailand not using a marketing approach (Mathews 1976).

In Mexico, family planners face a tougher challenge because traditional values oppose the idea of family planning, as did past government policy designed to increase the population. Manhood and womanhood have traditionally been measured by the number of children produced. The dominant Catholic culture and widespread ignorance of birth control further hamper family planning efforts. Yet in 1974 the Mexican government es-

tablished the National Population Council (NPC) to slow the country's galloping rate of population increase. The NPC adopted a classic social marketing approach with the following elements. All promotional materials feature a logo showing a mother, a father, and two children. The family planning messages are carried by posters, booklets, and radio and TV spots. Family planning commercials are broadcast virtually every half hour on the radio. Free contraceptives are available at about 950 hospitals and clinics operated by the Ministry of Health and at 930 clinics run by an affiliate of the International Planned Parenthood Foundation (Wille 1975).

The effectiveness of social marketing of family planning can be assessed by looking at sales data, distribution systems, changes in knowledge, attitudes, and practices of consumers, cost-effectiveness, and, at the macro level, changes in fertility and birth rates. The Population Information Program reports micro-level measures indicating positive results. Positive results also can be claimed at the macro level. Bogue and Tsui (1979), analyzing the effect of several different variables, found that family planning efforts explain much more of the birth rate reduction since 1968 than does any other factor, including changes in economic and social development which usually have been given most of the credit. According to their data, the recent decline in the world fertility rate has been primarily due to "the worldwide drive by Third World countries to introduce family planning as part of their national social-development services" (pp. 99–100).

Heart Disease Prevention

Coronary disease is a byproduct of "the good life." Though nearly nonexistent in most of the world, it has reached epidemic proportions in Western industrialized countries. Between 1972 and 1975 the Stanford Heart Disease Prevention Program carried out an interdisciplinary intervention to determine ways to reduce risk of coronary disease through long-term changes in health practices—decreasing dietary cholesterol consumption and cigarette use, and increasing exercise levels.

Though fundamentally a sophisticated use of social communication, carried out by public health and communications research specialists, the program embodied many of the elements of a social marketing approach. As in the case of family planning, the goal of long-term behavior change required carefully designed and implemented interventions. To facilitate evaluation, the program was carried out in three similar rural California communities: in one community a mass media campaign alone was used; in a second, a mass media campaign was combined with personal instruction for a sample of high-risk individuals; in the third, neither treatment was used.

The extensive media campaign in the first two communities consisted of radio and TV spots and minidramas; "doctor's columns" and columns on diet in local newspapers; printed items, including an information booklet, a heart health calendar, and a cookbook, mailed to all residents; and billboards and bus posters. Residents in the second community also received personal instruction utilizing modeling and reinforcement to encourage them to quit smoking, lose weight, and get more exercise. In each of the three communities a sample of people was selected and tested at the beginning of the program and followed up annually.

The mass media were used to teach specific behavioral skills whenever possible, rather than simply to exhort people to change. Maccoby and Alexander (1979) cite several other key features of the study which match marketing considerations, including:

· The establishment of specific objectives for each component of the campaign over time.
· Clearly defined audience segments.
· The creation of clear, useful, and salient messages through formative research and pretesting.
· Utilization of creative media scheduling to reach the audience with adequate frequency.
· Stimulation of interpersonal communication to encourage a synergistic effect of multiple channels.
· Promotion of clear and well-paced behavioral changes in messages.
· Use of feedback to evaluate the campaign's progress over time.
· The use of a long-term campaign to avoid threshold effect considerations.

The program demonstrated that long-term changes in habits and significant reduction in risk for heart disease could be assisted through communitywide interventions utilizing the mass media (Meyer and Maccoby 1978). Both interventions yielded a significant increase in knowledge of risk factors and of desirable practices and a significant reduction in overall risk, with the media-plus-direct-instruction intervention producing the greater changes.

A social marketer might consider ways of extending the effectiveness of the Stanford Heart Program. For example, participants might be given special incentives or reinforcements for conforming to good health habits. Grocery stores might participate by highlighting healthful foods, as is now being done by Giant Food Stores in the Washington, D.C., area. The direct support of local doctors and dentists could be enlisted because they are particularly likely to see high-risk individuals.

Other Applications of Social Marketing

A growing number of health improvement programs reflect or have been consciously developed with a social marketing approach:

1. The Cancer Information Office of the National Institutes of Health has produced and pilot-tested a "Helping Smokers Quit" kit to encourage physicians to use their influence with patients who smoke. The kit includes a brief guide for the doctor, patient education materials, and a followup letter and brochure to be sent to the patient after the office visit.

2. The U.S. Department of Agriculture is supporting a project to use mass media and other channels to improve children's eating habits. The project began with extensive consumer research—interviews with children about their food preferences and eating habits.

3. The American Hospital Association's Center for Health Promotion is working to encourage preventive health measures and healthy "life habits" through programs run by hospitals, businesses, and community organizations. The Center recently conducted a workshop for hospital decision makers on marketing health promotion programs to local industry.

4. When infant immunization levels in Missouri dropped to ominous levels, a marketing plan was designed on the basis of a statewide study of the social-psychological factors affecting the problem (Houston and Markland 1976). The market was segmented and promotional material was directed to parents and expectant parents, as well as to the staff of the Missouri Division of Health. The campaign spokesman, "Marcus Rabbit, M.D.," was created to link the program to children, but to appeal to adults.

5. Public health specialists are using new channels to provide diagnostic services. A team of homosexual male clinicians from the Denver Metro Health Clinic conducted weekly VD screening in one of Denver's three steam baths catering to homosexuals (Judson, Miller, and Schaffnit 1977).

6. The National Heart, Lung, and Blood Institute changed eating habits in a National Institutes of Health employee cafeteria through a "Food for Thought" game. Food information was presented on playing-card-like cards which employees received each time they went through the serving line. Small prizes were awarded to those who acquired sets of cards. An increase in purchases of skim milk and decreases in purchases of bread and desserts and in total calories consumed were measured with the aid of the existing inventory control cash register system which automatically recorded every food item selected (Zifferblatt, Wilbur, and Pinsky 1980).

Although many of these campaigns are still to be evaluated, especially in terms of benefit/cost criteria and long-term effects, the use of conscious social marketing planning by cause organizations is clearly on the up-swing.

What Are the Major Criticisms of Social Marketing?

Not surprisingly, the increasing application of social marketing has been accompanied by questions about its legitimacy and possible negative impacts. The following four classes of criticism have appeared.

Social Marketing is Not Real Marketing

Some marketers still feel that marketing is largely a business discipline with little or no application to social causes. They believe that marketing is valid only where there are markets, transactions, and prices. As stated by Laczniak and Michie (1979), marketers should "take enough pride in the scope of traditional marketing."

Every discipline has its orthodox group which is content to ply familiar waters, believing either that their discipline has nothing to offer in the new territory or that, if it does, others will resent the intrusion. However, we believe that scholars and practitioners have a right, indeed, an obligation, to venture out and look freshly at phenomena from their discipline's perspective. Such ventures have produced such new fields as political sociology, economic anthropology, social psychology, and quantitative geography. If the new framework or findings are accepted, then the discipline has made a contribution.

Social Marketing is Manipulative

Many of the issues in social marketing call for changing people's attitudes and behavior, urging them to give up or cut back on comfortable habits. In contrast, commercial marketing frequently supports and encourages present habits, including those that are potentially harmful. Given that commercial marketing is often accused of being manipulative (primarily in persuading people to buy more things or in convincing them that one brand will satisfy a given need better than another brand), it is not surprising that social marketing is charged with being even more manipulative. For example, Laczniak, Lusch, and Murphy (1979) believe that social marketing is potentially unethical in giving power to a group to influence public opinion on such contested issues as pornography and abortion.

The word "manipulative" is something of a red herring in this discussion. The word "manipulative" usually connotes hidden and unfair ends and/or means used in the influence process. We argue that if a cause is marketed openly with the purpose of influencing someone to change his or her behavior, then the process is not manipulative, any more than is the activity of a lawyer, religious leader, or politician trying to convince others. If the social marketer simply makes the strongest possible case in favor of a cause without distorting the facts, the approach is not manipulative. Social marketing, especially when used in countermarketing, can provide a voice for those with competing points of view.

Social Marketing is Self-Serving

Some critics might be distressed that some social marketers who are promoting a cause are also making a profit in the process. Consider the following examples.

- Seat belt manufacturers are major supporters of auto safety legislation, partly because they stand to gain.

- Bottled water manufacturers in France have backed efforts to influence French citizens to reduce their alcohol consumption.

- Condom manufacturers have lent support to campaigns against VD because they stand to gain through greater use of condoms.

- Life insurance companies are encouraging people to jog, cut down on fats and sugar, install smoke alarms, and in other ways reduce illness, accidents, and premature deaths, thus cutting insurance claims and raising company profits.

Clearly commercial enterprises will increasingly support social marketing programs as they see financial benefits accruing to their companies while they also promote beneficial social change. This development appears to us to be desirable because it increases the incentive for commercial marketers to consider the best interests of consumers. Too often, social marketing efforts are undertaken by underfinanced cause organizations which run the risk of creating excessive demands on their limited resources when they achieve a major success, a phenomenon which Houston and Homans (1977) term "the failure of success."

A more troublesome issue is the use of tax money by government agencies to promote politically motivated efforts. For example, a booklet on energy conservation measures was delivered to every home in New England at the start of the 1979–80 heating season, paid for by the Department of Energy and private corporate contributions. Critics pointed to the "coincidence" of the upcoming New Hampshire primaries and President Carter's need to improve his image as an effective leader on conservation. In contrast, most government-sponsored social marketing efforts are likely to be fairly uncontroversial when used to increase the effectiveness of legislatively mandated social programs. Social marketing is already being applied in this way by several federal agencies.

Social Marketing Will Damage the Reputation of Marketing

Some marketers fear that applications of social marketing might arouse negative public sentiment toward marketing. Social marketing might acquire a bad name in two ways. First, it might be attacked for promoting unpopular causes, such as abortion or family planning. Second, it might influence people to accept a new behavior that turns out not to be in their best interest. The public might ultimately turn against social marketing and call for its curbing or regulation. Such attacks might strengthen present criticisms of commercial marketing and result in a setback to both.

There is some irony in this scenario because social marketing should, if anything, add luster rather than disrepute to marketing's image as the public sees marketing used to enhance the quality of their lives.

What Are the Real Hurdles to Successful Social Marketing?

The most devastating blow to social marketing would be to demonstrate that it is ineffective, that it does not change anything. Ineffective marketing is wasteful of resources and may lead people to expect results which cannot be produced. Novelli (1980) notes that managers and planners looking for a panacea or a "quick fix" may rush to embrace social marketing with inflated expectations: "When these quick solutions are not forthcoming, they are disappointed and view marketing as having failed." Some social issues are not likely to be affected by social marketing because the costs, although mainly nonmonetary, are too great and because the level of consumer involvement is either too low to overcome inertia—e.g., antilittering campaigns—or so high that producing behavior change will require great facilitation effort—e.g., antismoking campaigns (Rothschild 1979).

Social marketing practitioners are the first to admit that social marketing will have a different degree of effectiveness with different social causes, and that most social marketing problems will be more formidable than the typical marketing problems facing commercial marketers. William Novelli, a leading social marketing practitioner, admits, "It's a thousand times harder to do social marketing than to do package goods marketing." He and Paul Bloom recently reviewed the major hurdles faced by social marketers, and their observations are summarized hereafter (Bloom and Novelli 1979).

First, the market is usually harder to analyze. Social marketers have less good quality secondary data about their consumers. They have more difficulty in obtaining valid and reliable measures of salient consumer attributes, and in sorting out the relative influence of various determinants of consumer behavior. They have more difficulty getting consumer research studies funded, approved, and completed in a timely fashion.

Second, target market choice is more difficult. There is often public pressure to attempt to reach the whole market rather than to zero in on the best target groups. Thus a family planning campaign is restrained from focusing on the families who have the most children because of charges of racial or religious discrimination. When the relevant groups can be targeted, these groups are usually the most negatively predisposed to adopt the desired behavior, and thus success is harder to achieve.

Third, formulating product strategy is more difficult. The antismoking crusader should really invent a safe cigarette but this is not easy to do, and therefore the range of product innovation options is smaller. For many causes the reformer must get people to do something that is unpleasant rather than offering them something that would be even more pleasant than their present behavior.

Fourth, social marketers have fewer opportunities to use pricing and must rely more on other approaches that would increase or decrease the cost to consumers of certain behavior. Thus getting people to stop littering is not accomplished as well through a fine (very difficult to enforce) as by reducing the cost of not littering by providing more refuse containers in parks and on busy thoroughfares.

Fifth, channels of distribution may be harder to utilize and control. For example, a family planning organization may be able to get many retailers to carry condoms but has less control over how they will display them, price them, sell them, and replace them when out of stock.

Sixth, communication strategies may be more difficult to implement. Some groups may oppose the use of certain types of appeals that otherwise would be very effective. The particular cause may require a longer explanation than is available within the confines of a short message. The budget may be too low to permit pretesting the message or to ensure its wide distribution or the evaluation of its impact.

Seventh, cause organizations are often backward in their management and marketing sophistication. Many cause organizations are small, rely mainly on volunteers, and have little familiarity with marketing concepts or planning approaches. They may not be able to handle a large demand for their service, should it arise. The staff may not really be committed to solving the problem, especially if they will lose their jobs when they succeed.

Eighth, the results of social marketing efforts are often difficult to evaluate. For example, should the success of a family planning campaign be measured by total births averted or by births averted in high fertility groups? Or should the measure be the number of people who become aware of family planning, or who begin to show an interest in adopting it? Even after an appropriate measure is determined, the contribution of the marketing program to the final outcome is often difficult to estimate.

The resolution of these problems will depend in part on the accumulation of additional experience in applying and evaluating social marketing, on continuing efforts to integrate and disseminate findings from social marketing programs, and on theoretical and empirical work to improve our understanding of factors that can be used to increase the impact of such programs (Bloom 1980; Cook and Campbell 1979; Cook and McAnany 1979; Fine 1979; Fox 1980; Rothschild 1979).

What is the Future of Social Marketing?

The 1980s outlook for social marketing is one of continued growth and application to an ever-widening range of issues. More and more cause organizations and government agencies will turn to social marketing in a search for increased effectiveness. Many will come to social marketing only by passing through the stages of social advertising and social communication first. Large and expensive advertising blitzes may be attempted, rather than integrated social marketing campaigns. The risk is that if such social advertising campaigns fail, critics may charge that marketing does not work when in fact it was not really tried.

Clearly there will be a need for more and better trained social marketers rather than simply social advertisers. The ideal training would have several components. Business marketing training which stresses market analysis, economic analysis, and management theory would be desirable. Because social marketers are involved in trying to change attitudes and behavior rather than simply to meet existing needs, they should study the social science disciplines, particularly sociology, psychology, and anthropology. They should also be trained in communcation theory. In addition, social marketers will need to acquire a social problem-solving perspective which will lead them to search for possible technological solutions that may eventually replace present solutions based on self-denial, regulation, or economic incentives.

Social marketers working in multicultural contexts in the United States and in overseas development projects will need particular sensitivity to cultural differences, a knowledge of relevant aspects of the cultures in which they work, and facility in language or in working with persons who have the necessary language competence. It is no wonder that many social marketers now working on overseas projects have been Peace Corps volunteers or have studied or worked overseas for extended periods. Courses in language, history, and anthropology contribute to this preparation.

Though at present many social marketers are outside consultants, a look into the future suggests that organizations may attract or develop their own "in house" social marketers. These people may already be educators, public health specialists, policy analysts, and communications experts, for example. Or organizations may attract business-trained marketers who are able to cross over by gaining an understanding of the specific issues and tasks that confront a specific organization or field, such as health promotion. In effect, social marketers will be dual specialists who can apply marketing to specific social causes.

Summary

What impact is social marketing likely to have on promoting beneficial social change in an effective manner? The evidence from the first decade of social marketing applications is promising. We have described social marketing as the application of marketing thinking and tools to the promotion of social causes, and have traced its evolution through social advertising and social communication. Cases from family planning, heart disease prevention, and other health areas are presented to illustrate the range and impact of social marketing applications, though we acknowledge that many are not fully elaborated examples of social marketing.

A growing number of cause organizations and government agencies are turning to social marketing. Groups that once relied on social advertising alone are now moving toward social communication and social marketing. Applications of social marketing have achieved some notable results and provide insights into the challenges confronting social marketers. We foresee that social marketing specialists, combining business marketing skills with additional training in the social sciences, will be working on a wider range of social causes with increasing sophistication. Advances in conceptualizing social marketing problems and in evaluating the impacts of social marketing programs will further enhance their effectiveness.

REFERENCES

Bloom, Paul N. (1980), "Evaluating Social Marketing Programs: Problems and Prospects," *1980 Educators Conference Proceedings,* Chicago: American Marketing Association.

———— and William D. Novelli (1979), "Problems in Applying Conventional Marketing Wisdom to Social Marketing Programs," paper presented at American Marketing Association Workshop, "Exploring and Developing Government Marketing," Yale University.

Bogue, Donald J. and Amy Ong Tsui (1979), "Zero World Population Growth?" *The Public Interest,* 55 (Spring), 99–113.

Cook, Thomas D. and Donald T. Campbell (1979), *Quasi-Experimentation: Design and Analysis Issues for Field Settings,* Chicago: Rand McNally College Publishing.

————— and Emile G. McAnany (1979), "Recent United States Experiences in Evaluation Research with Implications for Latin America," in *Evaluating the Impact of Nutrition and Health Programs,* Robert E. Klein et al., eds., New York: Plenum.

Fine, Seymour H. (1979), "Beyond Money: The Concept of Social Price," working paper, Rutgers University.

Fisher, Lucille (1977), "National Smoking Habits and Attitudes," American Lung Association.

Forbes (1979), 123 (September 17), 25.

Fox, Karen F. A. (1980), "Time as a Component of Price in Social Marketing, *1980 Educators Conference Proceedings,* Chicago: American Marketing Association.

Houston, Franklin S. and Richard E. Homans (1977), "Public Agency Marketing: Pitfalls and Problems," *MSU Business Topics,* 25 (Summer), 36–40.

————— and Robert Markland (1976), "Public Agency Marketing—Improving the Adequacy of Infant Immunization," in *Proceedings,* American Institute for Decision Sciences, 461–3.

Judson, Franklyn N., Kenneth G. Miller, and Thomas R. Schaffnit (1977), "Screening for Gonorrhea and Syphilis in the Gay Baths—Denver, Colorado," *American Journal of Public Health,* 67 (August), 740–2.

Kotler, Philip (1979), "Strategies for Introducing Marketing into Nonprofit Organizations," *Journal of Marketing,* 43 (January), 37–44.

————— and Gerald Zaltman (1971), "Social Marketing: An Approach to Planned Social Change," *Journal of Marketing,* 35 (July), 3–12.

Laczniak, Gene R., Robert F. Lusch, and Patrick E. Murphy (1979), "Social Marketing: Its Ethical Dimensions," *Journal of Marketing,* 43 (Spring), 29–36.

————— and Donald A. Michie (1979), "The Social Disorder of the Broadened Concept of Marketing," *Journal of Marketing Science,* 7 (Summer), 214–31.

Lazer, William and Eugene J. Kelley (1973), *Social Marketing: Perspectives and Viewpoints,* Homewood, Illinois: Richard D. Irwin, Inc.

Maccoby, Nathan and Janet Alexander (1979), "Field Experimentation," in *Research in Social Contexts: Bringing About Change,* R. F. Munoz, L. R. Snowden, and J. G. Kelly, eds., San Francisco: Jossey-Bass.

Mathews, Linda (1976), "What Makes Mechai Run, or How to Curb the Births of a Nation," *Wall Street Journal* (January 15), 1.

Meyer, Anthony J. and Nathan Maccoby (1978), "The Role of Mass Media in Maintaining Health," in *Vestinnan Virtauksia,* Erja Erholn and Leif Aberg, eds., Keruu, Finland: Delfiinikirkat.

Mikesh, Verna A. and Leona S. Nelson (1969), "Sugar, Sweets Play Roles in Food Texture and Flavoring," in *Food for Us All,* 1969 Yearbook of the United States Department of Agriculture, Washington, D.C.: Government Printing Office, 232–6.

Nickels, William G. (1974), "Conceptual Conflicts in Marketing," *Journal of Economics and Business,* 27 (Winter), 140–3.

Novelli, William G. (1980), personal communication, January 3.

Population Information Program (1980, "Social Marketing: Does It Work?", *Population Reports,* Family Planning Programs, Series J, number 21, The Johns Hopkins University.

Population Services International (1977), "Preethi Project Transferred to Sri Lanka FPA," *PSI Newsletter* (November/December), 4.

Post, James E. and Edward Baer (1978), "Demarketing Infant Formula: Consumer Products in the Developing World," *Journal of Contemporary Business,* 7 (4), 17–35.

Roberto, Edwardo (1975), *Strategic Decision-Making in a Social Program: The Case of Family-Planning Diffusion,* Lexington, Massachusetts: Lexington Books.

Rothschild, Michael L. (1979), "Marketing Communication in Nonbusiness Situations: or Why It's So Hard to Sell Brotherhood Like Soap," *Journal of Marketing,* 43 (Spring), 11–20.

U.S. Public Health Service (1979), *Healthy People: The Surgeon General's Report on Health Promotion and Disease Prevention,* Washington, D.C.: Government Printing Office.

Wiebe, G. D. (1951–52), "Merchandising Commodities and Citizenship on Television," *Public Opinion Quarterly,* 15 (Winter), 679–91.

Wille, Lois (1975), "Mexico Battles the Baby Boom," *Chicago Daily News* (December 3), 5.

Zifferblatt, Steven M., Curtis S. Wilbur, and Joan L. Pinsky (1980), "Changing Cafeteria Eating Habits: A New Direction for Public Health Care," *Journal of the American Dietetic Association,* 76 (January), 15–20.

Social Marketing of Health Behavior

by Philip Kotler

DISTINCTIONS AMONG TYPES OF SOCIAL CAUSES

Social marketing aims to produce an optimal plan for bringing about a desired social change. The fact that the plan is optimal, however, does not guarantee that the target change will be achieved. It depends on how easy or difficult the targeted health change is. Without social marketing thinking, it may be that the desired change has only a 10% chance of being achieved; the best social marketing plan may only increase this probability to 15%. In other words, some changes are relatively easy to effect, even without social marketing; others are supremely difficult to accomplish, even with social marketing.

I will distinguish among four types of health-related changes of increasing difficulty to effect, namely, cognitive change, action change, behavioral change, and value change.

Cognitive Change

There are many health causes that have the limited objective of creating a cognitive change in the target audience. They are called public information or public education campaigns. Many examples can be cited:

- Campaigns to explain the nutritional value of different foods
- Campaigns to expand awareness of Medicare and Medicaid benefits
- Campaigns to bring attention to pressing public health problems, such as those that accompany poverty or pollution

Cognitive change causes seem to be fairly easy to market effectively because they do not seek to change any deep-rooted attitudes or behavior. Their aim is primarily to create awareness or knowledge. The optimal marketing approach would

PHILIP KOTLER • J. L. Kellogg Graduate School of Management, Northwestern University, Evanston, Illinois 60201.

appear to be straightforward. In this case, marketing research would be used to identify the groups that most need the information. Their media habits are identified to serve as guides for distributing and timing effective messages. The messages themselves are formulated on the basis of target audience analysis. They are carried to the audiences through advertising, publicity, personnel, displays, exhibitions, and other means. The effectiveness of the campaign can be measured by postsampling members of the target groups to see how much increase in comprehension has taken place.

Although it may seem that information campaigns should succeed easily, the evidence is quite mixed. Hyman and Sheatsley (1947) give several reasons why information campaigns may fail:

1. There exists a hard core of "chronic know-nothings" who cannot be reached by information campaigns. In fact, "there is something about the uninformed that makes them harder to reach, no matter what the level or nature of the information."
2. The likelihood of being exposed to the information increases with interest in the issue. If few people are initially interested, few will be exposed.
3. The likelihood of being exposed to the information increases with the information compatibility with prior attitudes. People will tend to avoid disagreeable information.
4. People will read different things into the information that they are exposed to, depending on their beliefs and values. The bigot, for example, often does not perceive antiprejudice literature as such. People emerge with a range of different reactions to the same material.

Thus, much thought has to be given to planning the simplest of campaigns—those that are designed to produce cognitive change. The message must be interesting, clear, and consonant with the intended audience values (Douglas, Westley, & Chaffee, 1970).

Action Change

Another class of causes are those attempting to induce a maximum number of persons to take a specific action during a given period. Many examples can be cited:

- Campaigns to attract people to show up for a mass immunization campaign
- Campaigns to attract eligible people to sign up for Medicaid
- Campaigns to attract women over 40 to take annual cancer detection tests
- Campaigns to attract blood donors

Action causes are somewhat harder to market than cognitive change causes. The target market has to comprehend something *and* take specific action based on it. Action involves a cost to the actors. Even if their attitude toward the action is favorable, their carrying it out may be impeded by such factors as distance, time, expense, or plain inertia. For this reason, the marketer has to arrange factors that make it easy for target persons to carry out this action.

Mass immunization campaigns are a good example. Medical teams in Africa visit villages in the hope of inoculating everyone. Over the years a procedure to increase the number of villagers the teams attract has been developed. A marketing team is sent to each village a few weeks before the appearance of the medical team. The marketers meet the village leaders to describe the importance of the program so that the leaders in turn will ask their people to cooperate. The marketers offer monetary or other incentives to the village leaders. They drive a sound truck around the village announcing the date and occasion. They promise rewards to those who show up. Posters are placed in various locations. The medical team arrives when scheduled and uses inoculation equipment that is relatively fast and painless. The whole effect is an orchestration of product, price, place, and promotion—factors that are calculated to achieve the maximum possible turnout.

Behavioral Change

Another class of causes aims to induce or help people change some aspect of their behavior for the sake of their health. Behavioral change causes include the following:

- Efforts to discourage cigarette smoking
- Efforts to discourage excessive consumption of alcohol
- Efforts to discourage the use of hard drugs
- Efforts to help overweight people change their food habits

Behavioral change is harder to achieve than cognitive or one-shot action changes. People must unlearn old habits, learn new habits, and freeze the new pattern of behavior. For example, in the area of birth control, couples have to learn how to use new devices, such as a condom or diaphragm, and get into the habit of using them regularly, without anyone being around to help them or reinforce this behavior. In the area of safe driving, drivers who have a tendency to drink heavily at social gatherings must learn either to drink less or to know when they are not able to drive their own cars. Various campaigns have been directed at problem drivers to condition them to be aware of the problem and the penalties.

Change agents rely primarily on mass communication to influence changes in behavior. In some cases, mass communication can be counterproductive. In the late sixties when many young people were experimenting with hard drugs, advertising agencies, social agencies, and legislators felt that advertising could be a powerful weapon for discouraging hard drug usage. Much money was funded privately and by the government, with donations of time by advertising agencies and media organizations. Fear appeals were first tried, which were followed by informational advertising. Soon some people began to voice doubts about the good that this was doing. UN Secretary General Kurt Waldheim presented a drug evaluation study to the UN in 1972 and cautioned that "special care must be exercised in this connection not to arouse undue curiosity and unwittingly encourage experimentation" ("Wrong Publicity May Push," 1972). Antidrug messages, especially those on television, reach many young people who may never have thought about drugs. These young people do not necessarily perceive the message negatively and might in fact develop a strong curiosity about the subject. This is accompanied by the feeling that if the older generation is spending large amounts of money to talk them out of something, there must be something good in it. They start discussing drugs with their friends and soon learn where to obtain illegal drugs and how to use them. They also learn that drugs are not that dangerous if used carefully. Thus, mass advertising might provoke initial curiosity more than fear and lead the person into exploration and experimentation. The main point is that organizations of individuals often resort to advertising without sufficient knowledge of the audience or without testing the probable effects of their message upon the audience (Ray, Ward, & Lesser, 1973). They fail to create mechanisms that enable people to translate their motivation into appropriate action.

Value Change

The final class of causes attempts to alter deeply felt beliefs or values that a target group holds toward some object or situation. Examples include:

- Efforts to alter people's ideas about abortion
- Efforts to alter people's ideas about the number of children they should have
- Efforts to alter people's ideas about taking blood pressure medication for life

Efforts to change deeply held values are among the most difficult causes to market. People's sense of identity and well-being are rooted in their basic values. Their basic values orient their social, moral, and intellectual perceptions and choices. The intrusion of dissonance into their values creates heavy strain and stress. They will try to avoid dissonant information, rationalize it away, or compartmentalize it so that it does not affect their values. The human psychological system resists information that is disorienting.

Any effort to change people from one basic value orientation to another requires a prolonged and intense program of indoctrination. Even then, it is likely to succeed only to the smallest degree. Consider the classic case of the Chinese indoctrination program for American prisoners of war during the Korean War (Schein, 1956). The circumstances were most propitious for attempting to change the values of a target group. The Chinese had complete control over the informational, physical, and social environment of their captives. Their aim was to alter the beliefs and values of the prisoners toward communism and toward who was to blame for the war. The Chinese suffused their captives with their newspaper and radio propaganda so that the prisoners saw and heard only the Chinese point of view. They divided the prisoners into small groups without their friends and without the normal leadership of officers. They planted spies in the midst of each group to create fear and a lack of trust of other Americans. They lectured endlessly about American war crimes and rewarded the prisoners who gave the slightest positive response. They started with trivial demands for intellectual concession, and as the Americans acceded, they escalated the required responses. They presented photographs and experts as evidence for their point of view. They tailored their techniques to the intelligence, race, and political views of each man. In the end, they succeeded in persuading only 21 prisoners out of tens of thousands to refuse repatriation after the armistice, although many more underwent some alteration of beliefs.

The major factor limiting the success of the Chinese, in spite of their total control over the environment, was that they were a negatively regarded source. Because they were the enemy, the prisoners discounted their credibility. On the other hand, a totalitarian state can be effective if it has the trust of the people. Having control over all the instruments of information and reward, the totalitarian state can undertake to alter the value orientations of its people. Small-group experiments, conducted by Asch, Lewin, and others, confirm the readiness of participants in a group to go along with the group's judgment in spite of their initially resistant opinions (Asch, 1953; Lewin, 1952).

The values that people hold often are pragmatic as well as ideological, making them even more difficult to change. For example, the preference of rural farmers in India for large families makes economic sense. The farmer in his old age has protection in the form of male heirs who will take care of him. Of six children that his wife might bear, only three or four may reach adulthood. Of these, only one or two may be male. Thus, the father thinks in terms of six children to produce a living male heir when he is 65. Furthermore, birth delivery in the rural area costs virtually nothing, and the father can feed his children with scraps of food. At age 6, his child starts running errands, working in the field, or helping the mother, thus being productive. Consequently, when the rural farmer in India hears arguments that he should have fewer children because of overpopulation, it has no meaning for him in his particular life situation. Persuasive communication can have very little impact. In such cases, the state must resort to other measures if it is serious about bringing down the birthrate. Offering a positive economic incentive to have few children may not work because the value of the incentive is usually too small in relation to the value of having another child. The state may try negative economic incentives such as a tax on the number of children, compulsory schooling at the age of 6, which would reduce the productivity of children in rural areas, or a requirement that all children be born in hospitals, which would increase the cost of giving birth. These are harsh measures, but they may become necessary when it becomes clear that the major target groups for family planning—rural families who have many children—are the least likely to change their minds because of persuasive communication.

When values are highly resistant to change, many social planners prefer to use the law to require new behaviors, even if they are not accompanied by attitudinal change. The theory is that, as people have to comply with the new law, forces will be set into motion that will begin to produce the desired attitude change. Consider the case of nonsmoking rules in public buildings. Social attitudes reflecting the acceptance of smoking began to change when rules dictated new nonsmoking behavior. The passage of even a disliked law sets several forces in motion that may accelerate the adoption of the targeted change:

1. The new law helps the law's supporters gain new strength. They coalesce their forces and work harder for its implementation.
2. The new law stimulates more radical proposals, leading citizens to accept the original change in order to ward off the more radical proposals.
3. The new law creates sustained media attention and word-of-mouth discussion that leads people to examine their ideas and values more carefully.
4. The new law elicits conformity on the part of citizens who believe laws are to be obeyed. Conformity eventually leads from mere compliance to acceptance through processes of dissonance reduction.

Thus, when it comes to changing basic attitudes, the most effective means may be to pass laws requiring behavioral conformity, which set forces into motion that may accelerate the acceptance of new values. In this case, the marketer's role is to build a climate favorable to the passage and acceptance of the new law.

Application of Marketing Principles To Improve Participation in Public Health Programs

by Katherine Alexander and James McCullough

ABSTRACT: The application of marketing principles to develop a program aimed at increasing participation in a cervical screening program appears to be more effective than the use of sales techniques. Standard methods of promotion such as posters, direct mail, and flyers were generally ineffective. Direct personal contact produced the majority of program participants, and mass media approaches also resulted in significant participant response. A consumer orientation led to development of effective program features designed to satisfy specific consumer needs. Use of female health practitioners, for example, reduced cultural barriers to participation and insured adequate screening in Mexican-American populations.

Marketing is commonly defined as those activities undertaken to facilitate exchanges between buyers and sellers. Although many individuals view marketing as selling, or the use of slick promotional materials, it is, in fact, a broad-based approach to assessing consumer needs and satisfying them through development of effective programs. Kotler has clearly demonstrated the value of taking marketing principles developed in the business community and applying them to exchanges in the nonprofit sector.[1] In political campaigns and fund-raising programs, for instance, marketing techniques are being applied with varying degrees of success. As effective marketing programs are developed, some nonprofit organizations are finding they can use them to expand greatly the organizations' impact in the community. Public health programs are clearly exchange activities and should benefit from effective marketing programs.

Accordingly, the use of marketing to increase the effectiveness of social programs has recently generated considerable interest.[2-5] Unfortunately, however, most of the interest has focused on one facet of marketing—the use of selling and promotional techniques—rather than on developing a thorough

Ms. Alexander is with Pima Health Systems and Mr. McCullough is with the Department of Marketing, University of Arizona, Tucson, Arizona 85721. This research was supported by a grant from the National Cancer Institute through the Arizona Department of Health Services.

understanding of the potential consumer so that the marketing program can be adapted to a particular situation. As a result, many programs directed at public health issues have employed imperfectly integrated techniques, particularly mass media campaigns, and have failed to achieve the desired end: effective consumer participation in the public health program.

We can illustrate the problem as follows. Many health programs provide services at no direct monetary cost to the client. But participation often does require the consumer's cooperation, and the consumer sees the time and effort exchanged for the services of the program as a real price that must be paid. The development of a holistic, integrated program applying all the elements of marketing planning to insure satisfying the client's needs requires that the consumer's perceived value of the service is enhanced while the perceived cost is reduced. This involves far more than simply implementing a mass media campaign.

Ideally, the steps listed below should be followed to maximize chances of successfully marketing any product or service, whether offered by a profit or a nonprofit organization:

1. Marketing research: Analyze consumer needs and wants with regard to the type of product or service offered.
2. Marketing strategy: Design the product or service and select distribution points and price as compatible as possible with consumer needs and wants. Promote the product or service by emphasizing those attributes that will best satisfy consumer needs and wants.
3. Test marketing: Test the marketing strategy in a llimited area and monitor and evaluate the effectiveness of the strategy in the test area and revise as necessary.
4. Program management: Finally, implement the revised marketing strategy in the target area; monitor, evaluate, and revise strategy as necessary.

These principles can be seen in the management plan of the Cervical Cancer Screening Program (CCSP), a program to provide Pap tests to low-income women, minority women, and women who had not had a Pap test in the last three years. The program also examines the effectiveness of various marketing approaches in encouraging these target women to attend free Pap test clinics.

MARKETING RESEARCH

The marketing plan used in this project was based in an initial survey of approximately 200 women in households in the target areas. These sample households were selected from low-income census tracts. Sixty-six percent of the respondents were Hispanic. Twenty-one percent were 25 years of age or younger; 35% were between 26 and 45; 32% were 46–64; and 13% were over 65. The survey concentrated on product experience (awareness and previous use of Pap testing) and on access to communication media that might be used in a promotional campaign.

Many of the women showed no demand or negative demand for the cervical cancer screening. One group seemed uninterested or indifferent to the service. Since they did not perceive their risk of having cervical cancer as very high, they never thought about getting a Pap test. When no demand exists, it is necessary to devise a strategy to stimulate demand. The strategy used in this situation involved widespread distribution of information about the program, since it was thought that a lack of correct information was at least partly to blame for the lack of demand.

The women showing negative demand disliked Pap tests because they were embarrassed or uncomfortable during the exam and tried to avoid getting them. Negative demand is one of the most difficult situations any marketing manager faces. It requires first eliminating the negative attitude and then creating a positive demand for the service. This situation is often encountered in public health programs that attempt to encourage persons to get services that many consider undesirable, such as dental work, vaccinations, or vasectomies. A specific tactic to reduce negative demand devised for this program was to staff the pap test clinics with female nurse practitioners or physicians whenever possible, on the assumption that the women with negative demand for the service would feel less uncomfortable and embarrassed when examined by a woman.

Since communication is an essential part of any marketing program, the target population was asked about their use of various communication channels. The responses obtained in this initial survey are shown in column 1 of Table 1. The survey indicated that electronic media, friends, and print media should provide the best vehicles for reaching these groups.

MARKETING STRATEGY

According to Kotler, the marketing plan begins with a thorough understanding of the needs and wants of the potential consumer and is developed through decisions regarding four fundamental elements: product design, price, promotion, and place.[1] These four elements of the marketing mix should be tailored to match the characteristics of the target population.

On the basis of existing knowledge and the results of the preliminary survey, the following marketing program was developed.

Product

The basic product was the Pap test involving a fairly standard clinical procedure. Through the use of female examiners, this product was tailored to help meet some consumer needs and eliminate a source of potential embarrassment.

TABLE 1
Reported Sources of Community Program Information

Source	Initial Survey	Participant Survey
Television**	38	18
Radio**	38	6
Friends	24	24
Agency workers**	2	22
Other (print, direct mail, etc.)**	4	11

Note: Totals exceed 100% due to multiple responses.
**Differences are significant at the 0.01 level using a X^2 test based on the mean of all respondents.

Price

This test was provided free of charge. For the consumer, however, transportation costs, babysitting fees, and the time required to get the test represented real costs. Because these costs were known to the planners, clinics were conducted at locations near the women's homes to reduce time and transportation costs, and women were told they could bring their children to the clinic to eliminate babysitting costs.

Promotion

Since the survey had indicated heavy reliance on mass media for information, the program was widely publicized in the mass media, using public service announcements, appearances on local news programs and talk shows, and articles in major local newspapers. Other conventionally used promotional techniques were also tried. About 200 posters were distributed throughout the city on two separate occasions. One type of poster included a tear-off coupon with program information. Nearly 100,000 brochures were distributed through health agencies, given out along with staff presentations, and delivered by school children to their mothers. Several hundred coupons were distributed through a few private firms including a grocery store, health food store, and a welcome wagon service. Some health agencies distributed these also.

Inspired by success reported by Hulka,[6,7] the program also tried two mailings reaching over 18,000 households in low-income areas of the city. The first mailing was designed to test the effectiveness of two different messages. The second tested how effective a coupon for a free Pap test would be included in a packet with other coupons for free food and discounts on other products.

Place

Clinics were conducted at places convenient to the target population. Several clinics were used as regular sites, and special clinics were set up over 50 sites in either a two-exam-room mobile unit or in community buildings such as senior citizen centers or neighborhood area councils, which were converted into temporary clinics.

TEST MARKETING

The program was moderately successful in reaching the target population. During the 32-month program, 4,503 women were screened. It was estimated that there were 85,029 minority and low-income Anglo women in the program area in 1977. On the basis of the preliminary survey, 37% of this group were estimated to need a Pap test. Ten percent of these women attended a Cervical Cancer Screening Program clinic at least once.

CONCLUSIONS AND RECOMMENDATIONS

Information sources reported by the women who attended clinics are shown in column 2 of Table 1. Nearly half of all screenees (46%) mentioned a type of personal contact as their information source, i.e., either a friend and/or staff person of another agency told them about the clinics. Over one third (35%) mentioned one of the mass media as an information source. No other techniques appear to have recruited significant numbers of women. The response rates to all brochures, including mailings, were less than 1%.

With two interesting exceptions, these findings are fairly consistent with the projection made on the basis of the initial survey. The women interviewed during the initial survey reported mass media, particularly television and radio, much more frequently than did program participants. Two explanations are offered for this difference: 1) The surveyed women overrate the importance of the electronic media as sources of their information. About 7% of the women screened in a series of clinics in Phoenix reported learning about the program via television, although there was no known television coverage about these clinics. 2) Electronic media are less effective in informing women about Pap test clinics than about other types of community programs.

The other exception was the relative importance agency workers had in providing information. One fifth of the participants reported learning about the program from another agency, but only 2% of the women surveyed recalled this as a source of information about community programs. Apparently, these agencies play an important but unrecognized role in providing information.

Mailings were tried, although mail had not been mentioned as a source of information during the initial survey since it was assumed that few community programs used this method. The low response to both mailings was quite unexpected. Failure to pretest the effect of mailings resulted in unnecessarily high costs. Materials developed on the ''common sense'' of the staff often did not work and represented wasted resources.

On the basis of this study, several recommendations can be made to cervical cancer screening programs operating with goals and restrictions similar to the ones found in this project. First, solicit as much television, radio, and newspaper coverage as possible to publicize availability of services. Mass media are clearly a powerful tool to reach the women at risk to cervical cancer, and lack of awareness and information can be most effectively remedied with this method.

Second, word-of-mouth advertising is important in low-income areas; urge all screenees to tell their friends about the services. Establish strong referral links with all agencies whose staffs contact the target groups and also be willing to refer screenees to their programs. Contact these agencies periodically to let them know the services are still available and that screenees are reporting them as sources of information. Carefully test the effectiveness of mailing campaigns and brochure distribution, since such activities may be highly cost ineffective.

Third, pay particular attention to the nonpromotional aspects of the marketing mix. Product design, pricing policy, and distribution can be more effective and less expensive than elaborate mass media campaigns, for example, staff clinics with female physicians. If they are not available, employ nurse practitioners. Although few women said they attend the clinics because of the availability of a female examiner, most said after the exam that they would prefer a female examiner. Staffing the clinics with female examiners is expected more to increase the number of screenees who return for a repeat exam than to increase the number of initial visits.

Finally, establish several permanent screening sites throughout the target areas. Special clinics set up in facilities other than clinics, such as senior citizen centers and neighborhood area councils, were not particularly effective in attracting large numbers of target women, possibly because the women felt uncomfortable disrobing and being examined in places where they normally engage in other activities.

This screening program began by assuming that one of its results would be the discovery of specific promotional methods that were highly effective in motivating target women to attend clinics. Such methods were not discovered. Instead, the program reached its goals without an overly effective or costly promotional campaign because more attention was paid to a total marketing plan. The inclusion of product characteristics, pricing elements, and distribution alternatives that met particular previously unmet needs of the target market produced responses even when the promotional campaign was not effective.

Many of the more traditional approaches to the study of utilization patterns in public health note the wide range of factors that affect use of public health services.[8-11] A marketing perspective is useful in generating specific ideas about how to manipulate these factors and how to monitor and revise stratgegies to assure appropriate use of health services. A consumer orientation, understanding what the potential consumer wants and needs, can provide the basis for effective use of resources allocated for public health programs. Development of an effective marketing program may spell the differences between success and failure.

REFERENCES

1. Kotler P: *Marketing for Nonprofit Organizations*. Englewood Cliffs, NJ, Prentice-Hall, 1975.
2. El-Ansary AI, and Kramer OE: Social marketing: The family planning experience. *J Marketing* 37:1-7, 1973.
3. Burger P: Health care utilization: Marketing myopia and consumer behavior. In Sheth J, Wright P (eds): *Marketing Analysis for Societal Problems*. University of Illinois at Urbana, 1974. Pp 172-185.
4. Simon J: Strategy & segmentation of the birth control market. In Sheth J, Wright P (eds): *Marketing Analysis for Societal Problems*. University of Illinois at Urbana, 1974. Pp 123-147.
5. Fryzel RJ: Marketing nonprofit institutions. *Hospital & Health Services Administration* 23:8-16, 1978.
6. Hulka B: Motivation techniques in a cancer detection program. *Public Health Rep* 81:1009-1014, 1966.
7. Hulka B: Motivation techniques in a cancer detection program; Utilization of community resources. *Am J Public Health* 57:229-240, 1967.
8. Anderson R: A Behavioral Model of Families' Use of Health Services. Research Series No 25, Center for Health Administration Studies. Chicago, University of Chicago Press, 1968.
9. Green LW, Robert BJ: Toward cost benefit evaluations of health education: Some concepts, methods & examples. *Health Educ Monog* 2:34-64, 1974.
10. Rosenstock I: The health belief model and preventive health behavior. *Health Educ Mong* 2:354-386, 1974.
11. Rosenstock I: Public response to cancer screening and detection programs: Determinants of health behavior. *J Chronic Dis* 16:407-418, 1963.

Theories, Techniques, and Issues in Health
Behavior Change

Health Behavior, Illness Behavior, and Sick Role Behavior: I. Health and Illness Behavior

by Stanislav V. Kasl, Ph.D., and Sidney Cobb, M.D.

MUCH CONFUSION has been contributed to the study of diseases, "psychosomatic" illnesses in particular, by failure to recognize that the psychological component of the phenomenon under study was often the factor which brought the patient to the doctor, not the factor which brought on the disease. Further confusion has been added sometimes by failure to recognize and separate the three major aspects of behavior related to health and illness. It is our present purpose to review selectively the voluminous English literature, beginning with a classification scheme and gradually unfolding a theoretical framework in order to organize and illuminate already available findings, as well as to suggest future research.

We begin with three definitions. *Health behavior* is any activity undertaken by a person believing himself to be healthy, for the purpose of preventing disease or detecting it in an asymptomatic stage. *Illness behavior* is any activity, undertaken by a person who feels ill, to define the state of his health and to discover a suitable remedy. The principal

activities here are complaining and seeking consultation from relatives, friends, and from those trained in matters of health. *Sick role behavior* is the activity undertaken by those who consider themselves ill, for the purpose of getting well. It includes receiving treatment from appropriate therapists, generally involves a whole range of dependent behaviors, and leads to some degree of neglect of one's usual duties.

In this review, we seek to understand the pattern and the sequence of interacting social and psychological forces on the individual as he reacts to his state of health and the associated changes. These forces may be cumulative as the person moves from health to illness to sick role behavior. At each stage, the additional pressures make this tripartite division significant from a sociopsychological standpoint as well as from a health-illness viewpoint.

The proposed sociopsychological perspective broadens the traditional approach to the study of diseases begun under the aegis of social medicine.[1] The gradual evolution of the study of diseases from the germ theory and the doctrine of specific etiology to social medicine and medical sociology is ably described by King.[2] Clearly, a thorough

From the Survey Research Center, Institute for Social Research, The University of Michigan, Ann Arbor, Mich.
Reprint requests to Institute for Social Research, University of Michigan, Ann Arbor, Mich (Dr. Cobb).

understanding of the cause, course, and outcome of many diseases, and of the patient's behavior as he seeks out diagnosis and treatment, requires additional research carried out within this broad perspective.[3-6]

The Classification

Our framework seeks to clarify the behavioral accompaniments of changes in health which may be seen as a sequence of stages characterizing in a hypothetical schema the progression of most diseases:[7] (1) health, (2) asymptomatic disease susceptible to detection, (3) symptomatic disease not yet diagnosed, (4) manifest disease at the time of diagnosis, (5) course of disease as influenced by treatment, and (6) disease after therapy, ie, either cured, in chronic state, or having eventuated in death. At this level, illness is viewed as a disturbance of some normal function of body processes, marked by certain symptoms, and taking a certain course. These stages are presented as the bottom line in Fig 1.

In addition to the biologic level, we may also consider the stages of health and illness at the sociopsychological level, where they can be seen as the changes in the individual's capacity to carry out his normal social obligations. Being sick may be looked at as giving up, in part or totally, the performance of one's customary duties. This conforms rather well to popular conceptions [8,9] and is implicit in the working definition of illness in the US National Health Survey interviews.[10] Parsons [11,12] observed with great insight that when one becomes ill, one does not simply drop one's customary roles—the role of a parent, spouse, or provider; one actually adopts a new role which supersedes the others. Parsons called this the "sick role."

The concept of any role [13-15] implies two sets of expectations: how the individual in a certain role should behave and how the others should behave toward him. Such norms or rules of behavior indicate what behavior is prescribed, what is allowed, and what is proscribed. These rules apply both to the person in the role and to those who have to deal with him because he is in that role. When Parsons coined the term "sick role," he in effect suggested that in our society there are explicit and implicit rules about being sick. The individual is not held responsible for his incapacity and he is exempt from normal social obligations. On the other hand, the role of the sick is seen as undesirable, perhaps deviant. Therefore, the person should try to get well and is under an obligation to seek competent help. Parsons went on to describe the complementary role of the physician or therapist. This therapeutic role, designed as it is to reverse the disease process and enable the patient to resume his normal social duties, is characterized by permissiveness, support, denial of a reciprocal relationship, and by the power to manipulate rewards and sanctions.

Using the focal concept of role, we may now state the behavioral stages of health and illness as follows: (1) adequate performance in usual roles, (2) diminished capacity for such performance and preparing to enter the sick role, (3) adopting the sick role, and (4) leaving the sick role (Fig 1). In order to elaborate the second stage of the above schema, Mechanic [16-18] introduced the term illness behavior, which "refers to the ways in which given symptoms may be differentially perceived, evaluated and acted (or

Behavior	Health	Illness			Sick Role	
Identity	Healthy	Feel Sick			Am Sick	
Role Performance	Usual Social Roles	Diminished Function	Preparing to Enter Sick Role		Being in Sick Role	Leaving Sick Role
Health	Health	Asymptomatic Disease	Symptoms	Dx	Treatment	Outcome

Fig 1.—The continuum from health to disease, related to behavior, identity, and role performance.

not acted) upon by different kinds of persons." That is, in the presence of symptoms, an individual has at least three choices: he may seek diagnosis, enter into some treatment, or absent himself from work. He may do all of these, some of these, or none of these.

The reader will note that in Fig 1 another level of description is used, the level of self-identity. The concept of self-identity is introduced for two reasons. First, we want to be able to make a distinction between personal and situational (role) determinants of behavior;[19] an individual's action may be seen as a joint function of the role demands and of self-identity. In addition, we want to be able to study internalization of role demands, the process of identity formation or change which results from acceptance of the demands of one's major life roles as one's own rules of behavior.[20] Thus, a prolonged enactment of the sick role may lead to lasting identity changes. Second, a person's body image is an important component of his self-identity [21-23] which should be a useful variable in the study of diverse diseases,[21] the effects of physical disability,[24] or clinic consultation habits.[25]

Once we have delineated the several levels, it should be evident that the stages at the health level may or may not be accompanied by appropriate and corresponding stages in illness and sick role behavior. This discrepancy between health and behavioral levels and its determinants constitute the focus of our investigation. We shall address ourselves to three problems: (1) Under what circumstances, in the absence of symptoms, will individuals engage in health behavior or preventive health practices? (2) When will the presence of symptoms lead to seeking diagnosis and treatment? (3) When will the individual adopt the sick role and what are the determinants of the length of the sick role period; that is, what variables influence not only the acceptance of treatment but also the rate of convalescence and resumption of normal obligations?

The answers to these questions can be best formulated in a theoretical framework, a model of action, which is in large part based on the work of Hochbaum, Rosenstock, and collaborators.[26-29,39,40] This model can be used, with appropriate additions, in understanding each of the three kinds of health-related behaviors and appears to be somewhat more precise and specific than the suggestions of other writers in this area.[5,30-34]

The Theoretical Framework

The likelihood that an individual will engage in a particular kind of health, illness, or sick role behavior is a function of two variables: the perceived amount of threat and the attractiveness or value of the behavior. The amount of threat depends on at least three variables: (1) the importance of health matters to the individual, (2) the perceived susceptibility to the disease in question, and (3) the perceived seriousness of the consequences of the disease. The attractiveness of the contemplated action depends on: (1) the perceived probability that the action will lead to the desired preventive or ameliorative results, and (2) the unpleasantness or "cost" of taking the action compared with taking no action and suffering the consequences. We are talking, of course, about action possibilities of which the individual is aware.

This model of action is clearly a skeleton at best. It directs attention to a certain broad class of variables and suggests how these variables interact, but not the possible determinants of the variables themselves. For example, the dimension labeled "importance of health matters" may be influenced by age, sex, occupation, subcultural values, fluctuations in mood, and so on. The nature of these determinants is largely an empirical question and will be considered later.

Another limitation of the model is that one doesn't know within what limits it is operative. For example, is there a level of threat which is optimal to motivate health and illness behavior and beyond which psychological defenses begin to interfere? Rosenstock et al [27] suggest that moderately intense threat is most effective but do not offer any supporting evidence. Clearly this is an important issue with practical implications; for example, officials of the American Cancer Society need information concerning the optimal strength of fear appeal to motivate prompt health and illness behavior. We shall return later to this problem when the relevant studies have been examined.

While basically the same model is used to

describe health, illness, and sick role behavior, it should by no means be assumed that individuals who are more inclined to take preventive health measures will also show a greater propensity to seek diagnosis and treatment when symptoms appear, or to enter the sick role after diagnosis. This is partly because while the stimulus which initiates illness behavior will be generally the symptom itself, the stimulus of preventive health behavior may be unknown, may come from mass media, personal friends, or educational materials. It is also possible that some individuals are inclined to underestimate their susceptibility to a disease in the absence of symptoms, but to overestimate it once some symptoms do appear.

These factors in our conceptual model appear useful for describing all three kinds of health-related behavior. However, sick role behavior usually represents more lasting changes than either health or illness behavior and therefore requires additional variables for complete description. When will the person enter the sick role and how long will he remain in it? The decision to seek diagnosis and treatment may rather naturally be followed by the adoption of the sick role. However, one can enter the sick role without seeking medical aid or one can seek medical aid only as a way of legitimizing one's prior decision to adopt the sick role. Conversely, one can refuse to accept one's illness despite the doctor's recommendations.

Sick role behavior, then, appears to have some significant, nonmedical determinants which, when derived from a broad role theory viewpoint,[13-15] may be listed in the form of the following broad questions (see also Mechanic's discussion of this problem[35]):

1. What are the expectations, norms, or role pressures, with regard to sick role behavior? How well has the individual understood and internalized these norms? How are these norms influenced by such variables as occupational settings and subcultural values? How do these sick role norms complement or conflict with the norms of the individual's other roles?

2. Who are the significant individuals whose norms about sick role behavior are most influential and what power do they have? Do they send the sick individual consistent or conflicting norms? Does their influence increase in proportion to the importance to them of his customary duties, as Mechanic[35] has suggested? This would have implications for understanding the relationship between occupational status and illness absences.

3. How congruent are the sick role norms with the individual's self-identity, that is, his personality and need structure? Does the adoption of passive, compliant, and dependent behavior violate an individual's beliefs about what kind of a person he is and how he ought to behave?

4. What are the rewards and punishments which favor or impede adoption of the sick role, remaining in it, and resuming normal social obligations?

5. What are the supporting (enabling) and inhibiting behaviors of persons in reciprocal roles, such as doctors, nurses, family members, and employers? What is the availability of such persons?

This listing of environmental, interpersonal, and personality determinants is again merely an outline of a theory; it alerts us to some nonmedical variables thought to affect the occurrence of some particular behavior relevant to the sick role.

Sociomedical Studies of Human Behavior Dealing With Health and Illness

The following review of the literature will examine studies dealing with: (1) health behavior or preventive health measures, (2) illness behavior or seeking diagnosis and treatment, and (3) sick role behavior. Our presentation is organized with maximal relevance to the theory just outlined, but the fit between the theory and the data is far from perfect. Some findings involving variables such as demographic data are presented because they are relevant but do not support any particular hypothesis. On other occasions, empirical evidence is lacking for a particular proposition contained in the theory. Industrial studies of illness absences and company dispensary visits, representing a large, separate domain, are not included.

Studies of Health Behavior.—Preventive health measures available to an individual are, by and large, of two kinds: health examinations to find out about one's health and to detect a disease in its asymptomatic stage, and seeking to reduce the probability of future illness through immunization, prenatal care, and so on. (Other behaviors which promote or maintain health, such as exercising or dieting, will not be considered in this review.)

Studies [36-47] of participation in free health examinations reveal, in looking at a number of demographic and background variables, that high participation rates are more likely to occur in non-whites [36,45,46] (with the exception of one study [47] with a five year follow up), young [36,40,44,46] or middle-aged [36,47] individuals with high residential stability [47] and a past history of high utilization of medical services.[37,38,46] Veterans [36] and residents of rural communities [46] may also show higher participation rates. Knowledge about diseases and participation in community affairs seem to make little difference.[37] Women show higher participation rates in three studies [40,42,47] and no difference in a fourth.[46] Income, education, and socioeconomic status do not reveal consistent results.[36,38-40,42,45,47] Income and education possibly show a curvilinear relationship with highest participation in the intermediate range [46]—about the same distribution as that for favorable attitudes toward doctors.[36] However, in a study of frequency of physician contacts within a health insurance program,[48] the intermediate education group had the fewest contacts.

Second, if we look at subjects' attitudes, then frequent participants in free medical examinations consider health matters important,[36,45] see themselves as susceptible,[40,45] and would rather find out than not about illness they may have.[37] Moreover, they see the examination as reasonable [36] and important to medical research.[36,45] They believe that modern medicine can generally effect a cure.[45] They tend to report their health as poor and want a checkup without insisting on getting it from their own doctor.[37] Positive attitudes toward the medical profession are not more common among them, but they will more readily consult a physician in the presence of symptoms.[37] The examination is seen beneficial in two ways: they would profit from an early detection [40] and they realize that one

cannot always rely on the actual appearance of symptoms for early detection.[40,45] A most interesting finding appears to be that unless the above beliefs are applied by the respondent to himself, they do not result in higher participation. That is, subjects who agree that x-rays can detect tuberculosis before the appearance of any symptoms, but who believe that they could tell if they had tuberculosis themselves, do not show higher participation. This fits in with the finding [42] that subjects believe other people are more susceptible to diseases than they themselves are.

When the health examination is not offered free, financial considerations become a powerful determinant [42,49,50] and the proportion of individuals coming to a physician solely to obtain a health examination is low [50] and declines as we go down the socioeconomic scale.[51,52] Most recent data [42] show that about one-half of the respondents had visited a physician during the past five years for a checkup in the absence of symptoms.

There is an ongoing debate about the value of health examinations. The argument seems to revolve mainly around the frequency of "significant new pathology" which may be revealed by the examination. Estimates of the percentage of apparently healthy individuals who are found to have some pathology range from 30% to over 90%.[44,53-56] Such estimates do not appear very meaningful since the different studies are not comparable even on such basic variables as age, sex, and socioeconomic status. Moreover, "significant new pathology" can hardly be defined precisely and to everyone's satisfaction. For example, is "10% overweight" either significant or new? The important point is that only some proportion of newly detected pathology is generally interpreted by the subjects as requiring action. On the other hand, there is a strong indication [55] that of the new abnormalities detected, the anamnestic interview yields only 6% to 15% of the total and runs a poor third to physical examinations and laboratory tests.

Participation in free polio vaccine programs [28,57-63] shows that those accepting the vaccine are younger,[61] have more education [58,60] and income,[60,63] and come from higher social classes.[28,58,59,61] When social class is held constant, Negroes [63] and women [61] participate more. Moreover, foreign born participate more than native born if they come from the upper classes but less if they come from the lower classes.[63] Mass media are the best source of information about vaccines; [58,62] those informed about the vaccines participate more.[58,59] Private physicians are a source of information in 40% of largely upper class individuals.[62] Among those with little education, perceived susceptibility to poliomyelitis [28] or worry about it [58] is related to higher acceptance. Higher acceptance rates are also found in areas with a high frequency of recent cases of polio.[63] These generalizations, however, will not always hold. For example, when the vaccine is being introduced during a controversy over its safety, then the lower social class members show higher acceptance.[57]

The issue of acceptance of preventive health measures also applies to influenza immunizations.[64-69] When these are carried out on captive industrial populations to whom the immunization is offered free of charge, the acceptance rate runs between one-half [65,67,68] and two-thirds.[64,69] In only one study [65] were variables examined in relation to the extent of participation and no differences were found due to age, sex, job classification, or union status. In another study,[66] in which a follow-up questionnaire was used to find out how beneficial the employees considered the immunization program to be, those who participated expressed more positive attitudes. However, among the participants, more positive attitudes were found among those who did not have influenza subsequent to inoculation; whereas among nonparticipants, more positive attitudes were found among those who had influenza. Thus the understanding of the dynamics of voluntary participation is important not only in its own right, but may be necessary to interpret data on the effectiveness of such programs. For example, in one study [64] which included in its design participants who actually received no vaccine, effectiveness, measured by the admittedly inadequate criterion of absences due to respiratory conditions, depended on whether or not one chose to participate rather than whether or not one received vaccine. Even more

paradoxical findings are reported in another study [67] where lower absence rates from respiratory conditions were found among nonvaccinated nonparticipants. However, both studies were conducted under nonepidemic conditions and different results would probably have been obtained under epidemic conditions. In any case, our understanding of effectiveness seems to depend on a concomitant understanding of the dynamics of participation in a particular industrial setting.

Data on preventive dental health care, summarized by Kegeles,[29,70] support rather well the same general model of action which explained participation in physical examinations. However, more recent findings [41] suggest that the generality of the model depends on the design of a study. In a retrospective study, those who report many past preventive dental visits see themselves, at interview time, less susceptible to dental decay than those reporting few such visits.[41] In a prospective study, those who see themselves less susceptible are found subsequently to have fewer preventive dental visits than those who see themselves more susceptible.[29] To be sure, this reversal of association between perceived susceptibility and health behavior does not indicate any basic inconsistency of results.

The positive association of education, income, and occupational status with preventive dental visits [29,42,71,72] appears to be stronger and more nearly linear than the association with physical examinations. People see themselves more susceptible to dental decay than to tuberculosis or cancer,[42] but dental decay, while possibly painful and expensive, is neither seen as contagious, deadly, dramatic,[73] nor as very disrupting of one's social roles.[70] An interesting side issue here is the so-called fluoridation controversy where the attempts are to understand an active opposition rather than mere nonparticipation.[73-76] Opponents of fluoridation have lower income and occupational status, and show less upward mobility during the previous ten years.[76] Moreover, they have stronger feelings of helplessness [74] and a lower sense of political efficacy; [74,76] they do not see that an average citizen can do much about such problems as air pollution and flood control.[76] Finally, while opponents of fluoridation are not substantially more opposed to science as such, they are, nevertheless, quite concerned with the diffuse, unanticipated but threatening consequences of scientific advances.[75]

The findings on the adequacy of prenatal and postnatal care reveal a strong social class gradient: [71,77-79] mothers from upper classes come sooner for prenatal care, make more visits, receive considerably more postpartum care, and are more likely to be under the care of specialists rather than general practitioners. These findings, with the exception of one study,[77] are explicable on the basis of financial cost. However, when one controls for income, differences due to education are maintained.[78] Among the less educated, fewer believe in prenatal care within the first three months of pregnancy, fewer actually report for such care, and they show a larger opinion-performance discrepancy.[78] (That is, holding the right belief, or at least stating it to the interviewer, is less of a guarantee among the less educated that it will be accompanied by appropriate action.)

In summary, then, the findings on health behavior support a rather simple model of the relationship of perceived threat of disease to health behavior as depicted in Fig 2. Perceived value of preventive action is seen as the most important variable [41] mediating the influence of perceived threat. Furthermore, both kinds of perceptions, of the threat and of the remedial action, are

assumed to be influenced by diverse demographic and background variables. Conceptualized thus, the model in Fig 2 seems to describe satisfactorily the majority of findings. In pointing out the salient social and psychological determinants of health behavior, the model may also prove useful in the future teaching of preventive medicine.

Studies of Illness Behavior.—The basic problem of illness behavior is: in the presence of symptoms, what will the individual do and why will he do it? The answer is important, first, because successful treatment almost always depends upon the initiative of the patient in seeking diagnosis and treatment. Second, our understanding of many diseases is based on populations of self-referred sick patients. Systematic biases in self-referral, should they remain unknown, can seriously distort understanding of the disease process. To clarify the meaning and importance of the concept of illness behavior, we may briefly look at the voluminous literature on the role of emotion in the onset of disease. For example, it has been rather flatly asserted [80] that the onset of such chronic diseases as diabetes, rheumatoid arthritis, multiple sclerosis, and Parkinson's disease is frequently associated with emotional stress. Others emphasize the role of environmental stress and life crises in the development of tuberculosis [81-83] and cardiac diseases.[83,84] Another group of writers emphasize a particular kind of emotional stress: the loss of support and separa-

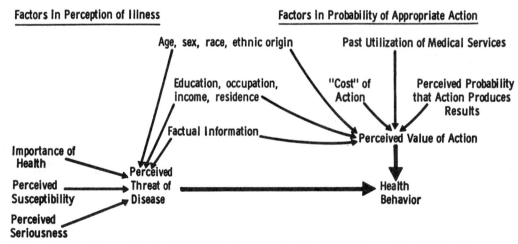

Fig 2.—The postulated relationship between perceived threat of disease and health behavior.

tion from some important person. They assert that such stress and the ensuing reaction of giving up and feelings of hopelessness-helplessness may be a factor in the onset of leukemia,[85,86] psychiatric illness,[87] and perhaps disease in general.[88] Finally, Hinkle and his collaborators [89-95] seek to demonstrate, on diverse populations working in different settings, the intimate relationship between an individual's lifetime and present social environment, his perceptions of and reactions to this environment, and his illnesses.

Many of these studies possess serious shortcomings. They tend to be uncontrolled, retrospective, and often the possibility of unconscious observer bias seems maximal. There is some doubt that the reported incidence of "separation" experiences is much higher than what one may find in normal, healthy adults.[96] However, the major point is that the above findings, no matter how sound or unsound, are open to the alternative interpretation that emotional stress in general or object loss in particular precipitates only illness behavior, not the illness as such. Psychological distress may sensitize a patient to already existing symptoms and directly influence his decision to seek medical care.

This point has been made by Mechanic [97] in his discussion of the implications of the concept of illness behavior for medical sampling as well as by Stoeckle et al.[98-102] The latter note that patients who seek medical aid on their own initiative very frequently exhibit psychological distress, mostly feelings of depression and grief, but sometimes also resentment. These findings agree with some clinical observations of Engel [103] on "pain-prone" individuals and with the psychological test data on industrial employees who come frequently to the company dispensary for reasons other than injury.[104,105]

Additional evidence supporting Stoeckle's observations comes from studies of the use of health services among college students and Army recruits.[17,18,25,96,106-109] Students with low self-acceptance [25] and those reporting frequent feelings of loneliness and nervousness [18,109] visit the college infirmary more often. Moreover, students who report on a questionnaire a higher propensity to seek

medical aid in the presence of specified symptoms come to the infirmary more often.[18] Furthermore, they come with complaints of illness which are common, relatively familiar, and with a predictable outcome.[17] Female students and those younger than their classmates also come to the infirmary oftener.[108] Another study [106] reveals generally inconsistent relationships between medical visits and many indices of adjustment, collected on several different populations of college students and Army recruits. It does not appear that either "separation" experiences [96] or hypochondriasis [107] (as measured by the MMPI [110]) is related to frequency of dispensary visits. Also relevant here is the finding [111] that mothers under stress tend to report more illness symptomatology for themselves and for their children, and are somewhat more likely to phone their doctor concerning their children's health.

A thorough understanding of the concept of illness behavior leads to a reexamination of other findings. Let us look at three such areas: 1. Studies [112-115] of the incidence of somatic disease in psychiatric patients show that a higher incidence of somatic illness accompanies a higher incidence of psychiatric illness. Speculation about "a healthy mind in a healthy body" should rule out the possibility that such a positive association is actually due to individual differences in readiness to admit to symptoms, be they physical or psychological. It is possible, as Mechanic [97] suggests, that "persons who are likely to bring mood and behavior complaints to a psychiatric clinic are also likely to be sensitive to physical symptomatology."

2. One of the conclusions drawn by Hinkle et al [89-95] is that those individuals "who had the greatest amount of sickness disability had experienced a wide variety of illnesses of various types, and various etiologies, involving a number of body systems"; [92] these authors believe that individuals exhibit differences in susceptibility not to specific diseases but to illness in general. A possible alternative conclusion would be that they are merely dealing with individual differences in propensity for illness behavior.

3. Finally, there are studies which attempt to link some social or psychological variable

with the rate of progression of a disease, notably cancer.[116-119] Any interpretation of such studies must first rule out the possibility that this social or psychological variable is not simply related to delay in seeking treatment so that the disease is more advanced when it comes to the physician's attention.

Since the problem of the possible role of emotional distress in illness behavior is so well covered by Stoeckle et al,[98-102] only a few additional comments will be made. The concept of illness behavior does not settle many arguments; it broadens our interpretive base, where appropriate, without ruling out possible effects of psychological distress on the illness itself. For example, some recent, better designed studies of tuberculosis [81,83] suggest a piling up of social stresses during the last two years before the onset of the disease itself; the fact that similar piling up of stresses also precedes pregnancy [83] requires careful interpretation of all of the findings. Moreover, if entrance to a home for the aged is interpreted as a separation experience, then data on higher death rates within the first year after admission [120] support the hypothesis that separation leads to illness rather than merely to illness behavior. The finding [121] that under the stress of an imminent medical school examination, the frequency of common cold increases for students given a placebo, but not for those receiving a regular dose of ascorbic acid and lemon bioflavonoid, again makes the illness behavior interpretation of this situation inappropriate.

Second, it is not known what proportion of individuals seek purely psychological help in coming to a physician or a dispensary. Third, it is not clear what effect physical symptoms have on psychological distress. A longitudinal design with follow-up data [25,96] may be necessary to untangle the possible relationships. Thus Roessler and Greenfield [25] discount the interpretation that bodily distress among college students leads both to low self-acceptance and to dispensary visits, for at the time when self-acceptance was assessed, the students did not experience or report bodily distress. Finally, if we attempt to apply to illness behavior basically the same theoretical model outlined in Fig 2 for health behavior, the role of psychological distress is not fully apparent: psychological distress may (a) increase the importance of health matters, (b) increase the perceived susceptibility, (c) make the consequences of disease look more threatening, or (d) raise the probability that action will lead to desired results. It is also possible,[52,101,102] that psychological distress generates symptoms from which the patient wants relief even though he does not believe them appropriate to present to the doctor.

In reading studies specifically concerned with determinants of illness behavior, an attempt to understand differences in seeking medical services, one quickly realizes that personal income is a less and less satisfactory explanatory variable.[122] In a study of a representative sample of families in London,[123] where a visit to a physician is free, over one-third of the families had a member who was suffering some pain or discomfort, but was not being treated. This compares quite well with earlier findings [124] that only 40% of those who had a diagnosed disorder and also expressed discomfort about it, were under any kind of medical care. Anderson [8] pointed out that:

> As health insurance became more widespread and family incomes increased, the economic factor became less and less important as a reason for not seeking services; consequently, other factors were clearly at work.

What are some of these other factors?

One set of factors may be grouped conveniently as variables affecting the perception of symptoms; the important ones are social class, subcultural values, age, sex, and attitudes toward self. Social class plays a prominent role in Koos' pioneering study of the health of a community.[52] Koos found a clear social class gradient in attitudes toward symptoms; the lower the class, the less likely was a specified symptom seen as requiring medical attention. For example, when presented with such a hypothetical symptom as "persistent pain in the back," then the lower the social class of the respondent, the less likely was he to indicate that such a symptom merits medical attention. It is not clear what factors underlie this gradient; Koos suggests that it not only reflects the felt need for treatment, but also the cost of the services and fear of treatment.

A number of studies suggest that the ethnic origin of an individual influences his perception and interpretation of symptoms. Zborowski's study of cultural components in response to pain [125] suggests that Americans of Italian origin are concerned mainly with the immediacy of pain experience, while Jewish Americans focus upon the symptomatic meaning of pain and its significance for their health and welfare. "Old stock" Americans also show future-oriented anxiety about pain, but are much more optimistic than the Jews. Zola [126-129] studied Italian, Irish, and Anglo-Saxon Americans and their decisions as to when to seek medical aid. He noted that, holding differences in objective symptoms constant, (1) Italian Americans seek aid when their symptoms interfere with social and personal relations. (2) Irish Americans tend to do so only after receiving the approval of others while (3) Americans of Anglo-Saxon origin see a physician when the symptom is considered to be interfering with some specific vocational or physical activity. Jewish college students seem to have a higher threshold for seeking medical attention than Protestant and Catholic students and appear at the student health service considerably less frequently [108] (it is not known to what extent the admission policy at this college, Cornell, is selective with regard to the prospective student's religion). On the other hand, Jewish members of the Health Insurance Plan of Greater New York had more physician contacts than Protestant or Catholic members.[48] Jewish subjects also stand out in a study of reactions to physical disabilities: [130] when asked to rank their preferences for drawings of children with various types of visible handicaps, Jewish children show a higher agreement among themselves than do non-Jewish children as well as a different order of preferences. The basis for such preferences was not investigated.

No studies have been found which specifically seek out effects of age and sex on perception of symptoms. However, reasonable inferences can be made from studies which compare physicians' evaluations of an individual's health with the latter's own evaluations.[131-136] Under-reporting of symptoms is a more prevalent problem than over-reporting.[131] Men [133,134] and older subjects [135,136] are more optimistic about their health than women and younger subjects. One study found no age or sex differences.[131] Since under-reporting varies with the nature of symptoms [131,133,135] and since many symptoms are age or sex-related, or both, more refined analyses than are presently available need to be made.

Three studies [132,134,135] were detailed investigations of elderly subjects. The most striking finding was the relative lack of agreement between physicians' and subjects' evaluations of the latter's health, in all three studies agreement was between 60% and 65%, where 50% agreement is chance. Two studies [132,135] permitted computation of tetrachoric correlations (estimated from a cosine-π table [137]) and both were in the neighborhood of 0.30. A number of the subjects' attitudes relating to personal happiness, worry about health, and feeling oneself young vs old were strongly related to self-assessed health but not to the doctors' ratings.[132,135] Those who were overly optimistic about their health came from non-manual occupations, had maintained their major lifetime work roles, and remained relatively active socially.[134] These findings on the relationship of self-assessed health to various attitudes among elderly subjects are supported by two studies of college students [138,139] which show that "body cathexis," the degree of feeling of satisfaction with various parts or processes of body, is positively related to satisfaction with various attributes of the self [138,139] and negatively related to symptom scores on the Cornell Medical Index Health Questionnaire.[138] Another study of college students [140] reveals that those who are aware of their body's autonomic activity (respiration, heart rate, perspiration, etc) do in fact show higher autonomic reactivity under conditions of intellectual stress.

Some implications of these studies are that, first, such differences in perception of symptoms influence an individual's readiness to seek medical aid and, possibly to accept treatment. Second, differences in perceptions of symptoms cast doubt on the results of studies which rely on interviews [141] or assessment techniques like the Cornell Medical Index.[142] These methods, which are surprisingly sensitive to the interpersonal aspects of the interview technique,[143] are probably vulnerable to the implied perceptual and self-report bias. This criticism of interview morbidity surveys is not new,[144,145] but we are beginning to learn something about the nature of the bias which may be present. Many of the studies are methodological investigations of the adequacy of reporting illness,[146-148] while "attempts to link illness attitudes and behavior to quality of reporting are rare."[144] One study[144] in this direction finds that college students who are disinclined to seek medical aid in the presence of specified symptoms[18] under-report more of their visits to a college infirmary the previous year. Third, can the known differences in the ways symptoms are perceived and acted upon teach us anything about a disease, its etiology, its course, or both? For example, Epstein et al[149,150] report that in a homogeneous group of clothing workers in New York City, manifest coronary heart disease was twice as frequent among Jewish men as among Italian men. Moreover, while the overall prevalence rate of the disease among the Italians was associated with serum cholesterol levels, blood pressure, and body weight, the same three variables had no appreciable effect on the rates among the Jewish men. Can the work of Zborowski[125] and Zola[126-129] on cultural factors in response to pain and interpretation of symptoms help us explain these puzzling findings? Clearly, at the moment one can only say that such work is a possible source for explanatory hypotheses.

In seeking diagnosis and treatment for symptoms possibly indicative of cancer, an example of illness behavior par excellence is available to us; such studies[151-156] afford a good look at some sociopsychological variables involved in causes of delay in the diagnosis and treatment of cancer. The concept of delay has two possible meanings, depending on whether delay is computed from the date of first appearance of symptoms or from the time a complaint is recognized by the patient as requiring medical attention. Kutner et al[155] call these unavoidable and avoidable delay. We are more concerned with "avoidable" delay, even though "unavoidable" delay may reflect a period of defense by denial. Not all studies make this distinction nor define delay in the same way. Cobb et al[152] define delay as waiting more than three months after cancer was sus-

pected, while Goldsen et al[153] call delayers those who waited at least three months between onset of symptoms and first attempts to seek diagnosis.

Persons who delay about cancer may be characterized as more likely to be older,[152,155] native Americans of Protestant religion[155] and lower socioeconomic status,[152-155] coming from families with some experience with cancer.[152] It is commonly asserted that delay for cancer is part of a more general habit of delay for other medical problems.[153,155] However, at least one study[154] talks about two types of delay patterns—for general medical symptoms and for cancer symptoms—which are differently related to social class. Holding other medical symptoms constant, presence of cancer symptoms tended to increase delay.[154] The nature of cancer symptoms does not seem to influence delay.[152,153] The site of the symptom, however, made a difference in one study[153] in which symptoms which were noticeable and apparent to others were associated with greater delay; in another study,[152] a comparison of internal vs. external sites yielded no differences. Better knowledge about cancer symptoms was associated with greater promptness in one study[152] but made little difference in another.[153]

The role of anxiety in cancer delay is rather complex. Cancer evokes more fear than other diseases, such as polio, arthritis, or tuberculosis;[156] patients awaiting an examination for cancer are clearly anxious.[151] Cancer is seen as less preventable than tuberculosis or dental decay and about 43% of adults see themselves susceptible.[42] And while respondents believe other people are more susceptible to diseases than they themselves are, this difference is considerably larger for cancer than it is for tuberculosis or tooth decay.[42] Rosenstock et al consider this differential in projected susceptibility indirect evidence of the greater anxiety aroused by cancer. Fear of cancer is higher among the less educated and those who know more about the disease and who consider it highly prevalent and expensive to treat,[156] but it is not clear how anxiety influences delay. Cobb et al[152] suggest that those who delay appear to be immobilized by the threat of the disease whereas those who are prompt in seeking diagnosis use their fear constructively to initiate action. Kutner et al [155] note that sometimes fear triggers positive action while at other times it inhibits it. They suggest that general anxiety about cancer will be associated with delay if accompanied by knowledge of the danger signals, a conclusion supported by the Goldsen study.[153] These authors also note that reticence about one's symptoms increases delay, perhaps because one cuts oneself off from social pressures. For a more comprehensive review of this literature see Blackwell.[190]

These studies lead to the conclusion that the role of anxiety in the delay of illness behavior is not yet clear. One possibility is that anxiety is curvilinearly related to such behavior. It was found [157] that moderately intense fear is most effective in stimulating a group of subjects to adopt certain dental health practices. Anxiety may also interact with a number of other variables not assessed in studies reviewed above: individual differences in thresholds for anxiety arousal, different ways of coping with anxiety, subcultural norms with regard to anxiety about one's health,[125-129] and so on. Cartwright et al [158] studied beliefs among smokers, quitters, and nonsmokers, and their results are a nice illustration of protective and anxiety-reducing distortions. They showed that smokers are less likely to believe that smoking affects health and if they believe it, they are more likely to think it affects health in others but not themselves. If asked about the level of smoking at which the danger of lung cancer starts, the more they smoke the higher they place the level. Festinger's theory of cognitive dissonance [159] appears to be the most suitable framework within which to see these relationships between practice and belief. In summary, data on anxiety and delay do not lead to rejection of the general viewpoint that individuals will adopt those behaviors most effectively reinforced by reduction in anxiety.[160] However, much more work is needed to determine what these behaviors are and whether they facilitate or interfere with prompt illness behavior. It is possible that, at moderate levels of anxiety, prompt action in seeking diagnosis most effectively reduces anxiety; however, at more intense levels, only maladaptive denial or arational medical practices [161] effectively reduce anxiety.

A review of illness behavior must also include an examination of variables influencing "utilization of medical services." [3] However, to illuminate the sociopsychological dynamics of illness behavior, utilization data possess a number of shortcomings. Since utilization rates presumably reflect both the person's actual state of health and his decision as to what to do about it, studies which do not hold the former constant yield ambiguous data: a relationship between a particular variable and utilization rates may be interpreted as an association of that variable with illness or with propensity toward illness behavior. Second, most utilization studies are conducted for the benefit of policy-makers, administrators, and health economists (see Anderson's recent review [3]). They are predominantly concerned with such variables as frequency and types of services provided and their costs, but evince little interest in the many possible sociopsychological variables which may affect utilization rates. Age, sex, and social class are generally the only variables related to utilization. Third, utilization studies generally omit two aspects of illness behavior: self-medication, Polgar's "self-addressed" phase of health action,[32] and the use of the various nonmedical functionaries, omissions which may not bother a public health official but are rather serious in trying to understand all of the sociopsychological aspects of illness behavior. Since little is known about self-medication, the consequences of this omission cannot be estimated. However, we do know something about the use of nonmedical personnel:[52,162,163] it is a phenomenon confined largely to the lowest social classes and frequently follows prematurely terminated medical treatment. The primary reasons for it do not appear to be economic but rather come from the nature of the doctor-patient relationship. Finally, we may note that in terms of our classification schema, "utilization of health services" can be viewed as illness behavior or sick role behavior. Stoeckle et al,[101] for example, assert that "most participation and utilization studies, while seemingly similar to the initial process of seeking medical advice, are really the repeated use or reuse of the doctor-patient relationship." This might imply that variables associated with initial seeking of medical aid need not be the same as those which keep the patient coming back.

Studies of rates of visits to physicians by non-members of health care plans [164-166] show consistently higher rates for females over age 10 which hold for both acute and chronic illnesses [164] and are not due to visits for conditions associated with pregnancy. Age shows a positive association with frequency of visits. In studies of members of health care plans, we find that these age and sex differences are replicated, both in visits to physicians [167,168] and in hospital admissions. [164,169,170] Men have higher rates of hospital admissions for chronic conditions [164] and their stay at the hospital per visit is longer. [169,170] Looking at marital status and hospital admissions, we find that being married is associated with the lowest rates among males and highest rates among females [170] (corrected for conditions associated with pregnancy). Short- and long-term longitudinal investigations [167,171] reveal a good deal of stability of utilization levels, probably a characteristic of individuals rather than of families because high utilizers are not concentrated in the same families. [167] Individuals over 60 are most likely to be either very high or very low level utilizers and the proportion of those with no physician visits increases with age. [167] Positive association between age and utilization rates found in cross-sectional studies is therefore rather misleading; the increasingly higher rates among older individuals seem to represent increased utilization, but for a decreasing proportion of individuals as successively higher age brackets are examined.

Social class data are not entirely consistent. One still finds positive association between social class and mean number of visits to physicians, [51] but more and more often one encounters no differences in frequencies of consulting a physician, when an illness is reportedly present. [172] The occasional curvilinear associations are not consistent. One study [48] reports fewest physician contacts for a group of intermediate status while another study [52] on a similarly intermediate group finds the most physician contacts (as derived from rates of reported illness and proportions of untreated illness). A British study of consultations in a total, self-contained community [168] shows that miners as an occupational group had more consultations but otherwise no social class differences were apparent. Another interesting study of a total community, a village in Israel, [173] contrasted those who wanted to stay in the community and, by consensus of village leaders should stay, with those who wanted to leave and by consensus ought to leave: the former had fewer visits to a free medical center than the latter.

Attitudes toward doctors and provided services do not seem to affect utilization rates. Feldman [174] reports that when one partials out statistically the effect of perceived medical needs, the correlation of attitude toward doctors with the number of times a doctor is seen per year is close to zero. A dissatisfied subscriber to a health plan may occasionally use an outside doctor but his level of utilization is not thereby strongly affected. [175] An upper class British patient may prefer home visits or telephone consultations to visits to surgery, but his consultations are not less frequent. [168] Thus, as long as we deal with so tenuous a form of the doctor-patient interaction as a consultation, attitudes toward doctors have relatively little influence on frequency of such interaction.

This brief review of the utilization literature confirms the suspicion that it provides little about the determinants of illness behavior. However, certain plausible arguments are possible from other data, such as a longitudinal study of children from birth to 18 years which revealed that at all ages boys, not girls, had a greater frequency of respiratory illnesses, which accounted for 83% of total illness experiences. [176] Yet women are more likely to follow recommended health practices, [42] have more physician visits [164-168] and more hospital admissions, [169-170] and college girls have more upper respiratory complaints. [108] Within the limits of comparing such discrepant age groups, this suggests that women have a lower threshold for illness behavior than men. This would fit the finding that men have fewer hospital admission but their stay per visit is longer. [169,170] If length of stay is an indication of severity, then men seem to seek hospitalization only for relatively more severe conditions. Finally, typical industrial illness absence data (eg, Blumberg and Coffin,[177] Enterline [178]) also are consistent with the interpretation that women have a lower threshold for illness behavior. While this conclusion is not surprising, it is nevertheless difficult to document from typical utilization data.

Let us next consider studies dealing with seeking help for psychological problems and symptoms. This form of illness behavior is examined separately, since here we can no longer talk, without considerable controversy, about two distinct levels of description: the disease process at the biological level and the accompanying behavior of the individual. The work of Stoeckle and his collaborators [98-102] suggests that an unknown, possibly large proportion of "medical" illness behavior may be in fact disguised seeking of help for primarily psychological problems. Thus, no sharp distinction can be made between these two forms of illness behavior and we must be satisfied with an admittedly inadequate measure of "psychological" illness behavior: seeking diagnosis and treatment from psychiatrists, psychologists, social workers, and so on.

Two survey studies, one on a national sample [179] and the other on residents of Manhattan,[180] have related help-seeking behavior to their questionnaire-based measures of mental health and to selected demographic variables. Gurin et al [179] found greater readiness for self-referral among women, younger and more educated respondents, and those admitting to worries, unhappiness, or approaching nervous breakdown. Moreover, subjects reporting symptoms indicative of psychological anxiety had a high readiness for self-referral whereas those reporting symptoms of poor physical health exhibited low readiness. Similarly, Srole et al [180] report that younger respondents and those from higher socioeconomic classes are more likely to have received treatment, though they are less likely to be rated as "impaired." If one considers only "impaired" subjects, then receiving treatment is unaffected by sex, age, or marital status—with the sole exception of very young single men who report higher rates of treatment.

Catholic and foreign-born respondents, when rated "impaired," are less likely to have received treatment but this is not adjusted for socioeconomic status. These results are consistent with the conclusions of other authors [181-183] that lower class patients tend to conceive of their problems in somatic terms, have a lower desire for psychotherapy, and are less likely to come to treatment on their own initiative. Other variables which facilitate the path to treatment are positive attitudes among friends and co-workers,[184] and the propensity to experience anxiety and dissatisfaction with oneself.[185]

A study of public attitudes toward mental health professionals [186] shows that they are less favorable than attitudes toward other medical specialists; moreover, they are most negative among those who need the help most, eg, older respondents of lower social class. This naturally aggravates the problem of treating those in need of therapy. One survey [187] estimated that 61% of "mentally ill" individuals received no treatment whatsoever and of the 39% treated cases, only one-half received treatment from appropriately trained professionals. Unfortunately, the authors do not make it clear what criteria of mental illness they used nor even the questions they asked. The problem of untreated cases is much more than a matter of attitudes. Lack of appropriate treatment facilities and services is another factor emphasized by many writers.[179,180,187,188] This lack, however, is a complex variable from the viewpoint of the needy individual: (1) He knows where to go but is not accepted for treatment. (2) He knows he needs psychiatric help but does not know where to get it. (3) He doesn't know he needs professional help of a special kind. For example, when survey respondents are faced with a hypothetical situation involving a behavior problem or a case of a mental illness, about half of them [180] or more [187] recommend no professional help whatsoever. Moreover, 61% knew of no psychiatric facility where they themselves could go.[187] Along similar lines, Gurin et al [179] report that of individuals who had sought help for mental health problems (14% of their total sample), fully 42% went to a clergyman, rather than a psychiatrist or a psychologist. And the results of a British study [189] show that general practitioners clearly differ in their inclination to refer their patients, irrespective of the presenting complaints, to a psychiatrist.

The studies of illness behavior which have been reviewed cannot be summarized easily. Many deal with superficial demographic and background variables rather than with fundamental, theoretically derived attitudes and subjective perceptions. This has an advantage in the area of measurement but the disadvantage that one does not always understand the meaning of such associations. Consequently, we cannot go much beyond the simple relationship depicted in Fig 3, which is meant as an addition to Fig 2 and, therefore, all the variables of that figure are still assumed to function. Two new major variables are introduced: psychological distress and the discomfort arising from the symptom. This is because we want to go beyond the purely cognitive significance of a symptom—what does the symptom indicate about one's present and future health and what should one do about it—in order to take into consideration the imperious quality of a painful symptom which demands prompt relief.

Figure 3 suggests that symptoms may cause psychological distress, that psychological distress may cause symptoms, and,

furthermore, psychological distress may influence the relation between symptoms and relevant illness behavior. Under psychological distress, a number of variables are included. At present, the depression syndrome and anxiety appear dominant but it seems likely that breaking the depression syndrome down into components such as resentment, low self-esteem, loss of sense of social support, guilt, sadness, etc, will prove profitable.

REFERENCES

1. Halliday, J.L.: *Psychosocial Medicine*, New York: W. W. Norton & Co., 1948.
2. King, S.H.: *Perceptions of Illness and Medical Practice*, New York: Russell Sage Foundation, 1962.
3. Anderson, O.W.: "The Utilization of Health Services," in Freeman, H.E.; Levine, S.; and Reeder, L.G. (eds.): *Handbook of Medical Sociology*, Englewood Cliffs, N.J.: Prentice-Hall, Inc., 1963, pp 349-367.
4. Gordon, G.: Needed Research on the Social-Psychological Aspects of Disease, *Amer Rev Resp Dis* 89:753-755, 1964.
5. Cassel, J.; Patrick, R.; and Jenkins, D.: Epidemiological Analysis of Health Implications of Culture Change: A Conceptual Model, *Ann NY Acad Sci* 84:938-949, 1960.
6. White, K.L.; Williams, T.F.; and Greenberg,

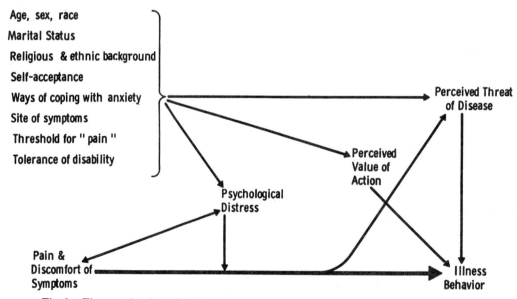

Fig 3.—The postulated relationship between symptoms and illness behavior (a supplement to Fig 2).

B.G.: The Ecology of Medical Care, *New Eng J Med* 265:885-892, 1961.

7. Hutchinson, G.B.: Evaluation of Preventive Services, *J Chron Dis* 11:497-508, 1960.

8. Apple, D.: How Laymen Define Illness, *J Health Hum Behav* 1:219-225, 1960.

9. Baumann, B.: Diversities in Conceptions of Health and Physical Fitness, *J Health Hum Behav* 2:39-46, 1961.

10. Woolsey, T.D.: The Concept of Illness in the Household Interview for the US National Health Survey, *Amer J Public Health* 48:703-712, 1958.

11. Parsons, T.: Illness and the Role of the Physician: A Sociological Perspective, *Amer J Orthopsychiat* 21:452-460, 1951.

12. Parsons, T.: "Definitions of Health and Illness in the Light of American Values and Social Structure," in Jaco, E.G. (ed.): *Patients, Physicians, and Illness*, Glencoe, Ill: The Free Press, 1958, pp 165-187.

13. Newcomb, T.M.: *Social Psychology*, New York: Dryden Press, 1950.

14. Rommetweit, R.: *Social Norms and Roles*, Minneapolis: University of Minnesota Press, 1954.

15. Gross, N.C.; Mason, W.S.; and McEachern, A.W.: *Exploration in Role Analysis*, New York: John Wiley & Sons, Inc., 1958.

16. Mechanic, D.: The Concept of Illness Behavior, *J Chron Dis* 15:189-194, 1962.

17. Mechanic, D., and Volkart, E.H.: Illness Behavior and Medical Diagnosis, *J Health Hum Behav* 1:86-94, 1960.

18. Mechanic, D., and Volkart, E.H.: Stress, Illness Behavior, and the Sick Role, *Amer Sociol Rev* 26:51-58, 1961.

19. Levinson, D.J.: Role, Personality, and Social Structure in the Organizational Setting, *J Abnorm Soc Psychol* 58:170-180, 1959.

20. Miller, D.R.: "The Study of Social Relationships: Situation, Identity, and Social Interaction," in Koch, S. (ed.): *Psychology: A Study of a Science*, New York: McGraw-Hill Book Co., Inc., 1963, vol 5, pp 639-737.

21. Fisher, S., and Cleveland, S.E.: *Body Image and Personality*, Princeton, NJ: D. Van Nostrand Co., Inc., 1958.

22. Jourard, S.M., and Remy, R.M.: Individual Variance Scores: An Index of the Degree of Differentiation of the Self and the Body Image, *J Clin Psychol* 13:62-63, 1957.

23. Schilder, P.: *The Image and Appearance of the Human Body*, Psyche Monograph No. 4, London: Kegan Paul, Trench, Trubner, & Co., Ltd., 1935 (New York: International Universities Press, 1950).

24. Barker, R.G.: The Social Psychology of Physical Disability, *J Soc Issues* 14:28-38, 1958.

25. Roessler, R., and Greenfield, N.S.: Personality Determinants of Medical Clinic Consultation, *J Nerv Ment Dis* 127:142-144, 1958.

26. Rosenstock, I.M.: What Research in Motivation Suggests for Public Health, *Amer J Public Health* 50:295-302, 1960.

27. Rosenstock, I.M.; Hochbaum, G.M.; and

28. Kegeles, S.S.: Determinants of Health Behavior, Unpublished data.

28. Rosenstock, I.M.; Derryberry, M.; and Carriger, B.: Why People Fail to Seek Poliomyelitis Vaccination, *Public Health Rep* 74:98-103, 1959.

29. Kegeles, S.S.: Why People Seek Dental Care: A Test of a Conceptual Formulation, *J Health Hum Behav* 4:166-173, 1963.

30. Caudill, W.: *Effects of Social and Cultural Systems in Reactions to Stress*, Pamphlet 14, New York: Social Science Research Council (June) 1958.

31. Holland, J.B.; Tiedke, K.E.; and Miller, P.A.: A Theoretical Model of Health Action, *Rural Sociol* 22:149-155, 1957.

32. Polgar, S.: "Health Action in Cross-cultural Perspective," in Freeman, H. E.; Levine, S.; and Reeder, L. G. (eds.): *Handbook of Medical Sociology*, Englewood Cliffs, NJ: Prentice-Hall, Inc., 1963, pp 397-419.

33. Rabinowitz, H.S., and Mitsos, S.B.: Rehabilitation As Planned Social Change: A Conceptual Framework, *J Health Hum Behav* 5:2-14, 1964.

34. von Mering, O.: Disease, Healing, and Problem Solving: A Behavioural Science Approach, *Int J Soc Psychiat* 8:137-148, 1962.

35. Mechanic, D.: Illness and Social Disability: Some Problems in Analysis, *Pacif Social Rev* 2:37-41, 1959.

36. Borsky, P.N., and Sagan, O.K.: Motivations Toward Health Examinations, *Amer J Public Health* 49:514-527, 1959.

37. Chen, E., and Cobb, S.: Further Study of the Nonparticipation Problems in a Morbidity Survey Involving Clinical Examination, *J Chron Dis* 7:321-331, 1958.

38. Cobb, S.; King, S.; and Chen, E.: Differences Between Respondents and Nonrespondents in a Morbidity Survey Involving Clinical Examination, *J Chron Dis* 6:95-108, 1957.

39. Hochbaum, G.M.: *Public Participation in Medical Screening Programs,* Public Health Service Publication No. 572, US Department of Health, Education, and Welfare, 1958.

40. Hochbaum, G.M.: Why People Seek Diagnostic X-rays, *Public Health Rep* 71:377-380, 1956.

41. Kirscht, J.P.: A National Study of Health Attitudes, Unpublished data.

42. Rosenstock, I.M., et al: A National Study of Health Attitudes, read before the 92nd Annual Meeting of the American Public Health Association, New York, October 5, 1964.

43. Steiner, S.D.: Management of Health Examination Program in General Motors, *J Occup Med* 3:424-428, 1961.

44. Tupper, C.J., and Beckett, M.B.: Faculty Health Appraisal—University of Michigan, *Industr Med Surg* 27:328-332, 1958.

45. *Attitudes Toward Co-operation in a Health Examination Survey,* Public Health Service Series D, No. 6, US Department of Health, Education, and Welfare: Health Statistics, 1961.

46. *Cooperation in Health Examination Surveys,* Public Health Service Series D, No. 2, US Depart-

ment of Health, Education, and Welfare: Health Statistics, 1960.

47. Wylie, C.M.: Participation in a Multiple Screening Clinic With Five-year Follow-up, *Public Health Rep* 76:596-602, 1961.

48. The Committee for the Special Research Project in the Health Insurance Plan of Greater New York: *Health and Medical Care in New York City*, Cambridge: Harvard University Press, 1957.

49. Thompson, C.E.; Zaus, E.A.; and Keller, P.R.: Some Observations on Periodic Executive Health Examinations, *J Occup Med* 3:215-217, 1961.

50. Collins, S.D.: Frequency of Health Examinations in 9000 Families Based on Nationwide Periodic Canvasses, *Public Health Rep* 49:321-346, 1934.

51. Ross, J.A.: Social Class and Medical Care, *J Health Hum Behav* 3:35-40, 1962.

52. Koos, E.L.: *The Health of Regionville*, New York: Columbia University Press, 1954.

53. Elsom, K.A.; Spoont, S.; and Potter, H.P.: An Appraisal of the Periodic Health Examination, *Industr Med Surg* 25:367-371, 1956.

54. Franco, S.C.: The Early Detection of Disease by Periodic Examination, *Industr Med Surg* 25:251-257, 1956.

55. Roberts, N.J.: "Periodic Health-Maintenance Examinations," in Hubbard, J. P. (ed.): *The Early Detection and Prevention of Disease*, New York: McGraw-Hill Book Co. Inc., 1957, pp 27-57.

56. Schenthal, J.E.: Multiphasic Screening of the Well Patient, *JAMA* 172:1-4, 1960.

57. Belcher, J.C.: Acceptance of the Salk Polio Vaccine, *Rural Sociol* 23:158-170, 1958.

58. Cassel, J.: Social and Cultural Considerations in Health Innovations, *Ann NY Acad Sci* 107:739-747, 1963.

59. Deasy, L.C.: Socio-Economic Status and Participation in the Poliomyelitis Vaccine Trial, *Amer Sociol Rev* 21:185-191, 1956.

60. Glasser, M.A.: Study of the Public's Acceptance of the Salk Vaccine Program, *Amer J Public Health* 48:141-146, 1958.

61. Ianni, F.A.J., et al: Age, Social and Demographic Factors in Acceptance of Polio Vaccination, *Public Health Rep* 75:545-556, 1960.

62. Ianni, F.A.J.; Albrecht, R.M.; and Polan, A.K.: Group Attitudes and Information Sources in a Poliovaccine Program, *Public Health Rep* 75:665-671.

63. Winkelstein, W., Jr., and Graham, S.: Factors in Participation in the 1954 Poliomyelitis Vaccine Field Trials, Erie County, New York, *Amer J Public Health* 49:1454-1466, 1959.

64. Collings, G.H.: Is Annual Influenza Immunization Worthwhile in Industry? *J Occup Med* 4:529-531, 1962.

65. Goldstein, D.H., and Benoit, J.N.: "A Study of the Influence of Immunization on the Clinical Course of Asian Influenza in an Industrial Community," read before the Thirteenth International Congress on Occupational Health, New York, 1960: *Proceedings* (New York, 1961) pp 266-270.

66. Greene, C.C., and Beaver, G.T.: A Study of Mass Influenza Inoculation in a Large Industry, *J Occup Med* 2:363-370, 1960.

67. Newquist, M.N., and Page, R.C.: Study of Absenteeism During a Five-month Period, *Industr Med* 15:676-677, 1946.

68. Sinclaire, H.A., et al: Inoculation Against Asian Influenza, *Industr Med Surg* 28:15-19, 1959.

69. Whitney, L.H.: The Control of Acute Respiratory Disease in Industry, *Industr Med Surg* 27:502-505, 1958.

70. Kegeles, S.S.: Why People Seek Dental Care: A Review of Present Knowledge, *Amer J Public Health* 51:1306-1311, 1961.

71. Rosenfeld, L.S., and Donabedian, A.: Prenatal Care in Metropolitan Boston, *Amer J Public Health* 48:1115-1124, 1958.

72. Yankauer, A., et al: A Study of Periodic School Medical Examinations: IV. Educational Aspects, *Amer J Public Health* 51:1532-1540, 1961.

73. Knutson, J.W.: Fluoridation: Where are We Today? *Amer J Nurs* 60:196-198, 1960.

74. Gamson, W.A.: The Fluoridation Dialogue: Is It an Ideological Conflict? *Public Opinion Quart* 25:526-537, 1961.

75. Kirscht, J.P., and Knutson, A.L.: Science and Fluoridation: An Attitude Study, *J Soc Issues* 17:37-44, 1961.

76. Simmel, A.A.: A Signpost for Research on Fluoridation Conflicts: The Concept of Relative Deprivation, *J Soc Issues* 17:26-36, 1961.

77. Brightman, I.J., et al: Knowledge and Utilization of Health Resources by Public Assistance Recipients: I. Public Health and Preventive Medical Resources, *Amer J Public Health* 48:188-199, 1958.

78. Donabedian, A., and Rosenfeld, L.S.: Some Factors Influencing Prenatal Care, *New Eng J Med* 265:1-6, 1961.

79. Yankauer, A., et al: Social Stratification and Health Practices in Child-Bearing and Child-Rearing, *Amer J Public Health* 48:732-741, 1958.

80. Travis, G.: *Chronic Disease and Disability*, Berkeley: University of California Press, 1961.

81. Hawkins, N.G.; Davies, R.; and Holmes, T.H.: Evidence of Psychosocial Factors in the Development of Pulmonary Tuberculosis, *Amer Rev Tuberc* 75:768-780, 1957.

82. Holmes, T.H., et al: Psychosocial and Psychophysiological Studies of Tuberculosis, *Psychosom Med* 19:134-143, 1957.

83. Rahe, R.H., et al: Social Stress and Illness Onset, *J Psychosom Res* 8:35-44, 1964.

84. Weiss, E., et al: Emotional Factors in Coronary Occlusion, *Arch Intern Med* 99:628-641, 1957.

85. Greene, W.A., Jr.: Psychological Factors and Reticuloendothelial Disease: I. Preliminary Observations on a Group of Males With Lymphomas and Leukemias, *Psychosom Med* 16:220-230, 1954.

86. Greene, W.A., Jr., and Miller, G.: Psychological Factors and Reticuloendothelial Disease: IV. Observations on a Group of Children and Adolescents With Leukemia: An Interpretation of Disease

Development in Terms of the Mother-Child Unit, *Psychosom Med* 20:124-144, 1958.

87. Adamson, J.D., and Schmale, A.H., Jr.: Object Loss, Giving Up, and the Onset of Psychiatric Illness, read before the Annual Meeting of the American Psychosomatic Society, Atlantic City, April 27-28, 1963, *Psychosom Med* 25:493, 1963.

88. Schmale, A.H., Jr.: Relationship of Separation and Depression to Disease: I. A Report on a Hospitalized Medical Population, *Psychosom Med* 20:259-277, 1958.

89. Hinkle, L.E., Jr.: Ecological Observations of the Relation of Physical Illness, Mental Illness, and the Social Environment, *Psychosom Med* 23:289-297, 1961.

90. Hinkle, L.E., Jr.: "Physical Health, Mental Health, and the Social Environment: Some Characteristics of Healthy and Unhealthy People," in Ojemann, R. H. (ed.): *Recent Contributions of Biological and Psycho-social Investigations to Preventive Psychiatry*, Iowa City: State University of Iowa Press, 1959, pp 80-103.

91. Hinkle, L.E., Jr., et al: An Investigation of the Relation Between Life Experience, Personality Characteristics, and General Susceptibility to Illness, *Psychosom Med* 20:278-295, 1958.

92. Hinkle, L.E., Jr., et al: Studies in Human Ecology: Factors Relevant to the Occurrence of Bodily Illness and Disturbances in Mood, Thought and Behavior in Three Homogeneous Population Groups, *Amer J Psychiat* 114:212-220, 1957.

93. Hinkle, L.E., Jr., and Wolff, H.G.: The Nature of Man's Adaptation to His Total Environment and the Relation of This to Illness, *Arch Intern Med* 99:442-460, 1957.

94. Hinkle, L.E., Jr., and Wolff, H.G.: "Health and the Social Environment: Experimental Investigations," in Leighton, A. H.; Clausen, J. A.; and Wilson, R. N. (eds.): *Explorations in Social Psychiatry*, New York: Basic Books, Inc., 1957, pp 105-137.

95. Hinkle, L.E., Jr., and Wolff, H.G.: Ecologic Investigations of the Relationship Between Illness, Life Experiences, and the Social Environment, *Ann Intern Med* 49:1373-1388, 1958.

96. Imboden, J.B.; Canter, A.; and Cluff, L.: Separation Experiences and Health Records in a Group of Normal Adults, *Psychosom Med* 25:433-440, 1963.

97. Mechanic, D.: Some Implications of Illness Behavior for Medical Sampling, *New Eng J Med* 269:244-247, 1963.

98. Stoeckle, J.D., and Davidson, G.E.: Bodily Complaints and Other Symptoms of Depressive Reaction, *JAMA* 180:134-139, 1962.

99. Stoeckle, J.D., and Davidson, G.E.: Communicating Aggrieved Feelings in the Patient's Initial Visit to a Medical Clinic, *J Health Hum Behav* 4:199-206, 1963.

100. Stoeckle, J.D., and Zola, I.K.: Views, Problems, and Potentialities of the Clinic, *Medicine* 43:413-422, 1964.

101. Stoeckle, J.D.; Zola, I.K.; and Davidson, G.E.: On Going to See the Doctor, the Contributions of the Patient to the Decision to Seek Medical Aid, *J Chron Dis* 16:975-989, 1963.

102. Stoeckle, J.D.; Zola, I.K.; and Davidson, G.E.: The Quantity and Significance of Psychological Distress in Medical Patients: Some Preliminary Observations About the Decision to Seek Medical Aid, *J Chron Dis* 17:959-970, 1964.

103. Engel, G.L.: Psychogenic Pain, *J Occup Med* 3:249-257, 1961.

104. Kasl, S.V., and Cobb, S.: Some Psychological Factors Associated With Illness Behavior and Selected Illnesses, *J Chron Dis* 17:325-345, 1964.

105. Kasl, S.V., and French, J.R.P., Jr.: The Effects of Occupational Status on Physical and Mental Health, *J Soc Issues* 18:67-89, 1962.

106. Fiedler, F.E., et al: Interrelations Among Measures of Personality Adjustment in Non-Clinical Populations, *J Abnorm Soc Psychol* 56:345-351, 1958.

107. Greenfield, N.S., and Roessler, R.: Hypochondriasis: A Re-Evaluation, *J Nerv Ment Dis* 126:482-484, 1958.

108. Summerskill, J., and Darling, C.D.: Group Differences in the Incidence of Upper Respiratory Complaints Among College Students, *Psychosom Med* 19:315-319, 1957.

109. White, C.; Reznikoff, M.; and Ewell, J.W.: Usefulness of the Cornell Medical Index Health Questionnaire in a College Health Department, *Ment Hyg* 42:94-105, 1958.

110. Welsh, G.S., and Dahlstrom, G.W.: *Basic Readings on the MMPI in Psychology and Medicine*, Minneapolis: The University of Minnesota Press, 1956.

111. Mechanic, D.: The Influence of Mothers on Their Children's Health Attitudes and Behavior, *Pediatrics* 33:444-453, 1964.

112. Gordon, R.E.; Singer, M.B.; and Gordon, K.K.: Social Psychological Stress, *Arch Gen Psychiat* 4:459-470, 1961.

113. Matarazzo, R.G.; Matarazzo, J.D.; and Saslow, G.: The Relationship Between Medical and Psychiatric Symptoms, *J Abnorm Soc Psychol* 62:55-61, 1961.

114. Roessler, R., and Greenfield, N.S.: "Incidence of Somatic Disease in Psychiatric Patients," in Roessler, R., and Greenfield, N. S. (eds.): *Physiological Correlates of Psychological Disorder*, Madison: The University of Wisconsin Press, 1962, pp 257-267.

115. Sainsbury, P.: Psychosomatic Disorders and Neurosis in Outpatients Attending a General Hospital, *J Psychosom Res* 4:261-273, 1960.

116. Blumberg, E.M.: "Results of Psychological Testing of Cancer Patients," in Gengerelli, J. A., and Kirkner, F. J. (eds.): *The Psychological Variables in Human Cancer*, Berkeley: University of California Press, 1954. pp 30-61.

117. Blumberg, E.M.; West, P.M.; and Ellis, F.W.: A Possible Relationship Between Psychological Factors and Human Cancer, *Psychosom Med* 16:277-286, 1954.

118. Krasnoff, A.: Psychological Variables and Human Cancer: A Cross-Validation Study, *Psy-*

chosom Med **21**:291-295, 1959.

119. Perrin, G.M., and Pierce, I.R.: Psychosomatic Aspects of Cancer, *Psychosom Med* **21**: 397-421, 1959.

120. Lieberman, M.A.: Relationship of Mortality Rates to Entrance to a Home for the Aged, *Geriatrics* **16**:515-519, 1961.

121. Dietz, N., Jr.: The Common Cold and Stress Conditions, *Industr Med Surg* **26**:229-233, 1957.

122. Stoeckle, J.D., and Zola, I.K.: After Everyone Can Pay for Medical Care: Some Perspectives on Future Treatment and Practice, *Medical Care* **2**:36-41, 1964.

123. Political and Economic Planning: *Family Needs and the Social Services,* London: G. Allen & Unwin, Ltd., 1961.

124. Pearse, I.H., and Crocker, L.H.: *The Peckham Experiment,* New Haven: Yale University Press, 1946.

125. Zborowski, M.: Cultural Components in Response to Pain, *J Soc Issues* **8**:16-30, 1952.

126. Zola, I.K.: *Socio-Cultural Factors in the Seeking of Medical Air,* PhD dissertation, Harvard University, Cambridge, 1962.

127. Zola, I.K.: Socio-Cultural Factors in the Seeking of Medical Aid: A Progress Report, *Transcultural Psychiat Res* **14**:62-65, 1963.

128. Zola, I.K.: Problems of Communication, Diagnosis, and Patient Care: The Interplay of Patient, Physician, and Clinic Organization, *J Med Educ* **38**:829-838, 1963.

129. Zola, I.K.: "Illness Behavior of the Working Class: Implications and Recommendations," in Shostak, A. B., and Gomberg, W. (eds.): *Blue-Collar World; Studies of the American Worker,* Englewood Cliffs, NJ: Prentice-Hall, Inc., 1964, pp 350-361.

130. Goodman, N., et al: Variant Reactions to Physical Disabilities, *Amer Sociol Rev* **28**:429-435, 1963.

131. Elinson, J., and Trussell, R.E.: Some Factors Relating to Degree of Correspondence for Diagnostic Information as Obtained by Household Interviews and Clinical Examinations, *Amer J Public Health* **47**:311-321, 1957.

132. Friedsam, H.J., and Martin, H.W.: A Comparison of Self and Physicians' Health Ratings in an Older Population, *J Health Hum Behav* **4**:179-183, 1963.

133. Leo, R.G.; Dysterheft, A.H.; and Merkel, G.G.: Health Profile of Lumber Mill Employees, *Industr Med Surg* **26**:377-379, 1957.

134. Maddox, G.L.: Self-Assessment of Health Status: A Longitudinal Study of Selected Elderly Subjects, *J Chron Dis* **17**:449-460, 1964.

135. Suchman, E.A.; Phillips, B.S.; and Streib, G.F.: An Analysis of the Validity of Health Questionnaires, *Social Forces* **36**:223-232, 1958.

136. Thompson, D.J., and Tauber, J.: Household Survey, Individual Interview, and Clinical Examination to Determine Prevalence of Heart Disease, *Amer J Public Health* **47**:1131-1140, 1957.

137. Guilford, J.P.: *Fundamental Statistics in Psychology and Education,* New York: McGraw-Hill Book Co. Inc., 1956.

138. Johnson, L.C.: Body Cathexis as a Factor in Somatic Complaints, *J Consult Psychol* **20**:145-149, 1956.

139. Secord, P.F., and Jourard, S.M.: The Appraisal of Body-Cathexis: Body-Cathexis and the Self, *J Consult Psychol* **17**:343-347, 1953.

140. Mandler, G.; Mandler, J.M.; and Uviller, E.T.: Autonomic Feedback: The Perception of Autonomic Activity, *J Abnorm Soc Psychol* **56**:367-373, 1958.

141. Schnore, L.F., and Cowhig, J.D.: Some Correlates of Reported Health in Metropolitan Centers, *Soc Prob* **7**:218-226, 1959-1960.

142. Felton, J.S.: The Cornell Index Used as an Appraisal of Personality by an Industrial Health Service, *Industr Med* **18**:133-144, 1949.

143. Jaffe, J., and Slote, W.H.: Interpersonal Factors in Denial of Illness, *Arch Neurol Psychiat* **80**:653-656, 1958.

144. Mechanic, D., and Newton, M.: Some Problems in the Analysis of Morbidity Data, *J Chron Dis* **18**:569-580, 1965.

145. Sanders, B.S.: Have Morbidity Surveys Been Oversold? *Amer J Public Health* **52**:1648-1659, 1962.

146. Feldman, J.: The Household Interview Survey as a Technique for the Collection of Morbidity Data, *J Chron Dis* **11**:535-557, 1960.

147. US National Health Survey: *Comparison of Hospitalization Reporting in Three Survey Procedures,* Series D-8, Public Health Service, January, 1963.

148. US National Health Survey: *Health Interview Responses Compared With Medical Records,* Series D-5, Public Health Service, June, 1961.

149. Epstein, F.H.; Boas, E.P.; and Simpson, R.: The Epidemiology of Atherosclerosis Among a Random Sample of Clothing Workers of Different Ethnic Origins in New York City: I. Prevalence of Atherosclerosis and Some Associated Characteristics, *J Chron Dis* **5**:300-328, 1957.

150. Epstein, F.H.; Simpson, R.; and Boas, E.P.: The Epidemiology of Atherosclerosis Among a Random Sample of Clothing Workers of Different Ethnic Origins in New York City: II. Associations Between Manifest Atherosclerosis, Serum Lipid Levels, Blood Pressure, Overweight, and Some Other Variables, *J Chron Dis* **5**:329-341, 1957.

151. Brown, F.; Katz, H.; and Kaufman, M.R.: The Patient Under Study for Cancer: A Personality Evaluation, *Psychosom Med* **23**:166-171, 1961.

152. Cobb, B., et al: Patient-Responsible Delay of Treatment in Cancer, *Cancer* **7**:920-926, 1954.

153. Goldsen, R.K.; Gerhardt, P.R.; and Handy, V.H.: Some Factors Related to Patient Delay in Seeking Diagnosis for Cancer Symptoms, *Cancer* **10**:1-7, 1957.

154. Kutner, B., and Gordon, G.: Seeking Care for Cancer, *J Health Hum Behav* **2**:171-178, 1961.

155. Kutner, B.; Makover, H.B.; and Oppenheim, A.: Delay in the Diagnosis and Treatment of Cancer: A Critical Analysis of the Literature, *J Chron Dis* **7**:95-120, 1958.

156. Levine, G.N.: Anxiety about Illness: Psychological and Social Bases, *J Health Hum Behav* 3:30-34, 1962.

157. Janis, I.L., and Feshbach, S.: Effects of Fear-Arousing Communications, *J Abnorm Soc Psychol* 48:78-92, 1953.

158. Cartwright, A.; Martin, F.M.; and Thomson, J.G.: Health Hazards of Cigarette Smoking: Current Popular Beliefs, *Brit J Prev Soc Med* 14:160-166, 1960.

159. Festinger, L.: *A Theory of Cognitive Dissonance,* Evanston, Ill. Row, Peterson & Co., 1957.

160. Dollard, J., and Miller, N.E.: *Personality and Psychotherapy,* New York: McGraw-Hill Book Co., Inc., 1950.

161. Lewis, L.S., and Lopreato, J.: Arationality, Ignorance, and Perceived Danger in Medical Practices, *Amer Sociol Rev* 27:508-514, 1962.

162. Koos, E.: "Metropolis"—What City People Think of Their Medical Services, *Amer J Public Health* 45:1551-1557, 1955.

163. Jaco, E.G. (ed.): *Patients, Physicians, and Illness,* Glencoe, Ill: The Free Press, 1958.

164. Downes, J.: Cause of Illness Among Males and Females, *Milbank Memorial Fund Quart* 28:407-428, 1950.

165. Standish, S., Jr., et al: *Why Patients See Doctors,* Seattle: University of Washington Press, 1955.

166. Public Health Service: *Health Statistics from the US National Health Survey,* Series B, No. 19, US Department of Health, Education, and Welfare, 1960.

167. Densen, P.M.; Shapiro, S.; and Einhorn, M.: Concerning High and Low Utilizers of Service in a Medical Care Plan, and the Persistence of Utilization Levels Over a Three Year Period, *Milbank Memorial Fund Quart* 37:217-250, 1959.

168. Kedward, H.B.: Social Class Habits of Consulting, *Brit J Prev Soc Med* 16:147-152, 1962.

169. Lerner, M.: *Hospital Use by Diagnosis,* Research Series No. 19, New York: Health Information Foundation, 1961.

170. Department of Public Health: *Annual Report of Saskatchewan Hospital Services Plan,* Province of Saskatchewan, Regina, 1959.

171. Smiley, J.R.; Buck, C.; and Hobbs, G.E.: A Short-Term Longitudinal Morbidity Investigation, *Milbank Memorial Fund Quart* 33:213-229, 1955.

172. Graham, S.: Socio-Economic Status, Illness, and the Use of Medical Services, *Milbank Memorial Fund Quart* 35:58-66, 1957.

173. Davies, A.M.: The Ecological Surveillance of Total Communities, *Milbank Memorial Fund Quart,* to be published.

174. Feldman, J.J.: What Americans Think About Their Medical Care, read before the annual meeting of the American Statistical Association, Chicago, Dec 27-30, 1958.

175. Freidson, E.: The Organization of Medical Practice and Patient Behavior, *Amer J Public Health* 51:43-52, 1961.

176. Valadian, I.; Stuart, H.C.; and Reed, R.B.: Contribution of Respiratory Infections to the Total Illness Experiences of Healthy Children from Birth to 18 Years, *Amer J Public Health* 51:1320-1328, 1961.

177. Blumberg, M.S., and Coffin, J.C.: A Syllabus on Work Absence, *Arch Industr Health* 13:55-70, 1956.

178. Enterline, P.E.: Work Loss Due to Illness in Selected Occupations and Industries, *J Occup Med* 3:405-411, 1961.

179. Gurin, G.; Veroff, J.; and Feld, S.: *Americans View of Their Mental Health,* New York: Basic Books, Inc., 1960.

180. Srole, L., et al: *Mental Health in the Metropolis: The Midtown Manhattan Study,* New York: McGraw-Hill Book Co., Inc., 1962, vol 1.

181. Brill, N.Q., and Storrow, H.A.: Social Class and Psychiatric Treatment, *Arch Gen Psychiat* 3:340-344, 1960.

182. Redlich, F.C.; Hollingshead, A.B.; and Bellis, E.: Social Class Differences in Attitudes Toward Psychiatry, *Amer J Orthopsychiat* 25:60-70, 1955.

183. Schaffer, L., and Myers, J.K.: Psychotherapy and Social Stratification, *Psychiatry* 17:83-93, 1954.

184. Grold, J.L., and Hill, W.G.: Failure to Keep Appointments With the Army Psychiatrist: An Indicator of Conflict, *Amer J Psychiat* 119:446-450, 1962.

185. Terwilliger, J.S., and Fiedler, F.E.: An Investigation of Determinants Inducing Individuals to Seek Personal Counseling, *J Consult Psychol* 22:288, 1958.

186. Nunnally, J., and Kittross, J.M.: Public Attitudes Toward Mental Health Professions, *Amer Psychol* 13:589-594, 1958.

187. Cole, N.J.; Branch, C.H.H.; and Shaw, O.M.: Mental Illness: A Survey Assessment of Community Rates, Attitudes, and Adjustments, *Arch Neurol Psychiat* 77:393-398, 1957.

188. Hollingshead, A.B., and Redlich, F.C.: *Social Class and Mental Illness,* New York, John Wiley & Sons, Inc., 1958.

189. Rawnsley, K., and London, J.B.: Factors Influencing the Referral of Patients to Psychiatrists by General Practitioners, *Brit J Prev Soc Med* 16:174-182, 1962.

190. Blackwell, B.: The Literature of Delay in Seeking Medical Care for Chronic Illnesses, *Health Educ Monograph* No. 16, pp 3-31, 1963.

Modifying and Developing Health Behavior

by Lawrence W. Green

Center for Health Promotion Research and Development, The University of Texas, Health Science Center at Houston, Houston, Texas 77225

INTRODUCTION

Public health has turned more and more in recent years to the social and behavioral sciences for a better understanding of the forces shaping lifestyle, conditioning health habits, influencing the diffusion of health knowledge, attitudes and practices, and providing support or pressure for the adoption of healthy and unhealthy behavior. This review examines recent developments specifically in those applications leading to interventions designed to modify or develop health behavior.

Modifying and developing health behavior both imply change of a conscious and planned nature, as distinct from change that occurs unconsciously in the natural history of growth and adaptation (51, 131, 132). This distinction has become blurred in modern societies that are conscious of and sophisticated about behavior, its causes, and ways to influence it. Individuals, families, health practitioners, health agencies, private organizations, and governments all have expanding repertoires of understanding and tools to modify and develop their own behavior and the behavior of their members, constituents, and consumers. At the same time, all of them may be developing conscious and unconscious repertoires of defense and resistance to the attempts of others to change them.

Because these repertoires have become so enriched and diverse, this review can only offer a superficial coverage of the major lines of recent advances. This is attempted first by outlining some alternative and complementary frameworks for organizing theory, research, policy, and practice in behavioral change for health. Second, some of these frameworks, notably those of the life span and the settings for health promotion, are used to present examples of the application of behavioral change strategies for health enhancement, and to highlight some issues of policy, ethics, and research confronting future applications of behavioral change in public health.

The author would like to thank for helpful comments Patricia Mullen and for assistance Blair Carter.

FRAMEWORKS TO ORGANIZE THE LITERATURE

Processes of Change

In an earlier attempt (58) to review and organize the diverse theoretical models and research literature related to change processes in health behavior, variables from psychology, sociology, anthropology, and their hybrids were arrayed under Kelman's (80) three processes of individual change: internalization, identification, and compliance. In returning to the literature for a similar review eight years later, one encounters again the problem of language: "One of the issues with which one must deal in the integration of models from the different disciplines, is not whether one or the other is more correct, but whether they are talking about the same thing in different languages" (58, p. 7). What Kelman called the "compliance" process of change, others refer to as environmental or economic contingencies, coercion, paternalism, passive controls on behavior, prescribed or proscribed norms or customs, and various neologisms (79, 99, 107, 111, 129, 131, 189). Kelman's "identification" process of change has been recast in social learning theory (6, 143) to include modeling, vicarious reinforcement, and the normative or social influence of significant others (25, 45, 47, 57, 98). Kelman's "internalization" process of change has come to be associated with terms and concepts such as value congruence, self-actualization, information processing, and informed consent (40, 49, 68, 86, 111, 112). All of these have served to describe and explain instances of behavioral change in relation to health, and some have been used as the theoretical rationale in the design of interventions.

Organizational and Theoretical Levels of Change

A second typology used to array the variables and concepts of change at several levels of aggregation considers organizational levels of change or units of analysis: the individual system, the group system, and the institutional or community system. The internal dynamics of the individual system are limited to psychological variables. Patient counseling, behavioral therapy, and mass media strategies in health have all derived largely from psychological theory and research. Changes in informal and membership groups resulting from individual and group effects are reflected primarily in the theories and variables of social psychology. Group instruction, social support strategies, and self-help groups have evolved with particular influence from social psychology. Changes at the institutional or community level include variables from sociology, anthropology, economics, and political science.

None of these levels or units of analysis has gone without theoretical and empirical scrutiny by one or more of the disciplines named, but the dominant contributions to the literature on interventions in health have been, perhaps regrettably, from psychology (6, 10–15, 26–29, 35–39, 43, 47, 54, 62, 70, 74, 75, 85, 101, 105, 106, 117–120, 156, 165–167, 184, 193, 194). Sociologists, whether for reasons of academic disdain or lack of opportunity, have contributed for the most part only indirectly to the development of interventions, though most of their theories and research are most significantly relevant to public health (155). Even in large-scale community interventions such as the Stanford three-community and five-community studies, the behavioral science contributions to planning the interventions have been made primarily by psychologists (41, 121). The result is that the behavioral change interventions have tended to emphasize the individual, and have been most useful in patient education (4, 10, 13, 29, 43, 54, 59, 64, 101, 113, 115, 116, 134, 135, 138, 162, 163, 165). This concentration of behavioral science applications is sometimes at the expense of action on needed change in organizational, institutional, environmental, and economic conditions shaping behavior.

Classification of Health-related Behavior

A third typology or framework for analysis of health behavior has emerged since Parson's (145) description of sick-role behavior in sociological terms, and since Kasl & Cobb (78) distinguished the sick role from illness behavior and health behavior. The call for finer distinctions has mounted. Baric (7) added the "quasi-sick role" or "at-risk" behavior, which has come to be associated in practice with risk reduction and "prospective medicine" (153, 137, 178). Others have struggled with the variety of overlapping forms of behavior, such that there has developed a specialized literature in "wellness" behavior (e.g. 1, 33, 177), one in self-care behavior (56, 102, 112), and one in "compliance" or adherance to medical regimens (10, 29, 64). Self-care and compliance behavior generally refer to the opposite extremes of dependency on therapists in sick-role behavior. When the relationships between patients and therapists are added to the delineation of behavior, the complexities of classification multiply (113, 114, 165).

Table 1, developed from Kolbe (88), defines nine distinguishable, though not entirely mutually exclusive, health-related types of behavior. Although greater specificity of this kind is helpful in the scientific measurement and

Table 1   A typology of health-related behaviors[a]

Behavior	Definition
Wellness behavior	Any activity undertaken by an individual, who believes himself to be healthy, for the purpose of attaining an even greater level of health.
Preventive health behavior	Any activity undertaken by an individual, who believes himself to be healthy, for the purpose of preventing illness or detecting it in an asymptomatic state.
At-risk behavior	Any activity undertaken by an individual, who believes himself to be healthy but at greater risk than normal of developing a specific health condition, for the purpose of preventing that condition or detecting it in an asymptomatic state.
Illness behavior	Any activity undertaken by an individual, who perceives himself to be ill, to define the state of his health and discover a suitable remedy.
Self-care behavior	Any activity undertaken by an individual, who considers himself to be ill, for the purpose of getting well. It includes minimal reliance on appropriate therapists, involves few dependent behaviors, and leads to little neglect of one's usual duties.
Sick-role behavior	Any activity undertaken by an individual, who considers himself to be ill, for the purpose of getting well. It includes receiving treatment from appropriate therapists, generally involves a whole range of dependent behaviors, and leads to some degree of neglect of one's usual duties.
Family planning behavior	Any activity undertaken by an individual to influence the occurrence or normal continuation of pregnancy.
Parenting health behavior	Any wellness, preventive, at-risk, illness, self-care, or sick-role behavior performed by an individual for the purposes of ensuring, maintaining, or improving the health of a conceptus or child for whom the individual has responsibility.
Health-related social action	Any activity undertaken by an individual singularly or in concert with others (i.e. collectively) through organizational, legal, or economic means, to influence the provision of medical services, the effects of the environment, the effects of various products, or the effects of social regulations that influence the health of populations.

[a]From Kolbe (88).

analysis, and in the programmatic targeting, of behavior, there may be a simultaneous need for pulling back to more generalized conceptualizations of complex, overlapping behavioral patterns related to health. This may be particularly needed in the analysis of statistical and practical interactions among the health practices making up the "lifestyle" risk factors for chronic diseases (e.g. 34, 76, 77, 87), for injuries and accidental death (e.g. 31, 65, 154, 161), for addictions, homicides, suicides, mental illness, and social well-being (3, 8, 9, 20, 32, 35, 45, 81, 94, 100, 114, 179–82, 185, 187, 192), as well as those making up the various aspects of parenting (60, 73, 97, 98, 108, 126, 150, 158), and use of health services across the spectrum of primary to tertiary care (97, 126, 164).

Life Transitions Requiring Adaptations of Health Behavior

A fourth dimension for the organization of theory and research, which is applied in this review, is a time dimension reflecting life transitions, particularly those of the life span (sometimes referred to as life cycle). This dimension has particular utility in public health, because no demographic marker, including sex or socioeconomic status, differentiates patterns of lifestyle and health more significantly than age. Other transitions, such as residential mobility, divorce, marriage, retirement, and sudden unemployment are comparable in their impact on the needs for lifestyle adjustment and problems of coping, but these too tend to be associated with stages in the life span.

Range of Interventions to Modify or Develop Health Behavior

A fifth dimension is the range of interventions for behavioral change. It has long been the contention of public health educators that policies directing their practice need to recognize that health behavior is shaped and buffeted by more than individual motivation and choice (e.g. 140). Education directed only at the individual has been used intentionally in some policies as an alternative to more appropriate interventions directed at organizations, industries, or environments that control the resources or conditions compelling or constraining health behavior (2, 40, 44, 47, 49, 55, 59–61, 90, 125, 152).

Since 1976, with the passage of P.L. 94–317 by the US Congress that year, the term "health promotion" has taken on new meaning in public health, and has breathed new life into health education. The Consumer Health Information and Health Promotion Act of 1976 gave the federal government a broader mandate for initiating programs and using a wider range of strategies to influence health behavior than previous policies in support of health education had provided in the United States. The informational role of government was still paramount, but the placement of the new initiative in the Office of the Assistant Secretary for Health opened new opportunities for policies to be promulgated in support of organizational, economic, and environmental factors, which health educators had always complained stood between their best efforts and effective development or modification of public health behavior.

Settings or Channels for Health Behavior Change

With these changes in the policies governing behavioral change strategies in public health, the subject now can be addressed with more than theoretical and political interest in the settings where economic and environmental factors influence health behavior. There is, consequently, a widening acceptance in practice of a definition of health promotion that encompasses these broader influences on lifestyle, rather than merely information directed at individual knowledge, attitudes, and behavior.

The definition of health promotion adopted for purposes of this review is "any combination of health education and related organizational, economic and environmental supports for individual, group and community behavior conducive to health" (51, 60). The behavior in question ultimately is that of the person whose health is at risk (or whose health enhancement is sought), but the processes of change often must include institutional decision-makers and collectivities of people acting in concert as groups, neighborhoods, organizations, communities, and electorates. Behavior at all of these levels and education through all of these channels is the object of health promotion. The settings in which health promotion may take place, then, become a primary consideration for this review.

Settings for health promotion include most notably schools, worksites, homes, and health care settings. They provide most of the services and resource supports for health behavior, simultaneously with serving their primary institutional functions. Channels for health promotion include the mass media, parents, teachers, counselors, physicians, nurses, self-help groups, and other individuals and media through which information, training, and persuasion may predispose, enable, and reinforce voluntary adaptations of behavior (55).

In addition to the organizational and educational components of the health promotion approach to the modification and development of behavior, there are aspects of the environment that require regulation beyond the voluntary control of individuals and organizations. These include physical, economic, social, and legal aspects of community life over which individuals may have little personal control and over which organizations may have limited control but may also have vested interests in not controlling, such as chemical wastes, or allowing workers to exercise on company time. Organizations might view their own gains from such reforms as too small to justify their costs. Regulation and incentives may be required in such cases.

Some of these environmental factors, like chemical wastes, have a direct effect on health; others, like facilities for employee fitness, influence health through their influence on behavior. Those that influence health through behavior are a part of health promotion. Those that influence health through the environment are referred to as health protection.

Figure 1 expresses the relationships among these and health services in the context of federal policy and the *Objectives for the Nation* in disease prevention and health promotion in the United States (48, 50, 72, 124, 170–172), which

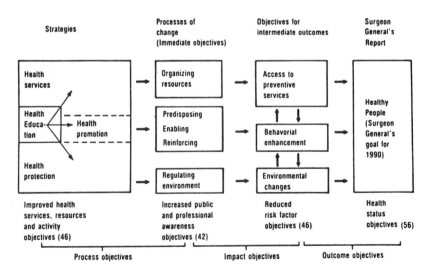

Figure 1 Structure and logical relationships of the objectives for the nation in disease prevention and health promotion.

represent a coordinated strategy of federal, state, local, voluntary, and private sector activities in health. The three components of organization, behavior, and environment in the United States' strategy approximate the "health field" components of the Lalonde report (96), which initiated a similar shift in health policy in Canada in 1974. Similar emphases on the behavioral or lifestyle component of health policy were introduced in Great Britain with the "red book" entitled *Prevention and Health: Everybody's Business, 1976* (46), and in Australia with *Health Promotion in Australia 1978–1979* (30).

Health promotion received its most global extension in policy with the joint declaration of the World Health Organization and UNICEF of a commitment to the development of policies in "primary health care," which they defined to include health education and participation of the public as essential elements (191). The so-called Alma-Ata Declaration set into motion a long-range strategy of "Health for All by the Year 2000," and a dedication of the World Health Assembly's Technical Discussions of 1982 to the topic of alcohol consumption (129) and in 1983 to the topic "New Policies for Health Education in Primary Health Care" (61). This was the first time in 22 years that the World Health Assembly Technical Discussions had been devoted to educational and behavioral aspects of health.

Figure 2 reflects the placement of health education and health behavior in the global strategy of WHO. The emphasis here is on participation of the public in planning and evaluating the primary health programs for their localities (61, 173, 191). The clear understanding is that participation is necessary to assure that the programs reflect the felt needs and cultural perspectives of the people for whom they are intended, and that health education is essential to the effective participation of people.

Some Cautious Generalizations

In summary, change in health behavior has been studied and attempted in public health from a variety of vantage points, theoretical inclinations, organizational levels, and disciplinary backgrounds; in a variety of settings; and with a variety of interventions. No single theory, method, or strategy has been found to hold any universal superiority over others. A few principles might be drawn from the elements common to most successful strategies, such as the principle of participation, which asserts that people are more likely to change and maintain the change in their behavior if they have participated actively in

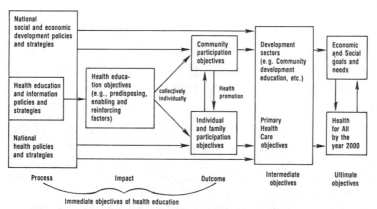

Figure 2 Logic and rationale for the assumed relationships among strategies and objectives for new policies in health education as related to primary health care and the global strategy for "Health for All by the Year 2000."

setting the goals and plans for the change. If one is seeking highly generalizable rules to guide public health programs directed at behavioral change, the principle of participation, like the principle of individualizing and tailoring interventions, is no generalization at all. It says, in effect, beware of generalizations. Idiosyncracy has reigned in most behavioral science applications to health, as it has in medicine. Hence, the majority of the contributions by behavioral scientists to the health literature have been by psychologists, whose business is individual behavior, and most of their publications are based on studies carried out in clinical and other highly controlled settings.

Public health seeks another level of generalization, or at least ways to apply the psychological generalizations to populations and in settings or institutions other than just clinical or medical settings. Renewed interest in worksites, schools, and other community settings and institutions that can affect behavior is evident. Such epidemiological, sociological, organizational, and environmental perspectives have been addressed in the most recent round of policy initiatives in disease prevention and health promotion in several English-speaking and European countries, and in the global policies of the World Health Organization.

The common elements of these new policies reflect some of the generalizations that have been drawn, with or without the explicit guidance of empirical evidence from the behavioral sciences:

1. Behavior, especially in its more complex lifestyle manifestations, accounts for a much larger proportion of the total mortality and morbidity of most societies than is reflected in the allocation of resources to modify or develop health behavior.

2. Effective programs to modify or develop health behavior in populations must include some combination of health education and organizational, economic, and environmental supports for the behavior.

3. Policies addressing health behavior cannot be made a substitute for the provision of basic, primary health care services or regulation of environmental factors influencing health. Instead, these components of health services and environmental health policy can support health behavior at the same time that they are directly addressing health through biomedical and environmental interventions.

These generalizations are summarized in Table 2 which combines some of the essential features of Figures 1 and 2 and much of the preceding discussion. It does not address questions of when or how to intervene to modify or develop health behavior. It also does not suggest who the target groups for intervention should be. These are unavoidable questions for any public health strategy and are taken up in the remainder of this review.

TIME-AND-PLACE STRATEGIES TO MODIFY OR DEVELOP HEALTH BEHAVIOR

The Life Span

The ideal intervention in public health in general, and in health promotion in particular, is one that anticipates health problems or needs and prepares the host to resist the problem or to provide for the need. If the environment can be structured to preclude the need for any action on the part of the host, so much the better. If the agent can be isolated and neutralized, better yet. Unfortunately, the agents of the new behavioral morbidities are pervasive and tightly woven parts of the fabric of modern living, such as rich foods, alcohol, drugs, sedentary work and leisure, stress, guns, and automobiles and other machinery.

Table 2 Essential elements of comprehensive policies combining organizational, educational, economic, and environmental supports for health behavior

Settings/channels	Interventions	Function	Impact	Outcome

Organizations
   Worksites
   Health care
   Schools
   etc.
	Services &
	resources
		To enable ──→	Biological
			development
			or adaptation	

Channels
   Parents
   Mass media
   Teachers
   Counselors
   Physicians
   Nurses
   Self-help groups
   etc.
	Education	To predispose──→	Behavioral ──→
			development
			and change
				Health,
				quality
				of life

Environments
   Political
   Physical
   Economic
   Social
   Legal
	Regulation
	& development
		To protect ──→
		and reinforce
			Environmental
			development
			& enhancement	

Few societies have been willing to turn back the clock on such agents. Some can be controlled through environmental regulation of their distribution, pricing, taxation, and public use, but most of these agents are used privately. There is little choice, then, but to supplement organizational, economic, and environmental strategies with interventions designed to build host resistance.

Anticipating potential health problems or needs of individuals or populations requires prediction of probabilities based on past experience with other people who have been exposed to the same agents under similar circumstances. As suggested in a preceding section, the best predictor of health or behavioral problems or needs is age. Transitions from one age range to another could be the most propitious times to intervene for purposes of primary prevention.

The life span is a natural—in the literal sense—approach to the study of human behavior (5, 16, 24, 57, 126). The life span has been applied in the US Surgeon General's Report (170) to the design of national goals and health policy. As shown in Table 3, the life span may be divided into numerous phases, demarcated by important transitions or events, each with a different set of coping tasks and health consequences if behavior is not adequately adapted. The number of stages and the specific boundaries of the stages will vary from one population or culture to another, and from one investigator or health professional to another. Vaillant (175, 176), Levinson (103), and Loevinger (109) have delineated in much greater detail the phases and stages of adult development, as Kohlberg & Mayer (86), and Piaget (147) have done with children.

The following discussion divides the life span, somewhat arbitrarily but in keeping with the Surgeon General's Report (170), into five stages: infancy (less than one year old), childhood (1–14 years), adolescence and young adulthood (15–24 years), adulthood (25–64 years), and older adults (65 years and older. Table 4 arrays these five age groups against the settings in which behavioral or health promotion interventions are possible, with examples in each intersect, based on an analysis by Mullen (130). Two points are illustrated by this matrix:

Table 3 Examples of issues for health promotion related to life span transitions

Developmental transitions	Major tasks of coping and adaptation	Health consequences
Infant → child	Avoidance of hazards	Safety and injury control
Preschool → school	Selection of foods	Dental caries, obesity, nutritional deficiencies
Elem. → jr. high (early adolescence)	Resistance to peer pressure; changing bodily functions	Smoking, alcohol, drugs, pregnancy
Jr. high → high school (middle adolescence)	Development of autonomous identity and confidence	Substance abuse, pregnancy, auto accidents, sexually transmitted diseases
High school → work or higher education	Development of autonomous function and role; coping skills; uprooting	Suicide, homicide, alcoholism, addictions
Single → married and/or pregnancy and parenthood	Curtailed freedom & increased responsibility for lifestyle; uprooting	Congenital defects, infant mortality, low birth weight, obesity
Young adult → middle age ("midlife" transition) Parent → "empty nest"	Reduced parenting roles, changing bodily function, reduced activity	Hypertension, digestive disease, atrophy, obesity, alcoholism
Working adult → retired adult or widowed	Reduced social roles; sedentary living; bereavement	Loneliness, reduced self-esteem, atrophy, loss of reasons for living and the will to live, or zest for living

first, none of the age groups are dependent on any single setting for intervention, and second, none of the settings is limited to a single age group in the opportunities it presents for health promotion interventions.

Two principal threats to infant health are low birth weight and congenital disorders including birth defects. Public health programs lay emphasis on strategies supporting prenatal health behavior, including the reduced misuse of alcohol, tobacco, and drugs during pregnancy, to reduce both of these problems. The behavioral change and health promotion issues in prenatal care and reproductive health are reviewed by Mullen et al (133). Some issues of measurement and evaluation on the impact of interventions to improve prenatal care are reviewed by Peoples & Siegel (146).

The primary preventable health threat to children 1–14 years is injuries. Injuries account for 45% of total childhood mortality: "By itself, a 50 percent reduction in fatal accidents would be enough to achieve the goal of fewer than 34 deaths per 100,000 by 1990" (170, p. 33). Another behavioral priority for this age group is improved exercise to enhance growth and development. The literature regarding behavioral change in this group was reviewed for the Select Panel on the Promotion of Child Health by Mullen (131, 132), for schools by Iverson & Kolbe (72) and Kolbe (88), Kreuter & Christianson (93), and in general by Bruhn & Parcel (23). Some recent evaluations (27, 42, 63, 67, 82, 110, 122, 127, 142, 148, 151, 174, 183) and meta-evaluations (39, 52, 69, 71, 104, 141, 157, 159, 168; L. J. Kolbe, in preparation) of school health education are more encouraging than earlier reports (cf 84, 160, 190). Programs, measurement instrumentation, and evaluation designs have all shown impressive development in recent years (53, 89, 149). Debates con- tinue on the appropriate outcome measures for school health interventions among cognitive, behavioral, and epidemiological criteria (89, 90, 93, 169, 186).

Table 4 Examples of health promotion activities in various settings for major age groups[a]

	Infants	Children	Adolescents and young adults	Adults	Older adults
Schools	• Support programs for adolescent parents • Parenting education in school curricula (for both boys and girls)	• Comprehensive health education curricula with emphasis on positive health behaviors • Physical fitness testing, training and awards programs • Health screening and immunization programs • Healthful snacks in vending machines	• Development of overall school climate of discipline and achievement • School health education curricula with emphasis on positive health behaviors • Establishment of peer-group counseling efforts	• Health education programs through community colleges and high school evening programs • Extension of high school exercise facilities for adult use • Health education classes through colleges and universities	• Extension of school meal programs to older adults • Volunteer service opportunities to promote interaction between older adults and children
Worksites	• Employer-sponsored day care programs, including parent education and support groups • Maternity/paternity leave and related programs that facilitate family formation • Policies that facilitate breastfeeding • Notification of employees about reproductive risks associated with work environments • Flexible work schedules for parents	• Family health and safety topics in health promotion programs	• Family use of worksite exercise facilities • Flexible work policies to maximize opportunities for adolescents	• Health promotion and employee counseling programs • High blood pressure detection and treatment programs • Provision of exercise facilities • Organization-wide policies designating nonsmoking areas • Cafeteria programs to promote good nutrition • Policies and programs to help ensure a safe and healthy work environment • Reduction of excessive stress in the work environment	• Expansion of worksite health promotion programs to retirees • Lifting mandatory retirement age • Flexible work schedules to ease retirement transition
Health care settings	• Nutrition counseling and guidance in risk reduction for pregnant women and parents of infants • Information and support for breastfeeding • Parent counseling on infant screening to identify high risk families • Poisoning prevention programs • Community outreach and education	• Counseling for parents on normal childhood growth and development • Education for parents on health habit formation and child safety • Classes for parents about home care of minor acute illness and injuries • Involvement of children in decisions about their health care	• Adolescent health counseling programs	• Education and counseling programs to reduce risk and maintain therapeutic regimens • Education about unnecessary surgery and procedures; second opinion programs • Self-care education	• Improved training of health care providers for geriatric practice • Development of home care alternatives to institutionalization
Communities	• Nutrition programs for pregnant and lactating women • Media campaigns such as "Healthy Mothers, Healthy Babies" • Support and education for parents • Injury control programs and ordinances	• Public service announcements countering advertisements directed at children • Assistance for parents in educating their children about sex and family life • After-school recreation programs	• Volunteer service opportunities • Targeted media programs, such as the 1982 Alcohol Abuse Prevention campaign • Adolescent health education programs sponsored by youth serving agencies	• National Health Promotion Training Network, e.g., health education and support programs sponsored by coalitions of local organizations • Media campaigns such as "HealthStyle" • Improved nutrition information through food labeling, print and electronic media, and advertising • Community intervention programs for specific health risks, such as the Trilateral High Blood Pressure Education Program	• Meals on Wheels and other nutrition support programs • Education on hypothermia and heat stress • Walking groups and exercise programs designed for older adults • Promotion of positive attitudes toward aging and the elderly • Bereavement counseling • Senior health promotion volunteer programs • Promotion of drug profile records

[a]From Mullen (130).

Adolecents entering the 15–24 year age range can be expected to face potential problems of motor vehicle crashes and temptations to take up alcohol, tobacco, and drugs (136). This is the only age group in the United States that has experienced an increase in mortality in the recent past. The modification and development of health behavior in this age group are reviewed most extensively and recently in Botvin & McAlister (19), Coates et al (28), Kolbe & Iverson (91), and Kovar (92). Brachman and associates (3) provide the most extensive longitudinal data on this critical transition.

Adulthood is the age of chronic disease. Substantial health promotion intervention is warranted for the reduction of mortality and morbidity resulting from heart disease, cancer, and strokes. These, together with accidental deaths, make up the four leading causes of premature death in the United States. The risk factors for all of these are primarily associated with behavior. Life span analyses of health behavior change in this age range include Breslow & Enstrom (21), Breslow & Somers (22), Green (57), and Vaillant (176). The most impressive advances in the development of population-based interventions to support behavior conducive to health in this age range, besides the patient education programs referred to in previous sections, have been in worksites (144).

As the elderly population grows, the health concerns of this age group are bound to become increasingly salient. Reducing premature death from influenza and pneumonia, reducing injuries due to falls, and increasing the population of very elderly who can function independently are high priority items for the promotion of health in this age range. Recent reviews of the research literature on health behavior modification and development in the elderly include Borgatta & McClusky (17), Borup & Gallego (18), Nickoley-Colquitt (139), and Windsor and associates (188). Contrary to the stereotypes held by many health workers, the elderly are found in evaluative research studies to be as much if not more responsive to behavioral change supports than younger patients or subjects (128).

Other Transitions

In addition to life span transitions, there are transitions from one status, role, or circumstance to another that require adaptations of lifestyle and problems of stress and coping similar to those of the life span. The high degree of mobility in American life presents individuals, families, social groups, organizations, and communities with problems of uprooting, discontinuity of social support, isolation, confusion, and economic insecurity. A general model for the distribution of health promotion concerns over the natural history of transitions in time, place or role is presented in Table 5. It is suggested as a framework to integrate the life-span approach and the life-events approach to the prevention of health problems by building host resistance and providing the necessary organizational, economic, and environmental supports for behavioral adaptations that are constructive rather than destructive.

The first row of Table 5 identifies stages in the natural history of coping with transitions or stressful events. The second row suggests the ways in which health promotion, as defined in this paper, can anticipate and intervene at each of the stages of the natural history. The third row states the objective of health promotion or behavioral interventions at each stage, from primary prevention through rehabilitation.

The major advantage of the life transitions or events approach to health promotion is that it is not specific to any particular disease, but can anticipate a great number of potential problems known to compromise host resistance and resources and to lead to risk factors for most of the leading causes of death and disability. Combined with the organization of interventions around settings for

Table 5 Proposed framework for analysis of problems in health behavior

	Primary prevention		Secondary prevention	
Natural history:	Critical transition or event	Environmental and internal demands on personal resources	Coping and adaptation	Health effects
Health promotion interventions:	Anticipatory guidance and education	Social support and self-care education	Professional and institutional response; organizational, economic and environmental supports	Patient education and mutual self-help groups
Objectives:	Prevent exposure or build "host resistance" to stress or risk	Strengthen personal resources	Compensate for inadequate personal resources, or reinforce successful adaptation	Treatment and rehabilitation to hasten return to maximum functioning

health promotion, this framework encompasses both the time and place dimensions of for public health strategies to modify or develop behavior.

SUMMARY

The literatures on both behavior modification and behavioral development have engendered innovations in public health programs, addressing problems of patient adherance to preventive and therapeutic regimens, delay in seeking diagnosis of illness symptoms, risk-taking behavior, and other aspects of lifestyle associated with health. Because most of this literature derives from psychology, there has been a distinct bias in the construction of interventions, pointing them directly at individuals, usually in a counseling or small group mode of delivery. These developments served public health well enough during a decade or so when the preoccupation was with utilization of health services and medical management of chronic diseases.

With the publication of the Lalonde Report in Canada in 1974, the passage of Public Law 94–317 in 1976 in the United States, and similar initiatives in other English-speaking and European countries, the recognition of the greater complexities of lifestyle development and modification in the absence of symptoms has taken hold. Policy makers and public health workers seek a more efficient and equitable set of strategies to meet the behavioral health challenges of modern society without placing the entire weight of responsibility for behavior on the individual or on therapeutic practitioners. Concurrently, on a more global scale and in the developing countries, a concern has emerged for strategies that give individuals, families, and communities a greater role in deciding their own health priorities.

The convergence of these two trends—one seeking to distribute responsibility for lifestyle more equitably and the other seeking to distribute responsibility for planning health programs more equitably—calls for policies, strategies, and interventions that will place similar emphasis on health education and organizational, economic, and environmental supports for health behavior. The combination of these elements of support for behavior calls, in turn, for research and more inventive applications of theory from sociology, political science, economics, and anthropology. Public health workers will need to become more conversant and facile in these social sciences, as they have in psychology and its applications in the recent past.

Literature Cited

1. Albert, M. P., Caughron, S. D. 1980. Developing a wellness model in family practice. *Phys. Patient Educ. Newslett.* 3:3–4
2. Allegrante, J. P., Green, L. W. 1981. When health policy becomes victim blaming. *N. Eng. J. Med.* 305:1528–29
3. Bachman, J. G., Johnson, L. D., O'Malley, P. M. 1981. Smoking, drinking and drug use among American high school students: Correlates and trends, 1975–1979. *Am. J. Public Health* (71(1)59–59
4. Bailit, H. L., Silversin, B., eds. 1981. Oral health behavior research: Review and new directions. *J. Behav. Med.* 4:243–379
5. Baltes, P. B., Brim, O. G. Jr., eds. 1980. *Life Span Development and Behavior.* New York: Academic
6. Bandura, A. 1969. *Principles of Behavior Modification.* New York: Rinehart & Winston
7. Baric, L. 1969. Recognition of the "at-risk" role: A means to influence behavior. *Int. J. Health Educ.* 12:24–34
8. Baric, L. 1979. Non-smokers, smokers and ex-smokers: Three separate problems for health education. *Int. J. Health Educ.* 22(1):1–20 Suppl.
9. Barnes, G. E. 1979. The alcholic personality: A reanalysis of the literature. *J. Studies Alcohol* 40(7):571–634
10. Becker, H. H., Maiman, L. A. 1980. Strategies for enhancing patient compliance. *J. Community Health* 6:113–35
11. Becker, M. H., ed. 1974. The health belief model and personal health behavior. *Health Educ. Monogr.* 2:324–473
12. Becker, M. H. 1979. Understanding patient compliance: The contributions of attitudes and other psychosocial factors. In *New Directions in Patient Compliance,* ed. S. J. Cohen. Lexington, Mass.: Lexington Books
13. Benfari, R. C., Eaker, E., Stoll, J. G. 1981. Behavioral interventions and compliance to treatment regimes. *Ann. Rev. Public Health* 2:431–71
14. Benfari, R. C., Ockene, J. K., McIntrye, K. M. 1982. Control of cigarette smoking from a psychological perspective. *Ann. Rev. Public Health* 3:101–28
15. Benfari, R. C., Sherwin, R. 1981. Forum: The multiple risk factor intervention trial (MRFIT). The methods and impact of intervention over four years. *Prev. Med.* 10(4) (whole issue)
16. Block, J. 1969. *Lives Through Time.* Berkeley: Bancroft Bowles
17. Borgatta, E., McCluskey, N., eds. 1980. *Aging and Society.* Beverly Hills: Sage
18. Borup, J., Gallego, D. 1981. Mortality as affected by interinstitutional relocation: Update and reassessment. *Gerontologist* 21:8–16
19. Botvin, G., McAlister, A. 1981. Cigarette smoking among children and adolescents. In *Advances in Diseases Prevention, Vol. 1,* ed. C. Arnold, L. Kuller, M. Greenlick, New York: Springer
20. Boyle, M. H., Chambers, L. W. 1981. Indices of social well-being applicable to children—A review. *Soc. Sci. Med.* 15E(3):161–71
21. Breslow, L., Enstrom, J. E. 1980. Persistence of health habits and their rela-

tionship to mortality. *Prev. Med.* 9:469–83
22. Breslow, L., Somers, A. R. 1977. The lifetime health monitoring program. *N. Eng. J. Med.* 296:601–8
23. Bruhn, J. G., Parcel, G. S. 1982. Current knowledge about the health behavior of young children: A conference summary. *Health Educ. Q.* 9:142–66
24. Brunswick, A. F. 1980. Health, stability, and change: A study of urban black youth. *Am. J. Public Health* 70:504–13
25. Catania, A. C., Brigham, T. A., eds. 1978. *Handbook of Applied Behavior Analysis: Social and Instructional Processes.* New York: Irvington
26. Chafetz, M. C. 1981. *Health Education: An Annotated Bibliography on Lifestyle, Behavior and Health.* New York: Plenum
27. Coates, T. J., Jeffrey, R. W., Slinkard, L. A. 1981. Heart healthy eating and exercise: Introducing and maintaining changes in health behaviors. *Am. J. of Public Health* 71:15–23
28. Coates, T. J., Perry, C., Peterson, A. C., eds. 1982. *Promoting Adolescent Health: A Dialog on Research and Practice.* New York: Academic
29. Cohen, S., ed. 1979. *New Directions in Patient Compliance.* Lexington, Mass: Lexington Books/Health
30. Davidson, L., Chapman, S., Hull, C. 1979. *Health Promotion in Australia, 1978–1979.* Canberra: Commonwealth of Australia
31. Douglas, R. L. 1982. Youth, alcohol and traffic accidents. *Alcohol and Health Monograph No. 4: Special Population Issues.* DHHS Pub. No. (ADM) 82–1193 Public Health Service. Rockville, Md.: Alcohol, Drug Abuse and Mental Health Admin.
32. DuPont, R. L., Basen, M. M. 1980. Control of alcohol and drug abuse in industry—A literature review. *Public Health Rep.* 95(2):137–48
33. Dunn, H. L. 1959. High-level wellness for man and society. *Am. J. Public Health* 49(6):786–92
34. Dwyer, T., Hetzel, B. S. 1980. A comparison of trends of coronary heart disease mortality in Australia, U.S.A. and England and Wales with reference to three major risk factors—hypertension, cigarette smoking and diet. *Int. J. Epidemiol.* 9(1):65–71
35. Eisenberg, L. 1981. A research framework for evaluating the promotion of mental health and prevention of mental illness. *Public Health Rep.* 96(1):3–19
36. Eiser, J. R., ed. 1982. *Social Psychology and Behavioral Medicine.* Chicester, NY: Wiley
37. Enelow, A. J., Henderson, J. B., eds. 1974. *Applying Behavioral Science to Cardiovascular Risk.* New York: Am. Heart Assoc.
38. Evans, R., Raines, B., 1982. Control and prevention of smoking in adolescents: A psychosocial perspective. In *Promoting Adolescent Health: A Dialog on Research and Practice,* ed. T. Coates, A. Peterson, C. Perry. New York: Academic
39. Evans, R. I., Hill, P. C., Raines, B. E., Henderson, A. H. 1981. Current behavioral, social and educational programs in control of smoking: A selective,

critical review. In *Perspectives on Behavioral Medicine*, ed. S. Weiss, A. Herd, B. Fox, pp. 261–84. New York: Academic

40. Faden, R. R., Faden, A. I., eds. 1978. Ethical issues in public health policy: Health education and life-style interventions. *Health Educ. Mono.* 6:177–257

41. Farquahr, J. W., Maccoby, N., Solomon, D. S. 1984. Community applications of behavioral medicine. In *Handbook of Behavioral Medicine*, ed. W. D. Gentry. New York: Guilford. In press

42. Feng, W. L. 1980. Evaluation of the effectiveness of a cardiovascular education pilot program. *Health Educ.* 11:34–38

43. Foreyt, J. P., Rathjen, D. P., eds. 1978. *Cognitive Behavior Therapy*. New York: Plenum

44. Freudenberg, N. 1978. Shaping the future of health education. *Health Educ. Monogr.* 6:372–77

45. Glassner, B., Berg, B. 1980. How Jews avoid alcohol problems. *Am. Sociol. Rev.* 45(4):647–64

46. Great Britain Expenditures Committee. 1977. *First Report from the Expenditures Committee, Session 1976–77, Preventive Medicine*. London: Her Majesty's Stationery Off.

47. Green, L. W. 1970. Should health education abandon attitude-change strategies? Perspectives from recent research. *Health Educ. Monogr.* 30:24–48

48. Green, L. W. 1980. Healthy People: The Surgeon General's Report and the prospects. In *Working for a Healthier America*, ed. W. J. McNerny. Cambridge, Mass: Ballinger

49. Green, L. W. 1981. National policy in the promotion of health. In *Medical Ethics and the Law: Implications for Public Policy*, ed. M. D. Hiller, pp. 135–48. Cambridge, Mass: Ballinger

50. Green, L. W., Wilson, R. W., Bauer, K. G. 1982. Data requirements to measure our progress on the Objectives for the Nation in health promotion and disease prevention. *Am. J. Public Health* 73:18–24

51. Green, L. W., Anderson, C. L. 1982. *Community Health*. St. Louis: Mosby. 4th ed.

52. Green, L. W., Heit, P., Iverson, D. C., Kolbe, L. J., Kreuter, M. W. 1980. The School Health Curriculum Project: Its theory, practice, and measurement experience. *Health Educ. Q.* 7:14–34

53. Green, L. W., Iverson, D. C. 1982. School health education. *Ann. Rev. Public Health* 3:321–38

54. Green, L. W., Kansler, C. C. 1980. *The Professional and Scientific Literature on Patient Education*. Detroit: Gale Res. Co.

55. Green, L. W., Kreuter, M. W., Deeds, S. G., Partridge, K. P. 1980. *Health Education Planning: A Diagnostic Approach*. Palo Alto, Calif.: Mayfield

56. Green, L. W., Werlin, S. H., Schaffler, H. H., Avery, C. H. 1977. Research and demonstration issues in self-care: Measuring the decline of medicocentrism. *Health Educ. Monogr.* 5:161–89

57. Green, L. W. 1975. Diffusion and adoption of innovations related to cardiovascular risk in the public. In *Applying Behavioral Science to Cardiovascular Risk*, ed. A. J. Enelow, J.

Henderson. New York: Am. Heart Assoc.

58. Green, L. W. 1976. Change-process models in health education. *Public Health Rev.* 5(1):5–33

59. Green, L. W. 1978. Determining the impact and effectiveness of health education as it relates to federal policy. *Health Educ. Monogr.* 6:28–66

60. Green, L. W., Johnson, K. W. 1983. Health education and health promotion. In *Handbook of Health, Health Care, and the Health Professions*, ed. D. Mechanic, New York: Free Press

61. Green, L. W., Kaplun, A., Moarefi, A. 1983. *New Policies for Health Education in Primary Health Care: Background Document for the World Health Assembly Technical Discussions*. Geneva: WHO

62. Griffiths, W. 1965. Achieving change in health practices. *Health Educ. Monogr.* 1(20):27–42

63. Gunderson, M., McCary, J. L. 1980. Effects of sex education or sex information and sex guilt, attitudes and behaviors. *Fam. Relat.* 29:375–79

64. Haynes, R. B., Taylor, D. W., Sackett, D. M., eds. 1979. *Compliance in Health Care*. Baltimore: Johns Hopkins Univ. Press

65. Helsing, K. J., Comstock, G. W. 1977. What kinds of people do not use seat belts? *Am. J. Public Health* 67:1043–49

66. Hochbaum, G. M. 1958. *Public Participation in Medical Screening Programs*. Washington, DC: PHS Pub. No. 572

67. Holcomb, J. D., Carbonari, J., Weinberg, A., Nelson, J. 1981. Evaluation of a comprehensive cardiovascular curriculum. *J. Sch. Health* 51:330–35

68. Horn, D. 1976. A model for the study of personal choice health behaviors. *Int. J. Health Educ.* 19:89–98

69. Iammarino, N., Weinberg, A., Holcomb, J. 1980. The state of school heart health education: A review of the literature. *Health Educ.* 298:320

70. Institute of Medicine, National Academy of Sciences. 1982. *Health and Behavior: Frontiers of Research in the Biobehavioral Sciences*, ed. D. A. Hamburg, G. R. Elliott, D. L. Parron. IOM, Pub. No. 82–010. Washington DC: Nat. Acad. Press

71. Iverson, B., Levy, S. 1982. Using meta-evaluation in health education research. *J. School Health* 52:234–39

72. Iverson, D. C., Kolbe, L. 1983. Evolution of the national disease prevention and health promotion strategy: The role of the schools. *J. Sch. Health* 53:294–302

73. Jason, L., Kimbrough, C. 1974. A preventive educational approach for young economically disadvantaged children. *J. Community Psychol.* 2:134–139

74. Jenkins, C. D. 1979. An approach to the diagnosis and treatment of problems of health-related behavior. *Int. J. Health Educ.* 22:3–24 (Suppl.)

75. Jenkins, C. D. 1980. Diagnosis and treatment of behavioral barriers to good health. In *Public Health and Preventive Medicine*, ed. J. M. Last, pp. 1095–1112. New York: Appleton-Century-Crofts 11th ed.

76. Kannas, L. 1981. The dimensions of health behavior among young men in Finland. *J. Health Educ.* 24:146–55

77. Kannel, W. B. 1971. Habits and heart disease. In *Prediction of the Lifespan*, ed.

E. Palmore, F. C. Jeffers, pp. 61–70. Lexington, Mass: Heath Lexington Books

78. Kasl, S., Cobb, S. 1966. Health behavior, illness behavior, and sick-role behavior. *Arch. Environ. Health* 12:246–66

79. Kazdin, A. E. 1979. Advances in child behavior therapy: Application and implications. *Am. Psychol.* 34:981–87

80. Kelman, H. C. 1969. Processes of opinion change. In *The Planning of Change: Readings in the Applied Behavioral Sciences.* ed. W. Bennes, K. Benne, R. Chin. New York: Holt, Reinhardt & Winston. 2nd ed.

81. Kessler, R. C., Cleary, P. D. 1980. Social class and psychological distress. *Am. Sociol. Rev.* 45(3):463–78

82. King, K. 1982. Selected behavioral strategies for the health educator. *Health Educ.* 13:35–37

83. Kirk, R. H. J., Hamrick, M., McAfee, D. 1980. Focus on health education and nutrition: Development of a guide for high school teachers. *Health Educ.* 11:21–24

84. Knowles, J. H., ed. 1977. *Doing Better and Feeling Worse: Health in the United States.* New York: Norton

85. Knutson, A. L. 1965. *The Individual, Society, and Health Behavior.* New York: Russel Sage Found.

86. Kohlberg, L., Mayer, R. 1972. Development as the aim of education. *Harvard Educ. Rev.* 42:449–96

87. Kok, F. J., Matroos, A. W., van den Ban, A. W., Hautvast, G. A. 1982. Characteristics of individuals with multiple behavioral risk factors for coronary heart disease: The Netherlands. *Am. J. Public Health* 72(9):986–91

88. Kolbe, L. 1983. Improving the health status of children: An epidemiological approach to establishing priorities for behavioral research. In *Proc. Natl. Conf. Res. & Dev. Health Educ. with Special Reference to Youth.* Southhampton, England: Southampton Univ. Press

89. Kolbe, L. J. 1979. Evaluating effectiveness: The problems of behavioral criteria. *Health Educ.* 10:12–16

90. Kolbe, L. J. 1982. What can we expect from school health education? *J. Sch. Health* 52:145–50

91. Kolbe, L. J., Iverson, D. C. 1981. Implementing comprehensive health education: Educational innovations and social change. *Health Educ. Q.* 8:57–80

92. Kovar, M. G. 1979. Some indicators of health-related behavior among adolescents in the United States. *Public Health Rep.* 94:109–18

93. Kreuter, M. W., Christianson, G. M. 1981. School health education: Does it cause an effect? *Health Educ. Q.* 8:43–56

94. Krondl, M. M., Lan, D. 1978. Food modification as a public health measure. *Can. J. Public Health* 69:39–48

95. Lairson, D. R., Swint, J. M. 1979. Estimates of preventive versus nonpreventive medical care demand in an HMO. *Health Serv. Rep.* 14:33–43

96. Lalonde, M. 1974. *A New Perspective On the Health of Canadians.* Ottawa, Canada: Ministry of Health and Welfare

97. Langlie, J. K. 1979. Interrelationships among preventive health behaviors: A test of competing hypotheses. *Public Health Rep.* 94:216–25

98. Langlie, J. K. 1977. Social networks, health beliefs, and preventive health behavior. *J. Health Soc. Behav.* 18:244–60

99. Lepper, M. R., Greene, D. 1978. *The Hidden Costs of Reward: New Perspectives on the Psychology of Human Motivation.* Hinsdale, NJ: Lawrence Erlbaum Assoc.

100. Lerner, M. 1973. Conceptualization of health and social well-being. *Health Serv. Res.* 8(1):6–12

101. Leventhal, H. 1983. Behavioral medicine: Psychology in health care. See Ref. 60

102. Levin, L. S., Idler, E. L. 1983. Self-care in health. *Am. Rev. Public Health* 4:181–201

103. Levinson, D. J. 1978. *The Seasons of a Man's Life.* New York: Ballantine

104. Levy, S., Iverson, B., Wahlberg, H. 1980. Nutrition-education research: An interdisciplinary evaluation and review. *Health Educ.* 7:107–26

105. Ley, P. 1980. The psychology of obesity: Its causes, consequences, and control. In *Contributions to Medical Psychology,* ed. S. Rachman, 2:181–213. Oxford: Pergamon

106. Lichtenstein, E., Antonussio, D. O. 1981. Dimensions of smoking behavior. *Addict. Behav.* 6:365–67

107. Lieberman, D. A. 1979. Behaviorism and the mind: A limited call for a return to introspection. *Am. Psychologist* 34:319–33

108. Litman, T. J. 1971. Health care and the family: A three-generational analysis. *Med. Care* 9:67–81

109. Loevinger, J. 1976. *Ego Development: Conceptions and Theories.* San Francisco: Jossey-Bass

110. MacPherson, B. V., Ashikaga, T., Dickstein, M. S., Jones, R. P. 1980. Evaluation of a respiratory health education program. *J. Sch. Health* 50:564–67

111. Mahoney, M. J. 1974. *Cognition and Behavior Modification.* Cambridge, Mass: Ballinger

112. Mahoney, M. J., Thoreson, C. E. 1974. *Self-Control: Power to the Person.* Monterey, Calif.: Brooks/Cole

113. Maiman, L., Green, L. W., Gibson, G., MacKenzie, E. J. 1979. Education for self-treatment by adult asthmatics. *J.A.M.A.* 241:1919–22

114. Marks, S. R. 1977. Multiple roles and role strain: Some notes on human energy, time and commitment. *Am. Sociol. Rev.* 42:921–36

115. Matarazzo, J. D. 1982. Behavioral health's challenge to academic, scientific and professional psychology. *Am. Psychol.* 37:1–14

116. Matarazzo, J. D. 1980. Behavioral health and behavioral medicine: Frontiers for a new health psychology. *Am. Psychol.* 35:907–17

117. McAlister, A. 1979. Tobacco, alcohol and drug abuse. In *Healthy People: Report of the Surgeon General on Health Promotion and Disease Prevention, Vol. 2, Background Papers,* pp. 197–206. Washington DC: GPO., DHEW (PHS) Pub. No. 79–55071A

118. McAlister, A. 1982. The development and prevention of substance abuse: An introduction to research and policy. In *Promoting Adolescent Health: A Dialog on Research and Practice,* ed. T. J. Coates, C. Perry, A. C. Peterson. New York: Academic

119. McAlister, A., Perry, C., Maccoby, N. 1979. Adolescent smoking: Onset and prevention. *Pediatrics* 63:650–58

120. McAlister, A., Bernstein, D. 1976. The modification of smoking behavior: Progress and problems. *Addict. Behav.* 1:89–102

121. McAlister, A., Farquhar, J., Thoreson, C., Maccoby, N. 1976. Applying behavioral science to cardiovascular health. *Health Educ. Monogr.* 4:45–74

122. McAlister, A., Perry, C., Killen, J. et al. 1980. Pilot study of smoking, alcohol and drug abuse prevention. *Am. J. Public Health* 70(7):719–21

123. McAlister, A. L., O'Shea, R. O. 1981. Community oral health promotion. *J. Behav. Med.* 4:337–49

124. McGinnes, J. M. 1982. Targetting progress in health. *Public Health Rep.* 97: 295–307

125. McKinley, J. B. 1975. A case for refocusing upstream: The political economy of illness. *Applying Behavioral Science to Cardiovascular Risk,* ed. A. Enelow, J. B. Henderson. New York: Am. Heart Assoc.

126. Mechanic, D. 1979. The stability of health and illness behavior: Results from a 16-year follow-up. *Am. J. Public Health* 69:1142–45

127. Mooney, C., Roberts, C., Fitzmahau, G. L. 1979. Here's looking at you—A school-based alcohol education project. *Health Educ.* 10:38–41

128. Morisky, D. E., Levine, D. M., Green, L. W., Shapiro, S., Russell, R. P. et al. 1983. Five-year blood pressure control and mortality following health education for hypertensive patients. *Am. J. Public Health* 73:153–62

129. Moser, J. 1980. *Prevention of Alcohol-related Problems: An International Review of Preventive Measures, Policies and Programmes.* Geneva: WHO

130. Mullen, P. D. 1983. Better health for Americans: A national health promotion program. In *Prevention '82.* Washington, DC: US Dept. Health Human Serv.

131. Mullen, P. D. 1981. Health related behavior: Natural influences and educational interventions. In *Better Outcomes for Our Children: A National Strategy, Vol. 4, Background Papers,* pp. 127–88. Washington DC: Select Panel for the Promotion of Child Health, DHHS, Public Health Serv.

132. Mullen, P. D. 1983. Promoting child health: Channels of socialization. *J. Family Community Health* 5(4):52–68

133. Mullen, P. D., Ottoson, J. M., Williams, T. B. 1981. *Health Promotion and Disease Prevention in a Reproductive Health Care Setting.* Rockville, Md: US Depart. Health and Human Serv., Public Health Serv.

134. Mullen, P. D., Zapka, J. G. 1981. Health education and promotion programs in HMOs: The recent evidence. *Health Educ. Q.* 8:292–315

135. Mullen, P. D., Zapka, J. G. 1982. *Guidelines for Health Promotion and Education Services in HMOs.* Washington DC: US Depart. Health and Human Services, Public Health Serv.

136. National Academy of Sciences, Institute of Medicine. 1978. *Adolescent Behavior and Health: A Conference Summary.* Washington DC: Nat. Acad. Sci.

137. National Health Information Clearinghouse. 1981. *Health Risk Appraisals: An Inventory.* Washington DC: DHHS(PHS) Pub. No. 81–50163

138. National Heart, Lung and Blood Institute. 1977. *Proc. Natl. Heart and Lung Inst. Working Conf. on Health Behavior.* Bethesda, Md: DHEW Pub. No. (NIH)77–868

139. Nickoley-Colquitt, S. 1982. Preventive group interventions for elderly clients: Are they effective? *Family Community Health* 167–85

140. Nyswander, D. B. 1942. *Solving School Health Problems.* New York: Oxford Univ. Press

141. Olsen, L., Redican, K., Krus, P. 1980. The School Health Curriculum Project: A review of research studies. *Health Educ.* 11:16–21

142. Parcel, G., Luttman, D., Meyers, M. P. 1979. Formative evaluation of a sex education course for young adolescents. *J. Sch. Health* 49:335–39

143. Parcel, G. S., Baronowski, T. 1981. Social learning theory and health education. *Health Educ.* 12:14–18

144. Parkinson, R. S., Green, L. W., McGill, A., Erikson, M., Ware, B., et al. 1981. *Managing Health Promotion in the Workplace: Guidelines for Implementation and Evaluation.* Palo Alto, Calif: Mayfield

145. Parsons, T. 1951. Social structure and dynamic process: The case of modern medical practice. In *The Social System,* ed. T. Parsons, New York: Free Press of Glencoe, Inc.

146. Peoples, M. D., Siegel, E. 1983. Measuring the impact of programs for mothers and infants on prenatal care and low birth weight: The value of refined analysis. *Med. Care* 21:586–605

147. Piaget, J. 1932. *The Moral Judgment of the Child.* London: Routledge and Kegan Paul

148. Podell, R. N., Keller, K., Mulvihill, M. N., Berger, G., Kent, D. F. 1978. Evaluation of the effectiveness of a high school course in cardiovascular nutrition. *Am. J. Public Health* 68:573–76

149. Popham, J. J. 1982. Appropriate measuring instruments for health education investigations. *Health Educ.* 13(3):23–26

150. Pratt, L. 1976. *Family Structure and Effective Health Behavior: The Energized Family.* Boston: Houghton-Mifflin

151. Redican, K. J., Olsen, L. K., Stone, D. B. 1978. Effects of a prototype health education curriculum on health knowledge of lower socioeconomic sixth-grade students. *Health Values* 2:84–91

152. Robbins, A. 1983. Can Reagan be indicted for betraying public health? *Am. J. Pub. Health* 73:12–13

153. Robbins, L. C., Hall, J. 1970. *How to Practice Prospective Medicine.* Indianapolis: Methodist Hospital

154. Robertson, L. S. 1981. Patterns of teen-aged driver involvement in fatal motor vehicle crashes: Implications for policy choice. *J. Health Polit. Policy Law* 6(2):303–14

155. Rogers, E. S. 1968. Public health asks of sociology . . . *Science* 159:506–8

156. Roskies, E., Lazarus, R. S. 1980. Coping theory and the teaching of coping skills. In *Behavioral Medicine: Changing Health Lifestyles,* ed. P. O. Davidson, S. M. Davidson. New York: Brunner/Mazel

157. Rothman, A., Byrne, N. 1981. Health education for children and adolescents. *Rev. Educ. Res.* 51:85–100
158. Schaefer, E. 1972. Parents as educators: Evidence from cross-sectional, longitudinal and intervention research. *Young Children* 27:227–39
159. Schaps, E., DiBartolo, R., Moskowitz, J., Polly, C., Churgin, S. 1981. A review of 127 drug abuse prevention program evaluations. *J. Drug Issues* 11:17–43
160. Smart, R., Fejer, D. 1974. *Drug Education: Current Issues, Future Directions.* Program Reports Ser. No. 3. Toronto: Addiction Res. Found.
161. Somers, R. 1981. Road user protection: Selected papers from the 8th International Conference on Accident and Traffic Medicine, Aarhus, Denmark, June 10–13. 1980. *Accident Anal. Prevent.* 13(1). New York: Pergamon
162. Squyres, W. D., ed. 1980. *Patient Education: An Inquiry Into The State of The Art.* New York: Springer
163. Stachnik, T. J. 1980. Priorities for psychology in medical education and health care delivery. *Am. Psychol.* 35:8–15
164. Steele, J. L., McBroom, W. H. 1972. Conceptual and empirical dimensions of health behavior. *J. Health Soc. Behav.* 13:382–92
165. Stone, G. C. 1979. Patient compliance and the role of the expert. *J. Soc. Issues* 35:34–59
166. Stuart, R. B. 1978. Weight loss and beyond: Are they taking it off and keeping it off? In *Behavioral Medicine: Changing Health Lifestyles,* ed. P. O. Davidson, S. M. Davidson, pp. 151–94. New York: Brunner/Mazel
167. Stunkard, A. J. 1981. The practice of health promotion: The case of obesity. In *Health Promotion Strategies for Public Health,* ed. L. K. Y. Ng, D. L. Davis, pp. 297–318. New York: Van Nostrand Reinhold
168. Thompson, E. L. 1978. Smoking education programs 1960–1976. *Am. J. Public Health* 68:250–57
169. US Center for Health Promotion & Education. 1982. *Teaching Parents to be the Primary Sexuality Educators of their Children: Volume 1—Impact of Programs.* Atlanta, Ga: CDC
170. US Dept. Health and Human Serv. 1979. *Healthy People: The Surgeon General's Report on Health Promotion and Disease Prevention.* Washington DC: GPO
171. US Dept. Health and Human Serv. 1981. *Strategies for Promoting Health for Specific Populations.* Washington DC: GPO, DHHS (PHS) Pub. No. 81–50169
172. US Dept. Health and Human Serv. 1980. *Promoting Health/Preventing Disease: Objectives for the Nation.* Washington DC: GPO
173. UNICEF/WHO. 1977. *Community Involvement in Primary Health Care: A Study of the Process of Community Motivation and Continued Participation.* Geneva: Joint Committee on Health Policy, UNICEF and WHO
174. Vacalis, T., Hill, E., Gray, J. 1979. The effect of two methods of teaching sex education on the behaviors of students. *J. Sch. Health* 49:404–9
175. Vaillant, G. E. 1977. *Adaptation to Life.* Boston: Little, Brown
176. Vaillant, G. E. 1979. Natural history of male psychologic health: Effects of mental health on physical health. *N. Engl. J. Med.* 301:1249–54
177. Vierki, S. 1980. The Lifestyling Program: Moving toward high level wellness. *Health Values* 4:237–41
178. Vogt, T. M. 1981. Risk assessment and health hazard appraisal. *Ann. Rev. Public Health* 2:31–47
179. Wan, T. T. H., Livieratos, B. 1978. Interpreting a general index of subjective well-being. *Milbank Mem. Fund Q.* 56(4):531–56
180. Ware, J. E. Jr., Davies-Avery, A., Brock, R. H., Johnston, S. A. 1979. *Associations Among Psychological Well-Being and Other Health Status Constructs.* Santa Monica: Rand
181. Ware, J. E., Johnston, S. A., Davies-Avery, A., Brook, R. H. 1979. *Conceptualization and Measurement of Health for Adults in the Health Insurance Study: Volume 3, Mental Health.* Santa Monica. Rand
182. Warr, P., Parry, G. 1981. Paid employment and women's psychological well-being. *Psychol. Bull.* 91(3):498–516
183. Way, J. W. 1981. Project Superheart: An evaluation of a heart disease intervention program for children. *J. Sch. Health* 51:16–19
184. Weiss, S., Herd, A., Fox, B., eds. 1981. *Perspectives on Behavioral Medicine.* New York: Academic
185. Wheaton, B. 1980. The sociogenesis of psychological disorder: An attributional theory. *J. Health Soc. Behav.* 21:10–124
186. Wickler, A. W. 1969. Attitudes versus actions: The relationship of verbal and overt behavioral responses to attitude objects. *J. Soc. Issues* 25:41–78
187. Williams, A. W., Ware, J. E. Jr., Donald, C. A. 1981. A model of mental health, life events, and social supports applicable to general populations. *J. Health Soc. Behav.* 22:324–36
188. Windsor, R. A., Green, L. W., Roseman, J. M. 1980. Health promotion and maintenance for patients with chronic obstructive pulmonary disease: A review. *J. Chron. Dis.* 33:5–12
189. Wolpe, J. 1981. Behavior therapy versus psychoanalysis: Therapeutic and social implications. *Am. Psychol.* 36:159–64
190. World Health Organization. 1969. Research in health education: report of a World Health Organization scientific group. *WHO Tech. Rep. Ser.* 432:430–41
191. World Health Organization. 1978. *Alma-Ata 1978: Primary Health Care.* Geneva: WHO *Health for All* Ser. 1
192. Zablocki, B. D., Kanter, R. M. 1976. The differentiation of life-styles. *Ann. Rev. Sociol.* 3:269–98
193. Zifferblatt, S. M. 1975. Increasing patient compliance through the applied analysis of behavior. *Prev. Med.* 4:173–82
194. Zifferblatt, S. M., Wilbur, C. S. 1977. Maintaining a healthy heart: Guidelines for a feasible goal. *Prev. Med.* 4:173–82

Selected Behavioral Strategies for the Health Educator

by Karen King

A significant and increasing proportion of contemporary morbidity is man-made. Because health education is no longer disease education, it is appropriate that health professionals are attempting to determine the role of cultural, sociological, and psychological variables as related to healthy and nonhealthy practices of living.

While Dr. Mayhew Derryberry, the renown public health educator, introduced the notion of compatibility between the behavioral sciences and health education as far back as 1954,[1] the use of behavioral learning principles by health educators has not been realized fully. For many the ultimate aim of health education is to help students achieve positive health and safety through their own actions and efforts, and health educators are seeking alternative methodologies to attain this objective. Traditional approaches, such as "telling and testing" and values clarification, have not been effective in helping pupils maintain or develop desirable health practices. This paper will present a rationale for the applied use of behavioral strategies in the practice of health education and describe selected examples of particular behavioral teaching strategies.

Karen King is an assistant professor in the Health Education Division at the University of North Carolina at Greensboro, North Carolina 27412.

Rationale

Since the most important objective of health education is to help people behave in as healthy a manner as possible,[2,3] it makes sense that health educators should use the empirically substantiated behavioral principles of behavioral psychology. Many health educators have long assumed that the acquisition of health knowledge would lead to an appropriate change in attitude, which in itself would precipitate a change in behavior and finally the acquisition of desirable health habits.[4] An unclear picture, however, exists of the exact relationship between beliefs and attitudes and either subsequent health or illness behavior.[5] Controlling man-made and chronic disease in the 1980s requires strategies above and beyond those focusing on knowledges and attitudes. Figure 1 represents the *assumed* dirrection that learning takes as it leads to behavior and habitual practices.

The following example illustrates that the relationships shown in Figure 1 are not operable. When 26 health education majors were asked what is the most important meal of the day, all correctly answered breakfast. When asked if they really felt that breakfast was the most important meal of the day, all but two answered yes. However, when asked how many ate breakfast at least four times a week, only four of the 26 an-

swered yes.

If the objective of health education is to change to, develop, and/or maintain desirable health practices, then the health educator should focus on actions and practices. While there is no way of influencing or convincing all people to behave in a healthful manner, there are behavioral techniques which have the potential to facilitate an effective health education program. Following are several such strategies and their application.

Behavioral Techniques Applicable to Health Education

Many behavioral strategies are available to the health educator. Selection of an appropriate technique depends on behavioral objectives, health education content areas, and characteristics of the target population. The success of a technique can only be measured in terms of its ability to develop, maintain, and/or change specific behaviors.

Positive Reinforcement

Positive reinforcement is probably the behavioral strategy most accessible to the health educator. In attempting to facilitate the development of a desirable behavior, it is generally recommended that positive reinforcement be either a primary intervention or a supplemental

Figure 1. Assumed Direction of Learning Leading to Acquisition of Behavioral Actions

Correct Knowledge	+	Positive Attitude	→	Behavior	→	Habitual Practices
Positive Attitude	+	Correct Knowledge	→	Behavior	→	Habitual Practices

strategy (see next section) in any program which defines outcome behaviors explicitly and objectively.[6] When given following the demonstration of a specific behavior, positive reinforcement is probably the most powerful technique available. There are a variety of reinforcers available: verbal and nonverbal praise, smiles, touches, social attention and grades.

The following example demonstrates the use of positive reinforcement alone in developing a positive health behavior—removal of plaque from the teeth as a desired outcome of dental health instruction. Brushing and flossing are two recommended health practices by which students can meet this objective.

Using plaque disclosing tablets prior to implementing the instructional program would accomplish three things. The teacher would see the existing plaque levels among all students. Students would see the amount of plaque on and around their own teeth and gums, and an observable criterion would be established for the importance of thorough brushing and flossing.

Next, a four-step program would be implemented.

The first step would be to explain and demonstrate brushing and allow individual practice time with individualized positive reinforcement for correct technique. In the second step a repeat of the disclosing test would permit the teacher to reinforce the efforts of students with lowered plaque levels and to illustrate that plaque still exists where the brush did not reach. The third step would be an explanation and demonstration of flossing followed by individual practice time with reinforcement of correct technique. The fourth step would occur the following day and would be a repeat of the disclosing test with appropriate reinforcement to those with lowered plaque levels.

To increase the chances that brushing and flossing be maintained over time, disclosing tests can be scheduled at least once a week to continue the appraisal and reinforcement of the desired practices. Through such a program, purposeful efforts must be made to reduce dental caries and gum disease and the management of dental care practices can be monitored and enhanced with the contingent use of positive reinforcement.

Modeling

One of the most effective techniques for teaching a desired behavior is modeling or observational learning. This technique provides students with a model, similar to them in age, sex, etc., who demonstrates the desired behaviors in person or on film. The use of modeling as a teaching strategy has been found to reduce the probability of incorrect responses[7] and can be more efficient than lecture, reading and discussion. While modeling alone results in learning,[8] it is necessary to provide reinforcement if students are to perform and practice the modeled behavior. Following is an example germane to health education.

A study attempting to teach 60 preschool age children how to make emergency phone calls compared three methods—behavioral training, instruction by the teacher and no training.[9] The behavioral strategy combined instruction, modeling, prompting, practice with help and alone, and reinforcement. The behavioral strategy resulted in statistically significant performance gains. The teacher instructed group performed better than the no-training group but not to a point achieving statistical significance. These results clearly show that behavioral training was more effective in developing emergency phone dialing skills among children aged three to six. Similar kinds of participation or guided modeling could readily be used in various health education areas such as nutrition, dental health, fitness and cardiovascular disease, etc.

Self-Control and Self-Monitoring

A relatively new concept that has made behavioral techniques more acceptable to health educators is self-management. Self-control is a process in which an individual, "in the relative absence of immediate external constraints, engages in behaviors whose previous probability has been less than that of alternatively available behaviors."[10] A self-managed approach to health education necessitates the active involvement of the person with an undesirable health behavior in the change process.

In order to make self-managed responses (e.g., not eating, not smoking, brushing one's teeth), individuals must first observe or monitor their own behavior.[11] Accordingly, increasing the regularity and frequency of self-monitoring should enhance the self-control process. Besides being a precursor to self-control, self-monitoring is a behavioral strategy that can also be used on its own as an agent for behavioral change. For example, self-monitoring has been found to reduce cigarette smoking rates[12] and to control alcohol consumption.[13]

In a study in which the behavioral objectives were to lose weight and maintain weight loss, participants were instructed to monitor their eating behavior daily before or after eating.[14] Both methods resulted in weight loss but those who monitored themselves before eating achieved the greatest weight loss and maintained it over time. Self-monitoring ultimately led to greater self-control of eating behavior. A health educator could easily use this strategy in a nutrition unit.

Stimulus Control

A fundamental behavioral concept is that "behavior is under stimulus control.[15] Many health behaviors are thought to be under the control of environmental stimuli. Examples are: watching TV and then getting a snack; having a cup of coffee and then lighting up a cigarette; seeing candy at the grocery store check-out and buying some; feeling stressed and anxious and taking a drink of alcohol; etc.

Health educators can use stimulus control strategies to facilitate the acquisition of healthful behaviors among students. In stimulus control, environmental conditions are planned to maximize and/or minimize the practice of specific target behaviors.

An illustration follows of the efficacy of stimulus control in achieving a desired health behavior. This study is valuable not just because it illustrates a strategy that worked, but also because it involved a school-age group. Most weight control/dietary change research involves adults. A group of 46 adolescents, all desirous of changing their eating habits and losing weight, were directed and voluntarily agreed to engage in predetermined stimulus control behaviors such as eating in only one setting, chewing each bite thoroughly, doing nothing else while eating, etc.[16] With no other intervention this group lost a significant amount of weight, changed their eating habits, and maintained the weight loss at least 50 weeks after the study had concluded.

Such a technique can be used easily by a health educator if: the students want to change their habits (eating or other habits); the teacher assesses the present environment and the frequency of the target behavior; and the environmental planning is discretely and objectively stipulated.

Habitual behaviors do not just occur; apparently they "appear when the environmental setting is very similar to past occasions when the behavior was exhibited and was reinforced."[17] Since many health behaviors are under stimulus control, a teacher could, when appropriate, help a student rearrange environmental stimuli to bring desired behaviors under specific stimulus control.

Conclusion

A fundamental principle of human behavior is that, in general, behaviors are cued and maintained. Cued behaviors are those triggered by some event, referred to as the stimulus, and maintained behaviors are those reinforced by events following their exhibition. "The fact that the principles of behavior are not confined to observable actions but also apply to thoughts and feelings is one of the most interesting and important recent discoveries of behavioral scientists."[18] This makes it even more relevant that health educators should begin to use behavioral teaching/learning strategies to facilitate the promotion of both healthy attitudes and practices.

If behavioral strategies are to be effective, students should help determine the objectives of instruction. Students should know where they stand, help select desired outcomes and be informed of progress. Involving the student directly will aid the success of the health instruction program.

The use of behavioral techniques is based on the systematic application of learning theory derived from experimental research to change behaviors. A behavioral approach to health education has the potential to facilitate a decrease in the prevalence and incidence of manmade diseases of civilization.

---

[1]Bureau of Health Education. *Focal points.* Atlanta, Georgia: United States Department of Health and Human Services, Public Health Service, Center for Disease Control, April, 1980.

[2]Green, L. W., *Determining the impact and effectiveness of health education as it relates to federal policy.* Prepared for the Office of the Deputy Assistant Secretary for Planning and Evaluation/Health, United States Department of Health, Education, and Welfare. Contract No. 5A-7974-75, April 30, 1976.

[3]World Health Organization. Research in health education: report of a World Health Organization scientific group. *World Health Organization Technical Report Series,* 1969, 430–441.

[4]Anderson, C. L. & Creswell, W. H., *School health practice.* St. Louis: The C. V. Mosby Company, 1980.

[5]Richards, N. D., Methods and effectiveness of health education: The past, present and future of social scientific involvement. *Social Science and Medicine,* 1975, 9, 141–156.

[6]Bellack, A. S. & Hersen, M., *Behavior modification: An introductory textbook.* Baltimore: The Williams & Wilkins Company, 1977.

[7]Ackerman, J. M., *Operant conditioning for classroom teachers.* Glenview, Illinois: Scott, Foresman and Company, 1972.

[8]Bandura, A., Influence of models' reinforcement contingencies on the acquisition of imitative responses. *Journal of Personality and Social Psychology,* 1965, 1, 589–595.

[9]Jones, R. T. & Kazdin, A. E., Teaching children how and when to make emergency telephone calls. *Behavior Therapy,* 1980, 11, 509–521.

[10]Thorensen, C. E. & Mahoney, M. J., *Behavioral self-control.* New York: Holt, Rinehart, & Winston, 1974.

[11]Kanfer, F. H. & Karoly, P., Self-control: a behavioristic excursion into the lion's den. *Behavior Therapy,* 1972, 3, 398–416.

[12]Lipinski, D. P., Black J. L., Nelson, R. O, and Ciminero, A. R., The influence of motivational variables on the reactivity and reliability of self-recording. *Journal of Consulting and Clinical Psychology,* 1975, 43, 637–646.

[13]Sobell, L. C. & Sobell, M. B., A self-feedback technique to monitor drinking behavior in alcoholics. *Behavior Research and Therapy,* 1973, 11, 237–238.

[14]Bellack, A. S., Rozensky, R., & Schwartz, J., A comparison of two forms of self-monitoring in a behavioral weight reduction program. *Behavior Therapy,* 1974, 5, 523–530.

[15]Bellock and Hersen, op. cit. p. 10.

[16]Weiss, A. R., A behavioral approach to the treatment of adolescent obesity. *Behavior Therapy,* 1977, 8, 720–726.

[17]Ackerman, op. cit. p. 83.

[18]Lanyon, R. I. & Lanyon, B. P., *Behavior therapy: A clinical introduction,* Reading, Massachusetts: Addison-Wesley Publishing Company, 1978.

Cancer Prevention Awareness Survey

from the National Cancer Institute

I. OVERVIEW OF STUDY FINDINGS

The Cancer Prevention Awareness Survey was conducted the week of June 20, 1983, to develop quantitative audience data concerning public knowledge, attitudes, and behavior related to cancer prevention and risk. The survey consisted of a national probability sample of 1,876 respondents interviewed one time by telephone.

Findings from the survey will provide baseline data for use in designing and targeting a National Cancer Prevention Awareness Program, to be initiated by the National Cancer Institute (NCI) in 1984. Highlights of findings and implications for the communications program are summarized below.

The results of the survey document the need for a program to improve public attitudes and awareness about cancer prevention. Results indicated that the public's view of cancer is confused and skeptical, that is, that myths and misperceptions exist, and that perceptions of risk and potential for personal control over cancer risk vary and are often pessimistic. Many people believe that "everything causes cancer" and that "there is not much a person can do to prevent cancer." These beliefs are more likely to be held by those with lower levels of education, with some geographic differences in evidence. Further, less than one-half of the population (38%) believe that cancer is related to lifestyle.

In spite of the beliefs that not much can be done to prevent cancer, most people did correctly identify tobacco, sunshine, and X-rays as items that can increase cancer risk. However, misconceptions were also prevalent. For example, nearly half the population believe that bumps and bruises can increase the chances of getting cancer.

The most frequently mentioned things that a person can do to reduce chances of getting cancer were changes in food choices or dietary habits and reduction or cessation of smoking. Fewer than one in five mentioned reduction in exposure to the sun. As might be expected, people with less education tended to be less knowledgeable about risk factors; for example, generally agreeing more often than others that bumps and bruises and foods that contain fiber increase cancer risk.

The most frequently reported sources of information about cancer were magazines, newspapers, and television, with only one-third of the adult population indicating radio or other sources of information. Some regional differences were evident among the sources cited. Those with more education frequently reported receiving information about cancer prevention from all three sources, while those with less than an eighth grade education reported magazines most frequently as a source of cancer information. Men reported television and radio as sources of information more often than women.

Nearly everyone said they had heard of the American Cancer Society (ACS) as a source of information about cancer. Three in five said they had heard of the National Cancer Institute, with one-half of the weighted sample aged 18 to 20 or with less than a ninth grade education unaware of NCI.

In general, the survey results demonstrated few major differences among demographic groups. The less educated, older respondent generally tended to have more misconceptions about cancer risks and prevention. Although there were regional differences, there were few consistent patterns. No significant gender differences were found.

II. BACKGROUND AND STUDY DESIGN

The Cancer Prevention Awareness Survey developed from a need to measure public attitudes and behavior regarding cancer risk and prevention and to aid in designing NCI's National Cancer Prevention Awareness Program. The activities described below contributed to this final report--focus group discussions (December 1982-January 1983); survey design, fielding, and data entry (June-August 1983); and data analysis and survey report preparation (September-November 1983).

FOCUS GROUP DISCUSSIONS

This presurvey activity was completed by Bonita L. Perry Associates for OCC under contract to Porter, Novelli and Associates. First, the study sought to understand consumer perceptions of risk and prevention of disease in general and cancer in particular. Second, it sought to test, among different target groups, the effectiveness of various formats for communicating information about cancer prevention.

Thirteen focus groups were conducted in Philadelphia, Pennsylvania, and Houston, Texas, between December 15, 1982, and January 6, 1983. There were seven groups of women and six groups of men. Ages ranged between 18 and 75 with various breakouts to provide fairly homogenous groups. The groups were structured by types to test whether various demographic or psychographic characteristics correlate with attitudes toward cancer prevention and risk.

Major topics of discussion in the focus groups were:

o Attitudes and behavior regarding health risks;

o Attitudes and behavior regarding prevention;

o Perceptions of disease susceptibility;

o Current attitudes, beliefs, and behavior patterns with respect to cancer;

o Reactions to the format for cancer risk assessment information.

Results obtained from the focus groups were used to develop the questions for this study.

SURVEY DESIGN, FIELDING, AND DATA ENTRY

The survey was designed by NCI's Office of Cancer Communications (OCC) and reviewed by an evaluation working group (experts in communication, advertising research, and survey research convened to advise on the evaluation component of the prevention program) formed by OCC. The survey was designed to collect information on:

o Respondents' description of their health;

o Awareness of health risks and substances or behaviors that increase the risk of cancer;

o Awareness of behaviors that decrease cancer risk;

o Attitudes associated with the chances of getting cancer;

o Sources of cancer information; and

o Demographics of the sample.

The survey design, fielding, and data entry phases were carried out by Westat, Inc., of Rockville, Maryland, a contractor to the FDA. A pretest of the instrument was conducted several days prior to the fielding of the principal study. On June 22, 1983, the final version of the questionnaire was fielded. A total of 2,479 eligible contacts were made--1,876 completions, and 603 refusals-for a response rate of 75.7 percent. Response choices for various closed-ended questions in the survey were rotated to prevent bias of first-mentioned items.

The findings contained in this report are based on telephone interviews conducted with a national probability sample of men and women over 17 years of age. Random digit dialing (RDD) techniques were used in the selection of the 1,876 survey respondents. The RDD method uses clusters or blocks of telephone numbers that are screened to identify sequences of telephone numbers having a relatively high proportion of residences. The method is designed to reduce the number of unproductive calls by taking advantage of the fact that a high percentage of nonworking and commercial numbers occur in consecutive sequences. Appendix 1 of the Technical Report contains specific details of the fielding methodology.

To improve the representativeness (demographic characteristics) of the sample and to increase the sample size (n) to the universe size (N), the data were weighted according to the following variables:

o Number of telephone numbers per household;

o Number of eligible respondents per household; and

o The demographic ratio of the population (i.e., sex, age, and educational attainment).

After superimposing a weight to each record, the sample of 1,876 was weighted to 170,281,000--the U.S. adult population.

DATA ANALYSIS AND REPORT PREPARATION

Data analysis and preparation of this report were completed by CDP Associates, Inc., Rockville, Maryland, for OCC under subcontract to Nancy Low & Associates, Inc. Approximately 600 crosstabulations of survey variables were computed to analyze the data. All variables in the questionnaire were crosstabulated by the four demographic characteristics (sex, age, education, and region of individuals participating, as developed by the Census Bureau) to determine whether sex or age, for example, influenced the responses given.

III. FINDINGS

A. HEALTH BELIEFS AND BEHAVIOR

Thirty-three percent of the adult population rated their overall health as excellent, 46 percent rated it as good, 16 percent rated it as fair, and 5 percent rated their overall health as poor. Younger people tended to rate their own health better than older people, and those with more education rated their health better than those with less education (with the exception of those with post-graduate degrees/training where the percentage dropped slightly). Males reported good or excellent health 5 percent more frequently than females.

Seven in 10 adults said they currently do or have done something to improve their health or to stay healthy. As a first response of the types of things they say they do, exercising was mentioned most frequently (43%), followed by changes in food and diet (26%), and changes in personal medical practices (12%) such as checkups, tests, taking medications, etc. Fifty-five percent described their overall health as good to excellent <u>and</u> do something to improve or maintain their health. Seven percent described their health as fair or poor <u>and</u> do nothing to improve their health.

B. PERCEPTIONS OF SERIOUS HEALTH PROBLEMS

Three questions in the survey addressed general health problems and the seriousness of each problem. Of the six health problems mentioned (high blood pressure, cancer, stroke, herpes, diabetes, and ulcers), cancer was considered to be serious by more people than any other health problem (98%). Cancer was also considered to be the most serious of all health problems. When asked if they believed that any of the health problems were caused by lifestyle, people tended to mention ulcers and high blood pressure most frequently (89% and 78%, respectively); diabetes and cancer were mentioned least frequently (34% and 38%, respectively).

The perception of cancer, high blood pressure, stroke, and diabetes as serious health problems showed little variance with respect to level of education. Every demographic subgroup (geographic region, age, sex, and education level) selected cancer as the <u>most</u> serious of the six health problems.

C. TYPES OF BEHAVIOR CONSIDERED RISKY

Respondents were asked "What are some things that people do that may be risky to their health?" The most frequently reported first response was smoking (41%), followed by poor food/diet choices (23%) and drinking alcohol (13%).

Drinking alcohol (as a first response) was reported almost 5 times more frequently among people over age 70 (24%) than among 18- to 21-year-olds (5%). Twice as many food/diet first responses were reported by those with some college education (31%) than those with just some high school education (15%). No significant gender differences were found among the adult population.

D. ATTITUDES TOWARD CANCER

Four statements were read to respondents for which they were asked to indicate their degree of agreement. About 9 out of 10 agreed that "people today seem more concerned about their health than ever before" and "the chances of being cured of cancer are better today than ever before." About half agreed that "it seems like everything causes cancer" and "there is not much a person can do to prevent cancer."

People from the New England region agreed 24 percent more frequently with these latter two statements than those from the Mountain region. The sex of an individual had no significant effect on the responses given to the four statements. Agreement or disagreement between males and females varied, at most, 5 percent. Thirty-five percent of the population age 31 to 40 agreed to some degree that "there is not much a person can do to prevent cancer," while 55 percent over 70 agreed to some degree with this statement. Also, the less educated (those who achieved less than a college degree) agreed 20 percent more frequently that "there is not much a person can do to prevent cancer."

E. BELIEFS AND BEHAVIORS
ASSOCIATED WITH CANCER RISKS

The survey asked people to indicate whether they believed a particular item could increase a person's chances of getting cancer. The following is a list of the items contained in this question and the percentage of people who believed that risk would be increased:

Evidence Indicates Increased Risk

   o Tobacco (87%)
   o Sunshine (75%)
   o X-rays (64%)
   o Alcohol (46%)
   o Marijuana (35%)
   o Herpes (26%)
   o Talcum powder (10%)

Evidence Indicates Decreased or No Risk

   o Foods with fiber (15%)
   o Bumps and bruises (46%)

Conflicting Research Opinion

   o Birth control pills (60%)
   o Coffee (20%)

The younger a person, the more likely that he/she believed that drinking coffee increases a person's risk of getting cancer. There was also a linear correlation between the age of an individual and the belief that bumps and bruises increase the risk of cancer (i.e., older people are much more likely to believe this). Men were less likely to agree that sunshine increases the risk of cancer. Less educated people generally agreed more often that herpes, marijuana, birth control pills, bumps and bruises, and foods that contain fiber increase the risk of cancer.

When people were asked to list things a person can do to reduce the chances of getting cancer, the most frequent first response was to reduce or to stop smoking (30%), followed by changing food and diet habits (21%) and changing personal medical practices (13%) (e.g., get more frequent check-ups, tests, examinations). Younger people were more likely to offer smoking-related responses than older people, and twice as many women than men reported changes in medical practices.

Following this question, people were asked what, if anything, they have done to reduce their chances of getting cancer. As in the previous question, the top three first responses were to reduce or to stop smoking (28%), followed by changing food and diet habits (16%) and changing personal medical practices (14%).

F. SOURCES OF INFORMATION

When asked to comment on whether they had received information about cancer from the television, the radio, a newspaper, a magazine, a family member, or a friend, magazines were mentioned by 64 percent, newspapers by 60 percent, and television by 58 percent. Regional differences were evident among the public's sources of information about cancer--more so among media sources (19%) than either family or friends (12%). People over 70 years of age received less information about cancer prevention than any other age group. Television and radio were reported by men 63 percent and 40 percent, respectively; women reported television 54 percent and radio 28 percent.

People were also asked whether they had ever heard of the various cancer organizations. Almost everyone said they had heard of the American Cancer Society (98%), three out of five said they had heard of the National Cancer Institute (61%), and just over one-third were familiar with the Cancer Information Service (CIS) (38%). No gender differences were found in these responses; however, individuals with post-graduate training claimed they had heard of NCI most often, and the CIS least often.

G. ATTITUDES TOWARD DOCTORS' ADVICE

When asked how likely they would be to follow a doctor's advice on ways to reduce chances of getting cancer, nearly 61 percent said they would be very likely and 30 percent said somewhat likely. Additionally, those over 60 years of age reported that they were likely to follow a doctor's advice more than did younger people. About 90 percent with excellent, good, or fair health said there would be some likelihood of their following a doctor's advice; only 77 percent of those with poor health gave the same response.

A crosstabulation of this question ("If a doctor told you about ways to reduce your chances of getting cancer, how likely would you be to try to follow his or her advice?") by ("What things do you do or have you done to improve your health or stay healthy?") was computed to determine whether engagement in a particular healthful activity or behavior influenced the likelihood of following a doctor's advice. Crosstabulation results indicated that for the two most frequently reported healthy behaviors--changes in food/diet and exercise--the behavior had no correlation with the self-reported likelihood of following a doctor's advice. Those who reported changing personal medical practices (e.g., getting more frequent check-ups, tests, examinations) to improve their health tended to be slightly more likely than others to heed the advice of a doctor.

When asked whether they had ever talked to a doctor about ways to reduce their chances of getting cancer, nearly 86 percent said "no" and only 14 percent said "yes." Those within each health group (excellent, good, fair, and poor) tended to answer similarly.

H. BELIEFS ABOUT PERSONAL RISK

When asked what they felt their chances were of getting cancer nearly 16 percent said "very likely," 45 percent said "somewhat likely," 28 percent said "not very likely," and 7 percent responded "no chance at all." Those with less education were more likely to believe their chances of getting cancer were very high, and females were slightly more likely (67%) to believe this than males (58%).

Food Habit Modification as a Public Health Measure

by M. M. Krondl, Ph.D., and D. Lau, M.Sc.

Inadequate knowledge of the motives influencing food selection is the main obstacle in food habit modification in the affluent society. It restricts the success of nutrition education which is an important public health measure.

Historical reasons are presented elucidating the development of the most influential motives for food choice. The motives are defined and categorized. The application of them as controlled variables in food habit analysis is discussed. They may be used in: a) ranking of food items according to the valency of the food choice motives; b) a comparison of the food valencies of food choice motives between different population groups; c) a comparison of the valency of food choice motives between one and other; d) a correlation between the food use frequency and food choice motives. The application of food choice motives in modification of frequency of use of individual food items is illustrated.

In the study of food choice motives, typifying population by the degree of internal/external control is indicated as different communication routes have to be used for different type of population groups if the modifying of food attitudes and changing of food use frequency (food habits) is to be successful.

M. M. Krondl, Ph.D., is Associate Professor, and D. Lau, M.Sc., is Research Assistant, at the Department of Nutrition and Food Science, Faculty of Medicine, University of Toronto.

The development of *Canada's Food Guide* and other similar eating patterns was viewed as a big step forward in nutrition education. As long ago as 1971, however, McClinton and his colleagues (1) concluded that it was inadequate for this purpose. Why? Food guides had been based on accredited research data obtained from a relatively stable environment which was characterized by little change in food resources, and only a gradual change in social and cultural values; their main purpose was to promote individual health knowledge and provide for a protective margin of nutrient intake. As far as was known, they answered all of man's physiological needs. Yet the results of nutrition surveys in both the United States and Canada made nutritionists and public health specialists painfully aware that people, in general, could not be following the eating patterns laid down in the food guides. Their poor nutritional status was powerful evidence that, if food guides were to be useful for the nutrition

education of the future, a missing ingredient must be added.

Production of any guide for food selection is a time-consuming process. Effective modification cannot be accomplished in a short period. Its resulting basic rigidity is therefore an obstacle to ready change when the time is ripe for expansion. Yet it is vital that public health approaches to the dissemination of nutrition education should be quickly reconstructed to meet modern nutritional needs. The fact that no mechanism existed for assessing or influencing individual motives for food choices has only recently been recognized. Perhaps we can solve the riddle of poor nutritional behaviour by trying to gain some understanding of the reasons for individual food preferences and the background meanings which man, consciously or unconsciously, attaches to certain foods.

For more than 90% of his evolutionary existence, man's food choices have been largely governed by the availability of his food resources (Figure 1). When as a nomad, he hunted for his food, his food selection was automatic. He ate whatever food he could

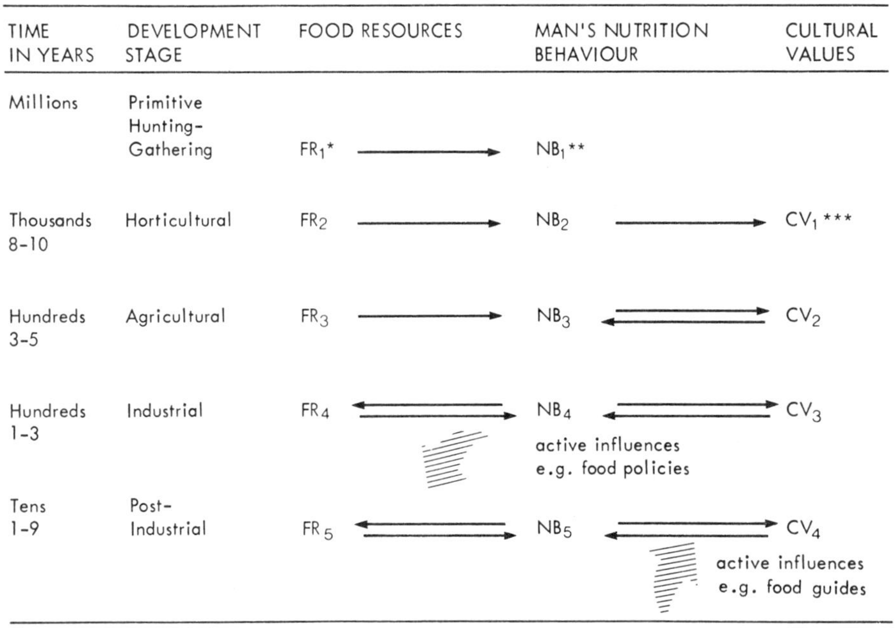

TIME IN YEARS	DEVELOPMENT STAGE	FOOD RESOURCES	MAN'S NUTRITION BEHAVIOUR	CULTURAL VALUES
Millions	Primitive Hunting-Gathering	FR_1* ⟶	NB_1**	
Thousands 8-10	Horticultural	FR_2 ⟶	NB_2 ⟶	CV_1 ***
Hundreds 3-5	Agricultural	FR_3 ⟶	NB_3 ⟵⟶	CV_2
Hundreds 1-3	Industrial	FR_4 ⟵⟶	NB_4 ⟵⟶ active influences e.g. food policies	CV_3
Tens 1-9	Post-Industrial	FR_5 ⟵⟶	NB_5 ⟵⟶	CV_4 active influences e.g. food guides

Figure 1. Development of Nutrition Behaviour

* FR_1 - FR_5 Degrees of development in food resources
** NB_1 - NB_5 Degrees of development in nutrition behaviour
***CV_1 - CV_4 Degrees of development in cultural values

Adapted from Quick (29).

find. When he entered the agricultural stage, about 8,000 years ago, food became more plentiful and he could often choose from an increasing variety. As a definite social organization began to emerge, his food selection pattern was still influenced by scarcity or plenty, but also by his personal tastes and by emphasis on the foods which the culture of his day considered desirable. Then populations began to increase and evolution proceeded toward industrialization. Man's nutritional behaviour, keeping pace with these ecological changes, now began to feel the effects of increasing food costs and new tastes resulting from scientific refining methods and the use of food additives. Pressurized advertising campaigns often made him spend more money on housing and material possessions than on his traditional food needs. He was forced to adjust to the crowding costs of spreading urbanization. The easy mobility of railway, automobile, and plane encouraged immigration, and he lost the security of being able to put down roots in the community where he lived. Where food and other resources were plentiful, he became indifferent to

waste, and ignored the hazards of pollution. Unconventional and disorganized mechanisms for food selection have begun to find their way into the nutritional scene as evidenced by the popular response to health food movements and food faddism. Modern man seems inclined to be blinded to the fact that he is still subject to biological bias in the complex environment of the post-industrial era. Perhaps it is not surprising that a functional gap currently exists between traditional public health schemes for nutrition education and much of the world's population.

It is fortunate that available food guides have established a data base for many foods; they have underwritten the need for more research in food composition; they have encouraged interest in increasing world food production. Changes in the concept of food as simply an energy substrate, and of nutrition as the process for generating body energy (including growth and reproduction) are becoming major issues in today's public health policies. Yet if we are to improve modern man's nutritional behaviour by increasing his adaptability to his environment, we

must learn more about what influences his food choices. And to study food choices we must begin by learning a new vocabulary. Nutritionists must recognize modern man's dependence not only on so-called "internal cues" such as hunger, but also on "external cues" related to man's ecological background, which may possibly play a larger part in influencing his individual nutritional behaviour than does the traditional satisfaction of his physiological needs.

A hypothetical model for interpreting nutrition behaviour in terms of a systems theory is hereby proposed. It has been developed from Brody's "Man Hierarchy Model" (2), and Schaefer's concept of socio-physiology (3). Based on this model, directions for further studies are indicated on the interrelationship of the socio-cultural, physical, and biological environments of man, and their influence on his food choices.

It is postulated that man's intellectual development, through countless generations of exposure to the implements, handicrafts, agriculture, economics, music, art, religious beliefs, traditions, language, and history of the society in which he lives, gradually produces certain attitudes toward food to which norms and values can be given (Figure 2). Thus, in a lifetime, it may be seen that food attitudes are learned through the influence of the society, the community, and the family by means of an exchange of symbols and goods (external cues). Personal food choice is the outcome of the learned food attitudes which are based on liking for a certain food, emotional response to it, or factual knowledge about it. Actual food choice is voluntary in contrast to the involuntary physiological processes of metabolism which are regulated by the neuroendocrine system (internal cues). It is influenced by feedback mechanisms which grow out of each individual's ecological background.

Individual feedback mechanisms which influence food choice have been well-documented by de Garine (4) and Lowenberg (5). In Figure 3, their influence may be expressed as part of a barrier which exists between environmentally and economically available foods and the consumer's food choice. It is obvious that the food supply may be adequate in terms of availability and cost, but the degree of biological hunger, long-term culturally-induced physiological adaptation, short-term influence of the society, and personal bias all influence individual food choice. These components may be present in varying proportions depending on the length of the adaptation period and the adaptability of the individual or group concerned. Thus each person concerned with choosing a food does so in terms of an individual "food meaning" which depends on the state of his "food barriers".

In Figure 4, the four components have been further divided into sub-units, designated as "food choice motives", which can be either "acquired" or "learned", and the food meaning picture becomes even more detailed. The acquired motives projected at the physiological systems level are typified by satiety, tolerance, and taste. At the cultural systems level some overlapping occurs: some acquired and some learned motives are present. At the societal systems level, overlapping occurs also, not only with the cultural systems level but with acquired and learned motives. Finally, on the personal systems level only learned motives influence eventual food choice.

It is obvious that so-called "food meanings" are derived by applying the postulated "food motives" to certain foods in terms of the individual's food choices. They reflect the degree to which his physiological and psychological needs are satisfied when the food in question is chosen. It is likely that some basic physiological needs are similar for everybody, but through versatile adaptive functioning of the human system, physiological differences among culturally-different populations have been shown to exist, not to mention differences in psychological and emotional needs (6).

The tie between psychological needs,

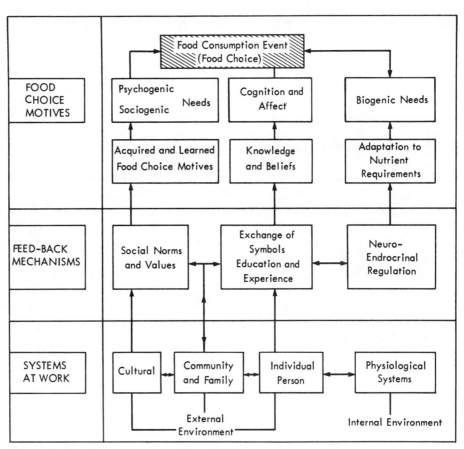

Figure 2. The Development of Food Choice Patterns

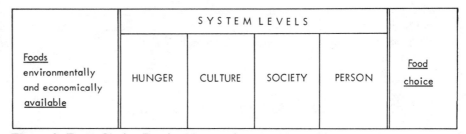

Figure 3. Food Choice Barrier. A model.

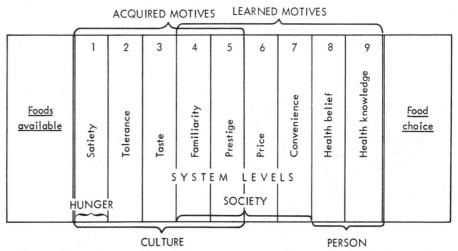

Figure 4. Food Meanings Expressing Food Choice Motives as Part of a Barrier. A model.

food choice motives, and food meanings was included in the postulated model on the basis of a study carried out by Fewster and his coworkers (7). A study of 383 societies by Moore (8) suggested the inclusion of the *satiety* effects of foods like rice, maize, and wheat. Intolerance to lactose was strikingly related to ethnic and racial differences of human subjects by Simoons (9), and Sowers and Winterfeldt (10). Intolerance to high-fibre foods has been studied by Koch and Donaldson (11) and by Donaldson (12). In 1975, Chau and Chang (13) demonstrated a cultural difference in fibre *tolerance* between Chinese and Anglo-Saxon Canadians. Patterns of food likes and dislikes were indicated in the work of Hall and Hall (14), Van Riter (15), Van Shaik (16) and Einstein and Hornstein (17). Frequency of intake, reflecting the degree of acceptance, was also found to have a relationship with food *familiarity* by Munn and Narang (18). *Taste* and flavour perception had been shown to influence food choice by Hall (14), Lee (19), Jellinek (20), and Weisberg (21). A recent study (18) showed cultural differences in the taste perception of sweetness. A report by Pangborn (22) demonstrated the cross-culture aspects of flavour preferences and food choice.

Illustrations also exist in the literature to indicate that social and economic factors may further limit the choice of food. Bock (23), Queen (24), McKenzie (25) and the Food Prices Review Board (26) have shown that food choice is directly related to income. The effect of *price, convenience,* and *prestige* on food choice has been studied by Reaburn (27). Her results suggest that certain foods are designated by society as being high or low in prestige, and that individuals, consciously· or unconsciously, tend to choose foods which will enhance their image and position and avoid foods which are considered to have low prestige. Wilson and Lamb (28) reported that a group of undergraduate and graduate college students were shown to accept questionable *beliefs* about food,

thus demonstrating that advanced general education does not necessarily ensure a more adequate diet. Finally, Bremer and Weatherholtz (29) found positive correlation between concern *about nutrition* and interest in choosing "healthful" foods.

Thus, food choice motives have been extensively studied. The main contribution of the proposed model is to identify the food choice motives as variables within a process of food choice and to categorize them. Once they had a defined role and could be related to food selection it was possible to assess them quantitatively. Scales patterned after semantic differential (7) are used to assess their valency. Table I summarizes examples of the scales.

Scoring of the answers provides quantitative measures of the motives for individual foods ascribed to them by a specific category of people. For example the score of the price motive for grapes assigned by low-income housewives is four, i.e., high, in spite of its comparatively low consumer price. The scores can be used for a number of approaches to food habit analysis: a) They can be used for ranking different foods and comparing the strength of the meaning between them. For example the relative degree of satiety of potatoes and rice can be assessed within one population. b) The scores of individual food meanings assigned to food items may be compared among different populations. For example an intensity of sweet taste of butterscotch tart can be

TABLE I.

Scales for testing the frequency of food use and food choice motives

Food Use Frequency

1	2	3	4	5
less than once a month	once a month	a few times a month	a few times a week	daily

Satiety

1	2	3	4	5
not satisfied			very satisfied	

Price

1	2	3	4	5
forbidding			bargain	

Tolerance

1	2	3	4	5
never tolerate			tolerate at all times	

Convenience

1	2	3	4	5
takes a great deal of time and effort to prepare			a ready food takes no time and effort to prepare	

Taste

1	2	3	4	5
tastes very bad			tastes very good	

Health Belief

1	2	3	4	5
extremely unhealthy			essential for health	

Familiarity

1	2	3	4	5
never ate it as a child			ate it often as a child	

Nutrition Knowledge

1	2	3	4	5
nitritionally undesirable			very nutritious	

Prestige

1	2	3	4	5
never offer to guests			always offer to guests	

compared between Canadian Caucasians and Chinese. c) Different food choice motives can be compared between themselves. For example the scores of taste and scores of familiarity can be correlated. d) All food choice motives or individual ones can be correlated with food use frequency. The application of food choice motive analysis is demonstrated in Figure 5. The example is taken from Reaburn's study of habits and food choice motives of low-class housewives. The three columns chosen for illustration indicate a) foods eaten daily, the staple foods; b) the foods eaten weekly or a few times per month; and c) foods eaten rarely. Within the arrows are motives strongly associated with the specific foods. The arrow prefixes of the motives indicate how these motives could be used as access points in modifying the frequency of their intake, if it would be desirable from the physiological point of view. In Figure 5 we see that price and prestige are the reasons why liver is eaten rarely. If it was desirable to increase the consumption of liver it would not be sufficient just to decrease the price of liver but it would mean enhancing its prestige value as well. This can be done by means so successfully used by advertisers, such as having

liver recommended by a respected personality.

If we accept the postulation that each person has unique psychological and emotional needs, and these influence his/her choice of food, it is evident that the personality differences may also be expected to affect the relative significance of individual meaning which are tied to a particular food. Thus any effort to modify nutrition behaviour and use the appropriate communication should include a prior personality assessment. In Figure 6, the categorization of personalities, or personality types, according to the degree of internal control is suggested. Type A represents mainly well-educated health-oriented persons; type B includes social types, highly influenced by existing norms and values; type C comprises the externally controlled. The hypothetical differences in the relative significance of food meanings are indicated. Type A is presumably guided mostly by "personal" motives, type B by "social" motives, and type C by motives categorized as "cultural".

The proposed model for the study of food habits is a basic structure for the systematic gathering of data on "food meanings" (i.e., food choice motives). A

wide range of opinions on foods held by different types of populations is represented. After solving the riddle why people choose the foods they eat, functional nutritional policies based on these food choice motives must be integrated with assessment of individual personalities. This information, supplementing the nutrient requirements, could be the means of fulfilling the objective of all health professionals in this country — better health for Canadians. Possible applications of this hypothetical model include the development of a new approach to nutrition education.

It is our belief that clarification of the reasons for man's food choices would influence economic and social institutions in the development of food consumption policies. In short, recognition of man's food choice motives can eventually lead to a more realistic standard of food needs, based not only on his organic needs, as at present, but also on his cultural and emotional heritage.

Acknowledgement

The premises for the proposed method have been developed with the aid of a Canada Council grant.

Thanks are due to Dean Emeritus, Iva L. Armstrong, for her helpful suggestions in preparation of this manuscript.

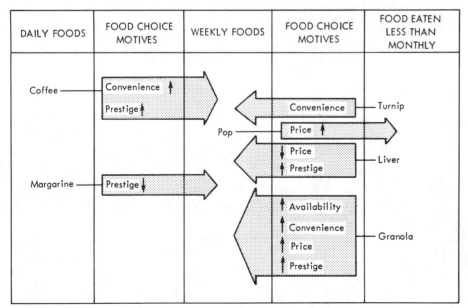

Figure 5. Food Choice Motives as Access Points to Food Habit Modification.

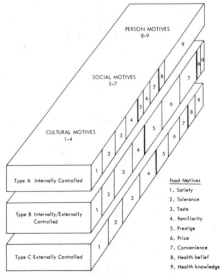

Figure 6. Hypothetical Personality Types and their Variations in Food Choice Motives.

Une connaissance insuffisante des motifs qui influent sur la sélection de nourriture constitue l'empêchement principal à la modification des habitudes alimentaires dans la société d'abondance. Elle limite la réussite de l'instruction en nutrition qui est une mesure importante de la santé publique.

On évoque des raisons historiques qui mettent en lumière l'évolution des motifs les plus influents dans la sélection de nourriture. On définit et on classe ces motifs. On discute leur application comme variables contrôlées

dans l'analyse des habitudes alimentaires. On peut les utiliser pour a) ranger les articles alimentaires selon la valence des motifs de sélection de nourriture; b) comparer les valences alimentaires des motifs de sélection de nourriture de différents groupes de la population; c) comparer les valences de motifs de sélection de nourriture entre elles; d) mettre la fréquence d'utilisation de nourriture en corrélation avec les motifs de sélection de nourriture. On illustre l'application des motifs de sélection alimentaire dans la modification de la

fréquence d'utilisation d'articles alimentaires particuliers.

Dans l'étude des motifs de sélection de nourriture, on signale la représentation de la population par le degré de contrôle interne et externe parce qu'on doit utiliser des voies d'intercommunication différentes pour des genres différents de groupes de la population. Ainsi, la modification des dispositions à l'égard de la nourriture et le changement de la fréquence d'utilisation de nourriture (habitudes alimentaires) pourront réussir.

REFERENCES

1. McClinton, P., Milne, H. and Beaton, G.H. An evaluation of food habits and nutrient intakes in Canada: Design of effective food guides. *Can. J. Public Health* 62: 139-46, 1971.
2. Brody, H. The systems view of man: Implications for medicine, science and ethics. *Perspect. Biol. Med.* 17: 71-91, 1973.
3. Schaefer, H. Sociophysiology. Das Medizinische Prisma. Ingelheim am Rhein, C.H. Boehringer Sohn, 1974.
4. De Garine, I. The social and cultural background of food habits in developing countries. *FAO Nutr. Newsletter* 8: 9, 1970.
5. Lowenberg. M.E. Social cultural-basis of food habits. *Food Technol.* 24: 751-6, 1970.
6. Jelliffe, D.B., Ifekwunigwe, A.E. and Jelliffe, F.P. Recommended dietary allowances for infants. *Ecol. Food Nutr.* 4: 53-5, 1975.
7. Fewster, W.J., Bostian, L.R. and Powers, R.D. Measuring the connotative meanings of food. *Home Econ. Res. J.* 2: 44-53, 1973.
8. Moore, F.W. Food habits in non-industrial societies. In: Dupont, J., Ed. Dimensions of nutrition. Denver, Colorado Associated University Press, 1970, pp. 181-221.
9. Simoons, F.J. The determinants of dairying and milk use in the Old World: ecological, physiological and cultural. *Ecol. Food Nutr.* 2: 83-90, 1973.
10. Sowers, M.F. and Winterfeldt, E. Lactose intolerance among Mexican Americans. *Am. J. Clin. Nutr.* 28: 704-5, 1975.
11. Koch, J.P. and Donaldson, R.M. A survey of food intolerance in hospitalized patients, *N. Engl. J. Med.* 271: 657-60, 1965.
12. Donaldson, R.M. The muddle of diets for GI disorders. *JAMA* 225: 1243, 1973.
13. Chau, E. and Chang, J. Fibre tolerance. A factor in food selection. B.Sc. Thesis. Faculty of Food Sciences, University of Toronto, 1975.
14. Hall, I. and Hall, C. A study of disliked and unfamiliar foods. *J. Am. Diet. Assoc.* 15: 540-8, 1939.
15. Van Riter, L.G. Acceptance of 26 vegetables. *J. Home Economics* 48: 771-3, 1956.
16. Van Schaik, T.F.S.M. Food and nutrition relation to family life. Ibid. 56: 225-32, 1964.
17. Einstein, M.A. and Hornstein I. Food preferences of college students and nutritional implications. *J. Food Sci.* 35: 429-36, 1970.
18. Munn, S. and Narang, P. Taste and familiarity as motives for food choice in Anglo-Saxon Canadians and Indian immigrants. B.Sc. Thesis. Faculty of Food Sciences, University of Toronto, 1975.
19. Lee, D. Cultural factors in dietary choice. *Am. J. Clin. Nutr.* 5: 166-70, 1957.
20. Jellinek, J.S. The meanings of flavour and textures. *Food Technol.* 27: 46-55, 1973.
21. Weisberg, S.M. Food acceptance and flavour requirements in the developing world. Ibid. 28: 48-52, 1974.
22. Pangborn, R.M. Cross cultural aspects of flavour preferences. Ibid. 29: 34-6, 1975.
23. Bock, J.K. Dietary intake and social characteristics. *Am. J. Clin. Nutr.* 4: 239-41, 1956.
24. Queen, G.S. Culture, economics and food habits. *J. Am. Diet. Assoc.* 33: 1044-6, 1957.
25. McKenzie, J. The impact of economic and social status on food choice. *Proc. Nutr. Soc.* 33: 67-73, 1974.
26. Food Prices Review Board. What Price Nutrition? Ottawa, Canada, Feb. 1975.
27. Reaburn, J. The effects of price, convenience and prestige on food choice. M.Sc. Thesis. Dept. of Nutrition and Food Sciences, Faculty of Medicine, University of Toronto, 1976.
28. Wilson, M.A. and Lamb, M.W. Food beliefs as related to ecological factors in women. *J. Home Economics* 60: 115-8, 1968.
29. Bremer, M. and Weatherholtz, W.M. Nutrition attitudes in a nutrition community. *J. Nutr. Educ.* 7: 60-4, 1975.
30. Quick, H.F. Geographic 'imensions of human ecology. In: Dupont, J. Dimensions of Nutrition. Colorado Associated University Press, 1970, pp. 133-152.

Nutrition Counseling in Private Practice: Attitudes and Activities of Family Physicians

by Thomas E. Kottke, Jane K. Foels, Cynthia Hill, Thomas Choi, and Douglas A. Fenderson

A community approach to cardiovascular disease control is advocated for the United States because of the high disease incidence and prevalence relative to other countries. The goal of this approach is to change nutrition behavior of all members of the community. As part of a program to identify barriers to physician participation, a survey of a random sample of family practice clinical faculty in a midwestern state was made to determine (a) if physicians agree that it is appropriate to give nutritional advice to a patient who came to the clinic for another reason, (b) the proportion of patients given nutritional advice, and (c) the barriers to giving nutritional advice. Most physicians report that giving nutritional advice to patients visiting them for other reasons is considered appropriate, but almost half the physicians give advice about dietary fat, dietary sodium, or dietary fiber to fewer than 20% of their patients. Only about 10% of physicians give advice to more than 80% of their patients. Absence of elevated risk factor levels or nutritional disease is the most common reason for not giving advice. Perceived lack of patient interest and expectation of patient nonadherence are also barriers. Unpalatability of the diet is occasionally a barrier. Cost of the diet is not a consideration. From these data it is concluded that family physicians consider it appropriate to give nutritional advice to patients who are not necessarily seeking it, but the perception that patients do not need or want, and would not follow, the advice inhibits physicians from delivering nutrition messages in private practice.

INTRODUCTION

Coronary heart disease (CHD), responsible for almost a million deaths in 1979, is the major cause of death in the United States (13). For each fatal event, two nonfatal coronary events occur, and clinical manifestations develop in 20% of all men under the age of 60 (13). Changes in care over the past two decades have

Thomas E. Kottke and Cynthia Hill are with the Cardiovascular Division, Department of Medicine, School of Medicine and Epidemiology Division, School of Public Health, University of Minnesota.

Jane K. Foels is with the North Memorial Medical Center, Minneapolis, Minnesota 55422.

Thomas Choi is with the Center for Health Services Research, School of Public Health, University of Minnesota.

Douglas A. Fenderson is with the Office of Continuing Medical Education, School of Medicine, University of Minnesota, Minneapolis, Minnesota 55455.

This work was supported by Preventive Cardiology Academic Awards 1K07-HL00662 and BRSG No. 2-S07-RR05448-20.

Address reprint requests to Thomas E. Kottke at Cardiovascular Division, Department of Medicine, Box 508 Mayo, 420 Delaware Street, SE, Minneapolis, Minnesota 55455.

done little to improve survival after a myocardial infarction (3). It is estimated that CHD cost $56.9 billion in 1983 (4).

Risk of cardiac disease clusters around factors such as elevated blood pressure and elevated serum cholesterol (10, 11). Dietary sodium appears to contribute to hypertension, and the proportion of dietary calories from saturated fat is strongly related to serum cholesterol levels. Clinical trials suggest that dietary modifications prevent CHD (5).

Although risk factors do tend to predict who will develop premature CHD, the lowest serum cholesterol levels in the United States are only as low as the highest serum cholesterol levels in Japan and Greece (7). As a result, CHD death rates in the United States are six to eight times those in Greece and Japan (7), and the majority of people dying of CHD have serum cholesterol levels at or only modestly above the population mean. Thus, optimal risk factor levels must be distinguished from normal levels. For example, a systolic blood pressure less than 160 is not considered abnormal. However, among the Framingham cohort, survival increased with systolic blood pressures as low as 120 mm Hg (1).

In the five studies combined for the Pooling Project, men with systolic blood pressure greater than 150 mm Hg had 1.9 times the risk of a coronary event as compared to men with blood pressure less than 129 mm Hg (10). However, 70% of the cardiac events in this population occurred in men with blood pressures less than 151 mm Hg—levels traditionally considered normal or borderline. Likewise, 68% of first coronary events occurred in men with serum cholesterol levels less than 268 mg/dl. Lower levels of risk factors, even within the normal range, are associated with increased survival, and the majority of events occur in people without markedly elevated risk factors.

Identifying high-risk patients is useful for defining risk factors, but for the reasons provided above, is less useful for preventing the diseases associated with the risk factors. Based on this observation, a World Health Organization expert committee has recommended the adoption of a community approach to cardiovascular disease control (16). The goal of the community approach is to shift population risk distributions downward by changing behaviors, expectations, and norms for whole communities. Another reason for *not* focusing on high-risk individuals alone is the finding of both the North Karelia Project and the Belgian Heart Disease Prevention Program that behavior change is no greater among individuals at high risk than it is among individuals at average risk (12, 2).

The public regards the physician as the primary source of dietary advice related to health (6, 8), and except for proprietary weight control programs or a registered dietitian in independent private practice, the registered dietitian is frequently available only through a physician. Physicians rarely include either nutrition counseling or referral to dietitians in their clinical repertoire. One reason for this low level of activity might be that physicians feel that it is inappropriate to make nutritional interventions if the patient does not ask for help. Other reasons can also be postulated as impediments.

As a planning tool for a program to increase physician dietary interventions and referrals to registered dietitians, we surveyed family practice clinical faculty to determine (a) whether the physician considers that initiating nutritional counseling is appropriate for the patient who is not necessarily seeking it, (b) the proportion of patients given nutritional counseling, and (c) the reasons for not providing nutritional counseling.

METHODS

A sample of 64 physicians was randomly selected from the University of Minnesota Family Practice Clinical Faculty. These physicians are in private practice throughout Minnesota. Family practitioners were the target population because a stated goal of family practice is to treat the entire patient.

One of two forms of a questionnaire about nutritional intervention practices for saturated fat, sodium, and fiber was mailed to each physician. Half of the physicians were randomly selected to receive a form with open-ended responses. The other half of the physicians received a form that offered several precoded choices for response and one opportunity for an open-ended response. A stamped, return envelope was included with the questionnaire. An identical questionnaire was mailed a second time to nonrespondents.

RESULTS

Of the 64 questionnaires mailed, 49 (77%) were returned with at least one question answered. The median year of graduation from medical school for the respondents was 1960; the range was from 1937 to 1978. As would be expected from the distribution of physicians throughout the state, the majority (63%) of the returned questionnaires came from physicians in Minneapolis, St. Paul, Rochester, and Duluth.

Sixty-two percent of physicians either agreed or strongly agreed with the statement that it is appropriate to give nutritional advice to a patient when the patient is at the doctor's office for a problem not directly related to nutrition. Twenty percent disagreed, and the remaining 18% were undecided (Table 1).

The majority of physicians reported giving dietary counseling to less than 40% of their male patients (Table 2). The pattern was similar for female patients. The most frequent response for not recommending a reduction in dietary saturated fat, given by half the physicians, was that the patient did not have an elevated serum cholesterol level (Table 3). Other reasons frequently cited included expectation of patient noncompliance and lack of need for dietary fat reduction because there was no weight problem. About one-third of physicians reported not being convinced of the value of saturated fat reduction, and an equal proportion indicated that a lack of patient interest in dietary information precluded their recommendations.

Lack of hypertension was the most frequently cited reason for not prescribing

TABLE 1

RESPONSES TO STATEMENT, "I believe that nutritional advice should be provided to patients visiting me for problems not related to nutrition"

Response	Percentage giving response
Strongly agree	7
Agree	54
Undecided	18
Disagree	14
Strongly disagree	7

TABLE 2

RESPONSES TO QUESTION, "For what percent of your adult male patients do you recommend a diet . . . ?"

Percentage of patients given diet	Type of diet		
	Low fat	Low sodium	High fiber
Less than 20	42	28	40
20 to 39	35	42	33
40 to 59	9	19	12
60 to 79	5	2	5
80 or more	9	9	10

TABLE 3

REASONS GIVEN FOR NOT COUNSELING ABOUT DIETARY FAT, SODIUM, AND FIBER

Response	Percentage giving response for each dietary component[a]		
	fat	sodium	fiber
The patient doesn't have . . .			
Elevated cholesterol	50		
High blood pressure		85	
Bowel problems			45
The patients would not comply with the diet	43	44	42
The patient is not interested in			
dietary information	30	26	32
I am not convinced of the value of the diet	30	8	32
The patient doesn't need weight reduction	35	13	3
The patient is elderly and probably won't			
develop heart disease	25	13	5
The diet is unpalatable	3	21	16
Dietary counseling is an			
inefficient use of my time	13	8	3
I don't have a dietitian or other			
resource person to help me	8	5	5
I'm not sure what to recommend to the patient	5	0	11
Nutrition education is not my responsibility	5	5	5
The diet is too costly for the patient	0	0	0

[a] Percentages total more than 100 because multiple responses were allowed.

sodium restriction (Table 3). Expectations of patient noncompliance and disinterest in dietary information were the next most frequent answers. A smaller proportion of physicians cited perceived unpalatability as a reason not to recommend sodium restriction. Other responses were selected with lower frequency.

Lack of bowel problems was the most commonly cited reason for not advising patients to increase their dietary fiber. As with fat and sodium, expectations of patient noncompliance and patient disinterest in increasing dietary fiber were also commonly selected reasons. The same proportion of physicians who mentioned patient disinterest stated they were not convinced of the value of the diet. A smaller proportion of physicians selected unpalatability as a reason for not recommending an increase in fiber intake.

The physicians who did not prescribe the diet tended to be the ones who did not agree that giving nutritional advice when the patient does not actively seek it is appropriate (for dietary fat $r = 0.32$; for both dietary sodium and dietary fiber $r = 0.24$). However, the majority of physicians who agreed that initiating a dietary intervention is appropriate even if the patient is not expressly seeking it gave nutrition counseling to less than 40% of their patients.

With responses of the physicians divided by those graduating from medical school before 1955, between 1955 and 1968, and after 1968, there was a trend for the earliest graduates to more frequently recommend a diet low in fat (Table 4). Physicians graduating after 1968 tended more frequently to recommend a diet low in sodium or high in fiber. However, the differences between groups was significant only for recommendations about fiber ($P < 0.05$).

DISCUSSION

As is typical for the United States as a whole, lifestyle contributes significantly to 7 of the 10 leading causes of death in Minnesota, and coronary heart disease,

TABLE 4

PERCENTAGE OF PATIENTS COUNSELED FOR THREE DIETARY COMPONENTS BY PHYSICIAN'S YEAR
OF GRADUATION

Dietary component	Year of graduation			All respondents	P value[a]
	Before 1955	1955–1968	After 1968		
Fat	36	33	22	31	.31
Sodium	30	33	41	35	.44
Fiber	23	28	47	33	.04[b]

[a] One-way analysis of variance.

[b] Percentage counseled by most recent graduates significantly differed from middle and least recent graduates.

stroke, and atherosclerosis are responsible for 60% of adult deaths (9). While the risk of disease is increased by certain behaviors, the majority of deaths occur in those persons at or only slightly above average risk. The absence of abnormal risk factor levels does not mean that an individual has no risk of premature disease.

Very few people in the United States have what might be considered optimal levels of cholesterol or blood pressure, and almost all clinicians come into contact with people who could clearly benefit from encouragement to lower dietary saturated fat and dietary sodium. A major reduction in cardiovascular disease deaths can only come about by controlling risk factor levels in people at average risk and lowering levels in those at high risk.

The public already looks to the physician for lifestyle advice (8), so the physician could play a role in changing both the individual patient's and the community's behavior. The physician who does not want to spend his or her time educating the patient has several options available: hiring a dietitian, contracting for a dietitian's services, using a hospital-based dietitian, or referring to a proprietary program.

We found that most physicians are not averse to initiating nutritional interventions—thus, this is not a barrier to care. However, the majority of physicians use the high-risk strategy to decide who is appropriate to receive care.

Anticipated lack of interest and anticipated lack of adherence are also significant barriers to intervention. As with anyone else, it is natural for physicians to avoid practices that are associated with negative reinforcement and are perceived to result in failure. It is not surprising that an intervention for which it is so hard to detect an effect and is sometimes unwanted by the patient is avoided.

It might be postulated that physicians learn to practice preventive medicine and nutritional interventions without formal medical courses. We found this not to be the case. Although the effects of dietary fat and serum cholesterol on death from CHD are the best documented of the three nutritional components (7, 11), recent graduates are even less likely to prescribe dietary fat modification and more likely to prescribe sodium restriction and fiber augmentation than are their earlier-trained counterparts. Wenger *et al.* also report that during the 1970s sodium-restricted diets were increasingly ordered for patients with CHD, but recommendations for fat- and calorie-restricted diets declined (15).

In this survey the major barrier to nutritional interventions was not conservatism in initiating care when the patient is not seeking treatment, but rather the belief that only a small proportion of patients would benefit from a nutritional intervention. Perceived lack of interest and expected nonadherence by the patient were also barriers. To play a role in reducing the CVD burden, physicians must be taught the rationale of the community approach to disease prevention. They must also be taught that patients are seeking nutritional information and will change their behaviors in response to an intervention.

REFERENCES

1. Dawber, T. R. "The Framingham Study: The Epidemiology of Atherosclerotic Disease," pp. 101–103. Harvard Univ. Press, Boston, 1980.
2. De Backer, G. "Studie van de omkeerbaarheid van risicofactoren voorbeschikkend tot coronaire hartziekten in een industriële bevolkingsgroep." Rijksuniversiteit, Gent, 1979.
3. Elveback, L. R., Connolly, D. C., and Kurland, L. T. Coronary heart disease in residents of Rochester, Minnesota. II. Mortality, incidence, and survivorship, 1950–1975. *Mayo Clin. Proc.* **56**, 665–672 (1981).
4. "Heart Facts" pp. 3–24. American Heart Association Office of Communications, Dallas, 1983.
5. Hjermann, I., Holme, I., Velve Byre, K., and Leren, P. Effect of diet and smoking intervention on the incidence of coronary heart disease. *Lancet* 1303–1310 (1981).
6. Inter-Society Commission for Heart Disease Resources. Atherosclerosis Study Group and Epidemiology Study Group. Primary prevention of atherosclerotic diseases. *Circulation* **42**, A55 (1970).
7. Keys, A. "Seven Countries. A Multivariate Analysis of Death and Coronary Heart Disease," p. 65. Harvard Univ. Press, Boston, 1980.
8. Levy, R. Progress in prevention of cardiovascular disease: A thirty-year retrospective. *Mod. Concepts Cardiovasc. Dis.* **47**, 103–108 (1978).
9. Minnesota Department of Health. Risks to good health: Behavior, *in* "Healthy People: The Minnesota Experience," p. 15. Minneapolis, 1982.
10. Pooling Project Research Group. Relationship of blood pressure, serum cholesterol, smoking habit, relative weight, and ECG abnormalities to incidence of major coronary events: Final report of the pooling project. American Heart Association Monograph Number 60. The American Heart Association, Dallas, 1978.
11. Rose, G. Incubation period of coronary heart disease. *Brit. Med. J.* **284**, 1600–1601 (1982).
12. Salonen, J. T., Heinonen, O. P., Kottke, T. E., and Puska, P. Change in health behavior in relation to estimated coronary heart disease risk during a community-based cardiovascular disease prevention programme. *Int. J. Epidemiol.* **10**, 343–354 (1981).
13. Stamler, J. Epidemiology of coronary heart disease. *Med. Clin. No. Amer.* **57**, 5–46 (1973).
14. Weinsier, R. L. Nutrition education in the medical school: Factors critical to the development of a successful program. *J. Amer. Coll. Nutr.* **1**, 219–226 (1982).
15. Wenger, N. K., Hellerstein, H. K., Blackburn, H., and Castranova, S. J. Physician practice in the management of patients with uncomplicated myocardial infarction—Changes in the past decade. *Circulation* **65**, 421–427 (1982).
16. World Health Organization. "Prevention of Coronary Heart Disease—Report of a WHO Expert Committee." World Health Organization Technical Report Series 678, Geneva, 1982.

Problems and Challenges in Social Marketing

by Paul N. Bloom and William D. Novelli

Introduction

MUCH has been written about social marketing since Kotler and Zaltman (1971) introduced the concept a decade ago. The literature has contained extended discussions about the definition of social marketing (Lazer and Kelley 1973, Sheth and Wright 1974), the ethics of social marketing (Laczniak, Lusch, and Murphy 1979), the appropriateness of broadening the marketing discipline to include social marketing (Luck 1974), and the potential of applying various social science theories in social marketing contexts (Swinyard and Ray 1977). In addition, several case studies of social marketing efforts have been reported (Blakely, Schutz, and Harvey 1977, Gutman 1978). However, there have been few attempts (Rothschild 1979) to move beyond the reporting of case studies toward the development of general knowledge about social marketing, including knowledge about the problems most organizations tend to find in applying conventional marketing approaches in social programs.

This article identifies a set of general problems that confront practitioners who attempt to transfer the marketing approaches used to sell toothpaste and soap to promote concepts like smoking cessation, safe driving, and breast self-examination. An awareness of these problems should allow social agency administrators or their marketing advisors to formulate more workable and effective social marketing programs. While the authors believe strongly in the contribution marketing can make to social programs, they feel compelled to temper the enthusiasm that many have shown for social marketing by pointing out the difficulties and challenges associated with its practice.

Note that the term social marketing is used throughout this article to mean "the design, implementation, and control of programs seeking to increase the acceptability of a social idea or practice in a target group(s)" (Kotler 1975, p. 283). Consequently, social marketing is treated as an endeavor that can be engaged in by profit making organizations (e.g., a liquor company program encouraging responsible drinking), as well as by nonprofit and public organizations. It is also treated as an endeavor that generally encourages people to do something that will be beneficial to more than just themselves (Lovelock 1979). For example, responsible drinking, safe driving, and smoking cessation can all reduce health hazards for others or lower the insurance premiums of others. This article is concerned with the marketing of social ideas and behaviors by any organization to any target group.

The problems discussed here have come to the

Paul N. Bloom is 1980–81 Visiting Research Professor, Marketing Science Institute, and Associate Professor of Marketing, University of Maryland. William D. Novelli is President, Porter, Novelli & Associates, Inc., Washington, DC. The authors would like to thank Alan Andreasen, Gerald Zaltman, Patrick Murphy, and Susan Watson for their comments and suggestions.

attention of the authors through work they have done with numerous social agencies and organizations. Problems are identified in eight basic decision making areas: market analysis, market segmentation, product strategy development, pricing strategy development, channel strategy development, communications strategy development, organizational design and planning, and evaluation. In each area an effort has been made to point out several problems encountered by social marketers that typically do not face the large commercial marketers who are the focus of most textbook examples. Admittedly, many of the cited problems may also confront small businesses and other less conventional marketers. But the discussion here will concentrate on how these problems manifest themselves for social marketers.

Market Analysis Problems

A basic tenet of marketing is that an organization builds its marketing program using research it has gathered on the wants, needs, perceptions, attitudes, habits, and satisfaction levels of its markets. The good marketer is supposed to examine previous research on his or her consumers and, if necessary, conduct original consumer research in order to design maximally effective marketing strategies. Although large commercial marketers surely have difficulty accumulating valid, reliable, and relevant data about their consumers, the data gathering problems facing the social marketer tend to be far more serious. Social marketers typically find that:

- *They have less good, secondary data available about their consumers.* Social marketers can rarely go to the shelf to get fast, inexpensive guidance from reports on previous consumer studies. Most social organizations have done little consumer research, and what has been done has been weakened by small budgets and, consequently, poor samples and simplistic analysis procedures. Moreover, there are no syndicated services or panels available that can provide reasonably priced data on health behavior, safety behavior, conservation behavior, etc. Perhaps the best source of secondary data is the academic or scholarly literature. Journals such as the *Journal of Health and Social Behavior, American Journal of Public Health, Health and Society,* and *Social Service Review* can sometimes be helpful. But many academic works tend to be narrowly focused and hard to tap for action-

able marketing ideas (especially by people with limited research backgrounds). Unfortunately, marketing academics—who have the capability of producing consumer studies that could be more readily used by social marketing planners—have given only limited attention to how consumers deal with social ideas and behaviors (Rothschild 1979, Swinyard and Ray 1977).

- *They have more difficulty obtaining valid, reliable measures of salient variables.* In doing primary data collection, social marketers must ask people questions about topics such as smoking, sickness, sex, and charity—topics that touch people's deepest fears, anxieties, and values. While people are generally willing to be interviewed about these topics, they are more likely to give inaccurate, self-serving, or socially desirable answers to such questions than to questions about cake mixes, soft drinks, or cereals. A recent study on how to ask questions about drinking and sex suggests that "threatening questions requiring quantified answers are best asked in open-ended, long questions with respondent-familiar wording" (Blair et al. 1977, p. 316). Using such methods can be extremely time-consuming and expensive.

- *They have more difficulty sorting out the relative influence of identified determinants of consumer behavior.* Social behaviors tend to be extremely complex and usually hinge on more than just one or two variables. The reasons patients drop out of antihypertensive drug therapy, for instance, may be related to an individual's limited self-discipline, lack of family support, drug side effects, physician/patient miscommunication, or any combination of these and other factors. It is extremely difficult for respondents to sort out these contributing variables in their own minds, and articulate them to a researcher in such a way that they can be recorded and analyzed for marketing planning. Furthermore, asking physicians to untangle patient behavior is often no more enlightening than asking the patients themselves. A recent study of physicians revealed, for example, that the reason patients were not on antihypertensive therapy was because they were not following the regimen that had been prescribed for them (U.S. Department of Health, Education, and Welfare 1979). This may be logical, in a self-evident sort of way, but not very helpful to the marketing planner.

- *They have more difficulty getting consumer research studies funded, approved, and completed in a timely fashion.* Social agencies typically have very limited funds, and the intangible output of a research study is often more difficult to justify to donors (e.g., Congress) than the more tangible output of a new program or publication. Furthermore, if the federal government is involved in some way in the proposed research, lengthy delays often will occur while the questionnaire and research design are approved by the agency doing the study, its Department, the Office of Management and Budget, and other parties. For example, the Office of Cancer Communications of the National Cancer Institute began the paperwork on a straightforward three stage study of knowledge, attitudes, and reported behavior related to breast cancer in April 1977. Red tape and the system delayed the completion of the analysis of the full study until July, 1980.

As a final comment on market analysis problems, it should be pointed out that the red tape that chokes and delays consumer studies can lead to some very unsound but highly original research tactics. One ploy is to conduct focus groups, always with fewer than nine respondents. This gets around the letter, if not the spirit, of the OMB clearance regulations concerning what constitutes a survey. However, this tactic, while it may provide some useful research hypotheses, can lead to misleading conclusions and poor planning. This is because the focus groups are often not followed by larger scale studies to quantify the preliminary findings and assess the hypotheses. The misuse of qualitative research as a substitute, rather than a precursor, to more definitive research appears to be a common problem among many social agencies.

Market Segmentation Problems

The process of dividing up the market into homogeneous segments and then developing unique marketing programs for individual target segments (while perhaps ignoring certain segments) is fundamental to modern marketing. Market segmentation is generally viewed as being more productive than treating the entire market in an undifferentiated manner. Although market segmentation is widely utilized and accepted by most profit making and many nonprofit (e.g., universities, hospitals) marketers, social marketers find that:

- *They face pressure against segmentation, in general, and especially against segmentation that leads to the ignoring of certain segments.* The notion of treating certain groups differently or with special attention while perhaps ignoring other groups completely, is not consistent with the egalitarian and antidiscriminatory philosophies that pervade many social agencies (particularly those within government). The social marketer is, therefore, frequently asked to avoid segmenting or to try to reach an unreasonably large number of segments (Lovelock and Weinberg 1975). If a marketing plan has only a few target markets identified, requests will be made to add to the list of targets until, with the limited funds that usually are available, only a very broad and very shallow marketing effort is authorized. This will produce the opposite of the rifle approach the marketer normally attempts to bring to bear.

An example of this problem occurred in a multiagency federal effort in 1978–79 to increase public understanding of the health risks of exposure to asbestos, and to persuade those exposed to get regular medical checkups, stop smoking, and seek prompt medical treatment for respiratory illness. The serious diseases associated with asbestos take from 15 to 35 years to develop, and workers exposed during World War II (especially ship yard workers) were identified as the primary target segment for the program. However, due to the mandates of some of the agencies involved, it became necessary also to target the effort to current workers. The characteristics of this segment differed substantially from the other, and throughout the planning and implementation of the program, there was a constant problem about whether to divide limited resources or simply take a general audience route.

- *They frequently do not have accurate behavioral data to use in identifying segments.* The data collection problems alluded to earlier impede segmentation attempts by making it difficult to separate users from nonusers. Utilizing self reports on behaviors like breast self-examination and contraceptive usage can be very misleading, and it may be impossible to obtain other behavioral measures (e.g., observational data).

- *Their target segments must often consist of those consumers who are the most negatively predisposed to their offerings*. Social marketers often segment on the basis of risk to the consumer. They will target their efforts at drivers who tend to avoid using seat belts, sexually active teenagers who tend to avoid using contraceptives, heavy smokers, etc. They may sometimes even target their efforts at segments facing greater legal risk, such as in a program recently formulated by William Novelli to persuade sheet metal contractors to recruit and accept more women into their field. This segmentation approach creates situations where social marketers face target markets having the strongest negative dispositions toward their offerings—the exact opposite of the situation faced by most commercial marketers. Moreover, as Rothschild (1979) has pointed out, these target markets are frequently highly involved with their negative feelings, making them much more resistant to changing their views than people who have negative attitudes toward low involved products like soap or bread.

Product Strategy Problems

Once the marketer has analyzed the market and determined target segments, he or she should then develop an offering that conforms closely to the desires of the target segments. Conventional marketers will typically adjust product characteristics, packaging, the product name, the product concept, and the product position to increase the likelihood of a sale to the target segments. However, social marketers find:

- *They tend to have less flexibility in shaping their products or offerings (Kotler 1975, Lovelock and Weinberg 1975).* They often find themselves locked into marketing a given social behavior that cannot be modified or changed. This could occur because the government might approve of only one way of doing the behavior. For example, social marketers may be able to market only one way to get a home insured against floods or one way to get a child immunized. On the other hand, they may be able to market several ways of quitting smoking, getting physically fit, or conserving energy.

- *They have more difficulty formulating product concepts.* They frequently find that the product they are selling is a complex behavior which may, in some cases, have to be repeat-

ed over a considerable period of time. It therefore becomes difficult to formulate a simple, meaningful product concept around which a marketing and communications program can be built. Effective concepts like a squeezably soft toilet paper and an extra thick and zesty spaghetti sauce do not come readily to mind when thinking about selling behaviors such as drug therapy maintenance or use of an in-home colon-rectal cancer detection test (i.e., the hemocult test). In addition, the problems associated with doing consumer research (discussed above) tend to hinder product concept development.

- *They have more difficulty selecting and implementing long-term positioning strategies.* Assuming the social marketer has some ability to shape the offering and to formulate a relatively simple product concept, he or she may still have major problems selecting a product position that will be attractive and/or acceptable to the extremely diverse publics that impact on the typical social agency. The current dilemma of the Asthma and Allergy Foundation of America (AAFA) illustrates this problem. The new executive director wants to revitalize the agency at the national headquarters level, to strengthen the existing 13 chapters, and to add new chapters throughout the country. She sees several positioning options open to help AAFA achieve these objectives, including presenting AAFA as a service organization, a research organization, or a public education organization. The best positioning approach is not clear, as each position has a positive appeal for some publics and a negative appeal for other publics. For instance, projecting a service position will probably help AAFA in its exchange relationships with patients and local chapter volunteers and personnel (who apparently favor this stance), but it might not be the best approach for attracting funds from donors or for generating public clamor for more congressional funding of research and public education.

Even if the social marketer can settle on a preferred positioning strategy, the implementation of this strategy over a lengthy period of time may be impossible. Social marketers frequently do not have the ability to communicate persistently and present a position—like Avis did with "We Try Harder"—for more than a few months. The result is often consumer confusion about what it is an agency or program is trying to accomplish. The short life of many positioning strategies is caused (in government agencies at least) by frequent budget shifts, sudden personnel changes, a desire to show that something new and different is being tried, and other forces. For example, the government rarely concentrates funds and effort on a single problem for an extended period, producing instead what seems like a disease of the month approach. A notable exception is the National High Blood Pressure Education Program, which has been unerring in its positioning for eight years and has made substantial progress in contributing to hypertension control in the United States (Ward 1978).

Because doing anything in the product strategy is difficult for social marketers, many will ignore this aspect of marketing planning and, instead, concentrate their efforts on developing advertising and promotion strategies for the product they have been told to sell. However, social marketers should recognize that although they may be unable to adjust the performance characteristics of their products, they may be able to adjust the perception characteristics of their products and achieve significant results. Through minimal amount of product testing research with consumers, and some creative concept development and positioning, social marketers can gain confidence that the signals being transmitted by their offerings are favorable. They can also avoid making the kind of product strategy mistake made by the Agency for International Development in a program designed to persuade Nicaraguan mothers to give their babies the proper treatment for diarrhea (a major cause of infant mortality). Problems occurred with this program because of lack of in-home product testing of the super lemonade (a rehydration solution) the program promoted. It was discovered after the program had begun, that the solution may not have been administered in some cases because some mothers who sampled it before giving it to their babies, thought it tasted bad. In addition, there was evidence that some women had difficulty measuring the ingredients and concocting the solution. The solution also caused the diarrhea to increase for a short time after first being administered, providing mothers with a potential signal that the product was ineffective or perhaps even harmful. In a new program in Honduras, extensive formative research, including product testing, is being applied (Smith 1980).

Pricing Strategy Problems

Marketers of most products and services find that the development of a pricing strategy involves primarily the determination of an appropriate (i.e., goal satisfying) monetary price to charge for an offering. On the other hand:

- *Social marketers find that the development of a pricing strategy primarily involves trying to reduce the monetary, psychic, energy, and time costs incurred by consumers when engaging in a desired social behavior.* Social marketers generally have much more complex objective functions than commercial marketers. They are primarily concerned with shifting birth rates, death rates, pollution levels, and the like, and are concerned with the financial consequences of their actions only to the extent that they want to insure their organization's financial viability. They do not price their offerings to maximize financial returns but instead try to price offerings to minimize any barriers that might be preventing consumers from taking desired actions. This task is made difficult because consumer research data are often not available to provide social marketers with information about the psychic, energy, and time costs consumers perceive as being associated with a particular action. In other words:

- *Social marketers have difficulties measuring their prices (Rothschild 1979).* In addition, the pricing task is made difficult because:

- *Social marketers tend to have less control over consumer costs.* Unlike commercial marketers who can readily change consumer costs by essentially adjusting monetary prices, social marketers often can do little to change the time costs involved with carpooling, the embarrassment costs involved with getting an examination for cervical cancer, or other nonmonetary costs. In some cases, all the social marketer can do is try to make sure that consumers perceive the various costs accurately and do not inflate them in their minds. In other cases, however, the social marketer may at least be able to cut some red tape or eliminate other inconveniences to lower the price. This last strategy is being employed in the food stamp program of New York State. They have made it easier to become enrolled and have eliminated the necessity of putting up any money with food stamps in the retail stores. Additional strategies for lowering time costs are discussed in a recent paper by Fox (1980).

Channels Strategy Problems

Developing a channels strategy usually gets an organization involved with selecting appropriate intermediaries through which to distribute its products or offerings, and formulating ways to control these intermediaries to make sure they behave in a supportive manner. Social marketers typically must distribute the idea of engaging in a social behavior and/or a place to engage in such behavior, rather than a tangible product. However, they find that, relative to more conventional marketers:

- *They have more difficulty utilizing and controlling desired intermediaries.* Social marketers often find that they cannot convince desired intermediaries, such as doctors or the television news media, to pass along and support an idea, nor can they control effectively what these intermediaries might say if they choose to cooperate. Control over clinics, community centers, government field offices, or other places where a social behavior might be performed or encouraged is also frequently lacking. Unfortunately, social marketers usually cannot provide incentives to desired intermediaries to get cooperation, as a business marketer would do, and they generally cannot afford to build their own distribution channels. To achieve a smoothly functioning distribution system of basically volunteers, they must rely primarily on the attractiveness of their offerings, the creativity of their appeals for assistance, and the quality of their intermediary training programs.

The problems associated with establishing, utilizing, and controlling distribution channels produce a major difference between social and more conventional forms of marketing. The following two examples illustrate just how serious these problems can be.

- The federal flood insurance program has had difficulty getting insurance companies' agents to add flood insurance to their product line. The agents have seen this insurance as being hard to learn about, hard to sell (with government forms and regulations to worry about), and low in profitability.

- A program designed to motivate physicians to teach their patients how to quit smoking ran up against the problem that, although the physicians wanted to cooperate, they did not know the most effective quitting skills, or benefits, or how to communicate them. It, therefore, became necessary to teach physicians how to teach patients—a task that was complicated by the beliefs held by many physicians that they are adept at all facets of patient management.

Communications Strategy Problems

There are several approaches that marketers use to communicate with their target markets. These include advertising, public relations, sales promotion, personal contact, and atmospherics. Social marketers, however, often find that their communications options are somewhat limited. As discussed in the previous section, social marketers sometimes find channels of distribution for their ideas unavailable or difficult to control. For instance:

- *They usually find paid advertising impossible to use.* This problem may arise because of advertising's cost or because of media fears of offending certain advertisers or audiences by carrying messages about controversial social issues. In addition, many voluntary organizations may see paid advertising as impossible to use because they fear the effects on all voluntary organizations. If the American Cancer Society pays for an anti-smoking campaign, then the media might ask the American Lung Association and others to pay for their campaigns also. Furthermore, government agencies may see paid advertising as impossible to use because they fear criticism about wasting taxpayer money and about having the media overly populated with government sponsored advertisements (e.g., military recruitment). Questions could arise about who controls the media if the government became the largest total advertiser.

An inability to use paid advertising restricts many social marketers to the use of public service announcements. Since the competition for PSA time and space is heated, social marketers often find they cannot control the reach and frequency of their messages among their target segments. Audience coverage, therefore, becomes much more uncertain.

Social marketers face several other communications problems:

- *They often face pressure not to use certain types of appeals in their messages (Houston and Homans 1977, Lovelock and Weinberg 1975).* Donors and other influential parties may not want to see a social change organization cheapened by the use of hard sell, fear, or humor appeals. The use of hard sell and fear appeals may also be unwise when target audiences are strongly predisposed against a social behavior. These appeals could backfire and solidify a person's feelings against behaviors such as seat belt usage, smoking cessation, or responsible drinking. In general, an audience reaction of they can't tell me how to run my life is much more likely to confront a social marketer than a more conventional marketer.

- *They usually must communicate relatively large amounts of information in their messages.* Social marketers typically need to say more to consumers in a media message than commercial marketers. A complex social behavior may need to be described, along with the benefits of the behavior (i.e., a reason why) and a time and a place for acting. Particular emphasis must be given to presenting benefits, since the benefits of behaviors like reducing salt in the diet or lowering one's thermostat might not be as obvious or personal to people as the benefits of buying a new car or piece of clothing (Rothschild 1979). Equally important is a message conclusion, which tells in specific terms what (and where and when) the consumer should do next. The social marketer cannot be like most commercial marketers and assume that consumers know this (e.g., pick up a six pack at the store and drink it). Unfortunately, the need to provide large amounts of information forces many social marketing messages to close with the old standby, For more information, please call or write. . . .

The need to communicate large amounts of information makes it imperative for social marketers to look beyond the use of public service announcements toward the use of nonadvertising channels of communication (Rothschild 1979, Mendelsohn 1973). One program that has clearly recognized this necessity is the breast cancer education program of the National Cancer Institute. They have recognized that communicating the benefits of doing breast selfexamination is very problematical, since unlike many other preventive health behaviors (e.g., exercise, taking blood pressure medication), the payoff is perceived by many women as the discovery of sickness rather than the improvement of one's health. This program has, therefore, shifted its emphasis away from media messages toward more personal forms of communication using health care professionals and other credible intermediaries.

- *They have difficulty conducting meaningful pretests of messages.* Given the problems social marketers tend to have with selecting appeals and communicating desired behaviors, it would seem essential for careful pretesting to be done on social media messages. However, pretests of social messages run up against the same funding and measurement problems discussed earlier. For example, in a recent test of a message on the need to take mental patients out of institutions and accept them into our communities, few respondents gave expected (but socially unacceptable) comments such as: "I don't like the message. These people are dangerous and unpredictable and I don't want them in my neighborhood."

Pretesting is also made less meaningful by the lack of any norms or standards against which newly tested social messages can be compared. Clearly, it would be instructive to the social marketer to know how his/her message performed compared to previously tested messages on measures of comprehension, recall, believability, personal relevance, etc. Fortunately, social marketers working in the health area can now get comparison data on pretest performances by using the newly established Health Message Testing Service. This service, funded and administered by the National Heart, Lung, and Blood Institute, National Cancer Institute, and several other Federal agencies, has now tested more than thirty-five television and radio messages with samples of up to 300 individuals. The service invites randomly selected subjects from specified target audiences to view pilot television programs that have health messages and other commercials appearing within them. During an experimental period that is still underway, the service has been conducting pretests for public and nonprofit organizations at no charge. The data accumulated by the service is also available at no charge. A print testing capability is now being added to the service (Novelli 1978, Bratic and Greenberg 1980).[1]

Organizational Design and Planning Problems

The well-managed marketing organization has a marketing person in a key position at the top of the organization chart and numerous well-trained marketing individuals throughout the organization. This organization has a carefully drawn marketing plan developed annually, with procedures set up to make sure the plan is implemented and monitored. However, social marketers typically find that while social organizations usually know something about management and organizational design, they rarely have an interest in setting up responsive marketing organizations with marketing planning and control procedures. Social marketers typically find that:

- *They must function in organizations where marketing activities are poorly understood, weakly appreciated, and inappropriately located.* Social organizations have a tendency to adopt marketing in small doses. The management may decide to try marketing by hiring a few employees or consultants with marketing backgrounds. These persons are generally assigned to work with public affairs or public information offices because management generally equates marketing with communications or promotion. The results the marketers can achieve in these positions are quite limited, since they have little influence over program development and administration and must restrict themselves primarily to informing the public about the features of the program. Thus, social marketers are often programmed for mediocre performance from the very beginning. They cannot convince management to give marketing the prominence it needs to be effective, and they cannot earn their way to prominence through outstanding performance. This dilemma may continue to confront social marketers as long as physicians, lawyers, scientists, law enforcement specialists, social workers, and others who often dominate social agencies and organizations feel uncomfortable and unfamiliar with marketing.
- *They must function in organizations where plans (if any are developed) are treated as archival rather than action documents.* Social organizations (particularly those in government) do not feel the competitive pressures that the business world feels. Employees do not lose their jobs or gain promotions based on how well the organization does. Consequently, it is more difficult to get them to take the time and effort needed to formulate and follow plans. This, of course, can seriously impede the social marketing effort.
- *They must function in organizations that suffer from institutional amnesia.* In trying to put together a comprehensive marketing plan for a social organization, it often is impossible to get guidance for present efforts from information on how past strategies worked. Unlike many commercial organizations, social organizations frequently do not have information about the past results of using free samples, contests, price cuts, and so on. This kind of forgetting occurs in social organizations because they tend to keep poor records and have high employee turnover.

  Two individuals involved in the high intensity national antismoking efforts of the late 1960's and early 70's recently remarked to the authors that none of the experience or lessons learned then seem to be applied to current programs. "They're starting from zero," remarked one official, "as if the earlier programs never existed."
- *They must predict how both friendly and unfriendly competitors will behave.* Marketing planning is made difficult in all organizations by the need to predict how competitors will behave over a planning horizon. Social marketers face this difficulty as much as anyone. The marketer of a smoking cessation program must assess what the tobacco companies and their trade association are likely to do, while the marketer of a nutrition program must give thought to the future activities of the grocery manufacturers and their associations. But social marketers must also be concerned about the impact of a type of competition that commercial marketers rarely face—the friendly competition provided by other social organizations fighting for the same cause. Thus, in developing a marketing plan for the smoking cessation program of the National Cancer Institute, it becomes necessary to consider the potential actions of the National Heart, Lung, and Blood Institute, the U.S. Office of Smoking and Health, the American

---

[1] For further information about this service contact Health Message Testing Service, Office of Cancer Communications, National Cancer Institute, Bethesda, Maryland 20205.

Cancer Society, the American Lung Association, the American Heart Association, and a host of others. Friendly competitors can help the social marketer in many ways, but they can also create fragmented efforts, funding problems, and other difficulties.

Evaluation Problems

Evaluating the effectiveness of a marketing program is difficult for all marketers. One must determine measures of effectiveness and then develop a research design capable of isolating the role the marketing program has had in shifting those effectiveness measures. Naturally, social marketers face the same problems in doing evaluation studies as in doing market analysis studies (see above). They have serious problems with measurement and with getting support and approval for the research. In addition, social marketers find that:

- *They frequently face difficulties trying to define effectiveness measures.* Unlike business firms having quantitative objectives stated in terms of profitability, sales, or market share, social organizations may merely have vaguely stated mission or goal statements from which measures of effectiveness are difficult to extract (Houston and Homans 1977). Even after lengthy discussions with management, social marketers often have difficulty deciding whether a program is designed to create awareness of an issue, change people's behavior, save lives, or do something else. Beyond this it is hard to identify constructs or variables that should be monitored to indicate whether program objectives are being achieved. Should one examine, for example, smoking quitting rates or cigarette sales to evaluate the success of a smoking cessation program? Should one examine measures that indicate something about the secondary or unintended effects of such a program, such as data on the consumption of junk food and alcohol by people who are persuaded to quit smoking?

- *They often find it difficult to estimate the contribution their marketing program has made toward the achievement of certain objectives.* Although the field of evaluation research has become increasingly sophisticated and precise (for reviews see Rossi and Wright 1977, Phillips 1978, Bloom and Ford 1979), social marketing programs do not typically lend themselves to evaluation using the more interpretable research designs that have been identified in the literature. Using randomized experiments or quasi-experiments is hard to do in social marketing, not only because they tend to be expensive but also because social marketing programs are hard to compress into neat packages that can be delivered to some people or regions and not to others. It is easy, for example, for a press release intended for an experimental group to be picked up by the media serving a control group.

As a result, much of the evaluation activity that has occurred with social marketing programs (see Bloom 1980 for a review) has taken the form of after only or before and after with no control group studies. While these types of studies can help to identify clearly ineffective programs and can provide management with an indicator that a program might be working, they cannot show an unambiguous cause and effect relationship between a program and an outcome. For instance, before and after studies have not been able to show that the sharp decline in hypertension related deaths that have taken place during the course of the National High Blood Pressure Education Program can be definitely attributed to the program. However, to discover the true impact of this program might cost more money and trouble than it would be worth.

Conclusion

The relationship between social marketing and more conventional commercial marketing may be somewhat like the relationship between football and rugby. The two marketing games have much in common and require similar training, but each has its own set of rules, constraints, and required skills. The good player of one game may not necessarily be a good player of the other.

In this article we have attempted to document why social marketing is the more difficult game to master. While success in the battles over market share in industries like detergents or automobiles may call for equal or even greater stamina and perseverance, success in the social marketing arena requires greater ingenuity and imagination. In spite of this, social marketing efforts can succeed, particularly if the problems cited in this article are anticipated and dealt with in a creative and logical manner. Social marketing clearly provides a difficult but potentially rewarding challenge for members of the marketing profession.

REFERENCES

Blair, Ed et al. (1977), "How to Ask Questions About Drinking and Sex: Response Effects in Measuring Consumer Behavior," *Journal of Marketing Research*, 14 (August), 316–21.

Blakely, Edward J., Howard Schutz, and Peter Harvey (1977), "Public Marketing: Policy Planning for Community Development in the City," *Social Indicators Research*, 4, 163–184.

Bloom, Paul N. (1980), "Evaluating Social Marketing Programs: Problems and Prospects," in *Marketing in the 80's: Changes and Challenges*, Richard P. Bagozzi et al., eds., Chicago: American Marketing Association, 460–463.

———, and Gary T. Ford (1979), "Evaluation of Consumer Education Programs," *Journal of Consumer Research*, 6 (December), 270–279.

Bratic, Elaine and Rachel H. Greenberg (1980), "An Approach to the Standardization of Pretesting Health Public Service Announcements," paper presented at the 30th annual conference of the International Communication Association, Acapulco, Mexico (May 19).

Fox, Karen F. A. (1980), "Time as a Component of Price in Social Marketing," in *Marketing in the 80's: Changes and Challenges*, Richard P. Bagozzi et al., eds., Chicago: American Marketing Association, 464–467.

Gutman, Evelyn (1978), "Effective Marketing of a Cancer Screening Program," in *Marketing in Nonprofit Organizations*, Patrick J. Montana, ed., New York: Amacom, 133–147.

Houston, Franklin S. and Richard E. Homans (1977), "Public Agency Marketing: Pitfalls and Problems," *MSU Business Topics*, 25 (Summer), 36–40.

Kotler, Philip (1975), *Marketing for Nonprofit Organizations*, Englewood Cliffs, NJ: Prentice-Hall.

———, and Gerald Zaltman (1971), "Social Marketing: An Approach to Planned Social Change," *Journal of Marketing*, 35 (July), 3–12.

Laczniak, Gene R., Robert F. Lusch, and Patrick E. Murphy (1979), "Social Marketing: Its Ethical Dimensions," *Journal of Marketing*, 43 (Spring), 29–36.

Lazer, William and Eugene J. Kelley, eds. (1973), *Social Marketing: Perspectives and Viewpoints*, Homewood, IL: Richard D. Irwin, Inc.

Lovelock, Christopher H. (1979), "Theoretical Contributions from Services and Nonbusiness Marketing," working paper 79–16, Harvard Business School.

———, and Charles B. Weinberg (1975), "Contrasting Private and Public Sector Marketing," in *1974 Combined Proceedings*, Ronald C. Curhan, ed., Chicago: American Marketing Association, 242–247.

Luck, David J. (1974), "Social Marketing: Confusion Compounded," *Journal of Marketing*, 38 (October), 70–72.

Mendelsohn, H. (1973), "Some Reasons Why Information Campaigns Can Succeed," *Public Opinion Quarterly*, 37 (Spring), 50–61.

Novelli, William D. (1978), "Health Messages: Milk Duds, Sunburns and Other Consumer Perspectives," working paper, Porter, Novelli and Associates, Inc., Washington, D.C.

Phillips, Lynn W. (1978), "Threats to Validity in Quasi-Experimental Evaluations of Consumer Protection Reforms: A Critical Review of Extant Research," technical report 78-102, Marketing Science Institute, Cambridge, Mass.

Rossi, Peter H. and Sonia R. Wright (1977), "Evaluation Research: An Assessment of Theory, Practice and Politics," *Evaluation Quarterly*, 1, 5–52.

Rothschild, Michael L. (1979), "Marketing Communications in Nonbusiness Situations or Why It's So Hard to Sell Brotherhood Like Soap," *Journal of Marketing*, 43 (Spring), 11–20.

Sheth, Jagdish and Peter Wright, eds. (1974), *Marketing Analysis for Societal Problems*, Champaign, IL: University of Illinois Press.

Smith, William A. (1980), "Mass Media and Health Practices-Implementation: Description of Field Activity in Honduras," working paper, Academy for Educational Development, Inc., Washington, D.C.

Swinyard, William R. and Michael L. Ray (1977), "Advertising-Selling Interactions: An Attribution Theory Experiment," *Journal of Marketing Research*, 14 (November), 509–516.

U.S. Department of Health, Education, and Welfare (1979), *Diagnosis and Management of Hypertension: A Nationwide Survey of Physicians' Knowledge, Attitudes, and Reported Behavior*, DHEW Publication No. (NIH) 79-1056.

Ward, Graham W. (1978), "Changing Trends in Control of Hypertension," *Public Health Reports*, 93 (January-February), 31–34.

A Critical Assessment of Marketing's Place in Preventive Health Care

by Godfrey M. Hochbaum

My familiarity with the field of marketing has, until yesterday, been restricted to the commercial realm. Yesterday, I was exposed for the first time to a broader concept of marketing, one that comes much closer to what I believe to be useful and desirable in preventive health and much more compatible, in fact, overlapping with my concept of health education. This paper does not consider this broader concept.

I am convinced not only that a great majority of marketing experts themselves see the field of marketing more as I saw it until yesterday, but that this is the almost universal concept among all people, including health educators and other health professionals. Therefore, the thoughts and concerns to be expressed about the role of marketing in preventive health care, are likely to reflect those of many, if not most, of my colleagues in the health professions.

If this supposition is correct, you must deal with it if you want to be welcomed into and fully accepted for your potential contributions to the health field. So, in a sense, I shall hold up a mirror in which you may see yourself as you are seen by many of my colleagues. It may help you market your own profession.

Those of us who have been addressing ourselves to the task of changing people's health behavior, are keenly aware that its problems are not exactly like those found in marketing commercial products or services. There are certain differences, some of them merely a matter of emphasis or degree but some quite substantive.

There is always a risk in taking concepts and techniques that have proven effective in solving <u>one</u> kind of problems in <u>one</u> context and applying them blindly to <u>another</u> kind of problems in <u>another</u> context. One must understand clearly the differences between the two kinds of problems and the contexts in which they occur. If one understands these differences, one

---

Godfrey M. Hochbaum is with the Department of Health Education, University of North Carolina.

can select from the arsenal of concepts and techniques that have proven effective in the one setting, those that seem appropriate to the other settings, and one can modify and adapt them to the special conditions that prevail.

My personal view of the term "marketing," until now, referred to a wide spectrum of decisions and actions, all of which are aimed in the long run at increasing the sales of a given product or the utilization of a given service. Marketing includes, therefore not only decisions about how to sell, but also decisions as to at what price it is to be sold, and where and how it is to be distributed.

In respect to each of these elements of marketing, certain differences exist between the health and the commercial areas. These differences do not decrease the usefulness of marketing concepts and techniques but may demand some modification and innovative developments in the application of marketing principles to the task of changing the public's health habits and practices.

WHAT IS TO BE MARKETED

In preventive health we sell very few products--that is, concrete goods. Seatbelts in automobiles are about as typical as any. We do sell some services such as immunizations, physical check-ups, dental services, and screening programs for early detection of diseases like cervical cancer, hypertension and glaucoma. But, with the exception of immunization, none of these services are really preventive. They only serve to detect disease processes early enough to permit medical intervention when prognosis is most favorable.

When we talk about true primary prevention, the emphasis is not really on services (again excepting immunization) but on actions to be taken by consumers. And what are such actions? Abstention from tobacco; restricting oneself in respect to taking substances like alcohol and certain drugs; dietary restrictions to control body weight; blood cholosterol level and other dietary risk factors; giving up the comforts of sedentary habits in order to engage in regular physical activity, etc.

I would like to point out that these actions (that is preventive behaviors) have certain striking characteristics in common: (1) They necessitate giving up things that many or most people like, (2) They are often unpleasant in themselves (at least for many people), and (3) They must last, not for a few days or even years - but a life time. Most of them mean changing an entire long-established, comfortable, and cherished living style. And, most of them are difficult to carry out for reasons to be mentioned later.

MARKETING IN THE COMMERCIAL AREA

Since the ultimate goal is to sell, the kinds and amounts of good produced for the commercial market depend usually on consumer demand. In fact, I cannot imagine that any reasonably smart manufacturers would ever deliberately produce any kinds of goods unless he has reason to believe that there exists a substantial demand for them, or that there is at least enough latent consumer interest which could be fanned into a demand.

Moreover, he will package, distribute, and display the product
in ways which he believes will attract the attention of potential purchasers. In other words, decisions as to what is to be
marketed, are based heavily on potential and expected consumer
demand.

In contrast, the health actions on which we try to "sell"
the public are given to us. They are prescribed by the medical
and other health professions. And these prescribed (or more
often, proscribed) health practices are defined rather exactly
and inflexibly. They can rarely (and even then only very little)
be tailored to consumers' desires, motives, or preferences. Instead of offering our consumers things they like and want, almost all the things we offer them in the health area, especially
in preventive health, are inherently unpleasant, inconvenient,
humiliating, and painful; they disrupt old, accustomed living
habits; and they necessitate depriving oneself of things one
wants and enjoys. Moreover, there is precious little we can do
to fit the product to the consumer's tastes or to package it
attractively. Almost the best we can do is to make the painful
a little less painful, the unpleasant a little less unpleasant,
the frightening a little less frightening.

In the commercial area, it is largely the potential consumer who determines what we produce and offer, and who influences
strongly the way it is packaged, distributed and sold. In the
health arena, it is the health professions who determine what
is produced or offered, and even where and in what form it is
offered, regardless of what the consumer wants and, as often as
not, against the consumer's desires and wishes. So we can see already that what we try to "market" in the area of health, especially in preventive health, is very different from most of
what we try to market in the commercial area, and that the decision of what to offer the public as well as in what shape and
form it is to be offered (its "packaging") are taken out of the
actual marketing process. --You, the market experts, have nothing to say about these vital aspects of marketing.

OTHER PROBLEMS UNIQUE TO THE HEALTH AREA

As a rule, the end points of the marketing process is the
sale of a product. What the consumer does with the product
once he has purchased it, is of little concern, except in as
much as it may relate to consumer satisfaction and future purchase of the same manufacturer's products. But, the seller
does not really care very much when and how the consumer uses
the product, or, indeed, whether he uses it at all.

In the health area, the concern with use after "purchase"
is as critical as and even more critical than the concern with
the purchase itself. The person who is sold on and goes through
disease screening procedures but does not follow through with
medical treatment for a diagnosed condition, is as much of a
failure as a person who did not avail himself of the screening
program to begin with. The obese individual who has been successfully sold on going on a medically prescribed diet but is
lured back to his candy jar and apple pie after one week, is
as much of a failure as if he never had been sold on the need
to lose and control his weight. The most challenging, most difficult, most perplexing problem is not how to sell people on
health-supportive practices, not even how to get them to initi-

ate such practices. We have been fairly successful with these. It is to persuade and help them to stick with new practices, to keep these up conscientiously and consistently for the rest of their lives. But which automobile salesman cares whether his customers drive their cars at all or how they drive them...as long as they bought them?

Let me once more illustrate by an example. We know that the single most prevalent and most powerful motive for giving up cigarettes is fear of disease, especially cancer. This has tempted health professionals to use the appeal to fear of disease, and very effectively. (The skills of marketing experts have, as a matter of fact, greatly contributed to this effectiveness.) Millions of smokers gave up smoking in response to this appeal. But what happens afterwards to most exsmokers? For days, weeks, months, perhaps years after throwing away the last pack of cigarettes, the ex-smoker experiences innumerable incidents when he suddenly craves a cigarette..A single cigarette..just one puff off a cigarette. What prompted him to quit to begin with was the fear of cancer, a disease caused by the accumulated consumption of thousands of cigarettes over many years. This one single cigarette which he craves right now, certainly would not contribute at all to this danger. So, the fear-motive that caused him to give up the habit at first, is rather powerless at such a moment against the strong conflicting motive to satisfy his intense and painful craving for this one cigarette.--He yields, and tomorrow this episode is repeated.. and again..and before he knows it, he is back in his old ways.

Similar processes can be observed in patients on prolonged regimens, such as long-term medication schedules, diets, and others. It is, to return once more to our automobile salesman, as if he had to worry not only about selling cars to his customers, but also about how, how often, where and when they drive them in subsequent months and years. And, the appeals, methods and techniques he would have to use to influence his customers' driving habits would obviously have to be very different from the sales techniques that led to the purchases to begin with. You can see that appeals, motivations, and methods that have proven effective for selling people on the idea of adopting the practices recommended by the health professions, are often relatively impotent in persuading people to persist in their new ways--and this is the critical issue. This is where the most critical challenge lies in preventive health.

THE PROBLEM OF PERSISTENT BEHAVIOR

Most people do prize health highly. Most anyone is eager to be and stay healthy, to lead a long life, to prevent disease and disability. We do not need to sell people on health. They are already sold on it. But, being even intensely motivated to remain healthy the rest of one's life does not necessarily mean being also motivated to do all the many things one should do to assure such lasting health. We all know, for example, that none of the millions of current smokers want to die of cancer. But this does not mean that they are also motivated to give up the one cigarette which they crave at a given moment. And the 40-year old man who knows that he could reduce his risk of heart disease (and surely wants to reduce it) by more physical activities and a more prudent diet, does not thereby necessarily want to jog or exercise daily or to give up his favorite dishes and still would want to spend his free time vigorously watching football or baseball on TV.

Of course, many people do engage in actions, even unpleasant ones, for the sake of assuring their present and future health, but very few do it systematically and conscientiously, and most people do it rarely, if at all. So, the challenge is how to persuade people to do things which most of them don't want to do but which they know that ought to do in order to get what they do want, namely that vague, illusive thing called, "health".

How often are you challenged in the <u>commercial</u> area to market a product or service which is actually counter to what people want? But, since this whole question of how to help people keep up the good works after they have started them, is itself too complex a subject to be covered here, I will proceed to still another critical difference.

THE DIFFERENCE IS IN THE PROMISE

One of the (if not <u>the</u>) most effective tools of commercial marketing is the persuasive (if not always truthful) promise of full satisfaction with a product or service. "Buy our pills, we promise, and your headache will disappear in 25 seconds;" "buy our toilet paper and it will be the softest ever;" "use Geratol and your husband will love you for ever and ever;" "let us handle your income tax return and you will save money." Note that each of these is the promise of a concrete, observable, directly experienced benefit, and that it is promised to accrue to the buyer immediately and in tangible form. The buyer is promised immediate, concrete, and assured reward for buying the goods.

But, in the health area such a promise can only be made relatively rarely because there is always a strong element of uncertainty in the outcome. We cannot, for example, promise the smoker that if he quits, he will never contract cancer of the lungs or emphyzema or heart disease; and, conversely, we cannot with any of these diseases. Only rarely can a physician promise for sure that a particular treatment, medication or surgery, will cure the patient.

Thus, people are often urged to give up long-standing comfortable, pleasurable, and deeply ingrained living habits, to sacrifice things and activities they cherish, to submit themselves voluntarily to all sorts of distasteful, unpleasant, even painful deprivations and experiences..and for what? For an uncertain and unpredictable outcome which in many cases even if it is as hoped for, may not be realized for many years. In fact, in most cases, the person will not know to the day he dies, if all these sacrifices had been worth it. Who in the commercial realm faces the task of selling people on a product like this?

OTHER STUMBLING BLOCKS

Obviously, the methods of Madison Avenue which are so predominantly based on promised consumer satisfaction, cannot be applied as universally or as simply in the health area without violating ethical principles to which the health professions adhere--or at least, to which they profess to adhere. In fact, when exaggerated claims for either preventive or therapeutic power of medicine have led first to unrealistic expectations and then to disappointment on the part of consumers (something that has happened all too often), the consequences have been deep disillusionment, refusal to follow even sound medical advice, and a turning to quackery.

Yet, here we are urging people to have periodic health examinations, to see their dentists every six months, and to engage in other preventive and health maintenance practices...but very few health insurance policies cover their considerable costs. We urge people to develop healthful dietary habits, but our entire food production, distribution and marketing system is designed to prevent or at least inhibit such habits. We urge people to become physically more active but our transportation technology, city planning, architectural designs, and other factors militate effectively against physical exercise.

I could give many more examples of cases where, even when we have effectively educated the public to engage in healthful practices, the social, economic and manmade physical environments make such practices difficult or impossible. In fact, our society and its technology--even our health care system itself--seem at times to be engaged in a giant conspiracy to prevent people from carrying out the very actions we try to sell them on. This is a problem that you face rarely if ever in commercial marketing because there, as a rule, you market things for which there is (or for which you suspect to be) a substantial number of consumers both ready and able to buy.

ADVERTISING EFFECTIVENESS IN THE COMMERCIAL AND HEALTH AREA

Advertising campaigns are as a rule intended less to create (and are less effective when they _try_ to create) _new_ desires for a given type of product in heretofore disinterested consumers, than they are designed to lure already interested consumers away from similar competitive products to one's own product. Advertisements for a given brand of, say, toothpaste or cigarettes or lawnmowers, only occasionally try deliberately to sell products to people who do not yet use them. Most such advertisements are designed to stress the advantages of one's own brand over other producers' brands. In the health area, this would be tantamount to physicians or hospitals publicly claiming that _their_ medical services are less painful or more effective than those offered by other physicians or hospitals.

Except for relatively few cases, there is little evidence that the mass media do generate new demands, and that they change public attitudes, values and behavior in a purposefully intended direction, even in respect to political views. Their effectiveness lies more in triggering latent audience desires, reinforcing and strengthening existing habits, and accelerating an already initiated spreading of new fads and practices.

But, even if we accept claims of effectiveness, the criteria by which such successes are evaluated, are not quite the same which we in the health area would apply. Consider a hypothetical manufacturing company whose product is bought by, say, 20 percent of its potential consumer population. If a sales campaign succeeded in increasing this volume by another five percent in one year, the company would probably be highly pleased. But, take a health program that tries to get all women at risk of cervical cancer to have yearly papsmear. If this program attracted only 20 or even 30 or 40 percent to begin with and succeeded only to add another five or ten percent to this number, the program would be regarded as a failure. Indeed, what would be proudly proclaimed as victory in the commercial arena, will often be bemoaned as defeat in the health arena. Thus, mass media sales campaigns are not quite as effective as is often claimed and believed when they are measured by standards used in the health area, and yet, even these limited gains by commercial campaigns are accomplished by enormous investments for an only slightly greater return. A large company may spend millions of dollars on sales promotion and would call the investment worthwhile if it leads to an increase in sales volume by a few percent.

In contrast, financial and other resources available in the promotion of desirable health behavior, are infinitesimal compared to those available in the commercial area. A case in point are the producers of Alka Seltzer who spent about seven times as much in 1975 to promote its use, as the entire annual budget of the federal Bureau of Health Education. (*)

CONCLUSION

By now you will understand why it was I said at the onset that the approaches, methods, and know-how that have proven so effective in commercial marketing, cannot be applied simply and blindly to the health area, especially to the areas of preventive health. Certain problems and situations have been pointed out that are peculiar to (or at least, more pronounced in) the health area than in the commercial area. They relate to what you are asked to market; to you consumers' perception of what they are urged to buy, use or do; to risks in using some of the most effective tools of traditional marketing; and to the fact that criteria of effective (or "cost-effective") marketing are more rigorous in the health area. There are other differences, too, which time limitations prevent me to discuss.

Finally, I would like to offer an observation I have often made when working with marketing experts. It has to do with the differences between health educators and these marketing experts in perception of what is to be marketed.

These marketing experts (possibly because they had been so tuned in on selling tangible things), tended to confuse two distinct concepts; promoting health behavior and promoting the use of particular agencies or facilities such as MHO's. Health administrators are likely to be much concerned with the last of these, but professionals concerned with the direct delivery of health services, with their utilization by consumers, and with people's health-related daily habits and practices, are more likely to be concerned with health behavior. Maybe, this is why marketing experts find themselves more heartily welcomed by health administrators than by, say, physicians or health educators.

---

*Report at the national conference on preventive medicine, fogarty international center, NIH, November 1975, page 53.

In any case, the distinction is an important one for reasons which hardly need spelling out. However, while the distinction exists, the problems are of such a nature that marketing know-how, skills and methods can apply to the health area.

Many examples could be given of how these have been used and have had considerable impact on promoting desirable health practices by our public. (Unfortunately, I could give <u>far</u> <u>more</u> examples of how they have had very <u>undesirable</u> impacts--but this is another matter.) In any case, there is not the slightest doubt that marketing concepts and methods do and can indeed make enormous contributions to our efforts to build sound preventive health habits and practices into the daily life of our population.

Dietary Intervention Studies Incorporating Social Marketing Techniques

Reducing the Risk of Cardiovascular Disease: Effects of a Community-Based Campaign on Knowledge and Behavior

by Nathan Maccoby, Ph.D., John W. Farquhar, M.D., Peter D. Wood, D.Sc., and Janet Alexander, M.A.

ABSTRACT: In 1972 the Stanford Heart Disease Prevention Program launched a three-community field study. A multimedia campaign was conducted for two years in two California communities (Watsonville and Gilroy), in one of which (Watsonville) it was supplemented by an intensive-instruction program with high-risk subjects. A third community (Tracy) was used as a control. The campaigns were designed to increase participants' knowledge of the risk factors for cardiovascular disease, to change such risk-producing behavior as cigarette smoking, and to decrease the participants' dietary intake of calories, salt, sugar, saturated fat, and cholesterol. Results of a sample survey indicate that substantial gains in knowledge, in behavioral modification, and in the estimated risk of cardiovascular disease can be produced by both methods of intervention. The intensive-instruction program, when combined with the mass-medica campaign, emerged as the most effective for those participants who were initially evaluated to be at high risk. The results after two years of intervention are reported for effects on knowledge and behavioral change for the total participant samples and for the high-risk subsamples in each of the three communities.

During this century, cardiovascular disease has become the greatest single killer in the developed countries. The United States ranks second highest, behind Finland, in its rate of morbidity and mortality due to cardiovascular disease.

Since 1968 mortality due to cardiovascular disease has declined slightly; even so, the death rate is still excessively high. The costs to society from cardiovascular disease continue to rise steadily; the medical costs alone command a larger and larger share of the gross national product. Future improvements in the health of Americans are not expected to come from improvements in their

Dr. Maccoby is Janet M. Peck Professor of International Communication and Director of the Institute for Communication Research, Stanford University, Stanford, California 94305; he is also Co-Director of the Stanford Heart Disease Prevention Program. Dr. Farquhar is Professor of Medicine, Stanford University, and Director, Stanford Heart Disease Prevention Program. Dr. Wood is Adjunct Professor of Medicine, Stanford University, and Deputy Director, Stanford Heart Disease Prevention Program. Ms. Alexander is Media Director, Stanford Heart Disease Prevention Program. This research was supported by grant HL-14174 to the Stanford Specialized Center for Research in Arteriosclerosis and contract NIH-71-2161-L to the Stanford Lipid Research Clinic from the National Heart, Lung, and Blood Institute.

medical care but rather from an increased attention to health promotion and disease prevention.[1] Surely, if prevention programs can be properly designed and implemented, they could result not only in sharp reductions in medical care costs but also in a considerable increase in the life span of many individuals.

Reducing the risk of premature cardiovascular disease will require that individuals reduce or eliminate the primary risk factors that are associated with increased risk of premature heart attack and stroke, e.g., cigarette smoking, high blood pressure, and high serum-lipid concentrations. Individuals will have to take action to avoid other potential contributors to risk, such as lack of exercise, obesity, or stress and tension. All of these risk factors can be reduced through changes in life style.[2-4] The behaviors associated with risk-factor modification have all been demonstrated to be potentially modifiable, at least by some individuals. People do stop smoking, maintain normal blood pressure, cut down on their intake of saturated fats, dietary cholesterol, sugar, and salt; they do reduce their weight to an optimal level, relative to their body structure, and take regular exercise. Some even achieve success in bringing their daily tensions under control.

Even though it is obvious that the behavioral changes required for risk reduction are potentially achievable, earlier reported attempts to reduce these risk factors systematically via life-style changes have typically not been successful. While initial changes are often made as a consequence of a medical consultation or clinical therapy, such programs have traditionally been unable to prevent the rapid regression to the risk-promoting status quo when treatment has ended. Anti-smoking and weight-control programs, in particular those reported from clinical settings, tend to follow this pattern of results. Also, even if effective clinical protocols are developed for risk-factor behavioral change, the problem remains as to how best to convey these risk-reduction techniques to a large heterogeneous population, in a successful and cost-effective way.

METHODS

In 1972 the prospects for achieving community-wide risk reduction were addressed by the Stanford Heart Disease Prevention Program when it launched a field study in three California communities. The aim was to combine biomedical expertise with that of the social sciences so as to find successful methods for reducing cardiovascular risk for the adult population at large.

The family-community model, rather than the medical-center model, was chosen because a community would be able to provide the milieu in which a consensus of support and mutual help could develop and become an essential and integral part of the behavioral change program. For example, as smoking was beginning to be considered unfashionable, or was being banned outright in many places, those who were attempting to change their smoking habits could find a variety of natural reinforcements and social supports throughout the community in their daily lives. The persistence of such environmental supports for non-smoking should accelerate others' efforts to quit or cut down.

In addition, a prevention program was needed that would provide training in the skills necessary to achieve the self-directed behavioral changes required to reduce risk in most areas. A family-community model could reduce the costs of such a program because both the mass-media and nonmedical personnel could contribute to the skills-training and behavioral counseling portions of a prevention-oriented campaign. Thus, such prevention programs would be more cost-effective because they would not be dependent on the more highly trained specialists and costly medical personnel.

Design

Because the media campaigns were to be directed at communities, the random assignment of individuals to treatment or control conditions was not feasible. Moreover, the alternative of treating a large number of populations as single units and randomly assigning them to treatment or control conditions was prohibitively expensive. Thus we chose the most realistic compromise between feasibility and rigor: a quasi-experimental research approach on a small number of experimental units.[5]

In this study, mass media were to be used alone in one community and in combination with a program of face-to-face intensive instruction in a second community so as to influence the adult population at large to change their living habits in ways that could reduce their risk of premature heart attack and stroke. Over a two-year period, the multimedia campaign was directed to two northern California communities, Watsonville (W) and Gilroy (G). Gilroy and Watsonville share some media channels (television and radio), but each town has its own newspaper. The community of Tracy (T) was selected as a control because it was relatively isolated from the media in the other communities.

Of the two intervention communities, Gilroy was selected for the media-only treatment. In Watsonville, the same mass-media program was used, but it was supplemented by an intensive program of face-to-face instruction for participants at higher-than-average risk. In the third community, Tracy, no preventive efforts were made; only the surveys took place.

To assess the effects of the interventions, sample surveys were conducted to gather baseline and yearly follow-up data from a random (or systematic probability) sample of adults ages 35–59 in all three towns. The first survey (S_B) took place just prior to the first campaign year, in the autumn of 1972. Follow-up surveys took place at the end of each of the two campaign years, in autumn 1973 (S_1) and autumn 1974 (S_2). Because the measurement process itself could cause some effects, an additional sample (an "after-only" sample) was surveyed in each community only at the end of the first year of study (S_1). Demographic characteristics of the communities and sample sizes and response rates for the total participant samples are presented in Table 1.

Each survey included a behavioral interview and a medical examination of each subject. The behavioral survey covered the subject's knowledge about the risk factors, his or her attitudes toward cardiovascular disease and towards modifying risk-promoting behavior in the areas of diet, weight, smoking, and exercise. The medical examination included measures of plasma cholesterol and triglyceride concentrations, blood pressure, relative weight, and electrocardiograms. These data were combined into a multiple logistic function of risk (based on the one developed by Truett, Cornfield, and Kannel in the long-term Framingham study[6]). This equation yields a prediction of the probability of a subject's developing cardiovascular disease within 12 years. A complete presentation of the effects of the campaign on physiological variables and on estimated risk is reported elsewhere.[7]

Those persons in all three communities who were found to be in the top

TABLE 1
Selected Town Characteristics and Baseline Sample Response Rates

Characteristic	Watsonville	Gilroy	Tracy
Entire town:			
Population (1970)	14,569	12,665	14,724
Population (age 35–59)	4,115	3,224	4,283
Mean age of 35–59 group	47.6	46.2	47.0
Male/female ratio of 35–59 group	0.86	0.88	0.96
Total community participant samples (age 35–59):			
Original sample	833	659	659
Subjects completing baseline	605	542	532
Percent of original sample	73	82	81
Subjects completing S_B, S_1, S_2	423	397	384

quartile according to this measure of risk were selected for special study. In Watsonville, a random subset of two thirds of these high-risk people (and their spouses) were selected for face-to-face intensive instruction; this group was designated W-I.I. The remaining one third of those in the quartile at highest risk not selected for W-I.I. were observed as controls and given the designation "randomized controls" (W-RC). A high-risk group in Gilroy also was followed and received the mass-media program. The high-risk subjects in Tracy received no additional attention other than their identification.

This assignment of the high-risk subjects in Watsonville to either an intensive-instruction treatment or to no treatment on a random basis created a true experimental condition that could compare high-risk subjects receiving media plus intensive instruction (W-I.I.) with a comparable high-risk group receiving the media educational programs only (W-RC). The demographic characteristics of these high-risk groups and their survey response rates are presented in Table 2.

In all, 12 partially overlapping study groups were defined: "total participants," a "high-risk" group, and an "after-only" sample in each of the three communities; within Watsonville, the intensive-instruction subsample (W-I.I.),

TABLE 2
Sample Response Rates for High-Risk Subjects at Baseline

Characteristic	Watsonville intensive instruction (W-I.I.)	Watsonville media-only (W-RC)	Gilroy media-only	Tracy control
High-risk sample completing baseline survey	113	56	139	136
Attrition due to death or migration	13	6	23	21
Potential participants	100	50	116	115
Subjects completing baseline S_B and S_2	77	40	94	95

the control high-risk group (W-RC), and the spouses of those in instruction groups were also selected out for observation. Also, in Watsonville, a "reconstituted" (with W-I.I. subjects replaced) sample of total participants (W-R) is observed. These 12 groups are defined in Table 3.

Intervention Techniques

Both the mass-media and the intensive-instruction programs were designed to incorporate the established psychological principles that govern the behavioral change processes, particularly those that relate to the self-management of such changes.

The aims of the intervention were to increase a person's awareness of the probable causes of cardiovascular disease and of the specific behaviors that may reduce risk. People were to be provided with the information and skills necessary

TABLE 3
Composition and Treatment of 12 Participant Groups in Three Communities

Participant group	N	Data collected at	Treatment given
Tracy (T)			
Total participants	384	S_B, S_1, S_2*	No intervention
High-risk†	95	S_B, S_1, S_2	No intervention
After-only	107	S_1	No intervention
Gilroy (G)			
Total participants	397	S_B, S_1, S_2*	Mass-media campaign
High-risk†	94	S_B, S_1, S_2	Mass-media campaign
After-only	102	S_1	Mass-media campaign
Watsonville (W)			
Total participants	423	S_B, S_1, S_2*	‡
Reconstituted (W-R)§	423	S_B, S_1, S_2	Mass-media campaign
High-risk participants:†			
Intensive instruction (W-I.I.)‖	77	S_B, S_1, S_2	Mass-media campaign and intensive instruction
Randomized control (W-RC)¶	40	S_B, S_1, S_2	Mass-media campaign
W-I.I. spouses (I.I.-spouse)	34	S_B, S_1, S_2	Mass-media campaign and intensive instruction
After-only	100	S_1	Mass-media campaign

*S_B = baseline survey; S_1 = first annual follow-up survey; S_2 = second follow-up survey.

†Participants in the baseline survey whose examination results placed them in the top quartile of risk of cardiovascular disease, according to a multiple logistic function of risk factors.

‡Of the 423 total participants, 312 received all three surveys plus media campaign; 77 of the high-risk participants and their 34 spouses also received the intensive instruction program.

§Weighted probability sample with I.I. group excluded. To correct for bias caused by the deletion of the intensively instructed subjects, i.e., the high-risk persons and their spouses, the means for the remaining subjects in the high-risk and lower-risk groups were weighted to compensate for the differential numbers of the deleted subjects in the two risk strata. The resulting weighted means were called "means of the reconstituted sample", and labeled W-R, i.e., the sample was reconstituted after the deletion of the intensively instructed subjects.

‖Two thirds of total high-risk group randomly assigned to receive intensive instruction.

¶One third of high-risk group randomly assigned *not* to receive intensive instruction.

to achieve the recommended changes to help them become self-sufficient in the maintenance of the new health habits and skills. They were advised to follow dietary habits that would lead to the prevention of weight gain or to a reduction in weight for those who were overweight. An increase in physical activity was advised for all, and cigarette smokers were educated on the need for ceasing or reducing their cigarette consumption and the ways to achieve these goals. Methods for self-assessment or self-scoring of risk-related habits were presented to provide a basis for self-directed behavior modification.

The mass-media campaign.   The media campaign was designed, as well, to take into account the participants' media habits and the specific behavioral changes the townspeople would have to make as indicated by the baseline survey. Care was taken to produce media items that would illustrate behavioral skills as well as inform and motivate the adult population.

Because of the sizeable Spanish-speaking population, the campaign was presented in both English and Spanish. A variety of media materials was produced for the campaign. Over the two years, about three hours of television programs and over 50 television spots were produced, as well as about 100 radio spots, several hours of radio programming, weekly newspaper columns, and newspaper advertisements and stories. Printed materials of many kinds were sent via direct mail to the participants, and posters were also used in buses, stores, and worksites.

The mass-media campaign was monitored while it was being presented and was revised in accordance with the information gained on its effectiveness in reaching goals. The various skilled professionals within the staff closely coordinated the instructional content, development, pretesting, application, and reformulations. Media development was therefore accomplished by a team of individuals skilled in the behavioral sciences, media production, and cardiovascular epidemiology.

The intensive-instruction program.   The purpose of the intensive-instruction program was twofold: First, it was designed to determine whether the addition of face-to-face intensive instruction of high-risk individuals (who, of course, were also subject to the mass-media campaign) would be superior to the mass-media treatment alone. The assumption was that the combination would be more efficacious. Second, it was hoped that the experience with the intensive-instruction program would provide a set of guidelines on how to improve future media-instruction programs by building in those ingredients discovered to be effective in the more costly face-to-face instruction.

The high-risk cohort was obtained from the baseline measure by the selection of the top 25% of the Watsonville sample on the multiple logistic function of risk. These 169 high-risk subjects were randomly subdivided into a treatment group ($N=113$) and a control group ($N=56$); 107 of the 113 were recruited into treatment. These 107 individuals with virtually all of their spouses took part in a ten-week program of weekly and then twice-a-month sessions. The face-to-face intensive instruction was provided to 63 of the 107 in small groups of 12 to 15 persons. Stanford counselors made at-home visits to conduct individual treatment sessions for the remaining 44 intensive-instruction participants. Due to death, migration, and dropout, 77 of the 107 high-risk participants remained by the end of the second follow-up survey (S_2).

The intensive-instruction treatment was administered under the guidance of the behavioral scientists and dieticians. Most therapists had college degrees in the liberal arts and were trained over a four-week period at Stanford in counseling methods. Two of the therapists were graduate students in the Department of Communication at Stanford who were well versed in the behavioral sciences and in the communication techniques needed for accomplishing these interventions. In its early phases, most of the educational program consisted of informational instruction. However, the content of the intensive-instruction program was one of behavior modification, representing a field application of the principles of social learning theory as outlined by Albert Bandura.[8] The results of a small-scale pretest of these methods have been reported elsewhere.[9]

The behavior modification principles applied in the intensive-instruction program follow these five general steps: (1) an analysis of the participants' behavior; (2) modeling of the new behaviors; (3) guided practice in the new behaviors; (4) artificial reinforcement in the new behaviors from instructions; and (5) maintenance of the new habits without artificial reinforcement. Individuals were given instructions that were specific to their own particular risk factors: smokers who were lean and had what were considered to be normal plasma cholesterol or triglyceride values were given supplemental instruction only about how to stop smoking. Individuals who had elevated blood pressure levels were given special instruction in salt restriction and weight loss, whereas individuals with elevated levels of plasma lipids were given supplemental instruction in qualitative dietary changes. A more detailed discussion of the methods used for achieving change in risk-taking behavior is presented elsewhere.[10]

RESULTS AND DISCUSSION

The results reflect changes in the participants' knowledge about risk factors and their changes in risk-related behaviors. Data are presented from each of the three communities: Gilroy, the mass-media-only town; Watsonville, the mass-media combined with intensive-instruction town; and Tracy, the no-intervention town. Also, for Watsonville, the results for a "reconstituted," or theoretical sample are presented to represent the effects of the mass media only (comparable to the Gilroy "total participant" sample). The Watsonville ("reconstituted" sample (designated W-R) was created by weighting techniques that preserve the ratio of high- to nonhigh-risk subjects in the sample while removing the effects of the intensive instruction. The baseline mean scores from the pre-campaign baseline 1972 survey (S_B) are presented; they are followed by the percentage changes that occurred by the end of the first year of intervention (year 1, S_1) as well as at the end of the second year (year 2, S_2). Unless otherwise specified, the data reported are for the subject groups that completed both the behavioral and medical portions of the first (S_B), second (S_1), and third (S_2) annual surveys from 1972 to 1975.

Knowledge of Risk Factors

Twenty-five items were used to test the participants' knowledge about cardiovascular disease and its risk factors at each survey: 14 items assessed the role of diet, 3 were concerned with smoking, 4 with physical activity, 2 with body weight, and 2 with general information. Table 4 lists these results. Statistically significant gains in the participants' knowledge about risk factors occurred in all three intervention conditions, and these gains were maintained through the second year. Thus the mass media in this case were effective in producing stable

TABLE 4

Changes from Baseline in Knowledge of Risk Factors
(25 Items) After One and Two Years of Risk-Reduction Campaign

| | *Total Community Participant Samples** | | | |
	Tracy (T)	*Gilroy* (G)	*Watsonville Reconstituted* (W-R)	*Watsonville* (W)
Baseline mean:†	11.42	11.16	11.15	11.15
Percentage change				
Year 1	1.7	18.1‡	30.9‡	36.3‡§
Year 2	6.3	26.5‡	36.0‡§	40.8‡§

| | *High-Risk Participant Samples** | | | |
	Tracy (T)	*Gilroy* (G)	*Watsonville Randomized Control* (W-RC)	*Watsonville Intensive Instruction* (W-I.I.)
Baseline mean:†	10.74	11.17	11.25	10.91
Percentage change				
Year 1	1.9	16.4‡	29.8‡	54.2‡‖
Year 2	5.2	27.7‡	30.4‡	54.2‡‖

*See Table 3 for definitions of participant samples. The names will be abbreviated in subsequent tables.

†Baseline mean is expressed as the numerical sum of the correct answers to the 25 knowledge-related questions.

‡Indicates a statistically significant difference ($p < 0.05$) for percent change values at Tracy (control) versus Gilroy, or versus Watsonville, study groups. Total participant groups (upper table) are compared with Tracy total participants as control; high-risk groups (lower table) are compared with Tracy high-risk participants as control. A one-tailed test was used to compare percent change values.

§Indicates a statistically significant difference ($p < 0.05$) for percent change values at Gilroy versus Watsonville total participants, or versus the Watsonville reconstituted groups (upper table).

‖Indicates a statistically significant difference ($p < 0.05$) for percent change values for Watsonville intensive-instruction group (W-I.I.) versus Watsonville randomized control (W-RC) (lower table).

knowledge gains. Where intensive instruction was added, the percentage gain was greatly improved.

We can rank the intensity of the treatment received by the several study groups as in Figure 1. The least intensive effort was with the Tracy "after-only" group (for whom the only contact was the second survey); the greatest effort was with the Watsonville intensive-instruction group (for whom contact included three surveys, the media campaign, and face-to-face instruction). This figure shows that the increases in knowledge about the dietary risk factors corresponded closely with the estimates of the intensity of the various interventions used in the three communities. This correspondence strengthens the inference that the changes were indeed related to the experimental treatments and not to chance differences among the study groups in the communities. The mere examination and interviewing of participants (note Tracy total participants' score) did very little to increase their knowledge, but the mass media alone and the

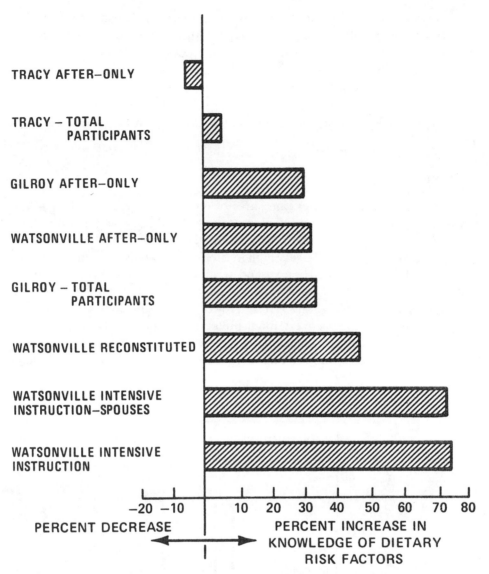

FIGURE 1: Percentage of change from the first to the second survey in participants' knowledge about dietary risk factors. The groups are ranked according to an estimation of the increasing intensity of the educational input. Groups are defined in Table 3. Knowledge of the dietary risk factors is based on the 14 items that concerned diet of the 25 items comprising the knowledge index reported in Table 4.

intensive-instruction campaign added to the mass media were powerful agents for increasing the participants' knowledge. This increase was greater among those Watsonville participants (Watsonville reconstituted) who received the mass-media programs and who lived in the same community as participants receiving face-to-face instruction than among those in Gilroy, where the intervention was limited to the mass media alone. This difference can possibly be best accounted for by the differences in the media channels that were available in the two treatment communities, particularly the newspapers. However, there is also evidence for some diffusion of the information from the intensive-instruction participants to the other Watsonville participants,[11] which could also account for the outcome.

Figure 2 shows the data for the increases in knowledge about the dietary risk factors among the Spanish- and English-speaking participants, with the estimated amount of educational effort being approximately constant for the two groups. Both the English and Spanish language groups showed impressive gains, and the noteworthy increase among the educationally less-advantaged Spanish group attests to the efficacy of the Spanish instruction, which was carefully tailored to the information-seeking habits of the Spanish-speaking community.

Behavioral Changes

In the area of behavior, measures of dietary behavior and of cigarette smoking are presented. A detailed report of the dietary and plasma lipid changes is presented elsewhere.[12] A representative finding reporting the eating of eggs, the yolks of which are very high in cholesterol, is presented in Table 5. It is evident that there is a definitive and significant secular trend in the non-intervention community. Clearly, national educational efforts, independent of our campaign, were having some effects. However, the reductions in the number of eggs eaten are very much greater in the intervention groups. By the end of the second year, the mass media alone (G) achieved almost as much of an influence as the maximum intervention community (W). In the high-risk participant sam-

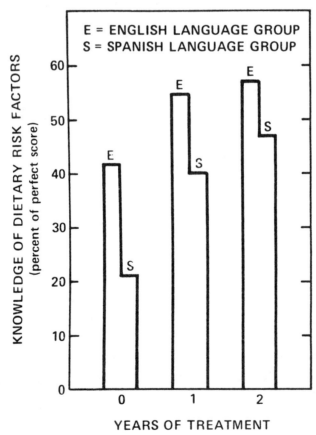

FIGURE 2: Knowledge of dietary risk factors (a 14-item subset of the total knowledge score) at baseline and after one and two years of health education among English- and Spanish-speaking participants in the two intervention communities.

ples, a secular trend also occurs in Tracy. Again the intensively instructed high-risk subjects (W-I.I.) evidenced a significantly greater reduction in their egg eating than did their mass-media-only counterparts (W-RC).

Table 6 presents the data reporting the number of cigarettes smoked per day. When the total community participant samples are considered, note that

TABLE 5
Changes from Baseline in Egg Consumption per Day After One and Two Years of Risk-Reduction Campaign

	Total Community Participant Samples*			
	T	*G*	*W-R*	*W*
Baseline mean:†	0.76	0.84	0.79	0.78
Percentage change				
Year 1	−14.9	−27.5‡	−37.1‡	−41.8‡§
Year 2	−15.9	−33.3‡	−42.2‡	−44.4‡
	High-Risk Participant Samples*			
	T	*G*	*W-RC*	*W-I.I.*
Baseline mean:†	0.88	0.93	0.74	0.70
Percentage change				
Year 1	−15.7	−34.5‡	−43.3‡	−61.9‡
Year 2	−19.3	−24.5	−49.3‡	−60.3‡

*See Table 3 for definitions of participant samples.
†Baseline mean is expressed as the number of eggs consumed per day.
‡§See Table 4 for definitions of these statistical symbols.

TABLE 6
Changes from Baseline in the Number of Cigarettes Smoked per Day After One and Two Years of Risk-Reduction Campaign

	Total Community Participant Samples*			
	T	*G*	*W-R*	*W*
Baseline mean:†	6.9	6.8	6.8	7.2
Percentage change				
Year 1	−1.1	−2.3	−6.9	−18.9‡§
Year 2	−2.5	−7.3	−13.7‡	−24.1‡§
	High-Risk Participant Samples*			
	T	*G*	*W-RC*	*W-I.I.*
Baseline mean:†	13.7	14.6	14.2	14.4
Percentage change				
Year 1	−8.5	−9.8	−5.8	−36.3‡‖
Year 2	−17.2	−13.8	−15.1	−42.3‡‖

*See Table 3 for definitions of participant samples.
†Baseline mean is expressed as the total number of cigarettes smoked per day.
‡§‖See Table 4 for definitions of these statistical symbols.

only for the community that includes intensive instructees (W) is there a substantial reduction in the mean number of cigarettes smoked per day, as compared with the non-intervention town (T). Among the high-risk samples, only among the intensive instructees (W-I.I.) was there a real decrease in cigarette smoking, as compared with the non-intervention town, and that difference holds up for the second year.

Particularly interesting to note is the evidence of an orderly relationship among the knowledge of risk, the changes in behavior, and the physiologic changes in risk at the end of the two years of intervention. Figure 3 presents the results of an analysis of the relationships between changes in the total participants' knowledge about the risk factors, other modification of smoking and eating habits, and the reduction in the multiple logistic function of risk for several participant groups. Apparently the more the study participants learned, the more they changed their behavior and, thus, their physiological risk of disease. The position of each group of study participants on the horizontal plane illustrates the correlation of the changes between knowledge and behavior. The vertical lines illustrate the percent changes in the multiple logistic function of risk and show that these changes are generally in the direction anticipated. Only one group increased in risk (the total participant sample in Tracy) and, in this group, essentially no changes occurred in their knowledge or behavior. At the other extreme, the greatest reduction in risk (-30%) occurred in the Watsonville intensive-instruction cohort. This group also had the greatest change in knowledge and in behavior. The other four groups are clustered within the midrange for risk reduction, and they are generally in the midrange for knowledge and behavior change. One interesting anomaly may be seen in the spouses of the high-risk participants, who also received intensive instruction. Although their knowledge gain was almost as great as that of their high-risk spouses, their behavior changes and risk scores were midrange. This finding is consistent with the hypothesis that exposure to instruction without a prior identification of being at high risk may limit the motivation to change.

Many cautions need to be observed in the interpretation of the above data. If, as should ideally be the case, we had had several communities in which to apply each treatment condition and if each community could have been assigned randomly to treatment, the results would be based on what could more clearly be characterized as a true experiment. Unfortunately, this procedure was not feasible, both because of staff and funding limitations and because of the difficulty of locating towns that met our media requirements. It would have been preferable to have used morbidity and mortality data as end points, but resources could not be extended to the selection and monitoring of large enough cities for a long enough period of time to make such analyses meaningful.

Nevertheless, with these limitations in mind, the findings are encouraging: mass-media risk-reduction programs, when appropriately conceptualized, pretested, and carried out, can help people to learn how to change their behavior so as to reduce their risk of cardiovascular disease.

As we have noted, the use of intensive instruction to supplement the mass-media campaign proved to be especially successful. We plan to explore means of even further enhancing the effectiveness of future mass-media risk-reduction campaigns by incorporating into the mass-media treatments some of the principles and methods found successful in the intensive-instruction program.

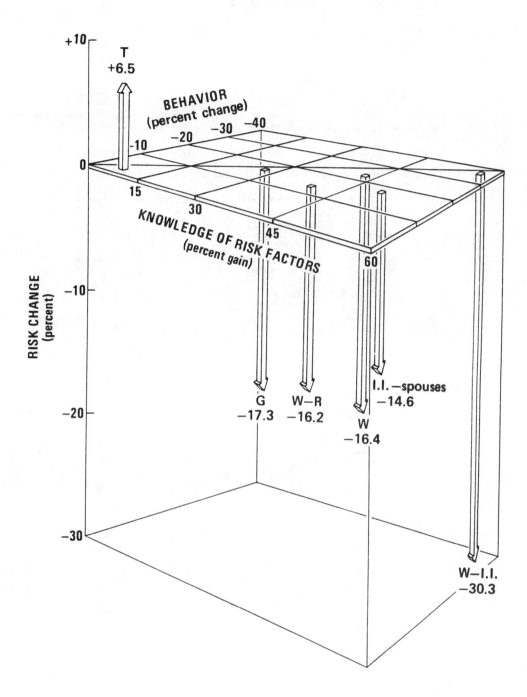

FIGURE 3: Relationship between changes in knowledge, behavior, and risk at the end of the two years of health education in various study groups. The groups are defined in Table 3. Harmful behavior is a composite of dietary intake of saturated fat and cholesterol and of smoking; dietary and smoking behavior were given equal weight. Knowledge of risk factors is derived from the 25-item questionnaire. Cardiovascular risk is measured by a multiple logistic function of risk factors; figures on the vertical axis represent the percentage of change in risk (T = Tracy total participants; G = Gilroy total participants; W = Watsonville total participants; W-R = Watsonville reconstituted sample; W-I.I. = intensive instruction group at Watsonville; I.I.-spouses = spouses of intensive instructees in Watsonville).

REFERENCES

1. Department of Health, Education, and Welfare, Public Health Service: *Forward Plan for Health,* 1976. DHEW Pub. No. (OS) 76-S0046; Washington, D.C.; Stock No. 017-000-00172-8. Pp 69–83.
2. Inter-Society Commission for Heart Disease Resources: Primary prevention of atherosclerotic diseases. *Circulation* **42**: A-55, 1970 (revised, April 1972).
3. Blackburn H: Progress in the epidemiology and prevention of coronary heart disease. In P Yu, J Goodwin (eds.): *Progress in Cardiology.* Philadelphia, Lea & Febiger, 1974. Pp 1–36.
4. Olefsky JM, Reaven GM, Farquhar JW: Effects of weight reduction on obesity: Studies of carbohydrate and lipid metabolism in normal and hyperlipoproteinemic subjects. *J Clin Invest* **53**:64–76, 1974.
5. Cambell DT, Stanley JC: *Experimental and Quasi-Experimental Designs for Research.* Chicago, Rand McNally & Company, 1967.
6. Truett J, Cornfield J, Kannel W: A multivariate analysis of the risk of coronary heart disease in Framingham. *J Chronic Dis* **20**:511–524, 1967.
7. Farquhar JW, Maccoby N, Wood PW, et al: Community education for cardiovascular health. *Lancet* I:1192–1195, 1977.
8. Bandura A: *Social Learning Theory.* Morristown, NJ, General Learning Press, 1971.
9. Meyer AJ, Henderson JB: Multiple risk factor reduction in the prevention of cardiovascular disease. *Prev Med* **3**:225–236, 1974.
10. McAllister AL, Farquhar JW, Thoresen CE, et al: Behavioral science applied to cardiovascular health: Progress and research needs in the modification of risk-taking habits in adult populations. *Health Educ Monogr* **4**:45–47, 1976.
11. Meyer AJ, Maccoby N, Farquhar JW: The role of opinion leadership in a cardiovascular health education campaign. *Communication Yearbook* (in press).
12. Stern MP, Farquhar JW, Maccoby N, et al: Results of a two-year health education campaign on dietary behavior: The Stanford three community study. *Circulation* **54**:826–833, 1976.

Heart Healthy Eating and Exercise: Introducing and Maintaining Changes in Health Behaviors

by Thomas J. Coates, Ph.D., Robert W. Jeffery, Ph.D., and Lee Ann Slinkard

Abstract: The Heart Healthy Program is a health education project developed for elementary school students. It was designed to 1) increase their consumption of complex carbohydrates, and decrease their consumption of saturated fat, cholesterol, sodium, and sugar; 2) increase their level of habitual physical activity; and 3) generalize these changes to other family members. The overall program and 12 class lessons were designed using informative instruction, participatory classroom activities, personal goal setting, parent handouts, feedback, and reinforcement. The program was evaluated using a time-series experimental design with all students in three 4th grade classes at School 1 and three 5th grade classes at School 2. Evaluation was conducted using direct observation of eating and activity, as well as paper-and-pencil assessments of knowledge and attitude. Results indicated substantial changes in eating behavior at school, knowledge about heart health, food preferences, and family eating patterns as reported by parents. Observed changes in exercise were minimal during treatment, and were related to seasonal sports activities at follow-up. Eating habit changes persisted over a four-month follow-up which spanned summer vacation. These outcomes suggest that school programs developed using specific techniques can be effective in facilitating important behavior changes at school and at home. (*Am J Public Health* 1981; 71:15–23.)

Elevated blood lipids and blood pressures among significant proportions of school-age children have been documented in large-scale epidemiological studies.[1-6] These "risk" factors for the development of cardiovascular disease may be influenced by habitual diet and activity patterns. The diets of children and adolescents in the United States share the same deficits and excesses characteristic of the entire population: over 40 per cent of calories eaten are from fat; saturated fat accounts for 15 to 18 per cent of the calories; and average dietary cholesterol is well in excess of 300 mg per day.[7-10] Some young persons are also quite sedentary.[11]

Changing children's health habits may be a key element in promoting widespread adoption of a healthier life style that could lead to reduction of cardiovascular risk behavior and disease events in the population. At the same time, working with children in schools might prove beneficial in helping the adults around them change as well. Primary prevention of cardiovascular disease may be dependent upon health education programs capable of promoting meaningful behavior changes.[12, 13]

We evaluated the effectiveness of a school-based program in changing elementary students' eating and exercise habits. The Heart Healthy Program was designed to accomplish three objectives: 1) increase elementary students' consumption of complex carbohydrates, and decrease their consumption of saturated fat, cholesterol, sodium, and sugar; 2) increase their physical activity; and 3) generalize these changes to other family members. The program was developed using social learning techniques to encourage behavior, knowledge, and attitude change. The program was implemented in 4th and 5th grades in two elementary schools. Evaluation consisted of direct observation of eating and exercise behaviors, as well as paper-and-pencil measures of

Address reprint requests to Thomas J. Coates, PhD, Division of Pediatric Cardiology, Johns Hopkins Hospital, 600 N. Wolfe Street, Baltimore, MD 21205. Dr. Jeffery is with the Laboratory of Physiological Hygiene, University of Minnesota; Ms. Slinkard is with the Program in Health Psychology, University of California School of Medicine, San Francisco.

nutritional knowledge, and preferences for specific foods and activities. Improvements obtained during the program were maintained at follow-up after summer vacation.

Materials and Methods

Subjects

Participants were all 4th grade students in three classes at School 1 (72 students) and all 5th grade students in three classes at School 2 (89 students) from the same school district near Stanford University. Two grade levels were used to obtain some estimate of the generalizability of results beyond one age group. Families living in this area are nearly all Caucasian and have mean education and income levels above national averages. All parents consented in writing to their child's participation. There were relatively equal numbers of males and females in each school, and the students were equally divided among the classes.

Study Design

The initial study was completed in the Spring 1978, with follow-up during the following September and October. A time-series design with multiple baselines and lagged replication was employed.[14, 15] Daily observations of eating and exercise behaviors were begun simultaneously in both schools to collect baseline data. After one week, the nutrition program was introduced in School 1 while baseline data collection continued in School 2. The nutrition program was introduced in School 2 one week later. The exercise program was introduced in each school two weeks after the beginning of the nutrition program in that school. Behavioral observations were conducted continuously during the program and continued at both schools until two weeks after the program was completed at School 2. Long-term follow-up observations were conducted four months later, after summer vacation, at the beginning of the following school year. The lagging of School 2 behind School 1 made it possible to control partially for temporal factors unrelated to treatment possibly causing changes in eating and exercise.

A second design feature involved separating the exercise program from the nutrition program. This permitted us to determine separately the efficacy of the instructional techniques for nutrition and exercise, as physical activity measures would not be expected to change until the exercise curriculum was introduced.

The Autoregressive Integrated Moving Averages (ARIMA) analysis, appropriate to time series data, was used to evaluate the statistical significance of eating and activity changes.[16]

Instructional Procedures

Instruction was given by undergraduate students from Stanford University while regular teachers were present in the classroom. The teachers were prepared for teaching by reviewing a written curriculum, modeling, role playing, and group discussion. Teacher preparation meetings were held twice weekly during the study.

Classes were scheduled as part of the school science curriculum; they occupied three 45-minute periods per week for four weeks. Each class emphasized a different meal and

target for behavior change. The class sequence was as follows: 1) snacks, using fruits and vegetables; 2) how to prepare a heart-healthy breakfast, reducing sugar and cholesterol; 3) how to prepare a heart-healthy lunch, reducing saturated fat and salt; 4) how to prepare a heart-healthy dinner, reducing saturated fat, salt, and cholesterol; 5) shopping, how to read labels; and 6) summary—fat, sugar, salt, cholesterol, and the heart. Table 1 presents "Heart Healthy" or foods encouraged by the program (everyday foods) and foods discouraged in the program (termed "sometimes" food to avoid the connotation that any food would be considered bad).

The next six classes were designed to meet the explicit objective of increasing levels of physical activity on the playground at the 45-minute lunch recess. These class sessions were: 7) pulse rate, warm-ups, the importance of exercise; 8) strength exercises; using the Parcourse; 9) skill exercises; 10) heart healthy exercises, using the Parcourse; 11) practicing the Parcouse; and 12) review and integration.*

The overall program and each class lesson were designed to incorporate five social learning strategies to encourage behavior change: models of desired behaviors, behavioral rehearsal, goal specification, feedback of results, and reinforcement for behavior change. In each class session, students were first taught one specific concept relative to the ways in which nutrition or exercise influence cardiovascular health (e.g., the relationship between dietary fat and atherosclerosis). This was followed by a demonstration of ways to change eating or exercise habits in accordance with the concept (e.g., substitute a low fat item such as chicken for a high fat item such as pork). Included in this part of the lesson was behavioral modeling of ways to ask parents to buy the recommended foods, to serve them at home, and to pack them in the student's lunch. Finally, students were encouraged to change one specific eating or exercise habit. They set a specific eating and exercise goal to be accomplished before the next class. The goal was written on specially prepared forms, reviewed by the teachers, and retained by the students in their desk.

As an example, the third class session introduced the concept of saturated fat and its relationship to atherosclerosis with lecture. Two models were then presented; a lunch high in saturated fat and a lunch low in saturated fat. Food items high in each category were identified and described. Students then divided into groups, inspected each others' lunches, and discussed the relative amounts of saturated fat contained in each lunch. At this point, the relationship between saturated fat and atherosclerosis was elaborated through group discussion and diagrams. Students were given a handout to take home specifying food substitute recommendations for families. Finally, each student chose a personal behavior change goal, indicating how to decrease saturated fat content in his or her lunch by substituting food items (e.g., chicken instead of bologna) and by goal setting.

The exercise classes were conducted using the same format: lecture, models of desired activities, behavioral re-

---

*The Parcourse[18] consists of a series of exercise stations. The participant jogs between stations, stopping at each one to perform the exercises indicated there. The exercise is designed to increase flexibility and stamina in a fun and enjoyable way.

TABLE 1—Heart Healthy Food Items Were Encouraged by the Program and "Sometimes" Foods Were Discouraged

Heart Healthy Food Items	"Sometimes" Foods
Home-cooked lean beef	Beef lunch meat
Chicken	Bologna
Corned beef	Hard cheese
Tuna	Ham
Turkey	Hamburger
Whole grain bread	Jelly
Low-fat cheese	Salami
Low-fat or skim milk	Tacos
Graham crackers	Eggs
Unsalted nuts	Hot dogs
Home-made pastry	White bread
Unsalted popcorn	Whole milk
Space food	Candy
Dried fruits	Pretzels, potato chips
Fresh fruits	Fruit roll
Unsweetened fruit juice	Jello
	Ice cream
	Juice bar
	Salted nuts
	Packaged pastry
	Pizza
	Salted popcorn
	Sweetened juice
	Canned fruits

These items represent common foods brought in students' lunches and were the foods emphasized in class lessons. Other food items were discussed and categorized according to p. 115 in Farquhar.[17]

hearsal (e.g., practicing the Parcourse), and goal setting (students indicated activity goals for the following noon recess).

Feedback and reinforcement were important components of the program. Graphs were prepared and posted weekly to show students their progress in changing the contents of their lunches and activity changes at lunchtime. To provide reinforcement for changes, the instructors circulated intermittently on the playground during lunch and gave stickers with red hearts (the logo of the Stanford Heart Disease Prevention Program) to students whose lunches were predominantly heart healthy and/or who were engaging in heart-healthy exercises.

This latter feature allowed us to give reinforcement at school for changes at home. Students could not receive positive feedback or earn token reinforcers at school unless lunches, packed at home, changed. It was hoped that this strategy, in combination with handouts, would stimulate parents to change home buying and eating patterns in directions encouraged by the program.

In addition to the school program, three educational meetings were held with teachers and principals, one with parents, and one with the Parent-Teachers Association (PTA) of each school. These activities were intended to answer questions about the program and to assure a supportive environment for changed health habits at home and in school.

Following summer vacation, the classroom teachers conducted three booster sessions to review the major elements of the curriculum and to encourage additional nutri-tion and activity changes. Follow-up observations were made prior to these booster sessions.

Measures

Direct observation was used to measure foods in lunches, foods that were deposited in the trash, and physical activity on the playground during the lunch recess.

Training of Observers—We followed standard quality control procedures for training and maintaining reliability among observers.[19] Five observers completed all observations at both schools throughout the study. A sixth observer served as supervisor and criterion observer. Observers were supplied first with forms and written operational definitions of the behaviors to be measured and the procedures for measuring them. These observers were not told the true purposes of the study and the research design that was employed. They were warned about the problems of observer bias and were asked not to guess or inquire either about design or purposes of the study. Role plays followed, until inter-rater agreements among all pairs of observers exceeded 95 per cent. In these role plays, criteria behaviors were acted out and the observers rated the behaviors observed. Observation in a practice school followed, until inter-rater agreements among all pairs of observers exceeded 95 per cent. Inter-rater agreements were always computed by dividing agreements by agreements plus disagreements and multiplying by 100.

Once training was completed, all observers observed independently on randomly selected days. Once per week, each observer's ratings were checked for reliability. Each observer was paired with one other observer and the supervisor; they observed the same students at the same time to determine reliability between pairs of observers and with the criteria.

Eating at lunch—Students were observed at lunchtime by the trained non-participant observers three or four times per week throughout the study. While the students were eating lunch, the observers approached each student individually and asked him or her to show the contents of his/her lunch. Each food item was recorded on a standardized form. No food item was marked down unless the observer actually saw it in the student's lunch.

Time constraints precluded inspection of all students each day. Observers began each observation period by following a student who was randomly preselected for observation before the period began. This student was followed to the lunch area where the contents of his/her lunch were observed and recorded. Students adjacent to this student were observed until two consecutive students were approached who had already finished one food item.

The food observation periods lasted only 10 minutes because students ate lunches hurriedly. An average of 22 students were observed each day over the course of the study. Inter-rater reliability was checked once weekly for each observer. Pairs of observers independently observed the same students at the same time; the average per cent agreement across observers was 99 per cent (S.D. = 2 per cent).

Playground Activity—Following lunch, the observers stationed themselves on the playground. They randomly selected 4th grade students at School 1 and 5th grade students at School 2 to observe. Each student was observed 10 times over a one-minute period. At each 5-second interval during the minute, indicated to the observer via a tape-recording, the observer recorded the student's activity: sitting, standing, walking, climbing, standing still but moving upper trunk, or running. Inter-rater agreements were consistently high (mean = 97 per cent, S.D. = 2 per cent). Observers also noted the student's specific activity (e.g., football, tag). An average of 15 students were observed each day for activity.

Trash—Following lunch and after the students had returned to the classroom, the observers inspected trash discarded by the 4th graders at School 1 and by the 5th graders at School 2. Students from each class ate in separate areas making it easy to examine trash discarded by separate classes. They tabulated the items found in the trash. No attempt was made to estimate the amount of each item that was consumed. Rather, an item was tabulated as being in the trash if 25 per cent or more of it remained unconsumed. Students were not told that the trash was being checked for items not eaten.

It might be argued that observation on the playground provided only a small sample of these students' activities during the day. We chose this measure over others (e.g., questionnaires about typical activity levels) for two reasons. First, our curriculum was designed to increase activity on the playground during recess; therefore, it seemed reasonable to measure that which was of greatest interest in evaluating our program. Second, direct observations may be more sensitive to small but important variations of physical activity than other measures. For example, it was not well documented that obese adolescents were less active than normal weight adolescents until Bullen, Reed, and Mayer[20] provided direct observations of obese girls during physical activities. Similarly, Waxman and Stunkard[21] found caloric

intake differences and physical activity differences (at home and not at school) between obese children and their siblings and peers. Again, these observations had not been documented using less sensitive self-report measures.

Knowledge and Preference—A 30-minute paper-and-pencil test containing 28 items in a forced-choice format, administered before and after the program and at follow-up, assessed knowledge of heart-healthy foods and heart-healthy concepts. A 20-minute, 28-item test using a forced-choice format was used to assess students' preference for heart healthy foods and exercises.

Family Interview—Randomly selected families were interviewed by telephone. The respondent (usually the mother) was asked to report food eaten by each family member on the previous day. Families at School 1 (n = 44) were interviewed before and after the program, while families at School 2 (n = 36) were interviewed both before the program and at follow-up.

Foods in Lunches

For analysis purposes, foods recorded by observers were later classified either as "Heart Healthy" or everyday foods (see Table 1). Presented in Figure 1 are the average number of heart-healthy food items in students' lunches before and throughout the program and at follow-up. Significant increases in the average number of target food items in students' lunches were found following the beginning of the classes. These levels increased even further following the end of the program (39 per cent increase at School 1 and 38 per cent at School 2). Most important, improvements were maintained at follow-up after summer vacation (35 per cent increase over baseline at School 1 and 26 per cent increase over baseline at School 2). As presented in Table 2 and Figure 1, students averaged four food items in their lunches pri-

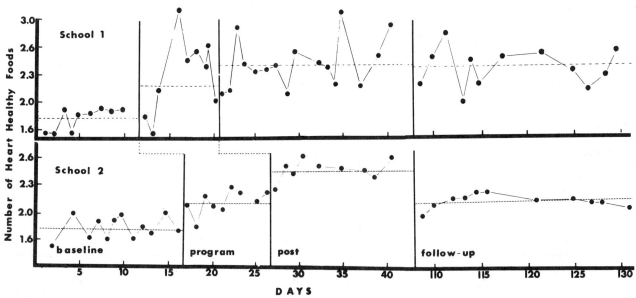

FIGURE 1—Average number of heart healthy food items in students' lunches during baseline, while the program was being taught, immediately following the program, and four months later after summer vacation.
Note: The dotted line in each phase represents the mean for that phase. time-lagging treatment for School 2 behind School 1 permitted some control over extraneous factors potentially responsible for change

TABLE 2—Heart Healthy Foods in Students' Lunches and Trash

	(1) Pre-Program	(2) Program	(3) Post-Program	(4) Follow-up	t-test for between period changes 1 vs 2 + 3	2 + 3 vs 4
Average Number of Heart Healthy						
Items per Student						
School 1						
Mean	1.69	2.12	2.36	2.28	+3.96**	0.22
S.D.	0.23	0.52	0.34	0.20		
School 2						
Mean	1.69	1.92	2.34	2.13	+4.24**	0.01
S.D.	0.33	0.21	0.13	0.19		
Percent of Foods in Trash Considered Heart Healthy						
School 1						
Mean	68.6	62.2	63.6	64.9	−2.25*	1.20
S.D.	4.4	6.2	8.2	7.3		
School 2						
Mean	56.8	63.7	63.3	62.4	+2.35*	0.16
S.D.	7.6	6.6	5.9	5.4		

***$p < .001$
**$p < .01$
*$p < .05$
t-tests were computed using the Autoregressive Integrated Moving Averages Analysis (using a 001 model) for time-series data.

or to and following treatment. Thus, the increases represent a change in target food items from less than to more than 50 per cent of the food items in lunches.

Trash—We next examined changes across phases in the proportion of food items in the trash that were categorized as Heart Healthy (Heart Healthy foods divided by total food items in trash × 100). These data are presented in Table 2.

The per cent of heart-healthy food items in the trash decreased from Baseline to Program by 5 per cent at School 1 and increased by 6.5 per cent at School 2. Thus, lunches were not being thrown away at higher rates during the program when compared to baseline. The per cent of the trash that was heart-healthy foods did not change from program to post-program or from program to follow-up. Statistically significant changes from baseline to post treatment were small in magnitude. The average number of items in the trash was 33.6 at School 1 and 30.8 at School 2. A 5 per cent decrease represents 1.6 items, while a 5.6 per cent increase represents 2.02 items.

Activity at Lunch

Figure 2 presents average per cent of time students spent sitting and standing through all assessments phases. Surprisingly, large amounts of playground time were spent in relatively sedentary activities. Boys at School 1 increased slightly the per cent of time spent sitting and standing during lunch, while boys at School 2 decreased slightly on this variable.

At follow-up, boys at both schools decreased in amount of time spent sitting and standing. We hypothesized that these changes were related to seasonal shifts in lunch activity (e.g., baseball in May and football in September).

Because our exercise intervention program was unsuc-

cessful, we decided to use our observations to explore relationships between typical playground activities and associated levels of physical activity. As noted before, observers recorded both behaviors (e.g., running, walking) and games (e.g., soccer, four square) for the individual students they were observing at any one time. Spearman rank-order correlations were computed to represent the association between number of time periods each day in which a given activity (e.g., football) was observed and the per cent of observa-

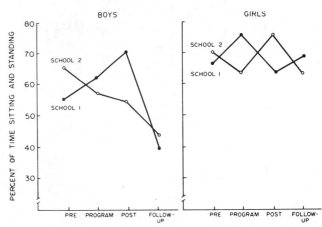

FIGURE 2—Per Cent of time boys and girls in Schools 1 and 2 spent sitting and standing during the program study period and at follow-up.
Note: The ARIMA analysis indicated significant changes for boys only:
School 1—Pre-Program vs Post Program (t = 2.13, p < .05), Post-Program vs. Follow-up (t = 6.70, p < .001).
School 2—Pre-Program vs Post-Program (t = 6.70, p < .001), Post-Program to Follow-up (t = 3.47, p. < .001)

tions for that day in which a given behavior (e.g., running) was observed. The results are presented in Figures 3 and 4. Clearly, running was associated with football for boys; four-square and handball were associated with still-moving, while baseball was decidedly sedentary. For the girls, chase and tag were associated with increased activity; tetherball, handball, and four-square were associated with still-moving, while other playground activities were associated with relatively little movement.

These results have important implications for the design of school programs to increase physical activity following lunch. Rather than focusing on physical activity, it would seem productive to design curricula to promote games associated with increased levels of physical activity.

Knowledge and Preferences

Students in both schools increased in knowledge of heart-healthy nutritional practices, activities, and concepts

from pre-program to post-program (1 vs 2 in Table 3). These results were maintained at follow-up (see 2 vs 3 in Table 3) except in School 1 in knowledge regarding heart-healthy activities. Reported preferences increased at post-treatment, but decreased at follow-up in both schools.

Reported Eating at Home

Three family members (father, mother, target child) at School 1 reported significant increases in per cent of foods in diet that were heart-healthy from pre- to post-program (cf. Table 4). Similar increases were noted from pre-program to follow-up at School 2. Families in both schools reported increases following the program in the percentage of foods bought that fell into heart healthy categories.

Parents were informed about the objectives of the program. Therefore, it is possible that some parents could have been inclined to respond consistently with what they thougnt we wanted to hear.

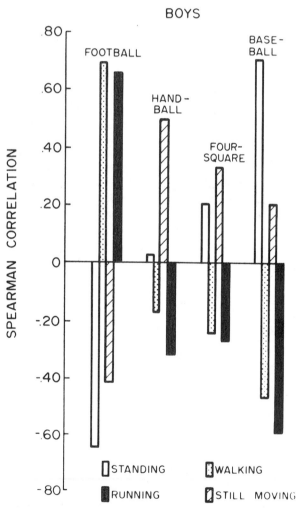

FIGURE 3—Spearman rank order correlation representing associations between per cent of time observed on a given day in which boys engaged in specific behaviors (running, walking) and percent of the time observed in specific games (football).

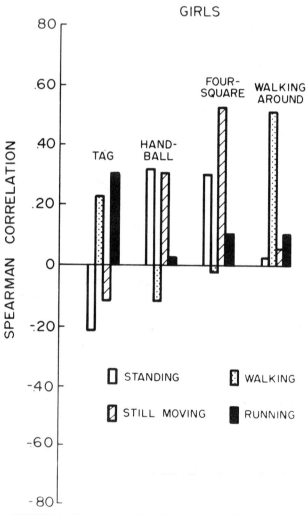

FIGURE 4—Spearman rank—order correlation for girls representing relationship between per cent of time observed in specific behaviors and per cent of time observed in specific games.

TABLE 3—Knowledge, Concepts, and Preferences

	(1) Pre-Program	(2) Post-Program	(3) Follow-up	1 vs 2	*t*-tests 2 vs 3
Knowledge Regarding Healthy Nutritional Practices					
School 1					
Mean	23.03	26.06	24.91	+8.11***	1.21
S.D.	3.15	1.54	5.46		
School 2					
Mean	22.37	25.36	25.83	+6.23***	1.05
S.D.	3.49	3.08	6.22		
Knowledge Regarding Exercise and Heart-Health					
School 1					
Mean	9.07	10.11	7.33	+4.81***	−3.03**
S.D.	1.11	1.47	4.43		
School 2					
Mean	8.92	10.09	9.17	+8.16***	0.87
S.D.	1.71	0.89	1.51		
General Concepts about Cardiovascular Health					
School 1					
Mean	6.26	7.69	6.54	+2.74**	0.53
S.D.	3.95	2.69	2.77		
School 2					
Mean	6.95	8.29	8.50	+6.58***	0.75
S.D.	1.69	1.61	1.86		
Reported Preferences for Heart Healthy Foods					
School 1					
Mean	12.89	17.97	9.18	+5.72***	−2.03*
S.D.	5.23	6.92	7.96		
School 2					
Mean	12.60	18.96	15.36	+7.78***	−3.28**
S.D.	4.83	6.41	6.73		
Reported Preferences for Heart Healthy Activities					
School 1					
Mean	12.51	13.87	8.50	+4.02***	−4.94***
S.D.	2.53	2.33	6.29		
School 2					
Mean	12.16	18.96	13.31	+7.78***	−3.01**
S.D.	5.29	6.41	4.48		

***p < .001
**p < .01
*p < .05

TABLE 4—Reported Eating at Home: Per Cent of Heart-Healthy Foods in Diet

	Pre-Program		Post-Program		
	Mean	S.D.	Mean	S.D.	
School 1					
Father	28%	28.32	49%	23.25	+2.65***
Mother	30	21.28	55	21.28	−2.58**
Target Child	27	28.85	44	18.37	+2.00*
Sibling	28	29.55	34	25.83	0.67
Food bought that was Heart Healthy	25	25.40	48	12.68	+3.97***
	Pre-Program		Follow-up		
School 2					
Father	47%	19.09	55%	26.94	+2.05*
Mother	49	18.06	59	4.08	+2.41**
Target Child	47	18.89	49	8.78	0.79
Sibling	49	17.14	62	19.56	+2.31*
Food bought that was Heart Healthy	52	10.66	57	14.67	+2.29*

***p < .001
**p < .01
*p < .05

Participant Reactions

Student, teacher, and parent reactions were extremely positive. When asked to estimate the importance of the Heart Health Curriculum, 88 per cent of the students, 67 per cent of the regular classroom teachers, and 63 per cent of the parents rated the program as "Very Important." All of the teachers, 72 per cent of the students, and 98 per cent of the parents indicated that they would like to see this kind of program repeated in the future. When the students were asked if they enjoyed the class, 80 per cent responded "Yes".

Discussion

The Heart Health Program resulted in some changes in students' lunches, knowledge about heart-healthy foods, and reported food habits of family members at home. The primary changes were documented using direct observation of eating behavior and discarded food items in the school trash receptacles. These measures are relatively free of expectancy bias.

There are some outcomes that remain perplexing: the decline in reported preferences for Heart-Healthy Foods at follow-up in School 1, the differences between Schools 1 and 2 in reported home eating at baseline, the lack of reported change at home for School 2 target children. These results make the measurement operations appear even more important, as they might not have emerged without multiple measures (observations, interview, self-report) on multiple dimensions (behavior, trash, knowledge, preference, reported behavior at home).

It was our impression that three elements of the program seemed essential for its success: behavioral commitment, feedback and incentives, and family involvement. Students at this (or any) age often have difficulty in translating general principles or even concrete recommendations into specific behavior changes. The daily goal sheets, in which students made a written commitment to substitute specific food items and to engage in specific playground activities, resulted in significant nutrition changes. The commitment appeared to focus students on changes needed for them to implement the program recommendations. The feedback system, in which students received information regarding their progress, provided students with objective information about changes they had made and further changes that were possible. An unplanned bonus was achieved when we presented data separately for boys and girls. The competition and interest in the feedback became keen at that point.

The reinforcement system proved to be enormously popular. Students who earned "heart stickers" pasted them on their lunch pails and notebooks. These motivated, and also cued, heart-healthy eating and exercise. Especially noteworthy were reported changes in family members' eating and food buying. Programs in schools may have potential in influencing other children and adults. The reward system at school may have facilitated family behavior and maintenance of change. It provided a method for rewarding at school changes that had to occur at home. The success of the program was contingent upon immediate and sustained changes in the home. This reward procedure in combination with handouts and parent meetings may have facilitated those changes.

Students' knowledge and preferences changed positively immediately following the program, but declined in some areas at follow-up. It is our impression that these declines at follow-up were due to students who failed to take the final assessments seriously.

The most disappointing, but also potentially most informative, results were the failure to observe changes in activity during the program. The correlational analysis, along with retrospection, pointed to some reasons for lack of change. The curriculum was developed using traditional cardiovascular fitness lessons. Activities emphasized in classes were quite similar to other programs with the same objective, but quite different from students' normal playground activities. As revealed in the correlational analysis, some student activities were associated with more movement than others. A better program to increase student activity might be to encourage increases in already existing vigorous playground activities.

A number of interesting questions for future research were raised by this study. Including physiologic measures (e.g., blood pressure and cholesterol) of children and their parents would help determine the health impact of such a program. Better delineation of socioeconomic, attitudinal and structural features of school populations might help to explain differences between school and age groups. The feasibility of having nutrition programs for prevention of disease adapted to ongoing school curriculum in a variety of settings, including those in which hot lunch programs are the rule, also needs to be treated. Further investigation of school-based preventive programs is clearly warranted and important.

REFERENCES

1. Lauer RM, Connor WE, Leaverton PE, *et al*: Coronary heart disease risk factors in school children. J Pediatr 1975; 86:697–700.
2. Lauer RM, *et al*: Coronary risk factors in children. The Muscatine Study, IN: *Atherosclerosis and the Child*, JGAT Hautvast and HA Valkenburg (eds). Rotterdam, Erasmus University, 1977.
3. Gilliam TB, Kotch VL, Thorland W, *et al*: Prevalence of coronary heart disease risk factors in active children, 7 to 12 years of age. Med Sci Sports 1977; 9:21–25.
4. Miller RA, Shekelle RB: Blood pressure in tenth grade students. Circulation 1976; 54:993–1000.
5. Keys A: Coronary heart disease in seven countries. Circulation 1970; 41:1–211 (Supplement).
6. Frerichs RR, Srinivasan SR, Webb LS, *et al*: Serum cholesterol and triglyceride levels in 3,446 children from a biracial community: The Bogalusa heart study. Circulation 1976; 54:302–308.
7. Glueck CJ, Mattson F, Bierman EL: Diet and coronary heart disease: Another view. N Engl J Med 1978; 298:1471–1474.
8. Fryer BA, Lamkin GH, Vivian VM, *et al*: Diets of preschool children in the North American region. J Am Diet Assn 1971; 50:228–232.
9. Frank GE, Voors AW, Schilling PE, *et al*: Dietary studies of rural school children in a cardiovascular survey. J Am Diet Assn 1977; 72:31–35.
10. Eppright ES, Sidwell VD, Swanson PP: Nutritive value of the

diets of Iowa school children. J Nutr 1954; 54:371–388.

11. Hovell M, Burrick J, Sharkey R, *et al*: An evaluation of elementary students' physical activity during recess. Res Quart 1978; 49:460–474.

12. Coates TJ, Thoresen CE: Obesity in children and adolescents: The problem belongs to everyone, IN: Advances in Clinical Child Psychology, Lahey B and Kazdin A (eds). New York: Plenum, 1980.

13. Farquhar JW: The community-based model of life style intervention trials. Am J Epidem 1978; 108:103–111.

14. Kratochwill T: Single-subject experiment: Design and analysis. New York: Academic Press, 1978.

15. Hersen M, Barlow DH. Single case experimental designs. New York: Pergamon, 1976.

16. Glass GV, Willson VL, Gottman JM: Design and analysis of time series experiments. Boulder, CO: Associated Universities Press, 1975.

17. Farquhar JW: The American Way of Life Need Not Be Hazardous to Your Health. Stanford, CA: Stanford Alumni Association, 1979.

18. Parcourse, Ltd., 3701 Buchanan, San Francisco, CA 94123.

19. Goodwin DC, Coates TJ: The teacher-pupil interaction scale: An empirical method of studying the interactive effects of teacher and pupil behavior. J School Psychol, 1977; 15:51–59.

20. Bullen BA, Reed RR, Mayer J: Physical activity of obese and nonobese adolescent girls appraised by motion picture sampling. Am J Clin Nutri 1964; 14:211–223.

21. Waxman M, Stunkard AJ: Caloric intake and expenditure of obese boys. J Pediatr, 1980; 96:187–193.

ACKNOWLEDGMENTS

This study was supported in part by Grant No-NIH HL 21906-01A1 from the National Heart, Lung and Blood Institute to the Stanford Heart Disease Prevention Program, and by Young Investigator Grant No-1-R23-HL24297 from the NHLBI to Thomas J. Coates.

The Multiple Risk Factor Intervention Trial (MRFIT): III. The Model for Intervention

by Robert C. Benfari (for the MRFIT)

Department of Behavioral Science, Harvard School of Public Health,
677 Huntington Avenue, Boston, Massachusetts 02115

The design, planning, and implementation steps taken to develop the MRFIT intervention model are discussed. The objective of the MRFIT program, which extends from 1974 to 1982, was to intervene on the primary risk factors for CHD: cigarette smoking, elevated blood pressure, and elevated cholesterol. Participants in the program are at high risk of developing CHD although initially free of clinical signs of CHD. The assumptions underlying the behavioral model, the use of group techniques, and other behavioral techniques over the life of the trial are discussed here. Overall intervention objectives and specific risk factor objectives of the MRFIT program are outlined. Brief descriptions of the roles and responsibilities of the intervention staff and the training programs used to achieve standardization and of the MRFIT intervention program are given.

A. BACKGROUND

The fundamental problem facing the MRFIT planning groups, including the Behavioral Factors and the Intervention Committees, was to develop a model for intervention to facilitate change of the primary risk factors for coronary heart disease (cigarette smoking, elevated blood cholesterol levels, and elevated blood pressure). Since a multiple intervention program on this scale had never been tried before, this attempt represented state-of-the-art development. The scientific literature contained numerous studies devoted to lowering of blood cholesterol levels, cessation of smoking, and lowering of blood pressure (8, 14, 15, 23, 25, 29, 31, 33–35). Most of them, however, were single-focus trials or experiments. Furthermore, the samples were of diverse demographic composition and sometimes included patients who were acutely or chronically ill. A multiple community-based study conducted at Stanford University began in 1972, but its methods were not applicable to the individual focus of MRFIT (10, 22). The Intervention Committee of MRFIT accepted the charge to devise an intervention program that would achieve *simultaneous* reduction in all three risk factors in order to achieve maximum risk factor change in as short a period of time as possible and to ensure the maximum preventive effect over the duration of the trial (24).

Because there were few models to emulate, the Intervention Committee looked at the behavioral science literature with the goal of extrapolating to the MRFIT

Program the best model or models and techniques for an integrated program. Since selection into the trial was based upon a multiple logistic function, a number of risk factor configurations were possible and, therefore, integrated intervention was slightly different for separate classes of individuals. Not everyone had the same risk factor profile. The overriding theoretical model adopted is broadly described as Behavioral Therapy or Intervention, as defined by Bandura (3) and Krasner (20). In this context, the term "Behavioral Intervention" encompasses the following elements:

- functional analytical approach to clinical data, and
- the treatment of observable activity.

Behavioral intervention consists of a series of activities which imply a contractual agreement between the interventionist and the participant in order to alter the problem behavior(s). Bandura has emphasized the role of cognitive processes in both acquisition and change of behavior. He postulates that cognitive processes mediate change and that they are altered by experiencing mastery arising from effective performance. In this context, a functional analysis of behavior includes the interaction between the person and the situation.

It was clear from the social psychological literature that attention must be given to the demand characteristics of any experimental design in order to achieve optimal results (27). The demand characteristics include: the complexity of the regimen, the propriety of the change to the interventionist and the participant, interventionist/participant interaction behavior, the motivation of the participant, and complications or side effects. It is these demand characteristics that are perceived and interpreted by the participant and will influence the outcome of the intervention effort.

One of the motivation problems faced by MRFIT was the fact that the men selected into the trial were essentially symptom free of coronary heart disease. They were men at risk who were not sick.

It was believed that this distinction is based upon real differences in the demand characteristics of the regimen, and has profound implications in consequences for outcomes. In dealing with change in risk factor status, a participant in MRFIT is not a patient in the usual sense of the word. The individual does not have symptomatic disease and is able to perform most social and occupational duties. The behavior change involved is the cessation or reduction of one form of activity and/or the substitution of another activity. Good examples are cigarette smoking cessation and dietary changes in which the responsibility for the change rests mostly with the individual.

On the other hand, compliance to prescribed treatment involving patients fits the criteria of Parsons' (28) sick role:

- there is sickness and incapacity,
- some curative process must take place, and
- the responsibility of a cure is usually in the hands of a trained physician.

Kasl and Cobb (18) point out that this theoretical framework of the sick role has limitations for studies in which the purpose is to understand the many aspects of risk reduction behavior. A number of health scientists have coined the term "risk role" as separate from "sick role." The "risk role" has been characterized by Baric (4) as the following:

- The role is not institutionalized, only duties are attached, and no privileges are afforded.
- It endures for an indefinite time span.
- It has no continuous reinforcement from the health care system and the social environment.

- It does not provide feedback from changes in symptomology or treatment procedures.

In MRFIT, committees responsible for each modality were charged with the development of an intervention program for that specific risk factor. These separate modules were then integrated into the intensive intervention program. Although the demand characteristics for each modality could be analyzed for effects upon outcome, no one knew at the outset the effects of simultaneous intervention on all the risk factors. Since that time, some light has been shed on this and it is clear that the following, among other problems, exist:

- Some interventions are antagonistic to others—smoking cessation vs weight loss, blood pressure control vs cholesterol lowering (2, 6, 12, 32).
- Participants may set priorities for change based upon ease of attainment.
- Intervention overload on some participants can cause motivational problems and lead to failure.

As a result of numerous meetings, the specific recommendations from the Intervention Committee were:

- Ten group sessions were to be the initial cornerstone of the integrated intervention program.
- The group team would be interdisciplinary in composition.
- The procedures in each of the sessions would be standardized for all clinical centers.
- A behavioral diagnosis would be used to facilitate the intervention process during and after the group sessions.
- All risk factors would be altered simultaneously.
- A national training program would be conducted to standardize procedures for training and evaluation.
- An extended intervention program would be devised for the duration of the trial to fill the further intervention and maintenance needs of the participants after the intensive group sessions were completed. This program would take into account the progress on risk factor alternatives to date and would define the next steps for intervention including frequency of contact, techniques or methods of individual counseling, and priority of the risk factor modalities.

A task force of the Intervention Committee was formed for the development, implementation, and evaluation of the training programs. A series of training programs were carried out in the first 5 years of the trial. Each training session had specific foci dependent upon the intervention needs of the trial at that time. The first training sessions were conducted in 1973–1974. The next major national training session was held in 1976. The objectives of these training sessions were to indoctrinate the intervention staffs at the clinical centers in the methods and procedures of the Intensive Intervention Program and to standardize the process. A final series of training programs were held in 1978, but this time they were done on a regional basis, i.e., east, west, and central areas. The objectives of regional training sessions were to familiarize the intervention staffs with a phase II portion of the Extended Intervention Program, with particular emphasis on maintaining and increasing intervention results in the areas of nutrition and smoking.

An evaluation task force was also appointed by the Steering Committee in 1976 to evaluate the process and outcome of intervention and to determine if there were center differences in performance in risk factor change. The task force faced some difficult methodological problems such as (a) ascertaining the contribution of Center baseline differences to risk factor change; (b) distinguishing true Center differences from changes due to secular trends in the communities; (c) assessing contributions of aggregate psychosocial variables to change.

B. OBJECTIVES

1. Overall Intervention Objectives

The MRFIT Intervention Program had three levels of outcome as objectives:

- awareness and information acquisition on the part of the participants;
- behavioral change in any one or all of the intervention modalities; and
- change in risk factor level.

Experience and research in the field of intervention in other settings (organizations, communities, and groups like MRFIT) have shown that people usually resist change except when six conditions are present, namely, when an individual perceives that:

- he knows what change is desirable and why, and has the substantive knowledge required by the change;
- he has the skill to use his knowledge to operate effectively in implementing the change;
- the change is in his self-interest;
- the change is in the self-interest of the groups (families, etc.) with which he identifies;
- both internal and external environmental forces require change; and
- both internal and external "change agents" give their support to the change and provide feedback throughout the process (1, 5).

In MRFIT, the intensive integrated intervention attempted to create a learning environment in which all of these conditions were present.

If one accepts the interdependence of the three levels of intervention outcome—awareness, behavior change, and risk factor change—then the following primary tasks can be delineated for the intervention process:

- generation of valid information (CHD risk factors, smoking, nutrition) and of the opportunity for feedback;
- acceptance of freedom of choice on the part of the participant to assume responsibility for the change or alternatives; and
- generation of internal commitment for change on the part of the participant.

The primary task of the intervention team was the generation of valid information about risk factors, coronary heart disease, and the development of alternative life patterns for the participants.

2. Specific Intervention Objectives

The MRFIT Special Intervention Program was based upon an integrated approach to life-style changes, but each risk factor modality had specific objectives and means for achieving life-style change and risk factor reduction.

The Nutrition Intervention Program was structured to modify the participant's eating habits to obtain a reduction in percentage of calories from total fat, a decrease in percentage of calories from saturated fats, an increase in percentage of calories from polyunsaturated fats, a decrease in dietary cholesterol intake, and modification of carbohydrate and alcohol intake. These basic nutritional goals were modified in later stages of the program (7).

The Hypertension Intervention Program involved a stepped-care system, which specified drugs, dosage ranges, duration of treatment, and methods for monitoring compliance and side effects for those participants who had elevated diastolic blood pressure. Weight loss and sodium restrictions were also encouraged (9).

The Smoking Intervention Program used behavioral techniques including focal groups, systematic desensitization, contingency contracting, and dissonance reduction in order to seek cessation in cigarette smoking (13).

The participants randomized into the Special Intervention (SI) Program were followed according to an established protocol in order to reinforce change and to isolate problem areas. Those men not randomized to the SI Group were classified as belonging to the Usual Care (UC) Group. Both the UC and SI groups were given annual examinations for the duration of the study. At these visits, risk factor status and clinical endpoints were measured for both groups. The specific methods and procedures for each intervention modality are presented elsewhere in this issue (7, 9, 13).

C. BEHAVIORAL METHODS

The MRFIT intervention program was based upon the adaptation of four behavioral methods:

- the use of group techniques;
- behavioral diagnosis;
- individual behavioral techniques;
- the use of support systems, e.g., the role of the homemaker.

1. The Rationale for Groups

A 10-week integrated intervention program was devised as the initial contact with the participants. Such a program cannot assure total success, but it seemed the minimum necessary for information dissemination and behavioral and social diagnosis, and it set the stage for the initiation of changes in life patterns.

The use of groups in MRFIT, as the preferred mode of intervention, was based on the assumption that groups were both efficient and effective for our purposes. The use of groups to effect change has become widespread. The types of groups can range widely including, for example, Alcoholics Anonymous, psychoanalytic groups, family therapy groups, Synanon, and others. Yalom *et al.* (37) point out that the goals of a group may vary from support and inspiration, reality testing, and building new defenses or reinforcing old ones, to changing coping style and character structure (38). Not only do the goals of groups vary, but so do, what Yalom calls, "the front." This consists of the trappings, form, techniques, jargon, and aura surrounding each type of group. Unlike "the front," which can be quite different from group to group, the "core" represents those aspects of the experience that are intrinsic to the therapeutic process. Groups may differ in form, but the actual mechanisms are limited in number and are similar across groups.

One primary concern was to ascertain if certain recognized "core" aspects of experience or "curative factors" would indeed act as mechanisms for behavior change within the MRFIT intervention population.

Aspects of the group that have been linked to therapeutic outcome are attendance at group sessions and group cohesiveness; Yalom and Rand have pointed out that group cohesiveness also influences group attendance (36). Lieberman *et al.* found that low cohesiveness eventually leads to people dropping out of the group. They conclude that "continuation in the group is obviously a necessary, though not a sufficient, prerequisite for successful treatment" (21).

Frank also points out that feelings of cohesion with the group and self-esteem are interrelated (11). Each person gains confidence and encouragement from watching others improve; each then identifies with the others, a phenomenon which in turn seems to be a function of cohesiveness of the group. Kapp and his co-workers (17) also found that a feeling of group unity is important for the promotion of self-perceived personality change.

Although the group sessions formed the first and major thrust of the intensive intervention program, the work of intervention was carried beyond these meetings. In the next sequence of intervention, the emphasis was on the individual and the profile of behavioral risk factor changes achieved at the time of assessment. The behavioral diagnosis was the vehicle used to assess progress and future directions for individual intervention.

2. Behavioral Diagnosis

The initial 10 sessions functioned for participants as an orienting phase to the problems of being at risk, introducing the components for each modality, determining the strategies for change, and defining the psychological contracts for the future.

The cornerstone to the next stage of intervention was the behavioral diagnosis, assessed in the case conference, which was carried out after the initial 10 sessions at regularly prescribed intervals.

In MRFIT, the basis for the behavioral diagnosis was a series of case conferences which involved the physicians, nutritionists, and behavioral scientists in discussing the life situation of the participants (16). At one session before the initial group session, baselines were established for risk factor determination, self-image, life event contingencies, social factors, behavioral deficits and assets. This was an initial classification and the factors changed as the participant's life conditions and activities began to change. This was, however, a starting point for the behavioral diagnosis of the individual as intervention commenced.

As the 10 sessions progressed, additional information about each participant was accumulated and integrated into the ongoing functional analysis. The following outline was used as a guide:

- What are the problem areas of the participant?
- Which persons or groups object to these behaviors?
  Which persons or groups support them?
  Who persuaded or coerced the participant to come to MRFIT?
- What consequences does the problem have for the participant and for significant others?
  What consequences would removal of the problem have for the participant or others?
- Under what conditions (biological, symbolic, social, vocational, etc.) do the problematic behaviors occur?
- What satisfactions would continue for the participant if his problematic behavior were sustained?
  What satisfactions would the participant gain if, as a result of the intervention, his problematic behavior were changed?
  What positive or adverse effects would occur for others if the participant's problematic behavior were changed?
  How would the participant continue to live if intervention were unsuccessful, i.e., if nothing his behavior changed?
- What new problems in living would successful intervention pose for the participant?
- To what extent is the participant capable of helping in development of an intervention program?

Such an approach can be supported from a behavioristic viewpoint. Behavior modification is, however, often criticized for its negative potential for manipulation and control of someone's behavior. Defenders of a behaviorist approach reply that good, ethical behavior modification is done with the consent of the person involved (as in contingency contracting). All of the goals, and methods to be used to attain a goal, are spelled out clearly. Indeed, it is most difficult to produce permanent change in a habit pattern in an open environment without the person's consent and participation, unless the alternatives are more intrinsically rewarding than the old behavior (3, 19).

Because participants had different constellations of risk factors, varying capacities for change, and a unique set of environmental factors, it was necessary to base the next phase of the intervention upon these considerations. Once the behavioral diagnosis was accomplished, a strategy was proposed for future intervention in each modality based upon the following factors:

- the importance of the risk factor or its priority in relationship to other risk factors;
- the degree of behavioral goal attainment, or the degree of adherence to the intervention objectives;
- the degree of risk factor change.

3. Behavioral Techniques

Once the priorities for future intervention were established, then the specific behavioral techniques could be chosen. The process was based upon prior planning by the intervention staff, followed by a negotiation or contracting session with the participant and any other significant person in his life. Insofar as each intervention modality had unique demand characteristics which interacted with the participant's personal and environmental characteristics the program became highly individualized. At this point, the behavioral techniques employed included the following basic components:

Self-monitoring. The interventionist asked the participant to make a written record indicating each time the proscribed or prescribed behavior was performed. Very often, for behaviors such as cigarette smoking, a simple checklist form can be devised. It has been found that merely recording regularly the behavior in question improves the record of compliance. Monitoring is particularly helpful at the beginning of a program of behavior change, but it tends to lose its effectiveness over time. Repeated brief periods of self-monitoring provide an invaluable base of ongoing evaluation of the treatment program. If the self-monitoring assignment includes description of the circumstances surrounding the behavior, as well as its time and place, an experimental analysis of the predisposing feelings and precipitating environmental circumstances can provide insights for new approaches to management of the behavior.

Detailed analysis of the specific parts of the behavioral sequence, including environmental circumstances. For eating behaviors, this sequence begins at the grocery store and continues through food preparation and the times, places, and circumstances of eating. For cigarette smoking, the analysis includes purchase of tobacco, storing of cigarettes, where they are carried, and circumstances triggering lighting up of the cigarette. This analysis may reveal additional weak links in the chain of behavior where interventions can more effectively break the habit.

Goal setting and contracting. In consultation with the interventionist, the participant was encouraged to set an explicit goal for changes in behavior. The goal was to be realistically achievable in light of the participant's behavior pattern. Modest goals were set at first to assure a foundation of early successes. The goal that the participant and interventionist agreed upon was written down, with a copy for each of the two parties to the "contract." For a nutritional intervention, the goal may take the form of specific exclusions from the diet (e.g., no more eating while watching TV); for smoking, an agreed-upon rate of tapering off cigarette usage or setting a date to stop completely; or, for other health behaviors, setting up certain "memory prompters" to assist in maintaining the correct schedule.

Provision of basic information. Instructions were to be given regarding the mechanics of self-directed behavior change and the development of lifelong, healthful living habits.

Opportunity for frequent feedback as to the success of the attempted behavior changes. Feedback would include weigh-ins in obesity control programs, serum determinations in cholesterol-lowering efforts, and blood pressure measurement in antihypertension therapy. The feedback was not to be presented as a way of checking on the participant. Rather, it was an opportunity for timely delivery of positive rewards if success was being achieved, and constructive assistance if it was not. Behavior change research has found that greater changes can be achieved if the behavior (e.g., dietary adherence), rather than the result (e.g., weight loss), is monitored and reinforced.

Provision of support and positive reinforcement from the health worker or peer group. This followed directly from the "feedback" step, above. The variety of forms of positive support are discussed more fully elsewhere in this issue.

Training of spouse or other household members to provide positive encouragement and to assist in maintaining a favorable immediate environment for the participant (see subsequent section on Support Systems).

Development of a self-reward system. This included tangible, intangible, or simply verbal rewards by which the participant could reinforce his own correct behaviors without depending upon the interventionist.

"Stimulus control of environment." This involved controlling the individual's environment to enhance the achievement of the desirable behavior. It would include such simple things as not smoking in the presence of a family member who is attempting to stop the habit, or the subtle but effective strategy of never doing the grocery shopping on an empty stomach.

Modeling of the correct health behaviors. Observation of others performing the desired health behaviors and being rewarded would teach the participant the correct techniques and create an expectation of reward for performing them.

Guided participation. Participants needed the opportunity to practice their new behaviors. This can be done effectively in the controlled environment of a self-help group meeting or on a weekend retreat.

Self-presented consequences and cognitive strategies. Participants were encouraged to work through in their imaginations the positive consequences of adhering to the health regimen and the negative consequences of failure to adhere. They also were encouraged to practice first with the interventionist, and then among themselves, the arguments they would use to keep from "backsliding" into their old behavioral patterns. This might have included how one would argue against the tendency to cut down on prescribed medication because of a possibly exaggerated perception of the side effects.

Systematic desensitization and relaxation. These techniques were taught to persons by a behavioral scientist skilled in their use in those circumstances in which adherence to the prescribed health behaviors may be difficult without additional specialized approaches.

With all of these techniques of engineering comprehensive behavioral change, the participant must cooperate actively and freely. As Bandura argues, the determinants of behavior are largely under an individual's own control (3). A person can alter his level of arousal through self-generated imagery. He can apply foresight to situational cues in order to predict and then to modify sequences leading to future behaviors.

4. Support Systems—The Role of the Wife or Homemaker in the MRFIT Intervention Program

A function of the interview with each participant at the third screen visit, after randomization, was to elicit directly his feeling about having his wife or homemaker participate in the group. At this interview, effort was made to indicate clearly to the participant the value of having this person participate in the program.

It was expected that many participants would agree to having their wives or homemakers participate. They could then enter into the mainstream approach of intervention and participate fully in sessions of the intervention program along with the participants. For any participants who raised objections to having them participate, however, a great effort was made to stress how important the participation of the wife or homemaker was in the project. An effort was made to have this person attend at least the orientation session. The wives or homemakers of participants who could not be induced to participate in the group were not permitted to participate alone.

Some wives or homemakers thus were unable to participate in groups because their participants may not have chosen that mode of intervention, or they had time and scheduling problems, and/or they were disinclined to be involved in a group program. Because most of these persons attended at least the orientation session, a decision was made at that time about arranging contact with those few who did not continue in the group, to assess the wife or homemaker's own wishes about changing her/his own behavior, which would reinforce and help change the participant's behavior. To this end, data were gathered about the wife or homemaker's smoking, dietary, and food preparation habits. Intervention programs for nutrition and smoking that supported the intervention efforts of the participant were then made available to these people; however, no hypertension intervention program was offered to them.

Because it had been clearly established that wives or homemakers who smoked made it more difficult for men to give up cigarettes or to change their own smoking behavior, it became critical to try to involve these smokers in some intervention programs. A decision about the particular program to be offered was made by the senior scientists in the clinical center. Solo method, individual counseling, or a special group focused on smoking all could be employed to help wives or homemakers who need to modify their own smoking behaviors in order to achieve desired changes in the MRFIT participants. Similarly, at each of the Clinical Centers wives or homemakers who did not participate in groups also may have been offered a specialized program in nutrition, directed toward achieving the specific changes desired for the participants.

D. STAFFING—ROLES AND RESPONSIBILITIES

The emphasis of the MRFIT Intervention Program was to treat the participant as an organic whole. In order to achieve this desired mode of interaction and to minimize the emphasis on any one risk factor, an integrator for the intervention process and for staff coordination, called the Intervention Director, was appointed at each clinical center. This individual had professional training in some area of the behavioral or social sciences or equivalent backgrounds, and was responsible for local staff training and for adherence to the MRFIT protocol as outlined in the manual of operations.

In order to carry out the specific interventions, a specialist was designated at each clinical center for each modality and was to be responsible for the technical and clinical aspects of that phase of the intervention program.

The Chief Nutritionist at each clinical center managed the nutrition program and provided information, interpretation, and guidance to the rest of the intervention staff, including other nutritionists. All of the chief nutritionists in the study had a minimum of a master's degree in foods and nutrition and 2 years of responsible experience in these fields; or an equivalent combination of training and experience.

The Smoking Specialist directed the smoking cessation aspects of the study at each center. This person supervised all smoking-related intervention such as problem diagnosis or assignment to intervention approach, record keeping, development of the implementation of the smoking cessation program at the center within the intervention guidelines, participation in the national smoking subcommittee, and provision of consultation regarding smoking intervention to other staff members. The suggested qualifications for the smoking specialist included a social or behavioral education background, master's level degree or experience working in a smoking cessation program, and experience in counseling or interviewing.

The Intervention Physician was responsible for carrying out the stepped-care hypertension program and supervising other auxiliary personnel working in the hypertension regime, and was responsible for conducting the annual physical examination.

The Hypertension Coordinator was responsible to the Intervention Physician for implementing the hypertension protocol. The Hypertension Coordinators were usually registered nurses with experience in hypertension management.

The group process specialist was usually one of the above individuals and was responsible for supervising the group sessions carried out as part of the initial integrated intervention program. The minimal requirements were an M.A. or Ph.D. in either social work or small-group, social, or clinical psychology, or an M.D. with special training in psychiatry.

Each center not already having a psychologist on its staff was also encouraged to have access to a psychological consultant who would work with problem participants. This function included the evaluation and assessment of the progress or lack of progress of a problem participant, and consultation with participants having difficulty complying with the intervention methods prescribed or having repeated failures. The qualifications were a Ph.D. in clinical or counseling psychology or an M.D. with specialization in psychiatry.

Staff members were assigned to individual participants as health counselors responsible for assisting in the implementation of the total intervention program. There were no specific formal educational requirements but specialized training was given by staff of the local center as needed.

E. INTERVENTION PROCESS

1. Introduction

During this period, which was a continuation of the screening process, major emphases were on:

- obtaining the participant's consent for his wife or homemaker's participation in the program or, at the minimum, this person's attendance at the orientation session;
- completing the collection of baseline information needed for the initiation of an efficient management program for each participant during intervention;
- informing the participant of the broad plans of the intervention program and introducing him to the resource and operational staff available throughout the program; and
- assigning each participant to a style of intervention mutually agreeable to him and the staff.

Immediately after randomization at the third screen visit, the participant assigned to SI was asked for his consent to his wife or homemaker's participation in the intervention program. In addition, current cigarette smokers were urged by a MRFIT physician to stop smoking. An interview was conducted with each smoker, specifically with respect to the degree of commitment to quitting cigarette smoking and the problem he may have had or anticipated with regard to quitting. This interview may have been used to probe further, if there were questions concerning the participant's degree of involvement in the initial intensive group sessions. If the interviewer considered that the matter needed to be brought up at a case conference for further discussion, the participant's file was flagged at this time to signal the need to review the case before the orientation session. The *Quit Smoking Book* could be handed out at this time to participants who wished to stop smoking without further assistance from the program.

Also, after randomization at the third screen visit, a simple nutrition message was given to motivate the participant to initiate modest modifications in his eating pattern. This was done by drawing on pertinent information supplied by him in a dietary recall, such as substituting skim milk for whole milk, or an acceptable brand of margarine for butter. The participant also could be given the MRFIT *Guide* with the accompanying MRFIT *Brand Name Food List* and the *Datebook,* at the discretion of the clinical centers. These materials are discussed in greater detail in another paper (7).

For SI participants who were nonsmokers, but overweight, and particularly for those who may have been hyperlipidemic and hypertensive, a weight message, alerting these participants to the facts and hazards of being overweight, was given, preferably by a physician. Counseling, however, did not begin at this time.

2. Intensive Intervention Groups

An orientation session lasting approximately 2 hr was held within 3 to 5 weeks after the third screen visit and randomization. A senior investigator, the group leader, and specialists for each risk factor modality were present at this session as were all participants randomized into the SI group in the preceding 2 to 3 weeks. All participants were encouraged to bring their wives or homemakers. At this session, opened by the group leader, the participants and staff were asked to introduce themselves and the format of the session was explained. Both participants and intervention staff were encouraged to express their expectations about their participation in MRFIT. The group leader briefly explained the purpose of the intervention groups, the discussions that were expected to take place, the feedback to be provided, and the specific changes to be made by the participants. The role of the homemaker in the intervention program was stressed. Participants were encouraged to raise topics relevant to habit changes for discussion with other members of the group.

The importance of hypertension as a risk factor and the general concept that "the lower it is the better" were discussed. For participants who had a high diastolic blood pressure and qualified for drug therapy in the Stepped-Care Program, the Step-Up Schedule was initiated. In addition, there was an overview of both the Nutrition Program and its goals, and the major parts of the Smoking Cessation Program as described elsewhere in this issue (13). The MRFIT orientation film, "The Heart of the Matter," was shown and discussion of the film was encouraged.

At the end of the orientation session, all participants who chose the group mode of intervention were given a schedule of the sessions. For participants who did not choose to join a group, individual appointments were planned. For those in the Stepped-Care Program for hypertension, follow-up visits were scheduled as required by that program to coincide, if possible, with the group sessions schedule.

The participants and their wives or homemakers were encouraged to become familiar with the educational materials given out at the postrandomization or the orientation session and were asked to bring to the next session any questions they had. Finally, the participants were encouraged to begin behavioral changes in diet and smoking and, while studying their own habits, to identify some of their problem areas.

Nine sessions beyond the orientation session were planned in the initial intensive group intervention. The total time required per session was between 1½ and 2 hr. It was recommended that no more than *two* co-leaders conduct a set of sessions and that a nutritionist attend as many group sessions as possible and participate as an active member of the intervention team.

A considerable degree of flexibility was allowed in the sequence of the presentation of materials and topics to be covered in the nine sessions. This allowed the group leader to make use of the ongoing dynamics of the group to produce an atmosphere best suited to the aims of the initial intervention.

Some educational materials required during the nine sessions, including films, cassettes, brochures, and pamphlets, were to be used at the option of the group leader and the nutritionist. These included: four nutrition slide–tape units and accompanying brochures; a number of films on smoking, suggested for the second session of intervention; the hypertension film "What Goes Up," considered to be the most appropriate for the third or fourth session of group intervention; the smoking films from the American Heart Association and the American Cancer Society, to be used whenever appropriate; and "We Can't Go On Like This," an antismoking film cassette, recommended for presentation early in the intervention program. "The Ordeal of Arnold Hertz" and "Gambling," two other antismoking film cassettes, were recommended for showing after most participants had quit cigarette smoking. (These last two films were useful in the maintenance and in extended intervention phases of the program, as well.)

Suggested topics for discussion included:

Decision making
Goal setting
Learning process
The environment and habits
Consciousness raising
Addiction or habit
Past and current failures
External/internal control
Breaking habits
Substitute behaviors
Self-esteem
Stress
Deprivation effects

Irrational beliefs
Rationalizations
Coping
Short-term versus long-term satisfaction
Evaluations and referrals
Compliance
Nutrition topics (identified by the clinical center chief nutritionist)
Information specific to smoking
Information specific to hypertension pill-taking habits

The intervention staff participating in the groups obviously had to be knowledgeable about the above areas in order to guide the discussion and provide suitable assistance.

Some requirements were specific for participants who quit cigarette smoking during the initial or extended intervention. As soon as a smoker reported that he had completely stopped smoking, the interventionist who had worked with him advised him that he or she would be calling him within the next few days to see how things were progressing and to offer help if needed. The interventionist continued this practice at least once a week *for 1 month following cessation*. Although this procedure was strongly advised by the smoking cessation specialists both to indicate their continuing interest and to provide moral support during this initially difficult period, *in no way* was it *imposed* on participants who voiced objections. We recognized that although this procedure was desirable, the participant who rejected it forced the interventionist to find other strategies to maintain frequency of contact. One such strategy was to ask the participant to initiate the contacts with the interventionist. Another was to ask the participant to mail an addressed and stamped postcard or letter to the interventionist (furnished to him by the center), on which he indicated whether he was still a nonsmoker and whether he was encountering difficulties remaining one. The last alternative, however, had obvious drawbacks.

3. Other Options for Intensive Intervention

An option of intensive individual intervention was offered to individuals who could not participate in the group sessions because of aversion or scheduling problems. It should be emphasized that this option was used in a very small number of cases and that the group method was the usual mode of intensive intervention.

Intensive individual intervention sessions (also referred to as the individual counseling sessions) began approximately 1 week after the orientation session for those selecting this approach. Six to ten individual sessions were believed sufficient to produce the desired changes, although it was recognized that the number of sessions would vary from participant to participant, depending on the individual's needs, risk factor profile, and rate of progress. Each individual session was to last usually between 30 and 45 min. One counselor/interventionist conducted the individual counseling sessions for each participant and his wife or homemaker who were under this mode of intervention.

4. Beyond Intensive Intervention

Intensive intervention ended when all ten sessions had been completed for a given group. No specific time period for completing these ten sessions was set; however, the last session usually occurred around the time of the first 4-month follow-up visit. The Maintenance Program and the Extended Intervention Program were made available to SI participants after both a regular 4-month follow-up visit and a case conference had been held for these participants, and in some instances later.

It was anticipated that at the conclusion of the Intensive Intervention Program and in the interim period prior to the 4-month follow-up visit, a substantial number of the SI participants would have succeeded in lowering their risk factors. The Maintenance Program was designed to reinforce these successes within each modality. Its thrust was toward sustaining the newly acquired behaviors that had resulted in lowering a risk factor to its intervention goal. Through this reinforcement it was expected that recidivism would be minimized.

In some cases, SI participants were not able to reach all of their risk factor goals with intensive intervention, or may have become recidivists. The Extended Intervention Program, also specific to each modality, was aimed at this group of participants to continue the attempt to modify the risk factors until the desired goals were reached. An individual SI participant could be in the Maintenance Program for one modality and in Extended Intervention for another. A totally successful participant was in the Maintenance Program for all modalities germane to his risk factor profile.

F. CONCLUSION

The MRFIT Intervention program covering the period from 1974 to 1982 involved the following steps:

- planning of intensive intervention;
- implementation of intensive intervention;
- planning of extended intervention and maintenance phases;
- implementation of extended intervention and maintenance activities;
- evaluation of risk factor change at regular intervals during the trial.

The evaluation of the effectiveness of any of the specific interventions is difficult since the study design was based upon a total push for risk factor change rather than a multilevel treatment design. However, the analysis of overall results for these risk factor modalities at various points in time will reveal the relative effectiveness of some of the intervention methods used in these stages. Furthermore, the planning and implementation of the MRFIT Intervention Program were based upon the reality that the needs of the study would change as new factors emerged during the course of the trial. Therefore the Intervention Committee was faced with a dynamic situation that demanded purposeful responses to unanticipated changes. The development of the extended intervention program and a phase II intervention thrust represent such reactions. In a long-term program in which the goal is optimizing efficacy such an approach is not only justifiable but absolutely necessary.

The accompanying articles are devoted to the specific objectives, methodologies, and results at 4 years for the risk factors (7, 9, 13, 30, 39). A separate article deals with the interrelationships among risk factors and the difference between the UC and the SI risk factor changes (26).

Further evaluation of the process and the results of the MRFIT Program should be helpful in the future planning, design, and implementation of other intervention programs.

REFERENCES

1. Agras, W. S. The behavior therapies: Underlying principles and procedures, *in* "Behavior Modification: Principles and Clinical Applications" (W. S. Agras, Ed.). Little, Brown, Boston, 1978.
2. Ames, R. P., and Hill, P. Elevation of serum lipid levels during diuretic therapy of hypertension. *Amer. J. Med.* **61**, 748−757 (1976).
3. Bandura, A. Self-efficacy: Toward a unifying theory of behavioral change. *Psychol. Rev.* **84**, 191−202 (1977).
4. Baric, L. Recognition of the at-risk role: A means to influence health behavior. *Int. J. Health Educ.* **12**, 35−44 (1969).
5. Benfari, R. C. Lifestyle alteration and the primary prevention of CHD: The Multiple Risk Factor Intervention Trial, *in* "Heart Disease and Rehabilitation" (M. L. Pollack and D. H. Schmidt, Eds.), pp. 341−351. Houghton Mifflin, Boston, 1979.
6. Benfari, R. C., Eaker, E. E., Reed, R., and McIntyre, K. M. Components of risk factor change in CHD program. *J. Clin. Psychol.* **37**, 61−70 (1981).
7. Caggiula, A. W., Christakis, G., Farrand, M., Hulley, S. B., Johnson, R., Lasser, N., Stamler, J., and Widdowson, G. The Multiple Risk Factor Intervention Trial (MRFIT). IV. Intervention on blood lipids. *Prev. Med.* **10**, 443−475 (1981).
8. Christakis G., Rinzler S., Archer M., *et al.* The anti-coronary club: A dietary approach to the prevention of coronary heart disease—a seven year report. *Amer. J. Pub. Health* **56**, 299−314 (1966).
9. Cohen, J. D., Grimm, R. H., Jr., and Smith, W. M. The Multiple Risk Factor Intervention Trial (MRFIT). VI. Intervention on blood pressure. *Prev. Med.* **10**, 501−518 (1981).
10. Farquhar, J. W., *et al.* Community education for cardiovascular health. *Lancet,* 1192 (June 4, 1977).
11. Frank, J. D. Some determinants, manifestations, and effects of cohesiveness in therapy groups. *Int. J. Group Psychother.* **7**, 53−63 (1957).
12. Grimm, R. H., Jr., Leon, A. S., Hunninghake, D., *et al.* Diuretic effects on plasma lipids and lipoproteins. *Clin. Res.* **26**, 290A (1978).
13. Hughes, G. H., Hymowitz, N., Ockene, J. K., Simon, N., and Vogt, T. M. The Multiple Risk Factor Intervention Trial. V. Intervention on smoking. *Prev. Med.* **10**, 476−500 (1981).
14. Hypertension Detection and Follow-up Program Cooperative Group. Therapeutic control of blood pressure in the hypertensive detection and follow-up program. *Prev. Med.* **8**, 2−13 (1979).
15. Hypertension Detection and Follow-up Program Cooperative Group. Five year findings of the hypertension detection and follow-up program. *JAMA* **42**, 2562−2571 (1979).
16. Kanfer, F. H., and Salow, G. Behavioral diagnosis, *in* "Behavior Therapy: Appraisal and Status" (C. M. Franks, Ed.), pp. 417−444. McGraw−Hill, New York, 1969.
17. Kapp, F. T., *et al.* Group participation and self-perceived personality change. *J. Nerv. Ment. Dis.,* 139−255 (1964).
18. Kasl, S., and Cobb, S. Health behavior, illness behavior, and sick-role behavior. *Arch. Environ. Health* **12**, 246 (1966).
19. Kelman, H. C. Processes of opinion change. *Pub. Opinion Quart.* **25**, 57−78 (1961).
20. Krasner, L. On the death of behavior modification. *Amer. Psychol.* **31**, 387−388 (1976).
21. Lieberman, M. A., Yalom, I. D., and Miles, M. B. "Encounter Groups: First Facts," pp. 61−70. Basic Books, New York, 1973.
22. Maccoby, H., Farquhar, J. W., Wood, P. D., and Alexander, J. Reducing the risk of cardiovas-

cular disease: Effects of a community-based campaign on knowledge and behavior. *J. Community Health* **3**, 100 (1977).

23. Mojonnier, L., Hall, Y., Berkson, D., *et al.* Experience in changing food habits of hyperlipidemic men and women. *J. Amer. Dietet. Assoc.* **77**, 140–148 (1980).

24. The Multiple Risk Factor Intervention Trial Group. Statistical design considerations in the NHLI Multiple Risk Factor Intervention Trial (MRFIT). *J. Chron. Dis.* **30**, 261–275 (1977).

25. National Diet–Heart Study Research Group. The national diet–heart study final report. *Circulation* **38** (Suppl. I), 428 (1968).

26. Neaton, J. D., Broste, S., Fishman, E. L., Kjelsberg, M. O., and Schoenberger, J. The Multiple Risk Factor Intervention Trial (MRFIT). VII. A comparison of risk factor changes between two study groups. *Prev. Med.* **10**, 519–543 (1981).

27. Orne, M. T. On the social psychology of the psychological experiment: With particular reference to demand characteristics and their implications. *Amer. Psychol.* **17**, 776 (1962).

28. Parsons, T. Definition of health and illness in light of American values and social structure, *in* ''Patients, Physicians and Illness'' (E. G. Jaco, Ed.), pp. 165–187. Free Press, New York, 1958.

29. Schwartz, J. L. A critical review and evaluation of smoking control methods. *Pub. Health Rep.* **84**, 489–506 (1969).

30. Sherwin, R., Kaebler, C. T., Kezdi, P., Kjelsberg, M. O., and Thomas, H. E., Jr. The Multiple Risk Factor Intervention Trial (MRFIT). II. The development of the protocol. *Prev. Med.* **10**, 402–425 (1981).

31. Smith, W. M., Johnson, W. P., and Bromer, L. Intervention trial in mild hypertension, U.S. Public Health Service Hospitals Cooperative Study Group, *in* ''Epidemiology and Control of Hypertension'' (O. Paul, Ed.). Stratton Intercontinental Med. Book Corp., New York, 1975.

32. Smith, W. M. ''The Effect of Thiazides on Plasma Lipids—Multiple Risk Factor Intervention Trial.'' Presented at the Council on Epidemiology of the American Heart Association Meeting, Orlando, Florida, March 1978.

33. Stamler, J. Prevention of atherosclerotic coronary heart disease by change of diet and mode of life, *in* ''Ischaemic Heart Disease'' (J. H. de Haas, H. C. Hemker, and H. A. Snellen, Eds.), p. 311. Leiden Univ. Press, Leiden, 1970.

34. Veterans Administration Cooperative Study Group on Antihypertensive Agents. Effects of treatment on morbidity in hypertension. *JAMA,* **202**, 1028–1034 (1967); **213**, 1143–1152 (1970).

35. World Health Organization. ''Report on a Working Group: Methodology of Multifactor Preventive Trials in Ischaemic Heart Disease, Copenhagen (1973).''

36. Yalom, I. D., and Rand, K. Compatibility and cohesiveness in therapy groups. *Arch. Gen. Psychiat.* **15**, 267 (1966).

37. Yalom, I. D., *et al.* Prediction of improvement in group therapy. *Arch. Gen. Psychiat.* **17**, 159 (1967).

38. Yalom, I. D. ''The Theory and Practice of Group Psychotherapy.'' Basic Books, New York, 1975.

39. Zukel, W. J., Paul, O., and Schnaper, H. W. The Multiple Risk Factor Intervention Trial (MRFIT). I. Historical perspectives. *Prev. Med.* **10**, 387–401 (1981).

Theory and Action for Health Promotion: Illustrations from the North Karelia Project

by Alfred McAlister, Ph.D., Pekka Puska, M.D., Ph.D., Jukka T. Salonen, M.D., Ph.D., Jackko Tuomilehto, M.D., Ph.D., and Kaj Koskela, M.D., M.Pol.Sc.

Abstract: The North Karelia Project in Finland illustrates the fundamental goals of health promotion. Specific activities of the project serve as examples of how concepts from the social and behavioral sciences can be applied to achieve estimated reductions in predicted risk of disease. The results in North Karelia are not conclusive, but they are encouraging, and the investigation conducted there is an essential reference for future research in health promotion and disease prevention. (*Am J Public Health* 1982; 72:43–50.)

Introduction

The prevention of chronic diseases has emerged as a major focus of modern public health.[1,2] Present knowledge indicates that adoption of healthy life-styles and environments are key elements of such preventive action. "Health promotion" is the effort designed to reduce unhealthy behaviors, improve preventive services, and create a better social and physical environment.[3,4] The obvious potential for prevention of several major chronic diseases has led to many campaigns and actions. Disappointment with the frequently marginal or unsatisfactory results has increased demand for a sounder theoretical basis for these health promotion activities. There is also a need for more communication between those involved with action and experts in the behavioral sciences. We believe that "nothing is as practical as a good theory,"[5] and that a comprehensive framework of theorization is urgently needed to guide research and development activities in this important field.

The North Karelia Project[6] is a comprehensive community program for health promotion in North Karelia, a rural county with 180,000 inhabitants in Eastern Finland. Most of the inhabitants of the region reside in very small villages. The largest population center, Joensuu, is a small town. Chief occupations in North Karelia are farming and forestry. The Project was started in 1972 after a petition by the local population requesting the government to do something to reduce high cardiovascular disease (CVD) rates in the area.[7] The aims of the program have been to improve detection and control of hypertension, to reduce smoking, and to promote diets lower in saturated fat and higher in vegetables and low-fat products. The following sections provide conceptual and theoretical analyses of these goals with reference to activities of the North Karelia Project.

Activities of the Project were based on practical ideas of how to improve services and change behaviors and environments. However, most of the sub-programs that were conducted demonstrate the fundamental goals of health promotion and illustrate theoretical principles in action. This paper is not intended as a description of the North Karelia Project and its results; a comprehensive report has been published by the World Health Organization.[7] The aim here is to present a framework of general goals and theoretical principles for health promotion, and to illustrate their application with examples from the North Karelia Project. A chronological listing of selected publications in English is included as an Appendix to this report.

Address reprint requests to Alfred McAlister, PhD, Department of Behavioral Sciences, Harvard School of Public Health, Boston, MA 02115. Dr. Puska is with the Epidemiological Research Unit, National Public Health Laboratory, Helsinki, Finland; Drs. Salonen, Tuomilehto, and Koskela are with the North Karelia Project, University of Kuopio, Kuopio, Finland.

Program Objectives

There are several general models that may be applied to the design of health promotion programs.[8-11] The general framework presented here is compatible with these models, but our schemata emphasizes planning and analysis based on the classification of objectives:

- *Improved preventive services* to identify persons at abnormal risk of disease and provide appropriate medical attention;
- *Information* to educate people about their health and how it can be maintained;
- *Persuasion* to motivate people to take healthy action;
- *Training* to increase skills of self-control, environmental management, and social action;
- *Community organization* to create social support and power for social action;
- *Environmental change* to create opportunity for healthy actions and improve various unfavorable conditions.

The following sections provide conceptual and theoretical analyses of these goals with reference to activities of the North Karelia Project.

Improved Preventive Services

Provision of preventive services is a key function of any health care system. Detection and treatment of hypertension as a means of preventing cardiovascular disease is one of the best examples of this kind of activity.[12] Large-scale detection and control of hypertension has proven to be difficult. The greatest problems are accomplishing widespread blood pressure screening and inducing adequate adherence to indicated treatment and follow-up.[13,14]

The North Karelia Project approached these problems with the notion that it would be more feasible to reorganize preventive services than to induce the population to use existing services more effectively. The Finnish health care system provides primary care through community health centers serving and largely governed by local populations. Only a small minority receive routine care from private physicians. Sponsored by the National Board of Health, the North Karelia Project worked together with the County Health Administration and local municipal authorities to change the way in which hypertension was detected and treated.[15]

The central features of this reorganization were a sharp increase in the responsibility assigned to the local public health nurse and the establishment of new offices at each of the 12 community health centers in North Karelia. To provide the data base for the new activities a county-wide hypertension register was established. Screening for hypertension was integrated into routine contacts with the health center and also provided through mass screening programs at county fairs and village centers. Public health nurses were trained to refer those with elevated blood pressure to a physician for definite diagnosis and for possible initiation of appropriate pharmacological regimens. Then the public health nurse was given responsibility for long-term surveillance of those patients' blood pressure through regular follow-up, including personal instructions on adherence to the treatment and on necessary modification of dietary and other habits. The public health nurses paid special attention to individuals who seemed to experience difficulty in bringing their blood pressure under control. Meanwhile, media and community organizations were spreading the message that control of hypertension is an important goal and that individuals should cooperate with the new activities of the public health nurses. Regular mailings of highly salient reminders of follow-up visits were sent to all the persons recorded in the hypertension register maintained by the public health nurse.

At the baseline survey in 1972, the proportion of male hypertensives (systolic $\geq$ 175 mm Hg or diastolic $\geq$ 100 mm Hg) receiving anti-hypertensive drug treatment was about 13 per cent in both Karelia and a neighboring province which was used as a reference for comparison. In the 1977 survey conducted after five years of reorganized preventive health services in North Karelia, the proportion of male hypertensives under appropriate drug treatment had increased to 45 per cent.[16] In the neighboring province, where services for hypertension detection and treatment were beginning to be modeled after the new procedures in North Karelia, the corresponding change was from 14 per cent to 33 per cent. The proportion of hypertensives dropped sharply among North Karelian middle-aged men (30–64 years) while it increased slightly in the reference area. These findings are more completely described elsewhere.[7]

Information

Cooperation with any program or service designed to prevent disease depends on the extent to which the community is informed about the purposes and importance of the program. Thus a major objective of health promotion is to educate people about their health and how it can be maintained. Examples of this kind of activity are informing the public that cardiovascular disease may be prevented through appropriate measures and explaining the purpose and nature of these measures. However it is not always easy to adequately communicate new and somewhat complex ideas in a large population which is subject to information, sometimes conflicting, from many sources.

The design of effective information campaigns can be facilitated by the application of practical principles derived from communication research and theory. For example, research shows that mass media, especially news, powerfully influence what people talk and think about and how they judge the importance of various social problems or issues.[17] Theory suggests that new ideas often must travel through several steps of interpersonal communication to reach the general population.[18] The messages must be simple and frequently repeated if they are to be comprehended and retained.[19]

The North Karelia Project offers several illustrations of the implementation of these principles. Project staff were able to attract intense and frequent attention from the news media in the region, especially from newspapers and radio.

Between 1972 and 1977, a total of 1,509 articles related to cardiovascular risk factors, their management, and the program activities were printed in the local newspapers. This was three times as many articles as appeared in the reference area papers. During that same period, over one-half million bulletins, leaflets, posters, signs, stickers and other educational materials were distributed. To stimulate further interpersonal communication, many different groups and organizations were contacted and asked to distribute materials in their everyday work or to cooperate in organizing health education meetings. A total of 251 general meetings, reaching over 20,000 community members, were held. The community groups and organizations that were involved in these activities included worksites, schools, shops and places of commerce, clubs, and voluntary organizations.

Information about the program and its aims was disseminated rapidly.[7] According to population surveys, over a five-year period understanding of the risk factors for cardiovascular disease increased in both North Karelia and the reference area, but somewhat more in North Karelia. There were sharp baseline differences in knowledge between different educational and occupational groups, but members of all the different groups in North Karelia showed 10 to 15 per cent increases in the proportion of correct responses to survey questions designed to measure knowledge, awareness, and understanding of cardiovascular disease risk factors. However, there were no significant differences between such changes in North Karelia and in the reference area, probably because of increasing attention from the national media serving both countries.

Persuasion

It is well known that behavior cannot always be changed simply by providing information.[20] People need to be persuaded to act on the information that they have been given, to be convinced that new ideas are socially acceptable, that new foods are tasty, and that new life-styles are enjoyable. Thus, in order to promote health effectively, we must accept responsibility for shaping attitudes and behavior in what we believe to be the proper direction.

Much has been written concerning the ethical issues that arise in persuasive health promotion.[21] Debate has been centered on the right of public health activists to interfere with existing processes and on the question of whether individuals or groups should be held responsible for their own health.[23] The promotion of change in life-style or environment is a natural outgrowth of an improved understanding of the epidemiology of disease and injury. Given the many forces which already exert persuasive influences on individuals in our society, those concerned with public health should not shirk the duty of prudent advocacy. To do otherwise is to leave attitudes and behaviors to be shaped by the short-term contingencies of our market economy.

We are products of our environment, but we can change our environment through concerted action. Thus, we may be held collectively responsible for public health, and we must learn to use our political system more effectively to create a favorable environment for all segments of society if we hope to limit the current burden of illness. Efforts to persuade those whose options are limited and whose values are distorted by economic and social problems to accept responsibility for their own health may be futile. Yet many public health activists seeking basic social or economic change are acutely aware of the difficulty of winning popular support for their views and recommendations.

There is a broad accumulation of research and theory concerning the social psychology of persuasion.[24] Three general approaches can be described:

• The ''communication'' approach focuses on basic parameters of communication; it emphasizes the credibility of the source of a persuasive message and how the message form or content influences cognitive processes in a human receiver.

• The ''affective'' approach to persuasion concentrates on creating emotional associations.

• The ''behavioral'' approach centers on achieving a minor behavioral commitment with the expectation that attitudes and beliefs will follow.[25] Although attitude change was not a stated objective of the program in North Karelia, several basic principles were taken into account when different activities were conducted.

In communicating new ideas, Project staff arranged for their messages to be disseminated from many different sources—deliberately seeking a mix which would maximize perceived credibility. Explicit endorsements were obtained from prestigious institutions such as the World Health Organization. In addition, opinion leaders from both formal and informal groups were involved.[26] These individuals were targets of especially intense persuasive communication from respected medical and other experts and were then encouraged to spread and support the new ideas in the community. The physicians and public health nurses were an important part of the communication system. The surveys showed that during the five-year period both of these professional groups distributed more information and were much more involved in active contacts with decision-makers in various community organizations in North Karelia than in the reference area: eight per cent of the decision-makers in the reference area and over 20 per cent in North Karelia had been explicitly advised by a public health nurse to change dietary habits.[7]

The content of the messages was carefully constructed to anticipate and suppress counter-arguments. Since many local people, engaged in active occupations, strongly believed that a diet high in meat fat was necessary for hardworking individuals, messages aimed at decreasing fat intake often pointed out that there were hard-working vegetarian lumberjacks and that one of the most famous distance runners from Finland, H. Kolemainen, was a vegetarian. Reference was also repeatedly made to the fact that the recommended low-fat diet was more ''traditional'' for North Karelia than the present high-fat diet. Comparisons of changes in dietary habits in North Karelia and the reference area revealed that sizable and significantly greater reductions were observed in reported intake of fat in North Karelia than in the reference area.[7]

Realizing that any fear-provoking messages must be accompanied by clear and attainable recommendations for reducing that fear, the Project was careful with the "high-risk" concept. People with elevated blood pressure or serum cholesterol were told that their condition was potentially serious, but that simple steps could be taken to alleviate the problem. Practical dietary advice was given, and the high-risk individuals were systematically reassured at the follow-up. No distinction was made between "pathological" and "safe" levels of risk, and public health nurses and educators repeatedly pointed out that the general risk in the population was high—that everyone had reason for change. The surveys showed that the behavior changes were similar among population groups with varied initial risk levels, and that there was no tendency toward increased anxiety or psychosomatic complaints as a result of the efforts to identify and influence those with exceptionally elevated risk factors.[27]

The "emotional" approach to persuasion relies upon emotional association rather than argument. There was conscious effort by the Project to associate the goals of the project with the pride and provincial identity of the population. People were urged to participate and to make changes not only for themselves, but for "North Karelia." For instance, signs reading "Do not smoke here—we are in the North Karelia Project" were everywhere and fostered a kind of local patriotism.

The "behavioral" approach to persuasion also does not rely on rational argument. The Project staff became acquainted with hundreds of local influential people with whom problems of varying nature were discussed. Almost everyone directly contacted was asked to make at least some minor behavioral commitment in favor of the Project. Thousands of citizens cooperated with small actions such as the display of stickers and posters. Such actions undoubtedly influenced the involved individuals to take a more favorable view of the Project and its recommendations.

Training

Information and persuasion are often sufficient to promote simple behavioral change such as choices among similar, equally accessible consumer products like butter and margarine. But when complex changes in habit or lifestyle are recommended, it is not always easy to translate intention into action. For example, adding of more vegetables to the family diet may require the homemaker to change long-standing patterns of shopping and preparation. Even when the family is persuaded that such changes should be made, they may find the transition difficult. The cessation of cigarette smoking provides another example of the difficulty of some actions.[28]

There is a fairly well-articulated body of research and theorization that can guide the creation of training programs to facilitate the learning of new habits and skills.[20] Four basic steps appear necessary for optimal training: 1) modeling or demonstration of new responses and action patterns; 2) guided and increasingly independent practice in those thoughts and behaviors; 3) feedback concerning the appropriateness or accuracy of responses; 4) reinforcement in the form of support and encouragement that can be gradually withdrawn if the new habit or skill leads to naturally reinforcing consequences. Illustrations of these steps can be drawn from the training course in dietary change that was conducted in the North Karelia Project.

Especially in rural Finland, most women occupy the traditional role of homemaker and in Eastern Finland many women belong to a local housewives' association known as the "Martha" Organization. In order to teach new cooking and food preparation skills and thus to change family diet, the North Karelia Project worked in cooperation with Martha leaders. A major practical activity here was the introduction of "Parties for a Long Life." Housewives of the village gathered in the afternoon to learn how to cook a healthier type of meal with actual demonstration and participation. For example, women were shown how potatoes and other roots can replace meat fat in soups, while still producing acceptable appearance and consistency. Guidance and feedback was presented by the course leaders as the new skills were practiced. The rest of the families were invited in the evening to enjoy the meal with them, creating good opportunities for natural reinforcement. A pleasant social program was then organized in conjunction with the meal. To increase the perception of natural incentives, participants were shown that the cost of the meal was less than that of their traditional way of preparing those dishes.

Three hundred forty-four of these sessions were held with approximately 15,000 participants. At the 1976 follow-up survey, 9 per cent of the men and 18 per cent of the women in North Karelia had been involved at least once. Since then, the "Party for a Long Life" has become a part of the activities of the Martha Association on a national basis. A variety of other forms of training were conducted, including smoking cessation classes and special coronary rehabilitation groups. These are more completely described elsewhere.[7]

Community Organization

No matter how effectively a person has been educated, persuaded, and trained to make healthy changes in behavior, it is unlikely that the change will be maintained unless it is reinforced by the social environment. One of the central ideas, and probably the most important concept, of the Project in North Karelia was to involve the whole community in a broad effort to prevent cardiovascular diseases. A variety of supportive activities were organized. They provide good examples of how members of the community can be trained and organized to reinforce the changes that were being recommended.

Support within the family was created by involving the complete family unit wherever possible, e.g., inviting the husbands and children to share in the results of cooking classes, or enlisting the support of wives in their husbands' adherence to smoking cessation courses, anti-hypertensive regimens, or coronary rehabilitation courses. Wives of smokers were informed about how to deal with nervousness on the part of a recent ex-smoker and how to be patient and reinforcing as their husband learned to live without cigarettes.

Special efforts were made to create general support within the community, based upon the well known sociological phenomenon of natural leadership in social networks of the community.[29] The Project staff, jointly with the Heart Association, identified local leaders by informally interviewing shopkeepers and other knowledgeable persons. They inquired about individuals who regularly have influential contacts with a large number of practical activities. Those who agreed to participate in the "lay leaders" program were invited to a weekend program of training which included basic information about risk factors for cardiovascular disease and suggestions on how to encourage positive changes in day-to-day contacts with people. Participants in these brief courses were also educated about the new activities that were being conducted by the health centers and given advice on how to encourage cooperation among their families, friends, and acquaintances. Finally, these natural leaders were told that they were models for the rest of the community and urged to be positive examples by following various recommendations themselves. This activity was started toward the end of the five-year period and was continued after that. Over a four-year period more than 1,000 of the most influential members of the local communities in North Karelia were involved in this local organizational work.

Environmental Change

The environment is often a determining influence on behavior and may be a direct influence on health. Thus a very important goal of health promotion is the achievement of appropriate environmental changes. Community organization is an important element of such change. Both governmental and economic organizations tend to be most responsive to organized, collective actions.[30,31] Various concepts and theories of social influence and change suggest both direct influence and advocacy among decision-makers[32] and indirect influence through the organization of "grass-roots" support and action.[33]

The major environmental goals of the North Karelia Project were to increase the availability of low-fat foodstuffs and to introduce restrictions on smoking in many indoor spaces such as restaurants. Direct advocacy of those goals was accomplished through individual meetings with crucial individuals. For example, shop proprietors were individually asked to display signs which prohibited smoking in their shops. Management of a local sausage factory was particularly interested in cardiovascular disease prevention after two managers suffered heart attacks. The Project staff took advantage of their offer of cooperation by helping to create a new sausage product which replaced some meat and fat with mushrooms. Especially important was the assistance of the main county dairy in promoting the consumption of low-fat dairy products. Through this cooperation some entirely new products were created.

Indirect influence was organized out of the many contacts between North Karelia Project staff and influential members of the community. The weekend courses for natural community leaders involved discussions of how useful environmental changes could be accomplished, and participants in these meetings were asked to accomplish specific objectives. For example, local restaurants and shops were visited by local leaders, who asked the proprietors to offer additions to the food products on sale, to prohibit or restrict smoking, and to remove tobacco advertisements.

A particularly powerful form of indirect influence on environmental change is the creation of consumer demand for new products or services. The educational and persuasive activities of the North Karelia Project stimulated increased demand for low-fat food products. When a survey showed that more than half of the population of North Karelia would buy low-fat milk if it were available, that fact was persuasively communicated to those responsible for the production and distribution of dairy products. In response, the dairy agreed to produce nonfat milk and other new products and joined with the Project in promoting those new products. Dairy sales were sustained without increasing costs.

The proportion of people in North Karelia who regularly drink high-fat milk dropped by almost 40 per cent. However, this development took place in the whole country, so that in the reference area similar but smaller shifts away from high-fat milk consumption were observed. Other environmental changes that were stimulated by the North Karelia Project also spread throughout Finland. A special soft butter (mixed butter and vegetable oil), introduced by the Project in connection with the "Parties for Long Life," was made available to all Finns as a result of legislative actions in 1978. The voluntary restraint on tobacco promotion that was evoked in North Karelia became a national law in 1977 with the passage of national legislation prohibiting the promotion of tobacco products.

Summary of Five-Year Results

Selected examples of the results achieved in North Karelia have been mentioned throughout this paper and full reports of intermediate and primary outcomes are available elsewhere.[7] Only a brief summary of the risk factor changes that were observed will be presented here. Because of the tendency for longitudinal study of cohorts to exaggerate estimates of change in the whole community,[34] the project evaluation relied upon independent surveys of population samples drawn from the national population register. In 1972, a baseline survey was conducted in which a total of 5,115 men and women between the ages of 25 and 59 were sampled in North Karelia and 7,348 were sampled in the reference area (neighboring county). Excluding those who had died or migrated out of the area, well over 90 per cent of those asked to respond were studied. In 1977, a five-year follow-up survey was made in which 4,728 new persons were sampled from North Karelia and 6,776 were sampled in the reference area. Response rates were again around 90 per cent. Both of these surveys included similarly structured questionnaires and direct risk factor measurement using standardized techniques. Smoking was measured by a set of questions; the reported answers were validated at the terminal survey by analyzing the serum thiocyanate levels of a random half of subjects. Casual blood pressure was measured in sitting position using standardized techniques; the fifth phase was used as diastolic blood pressure. Serum cholesterol assessments were made in one central laboratory standardized against the WHO reference laboratory in Atlanta. An overall risk score was computed for each subject using a multiple logistic function based on their smoking, serum cholesterol and systolic blood presure values.[7]

Changes in risk estimates for smoking, serum cholesterol, blood pressure, and total risk are presented in Table 1, showing significant reductions in North Karelia when compared to the reference area. A more detailed discussion of the evaluation efforts of the project can be found in the WHO report.[7]

Five years is obviously not a long enough period of time to reduce cardiovascular morbidity and mortality, but some changes have been observed.[35] There are good data from national records of pension disability payment and a clear relative reduction in cardiovascular disease pension was observed in North Karelia as compared to the reference area.[7] Estimates from pension disability data already suggest that payment of over $4 million (US) dollars in disability payments may have been avoided by the less than $1 million expended on the Project's intervention activities.

We realize that the observation of only two statistical units (counties) and the absence of random assignment of the intervention limit the certainty of inferences that may be drawn from this study. Given the origin of the Project, randomization was clearly out of the question. However, the reference area was chosen in a "matched" way. Because the possible impact of the Project on the reference area is not taken into account, and a new medical school was opened in the reference area in 1972, the true impact of the Project may have been greater than estimated. Socioeconomic develop-

ment was equivalent in both areas. Health services increased considerably. There was negligible in or out migration among citizens above the age of 30.

Because the objective was to serve the entire province of North Karelia, different components of intervention were not differentially applied within North Karelia. Thus, we cannot state secure conclusions about the unique or relative contributions of different programs, sub-programs, or channels of action. The observed changes may have been due to any one or all of the several actions toward each specific objective. Furthermore, the changes that took place in North Karelia were at least partly the result of more general international trends toward cardiovascular risk reduction which are difficult to disentangle from the specific effects of the North Karelia Project. In spite of that, a few comments about the feasibility and coverage of different activities can be made.

The new preventive services developed gradually and required a fair amount of organizational effort and training of local personnel. Training was extensive but at times the number of participants was restricted because of conflicts with work duties or other meetings. Environmental changes were certainly effective, but their extent was limited by national legislation, other national rules, or economic realities. The extent and coverage of general anti-smoking advice certainly matched with initial expectations. Health personnel were attentive to patients' smoking, but the success of more intensive group support in smoking cessation was not great. The nutrition program resembled these experiences. General nutrition information and counseling was extensive and had wide coverage. Less developed was the system to

TABLE 1—Mean Risk Factor Levels for Men and Women in North Karelia and Reference Area in 1972 and 1977

Assessment Areas	Men	1972	1977	Change
Cholesterol	North Karelia	269.3	259.0	−10.3*
	Reference	260.4	261.2	+0.8
Cigarettes/day	North Karelia	9.9	8.1	−1.8*
(total sample)	Reference	8.9	8.1	−0.8
Systolic BP	North Karelia	147.3	143.9	−3.4*
	Reference	145.0	146.8	+1.8
Diastolic BP	North Karelia	90.8	88.6	−2.2*
	Reference	92.4	92.8	+0.4
Risk Score	North Karelia	4.1	3.4	−0.7*
	Reference	3.7	3.7	0.0
	Women	**1972**	**1977**	
Cholesterol	North Korelia	265.3	258.2	−7.1
	Reference	259.2	255.1	−4.1
Cigarettes/day	North Karelia	1.3	1.1	−0.2
(total sample)	Reference	1.4	1.3	−0.1
Systolic BP	North Karelia	149.4	143.5	−5.9*
	Reference	144.1	145.4	+1.3
Diastolic BP	North Karelia	90.7	86.8	−3.9*
	Reference	90.0	89.5	−0.5
Risk Score	North Karelia	3.3	2.9	−0.4*
	Reference	3.0	2.9	−0.1

*Significant difference ($p < .01$) between change in North Karelia and reference area (one-tailed t test).

provide intense individual nutrition counseling for the overweight or those with very high cholesterol levels. On the other hand it was felt that mass intervention to change nutrition habits was probably a better strategy in the situation where practically everybody had an elevated cholesterol level relative to world norms. The hypertension subprogram succeeded with what proved to be clear and practical programs to screen, treat, and follow the approximately 10–15 per cent of the adult population with hypertension. The reorganization of preventive services and organization of community support and action were probably the most effective aspects of the overall project.

Although the final epidemiological results concerning mortality-reducing effects of the program in North Karelia are still to be shown, the goals of health promotion were met to the satisfaction of those who initially requested the action. The general perception of "success" had led to rapid national adoption of innovations that originated in North Karelia. For example, a major smoking cessation television program was based upon the Project experiences and methods,[36] and a more comprehensive risk factor reduction program on national television has now been conducted. As mentioned previously, several of the new dairy products and health service models that were developed in North Karelia are now available throughout Finland. The North Karelia Project has become popular as a practical and positive example that health promotion and control of modern chronic disease epidemics is feasible.

North Karelia is a fairly large administrative area, and Finland is a relatively small country where public health resources are as scarce as they are elsewhere. The expenditures for an extensive investigation have been limited to a single geographic unit, with only one other unit provided as a matched reference. We feel that the North Karelia Project must be viewed as a promising case study rather than a critical test of the effects of health promotion. That test will depend upon further studies. Only by using the different resources available for intervention and measurement in different countries can enough experience be gained to draw final conclusions on the value of health promotion in modern public health work.

Implications

It is difficult to estimate the potential impact of similar activities in the United States. Stunkard and his colleagues in Pennsylvania are attempting an approximate replication of the North Karelia Project in a rural setting and several other research teams have begun parallel investigations of community health promotion for cardiovascular disease prevention.* The Stanford-Three-Community-Study[37] demonstrated significant risk reductions in a cohort study in rural California. However there are critical differences between the Finnish and North American cultures that probably

---

*Personal communications from J. Farquhan, Stanford University, A. Stunkard, University of Pennsylvania, July 1980; H. Blackburn, University of Minnesota, February 1981; and R. Carlton, Pawtucket Memorial Hospital, (Pawtucket, RI), June 1980.

make health promotion easier to implement in Finland. United States citizens do not uniformly perceive governmental agencies as credible sources of information, whereas Finns are generally more willing to accept public recommendations and to cooperate with community health workers. Thus, public health interests in Finland find it easier to regulate promotion and marketing of products such as tobacco cigarettes. The governmental regulation of medicine in Finland undoubtedly increases the extent to which preventive services can be shaped to serve the interests of public health. Cultural acceptance of the notion that health is a public responsibility in Finland facilitates perception of the wisdom of shifting investments toward the prevention of disease. Thus the North Karelia Project serves not only to demonstrate objectives of health promotion but also to illustrate a cultural setting favorable for the development of innovations in public health and preventive medicine.

REFERENCES

1. Hamburg D: Disease prevention: the challenge of the future. Am J Public Health 1979; 69:1026–1034.
2. Surgeon General's Report on Health Promotion—Background Papers. Washington, DC: Govt Printing Office, 1979.
3. Somers AR (ed): Promoting Health. Germantown, MD: Aspen Systems, 1976.
4. Stunkard AJ: Behavioral medicine and beyond: the example of obesity. IN Pomerleau O, Brady J (eds): Behavioral Medicine. Baltimore, MD: Williams & Wilkins, 1979.
5. Lewin K: Field Theory in Social Science. New York: Harper, 1951.
6. Puska P: North Karelia Project: A program for community control of cardiovascular diseases. Publications of the University of Kuopio, Community Health—Series A:1, Finland, 1974.
7. Puska P, Tuomilehto J, Salonen J, et al: The North Karelia Project: Evaluation of a comprehensive community program for control of cardiovascular diseases in 1972–1977 in North Karelia, Finland. Monograph. WHO/EURO, Copenhagen, 1981.
8. Kirscht JP: The health belief model and illness behavior. Health Education Monographs 1974; 2:387–408.
9. Rosenstock IM: Historical origins of the health belief model. Health Education Monographs 1974; 2:328–35.
10. Jessor R, Jessor S: Problem Behavior and Psychosocial Development. New York: Academic Press, 1977.
11. Green LW, Kreuter MW, Deeds SG, Partridge KB: Health Education Planning. Palo Alto: Mayfield, 1980.
12. Kannel W: Importance of hypertension as a major risk factor in cardiovascular disease. IN: Genest, et al, (eds): Hypertension. New York: McGraw-Hill Book Company, 1977.
13. Langfeld S: Hypertension: deficient care of the medically served. Ann Intern Med 1973; 78:19.
14. Stamler R, Stamler J, Civinelli J, et al: Adherence and blood pressure response to hypertension treatment. Lancet 1975; 11:1227.
15. Tuomilehto J: Feasibility of the community program for control of hypertension. A part of the North Karelia Project. Publications of the University of Kuopio, Community Health—Series A:2, Finland, 1975.
16. Nissimen A: An evaluation of the community-based hypertension program of the North Karelia Project with special reference to the awareness and treatment of elevated blood pressures and the blood pressure level. A part of the North Karelia Project. Publications of the University of Kuopio, Community Health—Series original: 2, Finland, 1979.
17. Flay BR, Ditecco D, Schlegel RP: Mass media in health promotion. Health Education Quarterly. 1980; 7, 127–143.
18. Katz E, Lazarsfeld PF: Personal influence. Glencoe, IL: Free Press, 1955.

19. Griffiths W, Knutson A: The role of mass media in pubilc health. Am J Public Health 1960; 50:515–523.

20. McAlister A, Farquhar J, Thoreson C, Maccoby N: Applying behavioral sciences to cardiovascular health. Health Education Monographs 1976; 4:45–74.

21. Mendelson H: Which shall it be: Mass education or mass persuasion for health? Am J Public Health 1968; 58:131–137.

22. Wikler DI: Ethical issues in governmental efforts to promote health. Washington, DC: Institute of Medicine, National Academy of Sciences, June 1978.

23. Crawford R: You are dangerous to your health: the ideology of victim blaming. Int J Health Services 1977; 7:663–680.

24. McGuire WJ: The nature of attitudes and attitude change. IN: Lindsay G, Aronson E (eds): Handbook of Social Psychology. Reading, MA: Addison-Wesley, Vol III, 1969.

25. Bandura A: Principles of Behavior Modification. New York: Holt-Rinehart, Winston, 1969.

26. Neittaanmäki L, Koskela K, Puska P, McAlister A: The role of lay workers in a community health education in the North Karelia Project. Scand J Soc Med 1981; 1980; 8:1–7.

27. Salonen JT: Smoking and dietary fats in relation to estimated risk of myocardial infarction before and during a preventive community program. Publications of the University of Kuopio, Community Health—Series original reports: 1, Finland, 1980.

28. Bernstein D, McAlister A: The modification of smoking behavior: progress and problems. Addictive Behavior 1976; 1:89–102.

29. Meyer AJ, Maccoby N, Farquhar JW: The role of opinion leadership in a cardiovascular health education campaign. IN: Ruben BD (ed): Communication Yearbook I. New Brunswick: Transaction Books, 1977.

30. McKnight JL: Organizing for community health in Chicago. Science for the People 1978; 10:27–34.

31. Olson M Jr: The Logic of Collective Action. Cambridge, MA: Harvard University Press, 1965.

32. Guskin AE, Ross R: Advocacy and democracy: the long view. Am J of Orthopsych 1971; 41:43–57.

33. Perlman JE: Grass-rooting the system. Social Policy 1976; 7:4–20.

34. Glasunov I, Dowd J, Jaksic Z, et al: Methodological aspects of the design and conduct of preventive trials in ischaemic heart disease. Int J Epidemiol 1973; 2:137–143.

35. Salonen JT, Puska P, Mustainin H: Changes in morbidity and mortality during a comprehensive community program to control cardiovascular diseases during 1972–1977 in North Karelia. Br Med J 1979; 2:1178–1183.

36. Puska P, McAlister A, Koskela K, et al: A comprehensive television smoking cessation program in Finland. Int J of Health Educ (supplement) 1979; 22:1–26.

37. Farquhar J, Maccoby N, Wood P, et al: Community education for cardiovascular health. Lancet 1977; 1:1192—1195.

ACKNOWLEDGMENTS

Preparation of this manuscript was supported by a grant to the first author from the Ruth Mott Fund.

APPENDIX
Selected English-Language Publications on the North Karelia Project

1973

Puska P: The North Karelia Project—an attempt at community prevention of cardiovascular disease. WHO Chronicle 1973;27:55.

1974

Virtamo J, Puska P, Rimpela M: Screening in community control of cardiovascular disease. Community Health 1974;5:312.

1976

Koskela K, Puska P, Tuomilehto J: The North Karelia Project: a first evaluation. Int J Health Educ 1976;19:59.

Puska P, Koskela K, Pakarinen P, et al: North Karelia Project: a program for community control of cardiovascular diseases. Scand J Soc Med 1976;4:57.

Tuomilehto J, Puska P, Nissinen A: Hypertension program of the North Karelia Project. Scand J Soc Med 1976;4:67.

Tuomilehto J, Rajala AL, Puska P: A study on the drop-outs of the hypertension program of the North Karelia Project. Community Health 1976;7:149.

1978

Nissinen A, Tuomilehto J, Puska P: The hypertension register of the North Karelia Project. Clin Sci Mol Med 1978;55:355.

Puska P, Tuomilehto J, Salonen J: Community control of acute myocardial infarction in Finland. Practical Cardiology 1978;4:94.

Puska P, Virtamo J, Tuomilehto J, et al: Cardiovascular risk factor changes in 5-year follow-up of a cohort in connection with a community program (The North Karelia Project). Acta Med Scand 1978;204:381.

Tuomilehto J, Koskela K, Puska P, et al: A community anti-smoking program: interim evaluation of the North Karelia Project. Int J Health Educ 1978;(suppl)31:4.

Tuomilehto J, Puska P, Virtamo J, et al: Coronary risk factors and socioeconomic status in Eastern Finland. Prev Med 1978;7:359.

1979

Björkqvist S, Tuomilehto J, Puska P, et al: Costs of the hypertension program of the North Karelia Project. IN: Thurm R (ed): Essential Hypertension. Chicago: Year Book Medical Publishers, 1979.

Kottke T, Tuomilehto J, Puska P, Salonen JT: The relationship of symptoms and blood pressure in a population sample. Int J Epid 1979;8:355–360.

Puska P, Björkqvist S, Koskela K: Nicotine-containing chewing gum in smoking cessation: a double blind trial with half year follow-up. Addictive Behavior 1979;4:141–146.

Puska P, Koskela K, McAlister A, et al: A comprehensive television smoking cessation program in Finland: background principles, implementation and evaluation. Int J Health Educ 1979;18:7–8.

Puska P, Tuomilehto J, Salonen JT, et al: Changes in coronary risk factors during comprehensive five-year community program to control cardiovascular diseases during 1972–1977 in North Karelia. Brit Med J 1979;2:1173–1178.

Salonen J, Puska P, Mustaniemi H: Changes in morbidity and mortality during comprehensive community program to control cardiovascular diseases during 1972–1977 in North Karelia. Brit Med J 1979;2:1178–1183.

Tuomilehto J, Nissinen A, Puska P: Advances in the management of hypertension in the community over four years of intervention of the North Karelia Project. Public Health 1979;93:143–152.

1980

Neittaanmäki L, Koskela K, Puska P, McAlister A: The role of lay workers in community health education: The North Karelia Project. Scand J Soc Med 1980;8:1–7.

Nissinen A, Tuomilehto J, Puska P: Management of hypertension and changes in blood pressure level in patients included in the hypertension register of the North Karelia Project. Scand J Soc Med 1980;8:17–23.

Tuomilehto J, Puska P, Virtamo J, Nissinen A: Hypertension control in North Karelia before the intervention of the North Karelia Project. Scand J Soc Med 1980;8:9–15.

Forthcoming

Puska P, Salonen J, Tuomilehto J, Nissinen A, Kottke T: Evaluating community-based cardiovascular disease programs: problems and experiences from the North Karelia Project (manuscript in preparation).

Cancer Prevention: A Program to Inform the Public About Cancer Risk and Risk Reduction

from the Office of Cancer Communications, National Cancer Institute

SOCIETAL EVIDENCE

In addition to the scientific evidence about cancer risk factors summarized above, there is substantial evidence that the public is confused and skeptical about cancer, its risks, and prevention, and that well-planned communications programs can have a positive effect on public knowledge, attitudes, and behavior.

Public Confusion About Cancer
Cause, Risk and Prevention

Myths and misconceptions about the causes of cancer reflect public confusion about cancer and cancer risks. Recent surveys indicate that the public believes that cancer is hereditary, caused by bumps or bruises, spread by surgery, and contagious (NCI, Cancer Prevention Awareness Survey, 1983; NCI, Group Depth Interview Report, 1982; NCI, National Survey on Breast Cancer, 1980). In a survey in which participants were asked to respond to the question "what things do you think cause cancer?" older people were more likely to mention incorrectly injuries (bumps, bruises, etc.) and/or to state that they did not know what caused cancer (Luther et al., 1982).

Results of a recent national survey indicate that the public's perceptions of risk and potential for personal control over cancer risk vary and are often pessimistic (NCI, Cancer Prevention Awareness Survey, 1983). About half the population believes that "everything causes cancer" and that "there is not much a person can do to prevent cancer." These beliefs are more likely to be held by those with lower levels of education. Further, only 38 percent of the population believes that cancer is related to lifestyle.

Myths and misconceptions about cancer can create obstacles to appropriate actions. For example, if individuals incorrectly believe that surgery spreads cancer, they may delay giving consent to a surgical procedure that could effectively treat their cancer. Unwarranted fears and misunderstandings may prevent individuals from seeking treatment altogether, delay their seeking medical care, or provoke them to consider unproven treatments. Moreover, a belief that "cancer is inevitable" would discourage an individual from attempting to reduce specific, controllable risks. Thus, messages to dispel these beliefs are being developed.

Reprinted with permission from *Cancer Prevention: A Program to Inform the Public About Cancer Risk and Risk Reduction*, National Cancer Institute, January 1984, pp. 13-31.

How do individuals perceive risk? Studies have addressed this question by asking people what activities they consider most "risky" and why they are so perceived. Among national survey respondents, more people (41 percent) thought smoking may be risky to their health than any other factor, followed by poor food/diet choices (23 percent) and drinking alcohol (13 percent) (NCI, Cancer Prevention Awareness Survey, 1983).

In another study, individuals were asked to rank a list of activities and behaviors from the most to least risky. Results indicated that any activity that was new, imposed on them, beyond their control, or unfamiliar was perceived as more risky. In contrast, ordinary living patterns--drinking alcohol and imprudent dietary habits--were not considered as risky (Slovic et al., 1979). Thus, messages designed to motivate people to change these habit patterns to reduce their risks of cancer when they may not consider the behaviors (such as drinking) to be risky must be developed with care and reinforced throughout the prevention awareness program.

Even those who have an accurate perception of their personal risk-taking behavior may become confused about cancer risks. A recent survey of public and worker attitudes toward carcinogens and cancer risks found that only 28 percent of those questioned felt well-informed about cancer risks (Shell Oil Company, 1978).

When national survey respondents were asked to list things a person can do to reduce chances of getting cancer, the most frequent first answer was to reduce or stop smoking (30 percent), followed by changing food and diet habits (21 percent) and changing personal medical practices (13 percent). Only 14 percent of all respondents mentioned reducing exposure to sunlight. As expected, people with less education tended to know less about risk factors; for example, they generally agreed more often than others that bumps and bruises or foods that contain fiber increase cancer risks (NCI, Cancer Prevention Awareness Survey, 1983).

Another study analyzed qualitative data from 1,500 in-depth interviews on citizens' attitudes toward cancer risks. Results identified public and worker perceptions of cancer-causing risks and found that two-thirds of the workers said they did not know enough to evaluate the possible cancer risks of various chemicals (Union Carbide Corporation, 1977).

The results of these studies and others suggest that people acknowledge that they are not well-informed about cancer risks. In addition, people have little confidence in their ability to evaluate potential risk factors. It appears that it will not be enough simply to inform the public about cancer risks; an effort will be made to interpret the existing information and suggest specific ways that individuals can reduce their risks to cancer.

Finally, consideration will be given to the public's perception of cancer, in general, as a health risk. Surveys have indicated that when all health threats are considered, cancer is the major health concern of Americans today (NCI, Cancer Prevention Awareness survey, 1983; General Mills, Inc., 1979). They seem to underestimate the incidence of cancer in the population but to overestimate the number of deaths from the disease (American Cancer Society, 1978). Few people realize the progress that has been made in cancer treatment; survey results show that the public is usually quite pessimistic about the chances of survival once a diagnosis of cancer is made (American Cancer Society, 1978). For instance, people reported that one in five persons would survive for 5 years, whereas the actual rate is nearly 50 percent.

Figure 2 shows the substantial progress made since 1960 in cancer survival rates. Similarly, figure 3 shows that U.S. cancer mortality rates have dropped dramatically for all major cancer sites except female lung cancer, an increase attributable directly to the sharp increase in recent decades of cigarette smoking among women.

It is particularly significant to NCI's cancer prevention awareness program that although people are confused about cancer and risk factors, they are interested in obtaining more information about cancer risks and ways to prevent the disease (NCI, Literature Search Report, 1982; NCI, Group Depth Interview Report, 1982). Evidence shows, however, that some of the cancer information obtained by the public through television, newspapers, and popular magazines has contributed to the confusion. A review of cancer articles from 50 of the Nation's largest newspapers led to several observations that have practical implications for the prevention awareness initiative. For example, less than 5 percent of total cancer news coverage was related to cancer prevention, detection, and ways to minimize cancer risks (NCI, 1980 Content Analysis, 1982). In addition, news stories rarely gave information about specific cancer sites, and the subject matter did not reflect actual incidence of cancer by site. For example, cancers of the colon and rectum are among the three highest in incidence but are rarely the subject of news coverage. As the study concluded, "Information that places the disease (cancer) in perspective—in terms of cancer incidence rates, prevention, and control—was included in few of the stories analyzed" (NCI, 1980 Content Analysis, 1982).

Because many people want more cancer information, and continue to acquire it through mass media channels, program efforts are directed to developing quality health messages on cancer risks and prevention. Media specialists, print and broadcast alike, play key roles as gatekeepers of information to the public about cancer. Health educators now realize that they "need to work closely with the mass media in the development of a favorable public attitude, so to speak, about cancer prevention" (James, 1980).

It appears that the public is often confused and skeptical about cancer prevention information because of the terminology used and the way information is disseminated. Health professionals may contribute to the confusion by using unnecessarily technical terms. To help solve this problem, NCI is using a common language of simplified terms about cancer risk factors in its communications to the public, health professionals, and the media.

The Potential for Behavior Change

Educational objectives of the cancer prevention awareness program are aimed at improving public knowledge and attitudes regarding cancer as well as at enabling people to change certain health-related behaviors to reduce their cancer risks. A person's knowledge, attitudes, and beliefs about cancer interact to produce his or her health-related behavior. Theorists have attempted to explain how much (if any) influence each of those variables has on individual behavior, but the evidence is not yet conclusive. Knowledge alone cannot ensure attitude or behavior change. Nevertheless, communications research has shown that well-planned information programs can achieve realistic objectives (Rice and Paisley, 1981).

In NCI's prevention awareness program, messages have been developed to create awareness about cancer risks and inform people about actions they can take to reduce their risks. Public attitudes about cancer are more likely to improve when people

Figure 2

Increase in 5-Year Relative Cancer Survival Rates
Between 1960-1963 and 1973-1979

WHITE PATIENTS

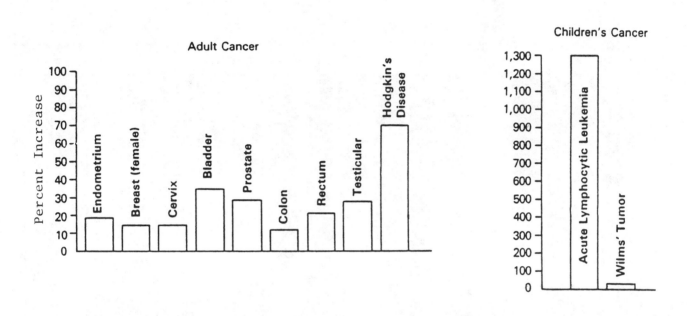

BLACK ADULT PATIENTS

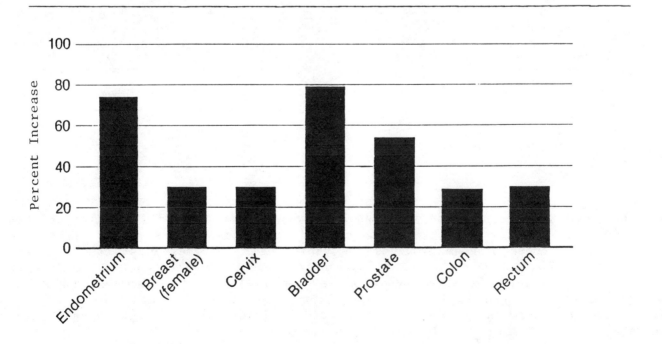

Figure 3

Changes in U.S. Cancer Mortality Rates, 1968-1979

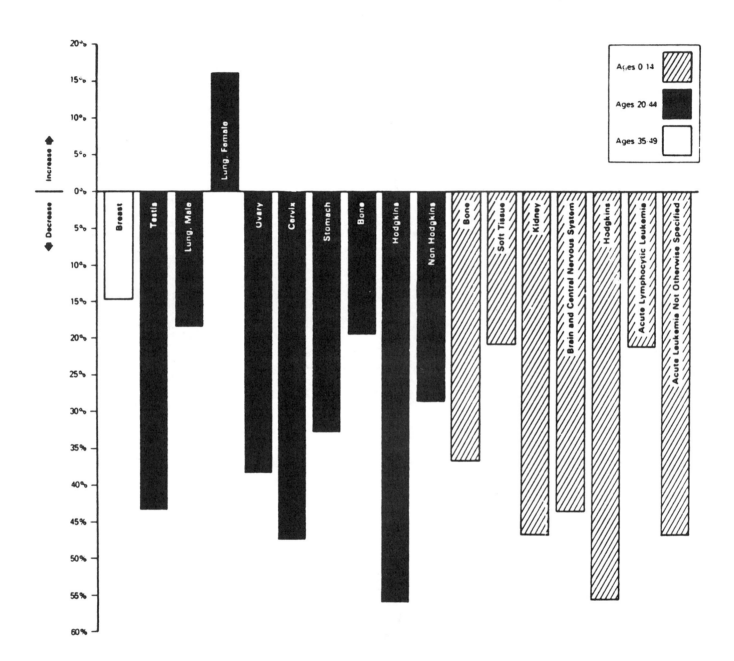

are made aware of the progress that has been made in treatment and survival and are informed about how they can exert some control over their cancer risks. Thus, the prevention awareness program provides the public with information on cancer risks, directions on how to reduce risks of developing cancer, and sources to contact for further information. In this manner, a favorable climate for behavior change is being created. As described in the next section, a variety of educational strategies, promoted by media efforts and reinforced by intermediaries, are being used to achieve the objectives of the NCI prevention awareness program.

III. DESCRIPTION OF THE NATIONAL CANCER
PREVENTION AWARENESS PROGRAM

The National Cancer Prevention Awareness Program is being developed over time and in two phases. This approach allows for a progressive development of program messages to reach specific target audiences through a variety of channels.

PROGRAM GOAL AND OBJECTIVES

The goal of the prevention awareness program is to improve public knowledge and attitudes related to cancer prevention in order to encourage individuals to adopt a healthful lifestyle. Specific program objectives are:

o To increase public <u>awareness</u> and <u>knowledge</u> that some risks to cancer are controllable;

o To increase public <u>awareness</u> and <u>knowledge</u> of healthful behaviors that afford personal control over cancer risks;

o To improve public <u>attitudes</u> regarding cancer incidence, treatment, and prevention; and

o To promote <u>behaviors</u> and <u>practices</u> that will help individuals protect themselves from cancer.

PROGRAM STRATEGIES

To achieve these objectives, NCI is implementing its communications activities in the context of the following strategies:

o Positioning all messages as one part of a <u>growing</u> body of <u>news</u> about cancer prevention;

o Establishing the concept that cancer prevention is, in fact, a <u>system</u> of healthful behaviors;

o Establishing that efforts at cancer prevention are, in reality, part of an overall system of <u>health promotion</u>;

o Establishing that the <u>National Cancer Institute</u> is an authoritative source of information on cancer prevention and health promotion; and

o Establishing that <u>every day individuals can do something</u> to protect themselves from cancer risks and promote a system of healthful behaviors.

TACTICS AND THEME

To assure that program tactics contribute to overall program objectives and strategies, each tactic:

o Reinforces the positive, <u>good news</u> theme, Cancer Prevention: The News Is Getting Better All the Time;

o Describes a <u>primary prevention</u> effort, some action that will reduce the likelihood of a cancer developing;

o Describes risk factors that an <u>individual can control</u>;

o Recommends a <u>positive</u> action; and

o <u>Eliminates message clutter</u> by focusing on information about major risk factors over which the individual can take specific actions--actions that
promote a system of healthful behaviors.

PHASE I ACTIVITIES

Initial, or Phase I, activities are directed to the general public primarily
through mass media channels and are focused on increasing knowledge and improving
attitudes, with the hope of encouraging the adoption of corresponding positive behaviors.

Phase I Messages

Messages during Phase I establish the underlying base of growing good news that
makes the prevention awareness program possible and feasible. They provide information about prevention, risk factors, and the ways in which eliminating or reducing
specific cancer risks promote a system of healthful behaviors.

General Prevention Messages

The <u>first</u> message of Phase I works to dispel negative and pessimistic attitudes
toward cancer. It establishes the base of legitimate optimism from which the prevention program arises with the:

GOOD NEWS: Everyone does <u>not</u> get cancer.
               2 out of 3 Americans will never get it.

The <u>second</u> message of Phase I helps promote a more positive attitude toward
cancer outcome. It builds momentum with the:

BETTER NEWS: Every day more and more people with cancer are cured.

The <u>third</u> general prevention message of Phase I introduces the news that individuals can take control of their own risks for cancer by putting into effect a
system of healthful behaviors for themselves. It encourages people to act in their
own behalf with the:

BEST NEWS: Every day you can do something to help protect yourself from can-
               cer. And the National Cancer Institute says, here's how!

Risk-Specific Messages

The general messages establish a momentum of increasingly positive news, building to messages about specific risk factors. During Phase I, specific messages
convey information that links reducing risks to overall systems of healthful behaviors.

For example, tobacco is a specific cancer risk factor. However, the information
that lung function returns to normal--and the risk of lung cancer to that of the

average nonsmoker--about 10 years after one stops smoking links smoking cessation to good health in general. Likewise, adequate protection from the sun prevents sun burning and sun blisters, thereby promoting health while it helps protect against skin cancer.

The specific risk factor messages are:

o Don't smoke or use tobacco in any form.

o If you drink alcoholic beverages, do so only in moderation.

o Eat foods low in fat.

o Include fresh fruits, vegetables, and whole grain cereals in your daily diet.

o Avoid unnecessary X-rays.

o Keep yourself safe on the job by using protective devices (respirators, protective clothing).

o Avoid too much sunlight; wear protective clothing; use sunscreens.

o Take estrogens only as long as necessary.

Phase I Channels

Messages in the first phase of the program have been developed for the general public and are being disseminated primarily through mass media channels. Radio and television public service announcements (PSA's) are being produced to create awareness of cancer risk factors and to announce the availability of the new cancer prevention booklet, <u>Good News, Better News, Best News: Cancer Prevention</u>, through promotion of the toll-free CIS telephone number, 1-800-4-CANCER. The booklet and the PSA's are being produced in both English and Spanish. Other electronic media programming is being developed to support and expand prevention messages.

Press kits, posters, and exhibits also are being developed during Phase I. Existing print materials, both from NCI and from other government and voluntary agencies, are being used to disseminate prevention-related messages, and new materials are being created as needed. In addition to the general prevention booklet, other publications created or adapted for the prevention awareness program include booklets on smoking cessation, diet and nutrition, X-rays, and estrogens; and fact sheets on each of the seven selected risk factors. Placement of articles and public service advertisements in major newspapers and magazines is a continuing activity.

People also acquire a great deal of cancer information from sources other than the mass media. In one recent survey individuals referred to physicians as their most reliable source of health information (Weinberg et al., 1982), and another study reported, "If there is any group that can have a profound impact on improving American families' attitudes toward preventive health and good health care, it is the family doctors . . ." (General Mills, Inc., 1979).

Because health professionals, especially primary care physicians, serve as both gatekeepers and sources of cancer prevention information for the public, they are being informed of the NCI prevention awareness program and asked to play a key role in Phase I promotion efforts. In addition, OCC is examining ways to incorporate cancer prevention education programs into physicians' practices. As Wakefield (1975) stated, "The success of cancer control programs may depend upon how seriously doctors and others in the medical profession take their responsibility to persuade and educate."

CCN offices, located at 21 comprehensive cancer centers across the United States, also support Phase I efforts. They are assisting by establishing appropriate state and local media channels and other networks for disseminating Phase I messages. As part of both Phase I and Phase II activities, a series of seven CCN area planning meetings in May and June 1984 will bring together representatives of regional and local organizations involved in programs related directly (for example, the American Cancer Society) or indirectly (for example, a youth organization) to cancer prevention. As information resource centers for these meetings, CCN offices will gain exposure, access to other organizations for wider outreach, and increased credibility as experts in the field of cancer information.

The "Challenge" Concept

To focus national attention on Phase I of the prevention awareness program, the "National Cancer Prevention Challenge" has been designed to heighten public awareness that every day people can do something to protect themselves from cancer. This 4-month campaign of national media exposure and key intermediary participation challenges the media, health professionals, other intermediaries, and the public to take positive steps toward cancer prevention. Challenge messages are aimed at making people aware of the new cancer prevention booklet, encouraging them to order it by calling 1-800-4-CANCER.

The Challenge is being launched at the Fifth National Cancer Communications Conference in February 1984 and will culminate during "Challenge Week" in June, a period of intensified mass media activity that will include both print and electronic exposure. The focus of "Challenge Week" will be a "quiz" designed to test the public's knowledge of cancer prevention.

PHASE II ACTIVITIES

Phase II activities are directed to targeted audiences at greater-than-average risk for any of the selected cancer risk factors. Efforts are focused on encouraging healthful behaviors through "how-to" messages and educational programs. These programs will be developed in cooperation with special media and intermediary organizations and will be used in a variety of settings (such as in worksite or community agency programs).

Primary care physicians, particularly those who specialize in family practice, obstetrics and gynecology, and internal medicine will play a significant role in Phase II efforts. Considered exemplars and educators for primary prevention, physicians will be encouraged to incorporate primary prevention in their practice settings.

Other health professionals, such as nurses, nurse practitioners, and occupational health specialists, will be asked to help reinforce Phase II efforts by disseminating cancer prevention information and encouraging healthful behaviors among their patients. Media channels to reach health professionals with cancer prevention messages (such as health and medical journals) will be used.

Other intermediaries include large organizations or corporations that have employee health care and education programs. These worksite programs present numerous opportunities for disseminating cancer information and sponsoring educational programs. For example, a slide-tape presentation may be used to describe to an employee audience the cancer risks related to nutrition. Posters, articles placed in trade journals, and other print materials with prevention-oriented messages also may be used.

CCN offices will serve three important functions during Phase II. They will be the main distribution points for all prevention-related print materials; they will promote cancer prevention messages to people who call the toll-free CIS number, 1-800-4-CANCER; and they will sponsor and/or coordinate special cancer prevention programs, pilot studies, evaluation efforts, and other education activities. These special initiatives will be formulated at the CCN area planning meetings.

PROGRAM PLANNING PHASE

Prior to the development of messages and communications strategies, NCI completed a number of planning activities related to the prevention awareness program:

o Reviewed the most current scientific literature and developed research summary reports for each selected risk factor: tobacco, alcohol, diet, radiation, estrogens, occupational exposures, and viruses. These reports provide the scientific foundation for developing appropriate and accurate messages and are available to health professionals and cancer prevention program planners.

o Developed a booklet of cancer prevention information, a program theme and messages, and a graphic format for the program. The material was pretested in a medical clinic setting with patients and health professionals and in individual interviews with 100 respondents in six U.S. cities.

o Convened various working groups of experts to advise OCC on developing messages related to the risk factors themselves and to different channels and audiences (electronic media; print media; health professionals; CIS promotion; worksite; youth audiences; black audiences). An evaluation working group has met twice to guide NCI's program evaluation planning and implementation.

o Analyzed recent media campaigns initiated by government agencies and state health departments and prepared a summary report highlighting approaches used in previous health promotion programs.

o Conducted a search of the Cancer Information Clearinghouse to identify existing print materials containing prevention-related messages.

o Conducted a search of the literature to identify previous studies of public knowledge, attitudes, and practices related to cancer.

o Conducted a series of 13 focus groups to study consumer perceptions of risk and prevention of disease in general and cancer in particular and to test, among different target groups, the effectiveness of various formats for communicating information about cancer prevention.

o   In cooperation with the Food and Drug Administration, completed a national survey of 1,876 respondents to develop quantitative audience data concerning public knowledge, attitudes, and behavior related to cancer prevention and risk.

o   In cooperation with the Maryland Center for Health Education, completed a review of the literature concerning physician involvement in cancer risk reduction and health promotion programs.

EVALUATION

Evaluation of the cancer prevention awareness program is necessary to provide information to aid in the design of individual program components, modify the program's direction, design future programs and program phases, and demonstrate effectiveness of the program to various audiences. In evaluating the program, NCI will develop a set of standards and procedures to assess the program's merits and to provide information about its objectives, process, outcome, impact, and costs.

NCI is evaluating program materials and messages using a variety of pretesting techniques. Both informative and promotional materials are pretested before they are put into use. National telephone surveys are being conducted throughout the program to track improvement in levels of public knowledge and awareness of cancer prevention. Other evaluation activities, including media tracking studies and special community studies coordinated through selected CCN offices, provide additional information about the success of the program.

REFERENCES

American Cancer Society. "A Study of Public Attitudes Toward the American Cancer Society and the Fight Against Cancer," conducted by the Gallup Organization, Inc., September 1978.

Centers for Disease Control. "Oral Contraceptive Use and the Risk of Endometrial Cancer: The Centers for Disease Control Cancer and Steroid Hormone Study," JAMA 249:1600-1604, March 25, 1983.

Doll, R. and R. Peto. "The Causes of Cancer: Quantitative Estimates of Avoidable Risks of Cancer in the United States Today," Journal of the National Cancer Institute 66:1191-1308, June 1981.

General Mills, Inc. "Family Health in an Era of Stress," The General Mills American Family Report 1978-79, Minneapolis, Minnesota, 1979.

Greenwald, P. "Assessment of Risk Factors for Cancer," Preventive Medicine 9:260-263, 1980.

James, W.G. "Health Education for Adults," Preventive Medicine 9:281-286, 1980.

Luther, S.L., J.H. Price, and C.A. Rose. "The Public's Knowledge About Cancer," Cancer Nursing 5:109-116, April 1982.

National Academy of Sciences. National Research Council. "Diet, Nutrition and Cancer," National Academy Press, 1982.

National Cancer Institute. "Cancer Prevention Awareness Survey: Technical Report," Office of Cancer Communications, Bethesda, Maryland, December 1983.

National Cancer Institute. "National Survey on Breast Cancer," Office of Cancer Communications, Bethesda, Maryland, November 1980.

National Cancer Institute. "1980 Content Analysis of Daily Newspaper Coverage of Cancer," Office of Cancer Communications, Bethesda, Maryland, March 1982.

National Cancer Institute. "Phase I of National Survey of Public Knowledge Attitudes and Practices Related to Cancer: Group Depth Interview Report," Office of Cancer Communications, Bethesda, Maryland, April 1982.

National Cancer Institute. "Phase I of National Survey of Public Knowledge Attitudes and Practices Related to Cancer: Literature Search Report," Office of Cancer Communications, Bethesda, Maryland, April 1982.

National Center for Health Statistics. "Current Estimates from the National Health Interview Survey: United States 1980," U.S. Department of Health and Human Services, Public Health Service, December 1981.

National Clearinghouse on Smoking and Health. "Adult Use of Tobacco, 1975," DHEW Publication No. (CDC) 21-74-520, June 1976.

Rice, R.E. and W.J. Paisley (eds). Public Communication Campaigns. Beverly Hills: Sage Publications, Inc., 1981.

Rothman, K.J. "The Proportion of Cancer Attributable to Alcohol Consumption," Preventive Medicine 9:174-179, 1980.

Shell Oil Company. "Public and Worker Attitudes Toward Carcinogens and Cancer and Cancer Risk," conducted by Cambridge Reports, Inc., March 1978.

Slovic, P., B. Fischoff and S. Lichtenstein. "Rating the Risks," Environment 21:14-20, 36-9, April 1979.

Union Carbide Corporation. "An Analysis of Citizen Attitudes Toward Cancer Risks," conducted by Cambridge Reports, Inc., June 1977.

Wakefield, J. "Education of the Public," In J.R. Fraumeni, Persons at a High Risk of Cancer. New York: Academic Press, 1975.

Weinberg, A.D., C.A. Spiker, R.W. Ingersoll and S.R. Hoersting. "Public Knowledge and Attitudes Toward Cancer: Their Roles in Health Decisions and Behaviors," Health Values: Achieving High Level Wellness 6:19-26, May-June 1982.

Vessey, M.P., M. Lawless, K. McPherson and D. Yeaks. "Neoplasia of the Cervix Uteri and Contraception: A Possible Adverse Effect of the Pill," Lancet 2:930-934, October 22, 1983.

Index

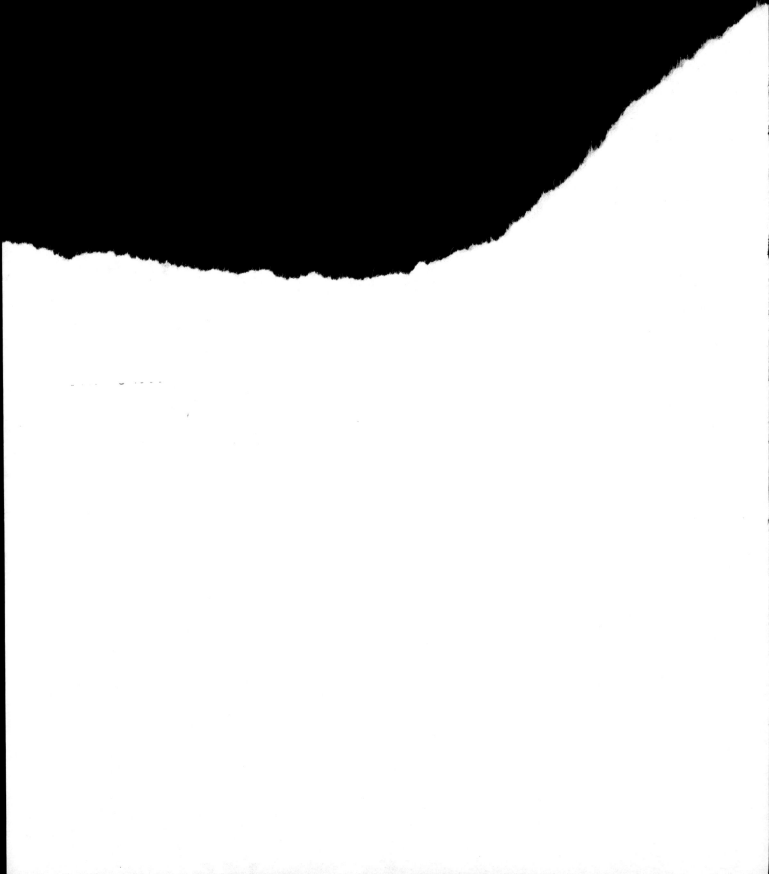